—THE— NeuroICU BOOK

THE NeuroICU BOOK

Editor

Kiwon Lee, MD, FACP, FAHA, FCCM

Assistant Professor of Neurology and Neurological Surgery
Columbia University College of Physicians and Surgeons
Department of Neurology, Division of Critical Care
Neurological Intensive Care Unit
New York Presbyterian Hospital
Columbia University Medical Center
New York, New York

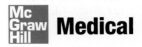

New York   Chicago   San Francisco   Lisbon   London   Madrid   Mexico City
Milan   New Delhi   San Juan   Seoul   Singapore   Sydney   Toronto

The NeuroICU Book

Copyright © 2012 by The McGraw-Hill Companies, Inc. All rights reserved. Printed in China. Except as permitted under the United States Copyright Act of 1976, no part of this publication may be reproduced or distributed in any form or by any means, or stored in a data base or retrieval system, without the prior written permission of the publisher.

3 4 5 6 7 8 9 0   CTP/CTP   16 15 14

ISBN 978-0-07-163635-3
MHID 0-07-163635-8

This book was set in Minion pro by Cenveo Publisher Services.
The editors were Anne M. Sydor, Christine Diedrich, and Karen G. Edmonson.
The production supervisor was Catherine Saggese.
Project management was provided by Sapna Rastogi at Cenveo Publisher Services.
The designer was Eve Siegel.
China Translation & Printing, Ltd., was printer and binder.

Library of Congress Cataloging-in-Publication Data

The neuroICU book / [edited by] Kiwon Lee.
       p. ; cm.
    Includes bibliographical references and index.
    ISBN-13: 978-0-07-163635-3 (softcover : alk. paper)
    ISBN-10: 0-07-163635-8 (softcover : alk. paper)
    1. Nervous system—Diseases.   2. Critical care medicine.   I. Lee, Kiwon.
    [DNLM: 1. Intensive Care.   2. Nervous System Diseases—therapy.   3. Intensive Care Units.   4. Perioperative Care. WL 140]
    RC346.N38354 2012
    616.8'0428—dc23

                                                                                    2011017374

McGraw-Hill books are available at special quantity discounts to use as premiums and sales promotions, or for use in corporate training programs. To contact a representative please e-mail us at bulksales@mcgraw-hill.com.

Contents

Contributors

Wissam Abouzgheib, MD, FCCP
Pulmonary, Critical Care and
    Interventional Pulmonary
Sparks Health System
Fort Smith, Arkansas
Chapter 40

Louis M. Aledort, MD, MACP
The Mary Weinfeld Professor of
    Clinical Research in Hemophilia
Division of Hematology and
    Medical Oncology
Department of Medicine
The Mount Sinai School of Medicine
New York, New York
Chapters 45, 46

Mireia Anglada, MD
Germans Trias i Pujol Hospital
Intensive Care Unit
Barcelona, Spain
Chapter 53

Neeraj Badjatia, MD, MSc, FCCM
Assistant Professor of Neurology and
    Neurological Surgery
Columbia University College of
    Physicians and Surgeons
Medical Director, Neurological
    Intensive Care Unit
Director, Neurocritical Care
    Training Program
NewYork-Presbyterian/Columbia
    University Medical Center
New York, New York
Chapters 4, 19, 50

Thaddeus Bartter, MD
Professor of Medicine
Director, Interventional Pulmonary
Division of Pulmonary and Critical
    Care Medicine
University of Arkansas for the Medical
    Sciences
Little Rock, Arkansas
Chapter 40

Rebecca Bauer, MD
Fellow, Division of Anesthesia and
    Critical Care
Department of Anesthesiology
Columbia University College of
    Physicians and Surgeons
NewYork-Presbyterian/Columbia
    University Medical Center
New York, New York
Chapter 11

H. Alex Choi, MD
Fellow, Division of Critical Care
Department of Neurology
Columbia University College of
    Physicians and Surgeons
NewYork-Presbyterian/Columbia
    University Medical Center
New York, New York
Chapters 9, 11

Jan Claassen, MD, PhD
Assistant Professor of Neurology and
    Neurological Surgery
Columbia University College of
    Physicians and Surgeons
Department of Neurology, Division of
    Critical Care
NewYork-Presbyterian/Columbia
    University Medical Center
New York, New York
Chapters 3, 13, 14, 16

Carlee Clark, MD
Assistant Professor of Anesthesia and
    Perioperative Medicine
Medical University of South Carolina
Charleston, South Carolina
Chapter 28

E. Sander Connolly, Jr, MD, FACS
Bennett M. Stein Professor of
    Neurological Surgery
Vice Chairman of Neurosurgery
Director, Cerebrovascular Research
    Laboratory
Surgical Director, Neuro-Intensive
    Care Unit
Columbia University College of
    Physicians and Surgeons
NewYork-Presbyterian/Columbia
    University Medical Center
New York, New York
Chapters 20 to 24

Celina Crisman, BS
College of Physicians and Surgeons
Columbia University
New York, New York
Chapter 20

Caroline Cromwell, MD
Assistant Professor of Medicine
Division of Hematology and
    Medical Oncology
Department of Medicine
The Mount Sinai School of Medicine
New York, New York
Chapters 45, 46

**Quinn A. Czosnowski, PharmD,
    BCPS**
Assistant Professor of Clinical
    Pharmacy
Department of Pharmacy Practice &
    Pharmacy Administration
Philadelphia College of Pharmacy
University of the Sciences
Philadelphia, Pennsylvania
Chapters 7, 48

Andrew Davenport, MD
University College London Center for
    Nephrology
University College London Medical
    School, Royal Free Campus
London, England
Chapter 42

Naman Desai, BA
Weill Medical College of Cornell
    University
New York, New York
Chapter 3

R. Phillip Dellinger, MD, FCCP
Professor of Medicine
Robert Wood Johnson Medical School
University of Medicine and
    Dentistry of New Jersey
Head, Division of Critical Care
    Medicine
Cooper University Hospital
Camden, New Jersey
Chapter 37

Amy L. Dzierba, PharmD, BCPS
Clinical Pharmacist, Medical
    Intensive Care Unit
Department of Pharmacy
NewYork-Presbyterian/Columbia
    University Medical Center
New York, New York
Chapter 18

Jennifer Frontera, MD
Assistant Professor of Neurosurgery
    and Neurology
The Mount Sinai School of Medicine
Division of Neuro-Critical Care
Mount Sinai Hospital
New York, New York
Chapter 6

Brian M. Fuller, MD
Assistant Professor of Anesthesiology
    and Emergency Medicine
Department of Anesthesiology
Division of Critical Care
Division of Emergency Medicine
Washington University School of
    Medicine
St. Louis, Missouri
Chapter 36

Maher Dahdel, MD
Post-Doctoral Fellow
Robert Wood Johnson Medical School
University of Medicine and Dentistry
    of New Jersey
Division of Pulmonary & Critical Care
    Medicine
Cooper University Hospital
Camden, NJ
Chapter 37

Mithil Gajera, MD
Postdoctoral Fellow, Critical Care
    Medicine
Department of Medicine
Division of Critical Care Medicine
Cooper University Hospital
Camden, New Jersey
Chapter 7

Jomy M. George, PharmD, BCPS
Assistant Professor of Clinical
    Pharmacy
Department of Pharmacy Practice &
    Pharmacy Administration
Philadelphia College of Pharmacy
    University of the Sciences
Philadelphia, Pennsylvania
Chapter 48

Paul Gigante, MD
House staff, Department of
    Neurological Surgery
Columbia University College of
    Physicians and Surgeons
NewYork-Presbyterian/Columbia
    University Medical Center
New York, New York
Chapter 22

Emily Gilmore, MD
Fellow, Division of Critical Care
Department of Neurology
Columbia University College of
  Physicians and Surgeons
NewYork-Presbyterian/Columbia
  University Medical Center
New York, New York
Chapter 13

Fredric Ginsberg, MD
Assistant Professor of Medicine
Robert Wood Johnson Medical School
University of Medicine and
  Dentistry of New Jersey
Director, Nuclear Cardiology
Director, Heart Failure Program
Cooper University Hospital
Camden, New Jersey
Chapter 33

Errol Gordon, MD
Assistant Professor of Neurosurgery
  and Neurology
The Mount Sinai School of Medicine
Division of Neuro-Critical Care
Mount Sinai Hospital
New York, New York
Chapter 16

Simon Hanft, MD, M Phil
House staff, Department of
  Neurological Surgery
Columbia University College of
  Physicians and Surgeons
NewYork-Presbyterian/Columbia
  University Medical Center
New York, New York
Chapter 8

Raqeeb Haque, MD
House staff, Department of
  Neurological Surgery
Columbia University College of
  Physicians and Surgeons
NewYork-Presbyterian/Columbia
  University Medical Center
New York, New York
Chapters 20, 21, and 24

Raimund Helbok, MD
Department of Neurology,
  Neurocritical Care Unit
Innsbruck Medical University
Innsbruck, Austria
Chapter 14

Brian Y. Hwang, MD
Neurosurgical Resident
Department of Neurosurgery
Johns Hopkins University Hospital
Baltimore, MD
Chapters 20, 21, 22, 24

Christopher Kellner, MD
House staff, Department of
  Neurological Surgery
Columbia University College of
  Physicians and Surgeons
NewYork-Presbyterian/Columbia
  University Medical Center
New York, New York
Chapter 23

Sang-Bae Ko, MD, PhD
Postdoctoral Research Fellow
Division of Critical Care
Department of Neurology
Columbia University College of
    Physicians and Surgeons
NewYork-Presbyterian/Columbia
    University Medical Center
New York, New York
Chapter 9

Ivan S. Kotchetkov, BA
College of Physicians and Surgeons
Columbia University
New York, New York
Chapter 21

Rose Kim, MD
Assistant Professor of Medicine
Cooper Medical School of Rowan
    University
Division of Infectious Diseases
Cooper University Hospital
Camden, New Jersey
Chapter 49

Dongwook Kim, MD
Clinical Nutrition and Obesity Fellow
Endocrinology, Diabetes & Nutrition
Boston University School of Medicine
Boston Medical Center
Boston, Massachusetts
Chapter 51

Pedro Kurtz, MD, MSc
Department of Intensive Care
    Medicine
Casa de Saúde São José
Rio de Janeiro, Brasil
Chapters 14 and 15

**Kiwon Lee, MD, FACP, FAHA,
    FCCM**
Assistant Professor of Neurology and
    Neurological Surgery
Columbia University College of
    Physicians and Surgeons
Department of Neurology, Division of
    Critical Care
New York-Presbyterian/Columbia
    University Medical Center
New York, New York
Chapters 1, 9, 10, 11, 12, 15, 52, and 53

Guillermo Linares, MD
Fellow, Division of Critical Care
Department of Neurology
Columbia University College of
    Physicians and Surgeons
NewYork-Presbyterian/Columbia
    University Medical Center
New York, New York
Chapter 53

Ramya Lotano, MD
Assistant Professor of Medicine
    Director, Pulmonary & Critical Care
    fellowship
Robert Wood Johnson Medical School
University of Medicine and
    Dentistry of New Jersey
Division of Pulmonary & Critical Care
    Medicine
Cooper University Hospital
Camden, New Jersey
Chapter 38

Frank Macchio, MD
Fellow, Division of Anesthesia and
    Critical Care
Department of Anesthesiology
Columbia University College of
    Physicians and Surgeons
NewYork-Presbyterian/Columbia
    University Medical Center
New York, New York
Chapter 29

Rishi Malhotra, MD
Neurointensivist
Department of Neurosurgery, North
    Shore University Hospital and
Long Island Jewish Medical Center
Cushing Neuroscience Institute
Manhasset, New York
Chapter 10

Stephan A. Mayer, MD, FCCM
Professor of Neurology and
    Neurological Surgery
Columbia University College of
    Physicians & Surgeons
Director, Division of Critical Care,
    Department of Neurology
NewYork-Presbyterian/Columbia
    University Medical Center
New York, New York
Chapters 2 and 12

Joanne Mazzarelli, MD
Postdoctoral Fellow, Cardiology
Robert Wood Johnson Medical School
University of Medicine and
    Dentistry of New Jersey
Department of Medicine
Division of Cardiovascular Diseases
Cooper University Hospital
Camden, New Jersey
Chapter 31

Christopher B. McFadden, MD
Assistant Professor of Medicine
Robert Wood Johnson Medical School
University of Medicine and Dentistry of
    New Jersey
Division of Nephrology
Cooper University Hospital
Camden, New Jersey
Chapter 44

Laura McPhee, DO
Postdoctoral fellow in Pulmonary and
    Critical Care Medicine
Maine Medical Center
Portland, Maine
Chapter 35

Joseph Meltzer, MD
Clinical Associate Professor
Department of Anesthesiology
Director, Cardiothoracic Intensive
    Care Unit
David Geffen Medical School
Ronald Reagan UCLA Medical Center
Los Angeles, California
Chapter 27

Daniel K. Meyer, MD
Assistant Professor of Medicine
Robert Wood Johnson Medical School
University of Medicine and
    Dentistry of New Jersey
Division of Infectious Diseases
Cooper University Hospital
Camden, New Jersey
Chapter 49

Philip M. Meyers, MD, FAHA
Associate Professor of Radiology and
    Neurological Surgery
Clinical Co-Director,
    Neuroendovascular Services
Columbia University College of
    Physicians and Surgeons
NewYork-Presbyterian/Columbia
    University Medical Center
New York, New York
Chapter 20

Samia Mian, MD
Postdoctoral Fellow, Nephrology
Robert Wood Johnson Medical School
University of Medicine and
    Dentistry of New Jersey
Division of Nephrology
Cooper University Hospital
Camden, New Jersey
Chapter 44

Steven Miller, MD
Assistant Professor of Anesthesiology
Department of Anesthesiology
Columbia University College of
    Physicians and Surgeons
NewYork-Presbyterian/Columbia
    University Medical Center
New York, New York
Chapter 25

Vivek K. Moitra, MD
Assistant Professor of Anesthesiology
Assistant Medical Director, Surgical
    Intensive Care Unit
Columbia University College of
    Physicians and Surgeons
NewYork-Presbyterian/Columbia
    University Medical Center
New York, New York
Chapter 18 and 25

Oliver Panzer, MD
Assistant Professor of Anesthesiology
Columbia University College of
    Physicians and Surgeons
NewYork-Presbyterian/Columbia
    University Medical Center
New York, New York
Chapter 30

Santiago Ortega-Gutierrez, MD
Fellow, Division of Critical Care
Department of Neurology
Columbia University College of
    Physicians and Surgeons
NewYork-Presbyterian/Columbia
    University Medical Center
New York, New York
Chapters 3 and 13

Joseph E. Parrillo, MD, FCCP
Professor of Medicine
Robert Wood Johnson Medical School
University of Medicine and
    Dentistry of New Jersey
Chief, Department of Medicine
Edward D. Viner MD Chair,
    Department of Medicine
Director, Cooper Heart Institute
Cooper University Hospital
Camden, New Jersey
Chapters 33 and 34

Melvin R. Pratter, MD
Professor of Medicine
Robert Wood Johnson Medical School
University of Medicine and Dentistry
    of New Jersey
Head, Division of Pulmonary Diseases
    and Critical Care Medicine
Cooper University Hospital
Camden, New Jersey
Chapter 40

Jean-Sebastien Rachoin, MD, FASN
Assistant Professor of Medicine
Robert Wood Johnson Medical School
University of Medicine and Dentistry
   of New Jersey
Department of Medicine, Division of
   Hospital Medicine
Cooper University Hospital
Camden, New Jersey
Chapter 41

Annette C. Reboli, MD, FACP, FIDSA
Vice Dean
Cooper Medical School of Rowan
   University
Professor of Medicine
Division of Infectious Diseases
Cooper University Hospital
Camden, New Jersey
Chapters 49 and 50

Fred Rincon, MD, MSc, FACP
Assistant Professor of Neurology and
   Neurological Surgery
Department of Neurological Surgery
Thomas Jefferson University Jefferson
   Medical College
Division of Critical Care and
   Neurotrauma
Jefferson Hospital for Neurosciences
Philadelphia, Pennsylvania
Chapters 2 and 7

Andrea M. Russo, MD, FACC, FHRS
Professor of Medicine
Robert Wood Johnson Medical School
University of Medicine and Dentistry
   of New Jersey
Department of Medicine
Division of Cardiovascular Diseases
Director of Cardiac Electrophysiology
Cooper University Hospital
Camden, New Jersey
Chapter 32

David Seder, MD
Assistant Professor of Medicine
Tufts University School of Medicine
Director of Neurocritical Care
Maine Medical Center
Portland, Maine
Chapters 35 and 39

David S. Seres, MD, ScM, PNS
Director of Medical Nutrition
Assistant Professor of Clinical Medicine
Department of Medicine
Columbia University College of
   Physicians and Surgeons
New York-Presbyterian/Columbia
   University Medical Center
New York, New York
Chapter 51

Michael J. Schmidt, PhD
Assistant Professor of Clinical
   Neuropsychology in Neurology
Director of Clinical Neuromonitoring
   and Informatics
Neurological Intensive Care Unit
Columbia University College of
   Physicians and Surgeons
New York, New York
Chapter 17

Shahzad Shaefi, MD
Fellow, Division of Anesthesia and
   Critical Care
Department of Anesthesiology
Columbia University College of
   Physicians and Surgeons
New York-Presbyterian/Columbia
   University Medical Center
New York, New York
Chapter 27

Hiren Shingala, MD
Postdoctoral Fellow
Robert Wood Johnson Medical
    School
University of Medicine and Dentistry
    of New Jersey
Division of Pulmonary & Critical Care
    Medicine
Cooper University Hospital
Camden, New Jersey
Chapter 38

Yousef Shweihat, MD
Instructor of Medicine
Pulmonary and Critical Care
    Medicine
Department of Internal Medicine
University of Arkansas for Medical
    Sciences
Little Rock, Arkansas
Chapter 40

Michael Sisti, MD, FACS
James G. McMurtry
Associate Professor of Clinical
    Neurosurgery, Radiation Oncology
    & Otolaryngology
Co-Director, The Center for
    Radiosurgery
Department of Neurological Surgery
Columbia University College of
    Physicians and Surgeons
New York-Presbyterian/Columbia
    University Medical Center
New York, New York
Chapter 8

**Robert N. Sladen, MBChB (Cape
Town), MRCP (UK), FRCP
(C),FCCM**
Professor and Executive Vice-Chair of
    Anesthesiology
Chief, Division of Critical Care
Department of Anesthesiology
Columbia University College of
    Physicians and Surgeons
New York-Presbyterian/Columbia
    University Medical Center
New York, New York
Chapter 18

Simon K. Topalian, MD, FACC
Assistant Professor of Medicine
Robert Wood Johnson Medical School
University of Medicine and Dentistry
    of New Jersey
Cooper University Hospital
Camden, New Jersey
Chapter 34

Constantine Tsigrelis, MD
Assistant Professor of Medicine
Cooper Medical School of Rowan
    University
Division of Infectious Diseases
Cooper University Hospital
Camden, New Jersey
Chapter 50

Thilagavathi Venkatachalam, MD
Postdoctoral Fellow, Nephrology
Robert Wood Johnson Medical School
University of Medicine and Dentistry
    of New Jersey
Division of Nephrology
Cooper University Hospital
Camden, New Jersey
Chapter 44

Tracy Walker, MD
Postdoctoral Fellow, Cardiology
Robert Wood Johnson Medical School
University of Medicine and Dentistry
    of New Jersey
Department of Medicine
Division of Cardiovascular Diseases
Cooper University Hospital
Camden, New Jersey
Chapter 32

Steven Werns, MD
Professor of Medicine
Cooper Medical School of Rowan
    University
Professor of Medicine
Robert Wood Johnson Medical School
University of Medicine and Dentistry
    of New Jersey
Director, Invasive Cardiovascular
    Services
Cooper University Hospital
Camden, New Jersey
Chapter 31

Lawrence S. Weisberg, MD
Professor of Medicine
Cooper Medical School of Rowan
    University
Professor of Medicine
Robert Wood Johnson Medical School
University of Medicine and Dentistry
    of New Jersey
Head, Division of Nephrology
Deputy Chief, Department of
    Medicine
Cooper University Hospital
Camden, New Jersey
Chapters 41 and 43

Joshua Z. Willey, MD, MS
Assistant Professor of Neurology
Columbia University College of
    Physicians and Surgeons
Department of Neurology, Division of
    Stroke
New York-Presbyterian/Columbia
    University Medical Center
New York, New York
Chapter 5

Teresa J. Wojtasiewicz, BA
College of Physicians and Surgeons
Columbia University
New York, New York
Chapter 24

Brian Woods, MD
Assistant Professor of Anesthesiology
Department of Anesthesiology
Columbia University College of
    Physicians and Surgeons
New York-Presbyterian/Columbia
    University Medical Center
New York, New York
Chapter 26

Jason A. Yahwak, MD
Clinical Instructor in Medicine
Tufts University School of Medicine
Division of Pulmonary and Critical
    Care Medicine
Maine Medical Center
Portland, Maine
Chapter 39

Moussa F. Yazbeck, MD
Postdoctoral Fellow
Robert Wood Johnson Medical School
University of Medicine and Dentistry
   of New Jersey
Division of Critical Care Medicine
Cooper University Hospital
Camden, New Jersey
Chapter 2

Sergio L. Zanotti-Cavazzoni, MD
Assistant Professor of Medicine
Robert Wood Johnson Medical School
University of Medicine and Dentistry
   of New Jersey
Department of Medicine
Division of Critical Care Medicine
Cooper University Hospital
Camden, New Jersey
Chapter 47

Moussa F. Yazbeck, MD
Postdoctoral Fellow
Robert Wood Johnson Medical School
University of Medicine and Dentistry
of New Jersey
Division of Critical Care Medicine
Cooper University Hospital
Camden, New Jersey
Chapter 4

Sergio L. Zanotti-Cavazzoni, MD
Assistant Professor of Medicine
Robert Wood Johnson Medical School
University of Medicine and Dentistry
of New Jersey
Department of Medicine
Division of Critical Care Medicine
Cooper University Hospital
Camden, New Jersey
Chapter 4

Foreword

This work is a dialogue. It could be between two colleagues from different disciplines, between a resident or fellow with a mentor, or between two neurointensivists trying to work through a challenging patient care dilemma. But, in any event, it is a dialogue.

Each chapter considers a case vignette or small number of vignettes. The patients presented illustrate the typical, common problems encountered in a NeuroICU. The vignettes are broken up and interspersed with the sort of discussions that occur every day in such a unit. In all cases, the discussion begins by establishing priority. What's the goal at this stage? What must we do *now*, to get to the next stage? The answers are as clear as the questions. Then, what else should we be thinking about? Question after question, answer after answer, the same straightforward dialogue occurs. What next? What is happening to the patient? What should we do about it? Why? Each question elicits a clear, practical response. The answer is supported by selected, pertinent evidence. Evidence is not presented as a mere list of data but rather as integrated information. The key data are explicitly stated but then there is also commentary based on subsequent studies and the subsequent collective experience of its accomplished authors. In other words, this is a dialogue. And finally, at the end of each section, as if asking "Still unsure how to proceed?", the answer comes back "Well let me tell you how we do it" and a step-by-step protocol follows.

This occurs over and over again, subject after subject and organ after organ. For this, work is not just about intensive care of the nervous system, it acknowledges and addresses all of the multiorgan problems that attend the complex diseases that can produce catastrophic injury of the nervous system.

This book is sure to be a favorite for many years to come. It is not a volume that will sit on an office shelf; it will live out in the ICU or the ED. One can only hope that the binding and pages are sturdy enough to handle the usage.

George C. Newman, MD, PhD

Preface

The field of medicine has always been in the state of constant evolution. Researchers have been relentlessly investigating challenging problems that appeared confusing and difficult to address both at the bedside as well as in the laboratories. As a result, clinicians have benefitted from learning new findings and elucidating previously equivocal and debatable issues. Along with remarkable advances in the recent years, particularly in the therapeutic aspect, the field of neurology is no longer considered merely a field of phenomenology and simply admiring the localization and neuronal circuits around it. Today, there are numerous acute and long-term therapies that are supported by scientific evidence of improving conditions of patients with illnesses in both central and peripheral nervous systems.

The idea of neurologic critical care is to provide acute medical therapies and appropriate interventions in a prompt fashion by monitoring the patients in one area by specially trained neurointensivists and nurses. It is by no means surprising to observe dedicated units with adequate staffing producing improved outcomes in both medical-surgical as well as neurologic intensive care units as people in critical condition require constant monitoring. As with many critical illnesses in general, acute brain injuries and other neurologic emergencies are complicated with time-sensitive matters. In order to provide adequate assessment and therapies without any delays, competency in being able to recognize acute changes in neurologic function cannot be overemphasized. By the same argument, other end organs in critical condition also require the same degree of close monitoring and rapid treatment. Patients with acute, severe brain injuries are often accompanied by other organ failures at the time of presentation and/or during the ICU stay. Priorities may differ between each case, but it is of paramount importance that all organs must be treated successfully in order to achieve favorable outcomes. For instance, it is physiologically impossible to improve brain oxygenation without addressing ARDS for a patient with both problems. It is true that as long as patients receive adequate care, it may not matter as to *who* is providing it. However, providing critical care medicine for a number of different injured organs by a system that requires consultants, who are not staffing the unit constantly, may possibly lead to delay in both diagnosis as well as providing therapy. Multiorgan failure needs a multidisciplinary team approach and adequate staffing. This text is written for that very reason. Readers will find that this book is not just about the brain. It is about *all* organ insufficiencies and failures along with neurologic illnesses in an effort to reflect the real-life challenges in a modern NeuroICU where care goes beyond the scope of classic neurology. The overall content is synthesized with another main concept: practicality. When an intensivist is faced with life-threatening neurologic and medical emergencies, pathophysiology and epidemiology are not as essential as step-by-step management plan. The flow of content is written with case-based, question-and-answer format in order to simulate the real life of making ICU rounds, which makes it easier and more interesting to read. By having 50 percent neuro and 50 percent critical care, this text may serve as a helpful tool in preparation for neurocritical care board certification examination, as well as for daily clinical work for anyone who provides critical care medicine for patients with acute brain injury and other organ failures.

Kiwon Lee, MD
New York City

Acknowledgments

This book is a proud product of many leading academic physicians at multiple medical institutions including Columbia University College of Physicians and Surgeons, UMDNJ Robert Wood Johnson Medical School, Mount Sinai School of Medicine, Thomas Jefferson University Jefferson Medical College, and University of California at Los Angeles David Geffen Medical School. First I would like to express my grateful heart to Anne Sydor, Executive Editor at McGraw-Hill, who has been supportive of the idea from the beginning and to the production staff Christine Diedrich, Karen Edmonson, and Catherine Saggese who worked diligently to bring the book to fruition. I would like to sincerely thank every contributing author especially those who served kindly as the section editors: Neeraj Badjatia, MD, Jan Claassen, MD, PhD, Stephan A. Mayer, MD, E. Sander Connolly, MD, Joseph Meltzer, MD, Joseph Parrillo, MD, R. Phillip Dellinger, MD, Lawrence S. Weisberg, MD, Louis Aledort, MD, and especially Fred Rincon, MD, who has been incredibly helpful to me throughout the entire process. Without the efforts from all the authors and section editors, it would not have been possible to successfully produce this textbook. I would like to also thank George C. Newman, MD, PhD who has kindly offered the Foreword.

Neurocritical Care Diseases

Section Editor: Neeraj Badjatia, MD, MSc

CHAPTER

1

Subarachnoid Hemorrhage

Kiwon Lee, MD, FACP, FAHA, FCCM

A 49-year-old man with history of hypertension and hyperlipidemia presents with a sudden onset of severe bifrontal headache followed by nausea. The patient vomited on his way to the nearby emergency department (ED) and became obtunded in the ambulance. On arrival to the ED, he was intubated for airway protection as his mental status continued to worsen. About 30 minutes after the onset of the initial symptoms, he progressed to stuporous mental status with minimal but intact withdrawal responses to painful stimulation. Brainstem reflexes were intact. Stat head computed tomography (CT) (Figure 1-1) revealed acute subarachnoid hemorrhage (SAH) filling the basal cistern, bilateral sylvian fissures with thick hemorrhages along with early radiographic evidence for hydrocephalus, and intraventricular hemorrhage (IVH) mainly in the fourth ventricle. The local ED physicians decided to transfer the patient immediately to the nearest tertiary medical center. During the emergent transfer, patient stopped responding to any painful stimuli and had only intact brainstem reflexes.

On arrival at the neurologic intensive care unit, the following is the clinical observation: Patient is intubated with endotracheal tube, in coma, decerebrate posturing on painful stimulation, intact corneal reflexes, pupils 5 mm in diameter briskly constricting to 3 mm bilaterally to the light stimulation, intact oculocephalic reflexes, and positive bilateral Babinski signs.

Vital signs: HR 110 bpm in sinus tachycardia, RR 20 breaths/min on the set rate of 14 breaths/min on assist control–volume control mechanical ventilation, temperature: 99.3°F, BP: 190/100 mm Hg by cuff pressure on arrival to the NeuroICU.

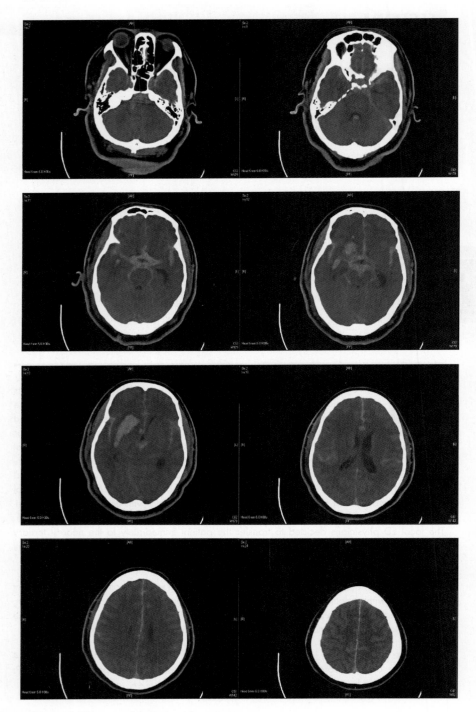

Figure 1-1. Axial CT images of the brain without contrast.

What are the initial steps for resuscitating acute aneurysmal subarachnoid hemorrhage in this case?

The clinical and radiographic presentation of this case is consistent with high-grade (initially Hunt and Hess [HH] grade IV, then quickly progressing to grade V in transit to the tertiary care center) acute SAH. Airway, breathing, and circulation (ABC) have all been addressed, although the blood pressure is high at this time. The very first step in managing this patient is ventricular drain, the second step is ventricular drain, and the third step is ensuring that the ventricular drain you have just placed is working (ie, draining the hemorrhagic cerebrospinal fluid [CSF] adequately when the drain is kept open, and maintaining good waveforms when the drain is clamped). After ABC, placing external ventricular drain (EVD) is the most crucial, lifesaving, important early step for managing the patients with *high-grade* acute SAH with poor mental status and IVH. The presence of IVH complicates the natural course of both intracerebral hemorrhage (ICH) as well as SAH cases. IVH is often associated with development of an acute obstructive hydrocephalus, which may lead to vertical eye movement impairment and depressed level of arousal by its mass effect on the thalamus and midbrain. IVH is also associated with elevated intracranial pressure (ICP), which lowers the cerebral perfusion pressure (CPP) (by the principle of the equation, $CPP = MAP - ICP$) if the mean arterial pressure (MAP) remains constant. IVH has also been reported to be an independent risk factor for increased risk of developing symptomatic vasospasm. The mass effect and cerebral edema may rapidly progress to herniation syndrome and death. As such, the presence of IVH has been recognized as a significant risk factor of poor outcome for both ICH and SAH.[1-3] Placing an EVD provides twofold benefits: (1) reliable (as long as the catheter tip is in the right location providing appropriate ICP waveforms without obstructing the ventricular catheter by any blood clot) measurements of the ICP, and (2) therapeutic drainage of the CSF in order to alleviate the intracranial hypertension (Figure 1-2).

It is important to note that the presence of IVH does not necessarily mean the ICP is abnormally elevated, and the placement of an EVD alone may not always lead to improved outcome even if the high ICP responds favorably to opening and lowering of the drain.[4] In the past, there were concerns regarding the potential harmful effect of EVD placement in treating the acute hydrocephalus in SAH cases. These concerns were mainly focused on the theoretical impact of suddenly lowering the ICP

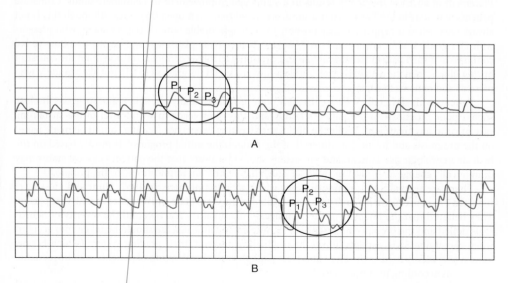

Figure 1-2. ICP waveforms and compliance. **A.** ICP waveform with normal compliance. **B.** ICP waveform with poor compliance.

by EVD placement and eliminating the tamponade effect on ruptured aneurysmal wall, leading to an increased risk of rebleed in the acute phase. However, the clinical studies have failed to prove such a hypothesis and there is not sufficient evidence to believe that the CSF diversion by an EVD in treating acute hydrocephalus after SAH leads to a higher incidence of rerupturing of the unsecured aneurysms.[5,6] It is wise, however, to avoid aggressively lowering the drain level immediately after placement. In managing SAH cases, whether to place an EVD or not is occasionally debatable. For instance, a patient with good-grade (eg, HH I or II) SAH who is awake, following commands with normal strength with no IVH, no acute hydrocephalus, and either absent or minimal volume of SAH (eg, classic Fisher groups 1 to 2) is *not* a candidate for EVD placement. On the other hand, a patient with a high HH grade, Fisher group 3 SAH, plus the radiographic evidence of severe IVH and acute hydrocephalus who is progressively getting worse in the level of arousal needs *emergent* placement of an EVD. These are extreme ends of the clinical spectrum of SAH, and the timing and indication for EVD could be debated for the cases that are somewhere in between these two extreme case scenarios. Acute hydrocephalus with IVH and clinical signs and symptoms of intracranial hypertension are all good indications for placing EVDs. It is also important to remember that even if the patient does not have any of the indications mentioned above, if the treating physician believes that there is a reasonable probability of developing these signs and symptoms in the near future, EVD placement should be considered. (Technical details and further management strategies are discussed in Chapter 22.) Despite the lack of "level 1" evidence of randomized data for improved outcomes, the use of an EVD is important as it can be helpful in managing ICP and CPP and is often lifesaving in certain SAH patients.

This patient's level of arousal improves a few minutes after placing the EVD (opening pressure 35 mm Hg). He is now able to localize to painful stimulations. Does the prognosis change with improved neuroexamination after EVD placement?

Changing Neurologic Status After EVD Placement

Placement of an EVD frequently results in a significant improvement in neurologic status. Comatose patients may start to localize to painful stimulation and may even open their eyes. Although this is not always seen, when it happens, it may possibly indicate a favorable outlook (eg, a patient, who presents with HH grade V after aneurysmal SAH, wakes up after EVD placement and begins to follow verbal commands: if such patient remains awake and continues to follow commands throughout the course of his/her illness, then the patient is behaving like a low-grade HH [ie, grades I to III], not like a grade V who presents and remains in coma).

Patients with HH grade V have extremely poor prognosis. Many physicians and surgeons disclose such a poor prognosis to the patient's family and this often leads to withdrawal of life-sustaining care prior to any treatment. While the decision of treating versus not treating should be made based on the prognosis and for the best interest of the patient, the initial prognosis is mostly based on the bedside neurologic assessment, and physicians should be aware that the patient's clinical status may dramatically change after placing an EVD, which has significant implications for the prognosis.[7]

There are several SAH grading systems worth mentioning here. In 1967, Hunt and Hess have reported 275 consecutive patients who were treated at the Ohio State University over a 12-year period. They believed that the intensity of the meningeal inflammatory reaction and the severity of neurologic deficit and the presence or absence of significant systemic disease should be taken into account when classifying SAH patients. From the original manuscript, their grading system (which is now known and widely used as the Hunt and Hess Grade) was a classification of patients with intracranial aneurysms according to surgical risk (Table 1-1).[8]

Higher grades are associated with increased surgical risk for the repair of ruptured intracranial aneurysms. The Hunt and Hess original report included the presence of significant systemic disease

Table 1-1. Hunt and Hess Grade for SAH[a]

Category	Criteria
Grade I	Asymptomatic, or mild headache and slight nuchal rigidity
Grade II	Moderate to severe headache, nuchal rigidity, no neurologic deficit other than cranial nerve palsy
Grade III	Drowsiness, confusion, or mild focal deficit
Grade IV	Stupor, moderate to severe hemiparesis, possibly early decerebrate rigidity and vegetative disturbances
Grade V	Deep coma, decerebrate rigidity, moribund appearance

[a]Classification of patients with intracranial aneurysms according to surgical risk.

(From Hunt W, Hess R. Surgical risk as related to time of intervention in the repair of intracranial aneurysms. J Neurosurg. 1968;28:14-20.)

(such as "hypertension, diabetes, severe arteriosclerosis, chronic pulmonary disease, and severe vasospasm seen on angiography") as a negative sign, and the presence of such disease resulted in placement of the patient in the next less favorable (higher surgical risk) grading category.[8] This grading system is not flawless as it can be challenging sometimes to differentiate between each category. For example, consider a patient with SAH with mild headache and nuchal rigidity versus another patient with moderate headache and nuchal rigidity (which means grades I and II, respectively, according to the original HH grading system). The only differentiating variable here would be the intensity of the headache, and that can be problematic as the intensity of headache is subjective and patients often cannot differentiate mild from moderate headache (most people would say "very bad" headache and cannot provide further details than that).

This criticism has been actually predicted, and the original authors have mentioned it in their journal article: "It is recognized that such classifications are arbitrary and that the margins between categories may be ill-defined."[8] For this reason, it has been pointed out that the HH system has poor interobserver reliability and reproducibility.[9] Nevertheless, the HH grading system is widely used and numerous studies have shown that the higher grade (or sometimes called poor grade, which usually refers to HH grades IV and V) is associated with a poor outcome.[10-13]

Another grading system to consider is the one that is the most universally accepted system for patients presenting with altered level of consciousness, the Glasgow Coma Scale (GCS). In 1975, Jennet and Bond, from the University of Glasgow, reported a scale called Assessment of Outcome After Severe Brain Damage, a Practical Scale (Table 1-2).[14]

The GCS is a more general grading system and was not developed specifically for SAH patients. However, studies show that for patients with aneurysmal SAH, the initial GCS score has positively correlated with long-term outcome.[15]

In 1988, the World Federation of Neurosurgical Societies (WFNS) developed a grading system that incorporated both the GCS and bedside neurologic assessment focusing on any focal deficit (Table 1-3).[16]

The HH and WFNS grading systems are by far the two most commonly used systems for grading patients with acute aneurysmal SAH. Despite the frequently raised criticisms regarding the interobserver variability, the HH grade is used even more commonly than the WFNS scale (71% of reported studies from 1985 to 1992 used the HH grade compared to 19% that used the WFNS scale),[17,18] and both grading systems have been shown to correlate reasonably well with the long-term outcome.[19]

In 1980, Fisher and colleagues reported the relationship between the amount of SAH and risk of developing severe vasospasm (defined as delayed clinical symptoms and signs, Table 1-4).[20]

The Fisher group's grading system is based on the description of CT findings mainly focusing on the actual volume of blood in the subarachnoid space. There is a linear relationship between the amount of hemorrhage and the rate of developing symptomatic vasospasm.[20] This grading system has

Table 1-2. Glasgow Coma Scale

Category	Score
Eye opening	
Spontaneous	4
To loud voice	3
To pain	2
None	1
Verbal response	
Oriented and converses	5
Confused, disoriented	4
Inappropriate words	3
Incomprehensive sounds	2
None	1
Best motor response	
Obeys commands	6
Localizes to pain	5
Withdraws (flexion)	4
Abnormal flexion posturing	3
Extension posturing	2
None	1

(From Jennett B, Bond M. Assessment of outcome after severe brain damage. Lancet. 1975;1:480-484.)

Table 1-3. World Federation of Neurosurgical Societies Scale for SAH

Grade	Criteria
I	GCS 15 without focal deficit[a]
II	GCS 13-14 without focal deficit
III	GCS 13-14 with focal deficit
IV	GCS 7-12 with or without focal deficit
V	GCS 3-6 with or without focal deficit

Abbreviations: GCS, Glasgow Coma Scale; SAH, subarachnoid hemorrhage.

[a]Focal deficit is defined as either aphasia and/or motor deficit.

(From Drake C. Report of World Federation of Neurological Surgeons Committee on a Universal Subarachnoid Hemorrhage Grading Scale. J Neurosurg. 1988;68:985-986.)

Table 1-4. Fisher Scale of SAH

Group	CT finding description
1	No detectable SAH
2	Diffuse SAH, no localized clot > 3 mm thick or vertical layers > 1 mm thick
3	Localized clot > 5 × 3 mm in subarachnoid space, or > 1 mm in vertical thickness
4	Intraparenchymal or intraventricular hemorrhage with either absent or minimal SAH

Abbreviation: SAH, subarachnoid hemorrhage. (From Fisher CM, Kistler JP, Davis JM. Relation of cerebral vasospasm to subarachnoid hemorrhage visualized by computerized tomographic scanning. Neurosurgery. 1980;6:1-9.)

been extensively studied and there are numerous clinical studies validating its usefulness.[21-25] In multiple studies, the risk of developing symptomatic cerebral vasospasm appears to increase along with the increasing amount of acute hemorrhage in the subarachnoid space. The original report by Fisher et al does describe the low risk of vasospasm, and yet there is a clearly observed risk of vasospasm even for patients with minimal blood in the subarachnoid space and for those with intraparenchymal or intraventricular hemorrhage.[20]

It is important to understand that the Fisher scale actually did report some incidence of vasospasm in groups 1, 2, and 4. The group 3 had the highest incidence of vasospasm, but other groups also had vasospasms, just much lower in frequency.[20] Like all other grading systems, the Fisher scale is not without limitations. There have been concerns in the literature reporting a low correlation between the Fisher grade and the incidence of symptomatic vasospasm (one of the recent studies showed about 50% correlation between the Fisher grade and vasospasm).[26] Another criticism about the Fisher scale is its inevitable interpresonal variability in assessing the estimated blood volume. Also, according to the scale, all cases of CT head showing SAH with greater than 1 mm of vertical thickness is categorized as grade III, but this includes vast majority of patients with SAH who may not in fact have the same risk of developing vasospasm.[26,27]

In light of these concerns, Claassen et al's group, from Columbia University, proposed another grading system (Table 1-5), the modified Fisher scale (mFS).[28,29]

Note that the mFS incorporates the presence or absence of IVH, and if a patient has IVH, even if there is no blood in the subarachnoid space, the scale is 2 (as opposed to 1 [no blood seen] or 4 [minimal SAH and the presence of intraparenchymal hemorrhage or IVH] in the original Fisher scale). This scale emphasizes that the presence of IVH increases the risk of developing symptomatic vasospasm. This emphasis is stronger but not completely different from that of the Fisher scale as the original Fisher scale does report some incidence (although low) of vasospasm in those with IVH and absent or minimal SAH. Furthermore, the mFS uses a subjective description and coding of the hemorrhage by the use of "thick" or "thin" clots in the subarachnoid space, and the description of IVH did not take the exact amount of IVH into account (this scale takes the "presence" versus the "absence" of IVH into account, not how much IVH there is). The mFS emphasizes the importance of IVH as well as it highlights how the amount of hemorrhage once again plays an important role. Its grading system is easy and intuitive (unlike the classic Fisher scale in which group 4 actually has a lower incidence of

Table 1-5. The Modified Fisher Scale

CT finding description	IVH	Modified Fisher Scale
Diffuse thick SAH	Present	4
	Absent	3
Localized thick SAH	Present	4
	Absent	3
Diffuse thin SAH	Present	2
	Absent	1
Localized thin SAH	Present	2
	Absent	1
No SAH	Present	2
	Absent	0

Abbreviations: IVH, intraventricular hemorrhage; SAH, subarachnoid hemorrhage.

(From Claassen J, Bernardini GL, Kreiter KT, et al. Effect of cisternal and ventricular blood on risk of delayed cerebral ischemia after subarachnoid hemorrhage: The Fisher Scale revisited. Stroke. 2001;32:2012-2020.)

vasospasm than lower grades), as the scale goes from 0 to 4, and the higher grade is the higher risk of developing delayed cerebral ischemia (DCI).

In order to minimize the interobserver variability in assessing the estimated volume of blood in the subarachnoid space, a volumetric quantification of Fisher grade 3 has been proposed and studied by Friedman and colleagues from the Mayo Clinic.[30] However, while quantification of SAH may provide a more accurate assessment of the volume of blood in the subarachnoid space, it requires *manual* outlining of the hemorrhage volume, which can be time consuming and less reliable.

In 2011, Ko and colleagues, from Columbia University, reported a study of volumetric analysis of SAH using a MIPAV (Medical Image Processing, Analysis, and Visualization; version 4.3; National Institutes of Heath, NIH) software package that *automatically* outlines the hemorrhage on CT at the click of a button.[31] This quantification analysis showed that patients with a higher volume of cisternal *plus* IVH clot burden developed a greater risk of developing DCI and poor outcome at 3 months (Figure 1-3). It also validated the modified Fisher scale as a reasonable grading system in predicting DCI that can be done easily at the bedside. However, it is important to note that although both the Fisher scale and the mFS have demonstrated the association between blood burden and DCI, a question still remained: Does the location and exact thresholds of blood volume matter? Ko and colleagues have reported:

> Our data show that the quantitative blood volume in contact with the cisternal space, whether directly in the cisternal subarachnoid space or intraventricular space, acts as *cumulative* blood burden and is associated

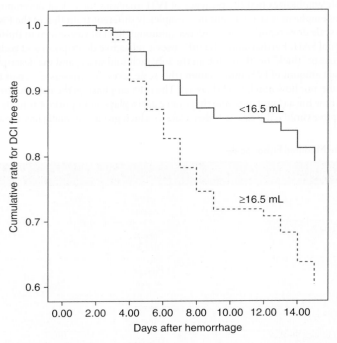

Figure 1-3. Survival plot for development of delayed cerebral ischemia. After dichotomization of patients' group based on cisternal plus intraventricular hemorrhage volume criteria, patients with higher blood burden (≥16.5 mL, dotted line) had earlier development of delayed cerebral ischemia compared to the less blood burden group (<16.5 mL, solid line; Cox regression analysis, $P < .024$). (*From Ko SB, Choi HA, Carpenter AM, et al. Quantitative analysis of hemorrhage volume for predicting delayed cerebral ischemia after subarachnoid hemorrhage. Stroke. 2011;42:669-674. Epub ahead of print Jan 21.*)

with an increased risk of DCI. The quantitative volume scale and the mFS were equivalent in predicting DCI, validating the accuracy of the mFS. However, volumetric analysis had no overlaps in the odds ratio for DCI in different blood burden groups, which may suggest more robust association between the total blood burden and DCI.

Klimo and Schmidt have eloquently summarized a historical review of the literature on the relationship between the CT findings and the rate of developing cerebral vasospasm after aneurysmal SAH using different scales[32]:

> The elucidation of predictive factors of cerebral vasospasm following aneurysmal subarachnoid hemorrhage is a major area of both clinical and basic science research. It is becoming clear that many factors contribute to this phenomenon. The most consistent predictor of vasospasm has been the *amount* of SAH seen on the postictal computed tomography scan. Over the last 30 years, it has become clear that the greater the amount of blood within the basal cisterns, the greater the risk of vasospasm. To evaluate this risk, various grading schemes have been proposed, from simple to elaborate, the most widely known being the Fisher scale. Most recently, volumetric quantification and clearance models have provided the most detailed analysis. Intraventricular hemorrhage, although not supported as strongly as cisternal SAH, has also been shown to be a risk factor for vasospasm.

Angiography shows an anterior communicating (A-comm) artery aneurysm and coiling was performed to secure the ruptured aneurysm. Patient returns to the ICU but now has elevated intracranial pressure (ICP) of 50 to 55 mm Hg with MAP of 100 mm Hg.

What is the stepwise approach for treating high ICP for SAH patients?

The early phase of high-grade SAH is often complicated by the presence of ICP crisis. An ICP value out of the normal range (0 to 20 mm Hg) is considered abnormal, but the ICP alone as an absolute value may not always signify the need for an urgent treatment. A good example would be people with pseudotumor cerebri and high ICP but having normal daily activities. ICP also rises when patients cough or get suctioned. Such a rise, if it is induced and transient, does not necessarily need any treatment. In the setting of acute, high-grade SAH, however, abnormally elevated ICP *is* a major concern owing to its direct, negative impact on the cerebral perfusion pressure (CPP). With persistently low or decreasing CPP, a certain degree of ischemic insult is inevitable. A step-by-step algorithm for managing refractory ICP crisis is outlined below. This is a recommendation that reflects the latest medical treatment available in the literature.

A Step-by-Step Algorithm for Intracranial Hypertension

ICP > 20 mm Hg for >10 min (EVD is functional and draining bloody CSF, and patient is not coughing, getting suctioned, or being agitated)

↓

Surgical Decompression

1. Consider placing the second EVD on the opposite side.
2. Decompressive craniectomy/craniotomy is the most effective way of reducing intracranial hypertension. If surgery is not an option, proceed to the following medical steps.

↓

Step 1: Sedation with Short-Acting Agents

(Patients should be on mechanical ventilation. The very first step in medically addressing an ICP crisis is sedation. LEAVE THE PATIENT ALONE. This is not the right time to pinch the patient to get the best examination every 10 min.)

If hemodynamically stable (no hypotension):

IV propofol: Repeat 20 mg IVP q20s up to 1-2 mg/kg for initial bolus, maintenance 5-50 µg/kg/min (0.3-3 mg/kg/h).

∗Dose higher than 50 µg/kg/min of IV propofol may be used but be aware of the rare but potentially fatal propofol infusion syndrome.

Refractory ICP crisis and status epilepticus are two important neuro-emergencies that may require a high-dose propofol often as high as 100-150 µg/kg/min.

OR

If hemodynamically unstable (hypotensive, poor cardiac output, intravascular volume depletion, etc.):

IV midazolam: Load 0.01-0.05 mg/kg over 2 min, maintenance 0.02-0.2 µg/kg/h.

AND

Consider adding an analgesic agent:

IV fentanyl: IV bolus 25-100 µg followed by maintenance 1-3 µg/kg/h.

∗Adding analgesic agent may synergistically lower the ICP more efficiently, but it takes longer for patient to wake up. This is not desirable during an active cerebral vasospasm as it is important to be able to follow patient's clinical examination closely. Analgesia is an important step in managing intracranial hypertension if pain is suspected component of agitation. Analgesia is especially helpful for SAH in trauma cases, but it may be helpful even for aneurysmal SAH cases. Pain can lead to agitation and agitation worsens ICP.

Step 2: Hyperventilation and Order Osmotic Agents

1. **Hyperventilation** (unless patient is already autohyperventilating over the set rate of mechanical ventilation) induces cerebral vasoconstriction and reduced cerebral blood flow (CBF), which leads to ICP reduction. Target end-tidal Pco_2 of 30 mm Hg.

*There are heated debates regarding whether to recommend hyperventilation or not as brain ischemia is a well-documented risk of hyperventilation. In the setting of refractory ICP crisis and brain herniation, hyperventilation is a rapid and effective way of controlling high ICP *temporarily*. This should be used only to buy time to initiate further therapies.

2. **Mannitol**: 1-1.5 g/kg 10%-25% solution IV bag infused over 30 min, q6h. Osm < 360, Osm gap < 10. Osm limit of "320" is a nonscientific, arbitrary number.

∗Avoid if intravascular volume depletion is present. Avoid underdosing and avoid blind dosing (eg, mannitol IV 25 g q6h round the clock, for all patients regardless of the body weight without assessing the intravascular volume or ICP). If the patients are showing signs and symptoms of ICP crisis and/or brain herniation, underdosing is not a good idea.

3. **Hypertonic saline (HTS)**: 30 mL of 23.4% IV push over 5 min, q4-6h. PRN. Avoid serum Na > 155.

∗Continuous infusion of 3% HTS all day, every day at high volume (eg, 3% HTS at 150 mL/h continuously for 5 days) frequently leads to severe *pulmonary edema* (remember, ICU patients are always receiving other medicine in high volume as well; this leads to liters of positive input and not enough output), and such blind infusion may not be effective in controlling high ICP as the intra-extracellular osmotic equilibrium occurs. It may be more effective to use the high concentration (23.4% bolus) on a prn basis. A recent small (N = 34) randomized trial demonstrated hypertonic saline (20% sodium lactate) showing more effective and longer-lasting control of ICP directly compared to an equivalent osmotic dose of mannitol in severe traumatic injury patients.[31]

Step 3: Barbiturate Coma

Pentobarbital: Load 10 mg/kg IV infusion over 1 h, maintenance 1-3 mg/kg/h, target 1-2 bursts per 10-s suppression on continuous EEG.

Many clinicians do not "like" using pentobarbital. Pentobarbital is notorious for suppressing the heart, leading to reduced cardiac output and systemic hypotension (get ready to use pressor/inotropes shortly after starting it). Due to its long elimination $t_{1/2}$ (15-50 hours), the loss of ability to follow the clinical examination is another serious (especially for high-grade SAH patients) downside. However, pentobarbital is effective in lowering ICP by its potent CNS suppression (lowers the metabolic demand).

*Avoid *prolonged* use of pentobarbital. The combination of prolonged use of high-dose pentobarbital and multiple pressors (Neo-Synephrine plus Levophed) is a cocktail for multisystem failure. (Kidneys will be injured first and then liver, followed by severe acidosis and irreversible shock, along with dark, necrotic distal fingers.) Yes, we are focusing on saving the brain, but brain also dies if everything else dies.

Step 4: Therapeutic Hypothermia

Target temperature = 32-34°C using either surface cooling or endovascular cooling device (IV infusion of cold saline is a cost-effective and efficient *induction* method)

- Surface devices are noninvasive with less complications.
- Endovascular devices are invasive but may achieve the target temperature more rapidly and are associated with less shivering.
- Use of advanced temperature modulation system is recommended over conventional methods (cooling blanket or ice packs) as temperature must be controlled during cooling and slow, passive rewarming in order to avoid rebound intracranial hypertension.
- A prolonged (> 7 days: the actual days for different devices' safety may vary) use of endovascular cooling devices increases the risk of developing thrombotic complication and catheter-related bloodstream infection.
- Hypothermia is a new and often effective method of reducing ICP in otherwise refractory intracranial hypertension.
- Shivering needs to be aggressively treated for three reasons:
  A. Shivering prevents the core body temperature from falling and leads to prolonged time to achieve the target temperature.
  B. Shivering can increase ICP and further worsen the intracranial hypertension.
  C. Shivering can increase the brain metabolism and increase the risk of developing brain hypoxia and cellular metabolic distress (decrease in partial pressure of brain tissue oxygen tension [$Pbto_2$] and increase in brain lactate/pyruvate ratio).
- Antishivering methods [33-38]:
  A. **Skin counterwarming**: warm, forced-air blankets and mattress
  B. **IV magnesium** (IV bolus 60-80 mg/kg, then maintenance 2 g/h) may reduce the shivering threshold but is not effective as a single agent to treat the shivering during full hypothermia (ie, 32-34°C)
  C. **Buspirone** 20-30 mg via nasogastric tube after crushing tid
  D. **IV dexmedetomidine** 0.4-1.5 µg/kg/h
  E. **IV meperidine** 0.4 mg/kg (usual dose 25-50 mg) IV q4-6
  F. **IV propofol** 50-100 mg rapid IV push, maintenance 0.3-3 mg/kg/h
  G. **IV clonidine** 1-3 µg/kg prn

With all other factors that are known to influence the ICP being constant, increasing the MAP leads to increased cerebral perfusion pressure. Increased cerebral perfusion pressure and blood flow may result in increased cerebral blood volume. Increased cerebral blood volume could lead to any one of the following scenarios:

1. Development of vasoconstriction would occur if autoregulation is intact in response to increased blood volume delivered. Such vasoconstriction may result in drop in ICP.

2. No vasoconstriction would occur if autoregulation is impaired (pressure-volume breakdown). Since blood volume is increased, there may be further rise in the ICP.

3. Mixed picture of all of the above as different parts of the brain have either impaired or intact autoregulation at a point prior to the pressure-volume breakdown.

Intracranial hypertension in SAH (ICP > 20 mm Hg)

↓ Should you increase the MAP?

CPP Optimization

This is important, but simply increasing the blood pressure with phenylephrine or norepinephrine may increase the volume of cerebral edema and may even worsen the ICP crisis. CPP optimization does not imply simply raising MAP, as CPP can be optimized by either increasing the MAP or reducing the ICP.

There may be a breakdown of the cerebral autoregulation curve (see right: blue curve, intact; red curve, impaired autoregulation) where every millimeter of mercury change in MAP leads to change in cerebral blood flow (CBF). Normally (the blue curve) the brain is able to self-regulate its vessels so that the CBF remains constant regardless of change in MAP. This capability may be impaired in severe brain injuries.

For example, if a SAH patient has ICP = 40 mm Hg, MAP = 90 mm Hg, CPP = 50 mm Hg, then the immediate next step is *not* to start the Neo-Synephrine in order to increase the MAP to 100-120 mm Hg to make the CPP 60-80 mm Hg and walk away. The right step is to focus on reducing the ICP without adding vasopressors, so that the CPP gets corrected by improving the ICP, not by bringing up the blood pressure without lowering the ICP. If ICP is controlled, then CPP must be kept above a certain

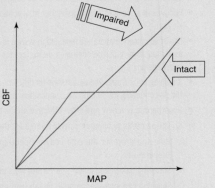

level (no class I evidence exists in SAH, but at least > 50-60 mm Hg). Of course, in the event of systemic hypotension + high ICP + low CPP, the first step is to improve MAP by using pressors. After making the MAP > 60 mm Hg, then the next step is to reduce the ICP (as opposed to just keep on increasing the MAP).

↓ Let's reduce the ICP!

1. *Adequate* sedation
2. Hyperventilation and osmotic therapy
3. Barbiturate coma
4. Therapeutic hypothermia

It is important to emphasize that increasing the blood pressure with phenylephrine may either make the ICP go up or down. Clearly, if the MAP is too low to the point that the patient is in a state of shock, it makes sense to increase the MAP in order to maintain adequate end-organ perfusion. However, if the MAP is already 90 mm Hg, then increasing the MAP to 130 mm Hg with Neo-Synephrine may have a deleterious effect on the ICP. Finally, it is important to remember that every effort needs to be made to avoid the worst combination that is associated with devastating results: systemic hypotension *and* uncontrolled ICP.

The $PbtO_2$ (partial pressure of brain tissue oxygen tension) monitoring system (Licox) is inserted in order to monitor the brain oxygenation. A jugular venous oximetry probe is also inserted.

What is the relationship between the DO_2 (delivery of oxygen), $PbtO_2$, and $SjvO_2$ (jugular venous oxygen saturation) (Figure 1-4)?

The cardiac output (CO), hemoglobin concentration [Hgb], and the arterial saturation of oxygen determine the delivery of oxygen from the heart to all the end-organ systems, including the brain. The $PbtO_2$ is significantly affected by the DO_2 and the blood flow to the brain. Flow, by definition, is blood volume per given time. Therefore, there is a positive correlation between the blood volume reaching the brain tissue and $PbtO_2$ measurements. DO_2 has a linear relationship with the CO and Hgb levels as well as SaO_2 (arterial oxygen saturation).

The oxygen content in the venous return from the brain back to the heart (measured by $SjvO_2$) depends on the DO_2 and VO_2 (oxygen consumption). The product of the DO_2 and O_{EF} (oxygen extraction fraction) determines the total VO_2:

$$VO_2 = DO_2 \times O_{EF}$$

Therefore, the oxygen extraction fraction is determined by the total consumption divided by the delivery of oxygen:

$$O_{EF} = VO_2/DO_2$$

Thus, the oxygen extraction decreases when the delivery increases while the consumption remains the same. As the consumption of oxygen decreases, the extraction decreases as not as much oxygen is needed to be extracted from the vasculature into the brain cellular tissues. Understanding this relationship is crucial in applying this principle to the bedside information. If a patient has $PbtO_2$, $SjvO_2$, and CO monitoring, one would observe that by increasing the cardiac output significantly, assuming

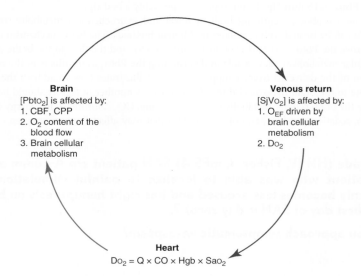

Figure 1-4. DO_2, $PbtO_2$, $SjvO_2$ relationship. CBF, cerebral blood flow; CPP, cerebral perfusion pressure; O_{EF}, oxygen extraction fraction; DO_2, delivery of oxygen; CO, cardiac output; Hgb, hemoglobin; SaO_2, arterial oxygen saturation; Q, a constant.

the brain cellular metabolism is constant (eg, under pentobarbital coma for ICP control), the O_{EF} will decrease, and as a result $Sjvo_2$ increases.

$$\uparrow CO \rightarrow \uparrow \text{brain } Do_2 \rightarrow \downarrow \text{brain } O_{EF} \rightarrow \uparrow Sjvo_2$$
(if brain oxygen consumption remains the same)

$$\uparrow CO \rightarrow \uparrow \text{brain } Do_2 \rightarrow \uparrow \text{brain } O_{EF} \rightarrow \downarrow Sjvo_2$$
(if brain oxygen consumption increases greater than Do_2)

As one can see above, the brain cellular metabolism plays an important role in brain oxygen consumption, and therefore extraction, and affects the $Pbto_2$.

ICP is finally controlled with the range of 5 to 15 mm Hg. MAP = 100 mm Hg, CPP > 85 mm Hg. However, the $PbtO_2$ is decreasing < 15 mm Hg, and the lactate/pyruvate ratio (LPR) is > 50. What could you do to improve the brain oxygenation and reduce the brain metabolic stress?

There are ongoing debates regarding whether the partial pressure of oxygen tension measured in the brain means anything in brain-injured patients (or what it means short- or long-term). Frequently encountered criticisms are focused on the fact that the location of the probe may not be in the perfect location for monitoring the injury. The probe provides direct information, but it only provides the local information, and whatever the number it gives may not be applicable to the rest of the brain. It is also criticized that the absolute value of $Pbto_2$ may not always correlate with the long-term outcome, making it difficult to determine what the critical or "dangerous" value is. From the traumatic brain injury literature, there are studies that have shown a positive correlation between the $Pbto_2$ level and mortality and outcome both in pediatric as well as in the adult population.[39,40] As long as the probe is not located in the isolated, dead brain tissue (eg, in the middle of a completed infarct, which will provide very low values of $Pbto_2$, but that does not necessarily mean the rest of the brain is critically ischemic), it is reasonable to believe that persistent, severe ($Pbto_2$ < 15 mm Hg) brain hypoxia is probably a bad sign.

As you can see above, significant brain hypoxia and neurochemical metabolic stress (lactate/pyruvate > 40) can be treated with a number of different methods. The basic mechanism of how these methods improve the $Pbto_2$ and LPR is by increasing the Do_2 and the flow to the brain. Another factor, brain cellular metabolism, plays a role in determining the $Pbto_2$ as it influences the consumption and extraction of the delivered oxygen supply. Figure 1-5 illustrates how to address the factors that may contribute to the brain hypoxia and metabolic stress. A number of factors should be considered for estimating the brain cellular metabolism: fever, shivering, CO_2 calorimetry for energy expenditure, pain/agitation, sedation/paralysis, and other variables that may affect the basic oxygen consumption and demand.

A high-grade (HH IV, Fisher 3, mFS 4) SAH patient s/p A-comm aneurysm coiling patient who was able to localize to painful stimulation bilaterally suddenly becomes less aroused and has right hemiparesis on bleed day (the very first day of SAH is day zero) 7.

How do you approach symptomatic vasospasm?

Transcranial Doppler (TCD)

TCD has been used for many years for monitoring SAH patients who are at risk for developing vasospasm. The TCD velocities rise in the segments of brain vasculature where vasospasm occurs. A mean

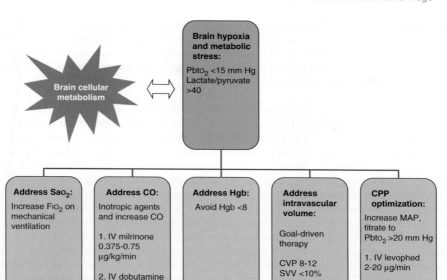

Figure 1-5. Addressing brain hypoxia after controlling ICP crisis. CO, cardiac output; CPP, cerebral perfusion pressure; CVP, central venous pressure; GEDVI, global end-diastotic volume index; Hct, hematocrit; Hgb, hemoglobin; MAP, mean arterial pressure; PAWP, pulmonary artery wedge pressure; SVV, stroke volume variation.

flow velocity greater than 120 cm/s is commonly used as a reference point for "TCD spasm."[41,42] Before firmly declaring whether TCD is useful or not, one should be aware of the frequent criticisms regarding the sensitivity and specificity of high velocities detected on TCD:

1. False positive: When the flow velocities rise, this does not necessarily mean the presence of true cerebral vasospasm. Hyperemia, a common cause of elevated velocity on TCD, is due to a number of different factors such as fever, hypervolemia, and even may be part of triple-H (hypertensive, hypervolemic, hemodilution) therapy. Consider a SAH patient who is getting 250 mL/h of normal saline infusion plus albumin 250 mL q6h for so-called prophylactic triple-H therapy for Fisher 3 with "lots of thick cisternal blood." This is bad medicine for two reasons: (1) prophylactic triple-H does not reduce the incidence of symptomatic vasospasm or improve outcomes, and may increase pulmonary complications (before saying that the heart and lungs can be abused in order to save the brain, we need to consider the following question: what would happen to the delivery of oxygen to the injured brain if we neglect to keep the lungs alive?) and (2) hypervolemia leading to high TCD velocities only increases the false-positive rate without having true cerebral vasospasm. This false rate then leads to more unnecessary and potentially harmful interventions. Hyperdynamic therapy may also increase the TCD velocities. There are physicians who utilize positive inotropic agents (eg, milrinone, dopamine, dobutamine, norepinephrine) and have a specific cardiac index goal for triple-H therapy. If you increase the cardiac output significantly, this will improve the flow, and an increase in flow leads to higher velocities. A recent article reports a poor correlation between the TCD spasm with clinically evident (symptomatic) spasm: ". . . of those with TCD spasm, only 28% had symptomatic spasm, and 34% had delayed cerebral ischemia."[41] Delayed cerebral ischemia (DCI) is defined as the presence of symptomatic vasospasm, infarction attributable to vasospasm, or both.[43]

2. False negative: The TCD is notorious for missing vasospasm occurring at the distal anterior cerebral artery (ACA) areas. The distal ACAs are technically challenging to insonate as they

are far away from the TCD probe to navigate (typically sonographers try to insonate the top of carotid, M1 A1, then A2, then A3, and so on). As the TCD probe follows the proximal ACA to the distal segment, there may be an increased amount of noise and other vessels interfering, which leads to poor reception of the distal flow. The TCD is user-dependent. As such, there may be significant interobserver variability.

Despite these well-known and documented limitations, TCD is widely used and can be useful in caring for patients with SAH. The statistical evidence of significantly high false-positive and false-negative rates of the TCD is not surprising: The TCD only detects the flow velocities, and from the waveform analysis, a number of different pulsitility indices may be obtained. Any narrowing in a vessel would lead to a higher velocity. Consider the following clinical scenario: A sonographer insonates a major vessel (eg, the M1 segment of the middle cerebral artery [MCA]), and the waveform is consistent with an M1, and the signal is strong and consistent with an M1. After documenting normal velocities of a SAH patient every day for 7 days, all of a sudden the same segment's velocity rises by 200% (or steadily increasing velocity over time); this is more likely to be true vasospasm, meaning the M1 segment's cross-sectional caliber is not as large as it used to be. This is particularly true in the absence of metabolic changes such as, for example, fever or hyperemia, and if the TCD has been performed by the same sonographer. In order to minimize the false-positive rate of TCD due to fever, hyperemia, and hyperdynamic status, a Lindegaard ratio (LR) has been described: LR = mean TCD velocity of MCA/mean TCD velocity of ipsilateral, extracranial internal carotid artery. A sudden rise in MCA mean velocity out of proportion to the rise in ipsilateral carotid artery mean velocity argues against hyperemia-induced, false-positive vasospasm. A normal LR is < 1.7, and a value > 2.0 might indicate higher risk of vasospasm. Different institutions use different threshold points of LR for categorizing TCD spasm. An example: LR < 1.5 normal, 1.5 to 2.5 hyperemia, 2.5 to 3.5 mild vasospasm, 3.5 to 4.5 moderate vasospasm, > 4.5 severe vasospasm. The literature lacks in terms of which of these LR cutoff points are more accurate. The criticism regarding the low correlation between high velocity and high LR on TCD with symptomatic vasospasm or DCI is also not surprising: just because the vessels are narrow, that does not mean the patient would become symptomatic neurologically. This all depends on the brain's margin of tolerability toward the ischemia. The cerebral ischemic cascade is complex, and the compensatory mechanisms, in the setting of ischemia due to vasospasm, leads to a variety of clinical findings: from normal to focal deficit. A high cerebral vessel velocity and LR on the TCD and yet no symptoms does not mean the TCD did not work. It could mean that the brain's compensatory mechanism is working and therefore no symptoms. Is everyone with narrow vessels on cerebral angiograph symptomatic? Of course not. Does that mean the angiograph lies and is useless? No. The TCD can be useful as long as one can interpret it appropriately and understands its limitations. Another aspect regarding the TCD is that it is more useful when the trend is followed, rather than focusing on any absolute value at any given day.

CT Angiography (CTA) and CT Perfusion (CTP)

CTA can provide a rapid, noninvasive method of visualizing the brain vasculature in patients suspected of having vasospasm (Figure 1-6). CTA can provide 2-D and 3-D images of the vessels and can be useful in detecting vasospasm and brain aneurysms without the risks that are associated with conventional angiography. It should be noted that the limitations of the CTA is that the false-negative rate can be significant for small brain aneurysms, particularly those that are < 3 mm in diameter. With the advent of the 64-section, multidetector CTA, however, the sensitivity of detecting small aneurysms, even for those that are < 3 mm in diameter, can be as high as 92%.[44] Recently, even higher resolution may be obtained with more than 300-slice, fine-cut CTA softwares. CTA can also be helpful in following patients for suspected vasospasm. CTA is not without potential risk, especially in elderly patients who might be intravascularly volume depleted or those with baseline renal impairment. Efforts should be made to prevent contrast-induced nephropathy (CIN). One single-center,

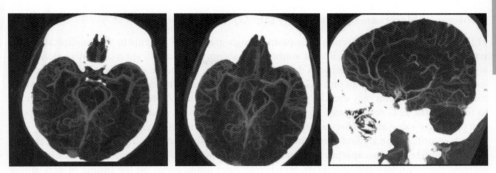

Figure 1-6. Computed tomographic angiography.

randomized trial revealed sodium bicarbonate showing a significantly reduced rate of CIN compared to sodium chloride infusion.[45,46] However, relevant data in the literature are mixed and the renal protective effect in preventing the CIN appears to be secondary to the additional volume, rather than the actual content of the IV fluid. The following is suggested protocol for preventing the CIN for high-risk ICU patients who need to undergo CTA or conventional angiography.

1. Sodium chloride 1 mL/kg/h for at least 12 hours, or
2. Sodium bicarbonate 3 mL/kg/h for at least 12 hours, and/or
3. *N*-acetylcysteine, 600 mg IV prior and then 600 mg PO bid postprocedure for 2 days.

CTP (Figure 1-7) provides three different perfusion maps.

1. Mean transit time (MTT) map: Time (in seconds) measured for the contrast material to reach the cerebral hemispheres. In the event of vasospasm, the areas that are supplied by the spasm vessel will have prolonged MTT.
2. Cerebral blood flow (CBF) map: The blood volume per given time. The areas that are supplied by the spasm vessel will have corresponding reduced CBF (usually the delayed MTT and reduced CBF occur concurrently).
3. Cerebral blood volume (CBV) map: The blood volume in the event of vasospasm shows either normal or increased blood volume if the cerebral autoregulation is intact (by compensatory self-dilatation of the brain vessels). This is the window of opportunity for appropriate medical and endovascular interventions. When and if the CBV map shows reduced volume, this may indicate complete infarction and hence irreversible ischemic injury.

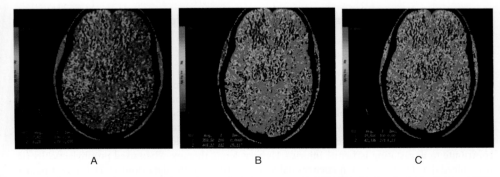

A   B   C

Figure 1-7. Computed tomographic perfusion. **A.** Mean transit time (MTT). **B.** Cerebral blood flow (CBF). **C.** Cerebral blood volume.

Continuous Electroencephalography (cEEG)

cEEG may be helpful in detecting vasospasm in high-grade SAH patients in whom clinical examinations may be of limited use. Recent studies have shown the quantification of relative alpha (RA)
signals on cEEG to be associated with detecting vasospasm—a positive association between the poor
variability of an alpha rhythm on EEG and symptomatic vasospasm—remarkably, the onset of symptoms due to vasospasm may even be preceded by the change in RA on cEEG.[47,48] Further details are
to follow in the EEG section later. Despite the small sample sizes, studies report a rather high positive predictive value and a false-negative rate. cEEG monitoring is required for all high-grade SAH
patients in order to be vigilant about the risk of nonconvulsive status epilepticus. Therefore, the use
of cEEG in detecting vasospasm can be used in conjunction with other diagnostic tests in order to
increase the sensitivity and specificity, which may have implications on the timing of performing
angiography.[49]

 A 30-year-old woman with aneurysmal SAH, HH III, F 3, mFS 3 becomes confused on
bleed day 5. cEEG shows significantly poor variability, TCD mean flow velocities have
increased to 160 cm/s in the right proximal MCA and distal ACA (with Lindegaard ratio
> 4). The patient appears to be in an euvolemic state. The patient becomes acutely left
hemiparetic with further depressed level of arousal on bleed day 7. Stat CTA and CTP reveal severe
narrowing on right M1 and right A1 and perfusion deficits with MTT prolongation affecting the entire
right cerebral hemisphere.

Any intensivist managing aneurysmal SAH patients in an ICU must be aware of when to call for
a conventional angiogram. The quick answer as to how to address this patient's acute hemiparesis and
obtundation is *stat* angiogram. It is important to acknowledge that this is a neurologic emergency. A
longer delay in getting the angiogram leads to a higher risk of irreversible ischemic damage. It is not
wise to delay the angiogram with the clinical scenario provided above. Clearly, cerebral angiography is
not a completely benign procedure. However, in an aneurysmal SAH patient, on day 7, who becomes
acutely hemiparetic and obtunded with TCD, EEG, CTA, and CTP evidence of severe vasospasm and
hypoperfusion, there should not be any delay in providing an angiogram. For clinically obvious cases,
even obtaining CTA prior to conventional angiogram may not be necessary and only delay an effective treatment. There is a role for obtaining CTA/CTP if the index of suspicion is not high enough for
severe vasospasm (ie, one can avoid getting an angiogram [which carries a potential risk] if the patient
does not really have treatable vasospasm).

What are currently available therapy options for symptomatic cerebral vasospasm?

Triple-H Therapy

Triple-H therapy has been used for many years to improve and maintain adequate brain perfusion
in patients with symptomatic vasospasm. Considering that SAH patients frequently tend to develop
natriuresis and intravascular volume depletion, it makes physiologic and intuitive sense to provide
adequate volume and avoid dehydration. This should be even more emphasized in the event of cerebral vasospasm and delayed cerebral ischemia as intravascular volume depletion could significantly
contribute to devastating ischemic injuries. Hypervolemic therapy, when used prophylactically (ie,
from bleed day 0 until day 14 in aneurysmal SAH regardless of the data from TCD, CTA, or neurologic examination), however, has failed to show improved CBF or CBV on a small (N = 82) but randomized clinical trial. In that study, the rate of developing symptomatic vasospasm was the same for

both hypervolemic and normovolemic groups.[50] There is a wide variety of clinical practice patterns regarding the use of triple-H therapy, but *prophylactic* hypervolemic therapy is not supported by any good evidence for any added benefit. Again, this does not mean that one should not provide adequate intravascular volume. It simply means, for a postoperative (clipping or coiling) SAH patient on bleed day 1, who is doing well without any signs of vasospasm, in an euvolemic state, adding additional fluid boluses is not likely to provide any additional benefit other than increasing the urine output. During the period of symptomatic vasospasm, however, nonrandomized studies indicate that additional fluid boluses can increase the CBF in the hypoperfused area even if the patient is considered to be in a euvolemic state.[51] Current diversity in clinical practice in using the triple-H therapy is secondary to the lack of "level 1" evidence in terms of when and how to use the therapy. However, it is not wise only to criticize the lack of data and not provide treatment. Until there are multiple randomized studies confirming what should be the gold standard, clinicians should be treating the patients with the best available knowledge, evidence, and, most of all, *good judgment* (because knowledge and evidence-based medical literature alone are often not sufficient to make a good decision).

One may conclude:

1. There are randomized data arguing *against* the use of prophylactic hypervolemic therapy in patients with no signs of vasospasm in SAH.[49]

2. There are no randomized data for use of triple-H therapy in improving the long-term outcome in SAH (regardless of whether triple-H therapy was used as a prophylaxis or as a treatment).

3. There are nonrandomized, observational studies showing augmentation of CBF in hypoperfused brain regions after triple-H therapy (or different parts of the triple-H therapy: ie, hypervolemic therapy alone [normal saline boluses],[51] or hyperdynamic therapy [increasing cardiac index without significantly increasing the blood pressure],[52] or hypertensive therapy alone, or a combination of all of the above).

The following is a reasonable algorithm for managing patients with risk of developing symptomatic vasospasm and delayed cerebral ischemia.

Intravascular Volume and Blood Pressure Management

Early Phase of SAH (typically bleed day 0-3, note the onset of symptomatic vasospasm may vary among patients)

Low HH grade (the patient is doing well clinically, intact neurologic examination, s/p securing of the ruptured aneurysm in the ICU):

1. Keep euvolemic (does *not* need induced hypervolemia)
   - Avoid persistently low CVP (0-3): Note that CVP is a poor surrogate for volume status. Keeping CVP greater than 12 is a blind approach and may not provide euvolemia. However, avoiding persistently low CVP is probably helpful.
   - Avoid severe anemia (Hgb < 7).
   - Avoid low PA (pulmonary artery) wedge pressure (< 10).
   - Avoid low GEDVI (global end-diastolic volume index) < 680 mL/m².
   - Avoid high SVV (stroke volume variation) and pulse pressure variation > 13%.
   - Avoid low SVI (stroke volume index) (< 40 mL/m²).
   - Avoid low urine output < 0.5 mL/kg/h.
2. Keep normal BP
   - MAP 60-90 mm Hg (does *not* need induced hypertension).
3. Normal cardiac output and index
   - CO 5-8 L/min
   - CI (cardiac index) 3-5 L/min/m²

(Proceed to the next box if the patient has any signs of vasospasm.)

High HH Grade (no examination to follow as patient is in stupor and coma to begin with):

1. Make sure patient is not having vasospasm by following other diagnostic studies other than clinical examination such as CTA/CTP, and/or TCD, cEEG, etc.
2. Do what is written above for volume, BP, and CO.

   (Proceed to next box if patient has any signs of vasospasm.)

Vasospasm Watch Period

This is typically bleed days 4-14, but symptomatic vasospasm with clinical deterioration can occur as late as day 21.

If the patient does not have any signs (clinical, TCD, CTA/P, or cEEG findings) of vasospasm, then manage the patient the same way as the early phase, targeting:

- Euvolemic
- Normotensive
- Normal cardiac performance

If the patient has any signs (clinical, TCD, CTA/P, or cEEG) of vasospasm, then:

- Hypervolemic
- Hypertensive
- Hyperdynamic cardiac performance

Optimizing Triple-H Therapy:

When the ICU team calls the interventional team for angiography for symptomatic vasospasm, one of the frequently asked (rightfully so) questions would be: "Have you maximized or fully optimized medical therapy for this patient?" This question is not unreasonable, as some patients with mild vasospasm may become asymptomatic and never really require any invasive procedure for their spasm.

How to Maximize or Fully Optimize Medical Therapy:

Use of either crystalloid or colloid is acceptable. It is highly recommended to consider using advanced dynamic variables such as stroke volume variation (SVV) and pulse pressure variation (PPV) in addition to commonly used stagnant variables such as central venous pressure (CVP) or pulmonary artery occlusion pressure.

Simply implementing CVP 10-14 would not be sufficient as CVP is a confounded variable with low reliability in terms of assessing preload responsiveness and other hemodynamic status. For patients who are *being mechanically ventilated, in the absence of arrhythmia*, the following recommendation is reasonable for active, symptomatic vasospasm:

- SVV < 10%
- PPV < 13%
- GEDVI > 680 mL/m^2
- SVI > 40 mL/m^2
- CI > 3 L/min/m^2
- Urine output > 0.5 mL/kg/h

- Reminder:
1. Reliability of advanced dynamic variables such as SVV and PPV requires controlled mechanical ventilation and the absence of arrhythmia.
2. Initiation of aggressive triple-H therapy does not mean one can delay providing more invasive therapy when necessary. For patients who do not respond to triple-H therapy, any delay in getting angiography for more definitive treatment may increase the risk of developing irreversible ischemic damage.
3. Symptomatic vasospasm is a time-sensitive emergency, and timely treatment with balloon angioplasty within 2 hours of symptom onset has been shown to have sustained clinical improvement.[53]

Invasive therapy options for symptomatic vasospasm

Cerebral Angiography (Figure 1-8)

There are a number of different vasodilators available for IA therapy of vasospasm in patients with aneurysmal SAH. These include papaverine, nicardipine, verapamil, and more recently milrinone. These vasodilators often produce an immediate result in increasing the vessel calibers, but there is a limitation: the positive effect may not last long. It is not uncommon to see patients with vasospasm who respond to initial IA vasodilators become symptomatic the same day or the next day, requiring further multiple angiographic treatments. Unless the interventional suite is located in the middle of the NeuroICU with the team actually staying in the angiography suite 24/7, there may be some delay between the redetection of the symptomatic vasospasm and the actual time of reangiography. If the patient has aspiration pneumonia on a high-maintenance ventilator setting with multiple vasopressors, the presence of an anesthesiologist is needed for reangiography, and this can be another source of delay. Balloon angioplasty (BA), despite being more aggressive and associated with potentially fatal complication, may provide a longer lasting effect. It is true that BA does not *guarantee* that the vasospasm will not ever occur again. There are clearly angioplasty-refractory vasospasms. However, it is usually fair to state that, in general, BA is superior in terms of the *durability* compared to injecting a few milligrams of any of the vasodilators mentioned above. It is difficult to quantify how long these vasodilators might work. Every practitioner has different thresholds for choosing different methods to address severe vasospasm. Ten milligrams of IA verapamil to the proximal M1 vasospasm may be perfectly fine for several days in some patients, but the positive effect may only last for 2 hours in others. Furthermore, the response rate among patients is unpredictable. IA infusion of vasodilation therapy may be considered safer in terms of performing the procedure compared to BA, as there is little to no risk of rupture of the vessel. However, if IA infusion of vasodilation therapy fails (and if it fails in the middle of night when no angiographic team members are available in-house), then there is a significant risk of stroke while preparing for repeat angiography. Another important aspect to consider is the operator's comfort level with each therapy. All of these pros and cons should be taken into account when choosing a therapy.

Intrathecal (IT) Infusion and Basal Cistern Implants of Calcium Channel Blockers

Recently, injecting L-type dihydropyridine calcium channel blockers such as nicardipine via EVD as an intrathecal (IT) therapy for vasospasm has been reported.[54-56] Although generally considered as a new therapy, one of the first human cases dates back to early 1990s when IT nicardipine was injected

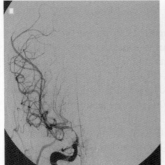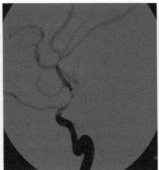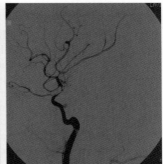

Figure 1-8. Cerebral angiography. Conventional cerebral angiography shows severe right-sided internal carotid artery vasospasm in the carotid terminus. In addition, there is a severe spasm in the right A1 segment of the ACA.

prophylactically with positive results.[54] These reports were case series with small sample sizes, and there is currently lack of good evidence at this time for routinely implanting this therapy. Given anecdotal reports of positive findings in both preventing and treating vasospasm, further studies are warranted to investigate the safety and efficacy of this therapy. As more $Pbto_2$ and other multimodality brain monitoring probes are used in clinical practice, there may be more information about how intraventricular use of vasodilators may improve the cerebral blood flow and whether it has more impact on the proximal versus distal vasculature. A recent randomized double-blind phase II study reported the use of prolonged-release implants of nicardipine and showed a reduced incidence of vasospasm and improved clinical outcome 1 year after SAH.[57] This study used nicardipine-releasing pellet implantation into the basal cisterns (10 implants placed directly onto the proximal vessels at the basal cisterns) after blood clots were washed out for both study and control groups. The implant group had a significantly reduced incidence of angiographic and symptomatic vasospasm with better short- and long-term outcome. Despite rather convincing data, it is important to remember that this therapy requires surgical clipping of the aneurysm, thorough washout of the fresh blood clots, followed by multiple implantation of nicardipine pellets.

Intra-aortic Balloon Counterpulsation Therapy

Patients with high-grade SAH may also have depressed cardiac function—a typical model for this is that of the neurogenic stunned myocardium phenomenon (sometimes described as neurogenic stress cardiomyopathy or takotsubo cardiomyopathy) with mid to moderately elevated troponin and severely depressed ejection fraction (EF) and reversible left ventricular wall motion abnormality (see below for further details). Depressed cardiac function poses an additional challenge in managing symptomatic vasospasm. Triple-H therapy (hypertensive, hypervolemic, hemodilution) can contribute to developing severe pulmonary edema, and yet patients require induced hypertension and hypervolemia, which increases the afterload and results in further cardiac injury. Intra-aortic balloon counterpulsation was first described in human cerebral vasospasm cases in the mid to late 1990s in order to "allow continuation of triple-H therapy and to maintain adequate cerebral perfusion."[58] Imaging studies of both animals and humans reported significantly augmented cerebral blood flow in vasospasm cases by using different methods of brain perfusion scans.[59,60] Inflation at the beginning of diastole and deflation at the end of diastole have been shown to increase the cardiac perfusion, reduce afterload, maintain cardiac performance, and optimize end-organ perfusion including the brain. This therapy is not used routinely, and there are no large studies demonstrating safety and outcome benefits in vasospasm patients. Nevertheless, it is reasonable to be aware and consider this therapy when patients are having severely depressed cardiac function and symptomatic vasospasm refractory to other less invasive medical therapy (for more details, refer to Chapter 35).

NeuroFlo Device

This is an intra-aortic catheter with two small balloons designed to augment CBF during the acute phase of ischemic brain injury. The distal balloon is placed above the renal arteries and the proximal balloon is placed below the renal arteries. Partial occlusion of the descending abdominal aorta by inflation of the balloons leads to redirected flow, providing increased CBF as a result (Figures 1-9 and 1-10).

In March 2005, the US Food and Drug Administration approved this device for clinical use under the humanitarian device exemption program after a pilot study in 2004 showed feasibility. In the pilot study, 1 hour of partial aortic occlusion in 17 patients with acute ischemic stroke led to improved blood flow and brain perfusion along with reduced neurologic deficits.[61] A randomized controlled trial, SENTIS (Safety and Efficacy of NeuroFlo for Treatment of Ischemic Stroke), is currently in progress for more data in acute stroke. A single-arm, observational study on symptomatic vasospasm after aneurysmal SAH has been reported in 24 patients, showing increased mean flow velocity and improvement in NIH stroke scale 20 minutes post-procedure with sustained clinical benefit on a 30-day follow-up in most patients.[62]

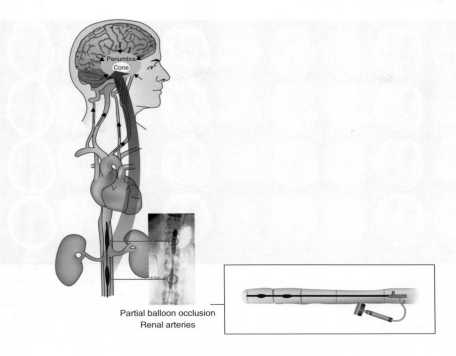

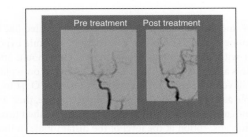

Partial balloon occlusion
Renal arteries

Pre treatment   Post treatment

Figure 1-9. NeuroFlo device. *(Reproduced with permission from Coaxia, Inc., and Richard Klucznik, MD.)*

A high-grade SAH (HH IV, F 3, mFS 4) patient survived the ICP crisis, brain hypoxia, brain metabolic stress, and vasospasm. On the regular floor, the patient is recovering well but develops hyponatremia (Na 125 mEq/L). It is bleed day 14 today. The patient is clinically stable but has had recurrent seizures in the past and the decision is made to treat the hyponatremia prior to transferring the patient to an inpatient rehabilitation facility. How would you approach this? What are the important points regarding cerebral salt wasting (CSW) versus syndrome of inappropriate antidiuretic hormone (SIADH)?

Cerebral (or Renal) Salt Wasting (CSW) Syndrome

Altered plasma and cerebrospinal fluid (CSF) concentration of natriuretic peptide has been thought to be the etiology of this syndrome, which is seen after any severe brain injury but more commonly described in patients with aneurysmal SAH. Sodium wasting is accompanied by free water loss leading

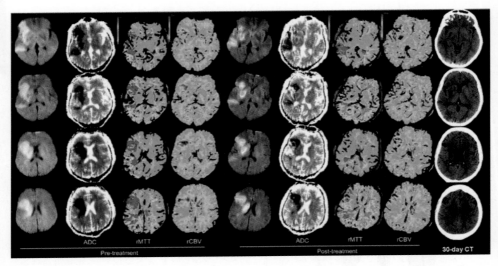

Figure 1-10. Magnetic resonance perfusion scan before and after placement of the NeuroFlo device. Diffusion-weighted imaging (DWI), apparent diffusion coefficient (ADC), relative mean transit time (MTT), and mean cerebral blood volume (CBV) maps obtained pretreatment and posttreatment. The 30-day CT images are in the far right column. Volumetric measurements reveal decreases of 27% and 45% in lesion volumes on the ADC and MTT maps, respectively, within the right MCA region posttreatment. The final infarct volume (30-day CT) was considerably smaller than the lesion volume observed on the pretreatment ADC maps and corresponds well to the lesion seen on the initial CBV maps. *With permission courtesy of Dr. Muhammad S. Hussain.*

to intravascular volume depletion. If CSW and intravascular volume depletion is treated like the syndrome of inappropriate antidiuretic hormone (SIADH) with water restriction, systemic hypotension and end-organ hypoperfusion may occur without improving hyponatremia. One should attempt to accurately assess intravascular volume status as the first step. Treatment should focus on replacing the sodium and targeting euvolemia for overall volume state. Oral salt tablets (2 to 4 g PO q4 to 8h) and isotonic saline via IV infusion is reasonable as the first step. If salt wasting gets worse, then 2% to 3% continuous IV infusion of hypertonic saline can be given (start 2% to 3% at 50 mL/h, then titrate up or down). Mineralocorticoids promote sodium absorption at the level of the distal tubule in the kidney and can be used to treat CSW (fludrocortisone 0.05 to 0.2 mg PO qd).

A wrong (and dangerous) fluid management would be to misdiagnose CSW as SIADH and perform water restriction with the use of a vasopressin receptor antagonist. Such therapy would lead to profound intravascular volume depletion in the setting of ICP crisis, brain hypoxia, brain metabolic crisis, and symptomatic vasospasm. This can lead to devastating ischemic brain injury. Recently, the term *cerebral* salt wasting syndrome has been challenged, with the term *renal* salt wasting syndrome being suggested as there have been cases where the same syndrome occurred in the absence of any brain disease.[63] In the setting of acute cerebral injury such as SAH, cerebral, or renal, salt wasting syndrome may be more common than what has been reported.

Syndrome of Inappropriate Antidiuretic Hormone Secretion (SIADH)

SIADH is another important differential diagnosis for hyponatremia in the NeuroICU. The same etiologies that can lead to CSW can also cause SIADH (eg, SAH, ischemic stroke, traumatic brain injury [TBI], tumor). Differentiating SIADH from CSW can be challenging. A traditional teaching regarding this is the concept of difference in volume status: SIADH has either a euvolemic or hypervolemic state and salt wasting syndrome has volume depletion.

Applying volume restriction and promoting free water loss (aquaresis) by antagonizing the vasopressin receptor (V2 receptors in the kidney) with IV conivaptan (20 mg IV loading over 30 minutes followed by 20 mg/day, may increase to 40 mg/day) or PO tolvaptan (15 mg PO qd, may increase to 30 mg/day with maximum of 60 mg/day) are appropriate therapies. As these aquaretic agents lead to effective free water loss, one needs to be cautious about aggressive fluid restriction.

With all the laboratory findings for both CSW and SIADH being similar, only volume status can be a hint for differentiating these two syndromes. However, there is no one gold standard parameter that is believed to be always accurate in assessing volume status. Assessing intravascular volume status is a daily challenge for any ICU. As such, for serum hyponatremia occurring in neurologic patients (eg, aneurysmal SAH), it should really be treated with one good old therapy: salt. Hyponatremia is often well tolerated and only patients who are symptomatic, or patients who have a low threshold for recurrent seizures, or patients with severe and worsening hyponatremia (< 125 mEq/L typically) should be treated. If hyponatremia is to be treated in a patient who needs adequate CPP and good intravascular volume (eg, in the middle of active symptomatic vasospasm), giving salt by hypertonic saline is preferred over aggressive volume management. Losing significant free water might be appropriate for SIADH, but can be harmful for patients without SIADH who really are experiencing CSW.

In general, the following tips can be helpful:

1. SIADH is a euvolemic or hypervolemic state due to free water retention, urine osmolality > 100 mOsm/kg, urine Na > 40 mmol/L.

2. FENa (fraction of sodium excretion) < 1% for volume depletion due to CSW, and > 1% for volume overloaded SIADH.

3. Serum uric acid level is normal (3.6 to 8.3 mg/dL) or high for hyponatremia due to dehydration without CSW or SIADH.

4. Serum uric acid level is low for both CSW and SIADH.

5. After successfully treating serum hyponatremia, the renal transport system problem may continue for CSW, so the serum uric acid level remains low (as fractional excretion of urate remains high) for CSW but may be normal for SIADH.

 A 32-year-old woman, SAH bleeds day 9, HH II, F 3, mFS 3, s/p right MCA aneurysm clipping is now transferred out of the ICU to a regular telemetry bed. Since bleed day 5, patient's TCD velocity was elevated on the right MCA at the depth of 55 mm with a mean velocity of 180 cm/s, and CTA showed mild vasospasm but never had any neurologic deficits other than headache. On the floor, her neurologic examination remained normal. On bleed day 10, she develops severe hyponatremia (Na = 117 mEq/L) and new-onset left arm pronator drift during the afternoon sign-out rounds. The following was the hemodynamic data:

1. CVP 3 mm Hg
2. SVI 35 mL/m²
3. Input and output 1.5 L net negative
4. Serum Na = 117 mEq/L, confirmed after recheck

Patient is emergently transferred back to the ICU for this new-onset left-sided hemiparesis.

You accept the patient back to the NeuroICU. What should you do next?

The most likely diagnosis for this patient is a vasospasm that has already been in progress since bleed day 5. When the trend of the TCD velocities of one vessel continues to rise along with corresponding

CTA evidence of luminal narrowing, it is reasonable to think that this patient has always had vasospasm—an *asymptomatic* vasospasm in this case—until now. She had had mild to moderate spasm that was not enough to cause any neurologic deficit. The hemodynamic and blood chemistry tests indicate that she has now developed severe serum hyponatremia and intravascular volume depletion. With reduced intravascular volume status, the CBF was reduced, and what was previously asymptomatic vasospasm is now becoming clinically significant. It is reasonable to think that the CSW syndrome is playing a major role here and as she lost sodium there was concurrent free water loss. The next thing to do for her is probably not an emergent angiogram. Angiography is not a completely benign procedure. Since she became symptomatic with salt and free water loss, the most logical and safe thing to do next is to provide salt and water (perhaps with a higher MAP target to augment CBF rather than ignoring it). With restoration of sodium, intravascular volume, and short-term hypertensive therapy, the patient's symptoms are likely to disappear rather rapidly.

A 35-year-old woman with no past medical history (PMH) presents after collapsing at home briefly after complaining of headache. Patient is admitted with HH III, F 3, mFS 4, and receives EVD for IVH and acute obstructive hydrocephalus. The patient gets endotracheal intubation and is admitted to the NeuroICU. In the unit, the BP is 60/40 mm Hg, sinus tachycardia at 110 bpm, SaO$_2$ drops to 70%, bilateral rhonchi and crackles on auscultation, on mechanical ventilator mode of assist control–volume control, set rate of 14, FIO$_2$ (fraction of inspired air) of 60%, PEEP (positive end-expiratory pressure) of 8. The electrocardiogram (ECG) shows nonspecific T-wave and ST changes, troponin = 2.5. Chest x-ray is consistent with acute pulmonary edema. Echocardiography showed ejection fraction of 20%.

- What is the diagnosis?
- How would you manage this?
- How do you differentiate neurogenic stunned myocardium from acute myocardial infarction?

Neurogenic stunned myocardium

Neurogenic stunned myocardium is a physiologically interesting phenomenon that is associated with a number of different disease states. For neurointensivists, a good example of this syndrome is in the setting of high-grade aneurysmal SAH. There are a number of terminologies that are considered synonymous with this syndrome and that share a similar proposed pathophysiology: neurogenic stunned myocardium, takotsubo cardiomyopathy, broken-heart syndrome, contraction band necrosis syndrome, and Gebrochenes-Herz syndrome among others. Despite different terms and variations between each of these syndromes, there is a common denominator that links all of these phenomena: mental stress. This type of stress is mediated by the brain—whether it is emotion driven (such as in broken-heart syndrome in which shocking news such as sudden death of a family member led to a cardiogenic shock and death, or literally "scared to death," either with good or bad emotions leading to a sudden onset of cardiac failure) with absolutely no structural brain pathology or with a structural abnormality such as acute SAH with intense ICP elevation, inflammation, and sympathetic surge; these are all cerebrally induced triggers. The condition is thought not to be induced by coronary artery atherosclerosis or plaque rupture as in typical acute coronary syndrome. The adrenergically mediated sympathetic surge has been pointed out as the main etiology and mechanism for stunning of the heart. Typically, patients present with clinical features that are consistent with a cardiogenic shock: systemic hypotension and forward/systolic failure with severely depressed ejection fraction (eg, new-onset heart failure with ejection fraction of 10% to 20% in a previously healthy young female). Unlike ST-elevation myocardial infarction (STEMI) cases, ECG may only show nonspecific T-wave ("cerebral T"; Figure 1-11) or ST-segment abnormalities. However, ECG *can* show ST-segment elevation that looks exactly the same as typical STEMI. Therefore, ECG alone cannot distinguish between STEMI/non ST-elevation myocardial infarction (NSTEMI) and neurogenic stunned myocardium.

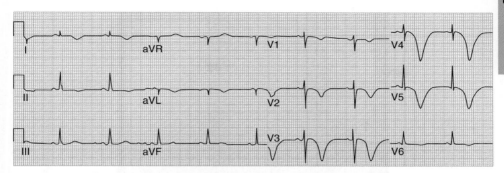

Figure 1-11. Cerebral T wave in neurogenic stunned myocardium syndrome (deep, inverted T waves with prolonged QTc intervals, so-called "cerebral" T waves are seen in this patient with aneurysmal SAH).

In the ED, this syndrome can be fairly challenging as the treatment for NSTEMI and neurogenic stunned myocardium is different. An echocardiogram can be helpful. What is typically seen is transient (as the clinical features, laboratory abnormalities, and ECG findings often resolve after several days) wall motion abnormality: the normal base of the left ventricle but akinetic everywhere else including the apex. *Normal base, abnormal apex* would not be a bad phrase to remember. The apex is not spared in classic takotsubo cardiomyopathy. On left ventriculogram (Figure 1-12), the apex of the left ventricle is diseased (not spared) and dilated—a classic description associates the shape of the heart in this syndrome to that of an octopus trap jar (in Japanese, "takotsubo"). Remember the apex of the heart is the left inferior and the base of the heart is the right superior portion. The regional wall motion abnormalities are to be seen in the nonvascular area. While variations do occur (eg, midventricular ballooning rather than apical ballooning and apical sparing pattern), it is important to remember the classic description and understand the pathophysiology behind it.

A recent study reported a retrospective analysis of 350 patients with acute SAH and highly abnormal cardiac enzymes.[64] This study revealed a few characteristic differences between a true coronary event versus a neurogenic event prior to obtaining an echocardiogram:

1. Troponins were at least 10-fold higher with infarcted heart than stunned myocardium (2.8 versus 0.22, $P < .001$).

2. Neurogenic stunned heart syndrome is reversible: usually within 4 to 5 days significant improvement can be seen in cardiac output, EF, and normalization of cardiac enzymes.

3. Echocardiogram showing significant inconsistencies with ECG abnormalities (ie, severely depressed EF but only nonspecific T wave inversions and cerebral T waves) is more consistent with neurogenic stunned myocardium.

4. Troponin < 2.8 ng/mL and EF < 40% in the setting of acute aneurysmal SAH is consistent with stunned myocardium rather than a true coronary event.

These tips are only true in general and, as such, care for each patient must be individualized. Nevertheless, it is helpful to remember how to differentiate these two entities in the emergency department in order to prioritize the procedures for managing the patients. Typical stunned myocardium patients should be treated with securing of the ruptured aneurysm in order to avoid rebleed and then providing appropriate hemodynamic support (avoid the use of pure alpha$_1$-adrenergic receptor agonist). The use of inotropic agents in order to support the reduced contractility and low EF while paying close attention to keep the patient euvolemic is essential (neglecting to address intravascular volume depletion in the setting of stunned myocardium would require a higher than necessary amount of vasopressors and may cause worsening of the cardiac injuries). Initiating prophylactic triple-H therapy in a patient with neurogenic stunned myocardium during the first few days of SAH may be more harmful than beneficial.

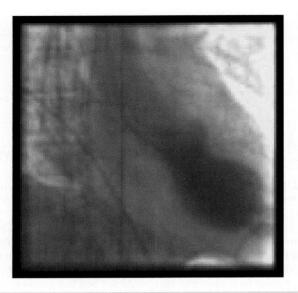

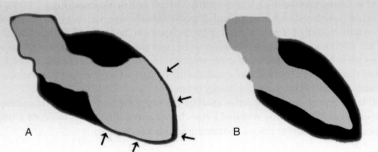

Figure 1-12. A. Apical ballooning on left ventriculogram, which is similar in shape to a *takotsubo* (Japanese octopus trap jar), demonstrating apical ballooning. B. Contraction of the heart is normal and hyperdynamic only at the base, and the apex is severely dilated and hypokinetic.

! CRITICAL CONSIDERATIONS

- Acute aneurysmal SAH is a dynamic (particularly true with poor grades) disease. Close neurologic observation and monitoring is required from the beginning and throughout the entire vasospasm precaution period. Just because patients are doing well, that does not necessarily mean he/she would continue to do well. Stopping TCD or neurochecks after 7 days for a Fisher group 3 patient who has been doing well is not recommended.

- Poor-grade SAH patients have stupor and coma examination, and therefore the value of the bedside clinical examination is limited. It is a good idea to perform a surveillance CTA and CTP for these patients in the middle of the peak vasospasm period even if examination remains the same.

- HH grade is associated with long-term clinical outcome and the Fisher scale is associated with risk of symptomatic vasospasm. The modified Fisher scale was developed in order to provide a more practical scale while incorporating the importance of IVH as an independent risk factor for DCI. The IVH alone, however, is not strongly associated with vasospasm, as it is uncommon to see vasospasm in patients with isolated IVH due to hypertension. Using more advanced, automatic outlining software to quantify the hemorrhage volume may provide useful information regarding the exact threshold of the volume in its relationship with the risk of DCI and outcomes.

- It is important to remember that the most consistent predictive variable for DCI is the amount of the hemorrhage.

- When a patient presents with high-grade SAH, IVH, and obstructive hydrocephalus with a large amount of cisternal blood burden (after ABC), the first thing to do is to place a ventricular drain, immediately. After placing the drain, it is important to ensure that the drain is working properly (provided that the full medical and surgical intervention is what the patient would want).

- ICP crisis is a major challenge in the acute phase (typically first week) of poor-grade SAH. Aggressive, timely intervention is necessary in order to avoid secondary neuronal injury. In addition to EVD placement, sedation, hyperventilation, mannitol/hypertonic saline, and pentobarbital have been the conventional therapies. Recently, therapeutic hypothermia has been reported in the literature and may be useful in treating the refractory cases.

- SAH management is not only about ICP and CPP. The brain oxygenation as well as the brain metabolic distress status may be important targets for successful resuscitation of the high-grade SAH cases.

- Goal-driven therapy of targeting the hemodynamic variables by optimizing the delivery as well as the perfusion of oxygen may help by reducing the damage mainly by avoiding secondary injury while giving the brain a chance to recover.

- Symptomatic cerebral vasospasm continues to be a major challenge—bleed days 3 to 14 are the usual peak period. Ultra-early vasospasm has been reported, but this is less common.

- Ictal infarction may occur in SAH, which represents the ischemic injury that occurs at the time of the rupture of an aneurysm rather than due to DCI.

- Vasospasm may be detected by using a number of different modalities: TCD, CTA, CTP, cEEG, and angiography (yes, of course you can and should do a good clinical examination, but understand this may be limited for high-grade SAH patients). Obtaining the angiogram quickly is the key, as delays in treatment by either IA vasodilators or balloon angioplasty may lead to irreversible ischemic damage. From the onset of acute, severe neurologic deficit, IA intervention should not be delayed by more than 2 hours, particularly if full medical support [triple-H] has already been initiated. Symptomatic vasospasm that is refractory to full medical therapy happening in the middle of the night should not and cannot wait until the next morning. This is a medical emergency and stat angioplasty must be done. Triple-H therapy is not an appropriate substitute for an angioplasty. (Yes, it is a good idea to make sure the patient is euvolemic with high blood pressure on board, but that does not mean the angioplasty can happen many hours later in a symptomatic patient just because the patient is being treated with triple-H therapy.)

- IA injection of nicardipine and verapamil (papaverine is not commonly used anymore; recently milrinone has been used) is useful in treating vasospasm but in some cases the positive effect may not last long. One may argue that such short-lasting IA nicardipine/verapamil is not necessarily consistent with "nicardipine/verapamil failure," as the therapy did work while the patient was in the angiography suite and the patient did well afterward for several hours. Regardless of what it is called, the bottom line is that the effort should be focused on minimizing and avoiding the stroke secondary to the vasospasm or recurrence of the vasospasm. If the IA injection of vasodilator therapy was only good for 6 hours, then another therapy of IA injection at that time or balloon angioplasty is needed in order to avoid stroke. If IA nicardipine or verapamil lasted 6 hours, and patient is symptomatic again, then another therapy is emergently needed at that time, not the next day.

- There is no evidence that opening up a spastic, symptomatic vasospasm leads to higher risk of reperfusion injury and hemorrhage—avoiding angioplasty and IA treatment for acute vasospasm may not be justified based on theoretical fear, as it is clear what the outcomes are when someone is acutely hemiparetic on full triple-H therapy due to severe vasospasm (the patient will most likely not be able to move that arm again if left untreated).

- If you have a three-strike rule (ie, vasospasm needs to be treated with IV nicardipine or verapamil *three times* [or twice for a two-strike rule] before any balloon angioplasty can be considered), it is important to remember that every time the patient becomes symptomatic there is a risk of having irreversible ischemic damage.

- For refractory, symptomatic vasospasm, both partial aortic occlusion and intra-aortic balloon counterpulsation therapy has been shown to improve CBF and reduce neurologic deficits based on anecdotal reports. Further studies are needed before recommending these therapies as routine treatment.

- CSW and SIADH can have very similar laboratory findings and therefore can be challenging to differentiate. A common therapy for both entities is to replace sodium. Hypertonic saline is a reasonable option for both. For aneurysmal SAH patients who develop symptomatic or significant serum hyponatremia, avoid aggressively promoting free water loss or severe fluid restriction as this may make CSW worse and can potentially be dangerous. IV conivaptan and PO tolvaptan should not be used for hypovolemic hyponatremia due to CSW as this can lead to severe intravascular volume depletion. Having intravascular volume depletion in the setting of symptomatic and angiographic vasospasm is a cocktail for ischemic injury.

- Assessing serum uric acid may be helpful in differentiating CSW versus SIADH after successfully reversing hyponatremia.

- Neurogenic stunned myocardium occurs not uncommonly after SAH (especially with high grades), and the troponin level may rise significantly.

- While the ECG alone cannot differentiate myocardial infarction (MI) from stunned myocardium, there are a few helpful tips: severely depressed EF with nonspecific, cerebral T waves 10-fold higher troponin values for MI and usually only mildly elevated troponin for stunned myocardium and quick reversibility of stunned myocardium with adequate hemodynamic support by judicious use of pressors and inotropic agents (eg, avoiding increased use of phenylephrine while the patient is severely volume depleted and having an EF of 20%: simply using IV Neo-Synephrine [phenylephrine] prophylactically to increase the blood pressure in the absence of symptomatic vasospasm is only going to make cardiac injury worse).

- High-grade SAH can be a dynamic disease, typically with multiple phases of challenges: first phase, ICP crisis; second phase, vasospasm; third phase, difficulty weaning the ventilator and ventricular drain needing ventriculoperitoneal shunt (VPS); fourth phase, dysautonomia and sympathetic storming.

- A patient with grade V SAH can potentially have a decent long-term neurologic outcome (modified Rankin score of 1 to 3 is possible) if aggressive medical and surgical care are provided. Premature withdrawal of care may be a self-fulfilling prophecy. While continuing medical care may not always lead to good outcomes (and the goals of care should be determined by the patient's known wishes and what would be the best interest for the patient), patients with HH grade IV and even V may have a chance to recover. Prognosis is not always accurate on high-grade SAH patients during the first few hours or during the first day of a bleed especially prior to performing an EVD placement.

- In patients with acute MI early administration of β blockers reduces the rate of reinfarction and chronic administration improves survival. However, β blockers, even with the ones with short-acting properties, should not be administered to patients who are hypotensive or with other signs of shock.

- Diltiazem and verapamil are contraindicated in patients with STEMI and associated systolic left ventricular dysfunction and CHF.

- An early invasive strategy (coronary angiography with possible percutaneous transluminal coronary angioplasty) is favored in patients with unstable angina or NSTEMI who have any of the following high-risk indicators: recurrent angina or ischemia despite intensive anti-ischemic therapy; elevated troponin; new or presumably new ST-segment depression; recurrent angina or ischemia with CHF or new or worsening mitral regurgitation; a high-risk noninvasive stress test; left ventricular ejection fraction less than 40%; hemodynamic instability; sustained ventricular tachycardia; PCI within the last 6 months; and prior coronary artery bypass graft surgery.

- Echocardiography is not useful in diagnosing ACS in patients with chest pain. However, it is essential in diagnosing mechanical complications of acute MI.

- Elevated serum cardiac biomarkers and ST-segment elevation and/or depression can occur in the absence of ACS.

- Post-myocardial complications include cardiogenic shock, CHF, left ventricular free wall rupture, ventricular septal rupture, ischemic mitral regurgitation, or papillary muscle rupture causing acute mitral regurgitation.

- ECG findings suggestive of ACS are often present in patients presenting with subarachnoid hemorrhage, cerebral infarction, and intracerebral hemorrhage even in the absence of underlying coronary artery disease.

REFERENCES

1. Gates PC, Barnett HJ, Vinters HV, et al. Primary intraventricular hemorrhage in adults. *Stroke.* 1986;17:872-877.

2. Mayfrank L, Hutter BO, Kohorst Y, et al. Influence of intraventricular hemorrhage on outcome after rupture of intracranial aneurysm. *Neurosurg Rev.* 2001;24:185-191.

3. Lisk DR, Pasteur W, Rhoades H, et al. Early presentation of hemispheric intracerebral hemorrhage: Prediction of outcome and guidelines for treatment allocation. *Neurology.* 1994;44:133-139.

4. Adams RE, Diringer MN. Response to external ventricular drainage in spontaneous intracerebral hemorrhage with hydrocephalus. *Neurology.* 1998;50:519-523.

5. McIver JI, Friedman JA, Wijdicks EF, et al. Preoperative ventriculostomy and rebleeding after aneurysmal subarachnoid hemorrhage. *J Neurosurg.* 2002;97:1042-1044.

6. Hellingman CA, van den Bergh WM, Beijer IS, et al. Risk of rebleeding after treatment of acute hydrocephalus in patients with aneurysmal subarachnoid hemorrhage. *Stroke.* 2007;38:96-99.

7. ter Laan M, Mooij JJA. Improvement after treatment of hydrocephalus in aneurysmal subarachnoid hemorrhage: Implications for grading and prognosis. *Acta Neurochir (Wien).* 2006; 148:325-328.

8. Hunt W, Hess R. Surgical risk as related to time of intervention in the repair of intracranial aneurysms. *J Neurosurg.* 1968;28:14-20.

9. Lindsay KW, Teasdale G, Knill-Jones RP, Murray L. Observer variability in grading patients with subarachnoid hemorrhage. J Neurosurg. 1982;56:628-633.

10. Hutchinson PJ, Power DM, Tripathi P, et al. Outcome from poor grade aneurysmal subarachnoid hemorrhage: Which poor grade subarachnoid hemorrhage patients benefit from aneurysm clipping? Br J Neurosurg. 2000;14:105-109.

11. Le Roux PD, Elliott JP, Newell DW, et al. Predicting outcome in poor-grade patients with subarachnoid hemorrhage: A retrospective review of 159 aggressively managed cases. J Neurosurg. 1996;85:39-49.

12. Mocco J, Ransom ER, Komota RJ, et al. Preoperative prediction of long-term outcome in poor-grade aneurysmal subarachnoid hemorrhage, Neurosurgery. 2006;59:529-538; discussion 529-538.

13. Wartenberg KE, Schmidt JM, Claassen J, et al. Impact of medical complications on outcome after subarachnoid hemorrhage. Crit Care Med. 2006;34:617-623.

14. Jennett B, Bond M. Assessment of outcome after severe brain damage. Lancet. 1975;1:480-484.

15. Oshiro EM, Walter KA, Piantadosi S, et al. A new subarachnoid hemorrhage grading system based on the Glasgow Coma Scale: A comparison with the Hunt and Hess and World Federation of Neurological Surgeons Scales in a clinical series. Neurosurgery. 1997;41:140-147.

16. Drake C. Report of World Federation of Neurological Surgeons Committee on a Universal Subarachnoid Hemorrhage Grading Scale. J Neurosurg. 1988;68: 985-986.

17. van Gijn J, Bromberg JE, Lindsay KW, Hasan D, Vermeulen M. Definition of initial grading, specific events, and overall outcome in patients with aneurysmal subarachnoid hemorrhage: A survey. Stroke. 1994;25:1623-1627.

18. Torres VE, Pirson Y, Wiebers DO. Cerebral aneurysms. Correspondence. N Engl J Med. 2006;355: 2703-2705.

19. Oshiro EM, Walter KA, Piantadosi S, Witham TF, Tamargo RJ. A new subarachnoid hemorrhage grading system based on the Glasgow Coma Scale: A comparison with the Hunt and Hess and World Federation of Neurological Surgeons Scales in a clinical series. Neurosurgery. 1997;41:140-147.

20. Fisher CM, Kistler JP, Davis JM. Relation of cerebral vasospasm to subarachnoid hemorrhage visualized by computerized tomographic scanning. Neurosurgery. 1980;6:1-9.

21. Gurusinghe NT, Richardson AE. The value of computerized tomography in aneurysmal subarachnoid hemorrhage. The concept of the CT score. J Neurosurg. 1984;60:763-770.

22. Qureshi AI, Sung GY, Razumovsky AY, et al. Early identification of patients at risk for symptomatic vasospasm after aneurismal subarachnoid hemorrhage. Crit Care Med. 2000; 28:984-990.

23. Davis JM, Davis KR, Crowell RM: Subarachnoid hemorrhage secondary to ruptured intracranial aneurysm: Prognostic significance of cranial CT. AJR Am J Roentgenol. 1980;134:711-715.

24. Suzuki J, Komatsu S, Sato T, et al. Correlation between CT findings and subsequent development of cerebral infarction due to vasospasm in subarachnoid hemorrhage. Acta Neurochir.1980;55:63-70.

25. Pasqualin A, Rosta L, Da Pian R, et al. Role of computed tomography in the management of vasospasm after subarachnoid hemorrhage. Neurosurgery. 1984;15:344-353.

26. Smith ML, Abrahams JM, Chandela S. Subarachnoid hemorrhage on computed tomography scanning and the development of cerebral vasospasm: The Fisher grade revisited. Surg Neurol. 2005;63:229-234.

27. Lindsay KW, Teasdale G, Knill-Jones RP, et al. Observer variability in grading patients with subarachnoid hemorrhage. J Neurosurg. 1982;56:628-633.

28. Claassen J, Bernardini GL, Kreiter KT, et al. Effect of cisternal and ventricular blood on risk of delayed cerebral ischemia after subarachnoid hemorrhage: The Fisher Scale revisited. Stroke. 2001;32:2012-2020.

29. Frontera JA, Claassen J, Schmidt JM, et al. Prediction of symptomatic vasospasm after subarachnoid hemorrhage: the modified fisher scale. Neurosurgery. 2006;59:21-27.

30. Friedman JA, Goerss SJ, Meyer FB, et al. Volumetric quantification of Fisher grade 3 aneurysmal subarachnoid hemorrhage: A novel method to predict symptomatic vasospasm on admission computerized tomography scans. J Neurosurg. 2002;97:401-401.

31. Ko SB, Choi HA, Carpenter AM, et al. Quantitative analysis of hemorrhage volume for predicting delayed cerebral ischemia after subarachnoid hemorrhage. Stroke. 2011;42:669-674. Epub ahead of print Jan 21.

32. Klimo P Jr, Schmidt RH. Computed tomography grading schemes used to predict cerebral vasospasm after aneurysmal subarachnoid hemorrhage: a historical review. Neurosurg Focus. 2006;15; 21:E5.

33. Ichai C, Armando G, Orban JC, et al. Sodium lactate versus mannitol in the treatment of intracranial hypertensive episodes in severe traumatic brain-injured patients. Intensive Care Med. 2009;35:471-479.

34. Kimberger O, Ali SZ, Markstaller M, et al. Meperidine and skin surface warming additively reduce the shivering threshold: A volunteer study. *Crit Care.* 2007;11:R29.

35. Elvan EG, Öç B, Uzun S, et al. Dexmedetomidine and postoperative shivering in patients undergoing elective abdominal hysterectomy. *Eur J Anaesthesiol.* 2008;25:357-364.

36. Wadhwa A, Sengupta P, Durrani J, et al. Magnesium sulphate only slightly reduces the shivering threshold in humans. *Br J Anaesth.* 2005;94:756-762.

37. Mokhtarani M, Mahgoub A, Morioka N, et al. Buspirone and meperidine synergistically reduce the shivering threshold. *Anesth Analg.* 2001;93:1233-1239.

38. Matsukawa T, Kurz A, Sessler DI, et al. Propofol linearly reduces the vasoconstriction and shivering thresholds. *Anesthesiology.* 1995;82:1169-1180.

39. Horn EP, Werner C, Sessler DI, et al. Late intraoperative clonidine administration prevents postanesthetic shivering after total intravenous or volatile anesthesia. *Anesth Analg.* 1997;84:613-617.

40. Figaji AA, Zwane E, Thompson C, et al. Brain tissue oxygen tension monitoring in pediatric severe traumatic brain injury: Part 1: Relationship with outcome. *Childs Nerv Syst.* 2009;25:1335-1343.

41. Rosenthal G, Hemphill JC, Sorani M, et al. The role of lung function in brain tissue oxygenation following traumatic brain injury. *J Neurosurg.* 2008;108:59-65.

42. Vora YY, Suarez-Almazor M, Steinke DE, Martin ML, Findlay JM. Role of transcranial Doppler monitoring in the diagnosis of cerebral vasospasm after subarachnoid hemorrhage. *Neurosurgery.* 1999;44:1237-1247; discussion 1247-1248.

43. Lysakowski C, Walder B, Costanza MC, et al. Transcranial Doppler versus angiography in patients with vasospasm due to a ruptured cerebral aneurysm: A systematic review. *Stroke.* 2001; 32:2292-2298.

44. Frontera JA, Fernandez A, Schmidt JM, et al. Defining vasospasm after subarachnoid hemorrhage: What is the most clinically relevant definition? *Stroke.* 2009;40:1963-1968. Epub 2009 Apr 9.

45. McKinney AM, Palmer CS, Truwit CL, et al. Detection of aneurysms by 64-section multidetector CT angiography in patients acutely suspected of having an intracranial aneurysm and comparison with digital subtraction and 3d rotational angiography. *Am J Neuroradiol.* 2008;29:594-602.

46. Merten GJ, Burgess WP, Gray LV, et al. Prevention of contrast-induced nephropathy with sodium bicarbonate: A randomized controlled trial. *JAMA.* 2004;291:2328-2334.

47. Baker C, Wragg A, Kumar S, et al. A rapid protocol for the prevention of contrast-induced renal dysfunction: the RAPPID study. *J Am Coll Cardiol.* 2003;41:2114-2118.

48. Vespa PM, Nuwer MR, Juhász C, et al. Early detection of vasospasm after acute subarachnoid hemorrhage using continuous EEG ICU monitoring. *Electroencephalogr Clin Neurophysiol.* 1997; 103:607-615.

49. Claassen J, Hirsch LJ, Kreiter KT, et al. Quantitative continuous EEG for detecting delayed cerebral ischemia in patients with poor-grade subarachnoid hemorrhage. *Clin Neurophysiol.* 2004; 115:2699-2710.

50. Lennihan L, Mayer SA, Fink ME, et al. Effect of hypervolemic therapy on cerebral blood flow after subarachnoid hemorrhage: A randomized controlled trial. *Stroke.* 2000;31:383-391.

51. Jost SC, Diringer MN, Zazulia AR, et al. Effect of normal saline bolus on cerebral blood flow in regions with low baseline flow in patients with vasospasm following subarachnoid hemorrhage. *J. Neurosurg.* 2005; 103:25-30.

52. Joseph M, Ziadi S, Nates J. Increases in cardiac output can reverse flow deficits from vasospasm independent of blood pressure: a study using xenon computed tomographic measurement of cerebral blood flow. *Neurosurgery.* 2003;53:1044-1051.

53. Rosenwasser RH, Armonda RA, Thomas JE, Benitez RP, Gannon PM, Harrop J. Therapeutic modalities for the management of cerebral vasospasm: timing of endovascular options. *Neurosurgery.* 1999;44:975-980.

54. Shibuya M, Suzuki Y, Enomoto H, Okada T, Ogura K, Sugita K. Effects of prophylactic intrathecal administrations of nicardipine on vasospasm in patients with severe aneurysmal subarachnoid hemorrhage. *Acta Neurochir (Wien).* 1994;131:19-25.

55. Suzuki M, Doi M, Otawara Y, Ogasawara K, Ogawa A. Intrathecal administration of nicardipine hydrochloride to prevent vasospasm in patients with subarachnoid hemorrhage. *Neurosurg Rev.* 2001;24:180-184.

56. Goodson K, Lapointe M, Monroe T, Chalela JA. Intraventricular nicardipine for refractory cerebral vasospasm after subarachnoid hemorrhage. *Neurocrit Care.* 2008;8:247-252.

57. Barth M, Capelle HH, Weidauer S, et al. Effect of nicardipine prolonged-release implants on cerebral vasospasm and clinical outcome after severe aneurysmal subarachnoid hemorrhage: a prospective, randomized, double-blind phase IIa study. *Stroke.* 2007;38:330-336. Epub 2006 Dec 21.

58. Apostolides PJ, Greene KA, Zabramski JM, et al. Intra-aortic balloon pump counterpulsation in the management of concomitant cerebral vasospasm and cardiac failure after subarachnoid hemorrhage: Technical case report. *Neurosurgery.* 1996;38:1056-1059.

59. Nussbaum ES, Sebring LA, Ganz WF, et al. Intra-aortic balloon counterpulsation augments cerebral blood flow in the patient with cerebral vasospasm: a xenon-enhanced computed tomography study. *Neurosurgery.* 1998;42:206-213.

60. Nussbaum ES, Heros RC, Solien EE, et al. Intra-aortic balloon counterpulsation augments cerebral blood flow in a canine model of subarachnoid hemorrhage-induced cerebral vasospasm. *Neurosurgery.* 199536:879-884.

61. Campbell MS, Grotta JC, Gomez CR, et al. Perfusion augmentation in stroke using controlled aortic obstruction: Pilot study results. *Stroke.* 2004;35:291.

62. Lylyk P, Vila JF, Miranda C, et al. Partial aortic obstruction improves cerebral perfusion and clinical symptoms in patients with symptomatic vasospasm. *Neurol Res.* 2005;27(suppl 1):S129-S135.

63. Maesaka JK, Imbriano LJ, Ali NM, et al. Is it cerebral or renal salt wasting? *Kidney Int.* 2009;76: 934-938.

64. Bulsara KR, McGirt MJ, Liao L, et al. Use of the peak troponin value to differentiate myocardial infarction from reversible neurogenic left ventricular dysfunction associated with aneurysmal subarachnoid hemorrhage. *J Neurosurg.* 2003;98: 524-528.

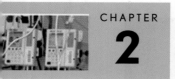

CHAPTER

2

Intracerebral Hemorrhage

Moussa F. Yazbeck, MD
Fred Rincon, MD, MSc, FACP
Stephan A. Mayer, MD, FCCM

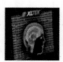

A 58-year-old African American man with a history of hypertension, mechanical mitral valve replacement, alcohol abuse, and atrial fibrillation (AF) suddenly developed nausea, vomiting, and left arm and leg weakness. He takes hydrochlorothiazide (HCTZ) 25 mg every morning for hypertension, metoprolol-XL 25 mg/day, and warfarin 5 mg/day. His wife promptly called 911 and the emergency medical services (EMS) arrived on the scene. The time of onset of symptoms was established to be approximately 20 minutes ago. A quick Cincinnati Pre-hospital Stroke Scale assessment shows left-sided weakness including face, arm, and leg and a Glasgow Coma Scale (GCS) of 12. Oxygen was applied through a nasal cannula and intravenous access was secured. The EMS personnel suspected a stroke and they notified the destination hospital.

On arrival at the emergency department, the patient was found to be more somnolent (GCS is 8) and responsive to painful stimulus. Vital signs are BP: 220/120 mm Hg, HR: 120 to 130 bpm, RR: 24, blood sugar by fingerstick: 182 mg/dL, and cardiac monitor shows a rapid AF. Initial computed tomographic (CT) scan showed a left frontoparietal intracerebral hemorrhage (ICH) (Figure 2-1) and the International Normalized Ratio (INR) was 5.8.

What are the risk factors for ICH?

Hypertension (HTN) is the most important and prevalent of the risk factors for ICH, leading to a form of vasculopathy termed *lipohyalinosis*. Nonmodifiable risk factors include advanced age, male gender, and African American and Japanese race/ethnicity.[1-4] Additionally, cerebral amyloid angiopathy (CAA), although usually asymptomatic, is an important risk factor for primary ICH in the elderly. CAA is characterized by the deposition of β-amyloid protein in small- to medium-sized blood vessels of the brain and leptomeninges, which may undergo fibrinoid necrosis as seen in chronic HTN. Other risk factors include cocaine use, low cholesterol levels, oral anticoagulants, and excessive alcohol abuse.[2,5-14]

How do we reliably establish the diagnosis of ICH?

The diagnosis of ICH is suggested by the rapid onset of neurologic dysfunction and signs of increased intracranial pressure (ICP), such as headache, vomiting, and decreased level of consciousness. The symptoms of ICH are related primarily to the etiology, anatomic location, and extension of the expanding hematoma. Abnormalities in the vital signs such as hypertension, tachycardia, or bradycardia (Cushing response) and abnormal respiratory pattern are common effects of elevated ICP. Confirmation of ICH cannot rely solely on the clinical examination and requires the use of an emergent CT scan (see Figure 2-1) or

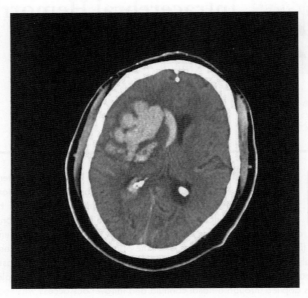

Figure 2-1. CT scan showing this patient's right basal ganglia ICH with small extravasation into the right lateral ventricle.

magnetic imaging (MRI) and will differentiate between ischemic and hemorrhagic strokes. The CT scan rapidly evaluates the size and location of the hematoma, extension into the ventricular system, hydrocephalus, degree of surrounding edema, and anatomic disruption.[4] Hematoma volume may be easily calculated from CT scan images by use of the ABC-2 method, a derived formula from the calculation of the volume of the sphere (Figure 2-2).[10,11] CT angiography (CTA) is not routinely performed in most centers, but may prove to be helpful in predicting hematoma expansion, outcome, and etiology.[15,16]

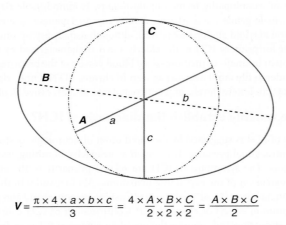

$$V = \frac{\pi \times 4 \times a \times b \times c}{3} = \frac{4 \times A \times B \times C}{2 \times 2 \times 2} = \frac{A \times B \times C}{2}$$

Figure 2-2. Calculation of the volume of the hematoma based on the volumetric formula for an ellipse. In this figure a, b, and c are the radius of the sphere; A, B, and C are diameters of the sphere; and $\pi = 3.14$. (*From Rincon F, Mayer SA. Intracerebral hemorrhage. In: Matta B, Mennon D, Smith M, eds. Core Topics in Neuroanaesthesia and Neurointensive Care. Cambridge University Press. Cambridge, UK. In press.*)

What is the explanation for the rapid deterioration seen in this patient?

Hematoma growth is an important cause of early neurologic deterioration, and ICH volume is a powerful predictor of the outcome after ICH.[17,18] However, the natural history and prognosis of ICH is not totally dependent on the volume of the hemorrhage.[19,20] An acceptable theory is that an expanding hematoma results from persistent bleeding and/or rebleeding from a single arteriolar rupture. Evidence from studies employing histopathology, CT analysis, single-photon emission computed tomography (SPECT), and both conventional and CTA suggest that secondary multifocal bleeding into the tissue at the periphery of an existing clot is more likely to occur in those cases of early hematoma enlargement. Analyses of brain tissue have indicated the presence of microscopic and macroscopic bleeds in the area surrounding the fatal hemorrhage, perhaps representing ruptured arterioles or venules.[21]

Other studies employing simultaneous CT and SPECT analyses have shown that, in some cases, early ICH growth relates to secondary bleeding in the periphery of the existing clot into ischemic, congested, perilesional tissue[22] (Figure 2-3). Similarly, the association between early hematoma growth and irregular clot morphology, which may reflect multifocal bleeding, has been reported, and in these studies, the incidence of hematoma growth was greater in patients with irregularly shaped hematomas compared with those with round hematomas, and it was postulated that the irregular shape indicated bleeding from multiple arterioles.[23,24] In one study involving CTA immediately after ICH, the presence of active contrast extravasation into the hematoma was associated with subsequent hematoma enlargement[25] and an increase in mortality rate[15] in 30% to 46% of patients.

Finally, bleeding from single and simultaneous bleeding from multiple lenticulostriate arteries have been demonstrated angiographically immediately after ICH,[26] and in a prospective study of 39 patients with spontaneous ICH, focal enhancing foci (contrast extravasation, "spot sign") seen in initial CTA were associated with the presence and extent of hematoma progression with good sensitivity (91%) and negative predictive value (NPV 96%) (Figure 2-4).[27]

Additionally, this patient was taking warfarin for mechanical valve replacement and AF. In the general population, warfarin increases the risk of ICH by 5- to 10-fold[13] and ICH in the setting of anticoagulation carries the worst prognosis.[28] Patients receiving oral warfarin should be reversed immediately with fresh-frozen plasma (FFP) or prothrombin-complex concentrates (PCCs) and vitamin K (Table 2-1). At least 8 units of FFP (15 to 30 mL/kg)[29] is required to immediately reverse

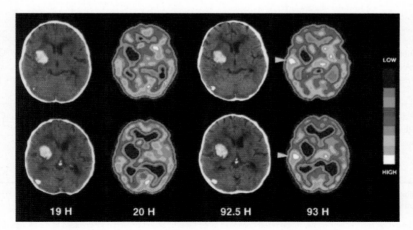

Figure 2-3. Early hematoma growth in a 71-year-old woman with left putaminal hemorrhage. The ICH volume increased by 80%, from 15 mL at 2.5 hours to 26 mL at 11.5 hours. Concurrent SPECT images indicate that the enlargement resulted from the addition of discrete hemorrhages within the no-flow zone around the existing clot (*yellow arrows*). (*From Mayer SA, Lignelli A, Fink ME, et al. Perilesional blood flow and edema formation in acute intracerebral hemorrhage: a SPECT study. Stroke. Sep 1998;29:1791-1798.*)

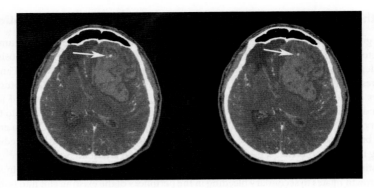

Figure 2-4. Contrast extravasation seen in the hematoma of a patient with acute ICH (*white arrows*). *(From Rincon F, Mayer SA. Clinical review: Critical care management of spontaneous intracerebral hemorrhage. Crit Care. 2008;12:237.)*

Table 2-1. Emergency Management of the Coagulopathic ICH

Scenario	Agent	Dose	Comments	Level of Evidence[a]
Warfarin	Fresh-frozen plasma (FFP) *or*	15 mL/kg	Usually 4-6 units (200 mL each) are given	B
	Prothrombin-complex concentrate *and*	15-30 U/kg	Works faster than FFP, but carries risk of DIC	B
	IV vitamin K	10 mg	Can take up to 24 h to normalize INR	
Warfarin and emergency neurosurgical intervention	*Above plus* Recombinant factor VIIa	20-80 μg/kg	Contraindicated in acute thromboembolic disease	C
Unfractionated or low-molecular-weight heparin[b]	Protamine sulfate	1 mg per 100 units of heparin, or 1 mg of enoxaparin	Can cause flushing, bradycardia, or hypotension, anticoagulation	C
Platelet dysfunction or thrombocytopenia	Platelet transfusion *and/or*	6 units	Range 4-8 units based on size; transfuse to > 100, 000 μL	C
	DDAVP	0.3 μg/kg	Single dose required	C

Abbreviations: DDAVP, desmopressin (1-deamino-8-D-arginine vasopressin); DIC, disseminated intravascular coagulation; FFP, fresh-frozen plasma; INR, International Normalized Ratio.

[a]Level A: based on multiple high-quality randomized controlled trials; Level B: based on single randomized trial or nonrandomized studies; Level C: case reports and series, expert opinion

[b]Protamine has minimal efficacy against danaparoid or fondaparinux.

(From Rincon F, Mayer SA. Clinical review: Critical care management of spontaneous intracerebral hemorrhage. Crit Care. 2008;12:237.)

the coagulation defect, but the associated volume load may exacerbate chronic conditions such as cardiac or renal disease.[30] High doses of intravenous vitamin K can fully reverse warfarin-induced anticoagulation but the effect may take up to 12 to 24 hours, during which time the ICH may continue to enlarge. A potential risk of anaphylaxis exists with IV vitamin[31]; therefore, infusion should be done slowly with attention to signs of allergy. Prothrombin-complex concentrates, which consist of the vitamin K–dependent coagulation factors (II, VII, IX, and X), may normalize the INR more rapidly than infusion of FFP or vitamin K alone in patients with ICH.[30,32]

An alternative to conventional warfarin anticoagulation reversal is the recombinant activated factor VII (rFVIIa, NovoSeven, Novo Nordisk A/S Copenhagen, Denmark).[33] Recombinant factor VIIa has been used to reverse warfarin-induced ICH,[33,34] but should be used in conjunction with FFP, PCCs, and vitamin K as rFVIIa corrects only the warfarin-induced deficit of factor VII, while PCC, FFP, and vitamin K correct the deficits in all of the vitamin K–dependent coagulation factors.[30] Heparin or low-molecular-weight heparin–induced anticoagulation should be reversed with protamine sulfate,[35] and patients with thrombocytopenia or platelet dysfunction can be treated with a single dose of DDAVP (1-deamino-8-D-arginine vasopressin), platelet transfusions, or both (see Table 2-1).[36]

Is there any role of activated factor VII (NovoSeven) in noncoagulopathic ICH?

No. Based on the results of the recently published phase III FAST trial, routine use of rFVIIa as a hemostatic therapy for all patients with ICH within a 4-hour time window cannot be recommended.

Describe the initial urgent steps to manage this deteriorating patient

A rapid deteriorating patient requires optimization of his/her ABCs, and a thorough laboratory panel should be obtained including hematologic, biochemical, and coagulation profiles; electrocardiogram (ECG); and chest radiographs.

Airway Management, Breathing, and Circulation

The rapid deterioration in this patient's neurologic examination mandates securing the airway. Failure to recognize imminent airway loss may result in complications, such as aspiration, hypoxemia, and hypercapnia. Preferred induction agents for rapid-sequence intubation (RSI) in the setting of suspected ICH include propofol[37] and etomidate,[38] although etomidate has less hemodynamic side effects and does not cause an abrupt drop in blood pressure. Both these agents are short acting and should not obscure the neurologic examination for a prolonged period of time. In certain circumstances like this one, neuromuscular paralysis may be needed as part of RSI. Succinylcholine is the most commonly administered muscle relaxant owing to its rapidity of onset (30 to 60 seconds) and short duration (5 to 15 minutes).[39] However, succinylcholine should be avoided in patients with renal disease because of the rare risk of life-threatening hyperkalemia; furthermore, succinylcholine causes theoretical elevation in the ICP in patients with intracranial mass lesions.[38,40] For this reason, in neurologic patients, nondepolarizing neuromuscular blocking agents such as *cis*-atracurium (preferred in renal disease), rocuronium,[38] or vecuronium are recommended.[41] In patients with increased ICP, premedication with lidocaine for RSI is frequently used, although this practice is of questionable use.[42]

Hypertension as well as hypotension should be immediately addressed to decrease hematoma expansion and to keep an adequate cerebral perfusion pressure. Isotonic fluid resuscitation and vasopressors may be indicated in those patients in shock.[43] Dextrose-containing solutions should be avoided as hyperglycemia may be detrimental to the injured brain[44].

Blood Pressure Control

Extreme levels of blood pressure after ICH should be aggressively but carefully treated to reduce the risk of hematoma expansion and to keep and maintain cerebral perfusion pressure (CPP = mean arterial pressure [MAP] – ICP). Controversy exists about the initial treatment of hypertension in patients with ICH. An expanding hematoma may result from persistent bleeding and/or rebleeding from a single arteriolar rupture. Some studies have reported evidence of hematoma growth from bleeding into an ischemic penumbra zone surrounding the hematoma but other reports have not confirmed the existence of ischemia at the hypoperfused area in the periphery of the hematoma.[45,46] In one study, no association was demonstrated between hematoma growth and blood pressure levels, although the use of antihypertensive agents may have negatively confounded this association,[47] and interestingly, the initial blood pressure level was not associated with hematoma growth in the Recombinant Activated Factor VII ICH Trial.[48]

On the other hand, aggressive blood pressure reduction after ICH may predispose to an abrupt drop in cerebral perfusion pressure (CPP) and ischemia, which in turn may be accompanied by elevations of ICP and further neurologic damage. Some studies have demonstrated that a controlled, pharmacologically based reduction in blood pressure has no adverse effects on cerebral blood flow in humans or animals.[49,50] The blood pressure level has been correlated with an increase in the ICP and volume of the hematoma, but it has been very difficult to explain if hypertension is the cause of hematoma growth or if this is just a response to elevated ICP in the setting of large-volume ICH. Results of the Intensive Blood Pressure Reduction in Acute Cerebral Hemorrhage Trial (INTERACT) suggested that early intensive blood pressure reduction seemed to attenuate hematoma expansion in patients with ICH,[51] and in an interim analysis of the Antihypertensive Treatment in Acute Cerebral Hemorrhage (ATACH) study, a nonsignificant relationship between the magnitude of systolic blood pressure (SBP) reduction and hematoma expansion and 3-month outcome was observed.[52] If more aggressive blood pressure reduction after ICH is safe is the subject of the ongoing National Institute of Neurologic Disorders and Stroke (NINDS)–supported ATACH pilot study.[53]

In general, the American Heart Association guidelines indicate that SBPs exceeding 180 mm Hg or MAP exceeding 130 mm Hg should be managed with continuous-infusion antihypertensive agents (Table 2-2).[54] The use of nitroprusside has drawbacks since this agent may exacerbate cerebral edema and intracranial pressure,[55] and oral and sublingual agents are not preferred because of the need for immediate and precise blood pressure control. In general, no matter how high the blood pressure is, the MAP should not be reduced beyond 15% to 30% over the first 24 hours.[49] In the setting of impaired blood flow autoregulation, excessive blood pressure reduction may exacerbate ischemia in the area surrounding the hematoma and worsen perihematomal brain injury.[22,56]

Is this patient at risk of further neurologic deterioration, and if so, how can we prevent it?

Observation in an ICU or a similar setting is strongly recommended for at least the first 24 hours, since the risk of neurologic deterioration is highest and because the majority of patients with brainstem or cerebellar hemorrhage have a depressed level of consciousness requiring ventilatory support.[57,58] Invasive arterial blood pressure, central venous pressure, and pulmonary artery catheter monitoring are invasive modalities that may be indicated in these patients. An external ventricular drain should be placed in patients with a depressed level of consciousness (GCS of 8 or less), signs of acute hydrocephalus or intracranial mass effect on CT, and a prognosis that warrants aggressive ICU care.[59] Additional acute physiologic derangements that require aggressive interventions include elevated ICP, hyperglycemia, hyperthermia, electrolyte imbalances, and seizure activity among others.

Management of ICH

Large-volume ICH carries the risk of developing cerebral edema and high ICP, and the presence of IVH further increases the risk of mortality[60,61] (see Figure 2-1). This effect is primarily related to the development of obstructive hydrocephalus and alterations of normal cerebrospinal fluid flow dynamics. Patients with large-volume ICH, intracranial mass effect, and coma may benefit from ICP monitoring,

Table 2-2. Intravenous Antihypertensive Agents After ICH

Drug	Mechanism	Dose	Cautions
Labetalol	α-1, β-1, β-2 Receptor antagonist	20-80 mg bolus every 10 min, up to 300 mg; 0.5-2.0 mg/min infusion	Bradycardia, congestive heart failure, bronchospasm
Esmolol	β-1 Receptor antagonist	0.5 mg/kg bolus; 50-300 μg/kg/min	Bradycardia, congestive heart failure, bronchospasm
Nicardipine	L-type calcium channel blocker (dihydropyridine)	5-15 mg/h infusion	Severe aortic stenosis, myocardial ischemia
Enalaprilat	ACE inhibitor	0.625 mg bolus; 1.25-5 mg every 6 h	Variable response, precipitous fall in BP with high-renin states
Fenoldopam	Dopamine-1 receptor agonist	0.1-0.3 μg/kg/min	Tachycardia, headache, nausea, flushing, glaucoma, portal hypertension
Nitroprusside[a]	Nitrovasodilator (arterial and venous)	0.25-10 μg/kg/min	Increased ICP, variable response, myocardial ischemia, thiocyanate and cyanide toxicity

Abbreviations: ACE, angiotensin-converting enzyme; BP, blood pressure; ICP, intracranial pressure.

[a]Nitroprusside may not be recommended for use in ICH because of its tendency to increase ICP.

(From Mayer SA, Rincon F. Management of intracerebral hemorrhage. Lancet Neurol. 2005;4:662-672.)

although this intervention has not been proved to benefit outcomes after ICH,[62,63] initial cerebrospinal fluid (CSF) drainage may be a lifesaving procedure, particularly in the setting of hydrocephalus and IVH.[64] This technique allows for rapid clearance of CSF, improvement of ICP, and ICP/CPP monitoring. As a general rule, an ICP monitor or external ventricular drain (EVD) should be placed in all comatose ICH patients (GCS of 8 or less) with the goal of maintaining ICP less than 20 mm Hg and CPP greater than 70 mm Hg, unless their condition is so dismal that aggressive ICU care is not warranted. Compared to parenchymal monitors, EVDs carry the therapeutic advantage of allowing CSF drainage and have the disadvantage of a substantial risk of infection (approximately 10% during the first 10 days).[65]

Sedation should be used to minimize pain, agitation, and decrease surges in ICP, and in general, many practitioners prefer sedative agents and nondepolarizing neuromuscular paralytic agents for RSI that do not have effects on ICP such as propofol, etomidate, cis-atracurium, and vecuronium.[37,41,66] Additionally, this patient's head should be positioned at 30-degree angle to minimize ICP and reduce the risk of aspiration or ventilator-associated pneumonia. In mechanically ventilated patients, the further need for head elevation should be guided by changing pulmonary and volume needs.

Additional advanced techniques for the management of elevated ICP have evolved from the experience in traumatic brain injury. Two different concepts for the management of ICP currently exist. The Lund concept assumes a disruption of the blood-brain barrier (BBB) and recommends manipulations to decrease the hydrostatic blood pressure and to increase osmotic pressures to favor the maintenance of the vascular compartment at the expense of a higher risk of ischemia.[67] The other concept, cerebral perfusion pressure (CPP) optimization (CPP = MAP − ICP) favors a maintenance of the CPP of 70 mm Hg or more to minimize reflex vasodilation or ischemia[68,69] at the expense of potentially aggravating ICP. There is no prospective control trial addressing the superiority of either of these two different methods for ICP management after ICH.

Hyperosmolar therapy and hyperventilation should be used after sedation and CPP optimization fail to normalize ICP.[70] The initial dose of mannitol is 1.0 to 1.5 g/kg of a 20% solution, followed by bolus doses of 0.25 to 1.0 g/kg as needed to a target osmolarity of 300 to 320 mOsm/kg. Additional doses can be given as frequently as once an hour based on the initial response to therapy with the anticipation of a transient drop in blood pressure (BP). Hypertonic saline (HS), such as 0.5 to 2.0 mL/kg of 23.4% saline solution, can be used as an alternative to mannitol, particularly in the setting of shock and when CPP augmentation is desirable through a central venous line.[71] Hyperventilation is generally used sparingly in the ICU and for brief periods in monitored patients because its effect on ICP tends to last for only a few hours. Good long-term outcomes can occur when the combination of osmotherapy and hyperventilation is successfully used to reverse transtentorial herniation.[72]

For cases of severe or intractable elevated ICP, barbiturates and induced therapeutic hypothermia are also effective tools to control refractory elevated ICP by decreasing cerebral metabolic activity, which translates into a reduction of the CBF, and fall of the ICP. These two techniques require expertise, advanced tools, and continuous monitoring of cerebral electrical activity, and it may be associated with significant complications.[73-75]

Hyperglycemia

Admission hyperglycemia is a potent predictor of 30-day mortality in both diabetic and nondiabetic patients with ICH.[76] In ischemic stroke, hyperglycemia occurs in 20% to 40% of patients and is associated with infarct expansion, worse functional outcome, longer hospital stays, higher medical costs, and an increased risk of death, and it is felt to be secondary to a catecholamine surge and generalized stress response.[77-79] In the critically ill population, hyperglycemia seems much more acutely toxic than in healthy individuals, for whom cells can protect themselves by downregulation of glucose transporters.[80] In a recent study, high serum glucose concentrations were related to lower scores on the admission GCS and to unfavorable clinical outcomes,[81] but episodes of hypoglycemia have also been associated with increased mortality[82] and worst outcomes in neurologic patients,[83] even though in strict clinical environments tight glucose control has been linked to reductions in intracranial pressure, duration of mechanical ventilation, and seizure activity in critically ill neurologic patients.[84] Thus, to minimize the risk of severe hypoglycemia and to avoid worsening possible neuronal damage related to hyperglycemia, it may be reasonable to have tight sugar control with targets between 100 and 150 mg/dL.

Temperature Control

Fever after ICH is common, particularly with IVH,[85] and should be treated aggressively. Sustained fever after ICH has been shown to be independently associated with poor outcomes.[86] A large body of experimental evidence indicates that even small degrees of hyperthermia can exacerbate ischemic brain injury[87,88] as brain temperature elevation has been associated with hyperemia, exacerbation of cerebral edema, and elevated ICP.[89,90] As a general standard, acetaminophen and cooling blankets are recommended for all patients with sustained fever in excess of 38.3°C (101°F)[73,91] despite the lack of prospective randomized controlled trials supporting this approach. Newer adhesive surface-cooling systems (Arctic Sun, Medivance Inc, Lousville, CO, USA) and endovascular heat exchange catheters (Cool Line System, Alsius, Inc, Chelmsford, MA, USA) have been shown to be much more effective for maintaining normothermia[92]; however, it remains to be seen if these measures can improve clinical outcome.

Fluids

Isotonic fluids such as 0.9% saline at a rate of approximately 1 mL/kg per hour should be given as the standard intravenous replacement fluid for patients with ICH and optimized to achieve euvolemic balance and an hourly diuresis of > 0.5 mL/kg. Free water given in the form of 0.45% saline or 5% dextrose in water can exacerbate cerebral edema and increase ICP because it flows down its osmotic gradient into injured brain tissue.[44] Systemic hyposmolality (> 280 mOsm/L) should be aggressively treated with mannitol or 3% hypertonic saline. A state of euvolemia should be maintained by monitoring fluid balance and body weight, and by maintaining a normal central venous pressure (range 5 to 8 mm Hg). Careful interpretation of the CVP should be done when analyzing its value in the setting of positive end-expiratory pressure (PEEP). The use of hypertonic saline in the form of a 2% to 3% sodium (50:50 chloride-acetate) solution (1 mL/kg per hour) has become an increasingly popular alternative to normal saline as a resuscitation fluid for patients with significant perihematomal edema and mass effect after ICH. The goal is to establish and maintain a baseline state of hyperosmolality (300 to 320 mOsms/L) and hypernatremia (150 to 155 mEq/L), which may reduce cellular swelling and the number of ICP crises. Potential complications of hypertonic saline use are encephalopathy, subdural hematomas, coagulopathy, fluid overload, hypokalemia, cardiac arrhythmias, and hyperchloremic metabolic acidosis.[93] The serum sodium level should never be allowed to drop more than 12 mEq/L over 24 hours, as rapid withdrawal of hypertonic therapy may result in rebound cerebral edema, leading to elevated ICP and/or herniation syndromes.[93,94]

Prevention of Seizures

Seizures should be treated with intravenous lorazepam (0.05 to 0.1 mg/kg) followed by a loading dose of phenytoin or fosphenytoin (20 mg/kg). Patients with ICH may benefit from prophylactic antiepileptic therapy (AED), but no randomized trial has addressed the efficacy of this approach. The American Heart Association guidelines have recommended antiepileptic medication for up to 1 month, after which therapy should be discontinued in the absence of seizures.[43] This recommendation may be supported by the results of a recent study that showed that the risk of early seizures was reduced by prophylactic AED therapy.[95] The 30-day risk for convulsive seizures after ICH is approximately 8%, and the risk of overt status epilepticus is 1% to 2%.[95] Lobar location and small hematomas are independent predictors of early seizures.[95] The argument for prophylactic anticonvulsant therapy in stuporous or comatose ICH patients is bolstered by the fact that continuous EEG monitoring demonstrates electrographic seizure activity in approximately 25% of these patients despite treatment.[96,97] The risk of late seizures or epilepsy among survivors of ICH is 5% to 27%.[95]

Deep Venous Thrombosis Prophylaxis

Patients with ICH are at high risk for deep vein thrombosis (DVT) and pulmonary embolism, a potentially fatal complication, due to limb paresis and prolonged immobilization. Dynamic compression stockings should be placed on admission.[98] A small prospective trial has shown that low-dose subcutaneous heparin (5000 U bid) starting after the second day significantly reduced the frequency of venous thromboembolism with no increase in intracranial bleeding.[99] Treatment with low-molecular-weight heparin (ie, enoxaparin 40 mg daily) is a reasonable alternative if renal function is normal. It is generally safe to initiate the DVT prophylaxis after ICH after the first 24 to 48 hours provided that there is no active bleeding or hematoma expansion in progress nor any underlying coagulopathy.

Nutrition

As is the case with all critically ill neurologic patients, enteral feeding should be started within 48 hours to avoid protein catabolism and malnutrition. A small-bore nasoduodenal feeding tube may reduce the risk of aspiration events.

What surgical interventions are currently available for the management of ICH?

Several surgical techniques have been studied in ICH patients and are currently under clinical investigation.

Craniotomy and Clot Evacuation

Craniotomy has been the most studied intervention for the surgical management of ICH. Two earlier smaller trials showed that for patients presenting with moderate alterations in the state of consciousness, surgery reduced the risk of death without improving the functional outcome[100] and that ultra-early evacuation of hematoma improved the 3-month National Institutes of Health Stroke Scale (NIHSS)[101] without effect in mortality rate, but a meta-analysis of all prior trials of surgical intervention for supratentorial ICH showed no significant benefit from this intervention.[102] The Surgical Trial in Intracerebral Haemorrhage (STICH) study, a landmark trial of over 1000 ICH patients, showed that emergent surgical hematoma evacuation by craniotomy within 72 hours of onset fails to improve outcome compared to a policy of initial medical management.[103] In a post-hoc analysis of STICH, the subgroup of patients with superficial hematomas and no IVH had better outcomes in the surgical arm.[104] This observation provided support for the STICH-II trial, which is currently enrolling patients. In contrast to supratentorial ICH, there is much better evidence that cerebellar hemorrhages exceeding 3 cm in diameter benefit from emergent surgical evacuation, as abrupt and dramatic deterioration to coma can occur within the first 24 hours of onset in these patients.[105] For this reason, it is generally unwise to defer surgery in these patients until further clinical deterioration occurs.

Emergency Hemicraniectomy

Hemicraniectomy with duraplasty has been proposed as a lifesaving intervention for several neurologic catastrophes such as malignant middle cerebral artery (MCA) infarction and poor-grade subarachnoid hemorrhage (SAH). No randomized controlled trial has been conducted in patients with ICH. In a report of 12 consecutive patients with hypertensive ICH and treated with hemicraniectomy, 92% survived at discharge and 55% had a good functional outcome at discharge.[106] These preliminary data support the need for better-controlled studies addressing the role of this surgical technique in ICH patients (Figure 2-5).

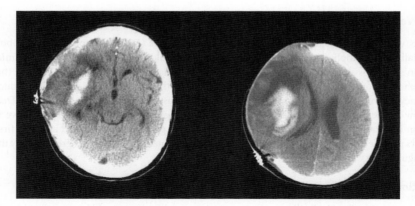

Figure 2-5. Lifesaving hemicraniectomy in a patient with lobar ICH considered otherwise lethal. *(From Rincon F, Mayer SA. Intracerebral hemorrhage. In: Matta B, Mennon D, Smith M, eds. Core Topics in Neuroanaesthesia and Neurointensive Care. Cambridge University Press. Cambridge, UK. In press.)*

Minimally invasive surgery (MIS)

The advantages of MIS over conventional craniotomy include reduced operative time, the possibility of performance under local anesthesia, and reduced surgical trauma. Endoscopic aspiration of supratentorial ICH was studied in a small single-center randomized controlled trial.[107] The study showed that this technique provided a reduction of mortality rate at 6 months in the surgical group, but surgery was more effective in superficial hematomas and in younger patients (younger than 60 years).[107] Similarly, a report from China evaluated the effects of minimally invasive craniopuncture versus medical therapy in a cohort of 465 patients with basal ganglia ICH. Improvement in neurologic outcome at 14 days and 3 months was better in the treatment group, although no differences were seen in long-term mortality.[108]

Thrombolysis and clot evacuation

Thrombolytic therapy and surgical removal of hematomas is another technique that has been studied in a single-center randomized clinical trial.[101] Patients in the surgical group had better outcome scores than the medically treated group. Finally, a multicenter randomized control trial examined the utility of sterotactic urokinase infusion when administered within 72 hours to patients with GCS score of 5 or more and hematomas 10 mL or more in size, provided a significant reduction in hematoma size and mortality rate at the expense of higher rates of rebleeding but no significant differences in outcomes measures were seen.[109]

Thrombolysis after IVH

Intraventricular hemorrhage (IVH) commonly results from extension of ICH into the cerebral ventricular system, and is an independent predictor of mortality rate after ICH.[20] Intraventricular administration of the plasminogen activator urokinase every 12 hours may reduce hematoma size and the expected mortality rate at 1 month.[110] Several small studies have reported the successful use of urokinase or tissue plasminogen activator (tPA) for the treatment of IVH, with the goal of accelerating the clearance of IVH and improving clinical outcome.[111] A Cochrane systemic review published in 2002 summarized the experience of several case series providing evidence of safety but no definitive efficacy.[112] The ongoing Phase III Clear IVH Trial (Clot Lysis Evaluating Accelerated Resolution of Intra Ventricular Hemorrhage) is designed to investigate the optimum dose and frequency of r-tPA administered via an EVD to safely and effectively treat IVH and will soon provide some insight on this issue. When used off-label, a dose of 1 mg of r-tPA every 8 hours (followed by clamping of the EVD for 1 hour) is reasonable until clearance of blood from the third ventricle has been achieved. Doses of 3 mg or more of tPA for IVH thrombolysis have been associated with an unacceptably high bleeding rate (D. Hanley, MD, personal communication, 2004).

What is this patient's prognosis and when can we restart his anticoagulation?

The mortality rate of ICH is 35% to 50% at 30 days and 47% at 1 year.[60,113] Factors that consistently predict mortality or adverse outcomes in ICH have been studied extensively. Independent predictors for 30-day and 1-year mortality rates include GCS and/or depressed level of consciousness, age, ICH volume, the presence of IVH, and infratentorial origin.[20,60] A simple clinical grading scale, the ICH score, permits calculation of mortality rate, allowing use of uniform terms and enhancing communication between physicians. Its usefulness has been validated in predicting 30-day mortality rate.[19] The mortality rates for scores of 0, 1, 2, 3, 4, and 5 are 0%, 13%, 26%, 72%, 97%, and 100%, respectively. Additional factors associated with high mortality rate after ICH include the presence of SAH, wide pulse pressure, history of coronary artery disease, and hyperthermia.[60] Factors associated with good outcomes include a low NIHSS score and low temperature on admission.[19] Restarting anticoagulation in patients with a strong indication, such as a mechanical heart valve or AF with a history of cardioembolic stroke, can be safely implemented after 10 days[114] (Table 2-3).

Table 2-3. The ICH Score

Component	Points	Total Points	30-Day Mortality (%)
Glasgow Coma Scale score			
3-4	2	5+	100
5-12	1		
13-15	0	4	97
ICH volume (mL)			
≥ 30	1	3	72
< 30	0		
Intraventricular hemorrhage			
Yes	1	2	26
No	0	1	13
Age (years)			
≥ 80	1	0	0
< 80	0		
Infratentorial origin			
Yes	1		
No	0		

(Adapted from Hemphill JC 3rd, Bonovich DC, Besmertis L, Manley GT, Johnston SC. The ICH score: A simple, reliable grading scale for intracerebral hemorrhage. Stroke. 2001;32:891-897.)

! CRITICAL CONSIDERATIONS

- Risk factors for ICH include age, male gender, African American and Japanese race/ethnicity, HTN, CAA, cocaine use, low cholesterol levels, oral anticoagulants, and excessive alcohol abuse.
- Hypertension as well as hypotension should be immediately addressed to decrease hematoma expansion and to keep an adequate cerebral perfusion pressure. Acute severe hypertension should be aggressively, but carefully, controlled with IV medications to reduce MAP more than 130 mm Hg by 15% to 30% of baseline, which corresponds to an approximate BP of 180/105 mm Hg. More aggressive blood pressure reduction may be preferable but is currently under study.
- Isotonic fluid resuscitation and vasopressors may be indicated in those patients in shock, and dextrose-containing solutions should be avoided as hyperglycemia may be detrimental for the injured brain.
- Suspected ICP elevations and symptomatic intracranial mass effect (ie, posturing, pupillary changes) should be treated emergently with head elevation, a large dose of 20% mannitol solution (1.0 to 1.5 g/kg) or HS 23.4% (0.5 to 2.0 mL/kg/bolus) and moderate hyperventilation (Pco_2 28 to 32 mm Hg).
- An EVD or ICP monitor should be placed in all patients in coma with evidence of intracranial mass effect or substantial IVH on CT, as long as their prognosis is such that aggressive ICU management is warranted.

- The use of rFVIIa within 4 hours of symptom onset of ICH is contraindicated in patients with spontaneous ICH, but may be an attractive alternative for patients with coagulopathic ICH, particularly from warfarin. Doses of rFVIIa ranging from 20 to 90 μg/kg can be given as an adjunct to expedite the reversal of anticoagulation as a treatment option. Additionally, FFP (15 U/mL), IV vitamin K (10 mg), or PCCs (15 to 30 U/kg) should be given as soon as possible.

- Observation in an ICU or a similar setting is strongly recommended for at least the first 24 hours based on the risk of neurologic deterioration.

- ICH patients are at high risk for thromboembolic disease. In addition to dynamic compression stockings, low-dose heparin (5000 U sc q12h) or enoxaparin (40 mg sc qd) can be safely started on day 2 after ICH.

REFERENCES

1. Broderick JP, Brott T, Tomsick T, Miller R, Huster G. Intracerebral hemorrhage more than twice as common as subarachnoid hemorrhage. *J Neurosurg.* 1993;78:188-191.

2. Qureshi AI, Mohammad Y, Suri MF, et al. Cocaine use and hypertension are major risk factors for intracerebral hemorrhage in young African Americans. *Ethn Dis.* 2001;11:311-319.

3. Arboix A, Vall-Llosera A, Garcia-Eroles L, Massons J, Oliveres M, Targa C. Clinical features and functional outcome of intracerebral hemorrhage in patients aged 85 and older. *J Am Geriatr Soc.* 2002;50:449-454.

4. Daverat P, Castel JP, Dartigues JF, Orgogozo JM. Death and functional outcome after spontaneous intracerebral hemorrhage. A prospective study of 166 cases using multivariate analysis. *Stroke.* 1991;22:1-6.

5. Iso H, Jacobs DR Jr, Wentworth D, Neaton JD, Cohen JD. Serum cholesterol levels and six-year mortality from stroke in 350,977 men screened for the multiple risk factor intervention trial. *N Engl J Med.* 1989;320(14):904-910.

6. Gill JS, Shipley MJ, Tsementzis SA, et al. Alcohol consumption—A risk factor for hemorrhagic and non-hemorrhagic stroke. *Am J Med.* 1991; 90:489-497.

7. Gill JS, Zezulka AV, Shipley MJ, Gill SK, Beevers DG. Stroke and alcohol consumption. *N Engl J Med.* 198623;315:1041-1046.

8. Gorelick PB. Alcohol and stroke. *Stroke.* 1987; 18:268-271.

9. Klatsky AL, Armstrong MA, Friedman GD. Alcohol use and subsequent cerebrovascular disease hospitalizations. *Stroke.* 1989;20:741-746.

10. Thrift AG, Donnan GA, McNeil JJ. Heavy drinking, but not moderate or intermediate drinking, increases the risk of intracerebral hemorrhage. *Epidemiology.* 1999;10:307-312.

11. Levine SR, Brust JC, Futrell N, et al. Cerebrovascular complications of the use of the "crack" form of alkaloidal cocaine. *N Engl J Med.* 199013;323:699-704.

12. Ariesen MJ, Claus SP, Rinkel GJ, Algra A. Risk factors for intracerebral hemorrhage in the general population: A systematic review. *Stroke.* 2003;4:2060-2065.

13. Wintzen AR, de Jonge H, Loeliger EA, Bots GT. The risk of intracerebral hemorrhage during oral anticoagulant therapy: A population study. *Ann Neurol.* 1984;16:553-558.

14. Amarenco P, Bogousslavsky J, Callahan A 3rd, et al. High-dose atorvastatin after stroke or transient ischemic attack. *N Engl J Med.* 2006;355: 549-559.

15. Becker KJ, Baxter AB, Bybee HM, Tirschwell DL, Abouelsaad T, Cohen WA. Extravasation of radiographic contrast is an independent predictor of death in primary intracerebral hemorrhage. *Stroke.* 1999;30:2025-2032.

16. Goldstein JN, Fazen LE, Snider R, et al. Contrast extravasation on CT angiography predicts hematoma expansion in intracerebral hemorrhage. *Neurology.* 2007;68:889-894.

17. Mayer SA. Ultra-early hemostatic therapy for intracerebral hemorrhage. *Stroke.* 2003;34:224-229.

18. Gebel JM Jr, Jauch EC, Brott TG, et al. Relative edema volume is a predictor of outcome in patients with hyperacute spontaneous intracerebral hemorrhage. *Stroke.* 200233:2636-2641.

19. Cheung RT, Zou LY. Use of the original, modified, or new intracerebral hemorrhage score to

predict mortality and morbidity after intracerebral hemorrhage. *Stroke.* 2003;4:1717-1722.

20. Hemphill JC 3rd, Bonovich DC, Besmertis L, Manley GT, Johnston SC. The ICH score: A simple, reliable grading scale for intracerebral hemorrhage. *Stroke.* 2001;32:891-897.

21. Fisher C. Pathological observations in hypertensive intracerebral hemorrhage. *J Neuropathol Exp Neurol.* 1971;30:536-550.

22. Mayer SA, Lignelli A, Fink ME, et al. Perilesional blood flow and edema formation in acute intracerebral hemorrhage: a SPECT study. *Stroke.* 1998;29:1791-1798.

23. Fujii Y, Takeuchi S, Sasaki O, Minakawa T, Tanaka R. Multivariate analysis of predictors of hematoma enlargement in spontaneous intracerebral hemorrhage. *Stroke.* 1998;29:1160-1166.

24. Fujii Y, Tanaka R, Takeuchi S, Koike T, Minakawa T, Sasaki O. Hematoma enlargement in spontaneous intracerebral hemorrhage. *J Neurosurg.* 1994;80:51-57.

25. Murai Y, Takagi R, Ikeda Y, Yamamoto Y, Teramoto A. Three-dimensional computerized tomography angiography in patients with hyperacute intracerebral hemorrhage. *J Neurosurg.* 1999;91:424-431.

26. Komiyama M, Yasui T, Tamura K, Nagata Y, Fu Y, Yagura H. Simultaneous bleeding from multiple lenticulostriate arteries in hypertensive intracerebral haemorrhage. *Neuroradiology.* 199;5 37:129-130.

27. Wada R, Aviv RI, Fox AJ, et al. CT angiography "spot sign" predicts hematoma expansion in acute intracerebral hemorrhage. *Stroke.* 2007;38: 1257-1262.

28. Hart RG, Boop BS, Anderson DC. Oral anticoagulants and intracranial hemorrhage. Facts and hypotheses. *Stroke.* 1995;26:1471-1477.

29. Chowdhury P, Saayman AG, Paulus U, Findlay GP, Collins PW. Efficacy of standard dose and 30 ml/kg fresh frozen plasma in correcting laboratory parameters of haemostasis in critically ill patients. *Br J Haematol.* 2004;125:69-73.

30. Hart RG. *Management of Warfarin Associated Intracerebral Hemorrhage.* Wellesley, MA: UpToDate; 2005.

31. Wjasow C, McNamara R. Anaphylaxis after low dose intravenous vitamin K. *J Emerg Med.* 200324:169-172.

32. Fredriksson K, Norrving B, Stromblad LG. Emergency reversal of anticoagulation after intracerebral hemorrhage. *Stroke.* 1992;23:972-977.

33. Sorensen B, Johansen P, Nielsen GL, Sorensen JC, Ingerslev J. Reversal of the International Normalized Ratio with recombinant activated factor VII in central nervous system bleeding during warfarin thromboprophylaxis: clinical and biochemical aspects. *Blood Coagul Fibrinolysis.* 2003; 14:469-477.

34. Freeman WD, Brott TG, Barrett KM, et al. Recombinant factor VIIa for rapid reversal of warfarin anticoagulation in acute intracranial hemorrhage. *Mayo Clin Proc.* 2004;79:1495-1500.

35. Wakefield TW, Stanley JC. Intraoperative heparin anticoagulation and its reversal. *Semin Vasc Surg.* 1996;9:296-302.

36. Mannucci PM, Remuzzi G, Pusineri F, et al. Deamino-8-D-arginine vasopressin shortens the bleeding time in uremia. *N Engl J Med.* 1983;6;308: 8-12.

37. Diringer MN. Intracerebral hemorrhage: pathophysiology and management. *Crit Care Med.* 1993;21: 152-157.

38. Reynolds SF, Heffner J. Airway management of the critically ill patient: rapid-sequence intubation. *Chest.* 2005;127:1397-1412.

39. Orebaugh SL. Succinylcholine: Adverse effects and alternatives in emergency medicine. *Am J Emerg Med.* 1999;17:715-721.

40. Booij LH. Is succinylcholine appropriate or obsolete in the intensive care unit? *Crit Care.* 2001;5:245-246.

41. Schramm WM, Strasser K, Bartunek A, Gilly H, Spiss CK. Effects of rocuronium and vecuronium on intracranial pressure, mean arterial pressure and heart rate in neurosurgical patients. *Br J Anaesth.* 1996;77:607-611.

42. Robinson N, Clancy M. In patients with head injury undergoing rapid sequence intubation, does pretreatment with intravenous lignocaine/ lidocaine lead to an improved neurological outcome? A review of the literature. *Emerg Med J.* 2001;18:453-457.

43. Broderick JP, Adams HP Jr, Barsan W, et al. Guidelines for the management of spontaneous intracerebral hemorrhage: A statement for healthcare professionals from a special writing group of the Stroke Council, American Heart Association. *Stroke.* 1999;30:905-915.

44. Passero S, Ciacci G, Ulivelli M. The influence of diabetes and hyperglycemia on clinical course after intracerebral hemorrhage. *Neurology.* 200325;61:1351-1356.

45. Siddique MS, Fernandes HM, Wooldridge TD, Fenwick JD, Slomka P, Mendelow AD. Reversible ischemia around intracerebral hemorrhage: a single-photon emission computerized tomography study. *J Neurosurg.* 2002;96:736-741.

46. Rosand J, Eskey C, Chang Y, Gonzalez RG, Greenberg SM, Koroshetz WJ. Dynamic single-section CT demonstrates reduced cerebral blood flow in acute intracerebral hemorrhage. *Cerebrovasc Dis.* 2002;14:214-220.

47. Brott T, Broderick J, Kothari R, et al. Early hemorrhage growth in patients with intracerebral hemorrhage. *Stroke.* 1997;28:1-5.

48. Broderick JP, Diringer MN, Hill MD, et al. Determinants of intracerebral hemorrhage growth: an exploratory analysis. *Stroke.* 2007;38:1072-1075.

49. Powers WJ, Adams RE, Yundt KD. Acute pharmacological hypotension after intracerebral hemorrhage does not change cerebral blood flow. *Stroke.* 1999;30:242.

50. Qureshi AI, Wilson DA, Hanley DF, Traystman RJ. Pharmacologic reduction of mean arterial pressure does not adversely affect regional cerebral blood flow and intracranial pressure in experimental intracerebral hemorrhage. *Crit Care Med.* 1999;27:965-971.

51. Anderson CS, Huang Y, Wang JG, et al. Intensive blood pressure reduction in acute cerebral haemorrhage trial (INTERACT): A randomised pilot trial. *Lancet Neurol.* 2008;7:391-399.

52. Qureshi AI, Palesch YY, Martin R, et al. Effect of systolic blood pressure reduction on hematoma expansion, perihematomal edema, and 3-month outcome among patients with intracerebral hemorrhage: Results from the antihypertensive treatment of acute cerebral hemorrhage study. *Arch Neurol.* 2010;67:570-576.

53. Antihypertensive Treatment in Acute Cerebral Hemorrhage. [02/27/2006]; Available from: http://www.strokecenter.org/trials/TrialDetail.aspx?tid=602

54. Broderick J, Connolly S, Feldmann E, et al. Guidelines for the management of spontaneous intracerebral hemorrhage in adults: 2007 update: A guideline from the American Heart Association/American Stroke Association Stroke Council, High Blood Pressure Research Council, and the Quality of Care and Outcomes in Research Interdisciplinary Working Group. *Stroke.* 200738:2001-2023.

55. Rose JC, Mayer SA. Optimizing blood pressure in neurological emergencies. *Neurocrit Care.* 2004;1:287-299.

56. Kuwata N, Kuroda K, Funayama M, Sato N, Kubo N, Ogawa A. Dysautoregulation in patients with hypertensive intracerebral hemorrhage. A SPECT study. *Neurosurg Rev.* 1995;18:237-245.

57. Mayer SA, Sacco RL, Shi T, Mohr JP. Neurologic deterioration in noncomatose patients with supratentorial intracerebral hemorrhage. *Neurology.* 1994;44:1379-1384.

58. Gujjar AR, Deibert E, Manno EM, Duff S, Diringer MN. Mechanical ventilation for ischemic stroke and intracerebral hemorrhage: indications, timing, and outcome. *Neurology.* 1998;51:447-451.

59. Mayer SA, Chong J. Critical care management of increased intracranial pressure. *J Intensive Care Med.* 2002;17:55-67.

60. Nilsson OG, Lindgren A, Brandt L, Saveland H. Prediction of death in patients with primary intracerebral hemorrhage: a prospective study of a defined population. *J Neurosurg.* 2002;97:531-536.

61. Tuhrim S, Horowitz DR, Sacher M, Godbold JH. Volume of ventricular blood is an important determinant of outcome in supratentorial intracerebral hemorrhage. *Crit Care Med.* 1999;27:617-621.

62. Bowers SA, Marshall LF. Outcome in 200 consecutive cases of severe head injury treated in San Diego County: A prospective analysis. *Neurosurgery.* 1980;6:237-242.

63. Unwin DH, Giller CA, Kopitnik TA. Central nervous system monitoring: what helps, what does not. *Surg Clin North Am.* 1991;71:733-747.

64. Liliang PC, Liang CL, Lu CH, et al. Hypertensive caudate hemorrhage prognostic predictor, outcome, and role of external ventricular drainage. *Stroke.* 2001;32:1195-1200.

65. Lozier AP, Sciacca RR, Romagnoli MF, Connolly ES Jr. Ventriculostomy-related infections: A critical review of the literature. *Neurosurgery.* 2002;51:170-181; discussion 81-82.

66. Schramm WM, Jesenko R, Bartunek A, Gilly H. Effects of cisatracurium on cerebral and cardiovascular hemodynamics in patients with severe brain injury. *Acta Anaesthesiol Scand.* 1997;41:1319-1323.

67. Lundberg N. Continuous recording and control of ventricular fluid pressure in neurosurgical practice. *Acta Psychiatr Scand Suppl.* 1960;36:1-193.

68. Chambers IR, Banister K, Mendelow AD. Intracranial pressure within a developing intracerebral haemorrhage. *Br J Neurosurg.* 2001;15:140-141.

69. Fernandes HM, Siddique S, Banister K, et al. Continuous monitoring of ICP and CPP following ICH and its relationship to clinical, radiological and surgical parameters. *Acta Neurochir Suppl.* 2000;76:463-466.

70. Qureshi AI, Suarez JI. Use of hypertonic saline solutions in treatment of cerebral edema and intracranial hypertension. *Crit Care Med.* 2000; 28:3301-3313.

71. Qureshi AI, Wilson DA, Traystman RJ. Treatment of transtentorial herniation unresponsive to hyperventilation using hypertonic saline in dogs: effect on cerebral blood flow and metabolism. *J Neurosurg Anesthesiol.* 2002;14:22-30.

72. Qureshi AI, Geocadin RG, Suarez JI, Ulatowski JA. Long-term outcome after medical reversal of transtentorial herniation in patients with supratentorial mass lesions. *Crit Care Med.* 2000;28:1556-1564.

73. Schwab S, Georgiadis D, Berrouschot J, Schellinger PD, Graffagnino C, Mayer SA. Feasibility and safety of moderate hypothermia after massive hemispheric infarction. *Stroke.* 2001;32:2033-2035.

74. Schwab S, Spranger M, Schwarz S, Hacke W. Barbiturate coma in severe hemispheric stroke: useful or obsolete? *Neurology.* 1997;48:1608-1613.

75. Rincon F, Mayer SA. Therapeutic hypothermia for brain injury after cardiac arrest. *Semin Neurol.* 2006;26:387-395.

76. Fogelholm R, Murros K, Rissanen A, Avikainen S. Admission blood glucose and short term survival in primary intracerebral haemorrhage: a population based study. *J Neurol Neurosurg Psychiatry.* 2005;76:349-353.

77. Baird TA, Parsons MW, Phanh T, al. Persistent poststroke hyperglycemia is independently associated with infarct expansion and worse clinical outcome. *Stroke.* 2003;34:2208-2214.

78. Capes SE, Hunt D, Malmberg K, Pathak P, Gerstein HC. Stress hyperglycemia and prognosis of stroke in nondiabetic and diabetic patients: A systematic overview. *Stroke.* 2001;32:2426-2432.

79. Williams LS, Rotich J, Qi R, et al. Effects of admission hyperglycemia on mortality and costs in acute ischemic stroke. *Neurology.* 2002;59:67-71.

80. Klip A, Tsakiridis T, Marette A, Ortiz PA. Regulation of expression of glucose transporters by glucose: a review of studies in vivo and in cell cultures. *FASEB J.* 1994;8:43-53.

81. Hansen TK, Thiel S, Wouters PJ, Christiansen JS, Van den Berghe G. Intensive insulin therapy exerts antiinflammatory effects in critically ill patients and counteracts the adverse effect of low mannose-binding lectin levels. *J Clin Endocrinol Metab.* 2003;88:1082-1088.

82. Finfer S, Chittock DR, Su SY, et al. Intensive versus conventional glucose control in critically ill patients. *N Engl J Med.* 2009;360:1283-1297.

83. Oddo M, Schmidt JM, Carrera E, et al. Impact of tight glycemic control on cerebral glucose metabolism after severe brain injury: a microdialysis study. *Crit Care Med.* 2008;36:3233-3238.

84. Van den Berghe G, Schoonheydt K, Becx P, Bruyninckx F, Wouters PJ. Insulin therapy protects the central and peripheral nervous system of intensive care patients. *Neurology.* 2005; 64:1348-1353.

85. Commichau C, Scarmeas N, Mayer SA. Risk factors for fever in the neurologic intensive care unit. *Neurology.* 2003;60:837-841.

86. Szczudlik A, Turaj W, Slowik A, Strojny J. Hyperthermia is not an independent predictor of greater mortality in patients with primary intracerebral hemorrhage. *Med Sci Monit.* 2002;8:CR702-707.

87. Baena RC, Busto R, Dietrich WD, Globus MY, Ginsberg MD. Hyperthermia delayed by 24 hours aggravates neuronal damage in rat hippocampus following global ischemia. *Neurology.* 1997;48:768-773.

88. Minamisawa H, Smith ML, Siesjo BK. The effect of mild hyperthermia and hypothermia on brain damage following 5, 10, and 15 minutes of forebrain ischemia. *Ann Neurol.* 1990;28:26-33.

89. Clasen RA, Pandolfi S, Laing I, Casey D Jr. Experimental study of relation of fever to cerebral edema. *J Neurosurg.* 1974;41:576-581.

90. Rossi S, Zanier ER, Mauri I, Columbo A, Stocchetti N. Brain temperature, body core temperature, and intracranial pressure in acute cerebral damage. *J Neurol Neurosurg Psychiatry.* 2001;71:448-454.

91. Mayer S, Commichau C, Scarmeas N, Presciutti M, Bates J, Copeland D. Clinical trial of an air-circulating cooling blanket for fever control in critically ill neurologic patients. *Neurology.* 2001;56:292-298.

92. Mayer SA, Kowalski RG, Presciutti M, et al. Clinical trial of a novel surface cooling system for fever control in neurocritical care patients. *Crit Care Med.* 2004;32:2508-2515.

93. Ziai WC, Toung TJ, Bhardwaj A. Hypertonic saline: first-line therapy for cerebral edema? *J Neurol Sci.* 2007;261:157-166.

94. Adrogue HJ, Madias NE. Hypernatremia. *N Engl J Med.* 2000;342(20):1493-1499.

95. Passero S, Rocchi R, Rossi S, Ulivelli M, Vatti G. Seizures after spontaneous supratentorial intracerebral hemorrhage. *Epilepsia.* 2002;43:1175-1180.

96. Vespa PM, O'Phelan K, Shah M, et al. Acute seizures after intracerebral hemorrhage: A factor in progressive midline shift and outcome. *Neurology.* 2003;60:1441-1446.

97. Claassen J, Jette N, Chum F, et al. Electrographic seizures and periodic discharges after intracerebral hemorrhage. *Neurology.* 2007;69:1356-1365.

98. Geerts WH, Pineo GF, Heit JA, et al. Prevention of venous thromboembolism: the Seventh ACCP Conference on Antithrombotic and Thrombolytic Therapy. *Chest.* 2004;126(suppl 3):338S-400S.

99. Boeer A, Voth E, Henze T, Prange HW. Early heparin therapy in patients with spontaneous intracerebral haemorrhage. *J Neurol Neurosurg Psychiatry.* 1991;54:466-467.

100. Juvela S, Heiskanen O, Poranen A, et al. The treatment of spontaneous intracerebral hemorrhage. A prospective randomized trial of surgical and conservative treatment. *J Neurosurg.* 1989;70:755-758.

101. Zuccarello M, Brott T, Derex L, et al. Early surgical treatment for supratentorial intracerebral hemorrhage: a randomized feasibility study. *Stroke.* 1999;30:1833-1839.

102. Fernandes HM, Gregson B, Siddique S, Mendelow AD. Surgery in intracerebral hemorrhage. The uncertainty continues. *Stroke.* 2000;31:2511-2516.

103. Mendelow AD, Gregson BA, Fernandes HM, et al. Early surgery versus initial conservative treatment in patients with spontaneous supratentorial intracerebral haematomas in the International Surgical Trial in Intracerebral Haemorrhage (STICH): A randomised trial. *Lancet.* 2005;29;365:387-397.

104. Bhattathiri PS, Gregson B, Prasad KS, Mendelow AD. Intraventricular hemorrhage and hydrocephalus after spontaneous intracerebral hemorrhage: results from the STICH trial. *Acta Neurochir Suppl.* 2006;96:65-68.

105. Ott KH, Kase CS, Ojemann RG, Mohr JP. Cerebellar hemorrhage: diagnosis and treatment. A review of 56 cases. *Arch Neurol.* 1974;31:160-167.

106. Murthy JM, Chowdary GV, Murthy TV, Bhasha PS, Naryanan TJ. Decompressive craniectomy with clot evacuation in large hemispheric hypertensive intracerebral hemorrhage. *Neurocrit Care.* 2005;2:258-262.

107. Auer LM, Deinsberger W, Niederkorn K, et al. Endoscopic surgery versus medical treatment for spontaneous intracerebral hematoma: a randomized study. *J Neurosurg.* 1989;70:530-535.

108. Wang WZ, Jiang B, Liu HM, et al. Minimally invasive craniopuncture therapy vs. conservative treatment for spontaneous intracerebral hemorrhage: Results from a randomized clinical trial in China. *Int J Stroke.* 2009;4:11-16.

109. Teernstra OP, Evers SM, Lodder J, Leffers P, Franke CL, Blaauw G. Stereotactic treatment of intracerebral hematoma by means of a plasminogen activator: A multicenter randomized controlled trial (SICHPA). *Stroke.* 2003;34:968-974.

110. Naff NJ, Carhuapoma JR, Williams MA, et al. Treatment of intraventricular hemorrhage with urokinase: effects on 30-day survival. *Stroke.* 2000;31:841-847.

111. Coplin WM, Vinas FC, Agris JM, et al. A cohort study of the safety and feasibility of intraventricular urokinase for nonaneurysmal spontaneous intraventricular hemorrhage. *Stroke.* 1998;29:1573-1579.

112. Lapointe M, Haines S. Fibrinolytic therapy for intraventricular hemorrhage in adults. *Cochrane Database Syst Rev.* 2002:CD003692.

113. Vermeer SE, Algra A, Franke CL, Koudstaal PJ, Rinkel GJ. Long-term prognosis after recovery from primary intracerebral hemorrhage. *Neurology.* 2002;59:205-209.

114. Ananthasubramaniam K, Beattie JN, Rosman HS, Jayam V, Borzak S. How safely and for how long can warfarin therapy be withheld in prosthetic heart valve patients hospitalized with a major hemorrhage? *Chest.* 2001;119:478-484.

CHAPTER

3

Status Epilepticus

Santiago Ortega-Gutierrez, MD
Naman Desai, BA
Jan Claassen, MD, PhD

Generalized convulsive status epilepticus. A previously healthy 19-year-old woman was brought to the emergency department (ED) for a witnessed "convulsion." She had suddenly stopped talking and stared into space in the middle of a conversation with her roommates. She then exhibited stereotypical picking behavior of her clothes followed by head deviation to the right and generalized tonic-clonic arm and leg movements lasting approximately 3 minutes. She was not incontinent but she did bite her tongue. Emergency medical services (EMS) were activated and immediately transferred her to the closest ED, where she was found to be lethargic with a temperature of 101.3°F. The rest of her vitals were within normal limits. She had bilaterally reactive pupils to light, an intact oculocephalic reflex, and intact corneal reflexes. She localized to painful stimulation with the left arm but did not move the right side. Her tone was decreased on the right side with a positive Babinski sign. The remainder of her neurologic examination was unremarkable. An admission chest radiograph and head computed tomography (CT) were unrevealing. On returning from the CT imaging, the patient had a second generalized tonic-conic seizure witnessed by the ED staff which lasted slightly more than 5 minutes.

What is the most likely diagnosis in this patient?

The clinical presentation is most consistent with secondary generalized convulsive status epilepticus (GCSE). For practical purposes, most practitioners would categorize any seizure lasting at least 5 minutes or two or more discrete seizures without recovery of consciousness in between seizures as status epilepticus (SE).[1-6] This cutoff is based on animal and human data suggesting irreversible neuronal injury[7] and pharmacoresistance[2,8,9] may occur after prolonged seizures and the observation that most clinical and electrographic seizures that do not progress to SE last less than 5 minutes.[1,10-12] The clinical presentation of GCSE is typically relatively characteristic; however, postanoxic myoclonus (see detailed discussion below), posturing during herniation, and psychogenic seizures may be considered in the differential diagnosis.

GCSE is a relatively common neurologic emergency with an overall estimated incidence of 41 to 61 cases per 100,000 patients per year.[13] Rapid diagnosis is crucial since untreated SE rapidly becomes refractory to therapy and carries significant morbidity and mortality rates. GCSE is defined as generalized convulsions that are associated with rhythmic jerking of the extremities.[14] Classic clinical features include generalized tonic-clonic movements or rhythmic jerking of the extremities and mental status impairment (coma, lethargy, confusion); additional neurologic findings may include aphasia, amnesia, staring, automatisms, blinking, facial twitching, agitation, nystagmus, eye deviation, and perseveration. After convulsions have ceased, focal findings such as focal motor impairment, also known as Todd paralysis, may persist.

A number of different classification schemes have been proposed to categorize SE into subtypes based on clinical and electrographic characteristics. For practical purposes, we will focus on convulsive and nonconvulsive SE (NCSE) since these are the most important to recognize for the emergency and intensive critical care (ICU) physician. Clinical features and differentiating characteristics of NCSE will be discussed in detail below.

When should the treatment of GCSE be started?

The most important principle in treatment of GCSE is initiating treatment as early as possible.[15,16] In one study, if therapy was begun within 30 minutes of onset, 80% responded to the first-line antiepileptic drug (AED), whereas only 40% responded if the therapy started beyond the 2-hour window.[15] Following this principle, studies were undertaken to study if initiation of SE treatment in the prehospital setting could be safely done and would lead to a better outcome.[6] Patients treated with lorazepam by EMS prior to reaching the hospital had better acute seizure control than those who received diazepam or placebo. Importantly, these practitioners found that respiratory compromise was more commonly seen in patients who received placebo than those who were given benzodiazepines, suggesting that administering AEDs as soon as possible is not only more efficacious but also safer than waiting. A number of studies investigated alternate routes of administrating benzodiazepines including diazepam per rectum and intranasal, buccal, or intramuscular midazolam. All of these routes of administration were shown to be effective alternatives to IV administration, and they should be considered in situations where the lack of IV access would delay initiation of benzodiazepine therapy.

What should be the first step in managing this patient?

Treatment of these patients should be guided by an institutional protocol to allow multiple team members to simultaneously initiate a series of steps including an assessment of airway, breathing, and circulation (ABCs), administration of AEDs, determination and addressing of underlying causes for seizures, and obtaining IV access. Initiation of treatment should begin within 3 to 5 minutes of seizure onset, depending on the circumstance. Most patients with GCSE will not be able to safely protect their airway because of ongoing seizures or the seizure treatment. Therefore, in most cases of GCSE, intubation should be initiated early. Good hemodynamic monitoring is mandatory since SE as well as an antiepileptic used to treat SE have been associated with arrhythmias and hypotension. Diagnose hypoglycemia rapidly since it will only respond to glucose administration and will result in permanent damage if not corrected rapidly (Table 3-1).

What should be the first AED that this patient receives?

In accordance with evidence from prospective randomized controlled trials, lorazepam (see Table 3-2 for dosing and pharmacokinetic information) should be given as the initial AED, with a success rate between 59% and 65%.[14] If IV access cannot rapidly be established, diazepam 20 mg per rectum (may use diastat or IV solution of diazepam), or midazolam 10 mg administered intranasally, buccally, or intramuscularly[6,14,17] may be chosen as alternatives.

Table 3-1. Initial Common Steps in the Management of Status Epilepticus

Immediate treatment
Preserve airway and oxygenation
Secure IV access with preferably two peripheral lines
Check vitals including oxygen saturation—treat hypotension with fluid and vasopressors if necessary (central line)
Measure fingerstick blood glucose. If < 60 mg/dL, administer 1 amp $D_{50}W$
$D_{50}W$ 50 mL IV and thiamine 100 mg IV unless adequate glucose known

Table 3-2. Doses and Pharmacokinetic Features of Initial Therapy for GCSE

Initial medication

1. **Lorazepam**
   Loading Dose: 4-8 mg IV (or 0.1 mg/kg)
   Onset of Action: 3-10 min
   Duration of Effect: 12-24 h
   Elimination Half-Life: 14 h
   Main Side Effects: Sedation, respiratory depression, hypotension

2. **Phenytoin**
   Loading Dose: 20 mg/kg IV, maximum infusion rate 50 mg/min (25 mg/min in elderly, patients with preexisting cardiovascular conditions).
   Maintenance: 5-7 mg/kg/day in 2-3 divided doses.
   Onset of Action: 20-25 min.
   Contraindications: Heart block; caution if hepatic and renal impairment.
   Main Drug Interactions: May displace other drugs that are protein bound and increase free level of other drugs. Induces hepatic metabolism of many medications, including other antiepileptic drugs (precipitates if given together with potassium, insulin, heparin, norepinephrine, cephalosporin, dobutamine).
   Main Side Effects: Cardiac arrhythmias, hypotension, hepatotoxicity, pancytopenia, phlebitis, soft tissue injury from extravasation, purple glove syndrome, allergy including Stevens-Johnson syndrome.
   Target Serum Level: Total 15-25 μg/mL, free level 2-3 μg/mL (monitor free level when on valproate, benzodiazepines, other highly protein-bound medications; low albumin; or critically ill), adjustments if free level not available: total level/ (Alb × 0.1) + 0.1 (in patients with renal failure: total level/[Alb × 0.2] + 0.1).

3. **Fosphenytoin**
   Loading Dose: 20 mg/kg IV, maximum infusion rate 150 mg/min. If patient continues having seizures after 20 mg/kg, an additional 5-10 mg/kg may be given.
   Maintenance: 5-7 mg/kg/day in 2-3 divided doses.
   Onset of Action: 20-25 min (can be given faster than phenytoin but needs to be converted to phenytoin prior to onset of action, which takes ~ 15 min).
   Main Side Effect: See phenytoin, additionally transient pruritus from solvent. No purple glove syndrome.
   Target Serum Levels: Same as phenytoin. Serum phenytoin levels should be measured more than 2 h after IV or 4 h after IM administration to allow complete conversion to phenytoin.

4. **Valproate**
   Loading Dose: 40 mg/kg IV over 10 min, if still seizing, additional 20 mg/kg over ~ 5 min (max rate 6 mg/kg/min).
   Maintenance: 1 g IV q6h (infusion dose range 2-8 mg/kg/h)
   Contraindications: Severe liver dysfunction, thrombocytopenia, active bleeding.
   Major Drug Interactions: Due to interactions between phenytoin and valproic acid, it is important to follow unbound levels, especially phenytoin to avoid toxicity. In combination with phenobarbital, valproate can cause severe impaired mental status. Meropenem decreases valproate concentrations dramatically.
   Main Side Effect: Hepatotoxicity, thrombocytopenia, pancreatitis, hyperammonemic encephalopathy (consider L-carnitine 33 mg/kg q8h), fibrinogen levels. Hypotension is rare but has been reported.
   Target Serum Levels: Total: 80-140 μg/mL, free: 4-11 μg/mL (only consider if toxicity suspected).

Abbreviation: GCSE, generalized convulsive status epilepticus.

In what circumstance should another AED be given and what medication should be chosen?

All patients with GCSE should be given a second AED since the initial benzodiazepine is not a long-term therapy to prevent recurrence of SE. Most physicians would not give first- and second-line AEDs in a sequential order. Although second-line therapy has not been prospectively evaluated, phenytoin or fosphenytoin (see Table 3-2) is recommended by most neurologists.[18] However, recent evidence has emerged from three small prospective, randomized, open-label trials to suggest that IV valproate is an efficacious and safe first- or second-line treatment (66% and 88% response rate, respectively) and perhaps superior to phenytoin (42% and 86%, respectively).[19] Other alternatives with even less data include levetiracetam and phenobarbital.

> Our patient received a total of 4 mg of lorazepam, was loaded with 20 mg/kg of fosphenytoin, and intubated for airway protection. The episode subsided after 7 minutes and once stable she was transferred to the Neuro-ICU for further care. On arrival, the patient was lethargic but no clinical evidence of seizures was noted.

What should be the next steps?

Management should focus on three aspects: (1) making sure that the patient is medically stable, (2) diagnosing and addressing the underlying cause of GCSE, and (3) determining if electrographic seizures are present. As a side note, avoid administration of paralytics for intubation whenever possible since they may mask ongoing convulsions.

1. Medical stability: Hypotension and arrhythmias may be seen during loading with phenytoin or fosphenytoin. Monitoring may include placing a central line or arterial line if not done already.

2. Diagnostic workup: The underlying differential is wide (Tables 3-3 and 3-4) and the diagnostic workup should be individualized depending on the clinical scenario (Table 3-5). In a general population-based study, the most common causes of SE were low levels of AEDs (in 34% of the cases), remote symptomatic etiologies (history of neurologic insults remote to first unprovoked seizures), and cerebrovascular disease.[20] Nevertheless, the causes of SE in critically ill patients may be different from those in the general population. In general ICUs, metabolic abnormalities and drug withdrawal represent 66% of the SE admissions.[21] In comatose patients admitted to general ICUs, anoxia-hypoxia followed by stroke and infection are the most common cause of NCSE and refractory status epilepticus (RSE).[22,23] Some of the diagnostic tests should be started in the ED and some may be completed once the patient is admitted to the floor or ICU. Most physicians would at least send basic blood and urine tests (including complete blood cell count [CBC], basic metabolic panel [BMP], calcium, magnesium, toxicology screens), get AED levels (ie, phenytoin, valproate, carbamazepine), and have a high suspicion to obtain imaging (head CT or magnetic resonance imaging [MRI]) and lumbar puncture. The presence of fever at presentation should raise the suspicion for central nervous system (CNS) infection, and empiric treatment with bacterial and viral coverage should be started until the results from the lumbar puncture and imaging ancillary testing are available.

3. Persistent electrographic seizures: The patient should be connected to computer-analyzed electroencephalography (cEEG) monitoring as soon as possible since electrographic seizures persist in 20% to 48% of clinically apparently successfully treated GCSE and 14% are in NCSE without any clinical signs of seizure activity.[14,24] These electrographic seizures in the aftermath of convulsive seizures are clearly associated with a worse prognosis,[24] while no study so far investigated if treatment of these patterns results in a better outcome. Currently, most practitioners would treat these electrographic seizures the same way they would treat clinical seizures.

Table 3-3. Etiology of Status Epilepticus

Etiology	Study Lowenstein Patients (%)	Study Towne et al. Patients (%)
Discontinuation of antiepileptic drugs	26	22.5
Cerebral vascular disease	4	22.5
Ethyl alcohol consumption	10	14.2
Idiopathic	4	14.2
Anoxia	4	11.9
Metabolic	4	11.5
Hemorrhage	?	5.1
Infection	8	5.1
Tumor	6	4.4
Trauma	5	4.0
Drugs	10	2.4
Central nervous system infection	8	0.8
Congenital disorder	?	0.8

(Adapted from Lowenstein DH. Status epilepticus: An overview of the clinical problem. Epilepsia. 1999:40 (suppl 1):S3-S8 and Towne AR, Pellock JM, Ko D et al. Determinant of mortality of status epilepticus. Epilepsia. 1994;35:27-34.)

Our patient's initial EEG showed continuous partial electrographic SE with occasional evolution to clinical seizures on the left hemisphere (Figure 3-1).

How should we approach this patient now?

Our patient has refractory status epilepticus (RSE), a neurologic emergency that should be managed in the ICU setting and requires cEEG monitoring. While some controversy regarding the exact definition persists, most experts classify SE that persists despite first- and second-line AED regardless of the elapsed time as RSE. Most commonly patients with RSE appear comatose and have subtle or no clinical manifestations of seizures.[25] Prior to the widespread use of cEEG, the incidence of RSE was estimated at 2000 to 6000 cases per year. It can occur at any age and both sexes are equally at risk.[26] Overall, the exact incidence and prevalence is readily underestimated because of the absence of population-based studies with cEEG monitoring. For instance, in a VA cooperative study, 38% of patients with "overt" SE and 82% with "subtle" SE continued seizing after receiving full doses of two AEDs.[24] Moreover, depending on sampling bias and utilization of cEEG monitoring after GCSE, 9% to 48% of patients continued to seize after initial therapy.[24,25]

What is the prognosis of patients with SE?

At hospital discharge, 9% to 21%[6,27,28] and at 30 days 19% to 27%[14,29] of adults with convulsive SE are dead. Among survivors, disability and particularly cognitive impairment are frequent.[6,15,30,31] Factors

Table 3-4. Precipitants of Seizures in the ICU

Common etiology and precipitants of seizures
Acute processes
Metabolic abnormalities
Renal
Liver
Electrolytes disturbances
Endocrine disturbances
Hypoxic/ischemia
Sepsis
Stroke
Primary CNS inflammation
Withdrawal
Delirium tremens
Benzodiazepine
Narcotics
Drugs
Antibiotics: imipenem, penicillins, cephalosporins, isoniazide, metronidazol
Antihistaminics, including over-the-counter diphenhydramine
Antipsychotics, especially clozapine and low-potency phenothiazines
Antidepressants: maprotiline, bupropion, tricyclics
Baclofen
Antiarrythmics: lidocaine, flecainide
Bronchodilators: theophyllineh
Fentanyl
Flumazenil
Ketamine
Lithium
Meperidine
Propoxyphene
Chronic processes
Preexisting epilepsy: breakthrough seizures or discontinuation of anticonvulsants
Central nervous system tumors
Remote central nervous system pathology such as stroke or abscesses that could potentially cause gliosis

(Adapted from Ortega-Gutierrez Wolfe T, Pandya DJ, et al. Neurological complications in non-neurological intensive care units. Neurologist. 2009;15:254-267.)

associated with poor outcome include older age, impairment of consciousness, duration of seizures, and the presence of medical complications.[27,32,33] Recurrent SE may be seen in up to one-third of patients according to one population-based study that followed patients for 10 years.[34]

RSE carries a dismal outcome with mortality rates close to 23% to 61%,[28,35-41] and it appears to be rather independent of the chosen therapeutic strategy.

What is the mechanism for RSE?

Exact mechanisms underlying the development of refractoriness are to date incompletely understood. Evidence has accumulated that impairment of gamma-aminobutyric acid (GABA)–mediated inhibition related to internalization of GABA receptors[42,43] and upregulation of excitatory AMPA (alpha-amino-3-hydroxy-5-methyl-4-isoxazolepropionate) and NMDA (N-methyl-D-aspartate) receptors[43] may play a role in the development of increasing refractoriness to treatment.

Table 3-5. Suggested Workup

All patients
1. Fingerstick glucose.
2. Obtain IV access.
3. Pulse oximetry, supplement prn.
4. Monitor BP, HR, O_2 sat, support if needed.
5. Cardiac monitoring.
6. Head CT (appropriate for most cases).
7. Order labs: Blood sugar, complete blood count, basic metabolic panel, calcium, magnesium, phosphorus, liver function tests, troponin, toxicology screen (urine and blood), ABG, anticonvulsant levels (at least for phenytoin, valproate, carbamazepine), type and hold, coagulation studies, inborn errors of metabolism.
8. cEEG monitoring: Notify EEG tech if available (as soon as available unless patient returns to pre–status epilepticus baseline).

Depending on clinical presentation
1. Brain MRI
2. Lumbar puncture
3. Comprehensive toxins that frequently cause seizures (ie, INH, tricyclics, theophylline, cocaine, sympathomimetics, alcohol, organophosphates, cyclosporine)

Abbreviations: ABG, arterial blood gas; BP, blood pressure; cEEG, continuous electroencephalography; CT, computed tomography; EEG, electroencephalography; HR, heart rate; INH, isoniazid; MRI, magnetic resonance imaging. (*Adapted from Walter M. Status epilepticus: An evidence based guide. BMJ. 2005;331:673-677.*)

How should this patient with RSE be treated?

There are no randomized controlled trials that have investigated this question, and practitioners do not agree on the best treatment for RSE. After standard treatment with two AEDs, the likelihood of responding to a third conventional medication regardless of the agent is only 2% to 5%, depending on the type of SE.[14] Despite these findings, half of the neurologists would still use a conventional AED as a third-line agent,[18] while most intensivists would choose continuous drips of midazolam, propofol, or pentobarbital (Table 3-6). If valproic acid has not been chosen already as a second-line agent,

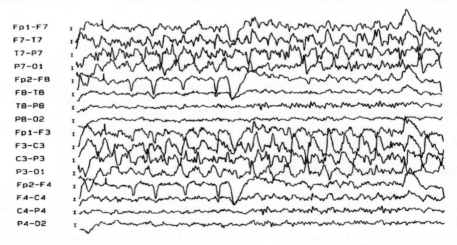

Figure 3-1. This patient's EEG reveals a continuation of a seizure from the entire left hemisphere despite first- and second-line treatment.

Table 3-6. Continuous IV Infusion Therapies Used in RSE

Medications

1. **Continuous IV Midazolam Infusion**

   Loading Dose: 0.2 mg/kg. Repeat 0.2-0.4 mg/kg boluses every 5 min until seizure stops, up to a maximum total loading dose of 2 mg/kg.

   Continuous IV: Initial infusion rate 0.1 mg/kg. Usual maintenance rate 0.05 mg/kg.

   Dose Range: 0.05-2.9 mg/kg/h. For breakthrough seizures, an additional bolus can be given and the continuous IV rate should be increased by approximately 20%.

   Time to Stop Status Epilepticus: Minutes, usually less than 1 h.

   Duration of Antiepileptic Effect: Minutes to hours.

   Elimination Half-Life: 1.5-3.5 h initially. With prolonged use, tolerance, tachyphylaxis, and significant prolongation of half-life can occur.

   Main Side Effect: Sedation of minutes to several hours and a possible day if prolonged use, respiratory depression, hypotension.

2. **Continuous IV Propofol Infusion**

   Loading Dose: 1 mg/kg. Repeat 1-2 mg/kg boluses every 5 min until seizure stops, up to a maximum loading dose of 10 mg/kg. Initial continuous IV rate: 2 mg/kg/h.

   Continuous IV Dose Range: 1-15 mg/kg/h. Do not exceed 5 mg/kg/h for > 48 h due to risk of propofol infusion syndrome.

   Time to Stop Status Epilepticus: Usually < 10 min.

   Contraindications: Allergy to soybean oil, egg lecithin, or glycerol. Use with caution in combination with carbonic anhydrase inhibitors, including zonisamide and topiramate, because of the risk of refractory acidosis.

   Main Side Effects: Sedation, large lipid load requiring adjustment of caloric intake, occasional pancreatitis, dose-dependant hypotension, potential fatal multiorganic failure and "propofol infusion syndrome" (metabolic acidosis, rhabdomyolysis, and circulatory collapse) with high dose or prolonged use.

   Monitor: CPK, triglycerides, amylase/lipase, blood gases, and lactic acid. Consider cardiovascular monitoring.

3. **Continuous IV Pentobarbital Infusion**

   Loading Dose: 5 mg/kg. Repeat 5 mg/kg boluses until seizure stops.

   Maximum Bolus Rate: 25-50 mg/min.

   Continuous IV Dose Range: Initial infusion rate 1 mg/kg/h. Usual maintenance range 0.5-10.0 mg/kg/h, traditionally titrated to suppression burst on EEG.

   Elimination Half-Life: 15-60 h.

   Main Side Effect: Prolonged coma (usually days after infusion stopped), hypotension (usually requires vasopressors), myocardial depression, immune suppression, ileus, allergy including Stevens-Johnson syndrome.

   Target Serum Levels: See phenytoin. Serum phenytoin levels should be measured > 2 h after IV or > 4 h after IM infusion to allow complete conversion to phenytoin.

Abbreviations: CPK, creatine phosphokinase; EEG, electroencephalogram; RSE, refractory status epilepticus.

particularly in patients with a "do not intubate" order, it may be a good alternative. All patients should be connected to cEEG at this point if it is available.

Traditionally, algorithms advocated for loading with phenobarbital with a success rate ranging between 2% and 58% depending on the previous AEDs, the length of SE, and cause of SE. Subsequently, a transition to pentobarbital followed if patients continued to seize.[44] Once started, pentobarbital infusion lowers cerebral oxygen demand, intracranial pressure (ICP), and lipid peroxidation, thereby stopping seizures almost invariably. However, barbiturates are heavily sedating agents with a long half-life, and many patients have complications including refractory acidosis due to propylene glycol toxicity and subsequent multiorgan failure.

Recently, a number of studies have reported the effectiveness of continuous drips of propofol or midazolam as alternative treatments for RSE. In a systematic review of published cases and small series, pentobarbital was found to be more effective in terminating seizures (acute treatment failure, breakthrough seizures, and posttreatment seizures) than midazolam or propofol but was also associated with more frequent side effects (ie, hypotension requiring pressors).[45] However, these results are to be interpreted with caution for a number of reasons: publication bias in small case series, most of the pentobarbital cases were reported a decade before those treated with the other two agents, cEEG monitoring was not available for the pentobarbital cases, no comparisons between medications, differences in underlying etiologies of SE, and the fact that some centers now use more than 10 times the doses for midazolam than those used in the reported case series.

Although some preliminary evidence in a small retrospective series have shown that propofol is associated with a higher mortality rate than midazolam,[41] a recent small single-center study suggested a decrease in mortality (22%) and morbidity rates (two-thirds of the patients had no sequelae) in a large series of 27 patients using the combination of propofol and benzodiazepine infusions to achieve burst suppression and subsequent maintenance on IV clonazepam.[46] Moreover, practitioners have recommended higher loading doses of midazolam infusions which may be more efficacious but are also associated with more side effects[46] (see Table 3-8). Interestingly, there was absolutely no difference in mortality rate (approximately 50%) when comparing the three agents.[41] It is conceivable that when a similar titration end point (ie, EEG end point) would be set for the three agents that the difference in side-effect and efficacy profiles would disappear.

What is the titration goal for continuous AEDs? Should the physician aim for seizure control, burst suppression, or complete background suppression? How long should the drip be maintained?

All of these treatment decisions are controversial since there are little or no data to base them on. The most recent European Federation of Neurological Societies (EFNS) guidelines recommend general anesthetic IV doses of sedative or barbiturates with the goal of burst suppression on EEG to be maintained for a minimum of 24 hours while conventional AEDs level are optimized.[47] A small study of 49 patients with RSE treated with propofol or pentobarbital drips (with or without additional midazolam) concluded that the outcome was independent of the choice of agent and the EEG titration goal. In the literature, cessation of nonconvulsive seizures,[48-53] achieving diffuse beta activity,[49,52,54] burst suppression,[55-57] and complete suppression of EEG[18,56] have been advocated. Most experts would recommend continuing IV AEDs for at least 24 to 72 hours after cessation of electrographic status to prevent recurrence of seizures.

Should additional diagnostic studies be initiated?

Yes. If the initial diagnostic tests do not identify the underlying cause of SE, a more comprehensive workup for less common causes of status needs to be initiated (Table 3-7).

Our patient was initially loaded with 20 mg/kg of valproic acid and continued on maintenance phenytoin and valproic acid (serum levels of phenytoin were 23 and valproic acid 96). MRI revealed left temporal hyperintensity with T-1 post–contrast enhancement. Cerebrospinal fluid polymerase chain reaction (CSF PCR) was positive for herpes simplex. At that time bacterial coverage was discontinued but acyclovir was continued. Owing to ongoing electrographic SE, she was started on a propofol drip for 24 hours with good seizure suppression. She required norepinephrine infusions for hypotension. After 24 hours on propofol, a slow taper was started but electrographic seizures recurred. At that point, a midazolam drip was added and maintained for 48 hours. Subsequently, slow titration was again attempted but frequent electrographic seizures were again noted.

Table 3-7. Potential Workup for Causes of RSE

Cerebrospinal Fluid (CSF) Test
    Bacterial and fungal cultures
    AFB smears and cultures
    Coxsackie complement fixation
    Encephalitis panel (PCR for HSV, VZV, CMV, EBV, enterovirus, SLE, EEE, CA encephalitis, Powassan virus, and WNV)
    ELISA for WNV
    Lyme titer and Western blot
    Crypto Ag
    Cytology, flow cytometry

Serum and Fecal Test
    Autoimmune: Anti-RBC antibodies, Rh factor, ANCA, anti-ENA, anti-DNA, ACE
    Viral: Dengue IgG; hepatitis A, B, C panel; NY State encephalitis panel (PCR for HSV, VZV, CMV, EBV, enterovirus, SLE, EEE, CA encephalitis, Powassan virus and WNV)
    Bacterial: Anaerobes and AFB smear and cultures from brain biopsy. *Legionella, Haemophilus* GPB, *Streptococcus pneumoniae,* streptococci group B, Meningo A, Y, B/E, C, W135, *Bartonella* titers.
    Parasitic and fungal: Stool for ova, parasites, *Protozoa, Cyclospora,* Cryptosporidia, *Isospora.* Blood for *Echinococcus, Histoplasma, Blastomyces, Aspergillus,* VDRL, Lyme titers.
    Paraneoplastic panel
    Flow cytometry
    Heavy metals

Abbreviations: ACE, angiotensin-converting enzyme; AFB, acid-fast bacilli; ANCA, antineutrophil cytoplasmic antibodies; CA, California; CMV, cytomegalovirus; Crypto Ag, cryptococcus antigen; EBV, Epstein-Barr virus; EEE, eastern equine encephalitis; ELISA, enzyme-linked immunosorbent assay; ENA, excitable nuclear antigen; HSV, herpes simplex virus; PCR, polymerase chain reaction; RBC, red blood cell; RSE, refractory status epilepticus; SLE, St Louis encephalitis; VDRL, Venereal Disease Research Laboratory; VZV, varicella zoster virus; WNV, West Nile virus.

What is a potential problem with using valproic acid and phenytoin at the same time?

Valproate produces inhibition of cytochrome P450 2C9 (CYP2C9), which leads to inhibition of the clearance of phenytoin.[58] In addition, valproate also displaces the drug from its protein-binding sites, thus increasing both the free fraction and the total amount of phenytoin present. The complex interaction between these two AEDs requires close monitoring, and following total levels as well as free phenytoin levels may be reasonable.[59]

What alternative treatment option can be tried in this patient?

There is a long list of medications used for RSE that have been described in small series or randomized trials (Table 3-8).

Alternative Treatment Options in RSE

Levetiracetam IV was initially approved in 2006 by the Food and Drug Administration (FDA) for patients with epilepsy who could not take oral medication. In a recent retrospective study, IV levetiracetam (mean loading dose of 994 mg over 30 minutes and maintenance dose of 2166 mg/day) was successfully used to treat 16 of 18 episodes of focal SE that were refractory to initial benzodiazepine trial.[60] In a second study of 24 critically ill patients with mainly focal-onset seizures and status, up to

Table 3-8. Alternative Options for Intractable SE

Antiepileptics	Immunotherapy	Others
Levetiracetam	High-dose steroids	Hypothermia
Ketamine	Immunoglobulins	Ketotic diet
Topiramate	Plasmapheresis	Vagal nerve stimulation
Lacosamide	ACTH	Deep brain stimulation
Inhaled anesthetics		Transcranial magnetic stimulation
Lidocaine		Neurosurgical removal
Verapamil		Electroconvulsive therapy

Abbreviations: ACTH, adrenocorticotropic hormone; SE, status epilepticus.

82% responded to mean IV loading dose of 1780 mg +/– 649 mg bid with the only side effect of transient thrombocytopenia (4% of the patients).[61]

Lacosamide, a new AED with both enteral and parenteral forms, was approved by the FDA in October 2008 as adjunctive therapy for partial-onset seizures in adults suffering from epilepsy. Successful use of lacosamide 200-mg bolus over 5 minutes has been reported in only one case of left-hemispheric NCSE.[62]

In the absence of ileus, enteric topiramate has been used successfully in dosages of 300 to 1600 mg/day to abort RSE to prevent the breakthrough and withdrawal seizures while tapering the continuous IV (cIV) infusions. Other adjunctive oral medications that we and others have used, especially while tapering off the drip, include oxcarbazepine, felbamate, pregabalin, and carbamazepine.

Ketamine is a NMDA-antagonist that has demonstrated positive results in abolishing self-perpetuating SE in animal models.[63] Moreover, it seems to have a synergistic effect when combined with benzodiazepines.[64] Although little experience exists in the adult population, the dosing has been extrapolated from the anesthesia literature (loading dose 1 to 2 mg/kg IV over 1 minute; maintenance 0.6 to 1.8 mg/kg per hour cIV). It is thought to possess other potential neuroprotective effects. Unlike most of the other agents used for RSE, it also increases blood pressure. Caution should be warranted in patients with elevated ICP, traumatic brain injury (TBI), ocular injuries, hypertension, chronic congestive heart failure (CHF), myocardial infarction (MI), tachyarrhythmias, and history of alcohol abuse.[65]

Few studies exist on using inhaled anesthetic including isoflurane, halothane, or desflurane. Although it seems to be highly efficacious in terminating RSE, hypotension, logistical issues in most ICU settings, and frequent seizure recurrence upon withdrawal make it a less attractive choice.

Hypothermia: Very little experience exists with this treatment option.[66,67] A very small case series of four patients has suggested that induced hypothermia with a target temperature 31°C to 35°C may have a potential antiepileptic effect in terminating SE. In all four patients, the treating physicians were able to stop the cIV midazolam, and two of them remained seizure-free. A potentially beneficial side effect of hypothermia is its neuroprotective properties. Disadvantages include shivering, electrolyte abnormalities, immunosuppression, and potential coagulopathy.

Immunomodulatory agents such as steroid IV, immunoglobulins, plasmapheresis, or adrenonocorticotropic hormone (ACTH) may be helpful; in selected cases of immunologic syndromes such as Rasmussen encephalitis, anti–voltage-gated potassium channel–related limbic encephalitis, acute disseminated encephalomyelitis, and paraneoplastic disorders have occurred. However, the role of these agents outside of identified immune processes is unclear.

Lidocaine (1.5- to 2.0-mg/kg bolus, maintenance dose 3 to 4 mg/kg per hour) was efficacious in terminating seizures in 75% of patients with refractory status after the initial bolus. However, narrow pharmacologic range and neurotoxic side effects (>5 μg/mL) limit its use.[68]

Some practitioners have also recommended using pyridoxine hydrochloride early on in patients with SE in an IV or enteral form at 100 to 300 mg/day, as it is a cofactor in the synthesis of the inhibitory neurotransmitter GABA, which may play a role in the initial phase of SE.

Surgery: Small series from the pediatric literature support that if a single, identifiable focus exists on EEG and imaging (single-photon emission CT [SPECT] or positron emission tomography [PET]), surgical removal of a focal structural lesion may be an option after intracranial mapping.[69]

In preparation of a second attempt to titrate the patient off cIV AEDs, levetiracetam 1000 mg IV was loaded and maintenance of 2000 bid was started. Propofol drip was first discontinued owing to hypotension and high norepinephrine requirements. With recurrence of electrographic seizures, ketamine was added and the Versed (midazolam) drip increased to 2 mg/kg per hour and a burst-suppression pattern was seen on cEEG.

When should an attempt be made to start tapering the continuous infusion? How rapidly should cIV AEDs be tapered?

There are no prospective studies to base these recommendations on. Most investigators agree that cIV AEDs should be continued for a minimum of 24 hours after control of seizure has been achieved, with some advocating for 48 hours and others 72 hours; few recommend continuing as long as 96 hours.[70] If prior tapers have failed, it might be necessary to treat longer and taper more slowly. A small retrospective study of 40 patients found no obvious difference in seizure control or survival comparing less versus more than 96 hours of pentobarbital infusions despite no obvious differences in underlying etiologies.

After 48 hours of EEG background suppression, ketamine and Versed infusions were slowly titrated over 24 hours. No further seizures were seen on cEEG, but diffuse bilateral rhythmic or semirhythmic fluctuating patterns appeared.

How would you describe the EEG seen in Figure 3-2? What does it represent? How should the patient be managed at this point?

The EEG in Figure 3-2 shows generalized periodic epileptiform discharges (GPEDs), which have been more recently labeled as generalized periodic discharges.[71] A range of periodic epileptiform discharges (PEDs) that do not meet formal seizure criteria are seen frequently in the aftermath

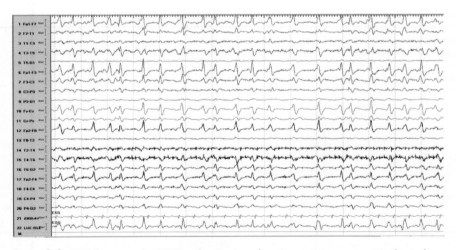

Figure 3-2. EEG demonstrating GPEDs after titration of continuous intravenous antiepileptic drug.

of convulsive or nonconvulsive SE.[14,24] PEDs are characterized by a spike, sharp wave, or sharply contoured slow wave that recurs at a rather regular interval (ie, every second). Discharges may be unilateral or generalized, and if generalized may be synchronous or independently asynchronous.

Patients may have PEDs with superimposed fast activity or other superimposed patterns or features.[71] While these still do not meet formal seizure criteria, many investigators would classify them on an ictal-interictal continuum, and the new classification guidelines identity these patterns with a "+."[71] These patterns may also be seen in acute brain injury without prior SE. One study investigated electrographic features of GPEDs in patients with and without SE. While there were some distinguishing features in the SE group (longer GPED duration and higher GPED amplitude), no generalizable conclusions regarding etiology, treatment, and prognosis could be made based on EEG.[72] In our practice, we consider treatment of PEDs if they have a frequency of two per second or more or are on the ictal-interictal continuum as described above. Supplemental information may be useful in some of these patients to support more aggressive antiepileptic therapy: (1) the clinical scenario and presumed underlying diagnoses, (2) benzodiazepine treatment trial (brief trial with small doses and sometimes a 1-day suppression [Table 3-9]), (3) serial neuron-specific enolase (including before and after the 1-day suppression trial), (4) results of invasive monitoring if available (elevated lactate-pyruvate ratio specifically from decreasing pyruvate levels, elevated glycerol and glutamate, and possibly a decrease in glucose), (5) brain SPECT (for focal increased blood flow at the site of EEG discharges), (6) MRI with diffusion-weighted imaging (DWI), especially at the foci of EEG discharges, and (7) spectroscopy (for increased lactate) (Table 3-10).[73] Of note, no study investigated if any of these supplemental tests is accurate in identifying patients that later have definitive seizures or if treatment decisions based on these tests impact outcome.

NCSE: A 66-year-old man with a history of recurrent glioblastoma multiforme undergoes his second left temporal lobe resection followed by intra-arterial bevacizumab. On arrival at the NeuroICU, he was neurologically intact. On postoperative day 3, the patient stopped following commands. Workup revealed no laboratory abnormalities, infectious workup was negative, and MRI showed mild left temporal lobe vasogenic edema and expected postoperative flair changes.

Table 3-9. Benzodiazepine Trial for the Diagnosis of Status Epilepticus

Benzodiazepine trial
Applies to: Patients with rhythmic or periodic focal or generalized epileptiform discharges on EEG with neurologic impairment.
Monitoring: EEG, pulse oximeter, blood pressure, ECG, respiratory rate.
Antiepileptic drug trial:
    Sequential small doses of rapidly acting short-duration benzodiazepine such as midazolam at 1 mg/dose.
    Between doses, repeat clinical and EEG assessment.
    Trial is stopped after any of the following:
        Resolution of EEG pattern (and exam repeated)
        Definitive clinical improvement
        Respiratory depression, hypotension, or other adverse effects
        A maximum dose is reached (such as 0.2 mg/kg midazolam)
    Test is considered positive if there is resolution of the potential ictal EEG pattern *and* either an improvement in the clinical state or the appearance of previously absent normal EEG patterns. If EEG improves, but patient does not, the result is equivocal.

Abbreviations: ECG, electrocardiogram; EEG, electroencephalogram. *(Adapted with permission from Hirsch LJ, Claassen J. The current state of treatment of status epilepticus. Curr Neurol Neurosci Rep. 2002;2:345-356.)*

Table 3-10. Approach to Periodic Epileptiform Discharges (PEDs)

Clinical approach to patients with PEDs
1. Investigate the cause: History, MRI, CSF, angiography, brain biopsy
2. Administer conventional AEDs for prophylaxis: Fosphenytoin, levetiracetam, and/or valproate
3. Consider a benzodiazepine trial to determine ictal nature
4. Continue cEEG monitoring for identification of definitive seizure or SE later during the hospitalization
5. Long-term management of these patients: PLEDs resolve in the absence of seizure: Taper AEDs after 1 mo PLEDs with seizures: Continue AEDs for 3-12 mo

Abbreviations: AEDs, antiepileptic drugs; cEEG, continuous electroencephalographic; CSF, cerebrospinal fluid; MRI, magnetic resonance imaging; PLEDs, periodic lateral epileptiform discharges; SE, status epilepticus.

What would be your next step in working up this patient?

The cEEG demonstrated NCSE (Figure 3-3), which is more common than previously recognized, particularly in the ICU setting. The exact prevalence of nonconvulsive seizures and NCSE is unknown because of a lack of population-based studies. In patients admitted to NeuroICUs, 18% to 34% and 10% have been reported to have nonconvulsive seizures (NCSz) and NCSE, respectively.[74-76] These frequencies are to be interpreted with caution since selection bias may be substantial as long as only a select subpopulation of patients undergoes the monitoring. In medical ICU settings, the incidence of NCSE is estimated to be near 10%[16] and is particularly prevalent in those with sepsis.[77] One prospective study conducted in the ER setting found NCSz in 37% of 198 patients that underwent urgent EEG for altered mental status.[78] The vast majority of seizures seen in the acute brain injury setting are electrographic and have no or minimal clinical signs (see Table 3-11). The large spectrum of clinical presentations for NCSz and NCSE can easily lead to misdiagnosis and delayed treatment (Tables 3-11 and 3-12).

Indications for cEEG include (1) recent clinical seizure or SE without return to baseline for more than 10 minutes, (2) coma, (3) epileptiform activity or periodic discharges on initial EEG, (4) acute brain injury with high likelihood of seizures, and (5) suspected nonconvulsive seizures and altered mental status.

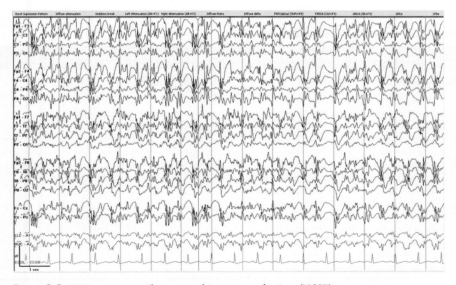

Figure 3-3. EEG consistent with nonconvulsive status epilepticus (NCSE).

Table 3-11. Semiologic Spectrum of Nonconvulsive Seizures and Nonconvulsive Status Epilepticus

Negative symptoms	Positive symptoms
Amnesia	Agitations/aggression
Anorexia	Automatism
Aphasia/mutism	Blinking
Catatonia	Crying
Coma	Delirium
Confusion	Delusions
Lethargy	Echolalia
Staring	Facial twitching
	Laughter
	Nausea/vomiting
	Nystagmus/eye deviation
	Perseveration
	Psychosis
	Tremulousness

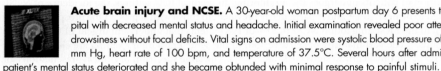 **Acute brain injury and NCSE.** A 30-year-old woman postpartum day 6 presents to the hospital with decreased mental status and headache. Initial examination revealed poor attention and drowsiness without focal deficits. Vital signs on admission were systolic blood pressure of 152/88 mm Hg, heart rate of 100 bpm, and temperature of 37.5°C. Several hours after admission, the patient's mental status deteriorated and she became obtunded with minimal response to painful stimuli.

What would be your first diagnostic test you order?

An imaging study such as a CT scan would be a good first step.

Table 3-12. Criteria for Nonconvulsive Seizure

Any pattern lasting at least 10 s satisfying any one of the following three primary criteria	
Primary criteria	**Secondary criterion**
1. Repetitive generalized or focal spikes, sharp waves, spike and slow-wave or sharp and slow-wave complexes at ≥ 3 s.	Significant improvement in clinical state of appearance of previously absent normal EEG patterns temporally coupled to acute administration of a rapidly acting antiepileptic drug. Resolution of the "epileptiform" discharges leaving diffuse slowing without clinical improvement and without appearance of previously absent normal EEG patterns would not satisfy the secondary criterion.
2. Repetitive generalized or focal spikes, sharp waves, spike and slow-wave or sharp and slow-wave complexes at < 3 s and the secondary criterion.	
3. Sequential rhythmic, periodic, or quasiperiodic waves at ≥ 1 s and unequivocal evolution in frequency (gradually increasing or decreasing by at least 1 s), morphology, or location (gradual spread into or out of a region involving at least two electrodes). Evolution in amplitude alone is not sufficient. Change in sharpness without other change in morphology is not enough to satisfy evolution in morphology.	

Abbreviations: EEG, electroencephalogram; EG, electrographic.

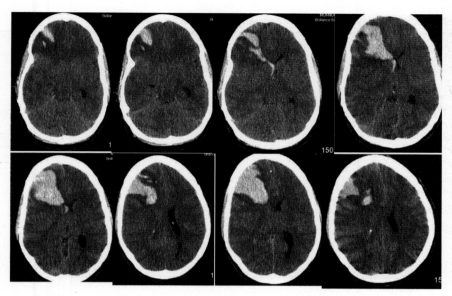

Figure 3-4. CT of head showing right frontal intracranial hemorrhage.

The head CT demonstrates a 60 mL right frontal intracranial hemorrhage (ICH) and intravascular hemorrhage (IVH) (Figure 3-4). An external ventricular drain (EVD) was placed and clot evacuation was performed, but the patient's mental status remained poor.

What would be your next diagnostic step?

As outlined above, unexplained alteration in behavior or mental status warrants an EEG as well as a consideration for NCSE. NCSz have been associated with coma, young age, epilepsy in the past medical history or remote risk factors for seizures, convulsive seizures prior to monitoring, periodic discharges (such as periodic lateral epileptiform discharges [PLEDs] or GPEDs), or burst-suppression, oculomotor abnormalities (ie, nystagmus, hippus, or eye deviation), cardiac or respiratory arrest, and sepsis.[76,77,79] NCSE and periodic EEG patterns are independently associated with poor outcome for patients with acute ischemic stroke, aneurysmal subarachnoid hemorrhage (SAH), central nervous system (CNS) infections, TBI, and nontraumatic ICH after controlling for other predictors of poor outcome.[80,81] Although some practitioners argued that NCSE can be a surrogate marker for severity of brain injury, there is a large body of accumulating animal and human data supporting that these EEG patterns may cause additional harm.[14,50-52,81] Interestingly, recently unilateral NCSz were associated with long-term hippocampal atrophy diagnosed on follow-up MRI.[53] There remains some controversy about how aggressively to treat NCSE, but currently most practitioners would agree that NCSE in the acute brain injury setting should be treated very similar to GCSE (Table 3-13).

The EEG demonstrates very frequent electrographic seizures arising from the right hemisphere which responded very well to treatment with levetiracetam and phenytoin. On angiography, bleeding of the arteries most consistent with Call-Fleming syndrome was seen. After control of her seizures, the patient woke up within hours and was successfully extubated 2 days later (Figure 3-5).

Table 3-13. Nonconvulsive SE Adult Treatment Protocol Recommendation

Preferred order of medication for nonconvulsive status, intermittent seizures, or later stages of RSE.

Continuous Infusions (respiratory depression)

1. Midazolam[a]
2. Propofol or pentobarbital[a]
3. Ketamine[a]: only if failure of or contraindications to midazolam, propofol, and barbiturates
4. Hypothermia

Noncontinuous Infusions (no respiratory depression)

1. Fosphenytoin/phenytoin or valproate[a]
2. Levetiracetam[b]
3. Lacosamide: only if failure or contraindications of the above[c]
4. Phenobarbital[a]

[a]Doses are similar to SE protocol table 3-6.

[b]Levetiracetam (Loading Dose: 2.5 g IV over 5 min give at 1-4 g over 15 min. Initial dose: 3-6 g/day divided in 3-4 doses. Maintenance: 2-12 g/day IV/PO in 3-4 divided doses).

[c]Lacosamide (Loading Dose: 300 mg IV over 30 min. Maintenance: 200-300 mg/day IV/PO over 30-60 min q12h).

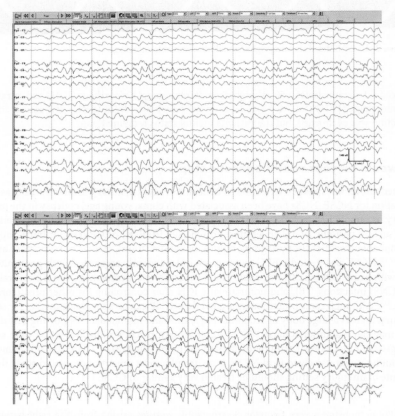

Figure 3-5. EEG demonstrates an evolving seizure originating in the right hemisphere.

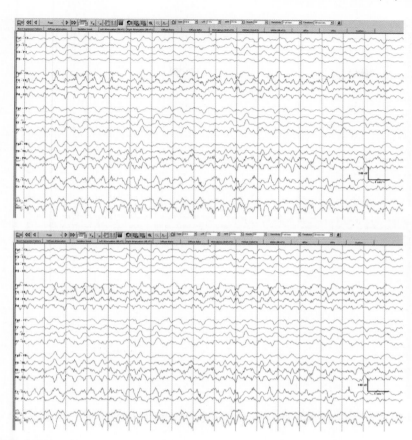

Figure 3-5. (*Continued.*)

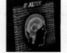

Acute brain injury and ICU-type seizures. A 68-year-old man with a history of hypertension and atrial fibrillation and who was not on Coumadin presented to the ED with decreased responses and left hemiparesis. An emergent head CT showed large right frontoparietal and left medial parietal infarction with mass effect and right-to-left midline shift. Neurologic examination did not improve after treatment of elevated ICP.

What would you do next?

Consider obtaining an EEG if the clinical examination is out of proportion to the imaging findings. As outlined in detail above, seizures are frequent in a number of acute brain injuries. These seizures are often slower frequency and have many patterns that do not clearly fulfill classic seizure criteria when compared to patients with epilepsy. Additionally, a number of poorly understood EEG findings such as periodic epileptiform discharges or stimulus-induced rhythmic, periodic, or ictal discharges (SIRPIDs) can be seen in the critically ill. These will be discussed in some detail in Chapter 13.

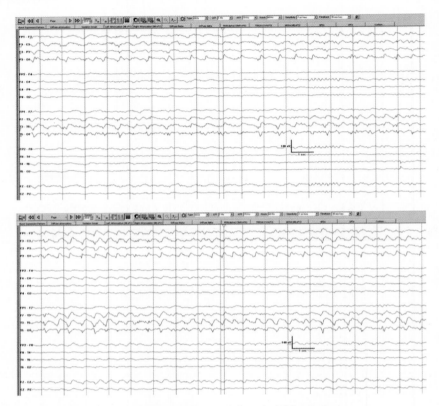

Figure 3-6. Slow-frequency electrographic seizure arising from the left hemisphere.

In our patient, EEG monitoring demonstrated left hemispheric seizures, which were rather typical for seizures seen after acute brain injury (Figure 3-6). The patient's mental status improved after loading with fosphenytoin.

Cardiac arrest and seizures. A 26-year-old woman with a history of asthma was found on the floor by her daughter at 10:36 AM. On arrival, EMS found her unresponsive and the electrocardiogram (ECG) revealed pulseless electrical activity (PEA).

Cardiopulmonary resuscitation was initiated and the patient received epinephrine 1 mg and atropine 1 mg each three times. Estimated time to return of spontaneous circulation (ROSC) was approximately 25 minutes. Her initial troponin level was normal and postresuscitation ECG demonstrated sinus tachycardia without ST-segment changes. She had a Glasgow Coma Scale score of 3 and intact brainstem reflexes on arrival at the NeuroICU. An intravascular cooling catheter was placed into the femoral vein and induction of hypothermia was started with a temperature goal of 33°C. EEG monitoring was started. Three hours after induction of hypothermia, she started to have sudden large-amplitude jerking movements involving the whole body. Her initial cEEG was mostly contaminated by muscle artifact, which made it difficult to determine the underlying rhythm. After administration of 50 mg of rocuronium, the cEEG shown in Figure 3-7 was recorded.

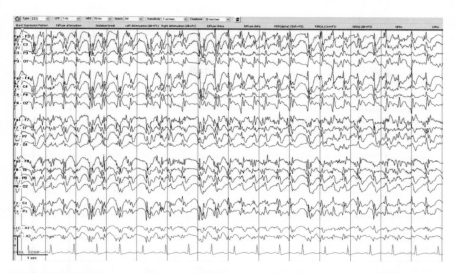

Figure 3-7. EEG demonstrates continuous generalized periodic rhythmic epileptiform discharges.

Interpret the cEEG findings? How would you treat this patient?

The EEG is consistent with SE and the clinical syndrome is called myoclonic SE (MSE). It is most frequently seen after cardiac arrest. In animal models of hypoxic-ischemic encephalopathy following cardiac arrest, isoelectric EEG is often followed by burst-suppression patterns, which may then evolve depending on the severity of hypoxia and the degree of neurologic recovery.[82] A distinction should be made between MSE and status myoclonicus, with only the former being epileptiform in nature. Both present with myoclonic jerks of the extremities but only MSE is associated with epileptiform electrical discharges on the EEG. Status myoclonicus can be seen in the setting of anoxic brain injury but also in any type of severe encephalopathy such as acute renal failure. The underlying pathophysiologic mechanism is related to subcortical white matter injury, specifically the corticospinal tract. EEG findings of status myoclonicus are slow waves or burst-suppression patterns but no epileptiform discharges.[83,84] Symptomatic treatments for this phenomenon include benzodiazepine, valproic acid, and levetiracetam. MSE is an epileptiform phenomenon and can be seen in the setting of epilepsy syndromes, but in the acute brain injury setting is most frequently related to hypoxia.[85] The EEG typically shows generalized polyspike and wave complexes on a nearly flat background. Patients with this EEG pattern are treated similarly to other patients with RSE, but the overall prognosis should be kept in mind.

What is the significance of MSE in terms of prognosis?

MSE on EEG in humans has traditionally been associated with a very poor prognosis.[86] However, most investigators agree that in the era of induced hypothermia for the treatment of patients with cardiac arrest,[87,88] this ominous fate is less established. Although a recent study confirmed the unfavorable prognosis associated with certain EEG features such as very low-voltage activity, burst-suppression, or generalized epileptiform patterns, these investigators did demonstrate that in the era of temperature modulation these EEG features as well as some clinical features previously associated with an invariably poor prognosis should be interpreted with caution.[89]

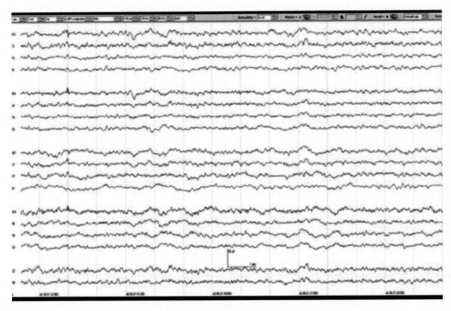

Figure 3-8. EEG without seizure activity after treatment with midazolam infusion.

The patient was treated with IV valproate and a continuous infusion of midazolam. Seizure activity subsided but an underlying rhythm showed diffuse attenuation with no reactivity of the background (Figure 3-8). After day 4 postarrest, the patient remained comatose and the family decided to transition to comfort care following with the patient's previous wishes. The patient died hours later.

EPC and focal brain injury. A 69-year-old female with history of hypertension and atrial fibrillation suffered from left frontal embolic stroke that caused mild hemiparesis in the right face and arm after being found to have subtherapeutic International Normalized Ratio (INR) levels. After 3 days of hospitalization, the patient was sent home with the appropriate Coumadin dose. Seven days later she returned to the ED presenting with 24 hours of continuous repetitive regular jerking with no impairment of consciousness.

What is the diagnosis of this patient? What is the appropriate therapeutic approach?

The presentation is most typical for a subtype of focal motor SE sometimes seen in the ICU called epilepsia partialis continua (ECP). This phenomenon can be very persistent, with epileptic focal jerking activity lasting days, weeks, or even decades.[90] Characteristically, a focal structural brain lesion can be identified including heterotopias, infectious lesions, vascular abnormalities, subdural hematomas, or neoplasms. Although long-term prognosis generally depends on the prognosis of the underlying lesion,[91] ECP may result in long-term morbidity due to weakness, sensory deficits, language dysfunction, or cognitive deficits.[92] AEDs, including benzodiazepines, may prevent secondary generalization but usually do not stop the seizure activity. Occasionally, it might resolve by itself without treatment, and surgery can be at times curative for intractable cases.[93] Of note, nonketotic hyperglycemia may be associated with EPC in patients with a concomitant focal cerebral lesion.[94] These patients may respond best to conventional AEDs in concert with correction of the metabolic disorder.

! CRITICAL CONSIDERATIONS

- Treat seizures in patients with generalized convulsive SE as soon as possible ("time is brain").
- First-line antiepileptic therapy should be a benzodiazepine, ideally intravenous lorazepam, but alternative benzodiazepines should be chosen if IV access cannot be secured quickly (ie, buccal midazolam).
- All patients with generalized convulsive SE should be given a second antiepileptic medication to prevent recurrence since the initial benzodiazepine is not a long-term therapy. Options include phenytoin/fosphenytoin or IV valproate; alternatively levetiracetam and phenobarbital may be chosen.
- Consider nonconvulsive seizures in patients who stop convulsing if they do not return to functional baseline. Diagnosis of nonconvulsive seizures requires EEG monitoring.
- Most seizures in the ICU are nonconvulsive.
- Initiate diagnostic workup to determine the cause of SE.
- Seizures that continue despite the first two AEDs are called refractory status epilepticus. Recommendations for treatment are not based on large randomized controlled trials but most would give intravenous valproate or continuous drips of midazolam, propofol, or pentobarbital. All patients with RSE should be managed in an ICU setting and undergo continuous EEG monitoring.

REFERENCES

1. Lowenstein DH, Alldredge BK. Status epilepticus. *N Engl J Med*. 1998;338:970-976.
2. Chen Chen JW, Wasterlain CG. Status epilepticus: pathophysiology and management in adults. *Lancet Neurol*. 2006;5:246-256.
3. Lowenstein DH, Bleck T, Macdonald RL. It's time to revise the definition of status epilepticus. *Epilepsia*.1999;40:120-122.
4. Meldrum BS. The revised operational definition of generalized tonic-clonic (TC) status epilepticus in adults. *Epilepsia*. 1999;40:123-124.
5. Knake S, Hamer HM, Rosenow F. Status epilepticus: A critical review. *Epilepsy Behav*. 2009;15:4-10.
6. Alldredge BK, Gelb AM, Isaacs SM. A comparison of lorazepam, diazepam, and placebo for the treatment of out-of-hospital status epilepticus. *N Engl J Med*. 2001; 30;345:631-637.
7. Meldrum BS, Brierley JB. Prolonged epileptic seizures in primates. Ischemic cell change and its relation to ictal physiological events. *Arch Neurol*. 1973;28:10-17.
8. Mazarati AM, Wasterlain CG, Sankar R. Self-sustaining status epilepticus after brief electrical stimulation of the perforant path. *Brain Res*. 1998;801:251-253.
9. Kapur J, Macdonald RL. Rapid seizure-induced reduction of benzodiazepine and Zn^{2+} sensitivity of hippocampal dentate granule cell GABAA receptors. *J Neurosci*. 199717(19):7532-7540.
10. Jenssen S, Gracely EJ, Sperling MR. How long do most seizures last? A systematic comparison of seizures recorded in the epilepsy monitoring unit. *Epilepsia*. 2006;47:1499-1503

11. Theodore WH, Porter RJ, Albert P. The second-arily generalized tonic-clonic seizure: a videotape analysis. *Neurology.* 1994;44:1403-1407.

12. Shinnar S, Berg AT, Moshe SL. How long do new-onset seizures in children last?. *Ann Neurol.* 2001;49:659-664.

13. DeLorenzo RJ, Hauser WA, Towne AR, et al. A prospective, population-based epidemiologic study of status epilepticus in Richmond, Virginia. *Neurology.* 1996;46:1029-1035.

14. Treiman DM, Meyers PD, Walton NY, et al. A comparison of four treatments for generalized convulsive status epilepticus. Veterans Affairs Status Epilepticus Cooperative Study Group. *N Engl J Med.* 1998;339:792-798.

15. Lowenstein DH, Alldredge BK. Status epilepticus at an urban public hospital in the 1980s. *Neurology.* 1993;43:483-488.

16. Young GB, Jordan KG, Doig GS. An assessment of nonconvulsive seizures in the intensive care unit using continuous EEG monitoring: an investigation of variables associated with mortality. *Neurology.* 1996;47:83-89.

17. Leppik IE, Derivan AT, Homan RW, et al. Double-blind study of lorazepam and diazepam in status epilepticus. *JAMA.* 1983;249:1452-1454.

18. Claassen J, Hirsch LJ, Mayer SA. Treatment of status epilepticus: a survey of neurologists. *J Neurol Sci.* 2003;211:37-41.

19. Misra UK, Kalita J, Patel R. Sodium valproate vs phenytoin in status epilepticus: A pilot study. *Neurology.* 2006;67:340-342.

20. DeLorenzo RJ, Towne AR, Pellock JM, et al. Status epilepticus in children, adults, and the elderly. *Epilepsia.* 1992;33(suppl 4):S15-S25.

21. Bleck TP. Convulsive disorders: status epilepticus. *Clin Neuropharmacol.* 1991;14:191-198.

22. Towne AR, Waterhouse EJ, Boggs JG, et al. Prevalence of nonconvulsive status epilepticus in comatose patients. *Neurology.* 2000;55:1421-1423.

23. Bleck TP, Smith MC, Pierre-Louis SJ, et al. Neurologic complications of critical medical illnesses. *Crit Care Med.* 1993;21:98-103.

24. DeLorenzo RJ, Waterhouse EJ, Towne AR, et al. Persistent nonconvulsive status epilepticus after the control of convulsive status epilepticus. *Epilepsia.* 1998;39:833-840.

25. Husain AM, Horn GJ, Jacobson MP. Non-convulsive status epilepticus: Usefulness of clinical features in selecting patients for urgent EEG. *J Neurol Neurosurg Psychiatry.* 2003;74:189-191.

26. Jagoda A, Riggio S. Refractory status epilepticus in adults. *Ann Emerg Med.* 1993;22:1337-1348.

27. Claassen J, Lokin JK, Fitzsimmons BF. Predictors of functional disability and mortality after status epilepticus. *Neurology.* 20028;58:139-142.

28. Novy J, Logroscino G, Rossetti AO. Refractory status epilepticus: a prospective observational study. *Epilepsia.* 2010;51:251-256.

29. Logroscino G, Hesdorffer DC, Cascino G, et al. Short-term mortality after a first episode of status epilepticus. *Epilepsia.* 1997;38:1344-1349.

30. Oxbury JM, Whitty CW. Causes and consequences of status epilepticus in adults. A study of 86 cases. *Brain.* 1971;94:733-744.

31. Aminoff MJ, Simon RP. Status epilepticus. Causes, clinical features and consequences in 98 patients. *Am J Med.* 1980;69:657-666.

32. Scholtes FB, Renier WO, Meinardi H. Generalized convulsive status epilepticus: causes, therapy, and outcome in 346 patients. *Epilepsia.* 1994;35:1104-1112.

33. Logroscino G, Hesdorffer DC, Cascino G. Time trends in incidence, mortality, and case-fatality after first episode of status epilepticus. *Epilepsia.* 2001;42:1031-1035.

34. Hesdorffer DC, Logroscino G, Cascino GD, et al. Recurrence of afebrile status epilepticus in a population-based study in Rochester, Minnesota. *Neurology.* 2007;69:73-78.

35. Young GB, Blume WT, Bolton CF, et al. Anesthetic barbiturates in refractory status epilepticus. *Can J Neurol Sci.* 1980;7:291-292.

36. Rashkin MC, Youngs C, Penovich P. Pentobarbital treatment of refractory status epilepticus. *Neurology.* 1987;37:500-503.

37. Krishnamurthy KB, Drislane FW. Depth of EEG suppression and outcome in barbiturate anesthetic treatment for refractory status epilepticus. *Epilepsia.* 1999;40:759-762.

38. Stecker MM, Kramer TH, Raps EC, et al. Treatment of refractory status epilepticus with propofol: clinical and pharmacokinetic findings. *Epilepsia.* 1998;39:18-26.

39. Classen J, Hirsch LJ, Emerson RG, et al. Continuous EEG monitoring and midazolam infusion for refractory nonconvulsive status epilepticus. *Neurology.* 2001;57:1036-1042.

40. Claassen J, Hirsch LJ, Emerson RG, et al. Treatment of refractory status epilepticus with pentobarbital, propofol, or midazolam: a systematic review. *Epilepsia.* 2002;43:146-153.

41. Rossetti AO, Reichhart MD, Schaller MD, et al. Propofol treatment of refractory status epilepticus: a study of 31 episodes. *Epilepsia.* 2004;45:757-763.

42. Goodkin HP, Yeh JL, Kapur J. Status epilepticus increases the intracellular accumulation of GABAA receptors. *J Neurosci*. 2005;25:5511-5520.

43. Naylor DE, Liu H, Wasterlain CG. Trafficking of GABA(A) receptors, loss of inhibition, and a mechanism for pharmacoresistance in status epilepticus. *J Neurosci*. 2005;25:7724-7733.

44. Meierkord H, Boon P, Engelsen B, et al. EFNS guideline on the management of status epilepticus. *Eur J Neurol*. 2006;13:445-450.

45. Claassen J, Hirsch LJ, Emerson RG, et al. Treatment of refractory status epilepticus with pentobarbital, propofol, or midazolam: a systematic review. *Epilepsia*. 2002;43:146-153.

46. Prasad A, Worrall BB, Bertram EH, et al. Propofol and midazolam in the treatment of refractory status epilepticus. *Epilepsia*. 2001;42:380-382.

47. Meierkord H, Boon P, Engelsen B, et al. EFNS guideline on the management of status epilepticus. *Eur J Neurol*. 2006;13:445-450.

48. Hirsch LJ. Continuous EEG monitoring in the intensive care unit: an overview. *J Clin Neurophysiol*. 2004;21:332-340.

49. Young B, Jordan K, Doig G. An assessment of nonconvulsive seizures in the intensive care unit using continuous EEG monitoring: An investigation of variables associated with mortality. *Neurology*. 1996;47:83-89.

50. Vespa P, Prins M, Ronne-Engstrom E, et al. Increase in extracellular glutamate caused by reduced cerebral perfusion pressure and seizures after human traumatic brain injury: a microdialysis study. *J Neurosurg*. 1998;89:971-982.

51. Vespa PM, McArthur D, O'Phelan K, et al. Persistently low extracellular glucose correlates with poor outcome 6 months after human traumatic brain injury despite a lack of increased lactate: A microdialysis study. *J Cereb Blood Flow Metab*. 2003;23:865-877.

52. Vespa P. Continuous EEG monitoring for the detection of seizures in traumatic brain injury, infarction, and intracerebral hemorrhage: "To detect and to protect." *J Clin Neurophysiol*. 2005;22:99-106.

53. Vespa P, McArthur DL, Glenn T, et al. Nonconvulsive seizures after traumatic brain injury are associated with hippocampal atrophy. *Neurology*. 2010; 75:792-798.

54. Jordan KG. Neurophysiologic monitoring in the neuroscience intensive care unit. *Neurol Clin*. 1995; 13:579-626.

55. Krishnamurthy KB, Drislane FW. Depth of EEG suppression and outcome in barbiturate anesthetic treatment for refractory status epilepticus. *Epilepsia* .1999;40:759-762.

56. Rossetti AO, Logroscino G, Bromfield EB. Refractory status epilepticus: effect of treatment aggressiveness on prognosis. *Arch Neurol*. 2005;62: 1698-1702.

57. Claassen J, Hirsch LJ, Mayer SA. Treatment of status epilepticus: a survey of neurologists. *J Neurol Sci*. 2003;211:37-41.

58. Lai ML, Huang JD. Dual effect of valproic acid on the pharmacokinetics of phenytoin. *Biopharm Drug Dispos*. 1993;14:365-370.

59. Rambeck B, Boenigk HE, Dunlop A. Predicting phenytoin dose—A revised nomogram. *Ther Drug Monit*. 1979;1:325-333.

60. Knake S, Gruener J, Hattemer K, et al. Intravenous levetiracetam in the treatment of benzodiazepine refractory status epilepticus. *J Neurol Neurosurg Psychiatry*. 2008;79:588-589.

61. Rüegg S, Naegelin Y, Hardmeier M, et al. Intravenous levetiracetam: Treatment experience with the first 50 critically ill patients. *Epilepsy Behav*. 2008;12:477-480.

62. Kellinghaus C, Berning S, Besselmann M. Intravenous lacosamide as successful treatment for nonconvulsive status epilepticus after failure of first-line therapy. *Epilepsy Behav*. 2009;14:429-431.

63. Mazarati AM, Wasterlain CG. N-methyl-D-aspartate receptor antagonists abolish the maintenance phase of self-sustaining status epilepticus in rat. *Neurosci Lett*. 1999;265:187-190.

64. Martin BS, Kapur J. A combination of ketamine and diazepam synergistically controls refractory status epilepticus induced by cholinergic stimulation. *Epilepsia*. 2008;49:248-255.

65. Mewasingh LD, Sékhara T, Aeby A, et al. Oral ketamine in paediatric non-convulsive status epilepticus. *Seizure*. 2003;12:483-489.

66. Corry JJ, Dhar R, Murphy T. Hypothermia for refractory status epilepticus. *Neurocrit Care*. 2008;9:189-197.

67. Orlowski JP, Erenberg G, Lueders H. Hypothermia and barbiturate coma for refractory status epilepticus. *Crit Care Med*. 1984;12:367-372.

68. Pascual J, Ciudad J, Berciano J. Role of lidocaine (lignocaine) in managing status epilepticus. *J Neurol Neurosurg Psychiatry*. 1992;55:49-51.

69. Alexopoulos A, Lachhwani DK, Gupta A, et al. Resective surgery to treat refractory status epilepticus in children with focal epileptogenesis. *Neurology*. 2005;64:567-570.

70. Treiman DM. Convulsive status epilepticus. *Curr Treat Options Neurol*. 1999;1:359-369.

71. Hirsch LJ. Continuous EEG monitoring in the intensive care unit: An overview. *J Clin Neurophysiol*. 2004;21:332-340.

72. Husain AM, Horn GJ, Jacobson MP. Non-convulsive status epilepticus: Usefulness of clinical features in selecting patients for urgent EEG. *J Neurol Neurosurg Psychiatry.* 2003;74:189-191.

73. Claassen J. How I treat patients with EEG patterns on the ictal-interictal continuum in the neuro ICU. *Neurocrit Care.* 2009;11:437-444.

74. Jordan KG. Nonconvulsive status epilepticus in acute brain injury. *J Clin Neurophysiol.* 1999;16:332-340.

75. Pandian JD, Cascino GD, So EL. Digital video-electroencephalographic monitoring in the neurological-neurosurgical intensive care unit: Clinical features and outcome. *Arch Neurol.* 2004;61:1090-1094.

76. Claassen J, Mayer SA, Kowalski RG, et al. Detection of electrographic seizures with continuous EEG monitoring in critically ill patients. *Neurology.* 2004;62:1743-1748.

77. Oddo M, Carrera E, Claassen J, et al. Continuous electroencephalography in the medical intensive care unit. *Crit Care Med.* 2009;37:2051-2056.

78. Privitera M, Hoffman M, Moore JL, et al. EEG detection of nontonic-clonic status epilepticus in patients with altered consciousness. *Epilepsy Res.* 1994;18:155-166.

79. Varelas PN, Spanaki MV, Hacein-Bey L. Emergent EEG: Indications and diagnostic yield. *Neurology.* 2003;61:702-704.

80. Claassen J, Hirsch LJ, Frontera JA, et al. Prognostic significance of continuous EEG monitoring in patients with poor-grade subarachnoid hemorrhage. *Neurocrit Care.* 2006;4:103-112.

81. Claassen J, Jetté N, Chum F, et al. Electrographic seizures and periodic discharges after intracerebral hemorrhage. *Neurology.* 2007;69:1356-1365.

82. Geocadin RG, Sherman DL, Christian Hansen H, et al. Neurological recovery by EEG bursting after resuscitation from cardiac arrest in rats. *Resuscitation.* 2002;55:193-200.

83. Celesia GG, Grigg MM, Ross E. Generalized status myoclonicus in acute anoxic and toxic-metabolic encephalopathies. *Arch Neurol.* 1988;45:781-784.

84. Jumao-as A, Brenner RP. Myoclonic status epilepticus: A clinical and electroencephalographic study. *Neurology.* 1990;40:1199-1202.

85. Hui AC, Cheng C, Lam A, et al. Prognosis following postanoxic myoclonus status epilepticus. *Eur Neurol.* 2005;54:10-13.

86. Wijdicks EF, Hijdra A, Young GB, et al. Practice parameter: Prediction of outcome in comatose survivors after cardiopulmonary resuscitation (an evidence-based review): Report of the Quality Standards Subcommittee of the American Academy of Neurology. *Neurology.* 2006;67:203-210.

87. Hypothermia After Cardiac Arrest Study Group. Mild therapeutic hypothermia to improve the neurologic outcome after cardiac arrest. *N Engl J Med.* 2002;346:549-556.

88. Bernard SA, Gray TW, Buist MD, et al. Treatment of comatose survivors of out-of-hospital cardiac arrest with induced hypothermia. *N Engl J Med.* 2002;346:557-563.

89. Rossetti AO, Oddo M, Logroscino G, et al. Prognostication after cardiac arrest and hypothermia: A prospective study. *Ann Neurol.* 2010;67:301-307.

90. Juul-Jensen P, Denny-Brown D. Epilepsia partialis continua. *Arch Neurol.* 1966;15:563-578.

91. Thomas JE, Reagan TJ, Klass DW. Epilepsia partialis continua. A review of 32 cases. *Arch Neurol.* 1977;34:266-275.

92. Cockerell OC, Rothwell J, Thompson PD. Clinical and physiological features of epilepsia partialis continua. Cases ascertained in the UK. *Brain.* 1996;119(pt 2):393-407.

93. Hart YM, Cortez M, Andermann F, et al. Medical treatment of Rasmussen's syndrome (chronic encephalitis and epilepsy): Effect of high-dose steroids or immunoglobulins in 19 patients. *Neurology.* 1994;44:1030-1036.

94. Singh BM, Strobos RJ. Epilepsia partialis continua associated with nonketotic hyperglycemia: Clinical and biochemical profile of 21 patients. *Ann Neurol.* 1980;8:155-160.

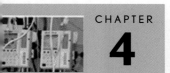

CHAPTER

4 Neurotrauma

Neeraj Badjatia, MD, MSc, FCCM

Traumatic brain injury (TBI). A 42-year-old man presents to your intensive care unit (ICU) with acute brain trauma. He reportedly has fallen from a ladder at home while trying to fix the roof. There has been a loss of consciousness immediately after the fall, and he remains in obtunded mental status. In the emergency department (ED), his eyes open to painful stimulation, makes incomprehensible sounds, localizes to pain on the left side but is paretic on the right side (Glasgow Coma Scale [GCS] of 9: eye 2, verbal 2, motor 5). Pupils were reactive to light, and other brainstem reflexes were intact. Patient was intubated with an endotracheal tube. Initial vital signs: heart rate 130 bpm, blood pressure 160/90 mm Hg, oxygen saturation 100% on assist control–volume control mechanical ventilation with FIO_2 of 0.4, tidal volume of 480 mL, at a rate of 12 times per minute. Body temperature is 37.5°C. A computed tomographic image of the brain without contrast is obtained (Figure 4-1).

What are the initial steps in the management of this patient?

This is a typical case of severe TBI with bilateral hemorrhagic contusions in the temporal lobes. Its proximity to the bony structures makes it a frequent location in the brain to be contused in trauma. Resuscitation of TBI patients varies widely, however, due to the heterogeneity of the disease itself. The aim of all good early resuscitation efforts is to begin as early as possible, with many efforts beginning in the prehospital setting, with an attention to airway, breathing, and circulation.

Three specific end points have been found to be independent predictors of poor outcome in the prehospital/emergency department setting: hypothermia, hypoxia, and hypotension.[1] Hypothermia is likely a marker of poor resuscitation, and most would agree that core body temperature should be passively supported during the resuscitation phase rather than actively warmed with a device. Aggressive volume resuscitation for hypotension and adequate ventilation are the primary focus of initial resuscitation efforts. Prehospital resuscitation with hypertonic saline in TBI has failed to demonstrate a long-term benefit,[2] and in a post-hoc analysis of the Saline versus Albumin Fluid Evaluation trial,[3] fluid resuscitation with albumin was associated with higher mortality rates than was resuscitation with saline. Therefore, the administration of isotonic crystalloids is the preferred method by which to volume resuscitate. All TBI patients should be ventilated to a goal of normal PCO_2 and be given supplemental oxygen to achieve SPO_2 greater than 90%. During the early resuscitation phase, it is important to realize that simple measures such as elevation of the head of the bed (30 degrees), midline positioning of the head (relieving any blockage of jugular venous drainage), and adequate pain control and sedation are very simple and effective methods to reduce intracranial pressure (ICP).

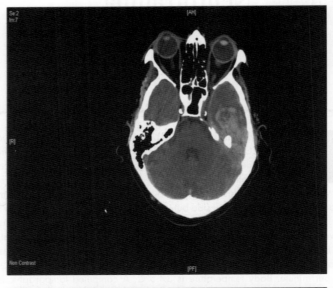

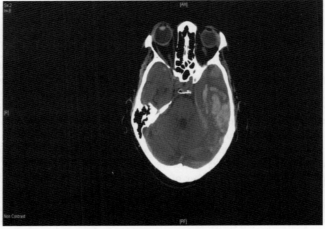

Figure 4-1. Noncontrast computed tomography of the brain.

The patient is now admitted to an ICU, and the repeat computed tomography (CT) of the brain 6 hours later confirms no expansion of the hemorrhagic contusion. His neurologic examination remains poor, being only partially responsive to painful stimulation. Remembering that the literature reports the combination of severe TBI plus status epilepticus (SE) carries a high mortality rate, you wonder whether he could have any nonconvulsive seizures.

How long should prophylactic antiepileptic drug (AED) be administered?

Reported risk factors for seizures include GCS score less than 10, cortical contusions, depressed skull fractures, wounds with dural penetration, prolonged length (longer than 24 hours) of coma, and posttraumatic amnesia. The majority of early posttraumatic seizures occur within the initial

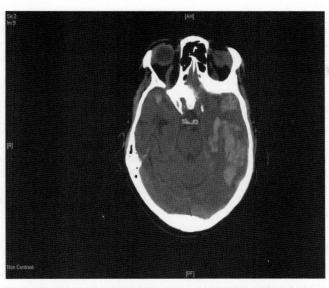

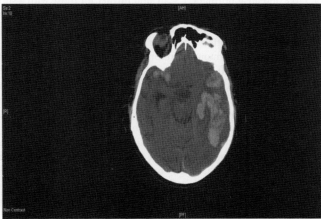

Figure 4-1. (*Continued.*)

48 hours of injury.[4] However, some seizures may escape clinical detection, and may be unnoticed in intubated sedated patients in the absence of electroencephalographic (EEG) monitoring. The presence of convulsive SE is associated with high mortality rate. Effective prophylaxis of early posttraumatic seizures reduces brain metabolic demands, thereby reducing intracranial pressure and neurotransmitter release. This in turn minimizes secondary brain injury. Furthermore, anticonvulsant treatment can minimize cognitive and behavioral sequelae.

Phenytoin is an established standard antiepileptic drug (AED) in the setting of acute TBI. The American Academy of Neurology suggests using phenytoin for seizure prevention only in the first 7 days after TBI.[5] If AEDs are given, it is important to remember that there is no added benefit of continuing beyond 7 days if it was given as a prophylaxis in the setting of trauma. The availability of newer AEDs questions the use of phenytoin as the first-line AED in this setting. Levetiracetam has gained favor in acute brain injury setting due to its tolerability, ease of use without the need to follow a drug level, and minimal drug-to-drug interactions. It has been used in the neurocritical care setting for several years now and numerous studies have reported on oral as well as IV use of this medication for the treatment or prevention of seizures in TBI. However, existing studies of levetiracetam regarding the safety and efficacy are not definitive, and do not provide enough evidence that levetiracetam has better short- and long-term outcomes when compared to phenytoin.[6]

What is the impact of steroids acutely after TBI?

High doses of steroids are greatly beneficial in experimental models, reducing lipid peroxidation and improving tissue recovery. Clinical studies with glucocorticoids have not shown similar benefit. The results from the large Corticosteroid Randomization After Significant Head injury (CRASH) trial demonstrated no benefit and increased mortality rate in TBI patients randomized to 3 g of methylprednisolone in the first 72 hours after injury. Currently, no data exist to support the use of glucocorticoid steroids acutely, and given the increased mortality rates seen in the CRASH trial, they are contraindicated acutely after brain injury.[7,8]

What type of intracranial monitoring is indicated after TBI?

The Brain Trauma Foundation guidelines state that ICP should be monitored in those with a postre-suscitation GCS of 3 to 8 and an abnormal CT scan, and further for those with a similar severity and a normal CT scan if two of the following are present: age older than 40 years, posturing, or hypotension. The first choice for monitoring should always be an external ventricular drain because it can be recalibrated after placement and also offers therapy in the form of cerebrospinal fluid (CSF) diversion. Parenchymal monitors provide continuous monitoring of ICP but can only be calibrated prior to placement and have an associated drift in their measurement.[9]

The ability to monitor brain tissue oxygen tension ($Pbto_2$) has added a dimension of monitoring that provides insight to cerebral metabolism. The preponderance of case series data indicate that a $Pbto_2$ level less than 15 mm Hg is associated with poor outcome, and may respond to either augmentation of mean arterial blood pressure (MAP), alteration in ventilation strategy, or transfusion of red blood cells. However, many questions regarding the utility of this monitoring technique have yet to be answered, such as timing, location, and pertinent treatment thresholds. Until such data become available, it is important to remember that the $Pbto_2$ value is a composite of various components of the content of oxygen in the arteries as well as an unknown quantity of passive diffusion. This value is also a very focal/regional measure and should be put into context of the entire clinical picture prior to embarking on therapeutic interventions.[10]

What is the role for antibiotics with intracranial monitoring?

There are sufficient data to support the use of periprocedural antibiotics, but the infusion must begin prior to the skin incision. The choice of antibiotic should be either cefazolin (1 g IV) or nafcillin (1 g IV). Vancomycin (1 g IV) can be utilized for those patients with a known penicillin allergy. The continued use of antibiotics for prophylaxis is controversial and has not been proven to reduce the rate of ventriculitis and may increase the incidence of drug-resistant bacterial infections.[11]

What is the goal cerebral perfusion pressure (CPP) for TBI patients?

The 2007 Brain Trauma Foundation (BTF) guidelines have indicated that CPP thresholds should be maintained within a range of greater than 50 mm Hg and less than 70 mm Hg. This threshold is based upon data that support CPP values lower than 50 mm Hg are associated with more cerebral insults, while achieving CPP more than 70 mm Hg on every TBI patient results in a fourfold increase in lung injury likely due to aggressive volume resuscitation and excessive use of pressors.[12] The use of $Pbto_2$ monitoring may help guide targeted CPP management so as to avoid tissue hypoxia while minimizing the risk of complications related to pressure augmentation.

When should hypothermia be utilized after TBI?

There have been two multicenter randomized controlled trials (RCTs) that have not demonstrated any benefit for the use of therapeutic hypothermia as a neuroprotectant.[13-15] However, therapeutic hypothermia can still be considered as an option in the treatment of raised intracranial pressure.[13] Owing to the lack of data and associated management complexities, therapeutic hypothermia has traditionally been reserved as a treatment option for patients who are either refractory or unable to receive osmotic therapy. The advent of modern temperature-modulating devices has allowed for a more safe and efficient delivery of therapeutic hypothermia, and as a result, this therapy may become more widely utilized in TBI patients. Since ICP is strongly dependent on core body temperature, any decrease in temperature less than 37°C will likely result in a reduction in ICP. However, this therapy has been traditionally targeted to lower core body temperature to 32°C to 34°C. The risk for infectious complications with therapeutic hypothermia is duration-dependent, with the rate of infectious complications rising sharply above 72 hours. Hypothermia will also result in a coagulopathy and increased risk of bleeding, although it is important to realize that there has not been any significant increase in intracranial bleeding due to hypothermia in any of the RCTs.

If hypothermia is utilized to control ICP, careful consideration should be also given to shivering, electrolyte imbalances, ventilator management, and rewarming. A commonly overlooked aspect of hypothermia's effect on normal physiology occurs in relation to the management of ventilation and blood-gas results. As a result of decreased metabolic activity, there is decreased production of carbon dioxide at lower body temperatures. If mechanical ventilation parameters are left unchanged during cooling, hyperventilation will occur, which may cause cerebral vasoconstriction and reduced cerebral blood flow. At lower temperatures, the solubility of gases in a liquid mixture increases. Most blood-gas analyzers warm the sample to 37°C prior to determining the values for pH, Pco_2, and Po_2. Without correcting for the patient's actual body temperature, this analysis will overestimate the Pco_2 during hypothermia because portions of the dissolved gases come out of solution on warming and contribute to the partial pressure detected. Two methods of blood-gas analysis exist with regard to changing patient body temperature: (1) alpha-stat management and (2) pH-stat management. Using alpha-stat ventilator management, the Pco_2 detected by the blood-gas analyzer at 37°C is targeted to 40 mm Hg regardless of body temperature. This method of blood-gas management may lead to hyperventilation due to the overestimation of Pco_2. In contrast, pH-stat management targets a temperature-corrected Pco_2 and pH. Using this method, as body temperature decreases, the total amount of CO_2 in blood will increase as solubility increases. This poses the risk for inducing hypercapnia, which may result in cerebral vasodilation and increased intracranial pressure.[16]

In the middle of a night, the ICU resident calls to notify you that the patient's left-side pupil has become enlarged (6 mm compared to 3 mm on the right) and is still reactive to light. Patient is right hemiplegic and the left side is not localizing to pain any longer. The overall mental status has been depressed further, and now painful stimulation does not lead to eye openings. Only minimal flexion to painful stimulation is seen in the left arm. Repeat CT reveals increased swelling and mass effect on the left temporal hemorrhagic lesion. ICP is 25 mm Hg, which is down from 40 mm Hg after 30 mL of 23.4% hypertonic saline injection given 4 hours ago. Patient is autohyperventilating himself with end-tidal CO_2 of 28 mm Hg. Licox monitoring shows $Pbto_2$ of 16 mm Hg in the left hemisphere frontal subcortical region where the probe is positioned.

Which patients should be considered for decompressive craniectomy?

Surgical decompression limits the damage caused by secondary injury (delayed brain injury) by reducing increased ICP with subsequent improvement in brain oxygenation. As with any surgical procedure, there are inherent risks. The decision to perform decompressive techniques is primarily based on the evacuation of a mass lesion, with temporal and frontal lesions more likely to result in decompression. There are no standard clinical criteria, although many institutions reserve this procedure for younger patients in coma who have failed at least one ICP-lowering measure. The key is not to delay the procedure since the primary benefit is as a result of reducing sequelae from secondary injury. Once decompression is decided upon, resection of a larger bone fragment is performed to allow for greater dural expansion with less risk of herniation. All clinical studies of decompression have demonstrated immediate reductions in ICP; however, there is conflicting evidence regarding the effects of craniectomy on long-term outcomes. As a result, this technique is not as widely utilized as medical interventions for lowering ICP.[17,18]

How does one clear the cervical spine in the setting of altered mental status?

The identification of any cervical spine injuries is part of the standard evaluation after the patient has been hemodynamically stabilized. The algorithm is straightforward in patients who are awake and alert. In this population, the need for additional radiographic evaluations is based upon the bedside examination. Those without pain (distracting, midline neck), no neurologic deficits localizing to the cervical spine, and not intoxicated are very unlikely to have significant cervical spinal injury and can be cleared without radiographs. If any of these signs or symptoms is present, then patients should undergo full C-T1 spine radiographs (including anteroposterior, lateral, and odontoid films) in addition to CT images from the occiput to T1. In patients with an alteration in mental status with a negative CT and gross motor function of extremities, flexion/extension radiography should not be performed. Many institutions have begun relying upon magnetic resonance (MR) images to look for ligamentous injury; however, the risk-to-benefit ratio of obtaining MR images in addition to CT is not clear, and its use must be individualized in each institution. If a decision is made to perform MRI, it must be done within 72 hours of injury in order to have reliable results. Most modern CT scanners in addition to plain radiographs likely identify nearly all significant cervical spine instabilities; however, there are no evidenced-based guidelines to support the practice of clearing cervical spines with only CT images in obtunded patients.[19]

When should anti-thrombotic therapy be initiated for the prevention of deep venous thrombosis (DVT)?

There is a high rate of DVT after TBI, indicating that this patient population should have prophylactic therapy. However, there is considerable concern that administering heparin and low-molecular-weight heparin will increase the risk for hematoma expansion.[20] In the absence of acquired coagulopathy, the risk for hematoma expansion decreases significantly after 48 hours. In addition, there is a very low risk for hematoma expansion with prophylactic doses of heparin or low-molecular-weight heparin resulting in hematoma expansion in this patient population. For these reasons, a reasonable, safe approach toward this patient population is to begin prophylaxis 24 hours after radiographic demonstration of hematoma stability. Others have advocated surveillance with weekly venous duplex ultrasound in addition to prophylaxis, although there is no evidence that this practice reduces the complications related to DVT after TBI.[21]

There are instances, such as the need for repeated surgeries or ongoing bleeding, where the use of DVT prophylaxis is not initiated for a prolonged period of time. In these cases, the use of temporary inferior vena cava (IVC) filters should be considered. However, it must be recognized that an IVC filter only provides incomplete prevention for only lower-extremity DVT and can pose a risk for future complications related to filter thrombosis, migration, and/or fracturing. Therefore, removing IVC filters once a patient is able to receive pharmacologic prophylaxis is an important step in the prevention of future complications.

In cases where a DVT has been diagnosed, the general recommendation is to wait for 7 days after intracranial surgery, although there are no clinical trial data to support any specific timeline. Decisions regarding timing should balance the risk for intracranial as well as systemic bleeding with the urgency for therapy.

What is the preferred osmotic therapy, mannitol or hypertonic saline?

Unfortunately, there is no level 1 evidence to support one therapy over another. In fact, owing to a paucity of prospective clinical trial data, there is a lack of level 1 data to support the use of any osmotic therapy after TBI. However, each therapy does have a slightly different physiologic impact, which may lead to a preferential use of one therapy over another.[22]

Mannitol

Mannitol is an osmotic agent that draws excess fluid from the cranial cavity, thereby decreasing ICP, and has also been associated with significant diuresis, acute renal failure, hyperkalemia, hypotension, and rebound increments in ICP. For these reasons, it has been recommended that mannitol only be used when signs of elevated ICP or deteriorating neurologic status suggest the benefits of mannitol outweigh potential complications or adverse effects. There remains considerable uncertainty regarding how and when it should be used but the recommended dose is 0.25 to 1.0 g/kg of body weight, with a goal to avoid hypotension due to intravascular volume depletion. Some clinicians have advocated replacement of urinary losses to avoid intravascular volume depletion. While improved outcomes may be obtained with higher doses, decisions regarding higher doses (higher than 1 g/kg) of mannitol administration should be made on a case-by-case basis.

Hypertonic Saline

Hypertonic saline is an osmotic agent that has traditionally been used as an adjunct to mannitol or in individuals who have become tolerant to mannitol. However, recent studies have examined hypertonic saline as a primary measure for ICP control. Hypertonic saline exerts its effect primarily by increasing serum sodium and osmolarity, thereby establishing an osmotic gradient. Water diffuses passively from cerebral intracellular and interstitial spaces into capillaries resulting in a reduction in ICP. Although mannitol works similarly, sodium chloride has a better reflection coefficient (1.0) than mannitol (0.9), making it a better osmotic agent. Hypertonic saline may also normalize resting membrane potential and cell volume by restoring normal intracellular electrolyte balance in injured cells. The dose and administration varies greatly, with boluses ranging between 30 mL of 23.4% NaCl and 150 mL of 3% NaCl, whereas others have advocated the use of a continuous infusion of either 2% or 3% NaCl to reach a goal Na of 150 mmol/L. Regardless of the choice of administration, therapy should be targeted to a specific ICP/CPP goal.

Based on this evidence, some general clinical guidelines regarding the use of mannitol and hypertonic saline:

1. Mannitol may be of added benefit when there is intravascular volume overload, but careful attention should be paid to urine output so that patients do not become intravascular volume depleted. The goal is euvolemic intravascular volume status.

2. Mannitol dosing should be done as a weight-based schedule ranging between 0.25 and 1.0 g/kg.

3. While there is no ceiling as to when osmotic therapies should be discontinued, the likelihood of developing renal insufficiency does increase with supranormal serum sodium levels.

4. Hypertonic saline should be administered with caution in patients with renal insufficiency or congestive heart failure.

5. Hypertonic saline may have an additional benefit of raising the MAP and therefore have a dual impact on improving CPP.

What is the optimal method by which to ventilate a patient with a TBI?

Regulation of blood carbon dioxide levels has a significant impact on cerebral blood flow and therefore intracranial volume and intracranial pressure. During mild hyperventilation, increased oxygen extraction can compensate for decreased blood flow and volume, allowing normal cellular metabolism to continue; however, prolonged hyperventilation may increase metabolic acidosis. In the short term, hyperventilation decreases cerebral blood CO_2, leading to an increase in pH, which may diminish the detrimental effects of acidosis. However, this process depends on the availability of bicarbonate in the cerebrospinal fluid. Prolonged hyperventilation may deplete bicarbonate levels, which may in turn result in ischemia and poorer outcomes. There have been four studies examining hyperventilation after TBI. The only RCT examining prolonged hyperventilation demonstrated poorer clinical outcomes, which were likely due to a depletion of cerebral bicarbonate supplies.[23] As a result, ventilation goals should be used to maintain arterial CO_2 within the range of normal (35 to 45 mm Hg). The use of hyperventilation should be reserved for rescue therapy (sudden surges in ICP), temporary reduction of ICP during procedures, and/or as an intermediate intervention until a more durable therapy can be initiated.

What are transfusion thresholds for brain injuries?

Among patients with severe TBI, the proportion of those who experience anemia and who receive a blood transfusion during the acute postinjury phase have not been carefully described, but recent series have described 40% to 50% of patients with moderate to severe TBI having at least one hematocrit less than 30%.[24,25] Clinical guidelines have recommended that anemia not be the sole consideration in decisions regarding transfusion. Instead, the decision to transfuse should be based upon reducing tissue ischemia. The TBI patient population is generally young and includes otherwise healthy people, and the Transfusion Requirements in Critical Care (TRICC) trial suggests that this particular subgroup of critically ill patients is at risk for harm from liberal transfusion. However, there is genuine disagreement and clinical equipoise as to whether brain-injured patients would benefit from more liberal (to maintain hemoglobin level greater than 10 g/dL) or more restrictive transfusion (to maintain hemoglobin level greater than 7 g/dL).[26]

> On ICU day 13, the same patient who recently received a tracheostomy and a percutaneous endoscopic gastrostomy is now having paroxysmal sympathetic hyperactivity episodes; sudden onset of periodic autonomic instability with sympathetic surge and dystonia. The patient is reported to have dilated pupils, hypertension, tachycardia, tachypnea, high fever, and increased body tones with periodic self-extensor posturing during these episodes. These are occurring in the absence of agitation or painful stimulation.

How do you address sympathetic storming after TBI?

Periodic sympathetic hyperactivity occurs up to 33% after severe TBI, although it has been reported with less frequency in other injury types as well.[27] These episodes are typically characterized as sudden onset of exaggerated sympathetic responses including hypertension, tachycardia, tachypnea, high fever, sweating, and papillary dilation, along with occasional dystonic posturing. Clinicians should be aware of this syndrome and understand that the first step of managing these episodes is to investigate and rule out other underlying medical conditions. DVT, pulmonary embolism, myocardial infarction, pneumothorax, and sepsis with a hyperdynamic phase can all lead to a syndrome at least partially similar to sympathetic storming. People with TBI are prone to infection such as aspiration pneumonia as well as volume overload, which often leads to total-body water overload. Pleural effusion and pulmonary congestion are not uncommon, and these conditions can mimic the syndrome as well. Bromocriptine, β blockers such as propranolol, morphine sulfate, dantrolene, and clonidine may be helpful. For severe refractory cases, continuous IV sedation and anesthetic medications are occasionally needed too. Central nervous system (CNS) storming can be challenging to manage and long-lasting. It is not uncommon to observe prolonged phases of sporadically occurring storming events even weeks after the initial injury.

 Spinal cord injury (SCI). A 34-year-old man was brought in by emergency medical services (EMS) from the ski resort where he was snowboarding. According to the report, he fell and hit the icy surface of an object during a challenging jump. He immediately lost the motor function of his legs and became numb below his waist.

How does one classify spinal cord injuries?

Easily reproducible classification schemes are important methods by which to assess severity of injury, facilitate communication between practitioners, and, more importantly, aid in the determination of prognosis. The American Spinal Injury Association (ASIA) assessment tool utilizes both disability-specific and functional-independence measures and is considered the gold standard for the assessment of SCI (Figure 4-2).[28]

What is the role for steroids after SCI?

There have been three randomized controlled trials in addressing this question: The National Acute Spinal Cord Injury Studies (NASCIS) I, II, and III.[29-31] NASCIS-I was a negative study showing no benefit with steroid. The main criticism for failure on NASCIS-I was underdosing, and as such the NASCIS-II used "high"-dose steroid, methylprednisolone 30 mg/kg IV bolus followed by 5.4 mg/kg per hour for total of 23 hours. Methylprednisolone was given to 162 patients, naloxone was given to 154 patients, and placebo was given to 171 patients.

Most (95%) of the patients who were randomized to the steroid group received the drug within the first 14 hours of the injury. There was no difference in the 6-month outcome between the groups. Therefore, NASCIS-II is considered a negative study. Only in a post-hoc subgroup analysis, which focused on the timing of the steroid administration, was there a positive 6-month outcome for some individuals who received the drug within the first 8 hours. This post-hoc analysis has been criticized and, in general, not considered class I or II evidence, as the original study's randomized groups did not show any differences. NASCIS-III randomized patients to nonbolus, methylprednisolone 5.4 mg/kg per hour for 24 hours versus 48 hours versus tirilazad 2.5 mg/kg every 6 hours for 48 hours. There was no difference between these groups at any point. Only positive reports are again based on the post-hoc analysis showing benefit in people who received the steroid between 3 and 8 hours of injury but no benefit in those who received the drug within the first 3 hours. As a result, the routine use of steroids remains controversial and is not recommended as a standard of care. It may be considered if the administration can be performed while minimizing the associated risks of high-dose steroids,[32] making it an option and not a strong recommendation.

What other treatments are considered for SCI?

The mainstay of ICU treatment of SCI is supportive for respiratory and cardiac systems and preventative for infections and DVTs.

A = Complete	No motor or sensory function is preserved in the sacral segments S4-S5.
B = Incomplete	Sensory but not motor function is preserved below the neurologic level and includes the sacral segments S4-S5.
C = Incomplete	Motor function is preserved below the neurologic level, and more than half of key muscles below the neurologic level have a muscle grade less than 3.
D = Incomplete	Motor function is preserved below the neurologic level, and at least half of key muscles below the neurologic level have a muscle grade of 3 or more.
E = Normal	Motor and sensory function are normal.

A

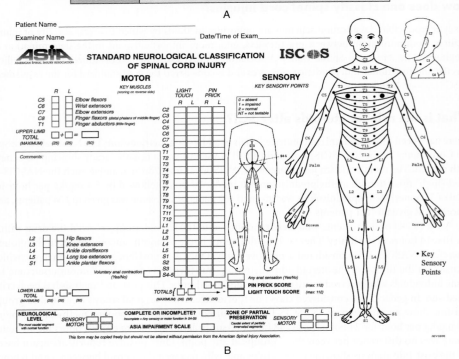

B

Figure 4-2. **A.** ASIA Impairment Scale. *With permission from www.asia-spinalinjury.org/publications/2006_Classif_worksheet.pdf.* **B.** Standard neurologic classification of spinal cord injury.

Respiratory System

Cervical cord injury is often associated with changes in respiratory patterns that are important to be aware of and can impact on ventilatory strategy. High-level cervical lesions result in the recruitment of accessory muscles with inspiration resulting in expansion of the upper rib cage with concomitant ascending diaphragm. This results in a paradoxical breathing pattern, reduction in all lung volumes (except residual volumes) but increased pulmonary and chest wall compliance and work of breath-ing.[33] Lower cervical lesions may result in less ventilatory difficulties but a significant inability to clear secretions. As a result, this population is at significant risk for developing aspiration pneumonia.

The main goals of respiratory management are to provide aggressive pulmonary hygiene, routine bronchodilator therapy, and aggressive attempts at ventilator weaning. Attempting intermittent ven-tilation with high tidal volumes (10 to 15 mL/kg), sighs, or adequate positive end-expiratory pressure (PEEP) may reduce the incidence and complications related to atelectasis.

Cardiac System

Hemodynamic instability is common after SCI. Lesions involving the cervical and upper thoracic cord result in sympathetic denervation, resulting in arteriolar vasodilation, venous pooling, bradycardia, and reduced myocardial contractility. The end result of this is a shock state that is characterized by hypotension, low systemic vascular resistance, and sinus bradycardia. However, given the impairment in myocardial contractility, hypotension cannot be overcome just with volume resuscitation and often requires additional vasopressor and/or inotropic agents. Some practitioners advocate for augmentation of MAP to maintain an adequate "cord perfusion pressure" greater than 60 mm Hg, although there is no reliable method to measure cord pressure and no clinical data support this practice.[34]

DVT Prophylaxis

SCI patients have a very high incidence of DVT, and while all agree this type of patient population should receive early prophylaxis, the regimen varies among institutions with regard to timing, dosing, and duration of pharmacologic intervention, as well as to the use of inferior IVC filters (see above). In general, there is no advantage to either subcutaneous low-molecular-weight heparin or heparin.[35]

Infectious Complications

Infectious complications are the leading cause for morbidity and mortality after SCI.[36] This may be due to a combination of acquired immunodeficiency from the injury itself as well as frequent use of high-dose steroids.[37] For reasons outlined above, this patient population is at very high risk for developing respiratory infections. Urinary tract infection risk is elevated due to neurologic dysfunction resulting in incontinence, high bladder pressures, and reflux. There should be a low threshold for investigating for GI tract infections in patients with persistent fever given the inability of patients to mount symptoms.

Is there a role for early surgical decompression?

Whether acute surgical intervention is needed in order to decompress the injured spinal cord contin-ues to be a controversial topic. This is mainly due to conflicting data in the literature with an absence of large randomized prospective studies demonstrating long-term outcome benefits. In some studies, when an early surgical decompression was performed, patients did not have better outcomes, and some of them had even worse outcomes.[38-40] Despites anecdotal reports of some benefits after early decompression, there is no strong evidence at this time for performing an early surgery. From a physi-ologic standpoint, an early intervention in correcting the malalignment of the spine structures makes at least intuitive sense. One of the frequently pointed out criticisms for these negative studies focuses on the timing of the decompression. Like the brain, the spinal cord may not tolerate a prolonged dura-tion of injury. So-called "early" surgical decompressions were done in days to weeks from the injury and not in the first few minutes or hours. By the time a decompression is done, typically 3 to 5 days or a week later, the injury has been completed, and no further intervention is likely to provide any long-term benefit. All of these criticisms point toward the need for a randomized controlled trial in order to better define the role and the timing of the surgical decompression.

!   **CRITICAL CONSIDERATIONS**

- Three specific end points have been found to be independent predictors of poor outcome in the prehospital/emergency department setting: hypothermia, hypoxia, and hypotension.
- During the early resuscitation phase, it is important to realize that simple measures such as elevation of the head of the bed (30 degrees), midline positioning of the head (relieving any blockage of jugular venous drainage), and adequate pain control and sedation are very simple and effective methods to reduce intracranial pressure.
- The American Academy of Neurology's practice guideline suggests using phenytoin for seizure prevention only in the first 7 days after TBI. Newer antiepileptic drugs with an improved safety profile may be a reasonable alternative. If prophylactic antiepileptics are used, they need to be discontinued after 7 days of use (if there has been no convulsive or nonconvulsive seizures).
- The significant head injury (CRASH) trial demonstrated no benefit and increased mortality rate in TBI patients randomized to 3 g of methylprednisolone in the first 72 hours after injury.
- The Brain Trauma Foundation guidelines state that intracranial pressure should be monitored in those with a postresuscitation GCS of 3 to 8 and an abnormal computed tomography scan, and further for those with a similar severity and a normal CT scan if two of the following are present: age older than 40 years, posturing, or hypotension. CPP thresholds should be maintained within a range of greater than 50 mm Hg and less than 70 mm Hg.
- CNS storming episodes are typically characterized as sudden onset of exaggerated sympathetic responses including hypertension, tachycardia, tachypnea, high fever, sweating, and papillary dilation, along with occasional dystonic posturing. Bromocriptine, β blockers such as propranolol, morphine sulfate, dantrolene, and clonidine may be helpful.
- The American Spinal Injury Association (ASIA) assessment tool utilizes both disability-specific and functional-independence measures and is considered the gold standard for the assessment of SCI.
- The routine use of steroids remains controversial and is not recommended as a standard of care. It may be considered if the administration can be performed while minimizing the associated risks, making it an option and not a strong recommendation.
- No clear data exist whether early surgical decompression is beneficial in SCI, especially in terms of timing. More data are needed before recommending early surgical intervention after SCI.

REFERENCES

1. Badjatia N, Carney N, Crocco TJ, et al. Guidelines for prehospital management of traumatic brain injury 2nd edition. *Prehosp Emerg Care.* 2008;12(suppl 1):S1-S52.
2. Cooper DJ, Myles PS, McDermott FT, et al. Prehospital hypertonic saline resuscitation of patients with hypotension and severe traumatic brain injury: A randomized controlled trial. *JAMA.* 2004;291:1350-1357.
3. SAFE investigators: Australian, New Zealand Intensive Care Society Clinical Trials Group, et al. Saline or albumin for fluid resuscitation in patients with traumatic brain injury. *N Engl J Med.* 2007; 357:874-884.
4. Temkin NR, Dikmen SS, Wilensky AJ, Keihm J, Chabal S, Winn HR. A randomized, double-blind study of phenytoin for the prevention of post-traumatic seizures. *N Engl J Med.* 1990;323: 497-502.
5. Chang BS, Lowenstein DH, Quality Standards Subcommittee of the American Academy of Neurology. Practice parameter: antiepileptic drug prophylaxis in severe traumatic brain injury: report of the Quality Standards Subcommittee of the American Academy of Neurology. *Neurology.* 2003;60:10-16.

6. Szaflarski JP, Sangha KS, Lindsell CJ, Shutter LA. Prospective, randomized, single-blinded comparative trial of intravenous levetiracetam versus phenytoin for seizure prophylaxis. *Neurocrit Care.* 2010;12: 165-172.

7. Edwards P, Arango M, Balica L, et al. Final results of MRC CRASH, a randomised placebo-controlled trial of intravenous corticosteroid in adults with head injury-outcomes at 6 months. *Lancet.* 2005;365:1957-1959.

8. Roberts I, Yates D, Sandercock P, et al. Effect of intravenous corticosteroids on death within 14 days in 10,008 adults with clinically significant head injury (MRC CRASH trial): Randomised placebo-controlled trial. *Lancet.* 2004;364:1321-1328.

9. Bratton SC, Chestnut RM, Ghajar, et al. VI. Indications for intracranial pressure monitoring. *J Neurotrauma.* 2007;24(suppl):S37-S44.

10. Bratton SC, Chestnut RM, Ghajar, et al. VII. Intracranial pressure monitoring technology. *J Neurotrauma.* 2007;24(suppl):S45-S54.

11. Bratton SC, Chestnut RM, Ghajar, et al. IV. Infection prophylaxis. *J Neurotrauma.* 2007;24(suppl): S26-S31.

12. Bratton SC, Chestnut RM, Ghajar, et al. IX. Cerebral perfusion thresholds. *J Neurotrauma.* 2007;24(suppl):S59-S64.

13. Bratton SC, Chestnut RM, Ghajar, et al. III. Prophylactic hypothermia. *J Neurotrauma.* 2007;24(suppl): S21-S25.

14. Clifton GL, Miller ER, Choi SC, et al. Lack of effect of induction of hypothermia after acute brain injury. *N Engl J Med.* 2001;344:556-563.

15. Clifton GLV, Zygun A, Cofey D, et al. Very early hypothermia induction in patients with severe brain injury (the National Acute Brain Injury Study: Hypothermia II): A randomised trial. *Lancet Neurol.* 2011;10:131-139.

16. Polderman KH. Mechanisms of action, physiological effects, and complications of hypothermia. *Crit Care Med.* 2009;37(suppl 7):S186-S202.

17. Ucar T, Akyuz M, Kazan S, Tuncer R. Role of decompressive surgery in the management of severe head injuries: Prognostic factors and patient selection. *J Neurotrauma.* 2005;22(11):1311-1318.

18. Compagnone C, Murray GD, Teasdale GM, et al. The management of patients with intradural post-traumatic mass lesions: A multicenter survey of current approaches to surgical management in 729 patients coordinated by the European Brain Injury Consortium. *Neurosurgery.* 2007;61:232-240; discussion 240-241.

19. Como JJ, Diaz JJ, Dunham CM, et al. Practice management guidelines for identification of cervical spine injuries following trauma: Update from the eastern association for the surgery of trauma practice management guidelines committee. *J Trauma.* 2009;67:651-659.

20. Bratton SC, Chestnut RM, Ghajar, et al. V. Deep vein thrombosis prophylaxis. *J Neurotrauma.* 2007;24(suppl):S37-S44.

21. Reiff DA, Haricharan RN, Bullington NM, et al. Traumatic brain injury is associated with the development of deep vein thrombosis independent of pharmacological prophylaxis. *J Trauma.* 2009;66:1436-1440.

22. Bratton SC, Chestnut RM, Ghajar, et al. II. Hyperosmolar therapy. *J Neurotrauma.* 2007;24(suppl): S14-S20.

23. Bratton SC, Chestnut RM, Ghajar, et al. XIV. Hyperventilation. *J Neurotrauma.* 2007;24(suppl): S87-S90.

24. Ariza M, Mataro M, Poca MA, et al. Influence of extraneurological insults on ventricular enlargement and neuropsychological functioning after moderate and severe traumatic brain injury. *J Neurotrauma.* 2004;21:864-876.

25. Salim A, Hadjizacharia P, DuBose J, et al. Role of anemia in traumatic brain injury. *J Am Coll Surg.* 2008;207:398-406.

26. Hébert PC, Wells G, Blajchman MA, et al. A multicenter, randomized, controlled clinical trial of transfusion requirements in critical care. Transfusion Requirements in Critical Care Investigators, Canadian Critical Care Trials Group. *N Engl J Med.* 1999;340(6):409-417.

27. Rabinstein AA. Paroxysmal sympathetic hyperactivity in the neurological intensive care unit. *Neurol Res.* 2007;29:680-682.

28. www.asia-spinalinjury.org/publications/2006

29. Bracken MB, Shepard MJ, Hellenbrand KG, et al. Methylprednisolone and neurological function 1 year after spinal cord injury. Results of the National Acute Spinal Cord Injury Study. *J Neurosurg.* 1985;63:704-713.

30. Bracken MB, Shepard MJ, Collins WF, et al. A randomized, controlled trial of methylprednisolone or naloxone in the treatment of acute spinal-cord injury. Results of the Second National Acute Spinal Cord Injury Study. *N Engl J Med.* 1990;322(20):1405-1411.

31. Bracken MB, Shepard MJ, Holford TR, et al. Administration of methylprednisolone for 24 or 48 hours or tirilazad mesylate for 48 hours in the treatment of acute spinal cord injury. Results of the Third National Acute Spinal Cord Injury Randomized Controlled Trial. National Acute Spinal Cord Injury Study. *JAMA.* 1997;277:1597-1604.

32. American Association of Neurological Surgeons. Pharmacological therapy after acute cervical spinal cord injury. *Neurosurgery.* 2002;50:S63-S72.

33. Scanlon PD, Loring SH, Pichurko BM, et al. Respiratory mechanics in acute quadriplegia. Lung and chest wall compliance and dimensional changes during respiratory maneuvers. *Am Rev Respir Dis.* 1989;139:615-620.

34. American Association of Neurological Surgeons. Blood pressure management after acute spinal cord injury. *Neurosurgery.* 2002;50:S58-S63.

35. American Association of Neurological Surgeons. Deep venous thrombosis and thromboembolism in patients with cervical spinal cord injuries. *Neurosurgery.* 2002;50:S73-S80.

36. Yeo JD, Walsh J, Rutkowski S, Soden R, Craven M, Middleton J. Mortality following spinal cord injury. *Spinal Cord.* 1998;36:329-336.

37. Nash MS. Immune dysfunction and illness susceptibility after spinal cord injury: An overview of probable causes, likely consequences, and potential treatments. *J Spinal Cord Med.* 2000;23:109-110.

38. Heiden JS, Weiss MH, Rosenberg AW, et al. Management of cervical spinal cord trauma in Southern California. *J Neurosurg.* 1974;43:732-736.

39. Horsey WJ, Tucker WS, Hudson AR, et al. Experience with early anterior operation in acute injuries of the cervical spine. *Paraplegia.* 1977;15:110-122.

40. Vaccaro AR, Daugherty RJ, Sheehan TP, et al. Neurologic outcome of early versus late surgery for cervical spinal cord injury. *Spine.* 1997;22:2609-2613.

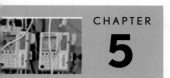

CHAPTER

5

Acute Ischemic Stroke

Joshua Z. Willey, MD, MS

A 62-year-old man with no known prior medical history presents to the emergency department (ED) after being found by emergency medical technicians (EMTs) for reportedly being intoxicated. Pedestrians had noted him walking on the street disoriented and "rambling," and he appeared to have difficulty walking. A local business owner, who had seen him on the streets before, thought this behavior was uncharacteristic and called 911 at 1300. The EMTs noted that he was unable to speak coherently, but his breath did not appear to smell of having alcohol in his system. As the EMTs were escorting the patient to the ambulance he developed acute-onset right face, arm, and leg weakness. The ED received notification of an acute stroke, and the stroke team was activated before the patient arrived at the ED. Upon arrival, his vital signs were blood pressure 142/78 mm Hg, heart rate 78 bpm in sinus rhythm, respiratory rate 14 breaths/min.

How common is stroke, and what is its public health burden?

Acute ischemic stroke is the most prevalent neurologic emergency in most of the world; one American has a stroke every 40 seconds. In the United States alone there are more than 780,000 strokes per year, with the majority being new events.[1] The number of hospitalizations in the United States continues to increase. The cost associated with the care of stroke patients in 2008 was $65.5 billion; the cost of care per patient is almost double for severe strokes. Stroke is the third leading cause of death in the United States, and among adults it is the leading cause of long-term disability. Stroke is disproportionately a disease of individuals of lower socioeconomic status, African Americans, the elderly, and women in the older age groups. Ischemic stroke accounts for the majority of stroke subtypes in case series from the United States.[1]

The majority of stroke survivors have some form of a residual disability, although 50% to 70% will nonetheless regain functional independence.[1] These patients remain at high risk for subsequent morbidity and mortality. A small proportion of acute ischemic stroke patients will be eligible for reperfusion therapy, and an even smaller proportion will actually receive it. In series from various locations in the United States the rate of thrombolysis varies when considering all stroke patients but remains low at 2.0% to 8.5%,[2] while analysis of data from the Nationwide Inpatient Service reveals this rate to be less than 2%.[3] The primary reason for not receiving reperfusion therapy is arrival outside of the appropriate time window.[4] Those who arrive by the appropriate window still have several reasons within the national guidelines for not being treated, and in some hospital series there are sizable numbers of patients who do not meet any exclusion criteria but are still not treated.[5] Prevention and treatment of the complications related to stroke remains the cornerstone of treatment for ischemic stroke.

Risk factors for ischemic stroke are somewhat similar to those of ischemic heart disease, with some notable exceptions. Hypertension remains the most important risk factor for ischemic stroke.[6] Dyslipidemia, while prominent for ischemic heart disease, is less important as a risk factor for ischemic stroke.[7] Large population-based cohort studies have failed to find a consistent association between dyslipidemia and ischemic stroke, although for the atherosclerotic stroke subtype, this may still be the case.[8]

Atherosclerotic disease of the extracranial or intracranial vessels is an important cause of ischemic stroke, most likely due to artery-to-artery emboli, or in a smaller proportion of cases due to flow failure.[9] Atrial fibrillation is an important risk factor, particularly for the older population, and frequently leads to more severe strokes and a poorer response to thrombolysis. Atrial fibrillation is more likely to be associated with large infarctions that could lead to malignant cerebral edema, as well as hemorrhagic infarcts/transformation.

What are the steps required to diagnose acute stroke in the ED before treatment can be initiated?

Stroke remains a clinical diagnosis, and in the acute setting a history and physical examination remain integral components of evaluation. In the triage area staff can activate the stroke team, if they have not already been activated based on a notification from the EMTs, and start the initial evaluation. This will include checking a fingerstick glucose level, vital signs, and a screening examination such as the Cincinnati Stroke Scale.[10] The latter can be used by nonphysician personnel with excellent reproducibility and sensitivity and involves checking for a facial droop, arm drift, and dysarthria. In patients with suspected stroke, two large-bore intravenous (IV) lines (at least 20 gauge) should be placed, and the following serum tests should be sent to the laboratory immediately: complete blood count, coagulation panel, basic metabolic panel, troponin, and type and hold. Our acute stroke pathway involves completing the history, carrying out an examination, and obtaining neurologic imaging (Figure 5-1).

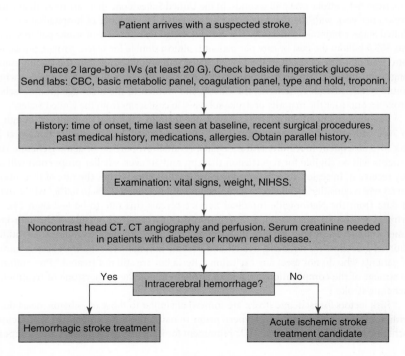

Figure 5-1. Suggested patient flow sheet for acute stroke patients. CBC, complete blood cell count; CT, computed tomography; G, gauge; NIHSS, National Institutes of Health Stroke Scale.

The history must be focused, and the initial goal should be to establish the exact time of onset. Frequently, patients such as the one above will not be able to provide an exact time of onset, and it is prudent to confirm the time of onset with friends or family. It is important to establish if there were minor symptoms present before the ones that caused the presentation, as well as whether the patient woke up with any deficits. For patients who wake up with a neurologic deficit, the time of onset is assumed to be the moment the patient went to sleep, or otherwise the last time they were seen at their baseline.

A complete neurologic examination is not often necessary in the initial evaluation in the ED; the National Institutes of Health Stroke Scale (NIHSS) is the initial examination of choice. It has excellent interexaminer reliability and sensitivity for most strokes,[11] can be performed quickly, and training in its use is available free of charge through the American Heart Association. Depending on the clinical scenario, more detailed examination may be required for suspected nondominant hemisphere injury, subtle aphasia, or cerebellar syndromes with a predominant astasia-abasia picture. Neurologic imaging is obtained before or after the examination, but should be completed within 20 minutes of arrival at the ED.

What is the preferred neurologic imaging modality in the acute setting? Are there other tests that may help with prognosis?

Given that stroke remains a clinical diagnosis, a noncontrast head computerized tomography (CT) scan is the initial test of choice for most patients.[12] The primary goal of the noncontrast head CT is to rule out intracerebral hemorrhage (ICH). In acute ischemic stroke the head CT will frequently be normal. Early infarct signs can be seen in the head CT and include loss of the insular cortical ribbon, sulcal effacement, and loss of the gray-white junction with blurring of basal ganglia nuclei differentiation. Occasionally, the dense middle cerebral artery sign, which likely represents intravascular dense clot material, is seen (Figure 5-2). Frequently, adjustment of the contrast may be required to visualize the early infarct signs.

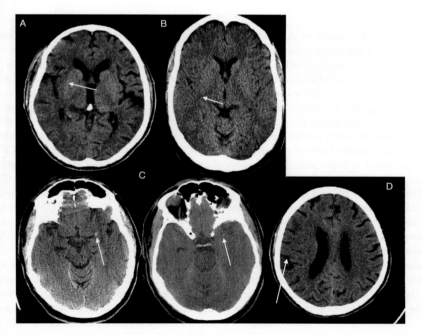

Figure 5-2. Computerized tomography images of the head showing early infarct signs. **A.** Loss of the insular ribbon **B.** Loss of the gray-white differentiation **C.** "Dense MCA sign." **D.** Sulcal effacement over the right hemisphere. MCA, middle cerebral artery.

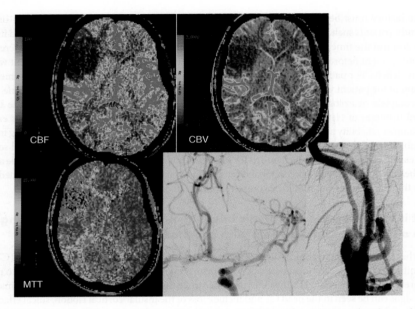

Figure 5-3. Computed tomography perfusion of the brain in a patient with a right carotid occlusion due to an acute dissection. CBF and CBV maps show an area of completed infarction in the right frontal lobe, with the MTT map showing a larger area of tissue at risk in the parietal lobe. CT, computed tomography; MTT, mean transit time; CBV, cerebral blood volume; CBF, cerebral blood flow.

In many stroke centers in the country, CT angiography and perfusion are routinely obtained in all acute ischemic stroke patients. CT angiography has the primary goal of identifying patients who have a major arterial occlusion, which may not respond well to intravenous thrombolysis, or which may portend risk of a large hemispheric infarction. CT perfusion is often obtained with CT angiography (Figure 5-3) and helps identify tissue that may be ischemic, but not yet infarcted, and therefore salvageable. CT perfusion allows the measurement of three parameters: cerebral blood volume (CBV), mean transit time (MTT), and cerebral blood flow (CBF). In early cerebral hemodynamic failure, the CBV will increase as distal arterioles vasodilate as a means of maintaining CBF in the face of dropping cerebral perfusion pressure (CPP). When this is insufficient, the CBV may remain increased or begin decreasing to normal or below, and the oxygen extraction fraction will increase; in the next stage, the cerebral metabolic rate of oxygen drops, and soon thereafter CBF will also drop.[13,14] The CBV and CBF maps are particularly useful in detecting potential tissue at risk, particularly when the CBF is low-normal and the CBV is increased. A very low CBV alternatively may indicate already infarcted tissue. The MTT is a useful adjunct, but there may be significant asymmetry in the MTT maps without having tissue at risk, and the optimal threshold for defining perfusion failure remains controversial.

Administering contrast remains a concern for many radiologists and ED physicians without knowing the patient's serum creatinine value. Unless there is a clinical history of renal disease or diabetes, the risk of developing contrast nephropathy is low,[15] and contrast can be administered without knowing the serum creatinine level; if there is still concern, isotonic sodium bicarbonate infusion can be administered. In one study, 3 ampules of sodium bicarbonate were mixed in 1 L of D_5W, and 1 hour before contrast the patient received 3 mL/kg, followed by 1 mL/kg for the 6 hours after the contrast is administered.[16] N-acetylcysteine 600 mg up to three times daily is frequently administered, but its clinical effectiveness may not be as high.

Transcranial Doppler (TCD) is commonly used in acute stroke evaluation to diagnose a major cerebral artery occlusion that may dictate advanced treatment, and may have a therapeutic benefit as well. The presence of a portable TCD machine in many institutions has made this a practical diagnostic tool. Magnetic resonance imaging (MRI) is available acutely in some centers, but in most centers it is not used before a decision to provide treatment in the acute setting. MRI can be useful to diagnose stroke mimics, distinguish TIA from stroke, and evaluate for the presence of a large infarction which may require a different degree of monitoring. MRI, however, is not necessary to make a recommendation on thrombolysis. The diffusion-weighted image (DWI) identifies areas of cytotoxic edema and infarction, although some DWI-positive lesions can be reversible. At the cellular level DWI identifies areas of impaired water molecule diffusion, frequently resulting from energy failure and an inability to maintain membrane gradients, such that brownian motion of water molecules is restricted.[17] Magnetic resonance angiography provides similar information to computed tomographic angiography (CTA), but it may overestimate the degree of stenosis. Magnetic resonance perfusion (Figure 5-4) may be useful in some clinical scenarios to establish a perfusion-diffusion mismatch, but the optimal parameters to define the penumbra remain an area of controversy.

The use of biomarkers in the diagnosis of stroke has received considerable attention in the literature, particularly for diagnosing ischemic stroke, but also for prognosis. Inflammatory markers (C-reactive protein) and measures of glial and endothelial cell injury (matrix metalloproteinase-9, S100B) have been associated with a diagnosis of ischemic stroke, although further data are required to validate their routine clinical use.[18]

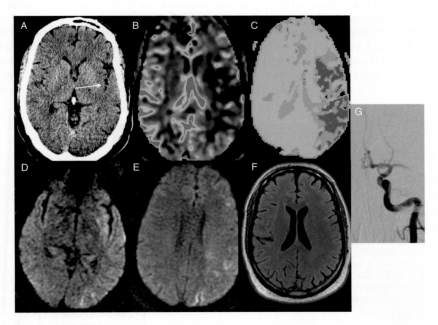

Figure 5-4. Computed tomography (CT), magnetic resonance imaging (MRI), and magnetic resonance perfusion imaging on a patient arriving 1 h from acute onset of global aphasia and right hemiparesis. **A.** CT head without contrast. The *arrow* points to the "spot sign," indicating a likely thrombus in M2 branches and loss of the insular ribbon. **B.** MR perfusion image, cerebral blood volume map, showing a large area of reduced volume in the left temporal-parietal region. **C.** MR perfusion image, mean transit time, showing a large area of delay in the left hemisphere. **D** and **E.** MRI diffusion-weighted images showing faint areas of restricted diffusion scattered in the left hemisphere. **F.** MRI FLAIR (fluid-attenuated inversion recovery) image showing no evidence of vasogenic edema. **G.** Digital subtraction angiography showing a left M1 occlusion.

The patient's parallel history is obtained when his family arrives and his last seen normal time was 2 hours ago. Head CT is normal, as are all of his laboratory values. The blood pressure is 196/118 mm Hg. His NIHSS is 18, and is notable for global aphasia, right hemiparesis, and a right visual field cut. What are the treatment options?

Intravenous Thrombolysis

Figure 5-5 outlines a suggested treatment paradigm for eligible patients. The only proven therapy to improve clinical outcomes for acute ischemic stroke is IV recombinant tissue plasminogen activator (r-tPA). The pivotal National Institute of Neurological Disease and Stroke (NINDS) r-tPA trial indicated that in patients treated within 3 hours of acute ischemic stroke there were significant clinical benefits.[19] The NINDS r-tPA trial did not demonstrate clinical effectiveness at 24 hours, although there was a trend toward benefit. The significant benefit was gleaned at 3 months where r-tPA was superior to placebo in the primary outcome of a composite of the NIHSS, modified Rankin Scale, Barthel Index, and Glasgow Outcome Scale. The treatment arm was associated with a 13% absolute benefit of attaining minimal to no disability after stroke (39% versus 26%), which translated to a number needed to treat of close to 8. There was no difference in mortality rate. The exclusion criteria for r-tPA need to be reviewed before administration and are summarized in Table 5-1.[20] There are several relative contraindications, such as hypodensity in greater than one-third of the middle cerebral artery (MCA) distribution and major deficits, age older than 80 years, and minor or rapidly resolving symptoms. The patient would be eligible for IV r-tPA, but his blood pressure should be lowered to less than 185/110 mm Hg before treatment with either IV pushes of labetalol or the use of an IV nicardipine drip.[20]

The NINDS r-tPA study differed from other acute stroke treatment trials by narrowing the therapeutic window to 0 to 3 hours from stroke onset, and using a dose of 0.9 mg/kg of r-tPA. Since then, analyses from this and other trials have pointed to a greater benefit to earlier treatment, particularly when r-tPA is started within 90 minutes of stroke onset.[21,22] Thrombolysis with r-tPA is beneficial in all subgroups and stroke subtypes, and its effectiveness has been proven in community cohorts.

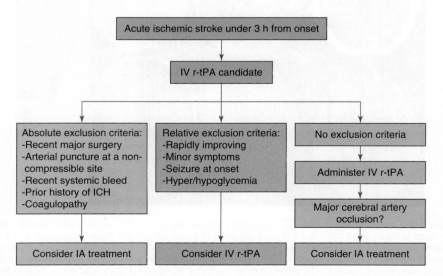

Figure 5-5. Clinical pathway for patients arriving under 3 h from ischemic stroke onset. IA, intra-arterial; ICH, intracranial hemorrhage; NIHSS, National Institutes of Health Stroke Scale; r-tPA, recombinant tissue plasminogen activator.

Table 5-1. Exclusion Criteria for Intravenous Tissue Plasminogen Activator in Patients Presenting Less 3 Hours from Ischemic Stroke Onset

Contraindications to r-tPA
Minor or rapidly improving symptoms
Seizure at stroke onset
Other stroke or trauma within 3 months
Major surgery within the last 14 days
History of intracerebral hemorrhage
Sustained blood pressure ≥185/110 mm Hg
Aggressive drug therapy needed to control blood pressure
Suspicion of subarachnoid hemorrhage
Arterial puncture at a noncompressible site within 7 days
Heparin received within the last 48 hours and PTT elevated
INR >1.7
Platelet count <100,000/μL
Plasma glucose level <50 mg/dL or >400 mg/dL

Abbreviations : PTT, partial thromboplastin time; r-tPA, recombinant tissue plasminogen activator; SAH, subarachnoid hemorrhage. (*From Tissue plasminogen activator for acute ischemic stroke. The National Institute of Neurological Disorders and Stroke rt-PA Stroke Study Group. N Engl J Med. 1995;333:1581-1587.*)

The typical protocol in the United States includes a door-to-needle time of no more than 60 minutes, with administration of r-tPA 0.9 mg/kg using a 10% bolus given over 1 to 2 minutes, followed by the rest of the infusion over 60 minutes. Consent is not required for IV r-tPA, as it is considered the standard of care, but the patient and family should be made aware that the treatment is being provided.[23] Thrombolysis can be safely and successfully administered via telemedicine, which is an attractive means for increasing treatment in rural and underserved hospitals.[24] Delays while waiting for the coagulation profile to return are common, but r-tPA can be safely administered without the coagulation profile.[25] After thrombolysis the blood pressure should remain less than 180/105 mm Hg, and any unacceptably high pressure should be promptly treated with easily titratable intravenous antihypertensive medications such as labetalol or nicardipine.

Intravenous treatment with thrombolysis is not effective in many individuals, and has a low likelihood of achieving vessel recanalization, particularly in individuals with an occlusion in one of the major intracranial arteries. Up to 34% of patients treated with r-tPA experience reocclusion after recanalization, with a subsequently high risk of neurologic worsening; these patients, however, still have better outcomes than those who do not recanalize.[26] Sonothrombolysis has been one proposed means of improving recanalization. High-frequency sound waves can cause cavitation and the formation of small bubbles that vibrate at a sufficiently high frequency to disrupt the fibrin network in thromboemboli, thereby facilitating entry of a thrombolytic into the clot. In the combined lysis of thrombus in brain ischemia using transcranial ultrasound and systemic tPA (CLOTBUST) phase II study, 126 patients who received IV r-tPA received placebo or a continuous insonation of the MCA via TCD probe.[27] The primary endpoint of vessel recanalization was achieved in 46% of the treatment arm versus 18% in placebo arm, with the benefit being maintained at 36 hours; in a secondary outcome there was a trend toward improved functional outcomes, and no differences in safety. Including microparticles to help break up the clot has been an active area of research. In one pilot study, microparticles were able to penetrate MCA thrombi and pass beyond,[28,29] while others have demonstrated improved recanalization rates with the use of microbubbles.[30] The type and composition of the microbubbles remain under investigation. Other investigators have attempted to combat the difficulties of vessel reocclusion or to potentiate the effects of r-tPA by adding pharmacologic adjuncts. The combined approach to lysis utilizing eptifibatide and r-tPA in acute ischemic stroke (CLEAR) trial randomized 94 patients to IV r-tPA at a reduced dose (0.3 mg/kg or 0.45 mg/kg) and eptifibatide versus IV r-tPA alone at full dose (0.9 mg/kg), with the primary end point being symptomatic intracranial hemorrhage (sICH) at 36 hours.[31] There was no statistically significant difference in the safety outcome or clinical effectiveness at 3 months, and until further trials are performed there is no evidence to support this approach. Holding antithrombotics for at least 24 hours after thrombolysis is currently advised.[20]

Before intravenous thrombolysis is administered, the patient is found to have an improvement in the NIHSS from 18 to 10. Should thrombolysis still be administered?

The benefit of r-tPA has been robust in routine clinical use, although there is still some resistance toward its use. Relative contraindications for r-tPA use include difficult to control blood pressure, "too good to treat" or rapidly improving syndromes, age older than 80 years, and seizure at onset. Blood pressure that requires aggressive control is not associated with increased rates of hemorrhage in at least one retrospective review,[32] while the benefit of aggressive glycemic control after thrombolysis remains under investigation. Several investigators have found that a substantial proportion (close to 20% in most case series) of the "too good to treat" patients end up with poor neurologic outcomes.[33-35] It remains an active area of research to identify which of these patients will worsen and which will not, although a more severe early benefit, primary motor symptoms, or the presence of a major cerebral artery occlusion appear to be notable risk factors for a poor outcome in the "too good to treat" group.[35-37] However, other case series have demonstrated that these patients may not have a poor outcome.[38] On the other hand, the safety of thrombolysis has been established for stroke mimics and these mild stroke patients.[39] Whether these "too good to treat" or rapidly improving patients should be treated remains a clinical decision on a case-by-case basis, with decision making being driven by the clinical impression of the disability the patient would have if left untreated. There is additional controversy as to whether individuals who are older than 80 years should be treated, although they still gain clinical benefit.[40,41] Several case series have reported an acceptable safety profile in the pediatric population,[42,43] although the clinical benefit in the pediatric population remains unknown.[44] Intravenous r-tPA remains beneficial even in patients with an initially severe deficit, and it appears to be safe in patients with cervical artery dissection, seizure at onset, and the presence of abnormality on CT; case series have documented it to be safe in patients with a known unruptured atrioventricular malformation (AVM) or aneurysm.[45] IV r-tPA should not be withheld for an otherwise eligible patient with an incidental finding of an unruptured aneurysm.

Whether IV r-tPA should be withheld from patients with other exclusion criteria is an additional area of controversy. A recent report demonstrated the safety at a single center of administering r-tPA to any patient arriving under 3 hours without a hemorrhage on head CT, while another report documented a high intracerebral hemorrhage rate after thrombolysis in patients taking warfarin with an International Normalized Ratio (INR) less than 1.7.[46] Regardless, the primary reason for not receiving intravenous thrombolysis remains arrival outside of the appropriate time window.[2] Interestingly, the bulk of the litigation cases in the United States related to r-tPA are related to failure to administer the medication.[47]

What are the expected complications from treatment with thrombolytics?

The most dreaded complication from r-tPA infusion is hemorrhage, of which ICH is the most serious. It will typically present with headache, nausea and vomiting, worsening of the neurologic deficit, and in more severe cases an altered level of alertness. In the NINDS tPA trial, the rate of symptomatic ICH (sICH), defined as the presence of hemorrhage on CT of the head with suspicion for hemorrhage or a decline in neurologic status, was present in 6.4% of those receiving r-tPA and 0.6% in those receiving placebo.[19] Of those who had sICH in the r-tPA arm, close to 50% had died at 3 months. Asymptomatic ICH was present in 4.4% overall. Major systemic hemorrhage was rare, while minor extracranial hemorrhage occurred in 23% of patients treated with r-tPA (compared to 3% in the placebo arm).

In the European Cooperative Acute Stroke Studies (ECASS), hemorrhages were classified as follows (Figure 5-6): Hemorrhage infarction type 1 (HI-1), small petechiae along the margins of the infarct; hemorrhage infarction type 2 (HI-2), more confluent petechiae within the infarcted area but without a space-occupying effect; parenchymal hematoma type 1 (PH-1), a hematoma in less than 30% of the infarcted area with some space-occupying effect; and parenchymal hematoma type 2 (PH-2), a hematoma in greater than 30% of the infarcted area with substantial space-occupying effect or as any hemorrhagic lesion outside the infracted area.[48] PH-2 is the only one associated with clinical

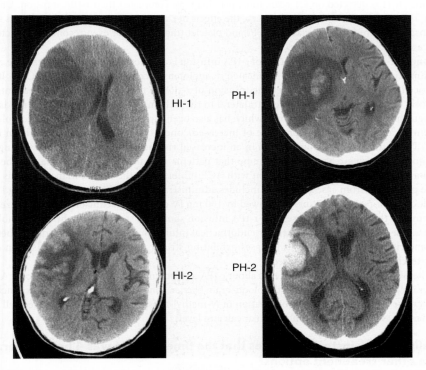

Figure 5-6. Computed tomography scans of the head showing the four subtypes of hemorrhagic conversion. HI-1, hemorrhagic infarction-1; HI-2, hemorrhagic infarction-2; PH-1, parenchymal hematoma-1; PH-2, parenchymal hematoma-2.

decline.[49] HI-1 and HI-2 are not predictive of a poor outcome, but their presence may indicate successful reperfusion and an association with subsequent clinical benefit from thrombolysis.[50]

The risk factors for development of sICH after thrombolysis have been variable, depending on the study. The most consistent risk factors across several studies include early hypoattenuation on head CT, elevated serum glucose and history of diabetes, hypertension,[51] increased stroke severity and size of stroke on DWI,[52] especially if there is reperfusion,[53] and protocol violations with treatment outside of the time window.[52, 54-56] It remains controversial whether treatment with antiplatelet agents before thrombolysis,[57,58] pretreatment with statins,[59,60] the presence of microhemorrhages on T2* sequence or gradient echo of MRI,[61,62] leukoaraiosis,[63] advanced age,[41] hemostatic factors,[64,65] early disruption of the blood-brain barrier via permeability imaging,[66] markers of endothelial cell injury (matrix metalloproteinase 9, S100B),[18] and persistent arterial occlusion[67] convey an additional risk for sICH. The presence of early infarct signs correlated with more severe stroke in the NINDS tPA trial, although they did not mitigate the clinical benefit of treatment or alter the safety outcomes.[68]

Perfusion studies may play an additional role in identifying those patients who are at high risk of sICH. The presence of a large area of reduced CBF as measured by xenon CT correlated well with an increased risk of sICH,[69] while a very low CBV may be a better predictor than absolute infarct size or relative ischemia.[70] There are insufficient data at this time to recommend withholding thrombolysis for patients with these characteristics, although they may be ones for whom more intensive monitoring in the first 24 to 48 hours is warranted.

Management of sICH after r-tPA infusion usually starts with discontinuing the infusion of thrombolytics in those patients for whom there is a clinical suspicion of hemorrhage, followed by immediate noncontrast head CT and full coagulation panel including fibrinogen and a complete blood count. By the time sICH is detected on CT scan, most patients have completed their r-tPA infusion. Unfortunately, there is no proven therapy to reverse the effects of r-tPA. However, if active bleeding is found, options include fresh-frozen plasma (FFP) and platelet transfusions or even recombinant factor VII on a case-by-case basis.

Another rare clinical complication of r-tPA infusion is angioedema, which appears to be caused by a similar pathway that has been implicated in angiotensin-converting enzymes (ACEs). It typically occurs 30 to 120 minutes after the infusion of r-tPA in typically 1% to 3% of patients, and curiously enough it tends to occur contralateral to the ischemic lesion.[71] Angioedema needs to be distinguished from tongue hematoma, which has also been reported. Activation of the complement and kinin cascades due to the presence of increased concentrations of plasmin have been implicated. This latter pathway is implicated in an increased risk being present in patients taking ACE inhibitors.[72] It seems reasonable to assume that patients who develop angioedema may be at an additional risk of the same complication with ACE inhibitors in the future. Management is based on the paradigms from case series, and includes administration of diphenhydramine 50 mg IV and H2-blocker as first-line treatment, followed by 100 mg IV of methylprednisolone or nebulized epinephrine. In the more severe cases, the r-tPA infusion should be stopped in light of a possible loss of the airway and the potential need for endotracheal intubation. The latter may require fiberoptic assistance in severe cases, such as in cases exhibiting stridor and airway compromise. An emergency tracheostomy may be required.

There are additional safety concerns about r-tPA as a potentially neurotoxic substance.[73] Animal studies indicate that r-tPA can cross the blood-brain barrier[74] and, once within the brain parenchyma, can increase ischemic injury via potentiation of N-methyl-D-aspartate (NMDA)–induced cell death and increase NMDA-mediated intracellular calcium levels.[75]

Parallel history instead indicates that the time of onset was 4 hours prior. Are there other treatment options?

The Alteplase Thrombolysis for Acute Noninterventional Therapy in Ischemic Stroke (ATLANTIS)[76,77] and ECASS I[78] and II[79] trials were notable for an attempt to try to expand the window for thrombolysis or alter the dose. In all of these cases, r-tPA was not associated with a clear clinical benefit when the time window extended beyond 3 hours, and appeared to increase the risk of ICH. The European Medicines Evaluation Agency approved r-tPA in 2002 under the condition that a trial of r-tPA be carried out and that a prospective registry include safety outcomes.[80] This registry tracked patients treated up to 4.5 hours, and there was no difference in complication rates between those who were in the less-than-3-hour window and those in the 3.0- to 4.5-hour window.[81]

In 2008, publication of the results from ECASS III revealed a statistically significant clinical benefit in a select group of patients between 3.0 and 4.5 hours from onset.[82] The trial excluded patients with an NIHSS greater than 25, those older than age 80, those taking oral anticoagulants regardless of prothrombin time, and those with a prior stroke and concomitant diabetes. The trial randomized 821 patients to r-tPA 0.9 mg/kg or placebo, with a primary outcome of mRS (modified Rankin Scale) at 90 days that was achieved in the treatment arm (52.4%) versus placebo (45.2%). Treatment was not associated with increased mortality rate, although there was a higher risk of hemorrhage (2.4% versus 0.3%). A science advisory from the American Heart Association/American Stroke Association recommended that IV r-tPA be administered up to 4.5 hours from stroke onset, but warned against prolonging time windows in the ED for those under 3 hours from stroke onset.[81] A proposed clinical pathway for patients between 3 and 8 hours from stroke onset is presented in Figure 5-7.

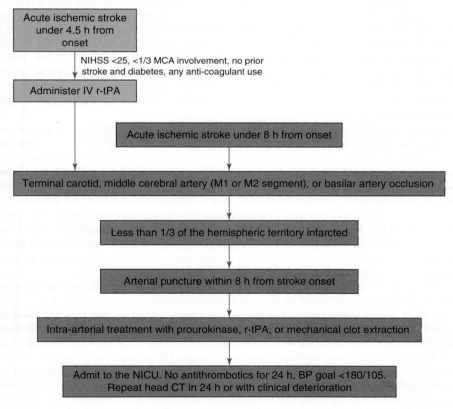

Figure 5-7. Proposed clinical pathway for patients arriving after 3 h from stroke onset. BP, blood pressure; CT, computed tomography; MCA, middle cerebral artery; NICU, neurologic intensive care unit; NIHSS, National Institute of Health Stroke Scale; r-tPA, recombinant tissue plasminogen activator.

In order to increase the proportions of individuals who receive intravenous thrombolysis, several strategies have been tried to date. Education of the public has achieved moderate success in improving arrival times at the ED, while the establishment of acute stroke teams and experience over time has led to reduced hemorrhagic complication rates and protocol violations and improved patient flow in EDs. The ischemic penumbra presented an attractive target beyond 3 hours based on retrospective reviews of clinical protocols of thrombolysis using perfusion-weighted imaging (PWI).[83,84] Moving toward a tissue-based window rather than the absolute time and "clock on the wall" window remains the most promising avenue of research to expand the treatment window.

Trials with other thrombolytics besides r-tPA have suggested a possible role of treatment beyond 4.5 hours in patients with perfusion-diffusion mismatch on MRI. Phase II trials have been carried out with desmoteplase, a chemical derivative from the saliva of vampire bats. Desmoteplase acts by a different mechanism of action, and has a high affinity for fibrin without having an effect on plasminogen or fibrinogen or apparent neurotoxicity.[73,75,85] In the Desmoteplase in Acute Ischemic Stroke trial (DIAS),[86] patients were randomized to placebo versus desmoteplase treatment if they presented in the 3- to 9-hour time window, had an NIHSS of 4 to 20, and evidence of MRI perfusion-diffusion mismatch. In the trial a non–weight-based dose led to excessive symptomatic hemorrhages (26.7%), with a rate that was significantly lower (2.2%) when it was switched to a weight-based algorithm. The treatment arm was associated with improved reperfusion and subsequent clinical outcomes. In the phase II Dose Escalation of Desmoteplase for Acute Ischemic Stroke (DEDAS)[87] study that included 37 patients, desmoteplase was associated with a trend toward improved clinical outcomes and a favorable safety profile in patients treated in the 3- to 9-hour time window. The findings were not confirmed in the phase III DIAS-2 trial, where desmoteplase treatment showed no improvement in clinical outcomes, and appeared to be associated with increased mortality rate.[88] In the Diffusion and Perfusion Imaging Evaluation for Understanding Stroke Evolution (DEFUSE) study, patients within 3 to 6 hours from stroke onset received r-tPA regardless of their baseline MRI profile. Patients with a favorable diffusion-perfusion pattern (small DWI lesion, with a perfusion-diffusion ratio of 2.6) and subsequent reperfusion had a favorable clinical response.[89-91] This study included only 74 patients and did not include a placebo arm.

In the larger Echoplanar Imaging Thrombolytic Evaluation Trial (EPITHET),[92] 101 patients were randomized to placebo versus r-tPA at 3 to 6 hours from stroke onset, with a primary hypothesis of clinical benefit in patients with a diffusion-perfusion mismatch. The primary outcome was infarct growth between baseline DWI and 90-day T2-weighted imaging for which there was a nonstatistically significant trend to benefit with r-tPA. Secondary outcomes included improved neurologic (NIHSS 0 to 1 or 8 or more point improvement at 90 days) or functional status (mRS 0 to 2 at 90 days) that was associated with reperfusion, which was defined as 90% or more improvement in PWI imaging volume at days 3 to 5. Reperfusion appeared to be more important than recanalization.[93] Criticisms of these studies relate to the technique used in measuring the penumbra. There are numerous difficulties with obtaining standardized processing of the perfusion sequences, as well as having them processed in a timely fashion for routine clinical use.

Additionally, the imaging of the penumbra was based on using the magnetic resonance perfusion (MRP) by examining the following parameters: mean time to enhance (mean transit time), negative enhancement integral (cerebral blood volume), and maximum slope of decrease (cerebral blood flow, calculated as CBV/MTT). Hypoperfused tissue on PWI has been primarily defined in EPITHET and DEFUSE as a greater than 2-second delay in the Tmax, analogous to the MTT, with reperfusion being defined as a greater than 90% improvement in this parameter. On the other hand, final infarct volume appears to correlate better with a Tmax of 6 to 8 seconds or more.[94] The other image maps are usually processed with a significant delay and are not readily available. In contrast, further understanding of the penumbra has led to the understanding that some portions of the penumbra will remain viable regardless of whether reperfusion occurs, while other will not, despite treatment.[83] The role of collateral flow, and imaging it, remains incompletely understood, as does the optimal parameters to define the penumbra. The correlations with quantitative CBF from other modalities also remain imperfect. It remains important to comprehend that recanalization, which thrombolytics may do, is not synonymous with reperfusion, although they tend to be correlated. The former is based on angiographic improvement in the appearance of the vessel, while the latter refers to an improvement in PWI parameters. A recent meta-analysis showed that reperfusion and recanalization rates improved using mismatch-guided thrombolysis and that recanalization improves outcomes; however, thrombolysis did not improve outcomes.[95] Currently, it remains controversial whether perfusion-diffusion imaging should be used in routine clinical care.[96,97]

Are there other acute treatment options for reperfusion if intravenous thrombolysis cannot be carried out? In the patient above, should we stop at intravenous thrombolysis?

Pharmacologic Treatment

Table 5-2 outlines the results of notable pharmacologic and device trials in acute ischemic stroke. Glycoprotein IIb/IIIa (GPIIb-IIIa) inhibitors have been an attractive target for pharmacologic treatment beyond thrombolysis. In a phase II dose-escalation study enrolling 74 patients, investigators found that the administration of abciximab was associated with a trend toward improved disability, with no significant increase in the rate of sICH.[98] The Abciximab in Emergency Treatment of Stroke Trial (AbESST), a phase II study using 400 patients, found similar results in terms of safety and a nonsignificant modest trend toward improvement in mRS at 3 months.[99] The phase III AbESST II study planned to enroll 1800 patients, with randomization to abciximab or placebo within 5 hours of stroke onset in those who did not receive thrombolysis. The phase III study failed to replicate these findings, as the study was stopped prematurely after 808 patients were enrolled by the data safety monitoring board. There was a significant increase in the rate of sICH in the treatment arm (5.5% versus 0.5%), with no difference in the prespecified primary outcome.[100] GPIIb-IIIa inhibitors have also been examined in combination with thrombolysis with the intent to improve recanalization rates based on experience with acute myocardial infarction.

Antithrombotic agents remain the most commonly used pharmacologic agent for acute stroke prevention. In the Chinese Acute Stroke Trial,[101] aspirin showed a modest absolute benefit over placebo in mortality and recurrent stroke risk. In the International Stroke Trial (IST),[102] aspirin again had a mild benefit over placebo in preventing stroke and improving mortality rate, while the heparin arm showed a trend toward a mild benefit in the 12,500 arm versus the 5000-unit arm that was offset by the hemorrhage risk. Danaparoid, a heparinoid, was found to be ineffective in grouping the acute setting for noncardioembolic stroke,[103] while low-molecular-weight heparin showed a similar lack of effectiveness in acute cardioembolic stroke.[104] Pilot data from the LOAD (Loading of Aspirin and Clopidogrel in acute ischemic stroke and transient ischemic attack) trial indicated a favorable safety profile in the acute setting for the combination of aspirin and clopidogrel, with a trend of reduced clinical worsening.[105] In the larger FASTER (Fast Assessment of Stroke and Transient ischemic attack to prevent Early Recurrence) trials, there was a reduction in clinical worsening with a combination of the two antiplatelet agents, which offset the slight increase in hemorrhage.[106] Currently, there are no phase III clinical trials proving the effectiveness of aspirin and clopidogrel in combination after acute ischemic stroke, although caution is warranted given the lack of clinical effectiveness in secondary prevention studies.[107] Heparin may be considered in the acute setting in the post–cardiac surgery stroke population, in selected cases of carotid dissection, and in patients with a mechanical heart valve.

Intra-arterial Treatment

Given the poor outcomes associated with not recanalizing the middle cerebral artery in particular, endovascular treatment has emerged as another option for acute stroke treatment. In the PROACT

Table 5-2. Summary of Completed Acute Stroke Clinical Trials

Trial and reference no.	Agent tested	Time window	Primary outcome	Positive? Effect size
NINDS tPA trial[19] Phase III	r-tPA (0.9 mg/kg) vs placebo	Under 3 h from onset	3-mo composite outcome of BI, NIHSS, mRS, and GOS	Yes. 39% vs 26%
CLOTBUST[27] Phase II	High-frequency ultrasound vs placebo in patients receiving IV r-tPA	Under 3 h from onset	Complete recanalization or dramatic neurologic improvement	Yes. 49% vs 30%
ATLANTIS[77] Phase III	r-tPA (0.9 mg/kg) vs placebo	3-5 h from stroke onset	NIHSS ≤ 1; composite of BI, NIHSS, mRS, and GOS	No for primary or secondary outcome. Significant increase in sICH rates
ECASS[78] Phase III	r-tPA (1.1 mg/kg) vs placebo	Up to 6 h from stroke onset	BI and mRS at 90 d	No
ECASS II[79] Phase III	r-tPA (0.9 mg/kg) vs placebo	Up to 6 h from stroke onset, and stratified at 0-3 h and 3-6 h	mRS at 90 d	No for the overall group
ECASS III[82]	r-tPA (0.9 mg/kg) vs placebo	3.0-4.5 h from stroke onset	mRS at 90 d	Yes. 52.4% vs 45.2%
DIAS[86] Phase II	Fixed (part 1) and then weight-based dosing (part 2) of desmoteplase	3-9 h from stroke onset with evidence of perfusion-diffusion mismatch	sICH. Secondary: MRI reperfusion and 90-d good outcome	Yes. 71.4% vs 19.2 % reperfusion for the highest weight-based dose; 60.0% vs 22.2% good clinical outcome for the highest weight-based dose compared to placebo
DEDAS[87] Phase II	Escalating dose 90-125 μg/kg desmoteplase vs placebo	3-9 h from stroke onset with evidence of perfusion-diffusion mismatch	sICH. Secondary: MRI reperfusion and 90-d good outcome	sICH not noted. Improvements in recanalization and clinical outcomes in the 125-μg/kg dose
DIAS-2[88] Phase II	90 μg/kg desmoteplase, 125 μg/kg desmoteplase, or placebo	3-9 h from stroke onset with evidence of perfusion-diffusion mismatch	90-d clinical composite outcome	No. 47% for lower dose and 36% for higher dose desmoteplase; 46% for placebo
EPITHET[92] Phase II	r-tPA (0.9 mg/kg)	3-6 h from stroke onset with evidence of perfusion-diffusion mismatch	Infarct growth	No siginificant change in volume of infarct, trend toward beneficial outcomes

Table 5-2. Summary of Completed Acute Stroke Clinical Trials (*Continued*)

Trial and reference no.	Agent tested	Time window	Primary outcome	Positive? Effect size
AbESTT-II[100] Phase III	Abciximab	Within 5 h, and in wake-up stroke	mRS	No. Stopped early due to lack of benefit and significant increase in hemorrhage
PROACT-II[109] Phase II	9 mg IA prourokinase and heparin vs heparin	Within 6 h of onset with angiographic documented MCA occlusion	mRS and recanalization	Yes. 40% vs 25% favorable outcome; 66% vs 18% recanalization; sICH in 10%
IMS-II[114] Phase II	0.6 mg/kg of r-tPA followed by IA treatment with further r-tPA or placebo	Within 3 h who received IV r-tPA	mRS, global outcome, and sICH	Similar sICH rates to PROACT II, with improvement in functional outcomes in the IA-treated patients
Multi-MERCI[121] Phase II	Merci device (multiple generations of devices), single arm	Within 8 h of stroke onset	Recanalization of the partner vessel	69.5% achieved recanalization, and 36% achieved a favorable mRS
Penumbra Pivotal Stroke Trial[122] Phase II	Penumbra device	Within 8 h of stroke onset	Safety profile	81.6% successful recanalization. 11.4 % sICH
CAST[101]	Aspirin 162 mg daily vs placebo	Within 48 h of stroke	Death or dependence at 4 weeks	Yes. 3.3% vs 3.9% mortality, and 1.6% vs 2.1% recurrent stroke
IST[102]	Heparin (5000 or 12,500 units bid), vs avoid heparin. The latter group randomized to aspirin 300 mg daily or placebo	As soon as possible	Death within 14 d, or death/dependency at 6 months	Yes. No difference in outcomes in heparin allocation. Aspirin had fewer recurrent strokes (2.8% vs 3.9%)
TOAST[103]	Heparinoid vs placebo in noncardioembolic stroke	Within 24 h of stroke	GOS and BI at 3 mo	No
HAEST[104]	Low-molecular-weight heparin vs aspirin in atrial fibrillation–related stroke	Within 30 h of stroke onset	Recurrent stroke at 14 d	No. 8.5% vs 7.5% in the heparinoid vs aspirin (nonsignificant)
Decompressive hemicraniectomy[142]	Hemicraniectomy in space-occupying MCA infarction vs medical management	Within 48 h of stroke onset	mRS favorable (0-4); mortality	Yes. 75% vs 24% for the favorable mRS. Mortality 78% vs 29% favoring surgery

Abbreviations: BI, brain injury; GOS, Glasgow Outcome Scale; IA, intra-arterial; MRI, magnetic resonance imaging; mRS, modified Rankin Scale; NIHSS, National Institutes of Health Stroke Scale; r-tPA, recombinant tissue plasminogen activator; sICH, symptomatic intracranial hemorrhage.

(Prolyse in Acute Cerebral Thromboembolism) study, 40 patients were randomized to intra-arterial (IA) infusion of prourokinase versus placebo. Treatment with prourokinase was associated with a statistically significant increase in the rate of recanalization, although there was a concomitant increase in the rate of sICH in the medication arm (15.4% versus 7.1%).[108] Much of the sICH could be attributed to the use of IV heparin.

Publication of the PROACT II study in 1999 significantly altered the paradigm for acute stroke care, and in specialized stroke centers throughout the country, treatment up to 6 hours from stroke onset became possible, if not part of routine clinical care. In PROACT II,[109] 180 patients were randomized to receive 9 mg of IA prourokinase plus heparin versus heparin alone. The main outcome was an mRS of 0 to 2, which was achieved in 40% of the treated patients versus 25% in the control group, with a 66% versus 18% success rate at recanalization with IA treatment. There was a statistically significant increase in the rate of sICH (10% versus 2%), although the investigators concluded that the benefits of the treatment outweighed the risks. The Middle Cerebral Artery Embolism Local Fibrinolytic Intervention Trial confirmed improved functional (mRS 0 to 1) and neurologic (NIHSS 0 to 1) outcomes at 90 days with intra-arterial urokinase, although the study's primary outcome of mRS 0 to 2 was not reached.[110] In PROACT II age, NIHSS, and initial head CT were all associated with a greater likelihood of clinical benefit from intra-arterial treatment, while experience at the University of Houston has identified age, NIHSS, and admission glucose as predictive of a poor outcome independently of recanalization.[111]

The Interventional Management of Stroke (IMS) trials further tested the hypothesis of combining intravenous and intra-arterial thrombolysis for patients who had major intracranial artery occlusions under the premise that these patients are unlikely to recanalize with intravenous treatment alone. The phase I Emergency Management of Stroke (EMS) bridging trial showed that this treatment paradigm was feasible and appeared to be safe.[112] In IMS I, 80 patients were treated with 0.6 mg/kg of IV r-tPA followed by intra-arterial r-tPA and were compared to historical controls.[113] The rates of sICH were similar to the treatment arm of the NINDS r-tPA trial (6.3%).

IMS II assigned 81 patients who received IV r-tPA (0.6 mg/kg) within 3 hours to intra-arterial r-tPA up to 22 mg or when recanalization was achieved, as well as the use of an intravascular sonothrombolysis device. Twenty-six patients were treated with IV r-tPA only, while the rest were treated with a combination of intra-arterial sonothrombolysis or microcatheter injections. Despite a nonsignificant trend toward a higher rate of sICH in the treatment arm compared to the NINDS tPA trial (9.9% versus 6.4%), there was a higher likelihood of achieving global outcomes in the endovascular treated group compared to the historical controls. There was an additional trend toward improvement in some of the outcomes in the endovascular treatment arm compared to the NINDS r-tPA–treated patients.[114]

IMS III is currently enrolling patients using IV r-tPA at a reduced dose (0.6 mg/kg) IV followed by the rest of the infusion in an IA fashion. A criticism of IMS III has been that patients are not receiving the optimal dose of IV r-tPA up front, although in one small clinical trial, patients also had a benefit from treatment with 0.6 mg/kg of r-tPA.[115] The optimal dose of IV r-tPA to be given before IA treatment remains controversial, although in at least one case series giving full-dose 0.9 mg/kg of IV r-tPA was safe and associated with successful recanalization.[116] The results are eagerly anticipated as there are reports that the combination of IV and IA r-tPA may increase the risk of sICH.[117] The risk factors for sICH remain the same for IV and IA r-tPA in many observational studies, with elevated serum glucose remaining a particularly important factor[118] and the number of microinjections during IA treatment being an additional factor.[119] Intra-arterial thrombolysis up to 6 hours from onset has class I, level B evidence for selected patients with MCA occlusion and class IIa, level C evidence for treatment in patients who cannot receive thrombolysis.[20]

In the meantime, industry has spearheaded the development of several devices for the endovascular treatment of acute ischemic stroke. These devices have used a combination of clot extraction, clot suctioning, and ultrasound-assisted thrombolysis. There are two currently approved devices by the US Food and Drug Administration for the mechanical clot extraction in an intracerebral artery—the Merci Retrieval System (Concentric Medical Inc, Mountain View, CA) and the Penumbra System (Penumbra, Inc, Alameda, CA). It is important to note that neither one of these devices has been approved to date to benefit patients but rather to recanalize the vessel. In the MERCI and Multi-MERCI studies, a corkscrew-type device was tested up to 8 hours from stroke onset in a nonrandomized fashion in 151 patients. Recanalization was achieved in up to 69.5% of patients, which is higher than in historical controls, with a comparable sICH rate (9.8%). Favorable clinical outcomes, defined as mRS of 0 to 2 at 90 days, were achieved more often in the patients who had successful recanalization.[120,121]

The Penumbra device uses continuous suction locally and was tested in 125 patients with an NIHSS greater than 8 and occlusion of a large intracerebral artery in a single-arm fashion. Recanalization was achieved in approximately 83% of participants, which the investigators mentioned was higher than with the Merci device, but there was a 12.8% procedural complication rate of which 2.4% was considered serious. The proportion of patients who had an asymptomatic ICH was 28%, while 11.2% had sICH; 90-day mortality was 32.8%, and 25% of individuals attained an mRS of 0 to 2.[122]

The window for treatment has been expanded by clinicians for patients who are neurologically devastated from basilar artery thrombosis up to 24 hours with the understanding that the patient's outcome is uniformally dismal, while the risk of hemorrhagic transformation is smaller in the brainstem. One recent research reported superior recanalization success and improved outcomes in patients with acute basilar artery occlusion who were treated with IA thrombolysis in combination with IV abciximab versus IA thrombolysis in a nonprospective manner, and these results cannot be generalized to non–basilar artery involvement.[123] A large international registry of patients with acute basilar artery occlusion that examined outcomes after IV r-tPA, antithrombotic treatment alone, and endovascular treatment has provided additional guidance.[124] In patients with a mild-moderate deficit, IV r-tPA appeared to be superior, while in a severe deficit, IV r-tPA in combination with IA treatment was a promising treatment modality. The investigators could not conclude on the optimal timing for when not to treat patients with IA modalities, although none of the patients treated after 9 hours from stroke onset had a good outcome.

Stenting for acute ischemic stroke, even in the setting of nonatherosclerotic strokes, has also received recent attention. In a 2009 published pilot trial, stenting performed less than 8 hours from stroke onset had an acceptable safety profile compared to other trials, with comparable recanalization rates to other modalities.[125] Further trials are required with this technology or other emerging modalities such as a retrievable stent.[126]

In patients with internal carotid artery, M1 or M2 segments of the middle cerebral artery, or vertebrobasilar artery occlusions, we will routinely perform catheter angiography after thrombolysis for endovascular treatment, and will consider it for patients up to 8 hours from stroke onset if there is no evidence of large cerebral infarction (more than one-third of the MCA distribution) (see Figure 5-7). In the case of intra-arterial treatment, informed consent is part of our routine clinical protocol, and we will explain thoroughly to the family the risks and benefits, as well as the quality of evidence available.

Nonthrombolytic Acute Stroke Treatment

Statins have shown a clear benefit in secondary stroke prevention, an effect that appears to be independent of the serum lipid panel. The cholesterol-independent effects of statins have been an attractive target in the acute stroke setting. Statins have the potential for being neuroprotectants independently of their effect on modification of dyslipidemia. Animal models have indicated that statins are associated with a reduction in infarct size, a result that was mediated in part by endothelial nitric oxide synthetase expression. Statins also appear to reduce inflammation and may increase angiogenesis, synaptogenesis, and neurogenesis. Lastly statins reduce membrane cholesterol synthesis in neurons, thereby rendering them more resistant to glutamate N-methyl-D-aspartate receptor–mediated excitotoxic effects, one of the principal mechanisms of neuronal death in ischemic brain.[127] Patients who were taking a statin in the Northern Manhattan Study at the time of their stroke were more likely to have a favorable outcome,[128] while withdrawal of a statin in the acute stroke setting is associated with worsening outcomes.[129] There are currently no phase III clinical trials that have enrolled patients in the acute stroke setting. Phase II studies of high doses of statins are currently ongoing.[130]

The American Heart Association (AHA) guidelines recommend that in patients not receiving thrombolysis the blood pressure should be allowed to remain as elevated as 220/120 mm Hg unless there is another medical reason not to do this. The rationale remains that autohypertension may maintain CBF in the face of impaired autoregulation after stroke, particularly in the penumbra. There is the associated belief that lowering the blood pressure could expand the size of the present infarct. The specific clinical trials that have demonstrated this are scant. Investigators have begun to examine this finding in rigorous clinical trials, though in the recently completed Scandinavian Candesartan Acute Stroke Study, treatment with candesartan was associated with a trend toward worse outcomes, primarily because of worsening neurologic status.[131] In phase II trials that enrolled both ICH and ischemic stroke patients, lowering of the blood pressure was not associated with worsening clinical deterioration.[132]

Salvaging the penumbra by improving blood flow to the region has been the rationale for many of the acute stroke trials. An alternative approach has been to reverse the biochemical pathways in the ischemic penumbra so as to prevent the progression to infarction, and thereby salvage more tissue than just with thrombolysis. Many of the agents have been successful in animal models. In specific G_{M1} calcium channel antagonists, anti–intercellular adhesion molecule 1 antibodies, G_{M1} ganglioside, γ-aminobutyric acid agonists, and sodium channel antagonists have all been tried unsuccessfully.[133] Preventing glutamate excitotoxicity at the level of the NMDA receptor has been a particularly attractive target, as has targeting free radicals. Gavistenel, a glycine antagonist of the NMDA receptor that reduces glutamate receptor depolarization, was not associated with improvement in clinical outcomes in two separate trials.[134,135] In the SAINT (Stroke Acute Ischemic NXY-059 Trial) I trial, patients were randomized to NXY-059 (a free radical scavenger) versus placebo, and there appeared to be a trend toward improvement in mRS at 3 months.[136] These findings were, however, not replicated in the SAINT II trial.[137] The reason for the failures of all these clinical trials points in part to the imperfect animal models for ischemic stroke.

The patient is found to have an M3 branch occlusion and as such does not receive acute IV thrombolysis or endovascular treatment. She is started on aspirin 325 mg daily. Her neuroimaging shows a final infarct size of less than one-third of the middle cerebral artery, and CT angiography shows 90% stenosis of the ipsilateral internal carotid artery (ICA) near its bifurcation. What is the next appropriate stage in management?

Carotid revascularization remains one of the most effective secondary prevention strategies for ischemic stroke in the setting of atherosclerotic stenosis of greater than 70%,[138] and in many centers carotid endarterectomy (CEA) remains the procedure of choice. Recent controversies have emerged regarding the timing of surgical intervention, and whether endovascular modalities are superior. The optimal modality for revascularization appears to be dependant on patient characteristics. In the recently completed Carotid Revascularization Endarterectomy versus Stenting Trial (CREST) investigators found that carotid angioplasty-stenting (CAS) had a similar rate to CEA for the composite end-point of stroke, myocardial infarction, or death.[139] Investigators found that CAS was associated with a higher risk of perioperative stroke, while CEA was associated with a higher risk of perioperative MI. Pooled data from United States and European trials support that the greatest clinical benefit is derived from revascularization performed within the first 2 weeks of ischemic stroke,[140] and recent guidelines support earlier treatment in patients with a minor stroke or transient ischemic attack (TIA).[6] In patients with a larger area of cerebral infarction, it may be reasonable to wait longer to minimize the risk of hemorrhagic conversion and allow the patient to recover. On the other hand, whether patients with symptomatic intracranial atherosclerotic stenosis should receive endovascular treatment remains in doubt given excessive stroke risk in the endovascular arm of the SAMMPRIS trial.[141]

The patient is instead found to have a carotid terminus occlusion. Intravenous and intra-arterial treatments are unsuccessful at recanalization. Follow-up head CT reveals complete infarction of the middle cerebral artery region. How would you manage the patient when he remains awake with symmetric and briskly reactive pupils?

The main life-threatening condition for this patient is malignant cerebral edema with subsequent herniation. Complete MCA infarctions can be found in up to 10% of all acute stroke patients, while malignant MCA comprises those patients who have a subsequent decline in their level of alertness and ventilatory capacity; this will typically occur in the first 24 to 48 hours and can peak at days 3 to 5 after the initial injury.[142] Treatment options for preventing malignant cerebral edema include at this point: (1) Monitoring his neurologic examination every 2 to 4 hours in the NeuroICU or stroke unit to assess for signs of elevated intracranial pressure (ICP); (2) starting hypertonic saline (23.4% boluses recommended as a rescue therapy over continuous infusion of 3% to achieve a certain sodium target) or mannitol boluses (1.0 to 1.5 g/kg); and (3) performing an early hemicraniectomy within 72 hours electively. A proposed clinical pathway for management of these patients is outlined in Figure 5-8.

Maintaining normoglycemia has been advocated by some to prevent malignant cerebral edema, but its effectiveness has yet to be proven. Prophylactic normothermia, or even hypothermia to 35.5°C, has also been carried out with the belief that this could spare the need for hemicraniectomy, although the clinical effectiveness remains unproven for prevention of edema. The potential for harm is substantial from shivering, infection, or coagulopathy when used empirically. Treatment with hypertonic saline is unlikely to be effective in preventing malignant cerebral edema in this case and holds the potential for harm.

In addition, although treatment with hypertonic saline may appear to be effective, the patient may become dependent on the treatment and it cannot be withdrawn without precipitating herniation. In addition, continued and prophylactic hypertonic saline may be associated with adverse medical outcomes, and specifically volume overload, lung injury, and hypernatremia, although not all groups have observed these adverse outcomes.[143] Hemicraniectomy is a viable option for this patient; however, the hemicraniectomy trials have required the presence of impaired alertness (most notably a score of at least 1 in the 1a item on the NIHSS) and an NIHSS greater than 15.[144] In the trials, treatment needed to be carried out within 45 hours from stroke onset, although there is heterogeneity in this criterion. The most prudent course of action in this case may be watchful waiting for at least 5 days, during which the maximum amount of cerebral edema is expected.

The patient becomes slightly more difficult to arouse, but still wakes up to a loud verbal stimulation and otherwise has no other signs of elevated ICP. There is no fever. What are the treatment options now?

At this time, it should be assumed that the patient has an elevated ICP and midline shift, and repeat a head CT to evaluate midline shift or the presence of hemorrhagic transformation. It has remained difficult to establish which patients with a complete MCA infarction will progress to have a malignant course (Figure 5-9), but it appears that those with first stroke, female gender, young age, heart failure,

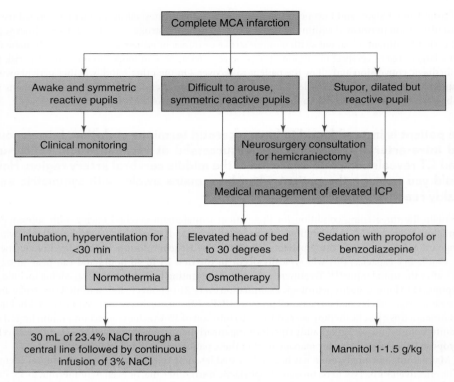

Figure 5-8. Proposed clinical pathway for management of elevated ICP due to ischemic stroke. ICP, intracranial pressure; MCA, middle cerebral artery.

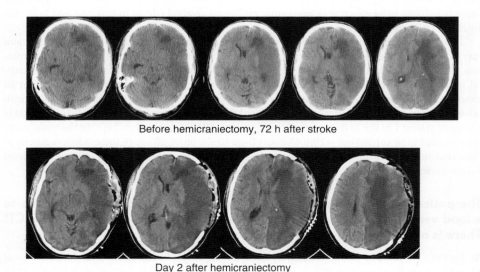

Figure 5-9. Computed tomographic scan of the head before and after hemicraniectomy in a patient with malignant middle cerebral artery infarction.

greater than 50% involvement of the MCA region, carotid occlusion and an abnormal ipsilateral circle of Willis, insufficient leptomeningeal vessels, involvement of the anterior choroidal artery region, and serum biomarkers correlating with infarct volume (such as S100B greater than 1.03 μg/L) are at higher risk.[145-148] The most important predictor may be the overall size of the infarct, and identification of the other factors should not be used to select candidates for hemicraniectomy before there is transtentorial herniation.[149]

The treatment options remain the same before the patient becomes somnolent. In this case, the clinical trial data clearly support the use of hemicraniectomy. A pooled analysis of three separate European clinical trials required the previously noted inclusion criteria, as well as greater than 50% involvement of the MCA distribution. In the trials, patients aged 18 to 60 years were randomized to early hemicraniectomy versus maximal medical management and followed for 1 year for the main clinical outcomes of a favorable mRS (0 to 4), as well as mRS of 3 or less and death. The surgical arm had an overwhelming benefit in all of the clinical outcomes. The number needed to treat in these studies was two, and there was a benefit regardless of which side the infarct was on.[144] The trial did not require an absolute cutoff of midline shift, and using an absolute cutoff to trigger hemicraniectomy is potentially dangerous. Predicting the outcome of surgical decompression remains difficult, and there have been no clear associations between outcome and size of the infarct, although in one case series age older than 50 years was a poor prognostic sign.[150] The trials leave many open questions, including the timing of when to operate and whether their outcomes are clinically meaningful to patients and their families. Depending on the patient's age, atrophy, and involvement of the medial temporal lobe, surprisingly small amounts of midline shift can be associated with injury to the thalamus and midbrain.

While awaiting surgery, the patient becomes unresponsive and his left pupil is dilated (but still reactive). What are the treatment options now?

Medical treatment has been advocated by many clinicians, but the clinical evidence is not particularly strong, and clinical trials and case series demonstrate no change in the high mortality rate in medically treated patients.[142] Treatment strategies in lieu of hemicraniectomy that have been suggested include osmotherapy (with mannitol, glycerol, or hypertonic saline), steroids, barbiturate coma, hyperventilation, and head elevation.[151-153] All of these therapies remain unproven (and transient in effect) in clinical trials, hold the potential for harm,[142] and should only be used as temporizing measures before surgery. Animal models and early studies indicate that hypothermia remains a promising medical treatment for patients with malignant MCA infarction, although it has yet to be tested in a blinded prospective clinical trial.[142]

The most effective treatment in this condition is emergent surgical decompression, with all other medical interventions being aimed at stabilizing the patient in preparation for the operating room. Rapid intubation is advised, both to prevent pneumonia as well as to help manage ICP. Hyperventilation can be effective at reducing ICP by reducing CBV via vasoconstriction of distal arterioles, although in the long-term this same process could precipitate cerebral injury. Hyperventilation is carried out with the help of an end-tidal CO_2 monitor, with a goal of 30 mm Hg, and for no longer than 30 minutes. After intubation the head of the bed should be maintained at 30 degrees, and sedation should be used to minimize agitation that might increase ICP; use of propofol may be helpful owing to its short half-life, although in select cases dexmedetomidine or midazolam may be considered. If surgery will not be carried out, sedation should be maintained, but at this point an ICP monitor is advisable. Discussion of the type of monitor is beyond the scope of this chapter.

Normothermia is an important component of medical treatment in preparation for surgery, although hypothermia may be necessary for intractable cases of high ICP; prevention of shivering in that case may be important to reduce ICP as well. Strategies to treat shivering will be covered in more detail in other chapters. For rapid lowering of ICP, osmotherapy is carried out at the same time as all of the above interventions. It is advisable to use either (or combination of) a 30-mL bolus of IV 23.4% sodium chloride given through a central line over 5 minutes or 1.0 to 1.5 g/kg of 10% mannitol solution, depending on the volume status. Hypertonic saline in the acute setting may be safer and per-haps more effective based on the trauma literature,[154] and has been associated with improvements in multimodality intracranial monitoring parameters[155,156] as well as reversal of transtentorial hernia-tion.[157] Hypertonic saline may be preferable because of a more rapid infusion time; how quickly each agent can be obtained and whether the patient has a central line frequently are the deciding factors in choosing one over the other.

The management of space-occupying infarcts in the posterior fossa is not as clear as in those with middle cerebral artery infarcts. Case series have pointed to a similar risk of cerebellar tonsilar herniation for infarcts of greater than 3 cm in size or those that involve the entire posterior-inferior cerebellar artery distribution, as in cerebellar hemorrhage. However, whether these patients should undergo prophylactic suboccipital decompression is unknown, but the differences in the herniation syndromes between cerebellar and cerebral edema should be considered.

A 61-year-old man with hypertension and coronary artery disease with a coronary bypass graft performed last year presents to the ED 12 hours after onset of left-sided weakness. Three days before he had developed transient visual loss in the right eye. His blood pres-sure on arrival at the ED was 168/78 mm Hg, heart rate 68 bpm, and respiratory rate 16 breaths/min. His examination revealed mild-left hemineglect, left hemiparesis, and a left visual field cut. His cardiac and pulmonary examinations were normal, and the electrocardiogram (ECG) showed normal sinus rhythm with no ischemic changes. The NIHSS was 12. CT head scan revealed small infarcts in the internal border zone region. Brain CTA showed complete occlusion of the right internal carotid artery. He was placed in Trendelenburg position and given 500 mL of intravenous saline. His examination improved to an NIHSS of 4. However, in the next few days he continued to worsen, despite treatment with pressors, up to a blood pressure of 220/120 mm Hg, and he developed a right middle cerebral artery infarction.

What is the next step in evaluation and treatment?

The patient was treated empirically in the ED with maneuvers to improve the blood pressure given the presence of an ICA occlusion. Currently, there are little clinical trial data to support such maneuvers, and many of the published case series are hindered by the lack of blinded neurologic assessments before, during, and after treatment with pressors. Early hypotension in some clinical trials and case series has been associated with poor neurologic outcomes and stroke-related mortality,[158] while the AHA guidelines recommend allowing blood pressure up to 220/120 mm Hg in the acute setting unless there is evidence of end-organ damage.[20] In the latter guidelines, pressor-induced hypertension for acute stroke was not recommended for most patients, while reviews indicate there is insufficient evidence for the routine induction of hypertension.[159] However, the cause and effect of hypotension after stroke with poor outcomes has not been established; for example, hypotension could be a mani-festation of poor cardiac function, which would predispose patients to adverse outcomes. On the other hand, animal and human studies have established the presence of an ischemic penumbra, where cerebral autoregulation is also impaired and where CBF and cerebral metabolic rate of oxygen can be improved with augmentation of the blood pressure.[158,160] In addition, the recently completed angio-tensin receptor blocker candesartan for treatment of acute stroke trial showed a trend toward poor neurologic outcomes in patients treated early with the study medication.[161]

Case series in the interim have shown improvements in NIHSS and other clinical measures by treatments with pressors.[162] Few trials of empirically raising the blood pressure in acute stroke have been done. It is important, however, to note that potential dangers do exist with raising the blood pressure, including inducing myocardial ischemia, potentiating pulmonary edema, or worsening neurologic outcome. The latter was explored in the DCLHb study, where ischemic stroke patients were treated in a placebo-controlled safety study with a hemoglobin-based oxygen-carrying solution (DCLHb) that induces brisk increases in blood pressure. In this study, participants treated with the study medication had greater odds of unfavorable outcomes (mRS 3 to 6) as well as medical complications and mortality.[163] This study has guided the latest *Cochrane Database System Review* to recommend against routine induction of hypertension,[164] although it is difficult to gauge if it was the actual agent used versus induction of blood pressure. It may be reasonable to consider inducing hypertension with vasoactive agents in patients who have evidence of a large area of perfusion deficit on imaging and no evidence of myocardial ischemia. In that instance, systematic examinations at pre-established time points with the NIHSS are important, especially those done by blinded adjudicators; these patients should be monitored carefully for cardiac and pulmonary complications.

Other promising areas of clinical care to enhance cerebral blood flow include transient partial aortic occlusion by the use of the NeuroFlo (CoAxia, Maple Grove, MN) device, which is occasionally used for refractory vasospasms after subarachnoid hemorrhage, although this device has yet to be formally tested in large clinical trials.[165]

What are the complications to expect after ischemic stroke?

Neurologic Complications

Patients with large cerebral infarctions may be at risk for other complications beyond herniation. Hemorrhagic conversion after ischemic stroke in patients who do not receive thrombolysis is most strongly associated with a cardioembolic etiology. Hemorrhagic transformation can peak at up to 2 weeks after ischemic stroke. Seizures and status epilepticus in the acute setting are unusual presenting symptoms or complications in ischemic stroke, but any patient with a more severe neurologic examination than the neuroimaging would suggest should be monitored. Antiepileptic medications are not routinely used in ischemic stroke patients, even in those with space-occupying infarcts, particularly due to the concern of the neurotoxic properties of some agents.

Infections

Infectious complications are some of the most likely outcomes in stroke patients and account for a significant proportion of the early morbidity in the care of stroke patients. Pneumonia, usually due to aspiration, is present in as many as 22% of stroke admissions at some point in their hospitalization[166] and is more likely in patients with dysarthria/dysphasia, age older than 65 years, cognitive impairment, and a failed bedside water swallow evaluation.[167] Urinary tract infections (UTIs) are also very common in stroke patients and present in up to 24% of patients during their inpatient admission.[166] Bladder dysfunction is very common in the acute period, although in our experience UTIs are more likely to occur as a result of inappropriately prolonged periods of indwelling urinary catheters. Both pneumonia and UTI have been associated with poorer functional outcomes in several studies.[168,169] Some clinicians have advocated prophylactic antibiotics early in the clinical course of patients with large ischemic strokes,[170,171] although this has not been proven in other clinical trials.[172] Admission to an organized inpatient stroke unit is one of the few interventions that reduces in-hospital mortality rate after stroke, and the mechanism appears to be through reduction of infectious complications.[173] Although less frequently documented in clinical studies, we have also observed occasionally life-threatening infections from peripheral IV lines. Our practice is to revisit on a daily basis whether patients require indwelling catheters and IV lines.

Cardiovascular Events

The incidence of ST-elevation myocardial infarction during the hospital stay is rare, but elevated troponins are observed in up to 18% of stroke patients.[174,175] Some myocardial infarctions will manifest as a non–ST-segment elevation event, and may not have associated chest pain, and as such it is often assumed to be secondary to neurocardiogenic origins. Troponin elevations from cardiac stunning are less likely in ischemic stroke than they are in hemorrhagic strokes, and they are most likely to occur in individuals with large hemispheric infarcts. It is still reasonable to assume based on epidemiologic data that patients with ischemic stroke also have atherosclerotic coronary artery disease. Treatment of myocardial infarction after ischemic stroke remains difficult when there are competing interests between the brain and the heart in relation to blood pressure management and antithrombotics. Unless there is an ST-elevation myocardial infarction, we avoid cardiac catheterization because of the possible need for multiple antithrombotic agents; for this same reason we also avoid IV heparin unless there is an imminent need for a cardiac catheterization. Decompensated congestive heart failure is an additional cardiac problem we have observed in our stroke patients, and in most cases it appears to be due to withholding diuretics to induce autohypertension. In general, it is reasonable to continue patients' diuretics and β blockers to prevent pulmonary edema or rebound tachycardia.

Pulmonary Complications

Pulmonary embolus (PE) remains one of the most preventable medical complications of any stroke subtype. The incidence of deep vein thrombosis (DVT) and pulmonary embolus is less than 3% in all stroke admissions.[166] Treatment with prophylactic heparinoids as early as possible is clearly warranted in all stroke patients unless there is a clear medical contraindication; HI-1 and HI-2 hemorrhagic transformation patients should probably not have their DVT prophylaxis withheld. It appears that the use of compression stockings alone is not sufficient after stroke to prevent DVT.[176]

Respiratory failure after stroke is not only associated with malignant MCA infarcts, but can also be present in other stroke subtypes and independent of cardiopulmonary injury. Independent risk factors for mortality in respiratory failure after ischemic stroke include age older than 60 years and a Glasgow Coma Scale (GCS) score less than 10, while respiratory failure is associated with a low probability of survival (33%) 2 years after stroke.[177] In a sample of patients with stroke and mechanical ventilation in Northern Manhattan Hospital mortality rate, was as high as 50% in ischemic stroke patients and higher in the hemorrhagic stroke subtypes.[178] It is unclear to what degree this is influenced by the decision to withdraw care in these patients by the family, and a cause and effect pathway is difficult to establish. As such, intubation should not be withheld for procedures, particularly when intubation is not felt to be permanently required.[179]

Death

In-hospital mortality rate after ischemic stroke is low overall, with one large series from Germany indicating a rate close to 5% and a higher rate being reported in other case series. The causes of death within 30 days after ischemic stroke is heterogeneous, but medical complications remain at the forefront, with pneumonia being a principal cause of death following stroke.[34,168,180] Case series have also described atrial fibrillation as a risk factor for in-hospital mortality, although it is not clear if this is related to the larger infarcts observed in this population or due to underlying cardiac disease.[181-183] Out of all the complications after stroke, the most likely one to be associated with mortality is elevated ICP and cerebral perfusion failure.[180]

! CRITICAL CONSIDERATIONS

- Stroke is the most common neurologic emergency in developed countries.
- Ischemic stroke is treatable, but only a small proportion of patients will receive IV r-tPA.

- IV r-tPA is indicated for eligible acute stroke patients within 3 hours from onset, but may be beneficial between 3.0 and 4.5 hours. The 2009 AHA/ASA scientific advisory board has class I (benefit is greater than risk) recommendations for those who meet the eligibility criteria and exclusion criteria set out by ECASS III (ie, excluding age older than 80 years, on anticoagulants regardless of INR, NIHSS greater than 25, and history of prior stroke and diabetes); and class IIB (benefit if either greater than or equal to risk) recommendation for those who do not meet the additional exclusion criteria. For class I recommendation, it is advisable that the treating physician gives the IV r-tPA therapy, and for class IIB, it is advisable that the treating physician "may consider" giving the IV r-tPA.

- Malignant cerebral edema is an important cause of early neurologic decompensation and mortality, and adequately powered and designed clinical trials document the effectiveness of hemicraniectomy in improving mortality rate and long-term outcome.

- Medical complications remain an important cause of morbidity and mortality in ischemic stroke patients and include infection such as hospital-acquired pneumonia, sepsis, DVT/PE, and cardiovascular diseases.

REFERENCES

1. Rosamond W, Flegal K, Furie K, et al. Heart disease and stroke statistics—2008 update: A report from the American Heart Association Statistics Committee and Stroke Statistics Subcommittee. *Circulation.* 2008;117:e25-146.

2. Kleindorfer D, Kissela B, Schneider A, et al. Eligibility for recombinant tissue plasminogen activator in acute ischemic stroke: A population-based study. *Stroke.* 2004;35:e27-29.

3. Schumacher HC, Bateman BT, Boden-Albala B, et al. Use of thrombolysis in acute ischemic stroke: Analysis of the nationwide inpatient sample 1999 to 2004. *Ann Emerg Med.* 2007;50:99-107.

4. Bambauer KZ, Johnston SC, Bambauer DE, Zivin JA. Reasons why few patients with acute stroke receive tissue plasminogen activator. *Arch Neurol.* 2006;63:661-664.

5. Cocho D, Belvis R, Marti-Fabregas J, Molina-Porcel L, et al. Reasons for exclusion from thrombolytic therapy following acute ischemic stroke. *Neurology.* 2005;64:719-720.

6. Furie KL, Kasner SE, Adams RJ, et al. Guidelines for the prevention of stroke in patients with stroke or transient ischemic attack. A guideline for healthcare professionals from the American Heart Association/American Stroke Association. *Stroke.* 2011;42:227-276.

7. Willey JZ, Xu Q, Boden-Albala B, et al. Lipid profile components and risk of ischemic stroke: The Northern Manhattan Study (NOMAS). *Arch Neurol.* 2009;66:1400-1406.

8. Shahar E, Chambless LE, Rosamond WD, et al. Plasma lipid profile and incident ischemic stroke: The Atherosclerosis Risk in Communities (ARIC) study. *Stroke.* 2003;34:623-631.

9. Sacco RL. Clinical practice. Extracranial carotid stenosis. *N Engl J Med.* 2001;345:1113-1118.

10. Kothari RU, Pancioli A, Liu T, Brott T, Broderick J. Cincinnati prehospital stroke scale: Reproducibility and validity. *Ann Emerg Med.* 1999;33:373-378.

11. Kasner SE. Clinical interpretation and use of stroke scales. *Lancet Neurol.* 2006;5:603-612.

12. Barber PA, Hill MD, Eliasziw M, et al. Imaging of the brain in acute ischaemic stroke: Comparison of computed tomography and magnetic resonance diffusion-weighted imaging. *J Neurol Neurosurg Psychiatry.* 2005;76:1528-1533.

13. Powers WJ. Cerebral hemodynamics in ischemic cerebrovascular disease. *Ann Neurol.* 1991;29:231-240.

14. Derdeyn CP, Videen TO, Yundt KD, et al. Variability of cerebral blood volume and oxygen extraction: Stages of cerebral haemodynamic impairment revisited. *Brain.* 2002;125:595-607.

15. Krol AL, Dzialowski I, Roy J, et al. Incidence of radiocontrast nephropathy in patients undergoing acute stroke computed tomography angiography. *Stroke.* 2007;38:2364-2366.

16. Merten GJ, Burgess WP, Gray LV, et al. Prevention of contrast-induced nephropathy with sodium bicarbonate: A randomized controlled trial. *JAMA.* 2004;291:2328-2334.

17. Srinivasan A, Goyal M, Al Azri F, Lum C. State-of-the-art imaging of acute stroke. *Radiographics.* 2006;269(suppl 1):S75-S95.

18. Foerch C, Montaner J, Furie KL, Ning MM, Lo EH. Invited article: Searching for oracles? Blood biomarkers in acute stroke. *Neurology.* 2009;73:393-399.

19. The National Institute of Neurological Disorders and Stroke rt-PA Stroke Study Group. Tissue plasminogen activator for acute ischemic stroke. *N Engl J Med.* 1995;333:1581-1587.

20. Adams HP Jr, del Zoppo G, Alberts MJ, et al. Guidelines for the early management of adults with ischemic stroke: A guideline from the American Heart Association/American Stroke Association Stroke Council, Clinical Cardiology Council, Cardiovascular Radiology And Intervention Council, and the Atherosclerotic Peripheral Vascular Disease and Quality of Care Outcomes in Research Interdisciplinary Working Groups: The American Academy of Neurology affirms the value of this guideline as an educational tool for neurologists. *Stroke.* 2007;38:1655-1711.

21. Hacke W, Donnan G, Fieschi C, et al. Association of outcome with early stroke treatment: Pooled analysis of ATLANTIS, ECASS, and NINDS rt-PA stroke trials. *Lancet.* 2004;363:768-774.

22. Marler JR, Tilley BC, Lu M, et al. Early stroke treatment associated with better outcome: The NINDS rt-Pa stroke study. *Neurology.* 2000;55:1649-1655.

23. White-Bateman SR, Schumacher HC, Sacco RL, Appelbaum PS. Consent for intravenous thrombolysis in acute stroke: Review and future directions. *Arch Neurol.* 2007;64:785-792.

24. Pervez MA, Silva G, Masrur S, et al. Remote supervision of IV-tPA for acute ischemic stroke by telemedicine or telephone before transfer to a regional stroke center is feasible and safe. *Stroke.* 2010;41:e18-24.

25. Rost NS, Masrur S, Pervez MA, Viswanathan A, Schwamm LH. Unsuspected coagulopathy rarely prevents IV thrombolysis in acute ischemic stroke. *Neurology.* 2009;73:1957-1962.

26. Alexandrov AV, Grotta JC. Arterial reocclusion in stroke patients treated with intravenous tissue plasminogen activator. *Neurology.* 2002;59:862-867.

27. Alexandrov AV, Molina CA, Grotta JC, et al. Ultrasound-enhanced systemic thrombolysis for acute ischemic stroke. *N Engl J Med.* 2004;351:2170-2178.

28. Alexandrov AV. Ultrasound enhancement of fibrinolysis. *Stroke.* 2009;40:S107-S110.

29. Alexandrov AV, Mikulik R, Ribo M, et al. A pilot randomized clinical safety study of sonothrombolysis augmentation with ultrasound-activated perflutren-lipid microspheres for acute ischemic stroke. *Stroke.* 2008;39:1464-1469.

30. Molina CA, Ribo M, Rubiera M, et al. Microbubble administration accelerates clot lysis during continuous 2-Mhz ultrasound monitoring in stroke patients treated with intravenous tissue plasminogen activator. *Stroke.* 2006;37:425-429.

31. Pancioli AM, Broderick J, Brott T, et al. The combined approach to lysis utilizing eptifibatide and rt-PA in acute ischemic stroke: The clear stroke trial. *Stroke.* 2008;39:3268-3276.

32. Martin-Schild S, Hallevi H, Albright KC, et al. Aggressive blood pressure–lowering treatment before intravenous tissue plasminogen activator therapy in acute ischemic stroke. *Arch Neurol.* 2008;65:1174-1178.

33. Smith EE, Abdullah AR, Petkovska I, Rosenthal E, Koroshetz WJ, Schwamm LH. Poor outcomes in patients who do not receive intravenous tissue plasminogen activator because of mild or improving ischemic stroke. *Stroke.* 2005;36:2497-2499.

34. Rajajee V, Kidwell C, Starkman S, et al. Early MRI and outcomes of untreated patients with mild or improving ischemic stroke. *Neurology.* 2006;67:980-984.

35. Nedeltchev K, Schwegler B, Haefeli T, et al. Outcome of stroke with mild or rapidly improving symptoms. *Stroke.* 2007;38:2531-2535.

36. Puetz V, Dzialowski I, Coutts SB, et al. Frequency and clinical course of stroke and transient ischemic attack patients with intracranial nonocclusive thrombus on computed tomographic angiography. *Stroke.* 2009;40:193-199.

37. Fischer U, Baumgartner A, Arnold M, et al. What is a minor stroke? *Stroke.* 2010;41:661-666.

38. van den Berg JS, de Jong G. Why ischemic stroke patients do not receive thrombolytic treatment: Results from a general hospital. *Acta Neurol Scand.* 2009;120:157-160.

39. Chernyshev OY, Martin-Schild S, Albright KC, et al. Safety of tPA in stroke mimics and neuroimaging-negative cerebral ischemia. *Neurology.* 2010;74:1340-1345.

40. Toni D, Lorenzano S, Agnelli G, et al. Intravenous thrombolysis with rt-PA in acute ischemic stroke patients aged older than 80 years in italy. *Cerebrovasc Dis (Basel).* 2008;25:129-135.

41. Pundik S, McWilliams-Dunnigan L, Blackham KL, et al. Older age does not increase risk of hemorrhagic complications after intravenous and/or intra-arterial thrombolysis for acute stroke. *J Stroke Cerebrovasc Dis.* 2008;17:266-272.

42. Amlie-Lefond C, deVeber G, Chan AK, et al. Use of alteplase in childhood arterial ischaemic stroke: A multicentre, observational, cohort study. *Lancet Neurol.* 2009;8:530-536.

43. Janjua N, Nasar A, Lynch JK, Qureshi AI. Thrombolysis for ischemic stroke in children: Data from the nationwide inpatient sample. *Stroke.* 2007;38:1850-1854.

44. Roach ES, Golomb MR, Adams R, et al. Management of stroke in infants and children: A scientific statement from a special writing group of the American Heart Association Stroke Council and the Council On Cardiovascular Disease in the Young. *Stroke.* 2008;39:2644-2691.

45. De Keyser J, Gdovinova Z, Uyttenboogaart M, Vroomen PC, Luijckx GJ. Intravenous alteplase for stroke: Beyond the guidelines and in particular clinical situations. *Stroke.* 2007;38:2612-2618.

46. Prabhakaran S, Rivolta J, Vieira JR, et al. Symptomatic intracerebral hemorrhage among eligible warfarin-treated patients receiving intravenous tissue plasminogen activator for acute ischemic stroke. *Arch Neurol.* 2010;67:559-563.

47. Liang BA, Zivin JA. Empirical characteristics of litigation involving tissue plasminogen activator and ischemic stroke. *Ann Emerg Med.* 2008;52:160-164.

48. Khatri P, Wechsler LR, Broderick JP. Intracranial hemorrhage associated with revascularization therapies. *Stroke.* 2007;38:431-440.

49. Fiorelli M, Bastianello S, von Kummer R, et al. Hemorrhagic transformation within 36 h of a cerebral infarct: Relationships with early clinical deterioration and 3-month outcome in the European Cooperative Acute Stroke Study I (ECASS I) cohort. *Stroke.* 1999;30:2280-2284.

50. Molina CA, Alvarez-Sabin J, Montaner J, et al. Thrombolysis-related hemorrhagic infarction: A marker of early reperfusion, reduced infarct size, and improved outcome in patients with proximal middle cerebral artery occlusion. *Stroke.* 2002;33:1551-1556.

51. Butcher K, Christensen S, Parsons M, et al. Postthrombolysis blood pressure elevation is associated with hemorrhagic transformation. *Stroke.* 2010;41:72-77.

52. Singer OC, Humpich MC, Fiehler J, et al. Risk for symptomatic intracerebral hemorrhage after thrombolysis assessed by diffusion-weighted magnetic resonance imaging. *Ann Neurol.* 2008;63:52-60.

53. Lansberg MG, Thijs VN, Bammer R, et al. Risk factors of symptomatic intracerebral hemorrhage after tPA therapy for acute stroke. *Stroke.* 2007;38:2275-2278.

54. Lansberg MG, Albers GW, Wijman CA. Symptomatic intracerebral hemorrhage following thrombolytic therapy for acute ischemic stroke: A review of the risk factors. *Cerebrovasc Dis (Basel).* 2007;24:1-10.

55. Derex L, Nighoghossian N. Intracerebral haemorrhage after thrombolysis for acute ischaemic stroke: An update. *J Neurol Neurosurg Psychiatry.* 2008;79:1093-1099.

56. Marti-Fabregas J, Bravo Y, Cocho D, et al. Frequency and predictors of symptomatic intracerebral hemorrhage in patients with ischemic stroke treated with recombinant tissue plasminogen activator outside clinical trials. *Cerebrovasc Dis (Basel).* 2007;23:85-90.

57. Uyttenboogaart M, Koch MW, Koopman K, Vroomen PC, De Keyser J, Luijckx GJ. Safety of antiplatelet therapy prior to intravenous thrombolysis in acute ischemic stroke. *Arch Neurol.* 2008;65:607-611.

58. Tanne D, Kasner SE, Demchuk AM, et al. Markers of increased risk of intracerebral hemorrhage after intravenous recombinant tissue plasminogen activator therapy for acute ischemic stroke in clinical practice: The multicenter rt-PA stroke survey. *Circulation.* 2002;105:1679-1685.

59. Uyttenboogaart M, Koch MW, Koopman K, Vroomen PC, Luijckx GJ, De Keyser J. Lipid profile, statin use, and outcome after intravenous thrombolysis for acute ischaemic stroke. *J Neurol.* 2008;255:875-880.

60. Meier N, Nedeltchev K, Brekenfeld C, et al. Prior statin use, intracranial hemorrhage, and outcome after intra-arterial thrombolysis for acute ischemic stroke. *Stroke.* 2009;40:1729-1737.

61. Fiehler J, Albers GW, Boulanger JM, et al. Bleeding risk analysis in stroke imaging before thrombolysis (BRASIL): Pooled analysis of T2*-weighted magnetic resonance imaging data from 570 patients. *Stroke.* 2007;38:2738-2744.

62. Kim HS, Lee DH, Ryu CW, et al. Multiple cerebral microbleeds in hyperacute ischemic stroke: Impact on prevalence and severity of early hemorrhagic transformation after thrombolytic treatment. *AJR Am J Roentgenol.* 2006;186:1443-1449.

63. Palumbo V, Boulanger JM, Hill MD, Inzitari D, Buchan AM. Leukoaraiosis and intracerebral hemorrhage after thrombolysis in acute stroke. *Neurology.* 2007;68:1020-1024.

64. Ribo M, Montaner J, Molina CA, et al. Admission fibrinolytic profile is associated with symptomatic hemorrhagic transformation in stroke patients treated with tissue plasminogen activator. *Stroke.* 2004;35:2123-2127.

65. Cocho D, Borrell M, Marti-Fabregas J, et al. Pretreatment hemostatic markers of symptomatic intracerebral hemorrhage in patients treated with tissue plasminogen activator. *Stroke.* 2006;37:996-999.

66. Kastrup A, Groschel K, Ringer TM, et al. Early disruption of the blood-brain barrier after thrombolytic therapy predicts hemorrhage in patients with acute stroke. *Stroke.* 2008;39:2385-2387.

67. Saqqur M, Tsivgoulis G, Molina CA, et al. Symptomatic intracerebral hemorrhage and recanalization after IV rt-PA: A multicenter study. *Neurology.* 2008;71:1304-1312.

68. Patel SC, Levine SR, Tilley BC, et al. Lack of clinical significance of early ischemic changes on computed tomography in acute stroke. *JAMA.* 2001;286:2830-2838.

69. Gupta R, Yonas H, Gebel J, et al. Reduced pretreatment ipsilateral middle cerebral artery cerebral blood flow is predictive of symptomatic hemorrhage post–intra-arterial thrombolysis in patients with middle cerebral artery occlusion. *Stroke.* 2006;37:2526-2530.

70. Campbell BC, Christensen S, Butcher KS, et al. Regional very low cerebral blood volume predicts hemorrhagic transformation better than diffusion-weighted imaging volume and thresholded apparent diffusion coefficient in acute ischemic stroke. *Stroke.* 2010;41:82-88.

71. Ottomeyer C, Hennerici MG, Szabo K. Raising awareness of orolingual angioedema as a complication of thrombolysis in acute stroke patients. *Cerebrovasc Dis (Basel).* 2009;27:307-308.

72. Hill MD, Barber PA, Takahashi J, Demchuk AM, Feasby TE, Buchan AM. Anaphylactoid reactions and angioedema during alteplase treatment of acute ischemic stroke. *CMAJ.* 2000;162:1281-1284.

73. Liberatore GT, Samson A, Bladin C, Schleuning WD, Medcalf RL. Vampire bat salivary plasminogen activator (desmoteplase): A unique fibrinolytic enzyme that does not promote neurodegeneration. *Stroke.* 2003;34:537-543.

74. Benchenane K, Berezowski V, Ali C, et al. Tissue-type plasminogen activator crosses the intact blood-brain barrier by low-density lipoprotein receptor-related protein-mediated transcytosis. *Circulation.* 2005;111:2241-2249.

75. Reddrop C, Moldrich RX, Beart PM, et al. Vampire bat salivary plasminogen activator (desmoteplase) inhibits tissue-type plasminogen activator-induced potentiation of excitotoxic injury. *Stroke.* 2005;36:1241-1246.

76. Clark WM, Albers GW, Madden KP, Hamilton S. The rtPA (alteplase) 0- to 6-hour acute stroke trial, part A (A0276G): Results of a double-blind, placebo-controlled, multicenter study. Thromblytic therapy in acute ischemic stroke study investigators. *Stroke.* 2000;31:811-816.

77. Clark WM, Wissman S, Albers GW, Jhamandas JH, Madden KP, Hamilton S. Recombinant tissue-type plasminogen activator (alteplase) for ischemic stroke 3 to 5 h after symptom onset. The ATLANTIS study: A randomized controlled trial. Alteplase thrombolysis for acute noninterventional therapy in ischemic stroke. *JAMA.* 1999;282:2019-2026.

78. Hacke W, Kaste M, Fieschi C, et al. Intravenous thrombolysis with recombinant tissue plasminogen activator for acute hemispheric stroke. The European Cooperative Acute Stroke Study (ECASS). *JAMA.* 1995;274:1017-1025.

79. Hacke W, Kaste M, Fieschi C, et al. Randomised double-blind placebo-controlled trial of thrombolytic therapy with intravenous alteplase in acute ischaemic stroke (ECASS II). Second European-Australasian Acute Stroke Study Investigators. *Lancet.* 1998;352:1245-1251.

80. Wahlgren N, Ahmed N, Davalos A, et al. Thrombolysis with alteplase for acute ischaemic stroke in the Safe Implementation of Thrombolysis In Stroke-Monitoring Study (SITS-MOST): An observational study. *Lancet.* 2007;369:275-282.

81. Del Zoppo GJ, Saver JL, Jauch EC, Adams HP Jr. Expansion of the time window for treatment of acute ischemic stroke with intravenous tissue plasminogen activator: A science advisory from the American Heart Association/American Stroke Association. *Stroke.* 2009;40:2945-2948.

82. Hacke W, Kaste M, Bluhmki E, et al. Thrombolysis with alteplase 3 to 4.5 h after acute ischemic stroke. *N Engl J Med.* 2008;359:1317-1329.

83. Darby DG, Barber PA, Gerraty RP, et al. Pathophysiological topography of acute ischemia by combined diffusion-weighted and perfusion MRI. *Stroke.* 1999;30:2043-2052.

84. Rother J, Schellinger PD, Gass A, et al. Effect of intravenous thrombolysis on MRI parameters and functional outcome in acute stroke <6 h. *Stroke.* 2002;33:2438-2445.

85. Lopez-Atalaya JP, Roussel BD, Ali C, et al. Recombinant *Desmodus rotundus* salivary plasminogen activator crosses the blood-brain barrier through a low-density lipoprotein receptor-related protein-dependent mechanism without exerting neurotoxic effects. *Stroke.* 2007;38:1036-1043.

86. Hacke W, Albers G, Al-Rawi Y, et al. The Desmoteplase in Acute Ischemic Stroke Trial (DIAS): A phase II MRI-based 9-hour window acute stroke thrombolysis trial with intravenous desmoteplase. *Stroke.* 2005;36:66-73.

87. Furlan AJ, Eyding D, Albers GW, et al. Dose escalation of Desmoteplase for Acute Ischemic Stroke (DEDAS): Evidence of safety and efficacy 3 to 9 h after stroke onset. *Stroke.* 2006;37:1227-1231.

88. Hacke W, Furlan AJ, Al-Rawi Y, et al. Intravenous desmoteplase in patients with acute ischaemic stroke selected by MRI perfusion-diffusion weighted imaging or perfusion CT (DIAS-2): A prospective, randomised, double-blind, placebo-controlled study. *Lancet Neurol.* 2009;8:141-150.

89. Albers GW, Thijs VN, Wechsler L, et al. Magnetic resonance imaging profiles predict clinical response to early reperfusion: The diffusion and perfusion imaging evaluation for understanding stroke evolution (DEFUSE) study. *Ann Neurol.* 2006;60:508-517.

90. Kakuda W, Lansberg MG, Thijs VN, et al. Optimal definition for PWI/DWI mismatch in acute ischemic stroke patients. *J Cereb Blood Flow Metab.* 2008;28:887-891.

91. Lansberg MG, Thijs VN, Bammer R, et al. The MRA-DWI mismatch identifies patients with stroke who are likely to benefit from reperfusion. *Stroke.* 2008;39:2491-2496.

92. Davis SM, Donnan GA, Parsons MW, et al. Effects of alteplase beyond 3 h after stroke in the Echoplanar Imaging Thrombolytic Evaluation Trial (EPITHET): A placebo-controlled randomised trial. *Lancet Neurol.* 2008;7:299-309.

93. De Silva DA, Fink JN, Christensen S, et al. Assessing reperfusion and recanalization as markers of clinical outcomes after intravenous thrombolysis in the Echoplanar Imaging Thrombolytic Evaluation Trial (EPITHET). *Stroke.* 2009;40:2872-2874.

94. Shih LC, Saver JL, Alger JR, et al. Perfusion-weighted magnetic resonance imaging thresholds identifying core, irreversibly infarcted tissue. *Stroke.* 2003;34:1425-1430.

95. Mishra NK, Albers GW, Davis SM, et al. Mismatch-based delayed thrombolysis: A meta-analysis. *Stroke.* 2010;41:e25-33.

96. Fiebach JB, Schellinger PD. MR mismatch is useful for patient selection for thrombolysis: Yes. *Stroke.* 2009;40:2906-2907.

97. Schabitz WR. MR mismatch is useful for patient selection for thrombolysis: No. *Stroke.* 2009;40:2908-2909.

98. The Abciximab in Ischemic Stroke Investigators. Abciximab in acute ischemic stroke: A randomized, double-blind, placebo-controlled, dose-escalation study. *Stroke.* 2000;31:601-609.

99. Abciximab Emergent Stroke Treatment Trial (AbESTT) Investigators. Emergency administration of abciximab for treatment of patients with acute ischemic stroke: Results of a randomized phase 2 trial. *Stroke.* 2005;36:880-890.

100. Adams HP Jr, Effron MB, Torner J, et al. Emergency administration of abciximab for treatment of patients with acute ischemic stroke: Results of an international phase III trial: Abciximab in Emergency Treatment of Stroke Trial (AbESTT-II). *Stroke.* 2008;39:87-99.

101. CAST: Randomised placebo-controlled trial of early aspirin use in 20,000 patients with acute ischaemic stroke. CAST (Chinese Acute Stroke Trial) Collaborative Group. *Lancet.* 1997;349:1641-1649.

102. The International Stroke Trial (IST): A randomised trial of aspirin, subcutaneous heparin, both, or neither among 19,435 patients with acute ischaemic stroke. International stroke trial collaborative group. *Lancet.* 1997;349:1569-1581.

103. Low molecular weight heparinoid, ORG 10172 (danaparoid), and outcome after acute ischemic stroke: A randomized controlled trial. The Publications Committee for the Trial of ORG 10172 in Acute Stroke Treatment (TOAST) Investigators. *JAMA.* 1998;279:1265-1272.

104. Berge E, Abdelnoor M, Nakstad PH, Sandset PM. Low molecular-weight heparin vs aspirin in patients with acute ischaemic stroke and atrial fibrillation: A double-blind randomised study. HAEST Study Group. Heparin in acute embolic stroke trial. *Lancet.* 2000;355:1205-1210.

105. Meyer DM, Albright KC, Allison TA, Grotta JC. LOAD: A pilot study of the safety of loading of aspirin and clopidogrel in acute ischemic stroke and transient ischemic attack. *J Stroke Cerebrovasc Dis.* 2008;17:26-29.

106. Kennedy J, Hill MD, Ryckborst KJ, Eliasziw M, Demchuk AM, Buchan AM. Fast assessment of stroke and transient ischaemic attack to prevent early recurrence (FASTER): A randomised controlled pilot trial. *Lancet Neurol.* 2007;6:961-969.

107. Diener HC, Bogousslavsky J, Brass LM, et al. Aspirin and clopidogrel compared with clopidogrel alone after recent ischaemic stroke or transient ischaemic attack in high-risk patients (MATCH): Randomised, double-blind, placebo-controlled trial. *Lancet.* 2004;364:331-337.

108. del Zoppo GJ, Higashida RT, Furlan AJ, et al. PROACT: A phase II randomized trial of recombinant pro-urokinase by direct arterial delivery in acute middle cerebral artery stroke. PROACT Investigators. Prolyse in acute cerebral thromboembolism. *Stroke.* 1998;29:4-11.

109. Furlan A, Higashida R, Wechsler L, et al. Intra-arterial prourokinase for acute ischemic stroke. The PROACT II Study: A randomized controlled trial. Prolyse in Acute Cerebral Thromboembolism. *JAMA.* 1999;282:2003-2011.

110. Ogawa A, Mori E, Minematsu K, et al. Randomized trial of intraarterial infusion of urokinase within 6 h of middle cerebral artery stroke: The Middle Cerebral Artery Embolism Local Fibrinolytic

Intervention Trial (MELT) Japan. *Stroke.* 2007;38: 2633-2639.

111. Hallevi H, Barreto AD, Liebeskind DS, et al. Identifying patients at high risk for poor outcome after intra-arterial therapy for acute ischemic stroke. *Stroke.* 2009;40:1780-1785.

112. Lewandowski CA, Frankel M, Tomsick TA, et al. Combined intravenous and intra-arterial r-TPA vs intra-arterial therapy of acute ischemic stroke: Emergency Management of Stroke (EMS) Bridging Trial. *Stroke.* 1999;30:2598-2605.

113. Combined intravenous and intra-arterial recanalization for acute ischemic stroke: The Interventional Management of Stroke Study. *Stroke.* 2004;35:904-911.

114. The Interventional Management of Stroke (IMS) II Study. *Stroke.* 2007;38:2127-2135.

115. Yamaguchi T, Mori E, Minematsu K, et al. Alteplase at 0.6 mg/kg for acute ischemic stroke within 3 h of onset: Japan Alteplase Clinical Trial (J-ACT). *Stroke.* 2006;37:1810-1815.

116. Shaltoni HM, Albright KC, Gonzales NR, et al. Is intra-arterial thrombolysis safe after full-dose intravenous recombinant tissue plasminogen activator for acute ischemic stroke? *Stroke.* 2007;38:80-84.

117. Singer OC, Berkefeld J, Lorenz MW, et al. Risk of symptomatic intracerebral hemorrhage in patients treated with intra-arterial thrombolysis. *Cerebrovasc Dis (Basel).* 2009;27:368-374.

118. Kase CS, Furlan AJ, Wechsler LR, et al. Cerebral hemorrhage after intra-arterial thrombolysis for ischemic stroke: The PROACT II Trial. *Neurology.* 2001;57:1603-1610.

119. Khatri P, Broderick JP, Khoury JC, Carrozzella JA, Tomsick TA. Microcatheter contrast injections during intra-arterial thrombolysis may increase intracranial hemorrhage risk. *Stroke.* 2008;39:3283-3287.

120. Smith WS, Sung G, Starkman S, et al. Safety and efficacy of mechanical embolectomy in acute ischemic stroke: Results of the MERCI trial. *Stroke.* 2005;36:1432-1438.

121. Smith WS, Sung G, Saver J, et al. Mechanical thrombectomy for acute ischemic stroke: Final results of the Multi MERCI trial. *Stroke.* 2008;39:1205-1212.

122. The Penumbra Pivotal Stroke Trial: Safety and effectiveness of a new generation of mechanical devices for clot removal in intracranial large vessel occlusive disease. *Stroke.* 2009;40:2761-2768.

123. Nagel S, Schellinger PD, Hartmann M, et al. Therapy of acute basilar artery occlusion: Intra-arterial thrombolysis alone vs bridging therapy. *Stroke.* 2009;40:140-146.

124. Schonewille WJ, Wijman CA, Michel P, et al. Treatment and outcomes of acute basilar artery occlusion in the Basilar Artery International Cooperation Study (BASICS): A prospective registry study. *Lancet Neurol.* 2009;8: 724-730.

125. Levy EI, Siddiqui AH, Crumlish A, et al. First Food and Drug Administration–approved prospective trial of primary intracranial stenting for acute stroke: SARIS (stent-assisted recanalization in acute ischemic stroke). *Stroke.* 2009;40:3552-3556.

126. Roth C, Papanagiotou P, Behnke S, et al. Stent-assisted mechanical recanalization for treatment of acute intracerebral artery occlusions. *Stroke.* 2010;41:2559-2567.

127. Willey JZ, Elkind MSV. HMG-CoA reductase inhibitors in the treatment of diseases of the central nervous system. *Arch Neurol* 2010;67: 1062-1067.

128. Elkind MS, Flint AC, Sciacca RR, Sacco RL. Lipid-lowering agent use at ischemic stroke onset is associated with decreased mortality. *Neurology.* 2005;65:253-258.

129. Blanco M, Nombela F, Castellanos M, et al. Statin treatment withdrawal in ischemic stroke: A controlled randomized study. *Neurology.* 2007;69:904-910.

130. Elkind MS, Sacco RL, MacArthur RB, et al. The Neuroprotection with Statin Therapy for Acute Recovery Trial (NEUSTART): An adaptive design phase I dose-escalation study of high-dose lovastatin in acute ischemic stroke. *Int J Stroke.* 2008;3:210-218.

131. Sanset EC, Bath PM, Boysen G, et al. The angiotensin-receptor blocker candesartan for treatment of acute stroke (SCAST): a randomised, placebo-controlled, double-blind trial. *Lancet.* 2011;26:741-750.

132. Potter JF, Robinson TG, Ford GA, et al. Controlling hypertension and hypotension immediately post-stroke (CHHIPS): A randomised, placebo-controlled, double-blind pilot trial. *Lancet Neurol.* 2009;8:48-56

133. De Keyser J, Sulter G, Luiten PG. Clinical trials with neuroprotective drugs in acute ischaemic stroke: Are we doing the right thing? *Trends Neurosci.* 1999;22:535-540.

134. Lees KR, Asplund K, Carolei A, et al. Glycine antagonist (gavestinel) in neuroprotection (GAIN International) in patients with acute stroke: A randomised controlled trial. GAIN International Investigators. *Lancet.* 2000;355:1949-1954.

135. Sacco RL, DeRosa JT, Haley EC Jr, et al. Glycine antagonist in neuroprotection for patients with

acute stroke: GAIN Americas: A randomized controlled trial. *JAMA*. 2001;285:1719-1728.

136. Lees KR, Zivin JA, Ashwood T, et al. NXY-059 for acute ischemic stroke. *N Engl J Med*. 2006;354:588-600.

137. Shuaib A, Lees KR, Lyden P, et al. NXY-059 for the treatment of acute ischemic stroke. *N Engl J Med*. 2007;357:562-571.

138. Beneficial effect of carotid endarterectomy in symptomatic patients with high-grade carotid stenosis. North American Symptomatic Carotid Endarterectomy Trial Collaborators. *N Engl J Med*. 1991;325:445-453.

139. Brott TG, Hobson RW 2nd, Howard G, et al. Stenting vs endarterectomy for treatment of carotid-artery stenosis. *N Engl J Med*. 2010;363:11-23.

140. Rothwell PM, Eliasziw M, Gutnikov SA, Warlow CP, Barnett HJ. Endarterectomy for symptomatic carotid stenosis in relation to clinical subgroups and timing of surgery. *Lancet*. 2004;363:915-924.

141. Chimowitz MI, Lynn MJ, Derdeyn CP, et al. Stenting versus aggressive medical therapy for intracranial arterial stenosis. *N Engl J Med*. 2011;365:993-1003.

142. Huttner HB, Schwab S. Malignant middle cerebral artery infarction: Clinical characteristics, treatment strategies, and future perspectives. *Lancet Neurol*. 2009;8:949-958.

143. Froelich M, Ni Q, Wess C, Ougorets I, Hartl R. Continuous hypertonic saline therapy and the occurrence of complications in neurocritically ill patients. *Crit Care Med*. 2009;37:1433-1441.

144. Vahedi K, Hofmeijer J, Juettler E, et al. Early decompressive surgery in malignant infarction of the middle cerebral artery: A pooled analysis of three randomised controlled trials. *Lancet Neurol*. 2007;6:215-222.

145. Ng LK, Nimmannitya J. Massive cerebral infarction with severe brain swelling: A clinicopathological study. *Stroke*. 1970;1:158-163.

146. Bounds JV, Wiebers DO, Whisnant JP, Okazaki H. Mechanisms and timing of deaths from cerebral infarction. *Stroke*. 1981;12:474-477.

147. Jaramillo A, Gongora-Rivera F, Labreuche J, Hauw JJ, Amarenco P. Predictors for malignant middle cerebral artery infarctions: A postmortem analysis. *Neurology*. 2006;66:815-820.

148. Kasner SE, Demchuk AM, Berrouschot J, et al. Predictors of fatal brain edema in massive hemispheric ischemic stroke. *Stroke*. 2001;32:2117-2123.

149. Hofmeijer J, Algra A, Kappelle LJ, van der Worp HB. Predictors of life-threatening brain edema in middle cerebral artery infarction. *Cerebrovasc Dis (Basel)*. 2008;25:176-184.

150. Gupta R, Connolly ES, Mayer S, Elkind MS. Hemicraniectomy for massive middle cerebral artery territory infarction: A systematic review. *Stroke*. 2004;35:539-543.

151. Bardutzky J, Schwab S. Antiedema therapy in ischemic stroke. *Stroke*. 2007;38:3084-3094.

152. Berrouschot J, Rossler A, Koster J, Schneider D. Mechanical ventilation in patients with hemispheric ischemic stroke. *Crit Care Med*. 2000;28:2956-2961.

153. Juttler E, Schellinger PD, Aschoff A, Zweckberger K, Unterberg A, Hacke W. Clinical review: Therapy for refractory intracranial hypertension in ischaemic stroke. *Crit Care (London)*. 2007; 11:231.

154. Kerwin AJ, Schinco MA, Tepas JJ 3rd, Renfro WH, Vitarbo EA, Muehlberger M. The use of 23.4% hypertonic saline for the management of elevated intracranial pressure in patients with severe traumatic brain injury: A pilot study. *J Trauma*. 2009;67:277-282.

155. Al-Rawi PG, Tseng MY, Richards HK, et al. Hypertonic saline in patients with poor-grade subarachnoid hemorrhage improves cerebral blood flow, brain tissue oxygen, and pH. *Stroke*. 2010;41:122-128.

156. Oddo M, Levine JM, Frangos S, et al. Effect of mannitol and hypertonic saline on cerebral oxygenation in patients with severe traumatic brain injury and refractory intracranial hypertension. *J Neurol Neurosurg Psychiatry*. 2009;80:916-920.

157. Koenig MA, Bryan M, Lewin JL 3rd, Mirski MA, Geocadin RG, Stevens RD. Reversal of transtentorial herniation with hypertonic saline. *Neurology*. 2008;70:1023-1029.

158. Mistri AK, Robinson TG, Potter JF. Pressor therapy in acute ischemic stroke: Systematic review. *Stroke*. 2006;37:1565-1571.

159. Geeganage C, Bath PM. Interventions for deliberately altering blood pressure in acute stroke. *Cochrane Database Syst Rev*. 2008:CD000039.

160. Shin HK, Nishimura M, Jones PB, et al. Mild induced hypertension improves blood flow and oxygen metabolism in transient focal cerebral ischemia. *Stroke*. 2008;39:1548-1555.

161. Sandset EC, Bath PM, Boysen G, et al. The angiotensin-receptor blocker candesartan for treatment of acute stroke (SCAST): A randomised, placebo-controlled, double-blind trial. *Lancet*. 2011;377:741-750.

162. Rordorf G, Koroshetz WJ, Ezzeddine MA, Segal AZ, Buonanno FS. A pilot study of drug-induced hypertension for treatment of acute stroke. *Neurology*. 2001;56:1210-1213.

163. Saxena R, Wijnhoud AD, Carton H, et al. Controlled safety study of a hemoglobin-based oxygen carrier, DCLHb, in acute ischemic stroke. *Stroke.* 1999;30:993-996.

164. Geeganage C, Bath PM. Vasoactive drugs for acute stroke. *Cochrane Database Syst Rev.* 2010: CD002839.

165. Liebeskind DS. Aortic occlusion for cerebral ischemia: From theory to practice. *Curr Cardiol Rep.* 2008;10:31-36.

166. Langhorne P, Stott DJ, Robertson L, et al. Medical complications after stroke: A multicenter study. *Stroke.* 2000;31:1223-1229.

167. Sellars C, Bowie L, Bagg J, et al. Risk factors for chest infection in acute stroke: A prospective cohort study. *Stroke.* 2007;38:2284-2291.

168. Aslanyan S, Weir CJ, Diener HC, Kaste M, Lees KR. Pneumonia and urinary tract infection after acute ischaemic stroke: A tertiary analysis of the GAIN International trial. *Eur J Neurol.* 2004;11:49-53.

169. Hong KS, Kang DW, Koo JS, et al. Impact of neurological and medical complications on 3-month outcomes in acute ischaemic stroke. *Eur J Neurol.* 2008;15:1324-1331.

170. Harms H, Prass K, Meisel C, et al. Preventive antibacterial therapy in acute ischemic stroke: A randomized controlled trial. *PLoS One.* 2008;3:e2158.

171. Schwarz S, Al-Shajlawi F, Sick C, Meairs S, Hennerici MG. Effects of prophylactic antibiotic therapy with mezlocillin plus sulbactam on the incidence and height of fever after severe acute ischemic stroke: The Mannheim Infection in Stroke Study (MISS). *Stroke.* 2008;39:1220-1227.

172. Chamorro A, Horcajada JP, Obach V, et al. The Early Systemic Prophylaxis of Infection After Stroke study: A randomized clinical trial. *Stroke.* 2005;36:1495-1500.

173. Govan L, Langhorne P, Weir CJ. Does the prevention of complications explain the survival benefit of organized inpatient (stroke unit) care?: Further analysis of a systematic review. *Stroke.* 2007;38:2536-2540.

174. Indredavik B, Rohweder G, Naalsund E, Lydersen S. Medical complications in a comprehensive stroke unit and an early supported discharge service. *Stroke.* 2008;39:414-420.

175. Kerr G, Ray G, Wu O, Stott DJ, Langhorne P. Elevated troponin after stroke: A systematic review. *Cerebrovasc Dis (Basel).* 2009;28:220-226.

176. Dennis M, Sandercock PA, Reid J, et al. Effectiveness of thigh-length graduated compression stockings to reduce the risk of deep vein thrombosis after stroke (CLOTS trial 1): A multicentre, randomised controlled trial. *Lancet.* 2009;373:1958-1965.

177. Schielke E, Busch MA, Hildenhagen T, et al. Functional, cognitive and emotional long-term outcome of patients with ischemic stroke requiring mechanical ventilation. *J Neurol.* 2005;252:648-654.

178. Mayer SA, Copeland D, Bernardini GL, et al. Cost and outcome of mechanical ventilation for life-threatening stroke. *Stroke.* 2000;31:2346-2353.

179. Foerch C, Kessler KR, Steckel DA, Steinmetz H, Sitzer M. Survival and quality of life outcome after mechanical ventilation in elderly stroke patients. *J Neurol Neurosurg Psychiatry.* 2004;75:988-993.

180. Heuschmann PU, Kolominsky-Rabas PL, Misselwitz B, et al. Predictors of in-hospital mortality and attributable risks of death after ischemic stroke: The German Stroke Registers Study Group. *Arch Intern Med.* 2004;164:1761-1768.

181. Kaarisalo MM, Immonen-Raiha P, Marttila RJ, et al. Arial fibrillation and stroke. Mortality and causes of death after the first acute ischemic stroke. *Stroke.* 1997;28:311-315.

182. Kimura K, Minematsu K, Yamaguchi T. Atrial fibrillation as a predictive factor for severe stroke and early death in 15,831 patients with acute ischaemic stroke. *J Neurol Neurosurg Psychiatry.* 2005;76:679-683.

183. Roquer J, Rodriguez-Campello A, Gomis M, et al. Comparison of the impact of atrial fibrillation on the risk of early death after stroke in women vs men. *J Neurol.* 2006;253:1484-1489.

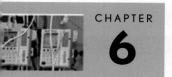

CHAPTER

6

Neuromuscular Diseases

Jennifer Frontera, MD

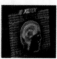

A 26-year-old woman with no past medical history presents to the emergency department (ED) with several days of fatigue, difficulty climbing stairs, and double vision. She has one-word dyspnea and appears to be using accessory muscles of respiration. Her chest radiograph is normal as are all her initial laboratory studies. She mentions having an upper respiratory infection 1 week ago. She does not take any medications and does not have any recent travel. Vital signs: HR 105 bpm, sinus tachycardia, BP 145/90 mm Hg, RR 30 breaths/min, temperature 37.2°C. Examination: The patient is in moderate respiratory distress and using accessory muscles of respiration. She has no rashes. She is drooling and has difficulty clearing her secretions. Her oropharynx is clear. Her neurologic examination is notable for ptosis, bilateral sixth nerve palsy, bilateral facial weakness, neck flexion 3/5, deltoids 3/5, biceps 3/5, triceps 3/5, wrist extensors and intrinsic hand muscles 5/5, iliopsoas 4+/5, quadriceps 4+/5, hamstrings 5/5, tibialis anterior 5/5, gastrocnemius 5/5. Her sensory examination is normal as are her reflexes.

What is the differential diagnosis for this patient?

Acute bilateral weakness can be due to either a central or peripheral lesion. When approaching such a patient, it is advisable to develop a methodology beginning with brain and spinal cord etiologies and moving peripherally, ruling out possibilities based on examination, imaging, and laboratory findings. The acuity of the presentation, symmetry, and pattern of weakness can be helpful. Generalized fatigue due to cardiopulmonary disease, anemia, malignancy, depression, and fibromyalgia, for example, can overlay objective muscle weakness. Similarly, pain can limit the motor examination. A broad overview of possibilities using the mnemonic VINDICATE is listed in Table 6-1.

The reflex examination can further assist with localization. Reflexes are brisk with central lesions of the brain and spinal cord, but can initially be absent or reduced with spinal cord lesions. Reflexes are preserved/normal with postsynaptic neuromuscular junction disease, but can be reduced with presynaptic disease. Reflexes are normal with myopathy. Fasciculations are specific to neuropathic disease.

Focusing on three common entities, a more specific differential diagnosis can be generated for each: myasthenia gravis, Guillain-Barré syndrome, and critical illness polyneuropathy/myopathy.

Myasthenia Gravis

1. *Myasthenic crisis* can present as a forme fruste of myasthenia gravis (MG). MG is an autoimmune disease of the neuromuscular junction characterized by a T-cell–dependent response targeted to the postsynaptic acetylcholine receptor or receptor-associated proteins. Weakness is confined to voluntary muscles (sparing smooth and

Table 6-1. Acute Motor and Sensory Weakness Differential Diagnosis

	Pure motor findings	Motor and sensory
Brain		
Vascular	Bilateral motor strip, centrum semiovale, corona radiata, internal capsule infarction, or hemorrhage; azygous ACA with ACA stroke; subdural hemorrhage; bilateral/central pontine infarctions, hemorrhage; MCA-ACA watershed infarction can cause "man in a barrel" syndrome with proximal arm and proximal leg weakness	Bilateral cortical or subcortical infarction, hemorrhage; bilateral brainstem infarctions, hemorrhage
Infection/Inflammation	Bilateral motor strip, centrum semiovale, corona radiata, or internal capsule abscess, demyelinating disease; bilateral/central pontine abscess, demyelinating disease, basilar meningitis, sarcoid	Bilateral cortical or subcortical infarctions; bilateral brainstem infarctions, abscess, demyelinating disease, basilar meningitis, sarcoid, rhombencephalitis
Neoplasm	Paramedian/falcine tumor; bilateral motor strip, centrum semiovale, corona radiata, internal capsule or pontine tumor, carcinomatous meningitis	Bilateral cortical, bilateral subcortical infarctions or brainstem tumor, carcinomatous meningitis
Drugs	Accidental ingestion: carbon monoxide poisoning (globus pallidus injury), methanol poisoning (putaminal injury)	
Idiopathic/Iatrogenic	Seizure with Todd paralysis	Bickerstaff-Cloake brainstem encephalitis
Congenital/genetic	Alternating hemiplegia of childhood, migraine with hemiplegia, progressive bulbar palsy	Leukodystrophy
Autoimmune		Bilateral MS lesions, ADEM, acute hemorrhagic encephalomyelitis, tumefactive MS, vasculitis, Behçet syndrome
Trauma		Bilateral trauma
Endocrine/metabolic	Central pontine myelinolysis	Global insult (typically accompanied by mental status changes): hypoxic ischemic encephalopathy, hypoglycemia
Spinal Cord		
Vascular		Infarction either due to embolic phenomenon or watershed infarction (greatest risk at level T4-8). Cardiothoracic and aortic surgery pose particular risks. Infarction in the territory of the artery of Adamkiewicz spares the dorsal columns. Vascular malformations

Table 6-1. Acute Motor and Sensory Weakness Differential Diagnosis (*Continued*)

	Pure motor findings	Motor and sensory
Infection/Inflammation	Poliomyelitis/postpolio syndrome, West Nile virus	Infectious myelopathy or intra-axial abscess (bacterial, fungal, mycobacterium, viral, parasitic), sarcoid, HIV, HTLV-1, -2, syphilis
Neoplasm		Tumor (metastatic, primary such as astrocytoma, or ependymoma), paraneoplastic syndrome
Drugs	Lead poisoning	Nitric oxide poisoning (mimics B_{12} deficiency, subacute combined degeneration)
Idiopathic/Iatrogenic	Motor neuron disease (ALS), Hopkins syndrome (acute postasthmatic amyotrophy), monomelic amyotrophy, progressive lateral sclerosis, progressive muscular atrophy	Radiation myelopathy
Congenital/genetic	Hereditary spastic paraplegia, familial spinal atrophy	Friedreich ataxia, adrenoleukodystrophy
Autoimmune		Immune-mediated myelopathy (transverse myelitis, multiple sclerosis, neuromyelitis optica), ADEM
Trauma		Direct trauma or nontraumatic compressive myelopathy (due to bony elements or extra-axial mass, tumor, abscess, hemorrhage)
Endocrine/metabolic		Vitamin B_{12}, vitamin E deficiency
Peripheral Nerve		
Vascular		Vasculitic neuropathy
Infection/Inflammation		CMV radiculitis, diphtheria, HSV, VZV, EBV, leprosy, sarcoid, *Bartonella*, Sjögren syndrome, Lyme disease, syphilis
Neoplasm		Paraneoplastic, myeloma, amyloid, carcinomatous meningitis
Drugs	Suramin, dapsone	Oxaliplatin, Taxol, aurothioglucose, arsenic, thallium
Idiopathic/Iatrogenic		CIP, radiation neuropathy
Congenital/genetic	Porphyria	Charcot-Marie-Tooth disease
Autoimmune	GBS	GBS, form fruste CIDP
Trauma	Compressive neuropathy (neurapraxia, axonotmesis, nerve transection (neurotmesis)	Compressive neuropathy (neurapraxia, axonotmesis, nerve transection, neurotmesis)
Endocrine/metabolic	Diabetic amyotrophy	

(*Contiuned*)

Table 6-1. Acute Motor and Sensory Weakness Differential Diagnosis (*Continued*)

	Pure motor findings	Motor and sensory
Neuromuscular Junction		
Vascular	-	
Infection/Inflammation	-	
Neoplasm	Lambert-Eaton syndrome	
Drugs/toxins	Botulism, organophosphate poisoning, penicillamine-induced myasthenia, tick paralysis, snake venom, hyper-magnesemia/hypocalcemia, neurotoxic fish poisoning	
Idiopathic/Iatrogenic	Prolonged neuromuscular blockade (particularly from amino steroid paralytic agents)	
Congenital/genetic	Congenital myasthenia	
Autoimmune	MG	
Trauma		
Endocrine/metabolic		
Muscle		
Vascular	Diabetic muscle infarction	
Infection/Inflammation	Polymyositis, dermatomyositis, inclusion body myositis, viral, bacterial, or parasitic myopathy	
Neoplasm	Paraneoplastic dermatomyositis, acute necrotizing myopathy, paraneoplastic neuromyotonia (Isaac syndrome), cachectic myopathy	
Drugs/toxins	Alcohol, glucocorticoids, cocaine, antimalarial drugs, antipsychotic drugs, colchicine, antiretroviral drugs	
Idiopathic/Iatrogenic	Critical illness myopathy, cachexia	
Congenital/genetic	Mitochondrial myopathy (MERRF), glycogen storage disease, disorders of lipid metabolism, adult-onset acid maltase deficiency, periodic paralysis	
Autoimmune	Interferon alpha, penicillamine-related myopathy	

Table 6-1. Acute Motor and Sensory Weakness Differential Diagnosis (*Continued*)

	Pure motor findings	Motor and sensory
Trauma	Rhabdomyolysis	
Endocrine/metabolic	Hyperthyroid/hypothyroid, Cushing, hyperaldosteronism with myopathy, hyperparathyroid myopathy, hypokalemic myopathy	

Abbreviations: ACA, anterior cerebral artery; ADEM, acute disseminated encephalomyelitis; ALS, amyotrophic lateral sclerosis; CIDP, chronic inflammatory demyelinating polyneuropathy; CMV, cytomegalovirus; EBV, Epstein-Barr virus; GBS, Guillain-Barré syndrome; HIV, human immunodeficiency virus; HSV, herpes simplex virus; HTLV, human T-lymphotropic virus; MCA-ACA, middle cerebral artery- anterior cerebral artery; MG, myasthenia gravis; MERRFR, myoclonus with ragged red fibers (syndrome); MS, multiple sclerosis; VZV, varicella-zoster virus.

cardiac muscles) and is variable in focus and degree. Breathing and swallowing may become significantly involved, with severe consequences leading to respiratory failure requiring mechanical intubation. Respiratory insufficiency due to MG is referred to as *myasthenic crisis*. It can begin with oropharyngeal weakness with or without appendicular symptoms and progress to crisis within hours to days, often in the context of infection or aspiration and occasionally following surgery. Half of patients with recently diagnosed MG will have a crisis within the first year and another 20% within the second year from diagnosis. Patients with long-standing MG are also at risk for crisis.

2. *Cholinergic crisis* can occur from excess acetylcholine esterase inhibitor. It is characterized by salivation, lacrimation, urination, diarrhea, gastrointestinal upset, and emesis (SLUDGE), miosis, bronchospasm, and flaccid weakness. Although a Tensilon (a solution of edrophonium chloride) challenge can distinguish cholinergic crisis from myasthenia, this test can be dangerous and often is not necessary.

3. *Lambert-Eaton myasthenic syndrome* is a presynaptic autoimmune attack of voltage-gated calcium channels, associated with cancer in 50% to 70% (typically small-cell lung cancer); limb symptoms more prominent than ocular/bulbar symptoms (5% with bulbar findings); facilitation with exercise; autonomic dysfunction; reduced reflexes; and respiratory failure uncommon.

4. *Botulism* is caused by a neurotoxin produced by *Clostridium botulinum* that permanently blocks presynaptic acetylcholine release at the neuromuscular junction. It is characterized by symmetric descending paralysis with dilated pupils (50%) and dysautonomia but no sensory deficit. It can be treated with trivalent equine antitoxin.

5. *Tick paralysis* results in presynaptic neuromuscular blockade. Associated ticks include Rocky Mountain wood tick, American dog tick, Lone Star tick, black-legged tick, Western black-legged tick, Gulf Coast tick, and Australian *Ixodes holocyclus* tick. It typically can present as ascending paralysis, ophthalmoparesis, bulbar dysfunction, ataxia, and reduced reflexes. It has a rapid course of progression (hours to days) and is accompanied by ataxia, but no sensory symptoms.[1] Complete cure can occur with tick removal.

6. *Snake venom* from the tiger snake, taipan snake, and Brazilian rattlesnake causes presynaptic blockade; and postsynaptic blockade is caused by alpha-bungarotoxin from the venom of kraits and is also due to the venom of cobras, mambas, coral snakes, and sea snakes. Other snakes with venom affecting the neuromuscular junction include copperheads, cottonmouths, moccasins, rattlesnakes, vipers, adders, boomslangs, and twig snakes. Snake venom initially affects cranial nerves resulting in ptosis, ophthalmoplegia, dysarthria, and dysphasia followed by progressive limb weakness.

7. *Organophosphate toxicity.* Organophosphates (eg, malathion, parathion, sarin, soman) inactivate acetylcholine esterase causing SLUDGE, miosis, bronchospasm, blurred vision, and bradycardia. It is characterized by confusion, optic neuropathy, extrapyramidal effects, dysautonomia, fasciculations, seizures, cranial nerve palsies, and weakness due to continued depolarization at the neuromuscular junction. Delayed polyneuropathy can occur 2 to 3 weeks after exposure. It is treated with atropine, pralidoxime (2-PAM), and benzodiazepines. Succinylcholine should be avoided.

8. *Guillain-Barré syndrome* can present with areflexia and ophthalmoplegia (Miller-Fisher variant) or ascending weakness, facial weakness, diplopia, and areflexia. It is often demyelinating, but can be axonal. Early loss of F waves is seen on electromyography (EMG). It is treatable with plasmapheresis or IV immunoglobulin.

9. *Neurotoxic fish poisoning* is caused by tetrodotoxin (from the puffer fish) and saxitoxin (from the organisms that cause red tide), both of which block neuromuscular transmission. Ciguatera toxin (from red snapper, grouper, barracuda) affects voltage-gated sodium channels of muscles and nerves and produces a characteristic metallic taste in the mouth and hot-cold reversal.

10. *Diphtheria,* caused by *Corynebacterium diphtheriae,* is associated with a thick gray pharyngeal pseudomembrane, atrioventricular (AV) block, endocarditis, myocarditis, lymphadenopathy, neuropathy with craniopharyngeal involvement, proximal to distal weakness, and decreased reflexes.

Guillain-Barré Syndrome

1. *GBS* is a heterogeneous group of immune-mediated polyneuropathies with motor, sensory, and dysautonomic features. It is the most common cause of acute flaccid paralysis in the United States with a frequency of 1 to 3 per 100,000 people and occurs in all age groups. The pathophysiology of GBS is thought to be related to molecular mimicry triggered by recent infection producing an autoimmune humeral- and cell-mediated response against the ganglioside surface molecules of peripheral nerves. A typical history involves acute symmetric ascending weakness, often beginning in the proximal legs. Weakness beginning in the arms or face occurs in 10%, but eventually 50% of patients have facial or oropharyngeal weakness. Paresthesias in the hands and feet are reported in 80% of patients, as is lower back pain. Diplopia occurs in 15% due to oculomotor weakness. Dysautonomia occurs in 70% (tachycardia/bradycardia, wide swings in blood pressure, orthostasis, tonic pupils, urinary retention, ileus/constipation, hypersalivation, and anhidrosis). Respiratory failure requiring intubation occurs in 30% (Table 6-2)

2. *Polyneuropathies* include the following:

   - Acute motor neuropathies due to arsenic, lead poisoning, or porphyria.

   - *N*-hexane (glue sniffing).

   - Peripheral nerve vasculitis (presents as, eg, mononeuritis multiplex and can be due to polyarteritis nodosa, Churg-Strauss syndrome, rheumatoid arthritis, lupus).

   - Neuropathy due to Lyme disease, sarcoidosis, paraneoplastic disease, and critical illness polyneuropathy.

   - Diphtheria, caused by *Corynebacterium diphtheriae,* is associated with a thick gray pharyngeal pseudomembrane, AV block, endocarditis, myocarditis, lymphadenopathy, neuropathy with craniopharyngeal involvement, proximal to distal weakness, and decreased reflexes.

   - Ciguatera toxin (red snapper, grouper, barracuda) affects voltage-gated sodium channels of muscles and nerves and produces a characteristic metallic taste in the mouth and hot-cold reversal.

Table 6-2. Acute Neuropathy Differential Diagnosis

Subtype	Comments
Acute inflammatory demyelinating polyradiculoneuropathy (AIDP)	Most common subtype in the United States (85%-90% of cases) 40% seropositive for *Campylobacter jejuni* Primarily demyelinating Progressive, symmetrical weakness, absent/depressed deep tendon reflexes
Acute motor axonal neuropathy (AMAN) Acute sensorimotor axonal neuropathy (AMSAN)	Primary axonal injury 5%-10% of US cases 70%-75% associated with preceding *Campylobacter jejuni* infection/diarrhea Up to 1/3 may be hyperreflexic Common in China, Japan, and Mexico GM1, GD1a, GalNac-GD1a, and GD1b antibodies
Miller-Fisher syndrome	Triad of ataxia, ophthalmoplegia, and areflexia 1/3 develop extremity weakness GQ1b antibodies in 95% 5% of cases in United States and 25% in Japan Bickerstaff-Cloake encephalitis: brainstem encephalitis with ophthalmoplegia, ataxia, encephalopathy, and hyperreflexia associated with GQ1b antibodies may be a related entity. It responds to IVIG and plasma exchange
Pharyngeal-cervical-brachial	Acute arm weakness and swallowing dysfunction May have facial weakness Leg strength and reflexes preserved
Paraparesis	Involvement limited to the lower extremities
Acute pandysautonomia	Sympathetic and parasympathetic involvement Orthostatic hypotension Urinary retention Diarrhea, abdominal pain, ileus, and vomiting Pupillary abnormalities Variable heart rate Decreased sweating, salivation, and lacrimation Reflexes diminished Sensory symptoms
Pure sensory	Sensory ataxia Reflexes absent GD1b antibody

(Courtesy of Frontera J, ed. Decision Making in Neurocritical Care. New York, NY: Thieme, 2009.)

3. *Neuromuscular junction disease.* There is no sensory involvement in any disorder of neuro-muscular transmission. This group of diseases includes the following:
    - MG
    - Lambert-Eaton myasthenic syndrome
    - Botulism
    - Organophosphate toxicity. Delayed polyneuropathy can occur 2 to 3 weeks after exposure. Treat with atropine, pralidoxime (2-PAM), and benzodiazepines. Avoid succinylcholine.
    - Neurotoxic fish poisoning. Caused by tetrodotoxin (from puffer fish), and saxitoxin (from organisms that cause red tide), both of which block neuromuscular transmission.

4. *Muscle disorders.* Critical illness myopathy and acute polymyositis can mimic GBS. Can differentiate with EMG/nerve conduction study (NCS).

5. *Spinal cord disorders.* Acute myelopathy can cause weakness, numbness, and acutely depressed deep tendon reflexes along with bowel and bladder dysfunction. Back pain is common in GBS and spinal cord disorders. Magnetic resonance imaging (MRI) can easily distinguish between the two (enhancement of nerve roots can occur with GBS).

6. *Brainstem disease with multiple cranial neuropathies* (stroke, Bickerstaff-Cloake brainstem encephalitis, rhombencephalitis, basilar meningitis, carcinomatous meningitis, Wernicke encephalopathy).

Critical Illness Polyneuropathy/Myopathy

1. Critically ill patients are at risk for developing severe weakness secondary to *critical ill-ness polyneuropathy* (CIP) and/or *critical illness myopathy* (CIM). Weakness may progress to severe quadriparesis and muscle wasting.[2] The incidence of CIP/CIM in critically ill patients has been reported as 33% to 44% of patients with prolonged admission to critical care settings. The incidence increases to nearly 70% when considering only patients with sepsis.[2-6]

2. *GBS.* Coincidental occurrence of GBS in a critically ill patient is relatively rare. However, if the history is suspicious, a lumbar puncture can be done (best yield is 1 to 2 weeks from symptom onset). Elevated protein without elevation in leukocytes would be suspicious for GBS. Cerebrospinal fluid (CSF) studies should be normal in CIP/CIM.

3. *Cachetic myopathy.* Critically ill patients can develop a subacute myopathy due to protein catabolism and disuse. Patients develop weakness and muscle atrophy. Type II muscle atrophy is seen histologically.

4. *Spinal cord lesions.* A lesion to the cervical spinal cord can result in tetraparesis and should be considered if the clinical setting is appropriate. Lesions in the cord can initially cause flaccid paresis with decreased reflexes, followed subacutely by hyperreflexia and increased tone. A sensory level may be evident in a patient who is able to participate in a sensory examination. If the history or examination is suspicious, an MRI of the cervical cord with and without contrast may be appropriate.

5. *Underlying neuropathy.* Toxins and medication effects: Often medications used in the intensive care unit (ICU) (ie, neuromuscular-blocking agents) can result in prolonged weakness and sedation. An NCS may help in this case. For patients who have been treated with neuromuscular-blocking agents, "a train of four" (slow repetitive stimulation at 2 to 3 Hz at the median or ulnar nerve) may be used to determine if the medication's effect is persisting.

What studies can be done to differentiate between possible diagnoses?

Electrophysiology

An electrophysiology examination consists of NCSs, needle EMG, and neuromuscular junction testing. Frequently, the EMG is not particularly useful for the first few weeks after symptom onset and many practitioners will wait at least 3 weeks prior to performing a needle study.

However, NCS examination can provide some insight early in the disease course. The NCS consists of peripheral motor nerve compound muscle action potential (CMAP) and sensory nerve action potential (SNAP). Decreased nerve conduction amplitude implies an axonal process, while slowed conduction velocities, distal latencies, temporal dispersion, and conduction block indicate a demyelinating process.

Late responses, F and H waves, can add additional information to the NCS. F waves represent the very proximal portion of the nerve and are generated by supramaximal stimulation of a motor nerve while recording over a muscle. An H reflex is typically a tibial reflex (patellar reflex arc) and represents the sensory and motor nerves of the entire reflex arc. Both amplitude and latency are measured bilaterally and greater than 50% difference between side-to-side amplitudes is considered abnormal.

The needle examination assesses muscle activity at rest, with mild voluntary contraction, and with maximal voluntary muscle contraction. During the needle examination the practitioner assesses for:

1. Insertional activity (increased in denervated muscle, decreased when muscle is replaced by fat or connective tissue)

2. Spontaneous activity (fibrillation potentials and sharp waves suggest recent denervation or muscle necrosis)

3. Recruitment (reduced recruitment with rapid firing occurs when there is damage to the axon, neuron, or when a large number of motor units are lost. Poor activation occurs with central disorders when there is a decreased number of motor units recruited and firing is slow. Early recruitment occurs in the context of myopathy.)

4. Motor unit potential duration (long duration is seen with lower motor neuron disorders, while short-duration motor units are common with myopathies, but may be seen in neuromuscular disorders and the early phases of reinnervation after neuropathy)

5. Motor unit potential amplitude (long-duration, high-amplitude motor units are seen with chronic neurogenic disorders, while small-amplitude, short-duration motor units are common to myopathic disorders)

6. Motor unit polyphasia (five or more phases constitute polyphasia, which can be seen in both myopathic and neurogenic disorders)

Electrophysiology, CSF, imaging, and serologic studies for MG, GBS, CIP/CIM are listed in Tables 6-3 and 6-4.

How can myopathy be diagnosed in a patient who cannot generate a motor unit/does not have any voluntary motor activity?

Direct muscle stimulation (DMS) has been suggested as a technique to differentiate CIP and CIM in patients who cannot generate a motor unit owing to extreme weakness or altered mental status.[7] Comparing CMAP amplitudes generated by motor nerve stimulation to CMAP amplitudes generated by direct muscle stimulation can help identify a myopathy as opposed to an isolated neuropathy. CMAP amplitudes derived from DMS may be inexcitable (absent) or decreased (less than 2 mV) in CIM,[8] while they remain normal in isolated CIP. When neuropathy alone is present, CMAP amplitudes produced by muscle stimulation are normal, but CMAP amplitudes produced by nerve stimulation are

Table 6-3. MG, GBS, and CIP/CIM Comparison —EMG and Nerve Conduction

	MG	GBS	CIP/CIM
NCS	Normal CMAP and SNAP amplitude, conduction velocity, and distal latency	*Demyelinating variant:* Nerve conduction velocity slowing to < 60% of normal, increased distal motor latency, prolonged or absent F waves, which indicate proximal nerve conduction velocity slowing, conduction block, low-amplitude SNAPs and CMAPs, multifocal demyelination. Sural sparing is typical, while median and ulnar sensory responses are affected. Particularly early in the course, 15%-20% of patients have normal NCS. During the first 2 weeks of illness, 50% fulfill diagnosis criteria compared with 85% by week 3. *Axonal variant:* Severe decrease in amplitude of CMAPs and SNAPs with relative preservation of conduction velocities and distal latencies. Very low CMAP amplitude (<20% of normal) portends a poor prognosis.	*CIP* is an acute axonal sensorimotor polyneuropathy. NCSs show amplitude reduction of both motor and sensory action potentials and normal or mildly slowed conduction velocities. Absence of conduction block or prolongation of F waves. *CIM* is an acute primary myopathy (ie, it is not due to muscle denervation). Routine electrodiagnositic studies often reveal nonspecific findings, including normal sensory nerve action potentials with small compound muscle action potentials.
EMG	The needle EMG study is typically normal. Single-fiber EMG is the most sensitive test for MG. Abnormal jitter can occur in other neuromuscular disorders, but is specific for a disorder of neuromuscular transmission when no other abnormalities are seen on standard EMG needle examination.	Needle examination reveals neuropathic changes with fibrillation potentials, large multiphasic motor unit potentials.	*CIP:* Needle examination reveals fibrillation potentials and PSWs; reduced recruitment patterns. Long-duration, high-amplitude motor unit potentials appear after weeks. There is an absence of decremental response on repetitive stimulation. *CIM:* Needle examination reveals fibrillation potentials and PSWs; complex repetitive discharges may be present; myopathic units (short-duration and polyphasic motor unit action potentials); early, normal, or reduced recruitment patterns. Fibrillation potentials and PSWs on EMG.

Table 6-3. MG, GBS, and CIP/CIM Comparison —EMG and Nerve Conduction (*Continued*)

	MG	GBS	CIP/CIM
Repetitive Stimulation	Slow repetitive stimulation at 2 Hz causes a decrement in CMAP amplitudes, and there is no increment of CMAP amplitude after exercise (an increase in CMAP amplitude after exercise implies a presynaptic neuromuscular defect.)	There is an absence of decremental response on repetitive stimulation.	There is an absence of decremental response on repetitive stimulation.

Abbreviations: CIP/CIM, critical illness polyneuropathy/critical illness myopathy; CMAP, compound muscle action potential; EMG, electromyography; GBS, Guillain-Barré syndrome; MG, myasthenia gravis; NCS, nerve conduction study; PSW, positive sharp wave; SNAP, sensory nerve action potential.

small. When CMAP amplitudes are low for both nerve and muscle stimulation, a myopathy is present and, thus, the ratio of nerve-evoked CMAP to muscle-evoked CMAP amplitude is greater than 0.5. When CIP is present alone, a ratio of nerve-evoked CMAP to DMS CMAP would be less than 0.5.

What are the risk factors for MG, GBS, and CIP/CIM?

The risk factors for MG, GBS, and CIP/CIM are given in Table 6-5.

What are the specific treatments for MG, GBS, and CIM/CIP?

Consider intubation early. MG and GBS patients can deteriorate rapidly. Check vital capacity (VC) and negative inspiratory force (NIF). If VC is less than 10 to 15 mL/kg or less than 1 L and/or the NIF is weaker than –20 cm H_2O or rapidly worsening, the patient should be intubated. Beware that patients with bulbar dysfunction often cannot form a proper seal for respiratory testing and results can sometimes appear worse than the patient's true respiratory status. Multiple VC/NIF measurements should be made to capture the patient's best effort. Poor pulmonary function assessment: Ask the patient to count as rapidly and as high as he/she can in one breath. Every 10 numbers counted roughly equates to 1 L of VC. If the patient cannot count to 10, intubation should be pursued. Similarly, oxygen saturation can be falsely reassuring. Most patients retain CO_2 prior to becoming hypoxia. Hypoxia is a late sign of respiratory failure in neuromuscular disease. If the patient is already hypoxic, the physician should proceed to intubation without delay. Patients with myasthenic crisis and many GBS patients should be monitored in an ICU setting (Tables 6-6 and 6-7).

Does bed rest lead to weakness? Can early mobilization improve neuromuscular weakness?

Every day of strict bed rest leads to a 1% decline in muscle strength.[9] Casting can lead to a 25% decline in muscle strength within 7 days.[10] As assessed by MRI or computed tomography (CT), muscle mass decreases by 1.5% to 2.0% per day after 2 to 3 weeks of bed rest.[11] A decrease in the size of muscle fibers is primarily responsible for this decrease in mass.[12] The underlying mechanisms of muscle atrophy and fiber injury are due to oxidative stress, down regulation of protein synthesis, and activation of calpain, caspase, and ubiquitin, which are involved in degradation of contractile fibers.[13] Mobility therapy has been shown to prevent muscle degeneration in healthy volunteers randomized to receive bed rest with or without resistance exercise training. Healthy volunteers who did not participate in an exercise regimen had a significant decrease in muscle protein synthesis as measured by needle biopsy

Table 6-4. CSF, Serology, and Imaging Findings of MG, GBS, and CIP/CIM

	CSF Studies	Serologies	Imaging/Other
MG	Lumbar puncture is typically normal.	Acetylcholine receptor antibodies are present in 85% of patients with generalized MG. Rare false positives can be seen in Lambert-Eaton syndrome, motor neuron disease, polymyositis, primary biliary cirrhosis, lupus, thymoma without MG, and in first-degree relatives of myasthenics. 15%-20% of patients with MG are seronegative. Of these patients, 40%-50% have MuSK antibodies. Since many patients with MG have other autoimmune diseases, testing for lupus, thyroid disease, and rheumatoid arthritis is suggested. Serologies specific to certain disease etiologies are listed: Lambert-Eaton syndrome—P/Q-type calcium channel binding antibodies; botulism—serum and stool botulism toxin assay; organophosphate toxicity—measure plasma and RBC cholinesterase levels. *Corynebacterium diphtheriae*—culture and PCR of toxin, serum diphtheria, antibodies.	Edrophonium (Tensilon) has a rapid onset and can be used to make the diagnosis of MG in patients with obvious ptosis. 2-mg doses can be administered every 60 s (up to 10 mg) while looking for a clinical response. Patients should receive ECG monitoring with atropine at the bedside while this test is being performed because of the risks of bradycardia. Since edrophonium has muscarinic effects, it can cause bronchospasm and increased secretions and is not recommended in those in crisis. Chest CT or MRI to screen for thymoma should be performed on all myasthenics. MRI of the brain may be necessary if a central brainstem etiology is suspected.
GBS	Albuminocytologic dissociation (elevated CSF protein with normal WBCs 10 cell/mm^3) appears in 80%-90% of patients within 1 week. CSF pleocytosis can occur with HIV-associated AIDP.	GQ1b (85%-90% of patients with Miller-Fisher variant); GM1, GD1a, GalNac-GD1a, and GD1b (associated with axonal variants); GT1a (associated with swallowing difficulty); GD1b (associated with pure sensory variant). Antibodies to *Campylobacter jejuni*, CMV, HIV, EBV, and *Mycoplasma pneumoniae* can be tested. Antibody tests are expensive and are not routinely used.	MRI is useful for ruling out, eg, cord compression and cauda equina syndrome. Spinal root enhancement can be seen in GBS (cauda equina nerve roots enhance in up to 83% of patients) and is due to disruption of the blood-CNS barrier.
CIP/CIM	CSF studies should be normal in CIP/CIM.	Serum CPK is usually normal or only mildly elevated in CIP/CIM	Although biopsy is the gold standard for diagnosis of CIM, it is not commonly necessary. Both fiber types I and II are generally affected, but type II myofibers are sometimes more affected. Atrophic myofibers (predominantly type II) with basophilic cytoplasm on H&E stain are seen under light microscopy. Electron

Table 6-4. CSF, Serology, and Imaging Findings of MG, GBS, and CIP/CIM (*Continued*)

CSF Studies	Serologies	Imaging/Other
		microscopy shows loss of myosin filaments with relative sparing of actin filaments (patchy thick filament loss). The presence of necrosis is variable, ranging from absent to diffuse lesions described in acute necrotizing myopathy. Inflammatory changes are usually absent and angulated fibers, rimmed vacuoles, and fatty degeneration may be seen. In patients with CIP, neuropathic features are seen on biopsy including grouped atrophy, fiber type grouping, and target fibers.

Abbreviations: AIDP, acute idiopathic demyelinating polyneuropathy; CIP/CIM, critical illness polyneuropathy/critical illness myopathy; CMV, cytomegalovirus; CNS, central nervous system; CSF, cerebrospinal fluid; CT, computed tomography; EBV, Epstein-Barr virus; ECG, electrocardiographic; H&E, hematoxylin and eosin; GSB, Guillain-Barré syndrome; HIV, human immunodeficiency virus; MG, myasthenia gravis; MRI, magnetic resonance imaging; MuSK, muscle-specific kinase; PCR, polymerase chain reaction; RBC, red blood cell; WBCs, white blood cells.

after infusions of radiolabeled phenylalanine.[14] Early mobility of ICU patients (including patients who were sedated and received passive stretch therapy) has been shown to shorten ICU and hospital length of stay, improve functional outcomes, and reduce delirium.[15,16] Based on histologic data,[17] passive stretching alone decreases muscle atrophy.

What is the most effective approach for ventilator weaning in patients with neuromuscular weakness?

Diaphragm weakness and dysfunction are very common in patients receiving mechanical ventilation due to the same mechanisms described above.[18-20] Strategies for expedited liberation from the ventilator have been suggested by the Centers for Disease Control and Prevention (CDC) and the Institute for Healthcare Improvement and Joint Commission.[21] Two major components of this strategy include daily sedation vacation and assessment for readiness to wean. Daily sedation interruption has been shown to reduce the duration of mechanical ventilation and length of stay in the ICU.[22] Daily spontaneous breathing trials or pressure support (PS) trials have also been shown to reduce the duration of mechanical ventilation.[23,24] Conversely, the use of a controlled mechanical ventilation mode, which does not allow for any patient respiratory effort, has been shown to cause muscle atrophy and severe diaphragm weakenss.[25,26] In animal models, PS ventilation has been shown to reduce mechanical ventilation–induced proteolysis and diaphragm weakness.[27] The coupling of sedation vacation and spontaneous breathing trials resulted in a shorter duration of mechanical ventilation, shorter ICU length of stay, and lower mortality rate in the Wake Up and Breathe Trial.[28]

Most ICUs use a PS mode for weaning. Although this mode, adjusted to a respiratory rate less than 25 breaths/min, was found to be inferior to a once-daily T-piece trial in one randomized study[23] a separate randomized trial found that a PS mode titrated to a respiratory rate less than 35 breaths/min was superior to T-piece trials in regard to reduction in mechanical ventilation time.[29] A meta-analysis revealed that both PS and T-piece modes are similar in time to ventilator liberation, but synchronized intermittent mechanical ventilation (SIMV) mode appears to be the worst method of mechanical ventilation weaning.[24,30] A PS mode may be safer than a T-piece mode because most ventilators provide back-up ventilation in patients who become apneic or fail their spontaneous breathing trial.

There is a paucity of literature addressing ventilation weaning in patients who undergo tracheotomy. Although early tracheotomy in a select group of patients projected to require mechanical ventilation for

Table 6-5. Risk Factors for MG, GBS, and CIP/CIM

MG	GBS	CIP/CIM

Infection	Bacterial infection:
	  Campylobacter jejuni
	  Haemophilus influenzae
	  Mycoplasma pneumoniae
	  Borrelia burgdorferi
		SIRS[3,4,6,31]

Tapering of immunosuppression	Viral infection:
	  CMV
	  EBV
	  HIV (seroconversion)
		Initiation of corticosteroids

Surgery	Vaccines:
	  Influenza vaccine
	  Oral polio vaccine
	  Menactra meningococcal conjugate
	  vaccine
		NMBAs

Aspiration	Medications:
	  Case reports related to streptokinase,
	  isotretinoin, danazol, captopril, gold,
	  heroin, and epidural anesthesia
		Hyperglycemia[32]

Worsening of other medical diseases (eg, cardiac, renal, autoimmune)		Multiple organ failure[33]
No apparent reason (30%-40%)		Muscle inactivity[33]
Medications[a]		

Abbreviations: CIP/CIM, critical illness polyneuropathy/critical illness myopathy; CMV, cytomegalovirus; EBV, Epstein-Barr virus; GBS, Guillain-Barré syndrome; HIV, human immunodeficiency virus; MG, myasthenia gravis; NMBAs, neuromuscular-blocking agents; SIRS, sepsis/systemic inflammatory response syndrome.

[a]Antibiotics: Aminoglycosides, fluoroquinolones (ciprofloxacin, levofloxacin, norfloxacin), macrolides (clarithromycin, erythromycin), ampicillin, clindamycin, colistin, lincomycin, quinine, tetracyclines

Anticonvulsants: Phenytoin, gabapentin

Antipsychotics: Chlorpromazine, lithium, phenothiazines

Anesthetics: Diazepam, chloroprocaine, halothane, ketamine, lidocaine, NMBAs (depolarizing agents such as succinylcholine have no efficacy in myasthenics), procaine

Cardiovascular: β Blockers, bretylium, procainamide, propafenone, quinidine, verapamil, calcium channel blockers

Ophthalmologic: Betaxolol, echothiophate, timolol, tropicamide, proparacaine

Rheumatologic: Chloroquine, penicillamine

Steroids: Prednisone, methylprednisolone, corticotropin

Other: Anticholinergics, carnitine, deferoxamine, diuretics, interferon alpha, iodinated contrast agents, narcotics, oral contraceptives, oxytocin, ritonavir and antiretroviral protease inhibitors, thyroxine

Table 6-6. Treatment for MG, GBS, and CIP/CIM

	Rapid therapy	Symptomatic therapy	Chronic therapy	Surgery
MG	Treat the underlying trigger for myasthenic crisis (eg, infection, change in medication) Plasmapheresis[a] IVIG[a]	Pyridostigmine	Prednisone Azathioprine Mycophenolate mofetil Cyclosporine	Thymectomy
GBS	Plasmapheresis[b] IVIG[b]	Lacrilube is useful in patients with facial nerve palsy to keep the cornea hydrated	No long-term therapy is necessary for AIDP	No surgical treatment
CIP/CIM	Treat the underlying trigger (steroid use, sepsis, etc)	Physical therapy. Avoid the use of NMBAs and corticosteroids	No long-term therapy is necessary	No surgical treatment

Abbreviations: AAN, American Academy of Neurology; AIDP, acute idiopathic demyelinating polyneuropathy; GBS, Guillain-Barré syndrome; IVIG, IV immunoglobulin; MG, myasthenia gravis; NMBAs, neuromuscular-blocking agents.

[a]Neither plasmapheresis nor IVIG has been compared directly to placebo in a randomized clinical trial. Since plasmapheresis has a shorter onset of action, it is often the initial therapy used. In a prospective randomized trial of plasmapheresis versus IVIG, 50% of patients reached a target improvement in the myasthenia muscle score by day 9 in the plasmapheresis group and by day 12 in the IVIG group, although there were no functional or strength differences by day 15, and there were fewer adverse events in the IVIG group.[34]

[b]AAN Practice Parameters[35]:
   Treatment with IVIG or plasma exchange speeds recovery.
   IVIG and plasma exchange are equivalent.
   Plasma exchange is recommended for GBS patients unable to walk who start treatment within 4 weeks of onset of symptoms.
   Plasma exchange is also recommended for ambulatory patients who start treatment within 2 weeks of symptom onset.
   IVIG is recommended for nonambulatory GBS patients who start treatment within 2 or possibly 4 weeks from symptom onset.
The time to onset of recovery is shortened by 40%-50% by plasma exchange or IVIG.
   Combining IVIG and plasma exchange is not beneficial.
   Steroids alone are not beneficial.[36]

(Courtesy of Frontera J, ed. Decision Making in Neurocritical Care. New York, NY: Thieme, 2009.)

more than 14 days has been shown to reduce mortality rate, pneumonia, mechanical ventilation time, and ICU length of stay,[37] there have been no studies addressing weaning strategies in tracheotomized patients. Most studies address extubation and require patients to either be noncomatose and/or able to clear their secretions prior to extubation. Most neurointensivists extrapolate from published weaning trials when addressing liberation from the ventilator in patients who have undergone tracheotomy. This means that even patients who are projected to undergo tracheotomy (owing to mental status or weakness) should undergo daily sedation vacation and spontaneous breathing trials. Daily spontaneous breathing trials may reduce diaphragm and muscle atrophy and allow patients to wean off the ventilator more rapidly than patients who are not afforded daily weaning trials.

What is the prognosis of myasthenic crisis, GBS, and CIP/CIM?

Myasthenic Crisis

Mortality rate from myasthenic crisis is less than 5%; however, the mean duration of mechanical ventilation is 2 weeks. Predictors for prolonged mechanical ventilation and ICU/hospital length of stay include preintubation HCO_3 greater than or equal to 30 mL/dL, peak VC on days 1 to 6 postintubation of less

Table 6-7. Details of Treatment Strategies

Type of treatment	Dose	Onset of effect	Maximal effect	Pros	Cons
Rapid Therapies					
Plasmapheresis	250 mL/kg total divided every other day x 5 treatments (3-5 L per treatment)	1-7 d	1-3 wk	Directly removes acetylcholine receptor antibodies from the circulation. Clinical efficacy correlates with reduction in antibody levels. Faster onset of action than IVIG. Improvement in 75% of cases after 2-3 exchanges.	Requires invasive line placement. Risk of line infection, hypocalcemia, hypofibrinogenemia, hypotension, dysautonomia, hypothermia, thrombocytopenia, thromboembolism. Should not be performed the day before surgery. Benefits last only a few weeks.
IVIG	400 mg/kg daily for 5 d (2 g/kg total)	1-2 wk	1-3 wk	No central line needed. Pretreatment with 250 mL of NS, acetaminophen (Tylenol), and diphenhydramine (Benadryl) can mitigate complications.	Risk of hypersensitivity with IgA deficiency (should check IgA levels before starting), aseptic meningitis, headache, fluid overload, renal failure (ATN), hyperviscosity syndrome (which can cause stroke or MI; caution with patients with cryoglobulinemia, monoclonal gammopathy, high lipoproteins, or preexisting vascular disease). Benefits last only a few weeks.
Symptomatic Therapy					
Pyridostigmine	60-120 mg PO q3-8h	10-15 min	2 h	Acetylcholinesterase inhibitor. Can be restarted after patient shows a response to rapid therapy.	Not given acutely during a crisis owing to increased secretions. Can cause cholinergic crisis, bradycardia, AV block, hypotension, diarrhea, nausea, vomiting, fasciculations, bronchospasm.
Chronic Immunotherapy					
Prednisone	60-80 mg/d	2-3 wk	5-6 mo	Can help prevent rebound in acetylcholine antibody levels. Faster immunosuppression than other drugs.	Can cause early worsening of MG, hyperglycemia, steroid psychosis, glaucoma, immunosuppression, ulcer, osteoporosis, weight gain.

Table 6-7. Details of Treatment Strategies (*Continued*)

Type of treatment	Dose	Onset of effect	Maximal effect	Pros	Cons
Azathioprine	1-3 mg/kg PO divided qd or bid (protocols vary)	4-10 mo	1-2 y	Steroid-sparing immunosuppression.	Neoplasia risk, immunosuppression, pancytopenia, pancreatitis, hepatotoxicity.
Mycophenolate mofetil	1 g PO bid (protocols vary)	2-4 mo	5-6 mo	Steroid-sparing immunosuppression.	Increased risk of lymphoma, immunosuppression, teratogenicity risk, pancytopenia, GI bleed risk, renal failure, acute interstitial lung disease, HTN.
Cyclosporine	2.5-4 mg/kg/d divided bid (protocols vary)	2-4 mo	7 mo	Steroid-sparing immunosuppression.	Neoplasia risk, skin malignancy risk, HTN, renal failure, immunosuppression, hepatotoxicity, seizures, posterior reversible leukoencephalopathy, seizures, increased ICP, tremor.
Surgery					
Thymectomy	Once 10%-15% of patients with MG have thymoma	1-10 y	1-10 y	Potential benefit to all patients with a life expectancy > 10 years. Can produce long lasting improvement and liberation from medical therapy. No known chronic side effects.	Operative morbidity and mortality, long delay before improvement. Total remission in 35%.

Abbreviations: ATN, acute tubular necrosis; AV, atrioventricular; GI, gastrointestinal; HTN, hypertension; IgA, immunoglobulin A; IVIG, IV immunoglobulin; MI, myocardial infarction; NS, normal saline.

(Courtesy of Frontera J, ed. Decision Making in Neurocritical Care. New York, NY: Thieme, 2009.)

than 25 mL/kg, and age older than 50 years. The need for more than 2 weeks of mechanical ventilation per number of risk factors is : 0/3 = 0%, 1/3 = 21%, 2/3 = 46%, 3/3 = 88%.[2]

GBS

The course of GBS is usually progressive for the first 2 weeks of illness, followed by 2 to 4 weeks of a plateau phase, and then a recovery phase. Disease progression for more than 8 weeks is consistent with the diagnosis of chronic inflammatory demyelinating polyneuropathy (CIDP). Poor prognostic factors include older age, rapid onset, preceding diarrheal illness, respiratory failure, and distal CMAP amplitudes less than 20% of normal. Overall, 85% of GBS patients achieve a full functional recovery within 6 to 12 months. The mortality rate is generally less than 5%, but up to 15% of patients may have neurologic sequelae. Of those who become ventilator-dependent, the mortality rate is 20%. Outcome depends on the GBS variant. Patients with acute idiopathic demyelinating polyneuropathy (AIDP) typically do better than axonal variants, with remyelination occurring over several weeks to months.

In a small fraction of AIDP patients there is superimposed axonal degeneration leading to incomplete or delayed recovery. Relapses occur in up to 10% of GBS patients, and 2% of patients develop CIDP.

CIM/CIP

Patients with CIP/CIM may be more difficult to wean from mechanical ventilation and require prolonged rehabilitation. The mortality rate of patients with CIP has been reported as ranging from 26% to 71% and may be significantly higher than for patients with similar underlying illness without evidence of CIP.[4,5] Patients who survive their underlying illness may recover some strength within weeks to months; however, many may have residual functional deficits. In one review, 68.4% of patients discharged from the ICU with CIP/CIM regained the ability to breathe and walk independently, while 28.1% had persistent severe disability.[5]

! CRITICAL CONSIDERATIONS

- Patients with myasthenic crisis or Guillain-Barré can deteriorate very rapidly and should be closely observed.
- Close monitoring for intubation depends on the clinical examination, VC, and NIFS.
- Rise in Pco_2 is an early sign of respiratory insufficiency. Neuromuscular failure is advanced once a patient becomes hypoxic.
- Elective intubation is recommended for a VC<10-15 ml/kg and NIF worse than -20 cm H_2O or steadily declining VC and NIF.
- Myasthenic crisis and Guillain-Barré are treated with rapid-acting agents (plasmapheresis, IVIG).
- EMG/NCS are the major elements of the diagnostic evaluation for myasthenic crisis, Guillain-Barré, and CIP/CIM. Serologies and CSF studies can add additional information.
- Have a high suspicion for CIP/CIM in patients with sepsis or SIRS.
- Failure to think of CIP/CIM may lead to errors in prognostication, as many patients with CIM/CIP may recover substantially over weeks to months.

REFERENCES

1. Felz MW, Smith CD, Swift TR. A six-year-old girl with tick paralysis. *N Engl J Med*. 2000;342: 90-94.

2. Garnacho-Montero J, Amaya-Villar R, Garcia-Garmendia JL, Madrazo-Osuna J, Ortiz-Leyba C. Effect of critical illness polyneuropathy on the withdrawal from mechanical ventilation and the length of stay in septic patients. *Crit Care Med*. 2005;33:349-354.

3. de Letter MA, Schmitz PI, Visser LH, et al. Risk factors for the development of polyneuropathy and myopathy in critically ill patients. *Crit Care Med*. 2001;29:2281-2286.

4. Hund E. Myopathy in critically ill patients. *Crit Care Med*. 1999;27:2544-2547.

5. Kane SL, Dasta JF. Clinical outcomes of critical illness polyneuropathy. *Pharmacotherapy*. 2002;22:373-379.

6. Latronico N, Fenzi F, Recupero D, et al. Critical illness myopathy and neuropathy. *Lancet*. 1996;347:1579-1582.

7. Rich MM, Bird SJ, Raps EC, McCluskey LF, Teener JW. Direct muscle stimulation in acute quadriplegic myopathy. *Muscle Nerve*. 1997;20:665-673.

8. Rich MM, Teener JW, Raps EC, Schotland DL, Bird SJ. Muscle is electrically inexcitable in acute quadriplegic myopathy. *Neurology*. 1996;46:731-736.

9. Bloomfield SA. Changes in musculoskeletal structure and function with prolonged bed rest. *Med Sci Sports Exerc*. 1997;29:197-206.

10. Muller EA. Influence of training and of inactivity on muscle strength. *Arch Phys Med Rehabil*. 1970;51:449-462.

11. Brower RG. Consequences of bed rest. *Crit Care Med.* 2009;37:S422-S428.

12. Adams GR, Caiozzo VJ, Baldwin KM. Skeletal muscle unweighting: Spaceflight and ground-based models. *J Appl Physiol.* 2003;95:2185-2201.

13. Petrof BJ, Jaber S, Matecki S. Ventilator-induced diaphragmatic dysfunction. *Curr Opin Crit Care.*16: 19-25.

14. Ferrando AA, Tipton KD, Bamman MM, Wolfe RR. Resistance exercise maintains skeletal muscle protein synthesis during bed rest. *J Appl Physiol.* 1997;82:807-810.

15. Morris PE, Goad A, Thompson C, et al. Early intensive care unit mobility therapy in the treatment of acute respiratory failure. *Crit Care Med.* 2008;36:2238-2243.

16. Schweickert WD, Pohlman MC, Pohlman AS, et al. Early physical and occupational therapy in mechanically ventilated, critically ill patients: A randomised controlled trial. *Lancet.* 2009;373:1874-1882.

17. Griffiths RD, Palmer TE, Helliwell T, MacLennan P, MacMillan RR. Effect of passive stretching on the wasting of muscle in the critically ill. *Nutrition.* 1995;11:428-432.

18. Chang AT, Boots RJ, Brown MG, Paratz J, Hodges PW. Reduced inspiratory muscle endurance following successful weaning from prolonged mechanical ventilation. *Chest.* 2005;128:553-559.

19. Laghi F, Cattapan SE, Jubran A, et al. Is weaning failure caused by low-frequency fatigue of the diaphragm? *Am J Respir Crit Care Med.* 2003;167:120-127.

20. Watson AC, Hughes PD, Louise Harris M, et al. Measurement of twitch transdiaphragmatic, esophageal, and endotracheal tube pressure with bilateral anterolateral magnetic phrenic nerve stimulation in patients in the intensive care unit. *Crit Care Med.* 2001;29:1325-1331.

21. Tablan OC, Anderson LJ, Besser R, Bridges C, Hajjeh R. Guidelines for preventing health-care–associated pneumonia, 2003: Recommendations of CDC and the Healthcare Infection Control Practices Advisory Committee. *MMWR Recomm Rep.* 2004;53:1-36.

22. Kress JP, Pohlman AS, O'Connor MF, Hall JB. Daily interruption of sedative infusions in critically ill patients undergoing mechanical ventilation. *N Engl J Med.* 2000;342:1471-1477.

23. Esteban A, Frutos F, Tobin MJ, et al. A comparison of four methods of weaning patients from mechanical ventilation. Spanish Lung Failure Collaborative Group. *N Engl J Med.* 1995;332:345-350.

24. Meade M, Guyatt G, Sinuff T, et al. Trials comparing alternative weaning modes and discontinuation assessments. *Chest.* 2001;120:425S-437S.

25. Levine S, Nguyen T, Taylor N, et al. Rapid disuse atrophy of diaphragm fibers in mechanically ventilated humans. *N Engl J Med.* 2008;358:1327-1335.

26. Sassoon CS, Caiozzo VJ, Manka A, Sieck GC. Altered diaphragm contractile properties with controlled mechanical ventilation. *J Appl Physiol.* 2002;92:2585-2595.

27. Futier E, Constantin JM, Combaret L, et al. Pressure support ventilation attenuates ventilator-induced protein modifications in the diaphragm. *Crit Care.* 2008;12:R116.

28. Girard TD, Kress JP, Fuchs BD, et al. Efficacy and safety of a paired sedation and ventilator weaning protocol for mechanically ventilated patients in intensive care (awakening and breathing controlled trial): A randomised controlled trial. *Lancet.* 2008;371:126-134.

29. Brochard L, Rauss A, Benito S, et al. Comparison of three methods of gradual withdrawal from ventilatory support during weaning from mechanical ventilation. *Am J Respir Crit Care Med.* 1994;150:896-903.

30. Brochard L, Thille AW. What is the proper approach to liberating the weak from mechanical ventilation? *Crit Care Med.* 2009;37:S410-S415.

31. Bird SJ. Diagnosis and management of critical illness polyneuropathy and critical illness myopathy. *Curr Treat Options Neurol.* 2007;9:85-92.

32. Van den Berghe G, Schoonheydt K, Becx P, Bruyninckx F, Wouters PJ. Insulin therapy protects the central and peripheral nervous system of intensive care patients. *Neurology.* 2005;64:1348-1353.

33. de Jonghe B, Lacherade JC, Sharshar T, Outin H. Intensive care unit–acquired weakness: Risk factors and prevention. *Crit Care Med.* 2009;37:S309-S315.

34. Gajdos P, Chevret S, Clair B, Tranchant C, Chastang C. Clinical trial of plasma exchange and high-dose intravenous immunoglobulin in myasthenia gravis. Myasthenia Gravis Clinical Study Group. *Ann Neurol.* 1997;41:789-796.

35. Hughes RA, Wijdicks EF, Barohn R, et al. Practice parameter: Immunotherapy for Guillain-Barré syndrome: Report of the Quality Standards Subcommittee of the American Academy of Neurology. *Neurology.* 2003;61:736-740.

36. Hughes RA, Swan AV, van Koningsveld R, van Doorn PA. Corticosteroids for Guillain-Barré syndrome. *Cochrane Database Syst Rev.* 2006:CD001446.

37. Rumbak MJ, Newton M, Truncale T, Schwartz SW, Adams JW, Hazard PB. A prospective, randomized, study comparing early percutaneous dilational tracheotomy to prolonged translaryngeal intubation (delayed tracheotomy) in critically ill medical patients. *Crit Care Med.* 2004;32:1689-1694.

CHAPTER 7

Bacterial Meningitis

Mithil Gajera, MD
Quinn A. Czosnowski, PharmD, BCPS
Fred Rincon, MD, MSc, FACP

An otherwise healthy 29-year-old man is brought in to the emergency department (ED) because of 2 days of headache, flu-like symptoms, fever, and change in sensorium. On arrival at the ED his vital signs were: temperature 103.3°F, heart rate 138 bpm, respiratory rate 24 to 32 breaths/min, blood pressure 88/48 mm Hg, saturation 88% (room air), and Glasgow Coma Scale (GCS) 10. The patient's general examination revealed a patient in mild distress, injected conjunctivae, erythematous throat, pallor without cyanosis, petechial rash in lower extremities, nuchal rigidity, and normal cardiac and lung examination. Abdomen was mildly tender but no peritoneal signs were elicited. He was stuporous but arousable to loud voice and strong painful stimulation, he was able to follow some simple commands but inconsistently. Cranial nerves were normal and fundus did not show papilledema. He was localizing briskly with the upper extremities and withdrawing appropriately with both lower extremities. Reflexes were three-fourths throughout. A Foley catheter was inserted, obtaining only 10 mL of dark urine.

What are the initial steps for the management of this patient?

This patient's clinical presentation indicates an infection of the central nervous system (CNS) and systemic compromise, as signs of sepsis and septic shock are evident by the initial assessment performed in the ED. The initial evaluation of patients with a suspected CNS infection should include a detailed clinical history, assessment of epidemiologic factors, risk factors for infection, and medical comorbidities. Initial neurologic assessment provides important prognostic information and allows for comparison of serial neurologic examinations. This patient should be isolated in the ED, and droplet precautions should be maintained until a final etiologic diagnosis is made. Following initial assessment and determination of a potential CNS infection, initial steps in the management of this patient should include an evaluation of the ABCs (airway, breathing, and circulation), assessment of the hemodynamic status, collection of blood and cerebrospinal fluid (CSF) samples, and initiation of appropriate antimicrobial therapy. Patients with suspected meningitis who present with abnormal mental status or neurologic deficits, especially those with a GCS of 12 or less, require intensive care unit (ICU) admission for observation (Table 7-1).

Airway

Rapid neurologic deterioration and ensuing loss of consciousness with impairment of reflexes that maintain the airway mandate permanent airway control (Table 7-2).[1] Failure to recognize imminent airway loss may result in complications such as aspiration, hypoxemia, and hypercapnia. Preferred induction agents for rapid sequence intubation (RSI)

Table 7-1. Indications for ICU Admission

Age older than 60 years
Change in mental status with depressed GCS ≤ 12
Clinical or radiographic evidence of brain edema and midline shift or hydrocephalus
New focal neurologic deficit or deterioration despite appropriate treatment
Seizures or metabolic complication
Septic shock and/or respiratory failure with need for mechanical ventilation

Abbreviation: GCS, Glasgow Coma Scale.

in the setting of suspected brain injury with high intracranial pressure (ICP) include propofol[2] and etomidate,[3] both of which are short-acting agents that will not obscure the neurologic examination for a prolonged period of time. Adverse effects of propofol include drug-induced hypotension that usually responds to fluid infusion.[3] Adverse effects of etomidate include nausea, vomiting, myoclonic movements, seizures (by lowering of seizure threshold),[3] and adrenal suppression.[4] Midazolam may be an alternative, but unfavorable effects on the ICP have been reported with the use of this agent.[2,5] Succinylcholine is the most commonly administered muscle relaxant for RSI owing to its rapidity of onset (30 to 60 seconds) and short duration (5 to 15 minutes).[6] However, side effects of succinylcholine include hyperkalemia, cardiac arrhythmias, exacerbation of neuropathy or myopathy, malignant hyperthermia, and elevation of ICP in patients with intracranial mass lesions.[3,7] For this reason, in neurologic patients, a nondepolarizing neuromuscular blocking agent such as cis-atracurium,[8] rocuronium,[3] or vecuronium is preferred if needed.[9] In patients with increased ICP, premedication with intravenous lidocaine for RSI is of questionable use but sometimes has been suggested.[10]

Breathing

The goal of treatment is to ensure oxygenation and ventilation at an adequate oxygen level and maintenance of normocarbia, as this is associated with good effects on the cerebral blood flow (CBF). Both hypoxia and hyercarbia are detrimental for the CBF and have the potential for increasing cerebral edema and development of high ICP (Figure 7-1).[11]

Circulation

Isotonic fluid resuscitation and vasopressors are indicated for brain-injured patients in shock.[12,13] Dextrose-containing solutions should be avoided as hyperglycemia may be detrimental to the

Table 7-2. Indications for Intubation (Permanent Airway)

Inability to protect airway
Glasgow Coma Scale score ≤ 8
Intracranial pressure management
Hypoxemia and impaired ventilation (respiratory failure)
Increased work of breathing
Need to safely complete a diagnostic test (computed tomography, magnetic resonance imaging, lumbar puncture)

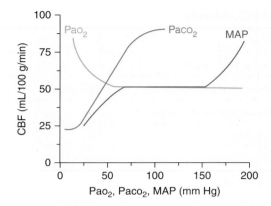

Figure 7-1. Effect of blood gases on cerebral blood flow (CBF) and intracranial pressure (ICP). (*Adapted from Miller RD, et al. Miller's Anesthesia, 7th ed, page 308.*)

injured brain.[14] Initial assessment of the volume status by placement of a central venous catheter for measurement of central venous pressure (CVP) is recommended by current Surviving Sepsis Campaign Guidelines to achieve a CVP of 8 to 10 mm Hg and a goal mean arterial pressure (MAP) of 65 mm Hg or more with crystalloids, colloids, or vasopressors.[13] The influence of such treatment on the CBF of these patients is unknown. In the healthy person, cerebral autoregulation maintains a constant CBF with MAP ranging from 60 to 130 mm Hg. However, when autoregulation is impaired, as it may in severe CNS infections, there is a risk of cerebral hypoperfusion as well as ischemia when MAP decreases, and a risk of hyperperfusion leading to vasogenic edema when MAP increases. An association between cerebral ischemia and poor neurologic outcome or death has been demonstrated in various studies of bacterial meningitis.[15,16] Cerebral perfusion pressures (CPPs) less than 30 mm Hg were strongly correlated with death or major neurologic sequelae in infants and children with meningitis.[17] Taken together, these findings suggest that maintenance of an adequate CPP, primarily by manipulating MAP, would prevent cerebral ischemia, attenuate brain damage, and improve the prognosis.

Dopamine, norepinephrine, and phenylephrine are frequently used to restore CPP by increasing the MAP in the ICU. Selection of the initial vasopressor is frequently guided by the clinical characteristics of the patient as well as the goals of therapy. Consideration should be given to the effect of vasopressors on cerebral hemodynamics (Table 7-3). The disruption of the blood-brain barrier (BBB) in

Table 7-3. Hemodynamic Effects of Vasopressors on Cerebral Circulation

Drug	Mechanism	CBF	ICP	$CMRO_2$	$PbtO_2$
Phenylephrine	Alpha-1 receptor agonist	⇑	⇑	⇔	⇔
Norepinephrine	Mixed alpha/beta-1 receptor agonist	⇑	⇔	⇔	⇑
Epinephrine	Mixed alpha/beta agonist	⇑	N/A	⇑	N/A
Dopamine	Dose-dependent agonist: dopa, beta, alpha	⇑	⇔	⇔	⇔
Vasopressin	V1 receptor agonist	⇑	N/A	⇔	⇑

Abbreviations: CBF, cerebral blood flow; ICP, intracranial pressure; $CMRO_2$, cerebral metabolic rate of oxygen; $PbtO_2$, brain tissue oxygen tension. (*Adapted with permission from Muzevich KM and Voils SA. Role of vasopressor administration in patients with acute neurologic injury. Neurocrit Care 2009;11:112-119.*)

CNS infections may allow for these agents to have direct effects on the cerebral vasculature, although this may be theoretical. Several studies have demonstrated that norepinephrine may increase the CBF with no net effect on ICP, global cerebral metabolism, and oxygen consumption, suggesting that the net effect on CBF is related to abnormal autoregulation (Table 7-3).[18] Both norepinephrine and dopamine have been recommended as first-line vasopressors in patients with septic shock; however, a recent study showed less side effects when using norepinephrine, making this the agent of choice in septic shock.[19]

Should antibiotics be delayed pending a lumbar puncture (LP) and when should a computed tomographic (CT) scan be performed?

A lumbar puncture is essential to obtain CSF and to make the definitive diagnosis of a CNS infection. Opening pressures are usually elevated and may be in the range of 20 to 50 cm H_2O.[20] Complications after LP are variable, but the most feared complication is life-threatening herniation. A theoretical pressure gradient with downward displacement of the cerebrum and brainstem can be triggered by an LP. However, studies addressing this phenomenon have found that herniation occurs more than 8 hours after the LP.[21] In a study of 129 adult patients with elevated ICP, 1% with papilledema and 12% without papilledema had unfavorable outcomes within 48 hours after LP.[22] This supports the possibility that herniation after LP in the setting of space-occupying lesion may occur in patients who are going to herniate even if the LP is not done. In a recent study of 301 adults with bacterial meningitis, abnormal findings in the physical examination associated with an abnormal head CT scan were age 60 years or older, history of CNS disease (tumor, stroke, focal infection), an immunosuppressed state (human immunodeficiency virus [HIV], acquired immune deficiency syndrome [AIDS], chemotherapy, and posttransplantation), history of new-onset seizures, abnormal level of consciousness, and abnormal neurologic examination (eg, gaze preference, visual field defects, paralysis).[23] On the basis of this study, the Practice Guideline Committee for the Treatment of Bacterial Meningitis recommends a CT scan of the brain in all patients with these abnormalities (Table 7-4).[20] CT scans are essential to evaluate for complications of CNS infections such as cerebral edema or collections (abscess or hemorrhage), and should be conducted in all patients even though some data suggest that CT scans are not very sensitive at predicting herniation following an LP.[24,25] The decision to obtain a CT scan prior to LP should not affect the timing of administration of antibiotics.

Table 7-4. Indications for CT Scan of the Brain Before LP in Suspected Bacterial Meningitis

Criteria	Indications
Depressed level of consciousness	Abnormal GCS
Focal or lateralizing neurologic examination	Papilledema, ophthalmoplegia, hemiparesis, abnormal motor response
New-onset seizures	Recent seizure
Immunosuppressed state	HIV/AIDS, chemotherapy for cancer or transplant, chronic high steroid use (>1 mg/kg/day, >1 week)
History of CNS pathology	Tumor, stroke, previous infections

Abbreviations: CNS, central nervous system; CT, computed tomography; GCS, Glasgow Coma Scale; HIV/AIDS, human immunodeficiency virus/acquired immune deficiency syndrome; LP, lumbar puncture.

What factors are important in the selection and delivery of an appropriate antibiotic treatment regimen?

The key to the treatment of CNS infections is early delivery of an appropriate empiric antibiotic regimen.[26] Selection of the empiric regimen will vary depending on the suspected organism and the local drug-resistance patterns for that organism. The suspected organism type varies based on several patient factors including age, immune status, predisposing conditions, and other comorbidities (Table 7-5). It is extremely important that patients are assessed for the most likely causative organisms and that intravenous treatment is delivered for those potential causes. Current guideline recommendations do not provide a recommended time frame from onset of symptoms to delivery of an appropriate antibiotic regimen owing to a lack of prospective data but experience in septic shock patients suggests the earlier the better.[13,27] Available studies demonstrate a reduced mortality rate and fewer neurologic complications in patients who received timely administration of antibiotics,[28,29] and retrospective observational data show that the delay in antibiotic therapy was independently correlated with unfavorable outcomes.[30] If antibiotics are administered prior to LP, they may diminish the yield of the bacterial Gram stain or culture of the CSF by 20%. Therefore, when LP cannot be conducted prior to antibiotic delivery, it should be performed as soon as possible after antibiotic administration to minimize the effect on Gram stain and culture.

In addition to timely administration of an appropriate antibiotic regimen, the dose of the antibiotic is extremely important. Transport of drugs across the BBB is dependent on several factors, including, but not limited to, lipophilicity, protein binding, and the presence of inflammation, and many commonly used antibiotics exhibit poor penetration into the CNS.[31] Owing to limited penetration and systemic toxicities associated with some intravenous therapies, some practitioners have utilized the intraventricular route of administration to treat severe infections.[20] After identification of the causative organism, the antibiotic regimen should be reviewed and adjusted to the most effective available antibiotic.

Empiric treatment regimens should also include treatment for viral encephalitis pending results of diagnostic testing. Numerous viruses have been reported as causes of encephalitis, although delivery of empiric antiviral therapy is typically limited to infections due to the herpesviruses. In addition, the empiric regimen may need to include doxycycline in patients who present with signs and symptoms suggestive of rickettsial or ehrlichial infections during the appropriate seasons (see Table 7-5). Empiric treatment regimens should not routinely include drugs for other causes of encephalitis. These treatment regimens should only be started once a specific viral cause is identified. Clinical practice guidelines are available for the treatment of encephalitis and should be used to determine the appropriate treatment for these infections.[32]

What is the role of systemic corticosteroids in the empiric treatment of patients with CNS infections?

Experimental models of bacterial meningitis have demonstrated that the inflammatory response in the subarachnoid space is a major contributing factor to the associated morbidity and mortality.[20] The majority of the data pertaining to corticosteroids in CNS infections comes from the pediatric population. A meta-analysis of all studies conducted in infants and children from 1988 to 1996 demonstrated reductions in hearing impairment in patients with infection due to *Haemophilus influenzae* and protection against severe hearing loss in patients with *Streptococcus pneumoniae* if corticosteroid therapy was started prior to or with the first dose of antibiotics.[33] To date, only one randomized, double-blinded, placebo-controlled trial has demonstrated a significant mortality rate reduction in adults.[34] In this study, patients received dexamethasone 10 mg IV every 6 hours for 4 days with the first dose being administered 15 to 20 minutes prior to antibiotics. Patients randomized to dexamethasone had significant reductions in unfavorable outcomes and death, but notably, the only subgroup of patients who experienced statistically significant reductions in unfavorable outcomes (26% versus 52%,

Table 7-5. Risk Factors, Common Pathogens, and Suggested Empiric Treatment Regimens

Risk Factor	Common Pathogens	Empiric Antibiotic/Antiviral Therapy and IV Dosing Recommendations[a]
Age		
<1 mo[b]	*Streptococcus agalactiae, Escherichia coli, Listeria monocytogenes, Klebsiella* species	Ampicillin plus cefotaxime or ampicillin plus an aminoglycoside
1-23 mo[b]	*Streptococcus pneumoniae, Neisseria meningitidis, S. agalactiae, Haemophilus influenzae, Escherichia coli*	Vancomycin plus ceftriaxone or cefotaxime
2-50 y[b]	*N. meningitidis, S. pneumoniae*	Vancomycin plus ceftriaxone or cefotaxime (Adult dosing: Vancomycin 20 mg/kg q8-12h plus either ceftriaxone 2 g q12h or cefotaxime 2 g q4-6h)
>50 y	*S. pneumoniae, N. meningitides, L. monocytogenes,* aerobic gram-negative bacilli	Vancomycin 20 mg/kg q8-12h plus ampicillin 2 g q4h plus either ceftriaxone 2 g q12h or cefotaxime 2 g q4-6h
Head trauma		
Basilar skull fracture	*S. pneumoniae, H. influenzae,* group A β-hemolytic streptococci	Vancomycin 20 mg/kg q8-12h plus either ceftriaxone 2 g q12h or cefotaxime 2 g q4-6h
Penetrating trauma	*Staphylococcus aureus,* coagulase-negative staphylococci, aerobic gram-negative bacilli (including *Pseudomonas aeruginosa* and *Acinetobacter baumannii*)	Vancomycin 20 mg/kg q8-12h plus either cefepime 2 g q8h or ceftazidime 2 g q8h or meropenem 2 g q8h
Postneurosurgery		
	Aerobic gram-negative bacilli (including *P. aeruginosa* and *A. baumannii*), *S. aureus,* coagulase-negative staphylococci	Vancomycin 20 mg/kg q8-12h plus either cefepime 2 g q8h or ceftazidime 2 g q8h or meropenem 2 g q8h
Cerebrospinal fluid shunt		
	Coagulase-negative staphylococci, *S. aureus,* aerobic gram-negative bacilli (including *P. aeruginosa* and *A. baumannii*), *Propionibacterium acnes*	Vancomycin 20 mg/kg q8-12h plus either cefepime 2 g q8h or ceftazidime 2 g q8h or meropenem 2 g q8h
Tick exposure		
	Ehrlichial, rickettsial	Doxycycline 100 mg q12h
Viral infection		
	Herpes viruses	Acyclovir 10 mg/kg q8h

[a]Dosage adjustments may be required based on renal function.

[b]Dosing varies for patients <18 years old.

(From Tunkel AR, Hartman BJ, Kaplan SL, et al. Practice Guidelines for the Management of Bacterial Meningitis. Clin Infect Dis. 2004;39:1267-1284.)

$P = .006$) and mortality rates (14% versus 34%, $P = .02$) were those with pneumococcal meningitis, although the other subgroups had relatively few patients.

Despite the available data, there is still controversy about the use of steroids in meningitis based on the fact that antibiotic penetration into the CSF relies on meningeal inflammation and administration of dexamethasone may decrease the inflammatory response. Nevertheless, current guidelines recommend the initiation of dexamethasone at a dose of 0.15 mg/kg IV every 6 hours for 2 to 4 days 10 to 20 minutes before or with antibiotic therapy in all infants, children, and adults with suspected bacterial meningitis. Steroids should not be administered following antibiotics as they are unlikely to be of benefit. In adults without evidence of pneumococcal meningitis on CSF Gram stain or blood culture, corticosteroids should be discontinued. Current data do not support a recommendation for their use in herpetic encephalitis.[32]

Should we be concerned about high ICP in this patient and is he a candidate for ICP monitoring?

Elevated ICP with herniation and compression of the brainstem is the most frequent cause of death in patients with CNS infections.[35,36] Increased ICP in bacterial meningitis is secondary to the development of cerebral edema. Additionally, high ICP could be the result of increased intracranial blood volume from venous congestion due to thrombotic venous occlusion of the cerebral sinuses or due to arteriolar dilation from impaired autoregulation and high CBF.[37,38] It is important to remember that neither CT scan nor papilledema can predict a high ICP in the acute setting, but intracranial hypertension may be suspected in stuporous or comatose patients, those who present acutely with clinical signs of brainstem herniation (ie, pupillary abnormalities or motor posturing), and those with abnormal CT scans suggesting brain shifts and mass effect.

If intracranial hypertension with imminent herniation is suspected, the head should be elevated to 30 degrees, 1.0 to 1.5 g/kg of 20% mannitol should be administered by a rapid infusion, and the patient should be hyperventilated to a $Paco_2$ of 26 to 30 mm Hg. As an alternative, or if the patient is relatively hypotensive, 0.5 to 2.0 mL/kg of 23.4% hypertonic saline (HS) solution can be administered through a central venous line,[39] but there is no evidence for the use of either agent in the treatment of high ICP in CNS infections, but HS has some advantages over mannitol in infection-related cerebral edema.

The osmotic reflection coefficient of the brain capillaries to sodium is 1.0 as compared to 0.9 in the case of mannitol, indicating that HS does not effectively cross the brain capillaries, and over the first few hours of a bolus of HS, the concentration of sodium in the CSF does not change; this forms the basis of efficacy of HS as an effective osmotic agent in brain edema.[40] Therefore, in infection-related cerebral edema, where permeability or integrity of the BBB is disturbed, less permeable agents like HS provide more osmosis than higher permeable agents like mannitol. HS has neuroprotective effects owing to its anti-inflammatory action,[41,42] whereas mannitol prevents biochemical injury owing to its free-radical scavenger effect.[43] Moreover, mannitol is relatively contraindicated in hypovolemic patients because of the diuretic effect, and HS is superior in hypovolemic and hypotensive patients and would be the preferred agent in this patient and those with severe sepsis or in septic shock. Adverse effects of HS include fluid overload, hematologic and electrolyte abnormalities, such as bleeding secondary to decreased platelet aggregation and prolonged coagulation times, hypokalemia, and hyperchloremic acidosis.[44] The serum sodium level should never be allowed to drop more than 12 mEq/L over 24 hours as rapid withdrawal of hypertonic therapy may result in rebound cerebral edema, leading to elevated ICP and/or herniation syndromes.[44,45] Additional adverse effects of mannitol include paradoxical cerebral edema and rebound high ICP based on its propensity to cross the BBB, drawing free water into the CNS. Other side effects include hyperosmolarity and renal failure specifically when serum osmolarities are greater than 320, which will wash out the renal medullary gradient.

An ICP of more than 20 cm H_2O (15 mm Hg) should be aggressively treated to prevent cerebral herniation and irreversible brainstem injury. Studies in patients with meningitis have shown that the mean ICP was significantly higher in nonsurvivors compared to survivors.[36] When an ICP monitoring device is in place, maintenance of an adequate CPP and a normal ICP should be attempted at all times. CPPs 50 mm Hg or less were found to be associated with a 100% death rate in patients with bacterial meningitis,[46] and when the initial ICP was higher than 40 mm Hg, death occurred in 75% of those patients.[36] Therefore, it is important to recognize signs of intracranial hypertension and institute adequate monitoring and aggressive treatment. High ICPs may be lowered successfully in most patients with bacterial meningitis by different measures and using unconventional volume-targeted (Lund concept) ICP management.[47]

For cases of severe or intractable elevated ICP, barbiturates and induced therapeutic hypothermia are also effective tools to control refractory elevated ICP by decreasing cerebral metabolic activity, which translates into a reduction of the CBF. These two techniques require expertise, advanced tools, and continuous monitoring of cerebral electrical activity and may be associated with significant complications.

Should we institute prophylactic anticonvulsant treatment in this patient?

The frequency of clinical seizures in bacterial meningitis is 5% to 27%[48] and in viral encephalitis is 62% to 67%,[49] and the presence of encephalitis and a GCS less than 12 were independent predictors for the occurrence of clinical seizure.[50] There are no data to suggest the role of prophylactic anti-seizure medication, but suspicion of ictal activity should be raised in those patients with abnormal movements, persistent coma, or altered sensorium.[51] Continuous electroencephalographic (EEG) monitoring may be indicated in these patients and may help with the identification of subclinical ictal activity and patterns associated with poor outcome such as periodic lateralizing epileptiform discharges (PLEDs),[52] but there is still no consensus on whether to treat these patterns and, if so, how aggressively.[53]

Once this patient is resuscitated in the ED, what would be the next step in the management?

This patient in septic shock requires admission to an ICU (see Table 7-1). Ongoing resuscitation should continue and systematic optimization of accompanying organ failure should be achieved. Measurements in the ICU indicated for the optimal cardiovascular monitoring of septic shock patients include invasive arterial blood pressure, CVP, and pulmonary artery catheter (PAC) monitoring. An external ventricular drain should be placed in patients with a depressed level of consciousness (GCS score 8 or less), signs of acute hydrocephalus or intracranial mass effect on CT, and a prognosis that warrants aggressive ICU care.[54] ICU monitoring of patients with CNS infections follows conventional guidelines for septic/septic shock patients.[13] Additionally, continuous EEG (cEEG) and measurements of Scvo$_2$, Pbto$_2$, and Jbo$_2$ can be accomplished but without a demonstrated change in patient's outcome.

Patient Positioning

To minimize ICP and reduce the risk of ventilator-associated pneumonia in mechanically ventilated patients, the head should be elevated 30 degrees. In mechanically ventilated patients, further need for head elevation should be guided by changing of pulmonary and volume needs.

Fluids

Isotonic fluids such as 0.9% saline at a rate of approximately 1 mL/kg per hour should be given as the standard intravenous replacement fluid for patients with meningitis and optimized to achieve euvolemic balance and an hourly diuresis of greater than 0.5 mL/kg. Free water given in the form of 0.45% saline or 5% dextrose in water can exacerbate cerebral edema and increase ICP because it flows down its osmotic gradient into injured brain tissue.[14] Systemic hyposmolality (less than 280 mOsm/L) should be aggressively treated with mannitol or 3% HS. A state of euvolemia should be maintained by monitoring fluid balance and body weight and by maintaining a normal CVP (range 6 to 8 mm Hg, or CVP 8 to 10 or more if in septic shock).

Sedation

Sedation should be used to minimize pain, agitation, and decrease surges in the ICP. In general, many practitioners prefer sedative agents that do not have effects on ICP. The main disadvantage is the inevitable loss of some elements of the neurologic examination required for clinical monitoring of these patients. Short-term sedation with propofol or midazolam plus either sufentanil or fentanyl is preferred.[2,8,9]

Management of Hyperglycemia

Hyperglycemia and insulin resistance are almost universal findings in patients with sepsis, although data on CNS infections are lacking.[55] In the critically ill population, hyperglycemia seems much more acutely toxic than in healthy individuals, for whom cells can protect themselves by downregulation of glucose transporters.[56] The acute toxicity of high levels of glucose in critical illness might be explained by an accelerated cellular glucose overload and more pronounced toxic side effects of glycolysis and oxidative phosphorylation.[57] In the Dutch Cohort Study, high serum glucose concentrations were related to lower GCS score on the admission and to unfavorable clinical outcome,[58] but episodes of hypoglycemia have also been associated with increased mortality[59] and worse neurologic outcomes,[60] even though in strict clinical environments tight glucose control has been linked to reductions in ICP, duration of mechanical ventilation, and seizures in critically ill neurologic patients as well.[61] Thus, to minimize the risk of severe hypoglycemia and to avoid worsening possible neuronal damage related to hyperglycemia, it may be reasonable to have tight sugar control with targets between 100 and 150 mg/dL.

DVT Prophylaxis and/or Full Anticoagulation

Critically ill patients are at high risk for deep vein thrombosis (DVT) and pulmonary embolism, a potentially fatal complication, due to limb paresis and prolonged immobilization. Alternatives include dynamic compression stockings, unfractionated heparin (UFH), or low-molecular-weight heparin (LMWH). Additionally, cerebrovascular complications like venous thrombosis or infarction occur in 15% to 20% of adults with bacterial meningitis. The possibility of thrombosis of the cerebral veins and sinuses should be considered in those patients who have deterioration of consciousness, seizures, fluctuating focal neurologic abnormalities, and stroke with nonarterial distribution. In this situation, full anticoagulation with UFH should be considered, as UFH has been found to modulate the inflammatory process in addition to its well-characterized effect on coagulation. Patients with bacterial meningitis who are treated with anticoagulant therapy are likely to have a higher risk of intracranial hemorrhage.[62,63]

Nutrition

As is the case with all critically ill neurologic patients, enteral feeding should be started within 48 hours to avoid protein catabolism and malnutrition. A small-bore nasoduodenal feeding tube may reduce the risk of aspiration events.

Therapy-Induced Hypothermia

The rise in ICP common to patients with meningitis often occurs within 12 hours of admission to the hospital, and this time coincides with the increase in the inflammatory response generated by the antibiotic enhancing the inflammatory response and worsening cerebral edema.[35] Recognizing the sequence of these events offers a window of opportunity to attenuate the inflammatory response and treat or prevent secondary neuronal damage. The application of moderate hypothermia in an animal model of severe meningitis preserved markers of BBB function, reduced release of excitatory amino acids, decreased CSF nitric oxide, decreased myeloperoxidase activity in brain tissue,[64] and reduced

ICP.[65] Mild therapy-induced hypothermia may be an effective adjuvant to conventional therapy in the management of severe meningitis.

Activated Protein C (APC)

A large multicenter, placebo-controlled trial reported the efficacy of APC in patients with severe sepsis and APACHE II score 25 or higher.[66] The number of patients with sepsis from meningitis who were included in this trial is unknown, but patients in this trial who were at increased risk of bleeding were excluded. Although life-threatening bleeds and intracranial hemorrhage (ICH) appeared to be uncommon in APC-treated patients,[66] there is still concern about intracranial bleeding in patients with meningitis. In a retrospective analysis of placebo-controlled, open-label, and compassionate-use trials, Vincent et al reported that the majority of patients with meningococcal meningitis had APACHE II scores of less than 22 and were not treated with APC.[62] However, those who received APC had a higher incidence of ICH, despite a lower 28-day mortality rate, and similar overall serious bleeding events. Thus, the safety of APC in patients with septic shock and CNS infections is questionable.

Are there any additional or promising therapies for patients with meningitis?

Yes, currently there are data suggesting that nimodipine and statins may play a role in the management of meningitis.

Nimodipine

In patients with bacterial meningitis, tissue-type plasminogen activator (tPA) and PA inhibitor-1 (PAI-1) concentrations in the CSF and serum are increased, indicating a decrease in fibrinolysis.[67] In one case series of 12 patients with bacterial meningitis, elevated serum urokinase and tPA protein concentrations correlated with adverse outcome.[68] Treatment with nimodipine in patients with subarachnoid hemorrhage (SAH) decreased the PAI-1 level, suggesting a role in fibrinolytic activity.[67] Nimodipine is already known to be neuroprotective and has some role in vasoconstriction or vasospasm. Although speculative, these findings indicate that impaired fibrinolysis might be an important factor in patients with bacterial meningitis and that nimodipine might be useful as an adjunctive therapy.[69]

Statins

These agents can attenuate leukocyte invasion into the CNS and completely abolish hyperthermia in bacterial meningitis. This neuroprotective effect can be explained by multiple pleiotropic and anti-inflammatory properties of the drug. Statins can downregulate the production of many acute-phase cytokines and chemokines, such as tumor necrosis factor-alpha (TNF-α) and the interleukins (ILs) IL-1β and IL-6. Statins increase the activity of endothelial NO synthase (eNOS) by upregulating eNOS expression, inducing eNOS phosphorylation and activating eNOS directly, which has a neuroprotective effect.[70]

! CRITICAL CONSIDERATIONS

- The initial evaluation of patients with a suspected CNS infection should include a detailed clinical history, assessment of epidemiologic factors, risk factors for infection, and medical comorbidities.

- Following initial assessment and determination of a potential CNS infection, initial steps in the management of this patient should include an evaluation of the ABCs, assessment of the hemodynamic status, collection of blood and CSF samples, and initiation of appropriate antimicrobial therapy.
- A lumbar puncture is essential to obtain cerebral spinal fluid (CSF) and to make the definitive diagnosis of a CNS infection. Although they may be contraindicated in certain subgroups, this should not delay the timely delivery of antibiotics.
- The key to the treatment of CNS infections is early delivery of an appropriate empiric antibiotic regimen, and selection of the empiric regimen will vary depending on the suspected organism and the local drug-resistance patterns for that organism.
- Steroids may be indicated in streptococcal meningitis and should be given prior to or with the first dose of antibiotics.
- A high ICP with herniation and compression of the brainstem is the most frequent cause of death in patients with CNS infections. Measures to lower ICP or prevent high ICPs should be instituted in patients with severe meningitis.

REFERENCES

1. Gujjar AR, Deibert E, Manno EM, Duff S, Diringer MN. Mechanical ventilation for ischemic stroke and intracerebral hemorrhage: indications, timing, and outcome. *Neurology.* 1998;51:447-451.
2. Diringer MN. Intracerebral hemorrhage: pathophysiology and management. *Crit Care Med.* 1993;21:152-157.
3. Reynolds SF, Heffner J. Airway management of the critically ill patient: rapid-sequence intubation. *Chest.* 2005;127:1397-1412.
4. Fellows IW, Bastow MD, Byrne AJ, Allison SP. Adrenocortical suppression in multiply injured patients: a complication of etomidate treatment. *Br Med J (Clin Res Ed).*1983;287(6408):1835-1837.
5. Papazian L, Albanese J, Thirion X, Perrin G, Durbec O, Martin C. Effect of bolus doses of midazolam on intracranial pressure and cerebral perfusion pressure in patients with severe head injury. *Br J Anaesth.* 1993;71:267-271.
6. Orebaugh SL. Succinylcholine: adverse effects and alternatives in emergency medicine. *Am J Emerg Med.* 1999;17:715-721.
7. Booij LH. Is succinylcholine appropriate or obsolete in the intensive care unit? *Crit Care.* 2001;5:245-246.
8. Schramm WM, Jesenko R, Bartunek A, Gilly H. Effects of *cis*-atracurium on cerebral and cardiovascular hemodynamics in patients with severe brain injury. *Acta Anaesthesiol Scand.* 1997;41:1319-1323.
9. Schramm WM, Strasser K, Bartunek A, Gilly H, Spiss CK. Effects of rocuronium and vecuronium on intracranial pressure, mean arterial pressure and heart rate in neurosurgical patients. *Br J Anaesth.* 1996;77:607-611.
10. Robinson N, Clancy M. In patients with head injury undergoing rapid sequence intubation, does pretreatment with intravenous lignocaine/lidocaine lead to an improved neurological outcome? A review of the literature. *Emerg Med J.* 2001;18:453-457.
11. Miller R. Anesthesia for neurosurgery. In: Firestone L, Lebowitz P, Cook C, eds. *Clinical Anesthesia Procedures of the Massachussetts General Hospital.* 3rd ed. Boston, MA: Little Brown; 1988.
12. Broderick J, Connolly S, Feldmann E, et al. Guidelines for the management of spontaneous intracerebral hemorrhage in adults: 2007 update: a guideline from the American Heart Association/American Stroke Association Stroke Council, High Blood Pressure Research Council, and the Quality of Care and Outcomes in Research Interdisciplinary Working Group. *Stroke.* 2007;38:2001-2023.
13. Dellinger RP, Levy MM, Carlet JM, et al. Surviving Sepsis Campaign: International guidelines for management of severe sepsis and septic shock: 2008. *Crit Care Med.* 2008;36:296-327.
14. Passero S, Ciacci G, Ulivelli M. The influence of diabetes and hyperglycemia on clinical course after intracerebral hemorrhage. *Neurology.* 2003;61:1351-1356.
15. Ashwal S, Stringer W, Tomasi L, Schneider S, Thompson J, Perkin R. Cerebral blood flow and

carbon dioxide reactivity in children with bacterial meningitis. *J Pediatr.* 1990;117:523-530.

16. Tauber MG. Brain edema, intracranial pressure and cerebral blood flow in bacterial meningitis. *Pediatr Infect Dis J.* 1989;8(12):915-917.

17. Tureen J. Cerebral blood flow and metabolism in experimental meningitis. *Pediatr Infect Dis J.* 1989;8:917-918.

18. Muzevich KM, Voils SA. Role of vasopressor administration in patients with acute neurologic injury. *Neurocrit Care.* 2009;11:112-119.

19. De Backer D, Biston P, Devriendt J, et al. Comparison of dopamine and norepinephrine in the treatment of shock. *N Engl J Med.* 2010;362:779-789.

20. Tunkel AR, Hartman BJ, Kaplan SL, et al. Practice guidelines for the management of bacterial meningitis. *Clin Infect Dis.* 2004;39:1267-1284.

21. Horwitz SJ, Boxerbaum B, O'Bell J. Cerebral herniation in bacterial meningitis in childhood. *Ann Neurol.* 1980;7:524-528.

22. Korein J, Cravioto H, Leicach M. Reevaluation of lumbar puncture; a study of 129 patients with papilledema or intracranial hypertension. *Neurology.* 1959;9:290-297.

23. Hasbun R, Abrahams J, Jekel J, Quagliarello VJ. Computed tomography of the head before lumbar puncture in adults with suspected meningitis. *N Engl J Med.* 2001;345:1727-1733.

24. Baker ND, Kharazi H, Laurent L, et al. The efficacy of routine head computed tomography (CT scan) prior to lumbar puncture in the emergency department. *J Emerg Med.* 1994;12:597-601.

25. Mellor DH. The place of computed tomography and lumbar puncture in suspected bacterial meningitis. *Arch Dis Child.* 1992;67:1417-1419.

26. Kumar A, Ellis P, Arabi Y, et al. Initiation of inappropriate antimicrobial therapy results in a fivefold reduction of survival in human septic shock. *Chest.* 2009;136:1237-1248.

27. Kumar A, Roberts D, Wood KE, et al. Duration of hypotension before initiation of effective antimicrobial therapy is the critical determinant of survival in human septic shock. *Crit Care Med.* 2006;34:1589-1596.

28. Miner JR, Heegaard W, Mapes A, Biros M. Presentation, time to antibiotics, and mortality of patients with bacterial meningitis at an urban county medical center. *J Emerg Med.* 2001;21:387-392.

29. Lu CH, Huang CR, Chang WN, et al. Community-acquired bacterial meningitis in adults: the epidemiology, timing of appropriate antimicrobial therapy, and prognostic factors. *Clin Neurol Neurosurg.* 2002;104:352-358.

30. Koster-Rasmussen R, Korshin A, Meyer CN. Antibiotic treatment delay and outcome in acute bacterial meningitis. *J Infect.* 2008;57:449-454.

31. Lutsar I, McCracken GH Jr, Friedland IR. Antibiotic pharmacodynamics in cerebrospinal fluid. *Clin Infect Dis.* 1998;27:1117-1127, quiz 1128-1129.

32. Tunkel AR, Glaser CA, Bloch KC, et al. The management of encephalitis: Clinical practice guidelines by the Infectious Diseases Society of America. *Clin Infect Dis.* 2008;47:303-527.

33. McIntyre PB, Berkey CS, King SM, et al. Dexamethasone as adjunctive therapy in bacterial meningitis. A meta-analysis of randomized clinical trials since 1988. *JAMA.* 1997;278:925-931.

34. de Gans J, van de Beek D. Dexamethasone in adults with bacterial meningitis. *N Engl J Med.* 2002;347:1549-1556.

35. Rennick G, Shann F, de Campo J. Cerebral herniation during bacterial meningitis in children. *BMJ.* 1993;306(6883):953-955.

36. Lindvall P, Ahlm C, Ericsson M, Gothefors L, Naredi S, Koskinen LO. Reducing intracranial pressure may increase survival among patients with bacterial meningitis. *Clin Infect Dis.* 2004;38:384-390.

37. Moller K, Larsen FS, Qvist J, et al. Dependency of cerebral blood flow on mean arterial pressure in patients with acute bacterial meningitis. *Crit Care Med.* 2000;28:1027-1032.

38. Moller K, Skinhoj P, Knudsen GM, Larsen FS. Effect of short-term hyperventilation on cerebral blood flow autoregulation in patients with acute bacterial meningitis. *Stroke.* 2000;31: 1116-1122.

39. Qureshi AI, Wilson DA, Traystman RJ. Treatment of transtentorial herniation unresponsive to hyperventilation using hypertonic saline in dogs: effect on cerebral blood flow and metabolism. *J Neurosurg Anesthesiol.* 2002;14:22-30.

40. Suarez JI. Hypertonic saline for cerebral edema and elevated intracranial pressure. *Cleve Clin J Med.* 2004;71(suppl 1):S9-S13.

41. Rhee P, Wang D, Ruff P, et al. Human neutrophil activation and increased adhesion by various resuscitation fluids. *Crit Care Med.* 2000;28: 74-78.

42. Rizoli SB, Kapus A, Fan J, Li YH, Marshall JC, Rotstein OD. Immunomodulatory effects of hypertonic resuscitation on the development of lung inflammation following hemorrhagic shock. *J Immunol.* 1998;161:6288-6296.

43. Mizoi K, Suzuki J, Imaizumi S, Yoshimoto T. Development of new cerebral protective agents: The free radical scavengers. *Neurol Res.* 1986;8: 75-80.

44. Ziai WC, Toung TJ, Bhardwaj A. Hypertonic saline: first-line therapy for cerebral edema? *J Neurol Sci.* 2007;261:157-166.

45. Adrogue HJ, Madias NE. Hypernatremia. *N Engl J Med.* 2000;18;342:1493-1499.

46. Gaussorgues P, Guerin C, Boyer F, et al. [Intracranial hypertension in comatose bacterial meningitis]. *Presse Med.* 1987;16:1420-1423.

47. Lundberg N. Continuous recording and control of ventricular fluid pressure in neurosurgical practice. *Acta Psychiatr Scand Suppl.* 1960;36:1-193.

48. Wang KW, Chang WN, Chang HW, et al. The significance of seizures and other predictive factors during the acute illness for the long-term outcome after bacterial meningitis. *Seizure.* 2005;4:586-592.

49. Skoldenberg B, Forsgren M, Alestig K, et al. Acyclovir versus vidarabine in herpes simplex encephalitis. Randomised multicentre study in consecutive Swedish patients. *Lancet.* 1984;2:707-711.

50. Kim MA, Park KM, Kim SE, Oh MK. Acute symptomatic seizures in CNS infection. *Eur J Neurol.* 2008;15:38-41.

51. van de Beek D, de Gans J, Tunkel AR, Wijdicks EF. Community-acquired bacterial meningitis in adults. *N Engl J Med.* 2006;354:44-53.

52. Carrera E, Claassen J, Oddo M, Emerson RG, Mayer SA, Hirsch LJ. Continuous electroencephalographic monitoring in critically ill patients with central nervous system infections. *Arch Neurol.* 2008;6:1612-1618.

53. Garcia-Morales I, Garcia MT, Galan-Davila L, et al. Periodic lateralized epileptiform discharges: etiology, clinical aspects, seizures, and evolution in 130 patients. *J Clin Neurophysiol.* 2002;19:172-177.

54. Mayer SA, Chong J. Critical care management of increased intracranial pressure. *J Intensive Care Med.* 2002;17:55-67.

55. Marik PE, Raghavan M. Stress-hyperglycemia, insulin and immunomodulation in sepsis. *Intensive Care Med.* 2004;30:748-756.

56. Klip A, Tsakiridis T, Marette A, Ortiz PA. Regulation of expression of glucose transporters by glucose: a review of studies in vivo and in cell cultures. *FASEB J.* 1994;8:43-53.

57. Van den Berghe G. How does blood glucose control with insulin save lives in intensive care? *J Clin Invest.* 2004;114:1187-1195.

58. Hansen TK, Thiel S, Wouters PJ, Christiansen JS, Van den Berghe G. Intensive insulin therapy exerts anti-inflammatory effects in critically ill patients and counteracts the adverse effect of low mannose-binding lectin levels. *J Clin Endocrinol Metab.* 2003;88:1082-1088.

59. Finfer S, Chittock DR, Su SY, et al. Intensive versus conventional glucose control in critically ill patients. *N Engl J Med.* 2009;360:1283-1297.

60. Oddo M, Schmidt JM, Carrera E, et al. Impact of tight glycemic control on cerebral glucose metabolism after severe brain injury: a microdialysis study. *Crit Care Med.* 2008;36:3233-3238.

61. Van den Berghe G, Schoonheydt K, Becx P, Bruyninckx F, Wouters PJ. Insulin therapy protects the central and peripheral nervous system of intensive care patients. *Neurology.* 2005;64:1348-1353.

62. Vincent JL, Nadel S, Kutsogiannis DJ, et al. Drotrecogin alfa (activated) in patients with severe sepsis presenting with purpura fulminans, meningitis, or meningococcal disease: a retrospective analysis of patients enrolled in recent clinical studies. *Crit Care.* 2005;9:R331-R343.

63. MacFarlane JT, Cleland PG, Attai ED, Greenwood BM. Failure of heparin to alter the outcome of pneumococcal meningitis. *Br Med J.* 1977;2:1522.

64. Irazuzta JE, Pretzlaff R, Rowin M, Milam K, Zemlan FP, Zingarelli B. Hypothermia as an adjunctive treatment for severe bacterial meningitis. *Brain Res.* 2000;881:88-97.

65. Angstwurm K, Reuss S, Freyer D, et al. Induced hypothermia in experimental pneumococcal meningitis. *J Cereb Blood Flow Metab.* 2000;20:834-838.

66. Bernard GR, Vincent JL, Laterre PF, et al. Efficacy and safety of recombinant human activated protein C for severe sepsis. *N Engl J Med.* 2001;344:699-709.

67. Roos YB, Levi M, Carroll TA, Beenen LF, Vermeulen M. Nimodipine increases fibrinolytic activity in patients with aneurysmal subarachnoid hemorrhage. *Stroke.* 200132:1860-1862.

68. Winkler F, Kastenbauer S, Koedel U, Pfister HW. Role of the urokinase plasminogen activator system in patients with bacterial meningitis. *Neurology.* 2002;59:1350-1355.

69. Hosoglu S, Ceviz A, Kemaloglu MS, et al. Effects of nimodipine on the cerebrovascular and neuronal changes during pneumococcal meningitis in the rat. *Acta Microbiol Immunol Hung.* 1997;44:271-279.

70. Winkler F, Angele B, Pfister HW, Koedel U. Simvastatin attenuates leukocyte recruitment in experimental bacterial meningitis. *Int Immunopharmacol.* 2009;9:371-374.

CHAPTER

8

Intensive Care Unit (ICU) Management of Brain Tumors

Simon Hanft, MD
Michael B. Sisti, MD

A 52-year-old woman with no significant past medical history presents with a headache and a subsequent fall without loss of consciousness. Over the next few days, the patient continued to have headaches of increasing intensity. On the day of admission, she complained of a particularly severe headache, which preceded another fall. It was at this time that the patient was brought to a nearby emergency department (ED), where a computerized tomographic (CT) scan of the head revealed a large space-occupying lesion, which was likely a parafalcine meningioma. The patient soon developed a seizure and then became obtunded, with newly documented pupillary asymmetry. After receiving mannitol, the patient was transferred to a neurologic ICU for further intervention.

On arrival at the neurologic intensive care unit (NICU), the patient was intubated with eyes closed and unable to follow commands. The right pupil was 5 mm and nonreactive, while the left pupil was 3 mm and reactive; corneal and gag reflexes were intact. The patient was able to briskly localize with the right arm and leg, while the left arm and leg were flexing to painful stimuli. Vital signs on admission were temperature of 99.7°F, HR 91 bpm in sinus rhythm, blood pressure of 120/67 mm Hg by cuff reading, and mechanical ventilation set to assist control–volume control.

What should be the first step in managing this patient?

This patient is clearly demonstrating clinical signs of herniation. The comatose examination with loss of airway protection requiring mechanical ventilation as well as the neurologic signs such as dilation and loss of reactivity of the right pupil and flexor posturing of the left arm/leg are strong indicators that the patient is suffering from right-sided brainstem compression. This constellation of neurologic signs is the most concerning issue in this patient's presentation and, as such, requires the most immediate attention from the treating physician.

A stat CT of the head (Figure 8-1) will demonstrate location of the mass, extent of midline shift, edema, hydrocephalus, lesional (with possible intraventricular) hemorrhage, and type of herniation. In this case, a large (5.5 × 5.6 × 5.7 cm), calcified, hyperdense mass is noted along the superior anterior falx associated with moderate surrounding edema and causing mass effect upon the right greater than left frontal horns. There is no associated hemorrhage or hydrocephalus. There is loss of sulcation indicative of elevated intracranial pressure (ICP), as well as acute infarcts in the bilateral occipital lobes, right greater than left, suggesting an ongoing process of transtentorial (uncal) herniation.

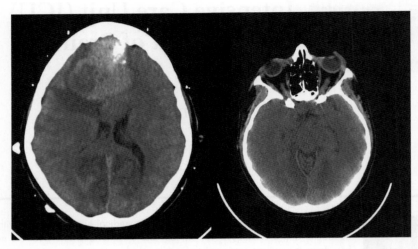

Figure 8-1. (Left) Noncontrast head CT revealing the large, midline hyperdense mass with calcifications along the anterior falx. Also noted is associated edema, bilateral compression of the frontal horns (right greater than left), and loss of sulcation suggestive of elevated ICP. (Right) Crowding of the ambient cisterns with medial displacement of the R temporal horn suggestive of downward (uncal) herniation. There are also bilateral hypodensities in the medial occipital lobes that may be an indicator of bilateral PCA infarction from herniation.

The immediate medical interventions are directed toward lowering the patient's elevated ICP. First, raising the head of the bed to at least 30 degrees will prevent cerebral venous outflow obstruction. Second, hyperventilating the patient to a goal $Paco_2$ of 25 to 30 mm Hg will provide transient lowering of ICP by inducing vasoconstriction of cerebral arteries and arterioles, which will lower cerebral blood volume (CBV). Third, administration of sedatives, analgesics, and potentially paralytic agents helps to control agitation and in particular cases, such as propofol (beginning at 10 mg/kg per minute), reduces CBV and slows cerebral metabolism, actions that contribute to lowering ICP.[1]

The next major intervention is the use of hyperosmolar therapy, typically with continuous infusion of 3% hypertonic saline coupled with boluses of 23.4% hypertonic saline (in 30-mL pushes), along with standard mannitol administration (25% solution given at 0.25 to 1 g/kg). Such agents work by increasing serum osmolality, which brings water from the extracellular space into the serum, thereby reducing brain swelling. The goal serum osmolality is typically greater than 320 mOsm/L and the goal plasma sodium level in such a patient is typically 150 to 155 with sodium checks every 4 to 6 hours, as a sodium level above 155 has not been shown to be of proven clinical benefit.[2] The side effects of hyperosmolar therapy include electrolyte imbalances (eg, hypokalemia), pulmonary edema (resulting from rapid intravascular volume expansion), coagulopathy, and intravascular hemolysis.[3] Despite the radiographic features of this lesion, which point to it being an extra-axial mass such as a meningioma, it is still causing significant vasogenic edema that should be treated with intravenous steroids. An immediate bolus of 10 mg IV dexamethasone (Decadron), followed by a maintenance dose of 8 to 32 mg/day, should be implemented.[4] Dexamethasone works by reducing the permeability of the cerebral capillaries.

Given the recent seizure, which likely precipitated the herniation event (seizures transiently elevate ICP, likely from increasing cerebral blood flow [CBF]), the patient should be maintained on antiepileptic medication, either phenytoin (Dilantin) (following a 20-mg/kg loading dose) or Keppra (following a 1-g loading dose).

There is also a discussion to be had regarding insertion of an ICP monitor in this patient. Typically, for patients with clinical signs of elevated ICP and a Glasgow Coma Scale (GCS) score less than 8 warrant direct, invasive monitoring of ICP.[5] Since this patient presented with a known intracranial mass causing elevated ICP, the indication for an ICP monitor is less cogent given that imminent surgery will remove the source of the elevated ICP. If the patient were to be stabilized and supported for an extended period of time, for example, in the case of an unresectable lesion or in the obvious case of traumatic brain injury, then the utility of an ICP monitor becomes clear. In this case, therefore, an ICP monitor was not inserted immediately given the plan for urgent operative decompression.

Following these interventions, the patient's right pupil becomes reactive and of equivalent size to the left pupil, and the patient's left side becomes more purposeful to deep stimulation. What are the current goals in management?

The initial interventions in this patient are directed at lowering ICP. But these interventions only solve part of the problem: edema and seizures as contributors to the herniation syndrome. Clearly, the next step needs to be aimed at expeditious resection of the intracranial mass lesion. Once the patient is stabilized, magnetic resonance imaging (MRI) of the brain with and without contrast must be performed to better characterize the lesion in terms of location, type, and precise anatomic relationships to surrounding structures including associated vasculature. This study will also aid in the decision of whether preoperative embolization is necessary, since this is likely a well-vascularized meningioma.

MRI of the brain was performed with magnetic resonance angiography (MRA) of the head and neck (Figure 8-2), revealing a 5.6 cm × 7.1 cm × 4.9 cm heterogeneously enhancing anterior falcine mass with evidence of internal necrosis and significant surrounding vasogenic edema and mass effect, which is consistent with a large parafalcine meningioma. The effacement of right greater than left frontal horns is again demonstrated. There is also diffusion-weighted imaging (DWI) restriction in bilateral medial temporal and occipital lobes suggestive of an acute infarct from bilateral posterior cerebral artery (PCA) compression during the recent herniation event (Figure 8-3).

At this point, the decision of preoperative embolization must be addressed. The major risk of embolization in a tumor of this size (which has very recently caused significant herniation) is causing

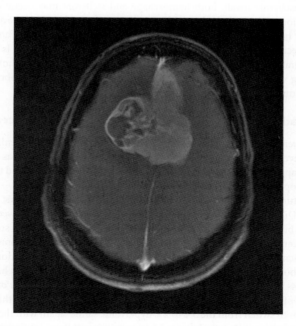

Figure 8-2. MRI of the brain with contrast (axial cut) revealing a heterogeneously enhancing parafalcine mass. Note the area of necrosis in the right frontal aspect of the tumor and the associated vasogenic edema (worse on the right). The MRI appearance of this lesion is suggestive of a more malignant meningioma subtype, and the final pathology confirmed this (World Health Organization [WHO] grade II, atypical meningioma).

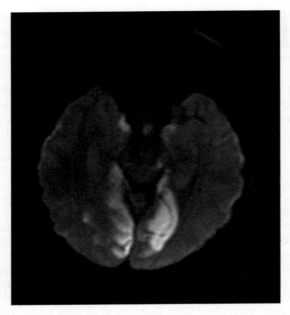

Figure 8-3. MRI of the brain, diffusion-weighted imaging (DWI). There is restricted diffusion in the bilateral medial temporal lobes as well as in the bilateral occipital lobes suggestive of bilateral PCA compression from a recent herniation event.

a hemorrhagic or ischemic insult; both hemorrhage and ischemia may occur in the intratumoral or peritumoral region, either of which could precipitate another herniation event.[6,7] There are no strict guidelines for making this decision, and therefore it is left to the cerebral angiographer and the neurosurgeon to decide on its safety and utility. The benefit of embolization is to minimize blood loss during the operation by injecting small particles (typically polyvinyl alcohol [PVA]) into major extracranial feeding vessels. In this case, the decision was made to forego embolization in favor of urgent open resection in the operating room.

Following operative resection, what are the postoperative concerns and goals?

The patient underwent a bicoronal craniotomy for resection of a parafalcine meningioma. The operation proceeded uneventfully; of note, the superior sagittal sinus was sacrificed as it was invaded with tumor and did not appear to be patent. A gross total resection was achieved, and the patient returned to the ICU for postoperative management.

The patient returned to the ICU ventilated, maintained on 3% hypertonic saline infusion, IV Decadron, and IV Dilantin. A postoperative CT scan was performed that showed complete removal of the meningioma but relatively significant residual edema. Now that the main source of the patient's elevated ICP has been removed, it is appropriate to begin weaning the hypertonic saline while keeping in mind that there is moderate to severe remaining edema. This must be done in slow, stepwise fashion to avoid rebound cerebral edema that could potentially incite another herniation event and with regular every 4- to 6-hour sodium checks.[8] Begin with decreasing the rate of the 3% hypertonic saline with the goal of keeping the sodium within 10 mEq of the plateau level within the first 24 hours. The following step is to switch from the 3% to 2% hypertonic saline, again with the goal of keeping the patient's sodium level above 140 over the next 24-hour window. After a minimum of 48 hours' post-surgery, it becomes possible to switch the patient to a normal saline infusion with the goal sodium in the normal range (135 to 145) for the remainder of the ICU stay.

The Decadron can be tapered off over a 2-week period, given the severity of the edema and the fact that this is a benign extra-axial lesion, while the patient should be maintained on a steady level of Dilantin for a minimum of 1 month and potentially for 3 to 6 months given that she presented with seizures.[9] There is also the option of transitioning the patient to Keppra from Dilantin in favor of a more benign side-effect profile at the discretion of the treating neurologist.[10] Ventilatory weaning and other intensive care interventions are left to the judgment of the critical care neurologist.

 A 60-year-old woman with hypertension presented on the day prior to admission with new-onset severe headache. On the day of admission, the patient still complained of headache but then developed significant nausea and vomiting that transitioned into leth-argy. Emergency medical services (EMS) were activated, and upon their arrival they found the patient awake before she rapidly declined and became minimally responsive. When the patient arrived in the emergency department (ED), the following clinical examination was noted: unarousable to stimuli; asymmetric pupils (left larger than right); intact corneal and gag reflexes; extensor posturing on the right side with purposeful movement on the left side. Following urgent intubation, a head CT was performed revealing a large left parietal mass with its apparent origin in the gray-white junction and a cystic component extending down into the left thalamus. There was a significant component of vasogenic edema involving the entire left hemisphere, although concentrated in the left temporoparietal region (Figure 8-4). The CT also showed evidence of uncal herniation and approximately 1.0 to 1.5 cm of midline shift. Once this mass lesion was identified, the patient was immediately given a large man-nitol bolus (1 g/kg is standard, but bolus amounts up to 1.5 g/kg can be utilized in urgent cases such as this); one bolus dose of 23.4% hypertonic saline through a recently established femoral central line; loading dose of fosphenytoin (Cerebyx, 20 mg/kg); and a large bolus of IV dexamethasone (100 mg). She was then transferred to the NICU.

On arrival at the NICU, the patient had improved neurologically. At this point, she was no longer extensor pos-turing on her right side and was able to minimally localize to stimuli. Her pupils also became symmetric. Over

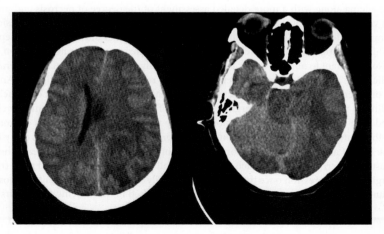

Figure 8-4. (Left) Noncontrast head CT identifying a large hypodensity in the left parietal region appearing to originate at the gray-white junction with a cystic component that extends into the left thalamus. There is severe surrounding vasogenic edema. (Right) Another cut of the head CT reveals significant effacement of the basal cisterns on the left consistent with uncal herniation. The temporal horn on the left is shifted with the uncus, and the vasogenic edema is apparent throughout the left temporal lobe as well.

the following 12 hours, the patient also began to open her eyes and attend to the examiner, although she remained unable to follow commands (likely due to transient damage to the reticular activating system).

Given this patient's neurologic improvement, what are the next steps in management?

Given the size and location of this malignant-appearing mass lesion, it comes as no surprise that this patient presented with a clinical herniation syndrome. Moreover, as is clear on the CT scan, another alarming radiographic feature of this lesion is its associated edema. In fact, the herniation event was most likely due to the edema and *not* to the mass itself, as evidenced by the patient's neurologic improvement from hyperosmolar therapy and the large IV corticosteroid bolus. There is also the possibility that the mass induced a seizure that transiently elevated her ICP, thereby precipitating the herniation episode.

So the question is whether this patient needs to undergo emergent operative decompression of this lesion or whether a delay is permissible in order to allow the steroids to take effect in terms of treating the edema. Such a brief delay would also allow for other interventions and studies to be pursued. With the observed neurologic improvement, the decision made in this case was to delay surgery. This was done at the risk of having the patient seize and perhaps transiently herniate again, as well as at the risk of developing intratumoral hemorrhage that could replicate the cascade of events that brought the patient to the ER in the first place. By delaying the surgery for 24 to 48 hours, important interventions were either initiated or continued: an MRI with gadolinium contrast was obtained; continuous electroencephalographic (cEEG) monitoring was begun to determine if the patient required more maintenance Dilantin or a second antiepileptic agent based on the presence or absence of seizure activity; hypertonic therapy in the form of 3% saline was infused with a goal sodium level of at least 145; and IV Decadron was continued at a dose of 10 mg every 4 hours. With the more reliable neurologic examination to follow, it was considered unnecessary at this point to insert an ICP monitor.

The contrast MRI allowed for better operative planning, especially because the noncontrast CT scan was somewhat difficult to interpret in this patient in terms of tumor origin. The MRI revealed that the tumor likely arose from the inferior left parietal lobe (Figure 8-5); there was also a better quantification of the edema along with a more detailed assessment of the degree of necrosis and proximity to important vasculature. All of this pointed to this tumor being a high-grade malignant lesion, likely a glioblastoma multiforme (GBM). In addition to the MRI, the cEEG did not reveal any epileptiform activity, while the patient's sodium level rose in response to the hypertonic saline infusion.

It is also important to note the surgical delay theoretically reduces the risk of intraoperative bleeding complications since the edema is given a chance to resolve with steroid therapy. An emergent operation on a very swollen brain that is actively herniating carries with it the risk of inducing significant bleeding as well as making the surgical resection of such a lesion more technically challenging when faced with such friable tissue. Therefore, surgery was performed in a 24- to 48-hour window following the acute herniation event, and in this case proceeded uneventfully. This delay is weighed against the risk of an intratumoral hemorrhage developing that could precipitate another, perhaps more devastating, herniation event. Such an intratumoral hemorrhage would need to be treated with urgent surgical decompression once the patient is medically stable. For this patient, the postoperative concerns and goals were essentially identical to those described in the aforementioned first case.

A 45-year-old man with no significant past medical history presents with 6 weeks of gradually worsening headaches and 2 weeks of intermittent nausea and vomiting. The patient brought himself to the ED, where on neurologic examination he demonstrated nystagmus on lateral gaze with left-sided dysmetria and was otherwise intact. A noncontrast head CT

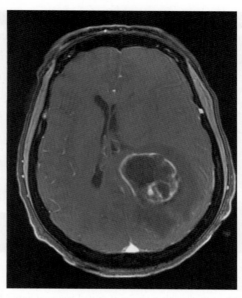

Figure 8-5. MRI of the brain with contrast (axial cut) shows a large, primarily rim-enhancing lesion with central necrosis situated in the left parietal lobe causing effacement of the left frontal horn. There is also midline shift of approximately 12 mm and significant surrounding vasogenic edema.

was performed, revealing a cystic lesion involving the left cerebellar hemisphere causing effacement of the fourth ventricle and dilatation of the lateral ventricles, third ventricle, and temporal horns consistent with hydrocephalus (Figure 8-6). Sulcation was preserved over the cerebral convexities, suggesting that the patient did not have significantly elevated ICP. Given the new discovery of a posterior fossa lesion with associated hydrocephalus, the patient was admitted to the NICU for close monitoring.

What major issue must be addressed first prior to proceeding with surgical resection?

Hydrocephalus is the most concerning issue in this patient. Intracranial mass lesions located in the posterior fossa as well as in the pineal region and third ventricle are prone to causing hydrocephalus due to obstruction of cerebrospinal fluid (CSF) outflow. In cases of hydrocephalus, there is a spectrum of clinical severity, ranging from mild headache to more severe headache with vomiting (as in this patient) to significant obtundation, loss of airway protection, and other signs of impending herniation. In this latter, more emergent scenario, the hydrocephalus must be treated immediately and can nearly always be controlled through placement of an external ventricular drain. This allows for external drainage of CSF prior to addressing the obstructive mass lesion.

In this case, ventricular drainage was considered unnecessary in light of the patient's clinical status (awake, interactive, orienting). Even in patients who demonstrate long-standing symptoms consistent with chronic hydrocephalus, they can present with an acute decline that may need to be treated with ventricular drainage.

What additional steps should be carried out prior to surgery?

MRI with and without contrast is the standard imaging study for all mass lesions of the posterior fossa. The MRI characteristics of the lesion in this case were most consistent with hemangioblastoma,

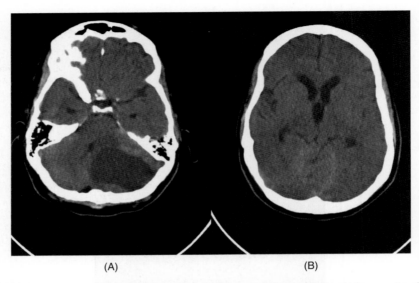

(A)   (B)

Figure 8-6. A. Noncontrast head CT reveals a cystic lesion in the left cerebellar hemisphere causing shift and mild compression of the fourth ventricle with evidence of dilated temporal horns. **B.** Another slice of the head CT reveals dilated lateral ventricles and a dilated third ventricle suggestive of early hydrocephalus given the lack of transependymal flow.

a benign well-vascularized central nervous system (CNS) tumor arising from stromal cells of small blood vessels and typically located in the cerebellum, brainstem, and spinal cord. In fact, 8% to 12% of all posterior fossa tumors are hemangioblastomas, although it accounts for only 1.0% to 2.5% of all intracranial mass lesions. It is commonly associated with Von Hippel–Lindau (VHL) disease (approximately 25% of all hemangioblastomas). As seen in the MRI here (Figure 8-7), the mass is avidly contrast enhancing with a characteristic mural nodule and a cystic core. There is also associated edema, and along with the hydrocephalus and headaches, it was considered prudent to start Decadron.

Since the MRI characteristics of this mass were very suggestive of hemangioblastoma, additional workup was conducted including ophthalmologic evaluation for retinal lesions (commonly found in VHL patients), a total spine MRI with and without contrast to search for spinal cord hemangioblastomas (may be performed postsurgery), and vanillylmandelic acid (VMA) and metanephrine levels (elevated with pheochromocytoma, which is also associated with VHL). Determining the presence of a pheochromocytoma preoperatively is a critical step given the anesthetic risks associated with this tumor; for example, hypertensive crisis and tachycardia from catecholamine release during anesthesia induction.[11] This patient had no retinal lesions, but was ultimately diagnosed with VHL; he also had a pheochromocytoma (elevated urine and plasma metanephrines coupled with an adrenal mass diagnosed on abdominal CT) and a T12-enhancing lesion suspicious for a spinal cord hemangioblastoma. In this circumstance, it is prudent to have an endocrinologist formally evaluate the patient and advise on preoperative and postoperative blood pressure management as well as alerting the anesthesia team to the presence of a pheochromocytoma. The endocrinologist is then in a position to follow the patient long-term once the surgery is finished.

There is also the question of preoperative angiography and embolization. Cerebellar hemangioblastomas are well-vascularized lesions that are occasionally embolized preoperatively in an effort to control intraoperative blood loss. Reports vary in terms of preoperative embolization success—more recent studies point to a high enough postembolization risk of hemorrhage such that embolization is not routinely recommended.[12]

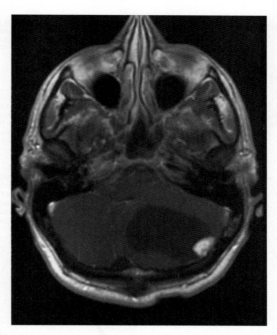

Figure 8-7. MRI of the brain with contrast (axial cut) showing an enhancing mural nodule on the posterior lateral aspect of the cystic lesion.

How should the hydrocephalus be managed in the perioperative period?

As noted earlier, there is no need to manage the hydrocephalus in this case in an urgent fashion. Therefore, the issue is how to manage the hydrocephalus both during and following the operation. In this case, the goal is obtain control of CSF drainage *prior* to operative decompression via a retrosigmoid suboccipital craniotomy approach. This will prevent cerebellar herniation through the dural opening made by the neurosurgeon while approaching the mass. Two interventions were made prior to the planned craniotomy: (1) an endoscopic third ventriculostomy (ETV) and (2) placement of a right frontal external ventricular drain (EVD). The ETV provides both short- and long-term control of hydrocephalus—by creating a new passage through the floor of the third ventricle into the prepontine cistern, the level of the obstruction caused by the hemangioblastoma (at the fourth ventricle) is essentially bypassed, allowing for CSF outflow and absorption to approach normal parameters (Figure 8-8). The EVD will provide continuous intraoperative control of CSF outflow and then will remain in place postoperatively to control the hydrocephalus while the patient recovers from the resection.

The hydrocephalus is expected to resolve following resection of the obstructive mass lesion, but it will not improve rapidly. Postoperative swelling will slow resolution of hydrocephalus, thus the EVD serves three functions in the recovery period: (1) ICP monitoring, (2) CSF drainage for control of hydrocephalus, and (3) CSF drainage to prevent leakage through the incision site and, therefore, to promote wound healing. The level at which the EVD is set is determined by the neurosurgeon; in this situation, the typical level is 10 cm H_2O above the external auditory meatus. Over the next few days, the EVD should be progressively raised above the 10–cm H_2O level, while the patient's symptoms (mainly headache, but also level of arousal), ICP readings, and wound must be assessed to determine whether the EVD wean is being tolerated. Exacerbation of headache, persistently elevated ICPs (typically above 20 is cause for concern), and leakage from the incision are

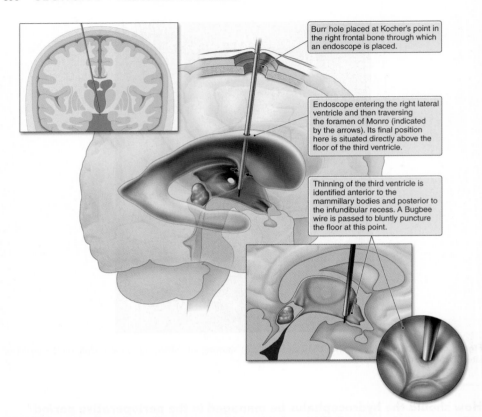

Burr hole placed at Kocher's point in the right frontal bone through which an endoscope is placed.

Endoscope entering the right lateral ventricle and then traversing the foramen of Monro (indicated by the arrows). Its final position here is situated directly above the floor of the third ventricle.

Thinning of the third ventricle is identified anterior to the mammillary bodies and posterior to the infundibular recess. A Bugbee wire is passed to bluntly puncture the floor at this point.

Figure 8-8. Schematic diagram of an endoscopic third ventriculostomy. The key concept is the opening of the floor of the third ventricle into the prepontine cistern, creating a new passage for cerebrospinal fluid outflow.

indications that the drain wean is not being tolerated and that the patient still requires additional CSF drainage.

Noncontrast head CT scans should also be intermittently performed to evaluate the patency of the fourth ventricle and the overall radiographic picture of hydrocephalus prior to planned bedside removal of the EVD. Although it is preferable to remove the EVD when the fourth ventricle appears patent on noncontrast head CT scan, the fact that an ETV was also performed here does not make a patent fourth ventricle an absolute requirement for drain removal. In those cases where an ETV is not performed, radiographic patency of the fourth ventricle is advisable prior to EVD removal (Figure 8-9). Once the EVD is removed, the patient is ready for discharge from the NICU to a floor bed.

Are there any other postoperative issues that need to be addressed while the patient remains hospitalized?

As is customary with lesions of the posterior fossa, a 2-week Decadron taper is prescribed immediately following the operation. There is no indication for antiepileptic therapy since tumors in this region are not associated with seizure formation. A postoperative MRI with and without contrast is typically done within 72 hours of the surgery to limit the artifact from normal postoperative changes. This study will provide a radiographic determination of the extent of resection, and it will also provide a clear image of the fourth ventricle and its patency. As mentioned earlier, an MRI of the total spine with and without

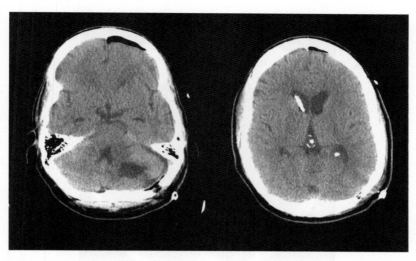

Figure 8-9. (Left) Postoperative noncontrast head CT showing that the fourth ventricle is more open than the preoperative CT. (Right) Improving hydrocephalus as compared to the preoperative CT with an external ventricular catheter terminating in the right frontal horn.

contrast to look for spinal cord hemangioblastomas can also be performed in the postoperative period and can conveniently be scheduled to coincide with the routine postoperative MRI of the brain.

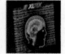 A 27-year-old woman with a history of recently diagnosed hypertension presented with sudden-onset severe headache that was initially accompanied by nausea and dizziness. The headache was mainly retroorbital. The headache did not respond to conventional analgesics (acetaminophen [Tylenol]). Approximately 1 to 2 hours following the initial headache, the patient began to experience visual changes, characterized mainly by diplopia as well as decreased peripheral vision. The patient was concerned enough by these new-onset symptoms to activate EMS. Upon arriving at her local ED, the patient's neurologic examination was notable for the following: impaired medial gaze of the R eye (adduction impairment suggestive of a third nerve palsy); mild ptosis of the R eye; and bitemporal hemianopia on visual field examination. Noncontrast head CT revealed a large sellar mass with evidence of acute blood (Figure 8-10). Given the neurologic findings and radiographic evidence of a pituitary mass with new hemorrhage, the patient was diagnosed with pituitary apoplexy and urgent transfer was arranged to the NICU.

What are the first steps in managing this case?

Pituitary apoplexy refers to a condition in which either hemorrhage or infarction of a pituitary tumor leads to the following clinical symptoms: abrupt-onset headache, visual changes (diplopia, loss of visual acuity, restriction of visual fields), nausea, vomiting, vertigo, and/or a decreased level of arousal.[13] The type of lesion most commonly associated with this condition is a pituitary adenoma, which makes up approximately 10% of all intracranial tumors. According to various studies, pituitary apoplexy arises in about 2% to 7% of all pituitary adenomas.[14] In fact, although adenomas make up only 10% of intracranial neoplasms, they give rise to 25% of tumor-associated hemorrhages.[13] An essential element of the definition of pituitary apoplexy is *acuity*: patients seek urgent medical

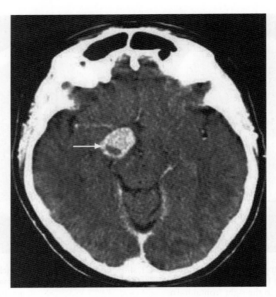

Figure 8-10. Noncontrast head CT reveals a large parasellar mass filled with hyperdense material suggestive of hemorrhage. There is also a hypodense area (*arrow*) that marks a cystic component. (*From Watt, A, Pobereskin L, Vaidya B. Pituitary apoplexy within a macroprolactinoma. Nat Clin Pract Endocrinol Metab. 2008;4:635-641.*)

attention for the abrupt onset of the symptoms described above. Importantly, these symptoms are due to an acutely enlarging mass in the sellar, parasellar, and/or suprasellar compartments.[15] The tumor expands because of edema from infarction or from the mass effect from hemorrhage into the tumor. Although it is an uncommon condition, prompt diagnosis of pituitary apoplexy is critical given the possibility that initial visual changes may progress to permanent visual deficits if not addressed by early surgery. In this case, the symptoms and neurologic findings were concerning enough to warrant urgent noncontrast head CT in the ED, which in turn located the pituitary mass. Oftentimes, the clinical picture of pituitary apoplexy mimics that of a ruptured intracranial aneurysm (as they both share headache and oculomotor palsies in their respective presentations), and so a head CT is a logical and important step in the evaluation of this symptomatology. Once the pituitary mass is identified on CT with associated hemorrhage, this activates a cascade of further steps as detailed below.

One of the initial concerns when a patient is diagnosed with pituitary apoplexy is the possibility of an adrenal crisis; the majority of these patients present with panhypopituitarism.[15] Therefore, the recommendation is to immediately administer 100 mg of IV hydrocortisone, followed by 100 mg IV hydrocortisone every 6 to 8 hours leading up to surgery.[13,16] As part of the endocrinologic workup, the patient should have blood sent for levels of all the relevant hormones (prolactin, growth hormone [GH], insulinlike growth factor 1 [IGF1], thyroid-stimulating hormone [TSH], adrenocorticotropic hormone [ACTH], luteinizing hormone [LH], follicle-stimulating hormone [FSH], free thyroxine [T_4], free triiodothyronine [T_3], and serum cortisol). Patients may also present with electrolyte disturbances such as hyponatremia (likely due to cortisol deficiency), so electrolytes must be monitored and managed accordingly by the NICU team. ICU management must also pay close attention to ophthalmologic, endocrine, and neurologic function while the patient awaits surgical intervention.

Beyond medical treatment and evaluation, the CT scan must be assessed for evidence of hydrocephalus. Some patients (not the one included here) present with a decreased level of consciousness and have evidence of hydrocephalus and/or ventricular hemorrhage. These patients must be considered for urgent EVD placement prior to or at the time of surgery.

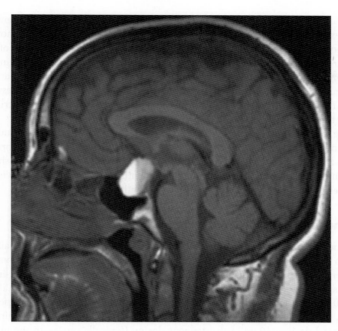

Figure 8-11. MRI of the brain without contrast, T1-weighted sagittal sequence revealing a hyperintensity within the sella consistent with hemorrhage. Note the fluid-fluid level within the tumor that is suggestive of different ages of hemorrhage. *(From Jane JA, Laws ER. Chapter 13: Surgical treatment of pituitary adenomas. In: Endotext. org, 2004.)*

In addition to the medical and procedural interventions described above, it is recommended that an MRI with and without contrast, including a dedicated pituitary protocol, be obtained prior to operative intervention. CT scan will detect hemorrhage and/or infarct anywhere from 20% to 30% of the time, while MRI will identify these features in pituitary tumors in more than 90% of cases (Figure 8-11).[13] Prior studies have established that contrasted MRI reveals evidence of hemorrhage, mainly as high-signal intensity on T1-weighted images; low- and high-signal intensity on T2-weighted images suggestive of old and recent hemorrhages; and various patterns of peripheral and heterogeneous tumoral enhancement on T1 sequences with gadolinium (with the nonenhanced areas suggestive of infarcted or necrotic tissue).[17] A recent study demonstrates that the additional MRI sequences, DWI and apparent diffusion coefficient (ADC) can help to identify areas of tumor infarction.[18] Moreover, and more importantly for the operating neurosurgeon, this study will provide significantly greater anatomic detail and, therefore, aid in surgical planning. It is possible that the lesion will require a craniotomy either in addition to or instead of the customary transsphenoidal approach, depending on location and extension of the hemorrhage among other factors.[13]

Should the patient undergo urgent surgery? If so, when?

Based on the severity and acuity of this patient's symptoms, urgent surgical decompression of the hemorrhagic pituitary mass is indicated. In any patient who presents with worsening visual acuity, expanding visual field deficits, declining level of arousal, or deteriorating oculomotor function, surgery is the recommended intervention.[13,19,20] Conservative management runs the risk of allowing the symptoms to worsen and perhaps become permanent since the processes of edema and ongoing bleeding may be at work. The decision to proceed with surgery, therefore, is based on the patient's symptoms once radiographic evidence of pituitary apoplexy has been established.

In the majority of cases, the transsphenoidal approach is adequate for tumor removal. As mentioned above, extension of hemorrhage to a hemisphere or a poorly aerated sphenoid sinus might prompt a craniotomy.[13] The transsphenoidal approach will permit decompression of the optic chiasm and the surrounding neural elements including the cranial nerves passing within the cavernous sinus. Recovery of oculomotor function occurs more often and more completely than improvement in visual fields and visual acuity, although expeditious removal has a very high success rate of restoring all of these functions.[19] Tumor removal may also help reestablish normal endocrine function by decompressing the functional pituitary gland.[13,14]

The timing of expeditious surgery varies according to different reports. Studies show that improvement in neurologic and endocrine function is achieved if surgery is performed anywhere from 48 hours to 1 week after symptom onset.[13-15,19] There are even studies that show significant improvement in oculomotor function and mild, but quantifiable, improvement in visual acuity and visual fields after 2 to 3 weeks and in one case up to 2 months.[21]

What are the postoperative goals of neurointensive care?

The patient should be monitored for diabetes insipidus (DI), which occurs in a small percentage of patients (2% to 3%) with pituitary apoplexy who undergo urgent surgery.[13] Sodium levels should be checked every 6 hours, while urine output should be monitored on an every-2-hour basis with accompanying specific gravities measured by urinalysis or urine dipstick. In general, if the urine output exceeds 250 mL per hour for two consecutive hours and is accompanied by a specific gravity of less than 1.005, the patient should be administered DDAVP (1-deamino-8-D-arginine vasopressin) by either intranasal dosing (10 µg), subcutaneous dosing (typically one-tenth the intranasal dose), or oral dosing (from 0.1 to 0.2 mg three times a day). An endocrinologist should be involved in the long-term management of this patient's hormonal issues, and it is reasonable to have such a specialist involved in the immediate postoperative management of this patient.

If the patient had hydrocephalus requiring EVD placement, this EVD should be rapidly weaned postoperatively based on the patient's neurologic status and the ICP readings. Progressive elevation of the drain by 5 to 10 cm H_2O per day from a likely initial level of 10 cm H_2O above the external auditory meatus (EAM) is a reasonable strategy given that surgical removal of the mass will allow for improved CSF outflow. If the hydrocephalus is secondary to ventricular hemorrhage, the patient may not tolerate a rapid wean, and so the goals must be titrated to the patient's symptoms (headache, level of arousal), ICP values, and interval CT scans to evaluate ventricular size. If the patient continues to fail attempts at raising and/or clamping the EVD, then placement of a ventriculoperitoneal shunt (VPS), although rare in cases of pituitary apoplexy, is likely.[15]

Outside of persistent hydrocephalus requiring EVD, even patients in active DI are typically stable enough to be managed on the floor. The goal is to transfer the apoplectic patient out of the NICU on the first postoperative day.

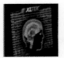

A 77-year-old man with a past medical history significant for hypertension, diabetes type II, chronic obstructive pulmonary disease (COPD), congestive heart failure (CHF), and small-cell lung cancer (lobectomy performed 20 years prior to admission) presented with sudden-onset confusion. According to the patient's daughter, he was speaking normally on the phone with her and then developed new word-finding difficulty and disorientation. She activated EMS, and upon their arrival the patient was found to be awake and alert but with significant slurred speech and disorientation. The patient was brought to a local ED, where a noncontrast head CT revealed multiple hemorrhagic brain lesions, with the most significant being two adjacent large left frontal lesions causing

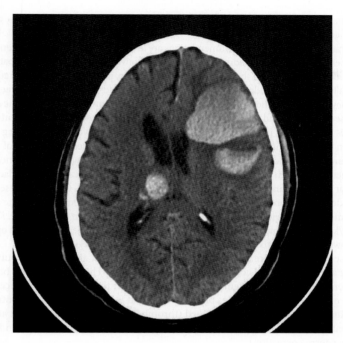

Figure 8-12. Axial noncontrast head CT reveals a large hemorrhagic lesion in the left anterior frontal lobe (5.1 cm × 4.3 cm) with a smaller hemorrhagic lesion (3.8 cm × 2.6 cm) immediately posterior to it. There is approximately 9 mm of midline shift. Also note the right thalamic hemorrhagic lesion.

midline shift (Figure 8-12). In addition, there was a right thalamic lesion and a right superior frontal lesion. The patient was then transferred to an NICU for further evaluation and treatment.

Upon arrival in the NICU, the patient was awake and alert, following commands, although oriented only to his name. The patient's speech was characterized by severe perseveration, anomia, and significant dysarthria. Otherwise the patient had intact cranial nerves and was full strength and symmetric on motor examination.

What are the next steps in managing this patient with multiple hemorrhagic brain lesions?

Due to the patient's distant history of lung cancer and the sudden-onset presentation of his symptoms, the guiding thought in the management of this case is that these hemorrhagic lesions represent brain metastases of his lung cancer. In addition to lung cancer (bronchogenic carcinoma), other primary cancers commonly associated with a hemorrhagic presentation include melanoma, renal cell and thyroid carcinoma, and choriocarcinoma.[22] Lung cancer, as the most common hemorrhagic metastasis to the brain and among the most likely to present with multiple lesions, fits in with this patient's history and presentation. It is, therefore, important to immediately implement the medical therapies associated with treating metastatic lesions: corticosteroids (typically Decadron) and anticonvulsants. A 10-mg bolus of IV Decadron, followed by maintenance dosing of around the same dose two to four times per day (typically dosed anywhere from 2 mg every 6 hours to 10 mg every 6 hours depending on the severity of the edema), is a well-accepted dosing range as noted in prior cases.[23] In this patient, the combination of vasogenic edema surrounding the left frontal lesion and its associated mass effect makes corticosteroid administration an important initial step.

In terms of anticonvulsants, the recommendations are less clear. In patients who present with a seizure (unlike the patient described here), administration of anticonvulsants is advised. For patients who first present with cerebral metastases in the absence of a clear seizure, prophylactic administration of anticonvulsants is actually *not* recommended. These medications have failed to demonstrate efficacy in preventing first seizures; they are often subtherapeutic when their plasma levels are measured; and the side-effect profile appears to be more profound in patients with brain tumors as opposed to those patients in the general population. This latter issue is in part due to the fact that many anticonvulsants, including the commonly utilized Dilantin, stimulate the cytochrome P450 system, which increases metabolism of corticosteroids and certain chemotherapeutic agents.[24] However, in the case of patients with multiple metastases and/or hemorrhagic metastases (both of which apply to our patient here), the efficacy of prophylactic anticonvulsants is less clear as these situations have not been systematically studied. Certainly, these patients are at higher risk for developing seizures and as such would seem to benefit from prophylactic administration of these medications.[5] In the end, it is left up to clinician preference, and in the case here, IV Dilantin was bolused (20 mg/kg) and then maintained at 100 mg IV every 8 hours. IV Keppra is also an option at a bolus dose of 1 g followed by 500 mg to 1 g every 12 hours as a maintenance regimen.

While these medications are administered, the patient should also undergo routine laboratory tests, including a complete blood count and coagulation profile. The patient should be evaluated for thrombocytopenia and elevated coagulation parameters given the presence of intracerebral hemorrhage. If either of these laboratory values prove abnormal, it is likely that they are contributing to the current condition and as such should be treated (thrombocytopenia through platelet administration, elevated International Ratio [INR] with fresh-frozen plasma [FFP] administration and possibly vitamin K for longer-term correction).

The question of blood pressure control should also be raised. In this case, the neurointensivist is functioning under the principle that this patient has multiple hemorrhagic metastases that have bled. In other situations, a patient may have multiple intracranial hemorrhages (ICHs) from cerebral amyloid angiopathy (CAA) or from hypertension, among the more likely etiologies. In these alternative cases, blood pressure control is necessary. In our patient, and in all patients with hemorrhagic cerebral metastases, there is no standard recommendation for blood pressure control. A guideline that may be applied here is to keep the systolic blood pressure (SBP) less than 140 mm Hg, which is the guideline typically used for postoperative patients and in patients with a presumed hypertensive ICH.

What are the appropriate imaging studies?

After the patient is transferred from the admitting facility to the tertiary-level NICU, it is recommended to repeat a noncontrast head CT to determine whether there is more midline shift or hemorrhage in the newly diagnosed metastatic lesions. In this case, the repeat head CT was read as unchanged compared to the prior CT obtained 6 hours earlier. Once the patient is considered stable for a longer imaging study, it is recommended to obtain an MRI with and without contrast with an MRA of the head and neck. The MRA will help to evaluate for a vascular malformation, such as an arteriovenous malformation (AVM), but is of less utility than the standard MRI with and without contrast, which can identify AVMs, cavernous malformations, and dural AV fistulas independent of an MRA sequence. In this case, an MRI with or without contrast may reveal an enhancing nodule adjacent to hemorrhage suggestive of an underlying neoplastic lesion. On gradient-echo sequencing, the MRI may also show heterogeneous signal changes within the lesion suggestive of hemorrhages of multiple ages; T2-weighted sequences may show a surrounding hypointense hemosiderin ring with increased peripheral signal suggestive of edema. Although MRI is quite often limited by the hemorrhage in identifying an underlying neoplastic growth, these findings point to metastasis as a likely diagnosis. Moreover, mass effect and edema out of proportion to

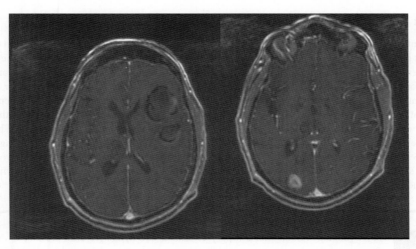

Figure 8-13. Axial T1-weighted image with contrast. (Left) Note the nodule of enhancement on lateral margin of the left anterior frontal lobe lesion. (Right) There is a right occipital lesion that was not present on noncontrast CT that avidly enhances. This lesion did not bleed so the uptake of contrast is clear and suggestive of a neoplasm.

what one would expect from an acute hematoma is a fundamental indicator of an underlying neoplastic process.[25] It is important to note any evidence of dural enhancement, which may represent meningeal seeding and carries a worse prognosis. This finding could impact the surgical management of the patient, perhaps leading to more palliative measures.

In this case, the patient underwent MRI, revealing vague ring enhancement of both left frontal lesions with central necrosis and hemorrhage; right thalamic lesion with hemorrhage and minimal ring enhancement; and a newly identified right occipital lesion with a heterogeneous enhancement pattern that was not seen on CT (Figure 8-13). The enhancement pattern of these three lesions is very suggestive of a metastatic process.

Additionally, the patient should undergo a CT with and without contrast of the chest, abdomen, and pelvis as part of a metastatic workup. Although the patient here has a remote history of lung cancer, it is important to establish whether there is diffuse multiorgan involvement of these metastases. Such a finding may factor into the overall prognosis for the patient and, therefore, may impact the decision among the neurosurgeon, neurointensivist, oncologist, and the patient's family regarding aggressive surgical intervention.

Given that this patient has multiple hemorrhagic lesions, how should he be treated?

In this situation where a patient has presented with multiple hemorrhagic metastases, the idea is to treat the lesion(s) that is causing the neurologic symptoms. The patient's clinical presentation, including dysarthria and disorientation, indicates that the twin left frontal lesions are to blame. The radiographic characteristics of these lesions are suggestive as well: the size (the anterior lesion is approximately 5 × 4 cm, the mid-frontal lesion is 4 × 3 cm), location (likely involving Broca's area through edematous extension and focal compression), and mass effect all point to the left frontal complex as the appropriate target for surgical intervention. Accordingly, the patient underwent a large left frontal craniotomy to allow for resection of both hemorrhagic left frontal lesions, and the surgery proceeded without incident. Subsequently, and typically beginning 1 to 2 weeks postoperatively, the patient underwent a chemotherapeutic regimen with whole-brain radiation (WBRT) under the care of a neurooncologist.

What are the postoperative concerns with this patient?

As mentioned above, postoperative systolic blood pressure control is of paramount concern in this patient given the existence of acute hemorrhage in his nonsurgically treated lesions. Also, the extent of the craniotomy and the size of the resected lesions increase the risk of postoperative hemorrhage. Therefore, strict SBP control between 90 and 140 mm Hg, coupled with a low threshold for urgent noncontrast head CT in the event of a neurologic change, are the necessary guidelines. Antiepileptic medications should be continued for at least a week, and probably maintained for a month if the patient remains seizure-free, although the recommendations remain vague. Decadron should be progressively tapered from a 10-mg oral dose every 6 hours for the first 24 hours down to 2 mg orally every 6 hours for the duration of WBRT (the duration of the taper typically extends well beyond the patient's stay in the ICU). The patient should remain in the NICU for at least 24 hours following surgery and then be discharged to the floor if no untoward events arise.

A 71-year-old woman with a history of asthma and hypothyroidism presented with 2 to 3 weeks of progressive cognitive difficulties and worsening left-sided weakness. Imaging conducted at an outside facility located a right frontal brain mass and she was referred for surgical resection. MRI of the brain with and without contrast revealed a large right frontal mass with ring enhancement; it extended into the right lateral ventricle and across the midline to the left frontal region (Figure 8-14). The patient underwent a right frontal craniotomy for what became a subtotal resection of a malignant glioma. Postoperatively, the patient was brought to the NICU and returned to her neurologic baseline within 2 hours of being extubated.

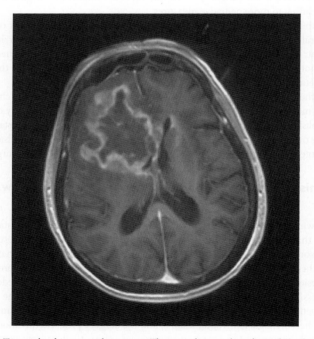

Figure 8-14. Axial T1-weighted image with contrast. There is a large right inferior frontal mass with heterogeneous enhancement. It extends into the right frontal horn and across the corpus callosum into the left frontal periventricular white matter. There is also approximately 4 mm of midline shift.

Approximately 6 hours after extubation, the patient was noted by the nurse to be more lethargic, dysarthric, and disoriented. Her postoperative examination documented a sleepy but easily arousable patient; orientation to name, place, and year; fluent speech; and greater than 4 out of 5 strength on the left side. Now, the patient was sleeping and difficult to arouse; oriented to name only; dysarthric; and barely lifting her left side off the bed with the aid of painful stimuli. What should be done?

There are two important time points here: (1) within a reasonable postoperative window, the patient was noted to return to her neurologic baseline and (2) a few hours beyond this initial time point, the patient was noted to have deteriorated to a neurologic state *worse* than her preoperative condition. This is suggestive of an active process, which could include the interval development of a hematoma, stroke or a new-onset seizure. The first step in evaluating a neurologic change in a postoperative tumor patient is to obtain an urgent noncontrast head CT. In this case, the CT revealed a sizable hemorrhage in the resection cavity with intraventricular extension (Figure 8-15). The presence of this hematoma and the patient's clinical decline warrants urgent surgical intervention for evacuation of the clot. Thus, the patient was taken back to the operating room for a reoperation and the hematoma was evacuated. A second postoperative CT revealed complete removal of the hematoma and interval resolution of the intraventricular hemorrhage (IVH) (see Figure 8-15). Following this second operation, the patient gradually returned to her preoperative neurologic baseline over the span of 2 to 4 hours.

It is important for neurointensivists to be cognizant of postoperative tumor patients who are at a higher risk for bleeding complications. This patient underwent a subtotal resection given the size and contralateral extent of the tumor. With residual tumor, there is great difficulty in achieving tumor bed hemostasis even when intraoperative coagulation strategies are rigorously employed, as was done in this case. It therefore behooves the neurointensivist to query the operating neurosurgeon regarding the extent of resection, the intraoperative blood loss, the friability of the tumor tissue, and the possible sacrifice of any important arteries or veins (distal middle cerebral artery [MCA] branch, superior sagittal sinus). All of these intraoperative issues can result in postoperative hemorrhage, as in the case presented here, or in postoperative stroke. Awareness of these issues will allow the neurointensivist to act swiftly and decisively in such cases.

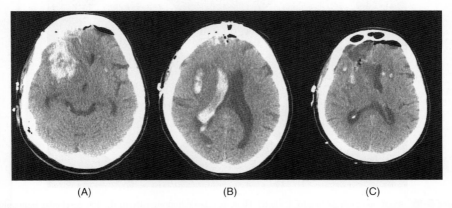

(A)   (B)   (C)

Figure 8-15. Axial noncontrast head CT. **A.** There is a hyperdense collection in the resection bed suggestive of postoperative hematoma. There is associated midline shift. **B.** Extension of the hemorrhage into the right lateral ventricle. **C.** Immediate postoperative noncontrast head CT reveals successful evacuation of the hematoma.

A 26-year-old man with no past medical history presented with intermittent headaches accompanied by some dizziness and left-sided hearing loss over the course of 1 to 2 months. Imaging at an outside facility revealed a 3-cm left cerebellopontine angle mass, which was likely an acoustic neuroma. Given the size of the lesion, extent of hearing loss, and health of the patient, the patient was referred for surgery. The patient underwent an uneventful left retrosigmoid suboccipital craniectomy for resection of acoustic neuroma.

After a routine 24-hour postoperative stay in the NICU, the patient was transferred to the floor. The patient was at his neurologic baseline, which was intact with the exception of the stable left-sided hearing loss and a new slight left-sided facial droop. On postoperative day 3, the patient became progressively lethargic throughout the day. On examination, he was sleeping but arousable to tactile stimuli; orienting to name, place, and year but requiring stimulation to remain awake; intact cranial nerves with the exception of the slight left-sided facial weakness; and symmetric with full strength on his motor examination. An urgent noncontrast head CT was performed revealing a hypodensity in the left cerebellar hemisphere; compression and near-total effacement of the fourth ventricle; hydrocephalus involving the lateral ventricles, the third ventricle, and the temporal horns; no evidence of hemorrhage (Figure 8-16). What is the next step in this patient's care?

The patient's clinical symptoms are suggestive of hydrocephalus and the CT scan confirms this diagnosis. Retraction injury of the cerebellum during surgery can cause delayed swelling, which is very similar to the process of an ischemic stroke. The swelling may take a few days before it causes significant compression of the fourth ventricle, thereby causing an obstructive hydrocephalus. Posterior fossa surgery

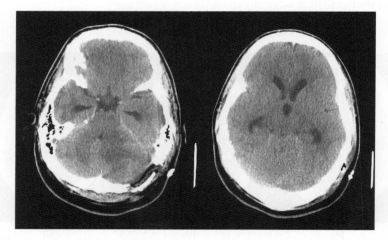

Figure 8-16. Axial noncontrast head CT. (Left) There is a large hypodensity in the left cerebellar hemisphere directly under the craniotomy site suggestive of retraction injury or infarct. The fourth ventricle appears patent on this slice but is shifted left to right. Also note the dilation of the temporal horns suggestive of hydrocephalus. (Right) Dilated frontal horns, a rounded and dilated third ventricle, and the previously noted enlarged temporal horns are radiographic signs of early hydrocephalus.

very often involves cerebellar retraction and, in certain approaches, involves sacrifice of some cerebellar veins.[26] The resulting edema can be significant enough to cause obstruction at the level of the fourth ventricle, leading to hydrocephalus as was seen in this case. Untreated hydrocephalus will progress to herniation and death, and so identification of this situation constitutes a clinical emergency.

This patient should be immediately transferred to the NICU for placement of an EVD. Beyond the lifesaving intervention of the EVD, it is also recommended to increase the patient's Decadron dosage to help combat postoperative edema; hypertonic saline is also an additional option (as is mannitol), with a goal sodium level greater than 140 (or serum osmolality greater than 320 in the case of mannitol). In this case, the patient's Decadron was increased from 6 mg orally every 6 hours to 10 mg orally every 6 hours, and 2% hypertonic saline was begun at an infusion of 75 mL per hour. Following EVD placement, the patient's level of arousal improved significantly. The EVD was maintained at 20 cm H_2O above the EAM for 2 to 3 days while the patient was weaned back to a Decadron dose of 6 mg every 6 hours and transitioned from 2% hypertonic saline to normal saline. The specific weaning parameters were the same as those utilized in an earlier case presented above. When a follow-up noncontrast head CT demonstrated adequate resolution of the cerebellar swelling and a patent fourth ventricle (Figure 8-17), the EVD was removed and the patient was considered ready for transfer to the floor. Since the EVD was kept at a high level above the EAM, weaning was not considered necessary in this case.

It is critical that the neurointensivist maintain awareness of postoperative tumor patients who have undergone approaches to the posterior fossa and the possibility of retraction injury giving rise to obstructive hydrocephalus. Although this complication may take days to unfold, more severe types of this injury and instances where a major stroke is induced may lead to earlier onset of hydrocephalus and its associated symptoms. Again, the threshold for a noncontrast head CT should be low, and the use of corticosteroids and hypertonic agents represent the key elements in the neurointensivist's armamentarium.

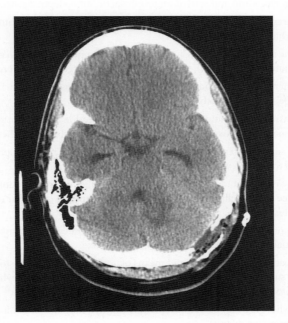

Figure 8-17. Axial noncontrast head CT. Significant interval resolution of the left cerebellar swelling. The fourth ventricle is now midline and more patent than noted on the prior CT. The temporal horns, although dilated, are smaller than in the previous CT.

! CRITICAL CONSIDERATIONS

- There are two stages in the intensive care of brain tumor patients: preoperative and postoperative.
- Patients who present preoperatively with a herniation event require emergent medical stabilization with the help of hyperosmolar agents, corticosteroids, and other interventions aimed at lowering ICP (eg, hyperventilation, sedation).
- Surgery should be viewed as urgent and potentially curative once the patient has been medically stabilized.
- Whenever possible in these patients, the best form of preoperative imaging (typically MRI) should be obtained to assist the neurosurgeon in achieving the safest maximum resection.
- Patients with posterior fossa tumors must have the issue of hydrocephalus addressed either preoperatively or perioperatively, with placement of an EVD when necessary.
- ETV is another surgical method of treating hydrocephalus from tumor compression of the fourth ventricle in the long-term.
- Patients with suspected pituitary apoplexy should undergo emergent CT scan followed by hydrocortisone administration if there is radiographic evidence of hemorrhage into a sellar lesion.
- MRI should also be performed on the apoplectic patient with an eye toward urgent operative decompression.
- Patients presenting with neurologic findings secondary to a hemorrhagic metastatic lesion should be given Decadron and started on prophylactic antiepileptic agents.
- MRI with contrast is useful for detecting a neoplastic lesion but can be limited by the presence of hemorrhage.
- If a hemorrhagic metastatic lesion is larger than 3 cm, symptomatic, and in a surgically resectable region (noneloquent cortex), the patient should undergo urgent operative resection.
- Postoperative hematoma is associated with residual tumor, patients with a known bleeding diathesis, and particularly bloody tumor types.
- The neurointensivist must inquire as to the extent of resection and any intraoperative bleeding issues that may predispose the patient to developing a postoperative hematoma.
- Posterior fossa surgery often involves cerebellar retraction that may precipitate swelling and compression of the fourth ventricle with resulting hydrocephalus.
- The neurointensivist must inquire as to the extent of retraction (eg, duration of surgery) and possible sacrifice of cerebellar veins, both of which may induce cerebellar swelling followed by hydrocephalus.
- The phenomenon of retraction injury applies to the supratentorial compartment as well, with the potential of inducing swelling that mimics stroke.
- Noncontrast head CT is a safe and rapid means of assessing nearly all postoperative complications, and as such, should be freely employed by the neurointensivist whenever there is a question of postoperative neurologic decline.
- In those cases where CT may be of limited utility, an MRI may also avail the neurointensivist (eg, early postoperative infarct).

REFERENCES

1. Girard F, Moumdjian R, Boudreault D, et al. The effect of propofol sedation on the intracranial pressure of patients with an intracranial space-occupying lesion. *Anesth Analg.* 2004;99:573-577.

2. Aiyagari V, Deibert E, Diringer MN. Hypernatremia in the neurologic intensive care unit: how high is too high? *J Crit Care.* 2006;21:163-172.

3. Bhardwaj A, Ulatowski JA. Hypertonic saline solutions in brain injury. *Curr Opin Crit Care.* 2004;10:126-131.

4. Kaal EC, Vecht CJ. The management of brain edema in brain tumors. *Curr Opin Oncol.* 2004;16:593-600.

5. Lin G, Keles GE, Berger MS. Management of patients with brain tumors. In: Andrews BT (ed). *Intensive Care in Neurosurgery.* New York: Thieme; 2003:197-205.

6. Carli DF, Sluzewski M, Beute GN, van Rooij WJ. Complications of particle embolization of meningiomas: frequency, risk factors, and outcome. *AJNR Am J Neuroradiol.* 2010;31:152-154.

7. Bendszus M, Monoranu CM, Schütz A, Nölte I, Vince GH, Solymosi L. Neurologic complications after particle embolization of intracranial meningiomas. *AJNR Am J Neuroradiol.* 2005;26:1413-1419.

8. Froelich M, Ni Q, Wess C, Ougorets I, Härtl R. Continuous hypertonic saline therapy and the occurrence of complications in neurocritically ill patients. *Crit Care Med.* 2009;37:1433-1441.

9. Sanai N, Sughrue ME, Shangari G, Chung K, Berger MS, McDermott MW. Risk profile associated with convexity meningioma resection in the modern neurosurgical era. *J Neurosurg.* 2010;112:913-919.

10. Usery JB, Michael LM 2nd, Sills AK, Finch CK. A prospective evaluation and literature review of levetiracetam use in patients with brain tumors and seizures. *J Neurooncol.* 2010;99:251-260.

11. Pacak K. Preoperative management of the pheochromocytoma patient. *J Clin Endocrinol Metab.* 2007;92:4069-4079.

12. Montano N, Doglietto F, Pedicelli A, et al. Embolization of hemangioblastomas. *J Neurosurg.* 2008; 108:1063-1065.

13. Verrees M, Arafah BM, Selman WR. Pituitary tumor apoplexy: characteristics, treatment, and outcomes. *Neurosurg Focus.* 2004;16: E6.

14. Arafah BM, Ybarra J, Tarr RW. Pituitary tumor apoplexy: pathophysiology, clinical manifestations, and treatment. *J Int Care Med.* 1997;12: 123-134.

15. Dubuisson AS, Beckers A, Stevenaert A. Classical pituitary tumor apoplexy: clinical features, management and outcomes in a series of 24 patients. *Clin Neurol Neurosurg.* 2007;109:63-70.

16. Lee CC, Cho AS, Carter, WA. Emergency department presentation of pituitary apoplexy. *Am J Emerg Med.* 2000;18:328-331.

17. Piotin M, Tampieri D, Rufenacht DA, et al. The various MRI patterns of pituitary apoplexy. *Eur Radiol.* 1999;9:918-923.

18. Rogg JM, Tung GA, Anderson G, Cortez S. Pituitary apoplexy: early detection with diffusion-weighted MR imaging. *Am J Neuroradiol.* 2002;23:1240-1245.

19. Bills DC, Meyer FB, Laws ER Jr, et al. A retrospective analysis of pituitary apoplexy. *Neurosurgery.* 1993;33:602-608.

20. Onesti ST, Wisniewski T, Post KD. Clinical versus subclinical pituitary apoplexy: presentation, surgical management, and outcome in 21 patients. *Neurosurgery.* 1990;26:980-986.

21. Muthukumar N, Rossette D, Soundaram M, Senthilbabu S, Badrinarayanan T. Blindness following pituitary apoplexy: timing of surgery and neuroophthalmic outcome. *J Clin Neurosci.* 2008;15:873-879.

22. Kamar FG, Posner JB. Brain metastases. *Semin Neurol.* 2010;30:217-235.

23. Nguyen T, DeAngelis LM. Treatment of brain metastases. *J Support Oncol.* 2004;2:405-410.

24. Soffietti R, Cornu P, Delattre JY, et al. EFNS Guidelines on diagnosis and treatment of brain metastases: report of an EFNS Task Force. *Eur J Neurol.* 2006;13:674-681.

25. Finelli, PF. A diagnostic approach to multiple simultaneous intracerebral hemorrhages. *Neurocrit. Care.* 2006;4:267-271.

26. Dubey A, Sung WS, Shaya M, et al. Complications of posterior cranial fossa surgery—An institutional experience of 500 patients. *Surg Neurol.* 2009;72:369-375.

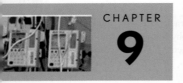

CHAPTER

9

Inflammatory and Demyelinating Central Nervous System Diseases

H. Alex Choi, MD
Sang-Bae Ko, MD, PhD
Kiwon Lee, MD, FACP, FAHA, FCCM

A 60-year-old man with a history of hypertension is admitted with several days of fever and generalized weakness. He complains of diplopia and anorexia and is found to have a low-grade fever of 100.1°F. Over the next few days he clinically deteriorates, developing progressive encephalopathy, worsening right arm weakness, bulbar weakness, and an inability to walk. A head computed tomography (CT) shows nonspecific white matter changes. He is intubated for airway protection and transferred to the neurologic intensive care unit (NICU). On presentation, his examination shows vital signs: temperature 100.2°F, HR 90 bpm, BP 130/90 mm Hg. He has intact cranial nerves except for an absent gag reflex. Motor examination reveals increased tone throughout, extensor posturing of the left arm, flexor posturing of the right arm, and no response in the lower extremities.

What is the differential diagnosis for this patient? And what are the essential next steps?

The constellation of fever, generalized weakness, and bulbar dysfunction can be from a multitude of diseases. Grouping them according to location of disease is useful in guiding diagnostic tests that are needed. Infectious etiologies for central nervous system (CNS) dysfunction (ie, meningitis, encephalitis, cerebral abscess) are important to diagnose and treat quickly. Given the emergent necessity of treating infectious etiologies of meningitis and/or encephalitis, it is prudent to begin treatment with antiviral and antibacterial agents while diagnostic testing proceeds. Intravenous acyclovir should be strongly considered as well as intravenous medication to treat bacterial meningitis, tuberculosis, and fungal infections, depending on clinical suspicion. Diagnosis and treatment of infectious diseases will be discussed in Chapter 7. To diagnose CNS infection, a lumbar puncture should not be delayed.

Although unlikely in this case, perhaps the most time-sensitive diagnosis would be a vascular etiology. In a patient with vascular risk factors and cranial nerve signs/symptoms, a posterior circulation ischemic event is most important to diagnose quickly. Although a noncontrast head CT is effective in diagnosing intracerebral hemorrhages, in this setting it is probably not very helpful. Magnetic resonance imaging (MRI) of the brain is the most effective tool for diagnosing ischemic strokes and also will help in diagnosing other diseases.

Once infectious and vascular etiologies are addressed, one must consider inflammatory diseases. The history of symptoms occurring after a viral prodrome, malaise, and low-grade fever is suggestive of a postinfectious inflammatory process. Acute disseminated encephalomyelitis (ADEM) is a disease that can cause rapid mental status changes and multifocal neurologic deficits. An MRI with and without gadolinium is necessary to diagnose ADEM.

Other possible parenchymal diseases include metastatic disease, other autoimmune inflammatory diseases such as tumefactive multiple sclerosis (MS), and CNS manifestations of systemic autoimmune diseases: lupus, Behçet syndrome, vasculitis, and paraneoplastic diseases.

Leptomeningeal processes can cause encephalopathy and multifocal neurologic symptoms. Again, infectious processes are the most urgent to diagnose. Other possibilities are inflammatory diseases such as sarcoid, neoplastisms, and carcinomatous meningitis.

Although the patient's encephalopathy suggests otherwise, another important location of disease can be in the peripheral nervous system. Demyelinating diseases such as Guillain-Barré syndrome (GBS) can progress over days and impair bulbar function. In fact, some diseases can affect both the central and peripheral nervous systems to produce this clinical syndrome. Bickerstaff encephalitis, a variant of GBS, involves ophthalmoplegia, ataxia, and encephalopathy. It is associated with peripheral motor axonal demyelination with brainstem encephalitis. The detection of the antiganglioside immunoglobulin G (IgG) GQ1b antibody is helpful in the diagnosis of this disease.[1] In a recent case series of patients with ADEM, 43% had polyradiculoneuropathy; mostly demyelinating.[2] If there is clinical suspicion for peripheral involvement, electromyography and nerve conduction studies (EMG/NCSs) are warranted. Patterns seen on EMG/NCS are discussed in Chapter 6.

The patient underwent a lumbar puncture that showed: 10 white blood cells (WBCs); 67% lymphocytes; 33% monophils; 0 red blood cells (RBCs); glucose 65; protein 80; albumin index 11.4 (elevated); herpes simplex virus polymerase chain reaction (HSV PCR) negative; no detected oligoclonal bands; bacterial cultures negative; encephalitis panel negative; paraneoplastic panel negative.

What is the differential diagnosis and what is the next step in management?

The MRI showed multiple bilateral lesions in the white matter of both hemispheres and large lesions affecting the basal ganglia and thalamus with minimal mass effect (Figure 9-1). This suggested a multifocal disease process affecting mostly white matter and deep gray matter.

ADEM is a disease of multifocal white matter demyelination. The typical clinical description of ADEM includes a rapid onset of progressive encephalopathy associated with multifocal neurologic deficits. The clinical syndrome is usually preceded by an antecedent infection or vaccination. A prodromal phase with fever, headache, and malaise may precede the full clinical syndrome.[3] Although more commonly seen in the pediatric population, it is also encountered in adults. The most commonly used definition has been published by the International Pediatric MS Study Group. ADEM: "A first clinical event with a polysymptomatic encephalopathy, with acute or subacute onset, showing focal or multifocal hyperintense lesions predominantly affecting the CNS white matter; no evidence of previous destructive white matter changes should be present; and no history of a previous clinical episode with features of a demyelinating event. . . ."[3]

MRI findings of ADEM have been extensively characterized. Lesions are typically large, multiple, asymmetric, and involve subcortical and central white matter, located at the gray-white junction in the hemispheres, cerebellum, and brainstem. Gadolinium enhancement is variable. Patterns can be complete ring enhancing, nodular, gyral, or spotty. As opposed to multiple sclerosis, the deep gray matter can be involved, especially the caudate head, globus pallidus, putamen, and thalamus. Four types of lesions have been described: (1) small lesions (less than 5 mm), (2) large, confluent, or tumefactive lesions, with edema and mass effect, (3) additional symmetric bithalamic involvements, and (4) acute hemorrhagic encephalomyelitis.[3-6]

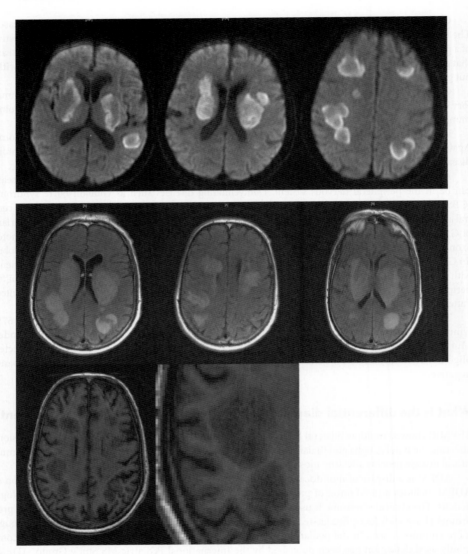

Figure 9-1. (Top row) DWI image showing restricted diffusion, predominantly in the bilateral cerebral white matter tracts, involving the basal ganglia. (Middle row) Fluid-attenuated inversion recovery (FLAIR) images showing hyperintensities in the bilateral cerebral white matter, bilateral basal ganglia, and bilateral thalami. (Bottom row) T1-weighted images showing hypointensities in corresponding white matter lesions.

In our patient, cerebrospinal fluid (CSF) analysis showed no evidence for an infectious process. A mild pleocytosis and an elevated protein with no oligoclonal bands are characteristic of ADEM.[3,6,7]

Another possibility is progressive multifocal leukoencephalopathy (PML). PML is a disease that is multifocal and involves mostly the white matter. As our patient is human immunodeficiency virus (HIV)-negative and has no history of immune suppression, PML would be exceedingly unusual. CSF testing for the presence of the JC virus is helpful with the diagnosis.[8]

What should be the first line of treatment for ADEM and what is the evidence for this?

No randomized clinical trials exist to guide our management for patients with ADEM. Most treatment options are extensions from experience with other demyelinating, autoimmune diseases. Intravenous, methylprednisolone 1 g per day for 3 to 5 days is the typical treatment of choice. The response to steroids can be dramatic, but up to one-third of patients may not respond. Patients with aggressive forms of ADEM may be less likely to respond to steroid treatment.[9,10]

The patient receives IV methylprednisolone for 5 days with no clinical improvements, what is the next step in management?

Aggressive ADEM with disease progression to the point of respiratory failure and admission to the NICU is infrequent occurring in less than 20% of ADEM cases.[6,11] As the complications of mechanical ventilation and immobility compound with time, the speed of recovery needs to be emphasized. This argues for an aggressive treatment strategy.

Immune-modulating treatments, intravenous immune globulin (IVIG), and plasmapheresis (PE) are the next steps in management. IVIG has been used more widely. The usual dose of 0.4 g/kg per day for 5 days has been shown to be efficacious in case series. Improvement usually begins within a week and progresses until 2 months.[9,10,12,13] Although the mechanism for the efficacy for IVIG is not fully understood, it is thought to work by blocking the Fc-receptor on macrophages and effectively decreasing the cell-mediated immune response.[14-16] In addition to direct immune effects, it may work by helping to normalize the blood-brain barrier.[17] Some have debated that in cases of severe disease with peripheral nerve involvement, IVIG along with IV steroids should be first-line therapy.[13]

PE has also been used in ADEM, and a number of case reports support its use. PE is thought to work by removing humoral factors and affecting the balance of B cells and T helper type 1 and type 2 cells.[15,18] In a randomized study of PE in patients with acute CNS inflammatory demyelinating disease, PE was associated with improved neurologic recovery.[19] Other case studies also support the use of PE in CNS demyelinating disease and specifically in ADEM patients. In general, about half of patients will respond. Factors associated with improvement are early treatment and male gender.[20,21]

If a patient does not improve after the first intervention regardless of whether IVIG or PE was performed, the other intervention in addition should be considered. Although no substantial evidence supports treatment with both PE and IVIG, some have suggested that it is more effective.[10,15]

In fact, for patients who are severely affected in the NICU, IV steroids should be started immediately. If little or no clinical response is observed in the first several days, PE should be started for a total of five to seven sessions. If the patient is still critically ill, IVIG should be instituted. PE should be attempted first because of the evidence of efficacy in CNS demyelinating disorders as opposed to the limited evidence behind IVIG. A secondary advantage of treating with PE first is the theoretical advantage of first removing humeral factors through PE and subsequently adding IVIG. Although IVIG is technically easier, if PE is added as a second agent, PE will wash out the previously administered IVIG. If no response to steroids is seen in the first several days of treatment, escalation to immune-modulating therapy should occur quickly as PE and IVIG are more effective the sooner they are started in the time course of the disease.

Other immune-modifying treatments including cyclophosphamide, interferon beta, glatiramer acetate, and rituximab have been suggested, but to date no large series of ADEM patients undergoing these treatments have been described. Owing to the rarity and refractory nature of ADEM in these patients, efficacy may be difficult to assess. Although treated with intravenous Solu-Medrol for 5 days, PE, and IVIG, this patient did not clinically improve. The MRI with diffusion tensor imaging showed atrophy of white matter tract across time (Figure 9-2).

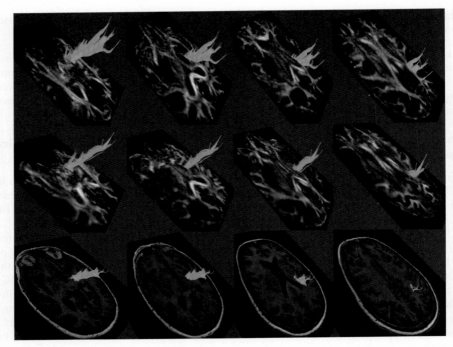

Figure 9-2. Serial diffusion tensor image (DTI), tractography showing decrease in number and density of longitudinal white matter tracts across time.

When do you biopsy a lesion?

Biopsy of the ADEM lesions is warranted when the disease does not respond to conventional treatments (ie, IV steroids, IVIG, or PE) and the presentation is atypical in that other infectious etiologies or neoplastic processes have not been ruled out. The hallmark of ADEM on biopsy is perivenous demyelination as opposed to confluent demyelination, which is seen in acute multiple sclerosis.[22]

 A 27-year-old woman presents with headache and bizarre behavior. About 1 week before presentation she tells family members that she does not feel well, but has no other specific complaints. Soon afterward she has auditory hallucinations and delusions of talking to God. She starts repeating phrases and stops recognizing family members. She is brought to a hospital where she is diagnosed with acute psychosis, started on an antipsychotic medication, and discharged home. At home she continues to have worsening hallucinations and difficult-to-control behavior. She has a witnessed seizure-like episode, and emergency medical services (EMS) is called. In the emergency department she is noted to have seizure-like movements with eyes jerking laterally and jerking movements of the arms and legs. She is treated with IV lorazepam for seizures and intubated for airway protection.

On arrival at the NICU, the patient is found to have rapid, repetitive, orofacial dyskinesias and rhythmic jerking movements of the face and neck. On examination, vital signs are: temperature 101°F, BP 170/90 mm Hg, HR 110 bpm. She is not following commands. She is intermittently localizing/withdrawing to pain in all four extremities. A CT of the head shows no abnormalities. A lumbar puncture is performed and shows 14 WBC; 10 RBC; protein 30; glucose 73; no organisms seen. An MRI with and without gadolinium shows no abnormalities.

What is the next step in management?

Although diagnostic studies are important, just as important in this case is treatment of seizures. Treatment of status epilepticus is discussed in Chapter 3.

In a patient who presents with altered mental status, fever, and seizure, infectious encephalitis is the most important disease to diagnose and treat. HSV encephalitis caused by herpesvirus should be presumptively treated with IV acyclovir. An extensive workup for other infectious encephalitides should be performed. Other noninfectious causes of encephalitis are inflammatory and paraneoplastic.

Paraneoplastic syndromes and autoimmune-mediated encephalitis are a group of disorders that can be challenging to diagnose and treat. The first step in managing a patient with a possible paraneoplastic syndrome is to identify the neoplasm and the associated autoantibody. CT of the chest, abdomen, and pelvis looking for masses; peripheral blood studies to diagnose hematologic neoplasms, and nuclear radiologic studies (positron emission tomography [PET], single-photon emission computed tomography [SPECT], and metaiodobenzylguanidine [mIBG] scans) can be preformed. A list of paraneoplastic neurologic diseases causing encephalitis is provided in Table 9-1.

A CT of the abdomen and pelvis looking for masses showed an ovarian mass suggestive of a teratoma. A transvaginal ultrasound confirms the findings.

What is the diagnosis?

Anti–N-methyl-D-aspartate receptor (NMDAR) encephalitis is a disease that has been recently characterized. Usually affecting women under 40 years of age, patients develop prominent psychiatric symptoms and

Table 9-1. Auto-antibodies and Associated Clinical Syndromes

Antibody	Predominant tumor	Comments
Hu (ANNA1)	Small-cell lung cancer (SCLC), thymoma	Brainstem encephalitis with bulbar signs and symptoms[23-25]
Ma2 (Ta)	Testicular	Limbic encephalitis, brainstem encephalitis, hypothalamic dysfunction[26]
AMPAR	Lung carcinoma	Memory loss, encephalopathy, seizures, tendency to relapse[27]
NMDAR	Teratoma	Limbic encephalitis, seizures, orofacial dyskinesias, autonomic instability[28]
VGKC	Variety of cancers	Memory loss, encephalopathy, seizures[29]
GluR3		Refractory epilepsy[30]
Ri (ANNA2)	Breast, SCLC	Brainstem syndrome (opsoclonus, myoclonus) cerebellar syndrome, Lambert-Eaton syndrome[31]
CV2 (CRMP5)	SCLC, thymoma	Cerebellar ataxia, movements disorders, myasthenic syndromes[32]
Amphiphysin	Breast, SCLC	Mostly peripheral neuropathy, stiff-person syndrome, myelitis[33]

behavior changes that progress to orofacial dyskinesias, seizures, encephalopathy, autonomic instability, respiratory failure, and a catatonia-like state. When first described, almost all patients had an associated ovarian teratoma. Now it is recognized that up to 60% of patients may not have a detectable tumor.[28,34] Although the prevalence is unclear, some suggest that NMDAR encephalitis may account for a significant number of unexplained new-onset epilepsy in women before the age of 40.[35,36]

NMDAR encephalitis is associated with antibodies against the NR1-NR2 heteromers of the NMDAR. The detection of these antibodies in the serum or CSF is diagnostic.[28,37] The disease is characterized by prominent microgliosis and deposits of IgG in the hippocampus, forebrain, basal ganglia, and spinal cord. NMDAR-expressing neurons with inflammatory infiltrates can be found in the teratomas. In addition, cytotoxic markers are extremely uncommon, suggesting that the antibody immune response is the primary mechanism of damage and cell death. Severity of disease is related to levels of antibody titers.[37,38]

Although intrathecal production of antibodies has been described, the antibodies to the NMDAR presumably start in the serum. How the antibodies cross the blood-brain barrier is unclear. The amygdala and hippocampus have the highest levels of NMDAR and are also the brain regions where the blood-brain barrier is the most vulnerable. It has been proposed that the dysautonomia with episodes of sympathetic overactivity and hypertension may weaken an already damaged blood-brain barrier and make these regions even more susceptible.[37]

MRI is nonspecific but approximately 55% of patients have increased fluid-attenuated inversion recovery (FLAIR) or T2 signal in brain parenchyma (Figure 9-3).[28] N-acetylaspartate (NAA) levels in the basal ganglia and thalamus have been shown to be reduced during involuntary movements. Diffusely the brain has a decreased NAA/Cr ratio, suggesting diffuse brain dysfunction. MR perfusion shows hyperperfusion diffusely.[39]

What is the treatment and prognosis?

Similar to other paraneoplastic diseases, tumor resection and immune suppression are the mainstays of treatment. Identification and removal of the teratoma is probably the most effective treatment.[34,40] In addition to tumor removal, immune suppression is commonly performed. Most patients receive IV corticosteroids and IVIG or PE depending on disease severity. For patients in the NICU

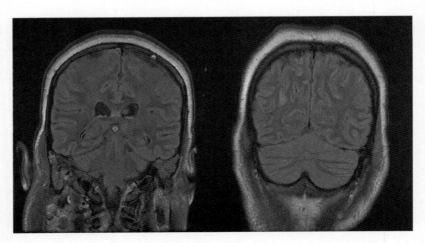

Figure 9-3. Coronal fluid-attenuated inversion recovery (FLAIR) images demonstrating bilateral posterior parieto-occipital cortex hyperintensities in a patient with prolonged seizures from anti–N-methyl-D-aspartate receptor (NMDAR) encephalitis.

we recommend early and aggressive treatment. Early detection and removal of the teratoma is paramount. For immune suppression, methylprednisolone 1 g IV for 5 days should be given. After tumor removal and steroids, if no clinical change is seen in the first few days, PE for five to seven sessions should be strongly considered. If no clinical change occurs after PE, serum and CSF should be reanalyzed for the presence and titers of anti-NMDAR antibodies. In addition, IVIG should be given at this time.[34,41,] If titers are still elevated and no clinical improvement is observed, rituximab or cyclophosphamide should be used.[34] Standard chemotherapeutic agents bleomycin, etoposide, and cisplatin have also been used successfully.[42,43] In patients without a detected teratoma, immune modulation/ suppression is needed with the same algorithm. In addition, routine monitoring for tumor occurrence with MRI of the pelvis is recommended.[44] In patients with refractory encephalitis not responsive to aggressive treatment, prophylactic bilateral ovariectomy without evidence of teratomas has been performed as a lifesaving intervention. The efficacy of this treatment has not been established.

Much attention has been given to the bizarre movements seen in this disorder as it can be very striking and difficult to control. Because many times the treatment of the movement disorder can be difficult and the side effects of medications substantial, treatment of movements should be treated with caution and only if medically necessary. Symptomatic treatment with benzodiazepines, usually long-acting agents such as clonazepam, typical neuroleptics including haloperidol, and atypical neuroleptics such as quetiapine have been used. In several patients, only induction doses of propofol and benzodiazepines effectively controlled the movements. In addition, because of the intense jaw clenching that occurs, botulinum toxin injections to the jaw have been performed.

As opposed to many of the other paraneoplastic diseases, the importance of identifying this disease is that the prognosis is generally good. Although tumor removal has been shown to be effective in treating NMDAR encephalitis, even without tumor removal full recovery after years of follow-up has been described.[44] In the most comprehensive case series of 100 patients, 75 patients recovered to normal or had only mild deficits.[28] However, cases severe enough to be admitted to the NICU most likely have a worse prognosis. Because of the evidence that early treatment improves outcomes and the high number of medical complications that occur in these patients, early and aggressive treatment is recommended.

In patients with refractory encephalitis, a devastating neurologic disease with significant brain atrophy and semi-vegetative state has been seen.

! CRITICAL CONSIDERATIONS

- CNS inflammatory and demyelinating diseases should always be kept in mind for a number of different clinical scenarios.
- A specific diagnosis is important to identify.
- Treatment with immune suppression and/or tumor removal should not be delayed. The severity of the disorder should dictate the aggressiveness of the treatment.

REFERENCES

1. Odaka M, Yuki N, Yamada M, et al. Bickerstaff's brainstem encephalitis: clinical features of 62 cases and a subgroup associated with Guillain-Barré syndrome. *Brain.* 2003;126(Pt 10):2279-2290.

2. Marchioni E, Ravaglia S, Piccolo G, et al. Postinfectious inflammatory disorders: subgroups based on prospective follow-up. *Neurology.* 2005;65:1057-1065.

3. Tenembaum S, Chitnis T, Ness J, Hahn JS. Acute disseminated encephalomyelitis. *Neurology.* 2007; 68(suppl 2):S23.

4. Singh S, Alexander M, Korah IP. Acute disseminated encephalomyelitis: MR imaging features. *AJR Am J Roentgenol.* 1999;173:1101-1107.

5. Kesselring J, Miller DH, Robb SA, et al. Acute disseminated encephalomyelitis. MRI findings and the distinction from multiple sclerosis. *Brain.* 1990;113 (Pt 2):291-302.

6. Tenembaum S, Chamoles N, Fejerman N. Acute disseminated encephalomyelitis: a long-term follow-up study of 84 pediatric patients. *Neurology.* 2002;59:1224-1231.

7. Dale RC, de Sousa C, Chong WK, Cox TC, Harding B, Neville BG. Acute disseminated encephalomyelitis, multiphasic disseminated encephalomyelitis and multiple sclerosis in children. *Brain.* 2000;123 (Pt 12):2407-2422.

8. Cinque P, Koralnik IJ, Gerevini S, Miro JM, Price RW. Progressive multifocal leukoencephalopathy in HIV-1 infection. *Lancet Infect Dis.* 2009;9: 625-636.

9. Ravaglia S, Piccolo G, Ceroni M, et al. Severe steroid-resistant post-infectious encephalomyelitis: general features and effects of IVIg. *J Neurol.* 2007;254:1518-1523.

10. Sahlas DJ, Miller SP, Guerin M, Veilleux M, Francis G. Treatment of acute disseminated encephalomyelitis with intravenous immunoglobulin. *Neurology.* 2000;54:1370-1372.

11. Wingerchuk DM. Postinfectious encephalomyelitis. *Curr Neurol Neurosci Rep.* 2003;3:256-264.

12. Marchioni E, Marinou-Aktipi K, Uggetti C, et al. Effectiveness of intravenous immunoglobulin treatment in adult patients with steroid-resistant monophasic or recurrent acute disseminated encephalomyelitis. *J Neurol.* 2002;249:100-104.

13. Straussberg R, Schonfeld T, Weitz R, Karmazyn B, Harel L. Improvement of atypical acute disseminated encephalomyelitis with steroids and intravenous immunoglobulins. *Pediatr Neurol.* 2001;24:139-143.

14. Kurlander RJ, Ellison DM, Hall J. The blockade of Fc receptor-mediated clearance of immune complexes in vivo by a monoclonal antibody (2.4G2) directed against Fc receptors on murine leukocytes. *J Immunol.* 1984;133:855-862.

15. Lu RP, Keilson G. Combination regimen of methylprednisolone, IV immunoglobulin, and plasmapheresis early in the treatment of acute disseminated encephalomyelitis. *J Clin Apher.* 2006;21:260-265.

16. Kurlander RJ, Hall J. Comparison of intravenous gamma globulin and a monoclonal anti-Fc receptor antibody as inhibitors of immune clearance in vivo in mice. *J Clin Invest.* 1986;77:2010-2018.

17. Pittock SJ, Keir G, Alexander M, Brennan P, Hardiman O. Rapid clinical and CSF response to intravenous gamma globulin in acute disseminated encephalomyelitis. *Eur J Neurol.* 2001;8:725.

18. Goto H, Matsuo H, Nakane S, et al. Plasmapheresis affects T helper type-1/T helper type-2 balance of circulating peripheral lymphocytes. *Ther Apher.* 2001;5:494-496.

19. Weinshenker BG, O'Brien PC, Petterson TM, et al. A randomized trial of plasma exchange in acute central nervous system inflammatory demyelinating disease. *Ann Neurol.* 1999;46:878-886.

20. Llufriu S, Castillo J, Blanco Y, et al. Plasma exchange for acute attacks of CNS demyelination: predictors of improvement at 6 months. *Neurology.* 22 2009;73:949-953.

21. Keegan M, Pineda AA, McClelland RL, Darby CH, Rodriguez M, Weinshenker BG. Plasma exchange for severe attacks of CNS demyelination: predictors of response. *Neurology.* 8 2002;58:143-146.

22. Dale RC, Branson JA. Acute disseminated encephalomyelitis or multiple sclerosis: can the initial presentation help in establishing a correct diagnosis? *Arch Dis Child.* 2005;90:636-639.

23. Saiz A, Bruna J, Stourac P, et al. Anti-Hu–associated brainstem encephalitis. *J Neurol Neurosurg Psychiatry.* 2009;80:404-407.

24. Graus F, Keime-Guibert F, Rene R, et al. Anti–Hu-associated paraneoplastic encephalomyelitis: analysis of 200 patients. *Brain.* 2001;124(Pt 6): 1138-1148.

25. Bataller L, Graus F, Saiz A, Vilchez JJ. Clinical outcome in adult onset idiopathic or paraneoplastic opsoclonus-myoclonus. *Brain.* 2001;124(Pt 2):437-443.

26. Dalmau J, Graus F, Villarejo A, et al. Clinical analysis of anti-Ma2–associated encephalitis. *Brain.* 2004;127(Pt 8):1831-1844.

27. Lai M, Hughes EG, Peng X, et al. AMPA receptor antibodies in limbic encephalitis alter synaptic receptor location. *Ann Neurol.* 2009;65:424-434.

28. Dalmau J, Gleichman AJ, Hughes EG, et al. Anti–NMDA-receptor encephalitis: case series and analysis of the effects of antibodies. *Lancet Neurol.* 2008;7:1091-1098.

29. Vincent A, Buckley C, Schott JM, et al. Potassium channel antibody-associated encephalopathy: a potentially immunotherapy-responsive form of limbic encephalitis. *Brain.* 2004;127(Pt 3):701-712.

30. Granata T, Gobbi G, Spreafico R, et al. Rasmussen's encephalitis: early characteristics allow diagnosis. *Neurology.* 11 2003;60:422-425.

31. Pittock SJ, Lucchinetti CF, Lennon VA. Anti-neuronal nuclear autoantibody type 2: paraneoplastic accompaniments. *Ann Neurol.* 2003;53:580-587.

32. Honnorat J, Antoine JC, Derrington E, Aguera M, Belin MF. Antibodies to a subpopulation of glial cells and a 66 kDa developmental protein in patients with paraneoplastic neurological syndromes. *J Neurol Neurosurg Psychiatry.* 1996;61:270-278.

33. Pittock SJ, Lucchinetti CF, Parisi JE, et al. Amphiphysin autoimmunity: paraneoplastic accompaniments. *Ann Neurol.*2005;58:96-107.

34. Ishiura H, Matsuda S, Higashihara M, et al. Response of anti-NMDA receptor encephalitis without tumor to immunotherapy including rituximab. *Neurology.* 2008;71:1921-1923.

35. Niehusmann P, Dalmau J, Rudlowski C, et al. Diagnostic value of N-methyl-D-aspartate receptor antibodies in women with new-onset epilepsy. *Arch Neurol.* 2009;66:458-464.

36. Kamei S, Kuzuhara S, Ishihara M, et al. Nationwide survey of acute juvenile female non-herpetic encephalitis in Japan: relationship to anti-N-methyl-D-aspartate receptor encephalitis. *Intern Med.* 2009;48:673-679.

37. Dalmau J, Tuzun E, Wu HY, et al. Paraneoplastic anti-N-methyl-D-aspartate receptor encephalitis associated with ovarian teratoma. *Ann Neurol.* J2007;61:25-36.

38. Tuzun E, Zhou L, Baehring JM, Bannykh S, Rosenfeld MR, Dalmau J. Evidence for antibody-mediated pathogenesis in anti-NMDAR encephalitis associated with ovarian teratoma. *Acta Neuropathol.* 2009;118:737-743.

39. Kataoka H, Dalmau J, Taoka T, Ueno S. Reduced N-acetylaspartate in the basal ganglia of a patient with anti-NMDA receptor encephalitis. *Mov Disord.* 2009;24:784-786.

40. Dalmau J, Bataller L. Limbic encephalitis: the new cell membrane antigens and a proposal of clinical-immunological classification with therapeutic implications. *Neurologia.* 2007;22: 526-537.

41. Breese EH, Dalmau J, Lennon VA, Apiwattanakul M, Sokol DK. Anti–N-methyl-D-aspartate receptor encephalitis: early treatment is beneficial. *Pediatr Neurol.* 2010;42:213-214.

42. Tang T, Tay KY, Chai J, et al. A multimodality approach to reversible paraneoplastic encephalitis associated with ovarian teratomas. *Acta Oncol.* 2009;48:1079-1082.

43. Seki M, Suzuki S, Iizuka T, et al. Neurological response to early removal of ovarian teratoma in anti-NMDAR encephalitis. *J Neurol Neurosurg Psychiatry.* 2008;79:324-326.

44. Iizuka T, Sakai F, Ide T, et al. Anti-NMDA receptor encephalitis in Japan: long-term outcome without tumor removal. *Neurology.* 2008;70:504-511.

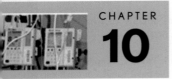

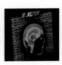

Cardiac Arrest and Anoxic Brain Injury

10

Rishi Malhotra, MD

A 62-year-old man with past medical history of hypertension was in a heated argument with his son when he suddenly complained of dizziness and collapsed to the floor. The son called 911, and paramedics arrived on the scene in 8 minutes. The patient was pulseless and cardiopulmonary resuscitation (CPR) was initiated. He was found to have ventricular fibrillation (VF). A 200-joule biphasic shock was delivered without success. Chest compressions were continued and intravenous (IV) vasopressin 40 units was given. After five cycles of chest compressions and breaths, a 360-joule (maximum for this unit) biphasic shock was delivered, with conversion to a wide-complex rhythm at 120 bpm. The blood pressure (BP) was 120/70 mm Hg. Amiodarone 300 mg was given IV. Estimated time from collapse to return of spontaneous circulation (ROSC) was 15 minutes. He was intubated at this point and then transported to the emergency department (ED) of a local hospital.

On arrival at the ED, the patient was in a narrow-complex sinus rhythm at 89 bpm, his BP was 149/85 mm Hg (without pressors) with a temperature of 36°C. SpO$_2$ 100% on a FlO$_2$ of 0.5. His electrocardiogram (ECG) did not reveal any ST-T changes, or bundle branch blocks. The QTc was normal and there were no Brugada-type changes. Initial labs were remarkable only for a negative troponin I (TnI). An echocardiogram revealed concentric left ventricular hypertrophy with high ejection fraction and no regional wall motion abnormalities. The chest radiograph was clear. A computerized tomographic (CT) scan of the head was unremarkable.

The patient's initial neurologic examination showed no response to verbal stimulation and no eye opening to noxious stimulation. He had reactive pupils, trace corneal reflexes, weakly present horizontal oculocephalic reflexes, no gag reflex, and a weak cough reflex. Upon noxious stimulation, he had extensor posturing of the arms and triple flexion in legs. The Glasgow Coma Scale (GCS) score was 4.

Does this neurologic examination exclude the possibility of a good outcome?

Many patients and their surrogates would consider limiting care if there is no hope for recovery. Therefore, it is important for medical providers to be aware of the prognostic possibilities at all stages of care so that accurate information can be provided to family and informed decisions can be made. Ideally, variables used for prognostication should produce few or no instances of "false positives." In other words, we want to make sure that close to 100% of those labeled as having a poor prognosis do in fact have no chance of recovery.

Unfortunately, most elements of the neurologic examination immediately after cardiac arrest (CA) lack sufficient predictive value to provide accurate outcome prediction.[1-3] Prognostication based solely on a "poor examination" in the hours after CA is inadvisable.

What happens to the brain when deprived of blood and/or oxygen?

After a complete cessation of cerebral perfusion, cerebral oxygen is depleted within 10 seconds and unconsciousness ensues.[4] Within 20 seconds, electroencephalography (EEG) shows electrocerebral silence.[5,6] Cerebral adenosine triphosphate (ATP) and glucose stores are consumed within 5 minutes, resulting in dysfunction of ion pumps and channels, and loss of transmembrane sodium, potassium, and calcium gradients.[6-8] Membrane depolarization results in excessive release of excitatory neurotransmitters, which in turn leads to further accumulation of intracellular calcium. Calcium overload results in the activation of lipases, proteases, nucleases, and other destructive enzymes.[9] Bulk inflow of ions brings with it water, which results in cell swelling. Free-radical production dramatically increases.[9] Systemic and local anaerobic metabolism results in neuronal acidosis, leading to deranged function of a wide variety of proteins.[10] Hyperglycemia can worsen this acidosis.[11,12] The process of cell death can begin as little as 1.5 to 5 minutes after complete cessation of cerebral blood flow (CBF), particularly within sensitive cell populations such as the CA1 hippocampal pyramidal neurons, cerebellar Purkinje neurons, medium spiny striatal neurons, and pyramidal neurons in layers 3, 5, and 6 of the neocortex.[13-15]

Reperfusion leads to a rapid increase in ATP levels[16] and reestablishment of ionic gradients- and is essential for the continued survival of neurons. Unfortunately, reperfusion also results in further damage. Arachidonic acid and other free fatty acids, which had been released by lipases during ischemia, undergo rapid oxidation. This leads to the production of superoxide radicals.[17-19] Xanthine dehydrogenase is converted to xanthine oxidase,[20] which results in additional superoxide radical production. Free iron released from damaged proteins[21,22] catalyzes the destructive peroxidation of membrane lipids by superoxide radicals. Superoxide also reacts with nitric oxide to form peroxynitrite, which is not a free radical but is a potent oxidizer. The damaging effects of peroxynitrite and xanthine oxidase may be particularly important in vascular endothelium,[23,24] leading to increased permeability of the blood-brain barrier and impairment of vascular reactivity.

Are there any therapies to protect the brain from the ongoing cascades after hypoxic-ischemic injury?

Numerous interventions have been studied to block the neurotoxic cascade after both global and local ischemic cerebral insults. Most of these have targeted specific steps in the cascade; for example, free-radical scavenging or calcium channel blockade. Despite promising animal studies, all drugs studied in humans have failed to show any clear benefit, including calcium channel blockers, barbiturates, benzodiazepines, magnesium, and glucocorticoids.[25-30] To date, only mild systemic hypothermia has been shown to improve outcome after CA.

Hypothermia after cardiac arrest (HACA) was initially studied in humans in the late 1950s, with some degree of possible success.[31,32] Peter Safar documents his use of HACA to 30°C in routine clinical practice during the 1950s and 1960s (Figure 10-1).[33] Despite this, additional human trials with HACA were not performed until the 1990s, when 3 small pilot studies showed mild HACA to be safe and feasible.[34-36]

In 2002, an Australian group published the results of a 77-patient controlled trial of hypothermia versus normothermia after out-of-hospital cardiac arrest (OHCA).[37] They included men older than 18 years and women older than 50 years whose initial rhythm was VF, and who remained comatose after spontaneous circulation was successfully reestablished. Coma was not defined. Patients were excluded if they had a systolic pressure less than 90 mm Hg despite pressors or if there was another possible cause

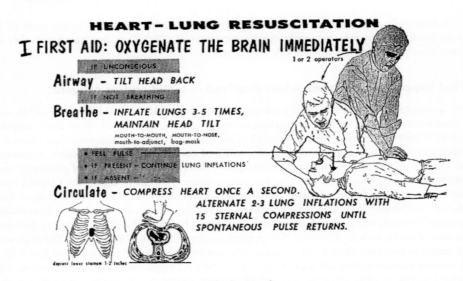

HEART - LUNG RESUSCITATION

I FIRST AID: OXYGENATE THE BRAIN IMMEDIATELY

1 or 2 operators

IF UNCONSCIOUS

Airway – TILT HEAD BACK

IF NOT BREATHING

Breathe – INFLATE LUNGS 3-5 TIMES, MAINTAIN HEAD TILT

MOUTH-TO-MOUTH, MOUTH-TO-NOSE, mouth-to-adjunct, bag-mask

• FEEL PULSE

• IF PRESENT – CONTINUE LUNG INFLATIONS

• IF ABSENT –

Circulate – COMPRESS HEART ONCE A SECOND. ALTERNATE 2-3 LUNG INFLATIONS WITH 15 STERNAL COMPRESSIONS UNTIL SPONTANEOUS PULSE RETURNS.

depress lower sternum 1-2 inches

for physicians only

II START SPONTANEOUS CIRCULATION

Drugs – EPINEPHRINE: 1.0 mg (1.0 CC OF 1:1000) I.V. OR 0.5 mg INTRACARDIAC. REPEAT LARGER DOSE IF NECESSARY
   SODIUM BICARBONATE: APPROXIMATELY 3.75 G/50 CC (1/2 DOSE IN CHILDREN) I.V. REPEAT EVERY 5 MINUTES IF NECESSARY

E. K. G. – • FIBRILLATION: EXTERNAL ELECTRIC DEFIBRILLATION. REPEAT SHOCK EVERY 1-3 MINUTES UNTIL FIBRILLATION REVERSED
   • IF ASYSTOLE OR WEAK BEATS: EPINEPHRINE OR CALCIUM I.V.

Fluids – I.V. PLASMA, DEXTRAN, SALINE
   Do not interrupt cardiac compressions and ventilation. Tracheal intubation only when necessary.
   AFTER RETURN OF SPONTANEOUS CIRCULATION USE VASOPRESSORS AS NEEDED, e.g. NOREPINEPHRINE (Levophed) I.V. DRIP

A.C.: 440 – 1000 V 0.25 sec
or D.C.: 150 W/sec 0.0025 sec

III SUPPORT RECOVERY   (physician - specialist)

Gauge   EVALUATE AND TREAT CAUSE OF ARREST

Hypothermia   START WITHIN 30 MINUTES IF NO SIGN OF CNS RECOVERY

Intensive Care SUPPORT VENTILATION: TRACHEOTOMY, PROLONGED CONTROLLED VENTILATION, GASTRIC TUBE AS NECESSARY
   SUPPORT CIRCULATION
   CONTROL CONVULSIONS
   MONITOR

Figure 10-1. A poster created by Peter Safar, outlining his approach to CA. (*Safar P. Community-wide cardiopulmonary resuscitation. J Iowa Med Soc. 1964;54:629-635.*)

of coma. There was no true randomization—on odd-numbered days, patients were assigned to hypothermia. Paramedics applied ice packs to the head and torso in the field. On arrival at the ED, all patients received initial doses of midazolam and vecuronium as well as lidocaine infusion to prevent recurrent ventricular arrhythmia. They maintained a mean arterial pressure (MAP) of 90 to 100 mm Hg, Pao_2 of 100 mm Hg, $Paco_2$ of 40 mm Hg, and glucose less than 180 mg/dL. Hypothermia patients had additional ice packs applied and maintained until core temperature reached 33°C. Additional midazolam and vecuronium were given as needed for shivering. At 18 hours, the patients began to be actively rewarmed with heated-air blankets. Normothermia patients were maintained at 37°C throughout this period.

Table 10-1. Cerebral Performance Categories (CPCs) Scale

CPC 1: Good cerebral performance: conscious, alert, able to work
CPC 2: Moderate cerebral disability: conscious, can carry out independent activities
CPC 3: Severe neurologic disability: conscious, dependent on others for daily support
CPC 4: Coma or vegetative state
CPC 5: Dead

(From Cronberg T, Lilja G, Rundgren M, Friberg H, Widner H. Long-term neurological outcome after cardiac arrest and therapeutic hypothermia. Resuscitation. 2009;80:1119-1123.)

The primary outcome measure was good neurologic outcome, defined as discharge home or to an acute rehabilitation facility. Significantly fewer patients in the hypothermia group received bystander CPR. Despite this, 49% of hypothermia patients had a good outcome versus 26% of normothermia patients ($P = .046$). Mortality (51% versus 68%) was not significantly different. There were no meaningful, deleterious laboratory or clinical consequences of hypothermia.

Holzer et al carried out a larger, more rigorous 275-patient trial of HACA conducted through nine centers in five European countries.[38] Patients 18 to 75 years old who had a witnessed OHCA were included if they had VF or nonperfusing ventricular tachycardia (VT) on paramedic arrival, 5 to 15 minutes of downtime before commencement of CPR, and no more than 60 minutes from CA to ROSC. Patents were excluded if they had a temperature below 30°C, sustained hypoxia or hypotension before randomization, or known impediments to long-term follow-up. No specific treatment was initiated before ED arrival. Randomization was via envelope-concealed, computer-generated treatment assignments. All patients received pancuronium, fentanyl, and midazolam for 32 hours. Hypothermia patients were placed in an air-cooling device that enveloped their body, with a goal temperature of 32°C to 34°C. Ice packs were added if needed. Hypothermia was maintained for 24 hours from initiation, and then patients were allowed to passively rewarm. Control patients had normothermia maintained.

The primary outcome measure was good neurologic outcome at 6 months, as defined by a Cerebral Performance Category (CPC) (Table 10-1) of 1 or 2. CPC scoring was determined by a blinded examiner. Just as in the Australian HACA trial, bystander CPR was performed on significantly fewer hypothermia patients. Good outcome was attained by 55% of hypothermia patients versus 39% of normothermia patients ($P = .009$). Fewer hypothermia patients were dead at 6 months (41% versus 55%; $P = .02$). There was no significant difference in any of the tracked complications.

After the publication of these two controlled trials, the International Liaison Committee on Resuscitation (ILCOR) Advanced Life Support Task Force published the following recommendations[39]:

> Unconscious adult patients with spontaneous circulation after out-of-hospital CA should be cooled to 32-34°C for 12-24 h when the initial rhythm was VF. Such cooling may also be beneficial for other rhythms or in-hospital CA.

Notice the ILCOR recommendation statement does include, "Such cooling may also be beneficial for other rhythms or in-hospital CA." Similar recommendations remain in the 2010 ILCOR CPR guidelines.[40] A Cochrane review pooling individual data from the above two RCTs, plus data from a 30-patient RCT of helmet cooling,[41] found an odds ratio of 1.55 (95% confidence interval 1.22 to 1.96) for good outcome at hospital discharge, with no significant difference in complications.[42]

How does hypothermia protect the brain?

Hypothermia has multiple effects on the brain and the toxic cascades after hypoxia-ischemia, which differentiates it from prior failed therapies. Polderman eloquently describes the numerous, interrelated effects of hypothermia on the injured brain, observed primarily in animal studies.[43] These are divided into early and late mechanisms of action, as summarized in Figure 10-2. At the target temperature for HACA, cerebral metabolic rate (CMR) is reduced by nearly 50%. The reduction in

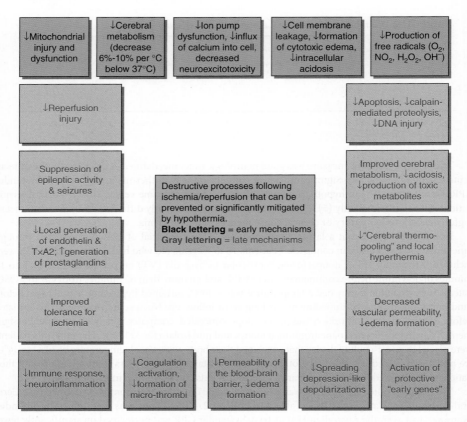

Figure 10-2. Mechanisms of neuroprotection from hypothermia after cardiac arrest. *(Polderman KH. Mechanisms of action, physiological effects, and complications of hypothermia. Crit Care Med. 2009;37:S186-S202.)*

CMR leads to decreases in the CBF threshold for ischemia, cerebral volume, and free-radical production. More energy is available for restoration and maintenance of neuronal ionic gradients, in turn reducing calcium overload, intracellular acidosis, and continued accumulation of glutamate. Oxidation from free radicals and peroxynitrite proceed at a slower rate. Hypothermia reduces disruption of the blood-brain barrier and improves endothelial function, thereby attenuating cerebral edema and, in turn, intracranial hypertension. Thromboxane A_2 and endothelin-1 levels are decreased, lessening vasoconstriction. A systemic inflammatory response[44] and activation of coagulation[45] normally occur after ROSC, and these are both attenuated by hypothermia. This may reduce cerebral microvascular thrombosis, in turn reducing ongoing ischemia. Activation of caspases is reduced, resulting in improved mitochondrial function and sparing some neurons from apoptosis. Finally, convulsive and nonconvulsive seizures occur commonly after CA, and hypothermia has been observed to have an antiepileptic effect in both animals and humans.[46]

The patient was regarded to be a good candidate for hypothermia. Two liters of ice-cold saline were administered. He was transferred to the neurologic intensive care unit at a nearby tertiary care center. On arrival, his temperature was 34.5°C, heart rate 86 bpm, BP 199/93 mm Hg. His examination revealed intermittent multifocal myoclonus and hyperventilation; otherwise the examination was the same as at the outside hospital. Propofol was started to control the hyperventilation and for the myoclonus in case it represented an epileptic phenomenon. Levetiracetam was also given. He was already nearly at the goal temperature of 33°C and was not shivering, so paralytics were not administered. Withholding paralytics would also avoid obscuring convulsive seizures. A microprocessor-controlled surface-cooling system was applied, with patient feedback from a bladder temperature catheter. The goal temperature was set at 33°C. Continuous EEG was requested.

What methods are currently available for induction and maintenance of hypothermia?

Table 10-2 lists some methods of cooling. Some modalities are suitable only for induction (eg ice-cold saline) or maintenance (eg, conventional cooling blankets). Some modalities are more likely to result in overcooling (eg, ice packs), which can lead to treatment complications such as bleeding

Table 10-2. Methods for Inducing and Maintaining Hypothermia

Method	Advantage	Disadvantage
Ice packs	Very low cost	Messy Prone to over- or under-cooling
IV ice-cold saline	Very low cost	Only suitable for induction Can lead to pulmonary edema
Conventional cooling blankets	Low cost	Limited effectiveness
Form-fitting cooling pads	Greater contact area compared with conventional cooling blankets Come with control units that automatically manage patient temperature More precise than other methods	High cost Slower induction than some other methods
Fan-assisted evaporative cooling	Low cost Rapid induction of hypothermia	Labor-intensive Can overcool
Liquid surface cooling	Rapid induction of hypothermia	Only suitable for induction High cost Hinders examination because all-enveloping
Nasopharyngeal evaporative cooling	Small, portable Enables cooling to commence during CPR	High cost No proven benefit of ultraearly cooling Only suitable for induction
Endovascular	Come with control units that automatically manage patient temperature More precise than other methods Some products provide rapid induction of hypothermia Some catheters provide lumens for infusions	High cost Requires placement of catheter before cooling can commence Invasive, with risk of vascular thrombosis and infection

and arrhythmias.[47] Cost, convenience, and effectiveness of each method need to be taken into consideration. Automated systems with patient temperature feedback are ideal from a convenience and effectiveness standpoint, but cost more.

What if he was shivering? Why is shivering harmful?

Shivering leads to an increase in metabolic rate, including CMR, which is counterproductive.[48-51] Severe shivering will prevent core body temperature from falling. The pivotal trials used sedation and paralysis throughout the hypothermia period to prevent shivering.[37,38] Paralysis is the most effective means of preventing or treating shivering, but obscures the detection of seizures.[52] EEG can be applied, but EEG would require frequent review by appropriately skilled professionals to detect seizures in a timely fashion. As a compromise, paralytics can be used solely in the induction phase to prevent shivering, and thereby speed cooling. Most patients do not shiver once at 33°C. Skin counter warming, buspirone, opioids, centrally acting α_2-agonists, and/or sedatives and anesthetics may be used to control shivering.[48]

Why 32-34 degrees celsius?

Levels of hypothermia are typically described as mild (32°C to 35.5 °C), moderate (26°C to 31°C), deep (20°C to 25 °C), and profound (less than 20°C). Experiments in cats and monkeys during the late 1970s found 48 hours of moderate hypothermia (29°C) to be neurologically detrimental in animals with focal cerebral ischemia and even in control animals.[53,54] It was speculated that increased blood viscosity might have impaired CBF. Using a dog model, Safar's team found 3 hours of moderate HACA to 32°C and 28°C resulted in less brain histologic damage compared with normothermia.[55] The 28°C group had more myocardial histologic damage, although this was not sufficient to impair cardiac function before sacrifice at 96 hours. In a separate study, they confirmed myocardial histologic damage in dogs after 1 hour of hypothermia to 15°C and 30°C compared with 34°C and 37.5°C.[56] Thereafter, the Safar group conducted all HACA studies using mild hypothermia.[57-59]

How long should I cool for?

Twenty-four hours of hypothermia is reasonable. The Safar group attained its best brain histology results with a 12-hour protocol of mild hypothermia.[59] Colbourne and Corbett conducted a series of experiments with gerbils, in which the best long-term histologic and functional outcomes were attained with 24 hours of mild hypothermia.[60,61] Prolonged hypothermia was also safe and efficacious in rats.[62] The aforementioned human pilot studies and subsequent phase III trials were based on these temperatures and durations.[34-38] The European HACA trial,[38] the larger and more rigorously conducted of the two pivotal trials, maintained mild hypothermia for 24 hours.

Are there any downsides to HACA?

RCTs of mild HACA have not shown any significant complications.[37,38] Hypokalemia, hyperglycemia, and cold diuresis are known to occur with mild hypothermia. Hypothermia less than 32°C can lead to bradycardia and ventricular arrhythmias, low cardiac function, immunocompromise, coagulopathy, and increased blood viscosity.[63] See Chapter 19 on therapeutic temperature modulation for further information.

What if he had pulseless electrical activity (PEA) or asystole as the initial rhythm? What if the CA was from a noncardiac cause?

Until further data are available, the best strategy may be to, *at least*, offer HACA to those PEA/asystole patients who are judged to have some chance of a recovery (eg, short time to ROSC, readily reversible cause of CA, younger or healthier patients).

Table 10-3. Summary of PEA/Asystole Outcome Data in Pre-HACA Era

Investigators	Design	Patients	N Admitted to ICU	Survival to discharge, n (%)	Survival at 1 y (%)
Niemann et al[71]	Retrospective	Cardiac-only, < 10 min downtime before paramedics arrive	39	10 (26)	
Böttiger et al[68]	Prospective	Cardiac-only	62	12 (19)	9 (15)
Engdahl et al[70]	Prospective	All causes	324	54 (17)	
Don et al[69]	Retrospective	All causes	191[a]	37 (19)	

[a]Number who survived to ED; includes patients who did not survive to ICU admission.

PEA and asystole are the initial rhythms in 60% of all OHCA[64,65] although the proportion has been as high as 93% in some series.[66] The two major trials of HACA included only VF and/or VT patients, essentially excluding the majority of OHCA patients.[37,38] The large trials focused on VF/VT because it has a better outcome than PEA/asystole, and therefore smaller sample sizes would suffice to show a treatment effect.

A word of caution before moving forward: One must be careful in interpreting outcome rates for OHCA, as this is heavily dependent on the choice of denominator.[67] Did the study in question include all patients encountered by EMS, most of whom did not obtain ROSC? This would create the largest possible denominator, and yield the poorest outcome rates. Other studies look only at those who attained ROSC and remained alive by ED arrival. Still others focus only on those who survived to ICU admission. Any data on neuroprotective strategies in PEA/asystole patients should be compared against the outcomes of this last subset of PEA/asystole patients, as other patients would not be amenable to neuroprotective treatment. In the pre-HACA era, 17% to 26% of these patients survived to discharge[68-71] (Table 10-3). In addition, one must be cognizant of the types of patients included in these series. Some studies include only patients whose arrest was cardiac in origin (ie, no drug overdoses, choking victims) or whose time to ROSC was within a certain limit.

Oddo et al prospectively collected data after the institution of a HACA program.[72] Of 74 consecutive patients (excluded age ≥80 years or known terminal disease), 36 had PEA/asystole, and all patients underwent HACA. Seventeen percent of PEA/asystole patients survived to discharge, which is in line with survival estimates in the pre-HACA era discussed above. Using stepwise logistic regression, only time to ROSC and lactate levels were found to be associated with poor outcome, whereas initial rhythm, shock, age, and gender were not. The investigators concluded that PEA/asystole carries a poorer chance of recovery compared with VF/VT because PEA/asystole generally has a longer time to ROSC, not because of anything inherent to the rhythms of PEA/asystole.

Nielsen et al published data from an international HACA registry.[73] PEA/asystole was the initial rhythm in 283 of 986 patients, and 30% of these survived to discharge (73% of these survivors with good function). The exclusion criteria were left up to individual centers, and these criteria were not disclosed, so these results may reflect a selection bias.

Don et al published their single-center experience before and after institution of a HACA protocol.[69] They found no difference in outcomes for PEA/asystole after they began cooling patients. However, there are several issues with the analysis. Patient ascertainment and data collection were done retrospectively, and all patients who presented to the ED were included even if they did not survive to ICU admission or receive HACA. The latter would certainly dilute any effect of hypothermia for PEA/asystole patients. It is stated that an analysis restricted to patients admitted to the ICU failed to show any difference for PEA/asystole patients, but further details were not provided.

Cronberg et al cooled consecutive CA patients[74] unless there was a comorbidity which assured a poor outcome or time to ROSC was long/unknown (T. Cronberg, MD, personal communication via email, January 17, 2011). PEA/asystole was the initial rhythm in 29 of 94 patients. Although outcome at discharge is not provided, 31% of PEA/asystole patients had good functional outcome at approximately 6 months. This is substantially better than even survival to discharge in the pre-HACA era.[68-71]

As it stands, there is no clear data to advocate one way or the other for HACA in PEA/asystole. Based on the above studies and others,[75-79] there is no hint that HACA is less safe in PEA/asystole patients compared with VF/VT. The 2010 ILCOR guidelines endorse HACA as an option for PEA/asystole.[40]

What if he was in shock? What if he had an ST-elevation myocardial infarction?

The European HACA RCT did not enroll patients with persistent shock. The Australian RCT did enroll such patients, but did not report results separately. Both trials included patients who received thrombolytics for acute myocardial infarction without apparent sequelae.[37,38] Subsequent data have not shown any significant adverse effects of HACA for patients requiring percutaneous coronary intervention, receiving thrombolytics, or in persistent shock.[69,72-74,80-86]

The patient was maintained at 33°C temperature until 24 hours from commencement of cooling. He did not shiver on a propofol drip. EEG did not reveal any seizures. Rewarming was device controlled at a rate of 0.25°C per hour to a goal of 37°C. Propofol was maintained until he reached 36°C to prevent shivering. Neurologic examination when propofol was off revealed no eye opening or command following, intact cranial nerve reflexes, no motor responses in the arms, and triple flexion of the legs.

What else can we do to provide neuroprotection after CA?

Cerebral autoregulation is known to be impaired after CA,[87,88] therefore higher MAPs may be needed to ensure adequate CBF and avoid secondary ischemia. Higher MAPs have been repeatedly correlated with better outcome, but no prospective data exists to demonstrate a causal association.[89-93] To avoid excessive strain on an already injured myocardium, the minimal MAP necessary to support CBF would be ideal. In this case, measuring surrogates of CBF, such as oxygen saturation at the jugular bulb ($Sjvo_2$)[88,94,95] or partial pressure of oxygen in brain tissue ($Pbto_2$) may aid in determining the appropriate MAP.

Many physiologic parameters other than MAP are known to affect CBF and cerebral oxygen supply and demand (Table 10-4). Hypocapnia has been found to cause cerebral ischemia in a number of disease states, including after the global cerebral insult of CA.[53,94-96] Intracranial pressure has been looked at prospectively after CA, and values > 25 mm Hg occur in at least 26% of patients.[97] Seizures and status epilepticus dramatically increase CMR, and are common after CA, occurring in up to 36%[98] and 12%[52,99] of patients, respectively. In the past, status epilepticus after CA was felt to guarantee a poor outcome, but anecdotal evidence and case reports[100] suggest that this may not be true after hypothermia, provided that status epilepticus is aggressively treated. Fever also increases CMR and is very common after CA.[101-103]

Hyperoxemia has been shown to exacerbate neurologic injury after CA in animals,[104-106] and has been correlated with worse outcome in humans. Kilgannon et al found even small increases in Pao_2 to be associated with poor functional outcome and mortality.[107] Each 25–mm Hg increment in Pao_2 was associated with a 6% increase in mortality rate.

Table 10-4. Suggested Management to Avoid Secondary Neurologic Injury

Parameter	Recommendation
CO_2	Strictly maintain $PaCO_2 > 35$
Hemoglobin	Optimal hemoglobin not defined; consider cerebral oximetry to guide therapy
$SjvO_2$ or $PbtO_2$	Maintain $SjvO_2 > 60\%$ or $PbtO_2 > 20$ mm Hg
Seizures	Continuous EEG as soon as possible, monitor for 48-72 hours. Treat seizures aggressively
ICP	Unclear if controlling ICP can improve outcome. Consider placement of a parenchymal ICP monitor and maintain ICP < 20 mm Hg
Fever	Maintain normothermia (after hypothermia period) via pharmacologic (eg NSAIDs) or non-pharmacologic means
Shivering	Shivering is known to increase cerebral metabolic rate. Use skin counter warming or medications to control shivering.
Hyperoxemia	Maintain minimum necessary PaO_2. Avoid $PaO_2 > 200$ mm Hg

The patient's examination was unchanged over the next 3 days. On day 4, he developed pneumonia and was treated with broad-spectrum antibiotics. Tracheostomy and gastrostomy were placed on day 10. The examination on day 10 showed eye opening only to noxious stimulation, no motor response in the arms, and extensor response in the legs. On day 13, he became hypertensive and developed pulmonary edema. Serum TnI rose to 20 ng/mL with ECG showing inferolateral T-wave inversions. Cardiology was consulted, and the cardiac ischemia was medically managed. At this time, the health care proxy was considering withdrawal of care. On day 16, he was made Do Not Resuscitate (DNR) and the proxy wanted to withdraw care in a few days. Examination at that time revealed spontaneous eye opening, roving eye movements, and intermittent head turning to the side of painful stimulation; arm and leg movements were unchanged. On day 18, after the goal of care had been shifted to comfort but mechanical ventilation was still ongoing, his neurologic examination unexpectedly improved. He spontaneously tracked bilaterally and had minimal but clear spontaneous movement of the arms. The lower extremities were still extensor posturing to noxious stimulation. Full medical support was resumed. On day 23, he started to mouth the word "ouch" with noxious stimulation and he became more active with his arms. Because of his improving neurologic status an automated implantable cardioverter-defibrillator (AICD) was implanted on day 25 to prevent recurrent ventricular arrhythmias. A cardiac catheterization revealed multivessel disease, so 3 coronary stents were placed. By discharge on day 35, he socially smiled, followed simple verbal commands, purposefully moved his arms against gravity, and was able to withdraw his legs from noxious stimuli.

What data can be used to prognosticate after CA?

Figure 10-3 shows the current American Academy of Neurology (AAN) evidence-based algorithm for prognosticating after CA.[108] It is important to note that this is based on data from the pre-HACA era, and these guidelines are NOT applicable to patients who were cooled. The presence of the following essentially guarantees poor functional outcome or death if the patient was not cooled:

1. Absent pupillary or corneal reflexes on day 3 (but not before)
2. Bilateral extensor posturing or absent motor responses on day 3 (but not before)

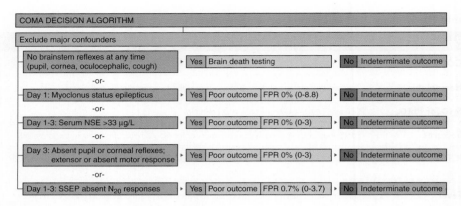

Figure 10-3. AAN decision algorithm for prognostication in comatose survivors of cardiac arrest. The numbers in parentheses are 95% confidence intervals. Confounding factors could diminish the accuracy of this algorithm. NSE, neuron-specific enolase; SSEP, somatosensory evoked potential; FPR, false-positive rate. *(Wijdicks EF, Hijdra A, Young GB, et al. Practice parameter: Prediction of outcome in comatose survivors after cardiopulmonary resuscitation (an evidence-based review): Report of the quality standards subcommittee of the American Academy of Neurology. Neurology. 2006;67:203-210).*

3. Myoclonus status epilepticus within 24 hours (Note: The AAN refers to multifocal jerking, not an electrographic phenomenon, to define this)

4. Serum neuron-specific enolase greater than 33 µg/L on days 1-3

5. Somatosensory evoked potentials (SSEPs) showing bilaterally absent N_{20} responses

For patients who underwent HACA, the following independent features CANNOT provide fool-proof prognostication:

1. Motor examination[109,110]

2. Serum neuron-specific enolase[111]

3. Early myoclonus[109]

4. Pupillary or corneal reflexes[109]

Rossetti et al prospectively looked at what factors can serve as accurate guides after HACA.[109] Bilaterally absent N_{20} responses on SSEPs, an unreactive EEG, or the combination of early myoclonus and absent pupillary or corneal reflexes provided certainty of a poor outcome with no false positives. However, a larger retrospective study did have 1 patient with bilaterally absent N_{20} responses who made an excellent functional recovery.[112] Until more prospective data is available on prognosticating in HACA patients, it would be prudent to proceed with caution.

! CRITICAL CONSIDERATIONS

- The neurologic examination immediately post-CA lacks sufficient predictive value to provide accurate outcome prediction. Prognostication based on a "poor examination" in the early hours after CA is inadvisable.

- Comatose patients with VF/VT CA who present within 6 hours should be cooled as soon as possible to 32-34°C for 24 hours. The ILCOR Advanced Life Support Task Force states: Such cooling may also be beneficial for other rhythms or in-hospital CA." As such, it is reasonable to cool selected patients with PEA/asystole and/or in-hospital CA (eg brief PEA arrest, young patients, etc). Given the safety of HACA, patients slightly past the 6-hour window should be offered HACA.

- Shock or planned coronary intervention are not contraindications to HACA. Cooling can and should be commenced in the cardiac catheterization lab to avoid delay in achieving goal temperature.

- Hypocapnia ($Paco_2$ < 35 mm Hg) and hyperoxemia are likely harmful after CA and should be avoided. Fever and shivering should be treated. Consider jugular bulb oxygen saturation and continuous EEG monitoring to prevent secondary injury.

- In patients who receive HACA, robust knowledge of prognostic factors is not yet available. Prognosticate with caution. In patients who are not cooled, any one of the following nearly guarantees a poor prognosis:

  - Absent pupillary or corneal reflexes by day 3

  - Bilateral extensor posturing or absent motor responses by day 3

  - Myoclonus status epilepticus within 24 hours (multifocal jerking, regardless of EEG findings)

  - Serum neuron-specific enolase greater than 33 µg/L on days 1-3

  - SSEPs showing bilaterally absent N_{20} responses

REFERENCES

1. Booth CM, Boone RH, Tomlinson G, Detsky AS. Is this patient dead, vegetative, or severely neurologically impaired? Assessing outcome for comatose survivors of cardiac arrest. *JAMA.* 2004;291: 870-879.

2. Levy DE, Caronna JJ, Singer BH, Lapinski RH, Frydman H, Plum F. Predicting outcome from hypoxic-ischemic coma. *JAMA.* 1985;253:1420-1426.

3. Rittenberger JC, Sangl J, Wheeler M, Guyette FX, Callaway CW. Association between clinical examination and outcome after cardiac arrest. *Resuscitation.* 81:1128-1132.

4. Kabat H, Anderson JP. Acute arrest of cerebral circulation in man: Lieutenant Ralph Rossen (MC), U.S.N.R. *Arch Neurol Psychiatry.* 1943;50: 510-528.

5. Hossmann KA, Grosse Ophoff B. Recovery of monkey brain after prolonged ischemia: I. Electrophysiology and brain electrolytes. *J Cereb Blood Flow Metab.* 1986;6:15-21.

6. Siemkowicz E, Hansen A. Brain extracellular ion composition and EEG activity following 10 minutes ischemia in normo- and hyperglycemic rats. *Stroke.* 1981;12:236-240.

7. Erecinska M, Silver IA. ATP and brain function. *J Cereb Blood Flow Metab.* 1989;9:2-19.

8. Lowry OH, Passonneau JV, Hasselberger FX, Schulz DW. Effect of ischemia on known substrates and cofactors of the glycolytic pathway in brain. *J Biol Chem.* 1964;239:18-30.

9. Neumar RW. Molecular mechanisms of ischemic neuronal injury. *Ann Emerg Med.* 2000;36:483-506.

10. Rehncrona S. Brain acidosis. *Ann Emerg Med.* 1985;14:770-776.

11. Pulsinelli WA, Waldman S, Rawlinson D, Plum F. Moderate hyperglycemia augments ischemic brain damage. *Neurology.* 1982;32:1239.

12. Siemkowicz E, Hansen AJ. Clinical restitution following cerebral ischemia in hypo-, normo and hyperglycemic rats. *Acta Neurol Scand.* 1978; 58:1-8.

13. Pulsinelli WA, Brierley JB, Plum F. Temporal profile of neuronal damage in a model of transient forebrain ischemia. *Ann Neurol.* 1982;11:491-498.

14. Kirino T, Tamura A, Sano K. Selective vulnerability of the hippocampus to ischemia—Reversible and irreversible types of ischemic cell damage. *Prog Brain Res.* 1985;63:39-58.

15. Vaagenes P, Safar P, Diven W, et al. Brain enzyme levels in CSF after cardiac arrest and resuscitation in dogs: Markers of damage and predictors of outcome. *J Cereb Blood Flow Metab.* 1988;8:262-275.

16. Siesjo BK, Ljunggren B. Cerebral energy reserves after prolonged hypoxia and ischemia. *Arch Neurol.* 1973;29:400-407.

17. Yoshida S, Abe K, Busto R, Watson BD, Kogure K, Ginsberg MD. Influence of transient ischemia on lipid-soluble antioxidants, free fatty acids and energy metabolites in rat brain. *Brain Res.* 1982;245:307-316.

18. Cao W, Carney JM, Duchon A, Floyd RA, Chevion M. Oxygen free radical involvement in ischemia and reperfusion injury to brain. *Neurosci Lett.* 1988;88:233-238.

19. Flamm E, Demopoulos H, Seligman M, Poser R, Ransohoff J. Free radicals in cerebral ischemia. *Stroke.* 1978;9:445-447.

20. Kinuta Y, Kimura M, Itokawa Y, Ishikawa M, Kikuchi H. Changes in xanthine oxidase in ischemic rat brain. *J Neurosurg.* 1989;71:417-420.

21. Komara J, Nayini N, Bialick H, et al. Brain iron delocalization and lipid peroxidation following cardiac arrest. *Ann Emerg Med.* 1986;15:384-389.

22. Krause GS, Joyce KM, Nayini NR, et al. Cardiac arrest and resuscitation: Brain iron delocalization during reperfusion. *Ann Emerg Med.* 1985;14:1037-1043.

23. Beckman JS. Peroxynitrite versus hydroxyl radical: The role of nitric oxide in superoxide-dependent cerebral injury. *Ann NY Acad Sci.* 1994;738:69-75.

24. Pritsos CA. Cellular distribution, metabolism and regulation of the xanthine oxidoreductase enzyme system. *Chem Biol Interact.* 2000;129:195-208.

25. Brain Resuscitation Clinical Trial I Study Group. Randomized clinical study of thiopental loading in comatose survivors of cardiac arrest. *N Engl J Med.* 1986;314:397-403.

26. Brain Resuscitation Clinical Trial II Study Group. A randomized clinical study of a calcium-entry blocker (lidoflazine) in the treatment of comatose survivors of cardiac arrest. *N Engl J Med.* 1991;324:1225-1231.

27. Jastremski M, Sutton-Tyrrell K, Vaagenes P, et al. Glucocorticoid treatment does not improve neurological recovery following cardiac arrest. *JAMA.* 1989;262:3427-3430.

28. Longstreth Jr W, Fahrenbruch C, Olsufka M, Walsh T, Copass M, Cobb L. Randomized clinical trial of magnesium, diazepam, or both after out-of-hospital cardiac arrest. *Neurology.* 2002;59:506.

29. Roine RO, Kaste M, Kinnunen A, Nikki P, Sarna S, Kajaste S. Nimodipine after resuscitation from out-of-hospital ventricular fibrillation: a placebo-controlled, double-blind, randomized trial. *JAMA.* 1990;264:3171-3177.

30. Thel MC, Armstrong AL, Mcnulty SE, Califf RM, O'connor CM. Randomised trial of magnesium in in-hospital cardiac arrest. *Lancet.* 1997;350:1272-1276.

31. Benson DW, Williams GR, Spencer FC, Yates AJ. The use of hypothermia after cardiac arrest. *Anesth Analg.* 1959;38:423-428.

32. Williams GRJ, Spencer FC. The clinical use of hypothermia following cardiac arrest. *Ann Surg.* 1958;3:462-468.

33. Safar P. Community-wide cardiopulmonary resuscitation. *J Iowa Med Soc.* 1964;54:629-635.

34. Bernard SA, Jones BMC, Horne MK. Clinical trial of induced hypothermia in comatose survivors of out-of-hospital cardiac arrest. *Ann Emerg Med.* 1997;30:146-153.

35. Yanagawa Y, Ishihara S, Norio H, et al. Preliminary clinical outcome study of mild resuscitative hypothermia after out-of-hospital cardiopulmonary arrest. *Resuscitation.* 1998;39:61-66.

36. Zeiner A, Holzer M, Sterz F, et al. Mild resuscitative hypothermia to improve neurological outcome after cardiac arrest : A clinical feasibility trial. *Stroke.* 2000;31:86-94.

37. Bernard SA, Gray TW, Buist MD, et al. Treatment of comatose survivors of out-of-hospital cardiac arrest with induced hypothermia. *N Engl J Med.* 2002;346:557-563.

38. The Hypothermia after Cardiac Arrest Study Group. Mild therapeutic hypothermia to improve the neurologic outcome after cardiac arrest. *N Engl J Med.* 2002;346:549-556.

39. Nolan JP, Morley PT, Hoek TLV, Hickey RW. Therapeutic hypothermia after cardiac arrest: an Advisory Statement by the Advanced Life Support Task Force of the International Liaison Committee on Resuscitation. *Resuscitation.* 2003;57:231-235.

40. Morrison LJ, Deakin CD, Morley PT, et al. Part 8: Advanced life support: 2010 International Consensus on Cardiopulmonary Resuscitation and Emergency Cardiovascular Care Science with Treatment Recommendations. *Circulation.* 2010;122(suppl 2):S345-S421.

41. Hachimi-Idrissi S, Corne L, Ebinger G, Michotte Y, Huyghens L. Mild hypothermia induced by a

helmet device: a clinical feasibility study. *Resuscitation.* 2001;51:275-281.

42. Arrich J, Holzer M, Herkner H, Müllner M. Hypothermia for neuroprotection in adults after cardiopulmonary resuscitation. *Cochrane Database Syst Rev.* 2009. Available at: *http://www.mrw.interscience.wiley.com/cochrane/clsysrev/articles/CD004128/frame.html.*

43. Polderman KH. Mechanisms of action, physiological effects, and complications of hypothermia. *Crit Care Med.* 2009;37:S186-S202.

44. Adrie C, Adib-Conquy M, Laurent I, et al. Successful cardiopulmonary resuscitation after cardiac arrest as a "sepsis-like" syndrome. *Circulation.* 2002;106:562-568.

45. Böttiger BW, Motsch J, Bohrer H, et al. Activation of blood coagulation after cardiac arrest is not balanced adequately by activation of endogenous fibrinolysis. *Circulation.* 1995;92:2572-2578.

46. Corry J, Dhar R, Murphy T, Diringer M. Hypothermia for refractory status epilepticus. *Neurocrit Care.* 2008;9:189-197.

47. Merchant R, Abella B, Peberdy M, et al. Therapeutic hypothermia after cardiac arrest: Unintentional overcooling is common using ice packs and conventional cooling blankets. *Crit Care Med.* 2006;34:S490-S494.

48. Badjatia N. Hyperthermia and fever control in brain injury. *Crit Care Med.* 2009;37:S250-S257.

49. Badjatia N, Kowalski R, Schmidt J, et al. Predictors and clinical implications of shivering during therapeutic normothermia. *Neurocrit Care.* 2007;6:186-191.

50. Badjatia N, Strongilis E, Gordon E, et al. Metabolic impact of shivering during therapeutic temperature modulation: The bedside shivering assessment scale. *Stroke.* 2008;39:3242-3247.

51. Badjatia N, Strongilis E, Prescutti M, et al. Metabolic benefits of surface counter warming during therapeutic temperature modulation. *Crit Care Med.* 2009;37:1893-1897.

52. Legriel S, Bruneel F, Sediri H, et al. Early EEG monitoring for detecting postanoxic status epilepticus during therapeutic hypothermia: a pilot study. *Neurocrit Care.* 2009;11(3):338-344.

53. Michenfelder J, Milde J. Failure of prolonged hypocapnia, hypothermia, or hypertension to favorably alter acute stroke in primates. *Stroke.* 1977;8:87-91.

54. Steen P, Soule E, Michenfelder J. Deterimental effect of prolonged hypothermia in cats and monkeys with and without regional cerebral ischemia. *Stroke.* 1979;10:522-529.

55. Leonov Y, Sterz F, Safar P, Radovsky A. Moderate hypothermia after cardiac arrest of 17 minutes in dogs. Effect on cerebral and cardiac outcome. *Stroke.* 1990;21:1600-1606.

56. Weinrauch V, Safar P, Tisherman S, Kuboyama K, Radovsky A. Beneficial effect of mild hypothermia and detrimental effect of deep hypothermia after cardiac arrest in dogs. *Stroke.* 1992;23:1454-1462.

57. Sterz F, Safar P, Tisherman S, Radovsky A, Kuboyama K, Oku K-I. Mild hypothermia cardiopulmonary resuscitation improves outcome after prolonged cardiac arrest in dogs. *Crit Care Med.* 1991;19:379-389.

58. Kuboyama K, Safar P, Radovsky A, Tisherman SA, Stezoski SW, Alexander H. Delay in cooling negates the beneficial effect of mild resuscitative cerebral hypothermia after cardiac arrest in dogs: A prospective, randomized study. *Crit Care Med.* 1993;21:1348-1358.

59. Safar P, Xiao F, Radovsky A, et al. Improved cerebral resuscitation from cardiac arrest in dogs with mild hypothermia plus blood flow promotion. *Stroke.* 1996;27:105-113.

60. Colbourne F, Corbett D. Delayed and prolonged post-ischemic hypothermia is neuroprotective in the gerbil. *Brain Res.* 1994;654:265-272.

61. Colbourne F, Corbett D. Delayed postischemic hypothermia: a six month survival study using behavioral and histological assessments of neuroprotection. *J Neurosci.* 1995;15:7250-7260.

62. Yanamoto H, Hong SC, Soleau S, Kassell NF, Lee KS. Mild postischemic hypothermia limits cerebral injury following transient focal ischemia in rat neocortex. *Brain Res.* 1996;718:207-211.

63. Polderman KH. Application of therapeutic hypothermia in the intensive care unit: opportunities and pitfalls of a promising treatment modality—Part 2: Practical aspects and side effects. *Intensive Care Med.* 2004;30:757.

64. Nichol G, Thomas E, Callaway CW, et al. Regional variation in out-of-hospital cardiac arrest incidence and outcome. *JAMA.* 2008;300:1423-1431.

65. Engdahl J, Axelsson Å, Bång A, Karlson BW, Herlitz J. The epidemiology of cardiac arrest in children and young adults. *Resuscitation.* 2003;58:131-138.

66. Cantineau JP, Lambert Y, Merckx P, et al. End-tidal carbon dioxide during cardiopulmonary resuscitation in humans presenting mostly with asystole: a predictor of outcome. *Crit Care Med.* 1996;24:791-796.

67. Eisenberg MS, Cummins RO, Larsen MP. Numerators, denominators, and survival rates: reporting survival from out-of-hospital cardiac arrest. *Am J Emerg Med.* 1991;9:544-546.

68. Böttiger BW, Grabner C, Bauer H, et al. Long term outcome after out-of-hospital cardiac arrest with physician staffed emergency medical services: the Utstein style applied to a midsized urban/suburban area. *Heart*. 1999;82:674-679.

69. Don CW, Longstreth WT, Maynard C, et al. Active surface cooling protocol to induce mild therapeutic hypothermia after out-of-hospital cardiac arrest: a retrospective before-and-after comparison in a single hospital. *Crit Care Med*. 2009;37: 3062-3069.

70. Engdahl J, Bång A, Lindqvist J, Herlitz J. Factors affecting short- and long-term prognosis among 1069 patients with out-of-hospital cardiac arrest and pulseless electrical activity. *Resuscitation*. 2001;51:17-25.

71. Niemann JT, Stratton SJ, Cruz B, Lewis RJ. Outcome of out-of-hospital postcountershock asystole and pulseless electrical activity versus primary asystole and pulseless electrical activity. *Crit Care Med*. 2001;29:2366-2370.

72. Oddo M, Ribordy V, Feihl F, et al. Early predictors of outcome in comatose survivors of ventricular fibrillation and non-ventricular fibrillation cardiac arrest treated with hypothermia: a prospective study. *Crit Care Med*. 2008;36:2296-2301.

73. Nielsen N, Hovdenes J, Nilsson F, et al. Outcome, timing and adverse events in therapeutic hypothermia after out-of-hospital cardiac arrest. *Acta Anaesthesiol Scand*. 2009;53:926-934.

74. Cronberg T, Lilja G, Rundgren M, Friberg H, Widner H. Long-term neurological outcome after cardiac arrest and therapeutic hypothermia. *Resuscitation*. 2009;80:1119-1123.

75. Arrich J. Clinical application of mild therapeutic hypothermia after cardiac arrest. *Crit Care Med*. 2007;35:1041-1047.

76. Busch M, Soreide E, Lossius HM, Lexow K, Dickstein K. Rapid implementation of therapeutic hypothermia in comatose out-of-hospital cardiac arrest survivors. *Acta Anaesthesiol Scand*. 2006;50:1277-1283.

77. Holzer M, Mullner M, Sterz F, et al. Efficacy and safety of endovascular cooling after cardiac arrest: cohort study and bayesian approach. *Stroke*. 2006;37:1792-1797.

78. Storm C, Steffen I, Schefold J, et al. Mild therapeutic hypothermia shortens intensive care unit stay of survivors after out-of-hospital cardiac arrest compared to historical controls. *Crit Care*. 2008;12:R78.

79. Sunde K, Pytte M, Jacobsen D, et al. Implementation of a standardised treatment protocol for post resuscitation care after out-of-hospital cardiac arrest. *Resuscitation*. 2007;73:29-39.

80. Indik JH. Hypothermia: Is it just for ventricular fibrillation? *Crit Care Med*. 2009;37:3175-3176.

81. Nilsson F, Höglund P, Nielsen N. On extending the indications for the use of therapeutic hypothermia. *Crit Care Med*. 2009;37:2865.

82. Oddo M, Schaller MD, Feihl F, Ribordy V, Liaudet L. From evidence to clinical practice: effective implementation of therapeutic hypothermia to improve patient outcome after cardiac arrest. *Crit Care Med*. 2006;34:1865-1873.

83. Skulec R, Kovarnik T, Dostalova G, Kolar J, Linhart A. Induction of mild hypothermia in cardiac arrest survivors presenting with cardiogenic shock syndrome. *Acta Anaesthesiol Scand*. 2008;52:188-194.

84. Hovdenes J, Laake JH, Aaberge L, Haugaa H, Bugge JF. Therapeutic hypothermia after out-of-hospital cardiac arrest: experiences with patients treated with percutaneous coronary intervention and cardiogenic shock. *Acta Anaesthesiol Scand*. 2007;51:137-142.

85. Wolfrum S, Pierau C, Radke PW, Schunkert H, Kurowski V. Mild therapeutic hypothermia in patients after out-of-hospital cardiac arrest due to acute ST-segment elevation myocardial infarction undergoing immediate percutaneous coronary intervention. *Crit Care Med*. 2008;36: 1780-1786.

86. Schefold JC, Boldt L-H, Pschowski R, Reinke P. Risk management after cardiopulmonary resuscitation—what is the real threat? *Crit Care Med*. 2008;36:3130-3131.

87. Sundgreen C, Larsen FS, Herzog TM, Knudsen GM, Boesgaard S, Aldershvile J. Autoregulation of cerebral blood flow in patients resuscitated from cardiac arrest. *Stroke*. 2001;32(1):128-132.

88. Nishizawa H, Kudoh I. Cerebral autoregulation is impaired in patients resuscitated after cardiac arrest. *Acta Anaesthesiol Scand*. 1996; 40(9): 1149-1153.

89. Kilgannon JH, Roberts BW, Reihl LR, et al. Early arterial hypotension is common in the post-cardiac arrest syndrome and associated with increased in-hospital mortality. *Resuscitation*. 2008;79(3):410-416.

90. Martin DR. Relation between initial post-resuscitation systolic blood pressure and neurologic outcome following cardiac arrest. *Ann Emerg Med*. 1993;22:206.

91. Müllner M, Sterz F, Binder M, et al. Arterial blood pressure after human cardiac arrest and neurological recovery. *Stroke*. 1996;27(1): 59-62.

92. Sasser HC, Safar P, BRCT Study Group. Arterial hypertension after cardiac arrest is associated

with good cerebral outcome in patients. *Crit Care Med.* 1999;27(12):A29.

93. Spivey WH. Correlation of blood pressure with mortality and neurologic recovery in comatose postresuscitation patients. *Ann Emerg Med.* 1991;20:453.

94. Buunk G, Van Der Hoeven JG, Meinders AE. Cerebrovascular reactivity in comatose patients resuscitated from a cardiac arrest. *Stroke.* 1997;28(8):1569-1573.

95. Pynnönen L, Falkenbach P, Kämäräinen A, Lönnrot K, Yli-Hankala A, Tenhunen J. Therapeutic hypothermia after cardiac arrest—cerebral perfusion and metabolism during upper and lower threshold normocapnia. *Resuscitation.* 2011;82(9):1174-1179.

96. Oku K, Kuboyama K, Safar P, et al. Cerebral and systemic arteriovenous oxygen monitoring after cardiac arrest. Inadequate cerebral oxygen delivery. *Resuscitation.* 1994;27(2):141-152.

97. Gueugniaud PY, Garcia-Darennes F, Gaussorgues P, Bancalari G, Petit P, Robert D. Prognostic significance of early intracranial and cerebral perfusion pressures in post-cardiac arrest anoxic coma. *Intensive Care Med.* 1991;17(7):392-398.

98. Krumholz A, Stem BJ, Weiss HD. Outcome from coma after cardiopulmonary resuscitation. *Neurology.* 1988;38(3):401.

99. Rittenberger J, Popescu A, Brenner R, Guyette F, Callaway C. Frequency and timing of nonconvulsive status epilepticus in comatose post-cardiac arrest subjects treated with hypothermia. *Neurocrit Care.* 2011:1-9.

100. Rossetti AO, Oddo M, Liaudet L, Kaplan PW. Predictors of awakening from postanoxic status epilepticus after therapeutic hypothermia. *Neurology.* 2009;72(8):744-749.

101. Cocchi MN, Giberson B, Farrell E, et al. Fever after rewarming: Incidence of pyrexia in post-cardiac arrest patients who have undergone mild therapeutic hypothermia. *Circulation.* 2010;122(21 Supplement):A236.

102. Takasu A, Saitoh D, Kaneko N, Sakamoto T, Okada Y. Hyperthermia: Is it an ominous sign after cardiac arrest? *Resuscitation.* 2001;49(3):273-277.

103. Zeiner A, Holzer M, Sterz F, et al. Hyperthermia after cardiac arrest is associated with an unfavorable neurologic outcome. *Arch Intern Med.* 2001;161(16):2007-2012.

104. Liu Y, Rosenthal RE, Haywood Y, et al. Normoxic ventilation after cardiac arrest reduces oxidation of brain lipids and improves neurological outcome· editorial comment. *Stroke.* 1998;29(8):1679.

105. Richards EM, Fiskum G, Rosenthal RE, Hopkins I, Mckenna MC. Hyperoxic reperfusion after global ischemia decreases hippocampal energy metabolism. *Stroke.* 2007;38(5):1578-1584.

106. Zwemer CF, Whitesall SE, D'alecy LG. Cardiopulmonary-cerebral resuscitation with 100% oxygen exacerbates neurological dysfunction following nine minutes of normothermic cardiac arrest in dogs. *Resuscitation.* 1994;27(2):159-170.

107. Kilgannon JH, Jones AE, Parrillo JE, et al. Relationship between supranormal oxygen tension and outcome after resuscitation from cardiac arrest / clinical perspective. *Circulation.* 2011;123(23):2717-2722.

108. Wijdicks EFM, Hijdra A, Young GB, Bassetti CL, Wiebe S. Practice parameter: Prediction of outcome in comatose survivors after cardiopulmonary resuscitation (an evidence-based review): Report of the quality standards subcommittee of the American Academy of Neurology. *Neurology.* 2006;67(2):203-210.

109. Rossetti AO, Oddo M, Logroscino G, Kaplan PW. Prognostication after cardiac arrest and hypothermia: A prospective study. *Ann Neurol.* 2010;67(3):301-307.

110. Al Thenayan E, Savard M, Sharpe M, Norton L, Young B. Predictors of poor neurologic outcome after induced mild hypothermia following cardiac arrest. *Neurology.* 2008;71(19):1535-1537.

111. Fugate JE, Wijdicks EFM, Mandrekar J, et al. Predictors of neurologic outcome in hypothermia after cardiac arrest. *Ann Neurol.* 2010;68(6):907-914.

112. Leithner C, Ploner CJ, Hasper D, Storm C. Does hypothermia influence the predictive value of bilateral absent N_{20} after cardiac arrest? *Neurology.* 2010;74(12):965.

CHAPTER
11

Fulminant Hepatic Failure

H. Alex Choi, MD
Rebecca Bauer, MD
Kiwon Lee, MD, FACP, FAHA, FCCM

A 42-year-old man with no past medical history presents with a 1-week history of sinus congestion. He was not getting adequate pain relief and took a total of 40 pills over 24 to 36 hours. The next day he developed right upper quadrant pain, nausea, and vomiting. He presented to the hospital for these symptoms. Examination is significant for jaundice and right upper quadrant abdominal pain but otherwise unremarkable. Labs are significant for aspartate aminotransferase/alanine aminotransferase (AST/ALT) 6180 U/L and 4860 U/L, respectively, total bilirubin 7.7 mg/dL, and International Normalized Ratio (INR) 4. Acetaminophen level was 108 µg/mL. He is started on an N-acetylcysteine drip and transferred to the neurologic intensive care unit (NICU) for close observation.

What are the most common etiologies of acute hepatic failure?

In this case, given the history of excessive acetaminophen intake, this is the most likely cause of hepatic failure. Acetaminophen is the leading cause of acute liver failure in the United States; approximately 18% to 39% of cases.[1] Other drug reactions including isoniazid, phenytoin, and others comprise 13% of cases. Viral hepatitis, specifically hepatitis A and B, accounted for a combined 12% of cases. In contrast, hepatitis E coinfection with hepatitis A is the leading cause of acute liver failure worldwide; reportedly up to 87%. Other more rare causes include autoimmune hepatitis, Wilson disease, *Amanita* spp (mushroom) poisoning, ischemic injury, Budd-Chiari syndrome, and pregnancy-associated acute liver failure. Importantly, in many cases, the cause of liver failure is not found, which is usually associated with a worse prognosis.[2]

Acetaminophen-induced fulminant hepatic failure (FHF) is associated with high mortality rate, approximately 50% without transplant.[3] Acetaminophen toxicity occurs in the setting of intentional overdose suicide attempt, unintentional overdose, or by ingestion of doses considered nontoxic in combination with other hepatotoxic substances (ethanol, ethylene glycol, antiepileptics). Symptoms of hepatotoxicity begin 24 to 28 hours after ingestion, and maximum prothrombin time occurs approximately 72 hours after ingestion. Acetaminophen can also be nephrotoxic, further complicating the clinical management.

Normally, acetaminophen is metabolized by the liver via three different pathways: sulfate conjugation (20% to 40%), glucuronidation (40% to 60%), and N-hydroxylation (15% to 20%) by the cytochrome P450 enzyme CYP2E1 to N-acetyl-p-benzoquinone imine (NAPQI). NAPQI is a toxic intermediate, and is conjugated with hepatic glutathione to a nontoxic final product. Glutathione stores can eventually become depleted, causing accumulation of NAPQI and subsequent hepatocellular necrosis[4,5] (Figure 11-1).

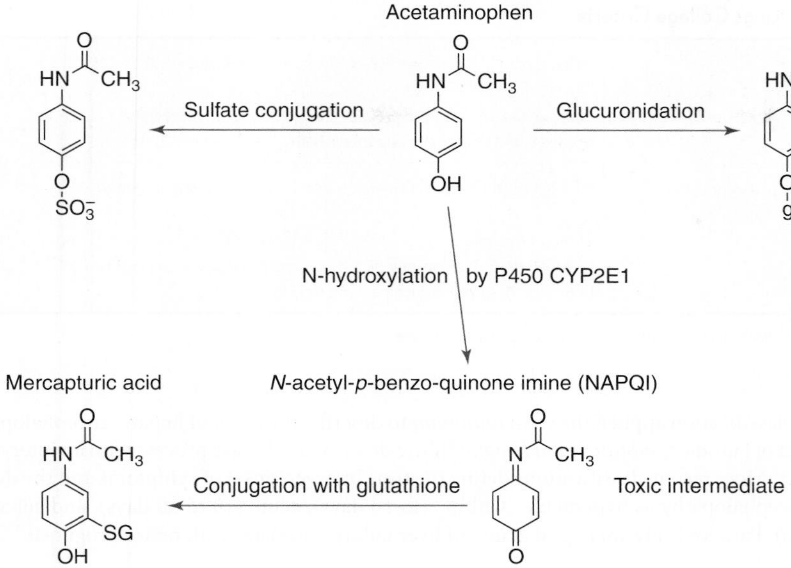

Figure 11-1. Metabolism of acetaminophen.

What are the relevant grading scales?

See Table 11-1. In the West Haven Criteria, high-grade (grades III and IV) encephalopathy distinguishes severe acute hepatic failure from FHF. High-grade encephalopathy predicts a higher mortality rate without transplantation. Patients with grade IV encephalopathy have an 80% mortality rate. Progression to grade III/IV encephalopathy can be rapid, and is a sign of intracranial hypertension and impending herniation.[6-8] Detection of high-grade encephalopathy often dictates the need for endotracheal intubation and institution of measures to lower intracranial pressure (ICP). Patients with grades III and IV encephalopathy are also at risk for subclinical seizure activity; a low threshold for continuous electroencephalographic (cEEG) monitoring is prudent.

The Kings College Criteria (Table 11-2) is used to estimate the prognosis of a patient in acute liver failure. The etiology of hepatic failure is emphasized, separating acetaminophen and non–acetaminophen-related hepatic failure.[9,10] Patients with acetaminophen-induced acute liver failure have a 50% mortality rate without transplantation, whereas patients in acute liver failure from other causes, such as hepatitis B, have an approximately 25% survival rate without transplantation.

Table 11-1. West Haven Criteria

Grade	Symptoms
I	Trivial lack of awareness; euphoria or anxiety; shortened attention span; impaired performance of addition or subtraction
II	Lethargy or apathy; minimal disorientation for time or place; subtle personality change; inappropriate behavior
III	Somnolence to semistupor, but responsive to verbal stimuli; confusion; gross disorientation
IV	Coma (unresponsive to verbal or noxious stimuli)

Table 11-2. Kings College Criteria

Acetaminophen	Arterial pH < 7.3 (irrespective of grade of encephalopathy)
	Or
	Combination of PT time > 100 s (INR > 6.5), serum creatinine > 3.4 mg/dL, grades II and IV hepatic encephalopathy
Non-acetaminophen-mediated liver injury	PT > 100 s (INR > 6.5) (irrespective of grade of encephalopathy)
	Or
	Three of the following variables: Age < 10 or > 40 y, non-A, non-B hepatitis, idiosyncratic drug reaction, jaundice > 7 d before onset of encephalopathy, PT > 50 s (INR > 3.5), serum creatinine > 3.4 mg/dL

Abbreviations: INR, International Normalized Ratio; PT, prothrombin time.

An early classification applied the term *fulminant* to describe the onset of hepatic encephalopathy within 2 weeks of jaundice; *subfulminant hepatic* failure described a disease process with an interval of 3 to 12 weeks.[11] More recent classifications define the time between onset of symptoms and the development of encephalopathy as hyperacute (within 7 to 10 days), acute (10 to 30 days), and subacute (4 to 24 weeks). Paradoxically, increased acuity of liver failure correlates with better prognosis.[12,13]

Why do patients with FHF develop encephalopathy?

Cerebral edema is a leading cause of death in patients with FHF.[1] Patients who have progressed to grade IV encephalopathy will invariably have evidence of cerebral edema. Many factors have been proposed to contribute to cerebral edema in FHF. Ammonia, glutamine, other amino acids, and proinflammatory cytokines cause cytotoxic edema and breakdown of the blood-brain barrier.

Ammonia, in particular, has been studied extensively in the pathophysiology of encephalopathy. Ammonia is a by-product of normal metabolism and is usually cleared by the liver. The accumulation of ammonia has been shown to lead to astrocyte swelling and dysfunction. Cortical astrocytes clear ammonia from the cerebral circulation by amidation of glutamate via glutamine synthetase to form glutamine. Extracellular transfer of osmotically active glutamine is limited by cell membrane transporter capacity. Hyperammonemia causes intracellular accumulation of glutamine, cellular edema, and intracranial hypertension.[14] High arterial ammonia levels are associated with cerebral herniation and poor outcomes.[15] Astrocyte edema can be exacerbated by hyponatremia, inflammatory cytokines, and benzodiazepine use. In addition to astrocyte edema, glutamine has a second effect on intracranial pressure. Glutamine accumulation in astrocytes also disrupts mitochondrial function, with ensuing oxidative stress and nitrosative stress, inducing vasodilation and cerebral hyperemia (Figure 11-2).

Arterial ammonia levels correlate with cerebral glutamine concentration, which correlates to ICP in patients in acute liver failure. Patients in FHF with persistently high ammonia levels (greater than 200 mol/L) are at risk for an increased intracranial pressure (Figure 11-2).[14] Note that increased ammonia levels may occur in chronic liver disease as well, but astrocytes are able to clear glutamine at a compensatory rate.

How should a patient be screened for increased ICP in this setting?

All patients with acute hepatic failure should be screened for signs of increased ICP. Patients should get frequent assessment of neurologic status at least every 2 hours. Basic assessment of attention: counting backward from 20 to 1, or saying months of the year backward from December to January, and checking for orientation is a quick and reproducible method of detecting slight changes in attention. A head

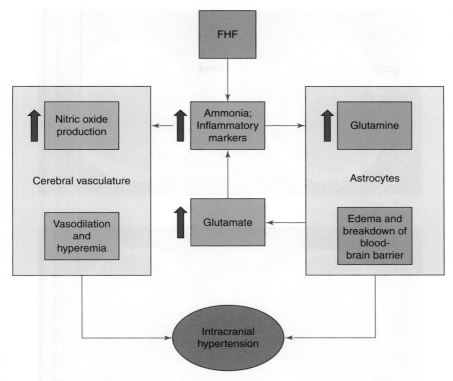

Figure 11-2. Pathophysiology of fulminant hepatic failure (FHF) causing intracranial hypertension.

computed tomographic (CT) or brain magnetic resonance image (MRI) may be helpful in predicting those who will go on to have cerebral edema, and a baseline study may be helpful in detecting changes in further studies. Transcranial Dopplers (TCDs) may also be helpful in detecting early increased intracranial pressure. The pattern associated with development of cerebral edema is that of lower mean flow velocities and higher pulsatility index. Given the many factors involved in TCD measurements, the information should not be used in isolation but in clinical context.[16,17] Ultimately, the clinical examination is the most important factor to base clinical decisions as the diagnostic cutoffs for studies are not well established.

> Overnight the patient progresses from being alert and fully oriented to becoming intermittently agitated and confused. Within hours he is lethargic and needs to be intubated for airway protection. On examination he has no response to painful stimuli. Cranial nerve examination is significant for blurred disc margins. A head CT is performed, which shows significant cerebral edema (Figure 11-3).

Once there is clinical evidence of elevated ICP, what is the next step?

An ICP monitor is essential for the treatment of intracranial hypertension. In the setting of a significant coagulopathy, the risk of placement of an ICP monitor is not to be overlooked.

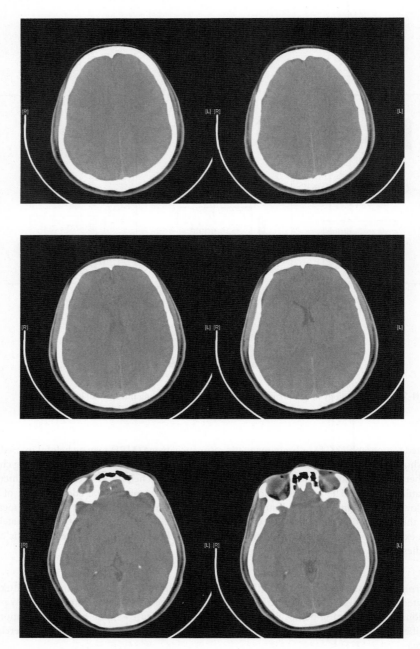

Figure 11-3. Computerized tomography of the head.

However, given the significant possibility of herniation with increasing encephalopathy, ICP monitoring is an essential tool to guide treatment. ICP monitoring can also be continued into the perioperative setting to guide management during transplantation. Because of the rapid course of encephalopathy progression, patients with stages III and IV encephalopathy should undergo placement of an ICP monitor.[18,19] More than 90% of patients in acute liver failure who fail medical management of intracranial hypertension will die within 12 hours.[9] In addition, placement of a jugular bulb catheter allows for calculation of arterial-jugular venous oxygen content differences, and therefore is an indirect measurement of cerebral blood flow and metabolism.

How do you minimize the risk of bleeding associated with placement of monitoring devices?

Coagulopathy associated with acute liver failure is due to lowered levels of clotting factors and thrombocytopenia.[20,21] Reduced levels of factors II, V, VII, IX, and X produce prolongation of the prothromin time (PT). Acute liver failure patients also have increased fibrinolysis and disseminated intravascular coagulation.[22] Because of the importance of PT values in prognosis, coagulation factor replacement is only recommended in cases of active hemorrhage or placement of invasive monitors.[23]

Recombinant activated factor VII (rFVII) may be a safer and more efficacious option for the rapid reversal of coagulopathy for the insertion of intracranial monitoring than fresh-frozen plasma.[18,23,24] For replenishment of factors II, VII, IX, and X, prothrombin complex concentrates may be used as well. Qualitative and quantitative defects in platelets may require correction in the same settings. For qualitative dysfunction from concomitant intake of antiplatelet agents, DDAVP (1-deamino-8-D-arginine vasopressin) should be considered.[18] In the setting of thrombocytopenia for platelets less than 50,000/mm^3, platelet transfusion may be necessary.[11]

This patient received the ICP monitoring probe after rFVII and platelets were given. How do you treat elevated ICPs in FHF?

The treatment of elevated ICP in FHF is similar to the treatment of ICP in other conditions (see Chapter 12). The differences lay in the cause of ICP elevation. As opposed to other types of ICP elevation, FHF is predominantly associated with hyperemia and global edema as opposed to ischemia.

Initial conservative treatment should be instituted including positioning of the head in a neutral, mildly elevated angle of 30 degrees. Adequate sedation should be given. Propofol is the preferred agent as it has the added effect of decreasing ICP, providing anesthesia, and has a short half-life, making it the ideal agent for following neurologic status. Hemodynamic parameters should be closely followed, however, as propofol may induce significant systemic hypotension. In the event of high ICP, frank systemic hypotension may be harmful as it will have a deleterious effect on cerebral perfusion. Other agents that are used are opiates and benzodiazepines. Given the hepatic metabolism of many of the medications and at times decreased renal clearance, medications should be adjusted appropriately.

If conservative methods are inadequate for ICP control, then osmotic agents should be considered next. Mannitol 1.0 to1.5 g/kg of body weight or 23.4% NaCl solution in a 30-mL injection are effective in treating elevated ICP.[25]

Given that cerebral vasodilation and hyperemia contribute to ICP issues in FHF, hyperventilation is a strategy often avoided in other types of ICP elevations but may be used in FHF. One must remember that prolonged hyperventilation can lead to ischemia due to cerebral blood flow (CBF) reduction, and its use therefore should be transient. Indomethacin is another agent that can be used to induce vasoconstriction to decrease ICP. Both hyperventilation and indomethacin should be considered in patients with evidence of vasodilation and hyperemia.[26]

In addition, therapeutic hypothermia to 33°C can be a useful adjunct to bridge patients to transplant. In addition to its effect in reducing intracranial hypertention, hypothermia lowers oxidative metabolism within the brain, reduces cerebral hyperemia, and decreases brain production of proinflammatory cytokines.[7] Therapeutic hypothermia reduces splanchnic production of ammonia, reducing the osmotic effect of ammonia via glutamine.[27,28]

However, therapeutic hypothermia is not without risk. Hypothermia is associated with hemodynamic instability, infection, and increased risk of bleeding, all of which are inherent issues of liver failure.[7]

What are other treatment considerations?

cEEG should be performed as patients with acute liver failure are at a significant risk of subclinical seizures warranting cEEG or prophylactic antiepileptics if cEEG is not available.[29] Seizures in the setting of increased ICP can lead to increased metabolic demand and clinical herniation[30] (Figure 11-4).

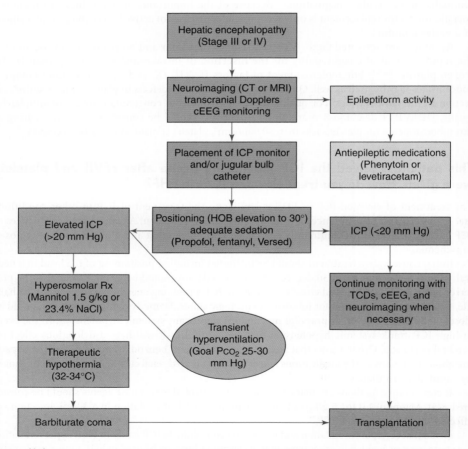

Figure 11-4. Treatment algorithm for neurologic management of fulminant hepatic failure. cEEE, continuous electroencephalography; CT, computerized tomography; HOB, head of bed; ICP, intracranial pressure; MRI, magnetic resonance imaging; TCDs, transcranial Dopplers.

! CRITICAL CONSIDERATIONS

- Acetaminophen-induced fulminant liver failure has a very poor prognosis without liver transplant.
- Etiology of disease, arterial pH less than 7.3, PT greater than 100 s, serum creatinine greater than 3.4 mg/dL are important prognostic markers.
- Patients should be monitored in an intensive care setting with frequent neurologic assessments for encephalopathy.
- Elevated levels of ammonia are associated with increased ICP.
- The development of stage III or IV hepatic encephalopathy is associated with a high risk of increased ICP.
- If stage III or IV encephalopathy develops, noninvasive monitoring with TCDs and neuroimaging should begin and intracranial monitoring should be strongly considered.
- Intracranial hypertension should be treated aggressively while awaiting transplant.

REFERENCES

1. Ostapowicz G, Fontana RJ, Schiodt FV, et al. Results of a prospective study of acute liver failure at 17 tertiary care centers in the United States. *Ann Intern Med.* 2002;137:947-954.

2. Bernal W, Auzinger G, Dhawan A, Wendon J. Acute liver failure. *Lancet.* 2010;376:190-201.

3. Makin AJ, Wendon J, Williams R. A 7-year experience of severe acetaminophen-induced hepatotoxicity (1987-1993). *Gastroenterology.* 1995;109:1907-1916.

4. Schiodt FV, Rochling FA, Casey DL, Lee WM. Acetaminophen toxicity in an urban county hospital. *N Engl J.* 1997;337:1112-1117.

5. Clark R, Borirakchanyavat V, Davidson AR, et al. Hepatic damage and death from overdose of paracetamol. *Lancet.* 1973;1:66-70.

6. Riordan SM, Williams R. Perspectives on liver failure: past and future. *Semin Liver Dis.* 2008;28:137-141.

7. Stravitz RT, Larsen FS. Therapeutic hypothermia for acute liver failure. *Crit Care Med.* 2009;37:S258-S264.

8. Larsen FS, Wendon J. Prevention and management of brain edema in patients with acute liver failure. *Liver Transpl.* 2008;14 (Suppl 2):S90-S96.

9. O'Grady JG, Alexander GJ, Hayllar KM, Williams R. Early indicators of prognosis in fulminant hepatic failure. *Gastroenterology.* 1989;97:439-445.

10. Shakil AO, Kramer D, Mazariegos GV, Fung JJ, Rakela J. Acute liver failure: Clinical features, outcome analysis, and applicability of prognostic criteria. *Liver Transpl.* 2000;6:163-169.

11. Bernuau J, Rueff B, Benhamou JP. Fulminant and subfulminant liver failure: definitions and causes. *Semin Liver Dis.* 1986;6:97-106.

12. O'Grady JG, Schalm SW, Williams R. Acute liver failure: redefining the syndromes. *Lancet.* 1993;342:273-275.

13. Tandon BN, Bernauau J, O'Grady J, et al. Recommendations of the International Association for the Study of the Liver Subcommittee on Nomenclature of Acute and Subacute Liver Failure. *J Gastroenterol Hepatol.* 1999;14:403-404.

14. Tofteng F, Hauerberg J, Hansen BA, Pedersen CB, Jorgensen L, Larsen FS. Persistent arterial hyperammonemia increases the concentration of glutamine and alanine in the brain and correlates with intracranial pressure in patients with fulminant hepatic failure. *J Cereb Blood Flow Metab.* 2006;26:21-27.

15. Clemmesen JO, Larsen FS, Kondrup J, Hansen BA, Ott P. Cerebral herniation in patients with acute liver failure is correlated with arterial ammonia concentration. *Hepatology.* 1999;29:648-653.

16. Abdo A, Lopez O, Fernandez A, et al. Transcranial Doppler sonography in fulminant hepatic failure. *Transplant Proc.* 2003;35:1859-1860.

17. Aggarwal S, Brooks DM, Kang Y, Linden PK, Patzer JF 2nd. Noninvasive monitoring of cerebral perfusion pressure in patients with acute liver failure using transcranial Doppler ultrasonography. *Liver Transpl.* 2008;14:1048-1057.

18. Raschke RA, Curry SC, Rempe S, et al. Results of a protocol for the management of patients with fulminant liver failure. *Crit Care Med.* 2008;36: 2244-2248.

19. Lidofsky SD, Bass NM, Prager MC, et al. Intracranial pressure monitoring and liver transplantation for fulminant hepatic failure. *Hepatology.* 1992;16:1-7.

20. Sass DA, Shakil AO. Fulminant hepatic failure. *Liver Transpl.* 2005;11:594-605.

21. Pereira SP, Langley PG, Williams R. The management of abnormalities of hemostasis in acute liver failure. *Semin Liver Dis.* 1996;16:403-414.

22. Pernambuco JR, Langley PG, Hughes RD, Izumi S, Williams R. Activation of the fibrinolytic system in patients with fulminant liver failure. *Hepatology.* 1993;18:1350-1356.

23. Le TV, Rumbak MJ, Liu SS, Alsina AE, van Loveren H, Agazzi S. Insertion of intracranial pressure monitors in fulminant hepatic failure patients: early experience using recombinant factor VII. *Neurosurgery.* 2010;66:455-458; discussion 8.

24. Shami VM, Caldwell SH, Hespenheide EE, Arseneau KO, Bickston SJ, Macik BG. Recombinant activated factor VII for coagulopathy in fulminant hepatic failure compared with conventional therapy. *Liver Transpl.* 2003;9:138-143.

25. Qureshi AI, Suarez JI. Use of hypertonic saline solutions in treatment of cerebral edema and intracranial hypertension. *Crit Care Med.* 2000;28:3301-3313.

26. Tofteng F, Larsen FS. The effect of indomethacin on intracranial pressure, cerebral perfusion and extracellular lactate and glutamate concentrations in patients with fulminant hepatic failure. *J Cereb Blood Flow Metab.* 2004;24:798-804.

27. Jalan R, Olde Damink SW, Deutz NE, et al. Moderate hypothermia prevents cerebral hyperemia and increase in intracranial pressure in patients undergoing liver transplantation for acute liver failure. *Transplantation.* 2003;75:2034-2039.

28. Jalan R, Olde Damink SW, Deutz NE, Hayes PC, Lee A. Moderate hypothermia in patients with acute liver failure and uncontrolled intracranial hypertension. *Gastroenterology.* 2004;127:1338-1346.

29. Ellis AJ, Wendon JA, Williams R. Subclinical seizure activity and prophylactic phenytoin infusion in acute liver failure: a controlled clinical trial. *Hepatology.* 2000;32:536-541.

30. Vespa PM, Miller C, McArthur D, et al. Nonconvulsive electrographic seizures after traumatic brain injury result in a delayed, prolonged increase in intracranial pressure and metabolic crisis. *Crit Care Med.* 2007;35:2830-2836.

Neurocritical Care Monitoring

Section Editor: Jan Claassen, MD, PhD

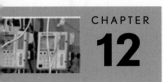

CHAPTER

12

Management of Increased Intracranial Pressure

Kiwon Lee, MD, FACP, FAHA, FCCM
Stephan A. Mayer, MD

A 38-year-old female tobacco smoker with no significant past medical history presents with sudden new-onset bifrontal headache. The patient describes sharp, constant frontal pain with nausea, photophobia, and neck stiffness. Noncontrast CT head and clinical examination reveal acute subarachnoid hemorrhage (SAH) with Hunt and Hess grade II, Fisher group 3, and modified Fisher group 4 with bilateral intraventricular hemorrhage (IVH). An emergent ventricular drain was placed when patient's mental status deteriorated to drowsy, difficult-to-arouse state along with radiographic evidence of worsening IVH and hydrocephalus.

What are the conditions associated with abnormally elevated intracranial pressure (ICP)?

Table 12-1 lists different classifications of medical conditions that are associated with high ICP. In a neurologic intensive care unit (NeuroICU, NICU) setting, common conditions that are frequently associated with elevated ICP include acute aneurysmal high-grade SAH, severe traumatic brain injury (TBI), large intraparenchymal hemorrhage either spontaneous (such as hypertensive bleed) or in the setting of underlying coagulopathy (atrial fibrillation on warfarin therapy or coronary artery disease with cardiac stents on dual-antiplatelet

213

TABLE 12-1. Conditions Associated with Increased Intracranial Pressure

Intracranial space-occupying mass lesions
• Subdural hematoma
• Epidural hematoma
• Brain tumor
• Cerebral abscess
• Intracerebral hemorrhage
Increased brain volume (cytotoxic edema)
• Cerebral infarction
• Global hypoxia-ischemia
• Reye syndrome
• Acute hyponatremia
Increased brain and blood volume (vasogenic edema)
• Hepatic encephalopathy
• Traumatic brain injury
• Meningitis
• Encephalitis
• Hypertensive encephalopathy
• Eclampsia
• Subarachnoid hemorrhage
• Dural sinus thrombosis
Increased cerebrospinal fluid volume
• Communicating hydrocephalus
• Noncommunicating hydrocephalus
• Choroid plexus papilloma

therapy), malignant middle cerebral artery infarction with herniation, and severe meningitis and/or encephalitis. Although medical centers around the country have different patient populations, a great majority of all NICU cases with high ICP would fall into one of these conditions, with severe TBI being the most common etiology for intracranial hypertension[1] at an annual incidence estimated to be 200 cases per 100,000 people.[2]

Describe the pathophysiology of ICP elevation and pathologic ICP waveforms reported in the current literature

Monro-Kellie Hypothesis

The Monro-Kellie hypothesis is a widely accepted concept for explaining the elevation of ICP. In 1783, Alexander Monro first articulated this in his *Observations on the Structure and Function of the Nervous System,* and later was supported by Kellie in 1824 by his observation in two humans: "Appearances observed in the dissection of two individuals; death from cold and congestion of the brain." The hypothesis explains that the human cranium has a fixed amount of space with three main components: cerebrospinal fluid (CSF), brain parenchyma, and blood. If any space-occupying

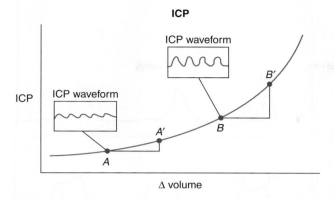

Figure 12-1. Intracranial pressure (ICP)–volume curve. At point **A**, on a flatter portion of the curve, the amplitude of the arterial reflection in the ICP waveform is small (*inset*), and the addition of the same amount of volume leads to a smaller increase in pressure (**A'**). At point **B**, on a steep portion of the curve, the intracranial compartment is relatively noncompliant, the amplitude of the arterial reflection in the ICP waveform is large (*inset*), and the addition of volume leads to a large increase in pressure. *(Redrawn from Mayer SA. Management of increased intracranial pressure. In: Wijdicks EFM, Diringer MN, Bolton CF, et al, eds. Continuum: Critical Care Neurology. Minneapolis, MN: American Academy of Neurology; 1997:47-61.)*

lesion or any of these constituents' volumes are increased beyond the compliance, an elevation of ICP is inevitable.[3]

Intracranial Compliance

Intracranial compliance is defined as the change in volume over the change in pressure ($\Delta V/\Delta P$). The relationship between pressure and volume in the brain is linear (Figure 12-1) in the beginning but exponential in the later phase. As volume increases, the ICP rises slowly (Figure 12-1, Point A), CSF is displaced into the spinal thecal sac, and blood is decompressed from the distensible cerebral veins. Once these compensatory and compliant redistribution mechanisms no longer continue, ICP can increase much more rapidly with just small increments of additional volume (Figure 12-1, Point B). The amplitude of the ICP pulse wave may provide a clue that compliance is reduced; as compliance falls, the ICP pulse amplitude increases (Figure 12-1, Point B, *inset*). During the high ICP crisis, ICP waveforms may show that the second peak (P2) may rise as high as (increased amplitude compared to normal waveforms) the first peak or even higher (Figure 12-2).

Cerebral Perfusion Pressure

The main negative consequence of elevated ICP is reduced cerebral blood flow (CBF) and secondary hypoxic-ischemic injury due to poor flow. Cerebral perfusion pressure (CPP) is calculated as mean arterial pressure (MAP) – ICP. CPP along with cerebral blood volume determines CBF; normally, autoregulation of the cerebral vasculature maintains CBF at a constant level between a CPP of approximately 50 and 100 mm Hg. Brain injury leading to impaired cerebral autoregulation may cause CBF to approximate a more straight-line relationship with CPP.[4] Although the optimal CPP for a given patient may vary, in general, CPP optimization should be greater than 60 (to avert ischemia) and below 110 mm Hg (to avoid breakthrough hyperperfusion and cerebral edema).[5,6]

Pathologic Pressure Waves

In patients with raised ICP, pathologic ICP waveforms may occur (Figure 12-3). Lundberg A waves (or plateau waves) represent prolonged periods of profoundly high ICP.[7] These waves do not refer

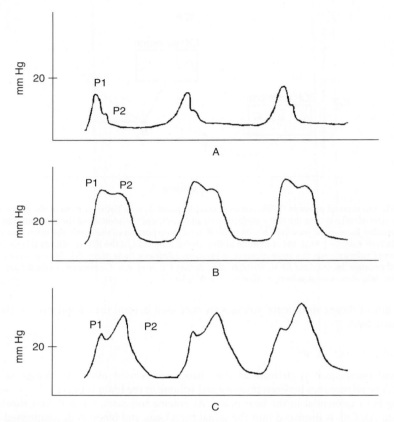

Figure 12-2. Intracranial compliance and intracranial pressure (ICP) waveforms. **A.** Normal ICP waves: higher P1, lower P2. **B.** Abnormal ICP waves: P1 and P2 with similar amplitudes. **C.** Abnormal ICP waves: P2 with higher amplitude than P1.

to the individual ICP waveform described in Figure 12-2, but rather a graphic representation of ICP values plotted over time. A plateau wave is considered a high risk of further (or ongoing) brain injury, with critically reduced perfusion as a result of a prolonged period of high ICP crisis. It often occurs abruptly when either CPP or intracranial compliance is low. Their duration may vary from minutes to hours, and pressures as high as 50 to 100 mm Hg may be seen and considered ominous in the setting of acute brain injury. Lundberg B waves are of shorter duration, lower amplitude elevations in ICP that indicate that intracranial compliance reserves are simply compromised. The important thing is not to memorize which is Lundberg A or B per se, but to understand the trend of the ICP elevations and figure out the overall picture as to why there is intracranial hypertension and how brain compliance is coping with the injury. Accurate assessment of the underlying etiology will help guide the clinicians to choose the right type and method of treatment.

The ICP of this high-grade SAH patient is now showing 40 to 50 mm Hg with CPP of 40-50 mm Hg. CPP optimization is being done by elevating the MAP and giving an osmotic agent to reduce ICP values, which are consistent with Lundberg B waves suggesting compromised brain compliance.

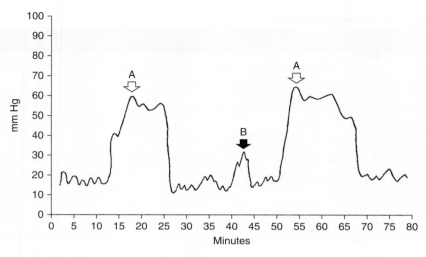

Figure 12-3. Pathologic intracranial pressure (ICP) waves. **A.** Lundberg A (plateau) waves. **B.** Lundberg B wave. Two classic A waves are shown (*open arrows*). Note that when the ICP falls after the A wave (*closed arrow*), it does not return to the baseline preceding the first wave.

What are typical clinical manifestations of persistent intracranial hypertension?

Clinical signs of intracranial hypertension may vary and depend on the underlying etiology. In general, the clinical manifestations are suggestive of global, or bilateral, hemispheric cerebral dysfunction rather than a focal finding such as arm weakness. Depressed level of consciousness, blurred vision, confusion, disorientation, nausea, vomiting, diplopia, and sixth cranial nerve palsy (false localizing sign) may be seen, especially if the rise in ICP is acute rather than chronic. It is important to once again emphasize that ICP as an absolute value by itself may not have much clinical significance. More importantly, it is the CPP and brain compliance. The Cushing triad, a well-known phenomenon of hypertension and bradycardia in the setting of critically elevated ICP, is more commonly seen with the late phase of intracranial hypertension such as near brain dead/herniation syndrome rather than in the beginning of an acute injury. ICP elevation may become a local phenomenon and compartmentalized as a result of the rigid boundaries formed by the falx and tentorium cerebelli. Compartmentalized mass effect and pressure differentials, in turn, can lead to herniation of brain tissue from the area of higher to lower pressure. Different herniation syndromes are each marked by characteristic signs (Table 12-2).

What is the indication of ICP monitoring? Is there a class I level of evidence for placing ICP monitoring in terms of improving long-term outcome?

Currently, the best level of evidence is the "level 2" recommendation of the Brain Trauma Foundation (2007 guidelines), which states that "treatment should be initiated with ICP >20 mm Hg." This is heavily driven by the large amount of observation data that showed poor outcome in TBI subjects with hypotension and ICP greater than 20 mm Hg (http://tbiguidelines.org). Systemic hypotension and high ICP leading to poor outcome further supports the theory that failure to optimize CPP is associated with an increased risk of poor flow and perfusion and, therefore, further injury.

Indications for ICP Monitoring

The diagnosis of increased ICP should not be made on clinical grounds alone as clinical signs are not reliable and vary. In acute brain injury, in order to accurately diagnose intracranial hypertension, ICP

TABLE 12-2. Herniation Syndromes

Type	Clinical Hallmark	Causes
Uncal (lateral transtentorial)	Ipsilateral cranial nerve III palsy Contralateral or bilateral motor posturing	Temporal lobe mass lesion
Central transtentorial	Progression from bilateral decorticate to decerebrate posturing Rostral-caudal loss of brainstem reflexes	Diffuse cerebral edema, hydrocephalus
Subfalcine	Asymmetric (contralateral > ipsilateral) motor posturing Preserved oculocephalic reflex	Convexity (frontal or parietal) mass lesion
Cerebellar (upward or downward)	Sudden progression to coma with bilateral motor posturing Cerebellar signs	Cerebellar mass lesion

must be directly measured. Because of the invasive nature of ICP monitoring, and the need for ICU management, patients should generally meet three criteria prior to placement of an ICP monitor: (1) brain imaging reveals a space-occupying lesion and severe cerebral edema suggesting that the patient is at risk for high ICP; (2) the patient has a depressed level of consciousness (this does not mean the patient must be comatose in order to meet the criteria, but clearly those with a Glasgow Coma Scale (GCS) score of 8 or higher would meet the criteria); and (3) the prognosis is such that aggressive ICU treatment is indicated. Although the literature supporting the use of invasive ICP monitoring originates from patients with severe TBI, it is not unreasonable to consider monitoring for other illnesses such as SAH, ICH, large ischemic strokes, and meningoencephalitis cases despite the lack of data.

ICP Monitoring Devices

Several types of ICP monitors exist (Figure 12-4). The external ventricular drainage (EVD) catheter is believed to be the gold standard; it consists of a catheter that is placed through a burr hole into the ventricle and connected to a pressure transducer set at ear level. It allows for both ICP monitoring and

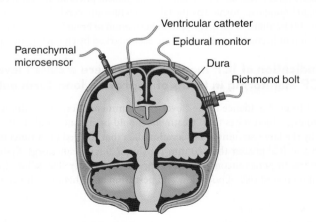

Figure 12-4. Intracranial pressure monitoring devices. *(Redrawn from Mayer SA. Management of increased intracranial pressure. In: Wijdicks EFM, Diringer MN, Bolton CF, et al, eds. Continuum: Critical Care Neurology. Minneapolis, MN: American Academy of Neurology; 1997:47-61.)*

therapeutic CSF drainage. Its major drawback is the risk of infection such as potentially life-threatening ventriculitis, which occurs in approximately 10% to 15% of patients and steadily increases until the 10th day of use.[8,9] As such, it is important to place the catheter with care using sterile technique as well as maintain the sterility thereafter. It is usually placed through a long subcutaneous tunnel in order to minimize the rate of infection. The best alternatives to EVD include fiberoptic transducers (Integra LifeSciences, Plainsboro, NJ) or pressure microsensors (Codman & Shureleff, Inc, Raynham, MA) placed through a burr hole into either the parenchyma or ventricle. These devices carry less risk of infection but do not allow therapeutic drainage of CSF.

An EVD is placed 10.5 cm posterior to the nasion and lateral 3.5 cm on the midpupillary line with a tunnel catheter technique. ICP reads 30 to 40 mm Hg when clamped, and it is set at 10 cm above the external auditory meatus that is open for drainage. What are appropriate steps in treating intracranial hypertension in this patient?

General Measures for ICP Control

These general measures apply to all patients at risk for or ongoing intracranial hypertension.

Head position

Elevation of the head to at least 30 degrees is advised in patients with raised ICP, with one study confirming that this degree of elevation produces consistent reduction in ICP.[10] Although some investigators advocate a head-flat position to preserve CPP, moderate elevation is safe as long as CPP is continuously maintained at greater than 60 mm Hg. For patients with large abdominal girth, it is also important to pay attention so that excessive head elevation is not causing abdominal distress, as increased abdominal pressure and pain may exacerbate ICP elevation.

Body temperature

Fever may potentiate ischemic brain injury and contribute to elevated ICP. It has been demonstrated that increases in brain temperature are correlated with ICP elevations, as CBF and cerebral blood volume (CBV) increase disproportionately in relation to the cerebral metabolic rate of oxygen consumption ($CMRO_2$).[11] Acetaminophen and cooling blankets are the first line of therapy and should be instituted when temperature is sustained over 101°F (38.3°C). Whether the prophylactic maintenance of mild hypothermia (34°C to 35°C) can reduce the number of ICP crises remains unknown at this time. Early mild-to-moderate hypothermia (32°C to 34°C) within 8 hours of onset has not been found to be effective for improving outcome after severe TBI even though a modest benefit on ICP was seen.[12] If fever is not adequately controlled with conventional methods, it would be wise to use advanced temperature-modulation devices—either surface or intravascular cooling catheters.

Seizures

Seizures cause an increase in $CMRO_2$ and hence CBV. These alterations tend to be abrupt and marked and, in patients with reduced cerebral compliance, can trigger plateau waves due to suddenly elevated flow and blood volume. For patients at risk for raised ICP, it is reasonable to administer prophylaxis with an intravenous anticonvulsant. This is not an absolute recommendation, but convulsion in the setting of ICP crisis would be devastating. In TBI patients, prophylaxis was shown to reduce the frequency of seizures during the first 7 days (with no evidence to continue beyond the first week) from 14% to 4%. Fosphenytoin or phenytoin (15- to 20-mg/kg bolus followed by 300 mg daily) has been recommended in this situation, but that is not because phenytoin is superior to other antiepileptic drugs. In fact, owing to multiple side effects, difficulty maintaining a therapeutic level, and numerous drug-to-drug interactions, it would be reasonable to use a newer agent such as levetiracetam or lacosamide, both of which are available in oral and intravenous formulations without the need for checking levels (as a prophylactic use anyway: this may be different in refractory status epilepticus management) or significant concerns of tolerability or drug-to-drug interactions.

Fluid management

Historically, raised ICP had been managed by fluid restriction. It was later found that this effort to dehydrate the brain actually worsened hypoxic-ischemic injury because the hypovolemia led to reduced CPP.[13] Patients with high ICP states should be kept *euvolemic* with isotonic saline. Hypotonic solution in any form (eg, 0.45% saline, D_5W, or enteral water) must be avoided because it will accumulate through an osmotic gradient in regions of injured brain and aggravate brain swelling. Some centers use a continuous infusion of 2% or 3% saline at 1 mL/kg as an alternative to normal saline for patients at risk for ICP, which is directed toward establishing and maintaining a hypernatremic (goal Na^+ approximately 155 mEq/L) hyperosmolar (goal osmolality approximately 320 mOsm/L) environment for the injured brain. However, whether this strategy is effective for reducing ICP crises or improving outcome is unknown. Continuing maintenance fluid intake at 2% to 3% hypertonic saline may not produce a sustained effect in controlling ICP crisis, and, if used, continuous infusion should only be used for a finite period of time. A higher concentration given in boluses (eg, 23.4% hypertonic saline in 30-mL boluses given as rapid IV push over 1 to 2 minutes) may be more effective in reducing high ICP.

Corticosteroids

Corticosteroids such as dexamethasone are *not* effective as a general measure to treat elevated ICP, with associated risk of developing or promoting nosocomial infection, hyperglycemia, impaired wound healing, muscle catabolism, and psychosis/delirium. Steroids are effective only for reducing the volume of mass lesions related to abscess or neoplasm, and the mechanism is based on its effect on vasogenic edema. A cytotoxic edema process such as acute ischemic stroke, therefore, would be a wrong indication to use this therapy.

Stepwise treatment protocol for ICP control in a monitored patient

Cranial Decompression

Whenever a sustained ICP elevation of 20 mm Hg or more occurs, the clinician should consider (or reconsider) surgical decompression. A CT scan should be considered, and if increased mass effect or CSF volume is detected, surgical intervention such as CSF drainage, mass evacuation, or hemicraniectomy may be performed.

By opening the cranial vault, hemicraniectomy can reverse brain tissue displacement and herniation, and effectively improve and usually normalize ICP. Hemicraniectomy is increasingly being used as a final salvage therapy for patients with malignant middle cerebral artery area infarction and other space-occupying mass lesions. It is considered as a definitive therapeutic option as an alternative to instituting barbiturate therapy or mild-to-moderate hypothermia. Several studies have found that hemicraniectomy definitely improves survival after malignant middle cerebral artery (MCA) infarction.[14] A meta-analysis of hemicraniectomy for MCA infarction found that survival with a good functional outcome is most likely among younger patients.[15]

Sedation

Agitation must be avoided because it can aggravate ICP elevation through straining (increasing thoracic, jugular venous, and systemic blood pressure) and increased $CMRO_2$. During an ICP spike, sedation must be maximized and may be all that is necessary to control the ICP. For this reason, adequate sedation must be the first pharmacologic intervention in managing ICP crisis. The preferred regimen is the combination of a short-acting opioid such as fentanyl (1 to 3 µg/kg per hour) or remifentanil (0.03 to 0.25 µg/kg per minute) to provide analgesia and propofol (0.3 to 3 mg/kg per hour) because of its extremely short half-life (despite its well-known side effect of systemic hypotension), which makes it ideal for periodic interruption for neurologic assessments. Bolus injections of opioids, however, should be used with caution in patients with elevated ICP because they can transiently lower MAP and increase ICP due to autoregulatory vasodilation of cerebral vessels.[16] Compared to an opioid-based sedation regimen, in one trial propofol was associated with lower ICP and fewer ICP interventions in patients with severe TBI.[17]

CPP Optimization

After adequate sedation, if ICP remains elevated, attention should be directed to optimizing CPP. CPP low enough to induce ischemia can trigger reflex vasodilation and aggravate ICP elevation. Conversely, a high CPP (greater than 110 mm Hg) can sometimes cause breakthrough cerebral edema and also potentially elevate ICP. For these reasons, in general, CPP should be maintained between 60 and 110 mm Hg. Appropriate vasopressors to raise blood pressure and CPP include phenylephrine (2 to 10 µg/kg per minute), dopamine (5 to 30 µg/kg per minute), or norepinephrine (0.01 to 0.6 µg/kg per minute). Useful agents to lower blood pressure and CPP include labetalol (5 to 150 mg per hour) and nicardipine (5 to 15 mg per hour); nitroprusside should be avoided because of its dilating effects on all cerebral vasculature, which may exacerbate the ICP. Sodium nitroprusside is also difficult to titrate compared to other agents.

Numerous studies have attempted to define optimal CPP management in acute TBI, with various conclusions. In recent years, two distinct approaches have developed with differing views on whether CPP should be maintained at a higher or lower level. The high-CPP approach, popularized by Rosner et al, focuses on pharmacologic means to elevate MAP and CPP in order to maintain adequate CBF.[18,19] Support for this method comes from case series demonstrating good clinical outcomes and higher brain tissue oxygen levels with this management approach, and clinical examples demonstrating that induced hypertension can lead to the termination of plateau waves, presumably by causing reflex vasoconstriction.[20] The main argument against the high-CPP approach comes from a randomized trial by Robertson et al that found no clinical benefit with CPP-targeted therapy (CPP greater than 70 mm Hg) compared with traditional ICP-targeted therapy (CPP greater than 50 mm Hg). In this study, the high-CPP approach led to fewer jugular venous desaturations, but a fivefold increase in the risk of acute respiratory distress syndrome (ARDS).[21]

The low-CPP approach, popularized in Lund, Sweden, concentrates on ICP reduction by minimizing CPP and reducing CBV and intravascular hydrostatic pressure.[22] The fundamental principles of the Lund approach include the maintenance of normal colloidal pressure to prevent extravascular fluid shifts, reduction of intracapillary hydrostatic pressure through systemic blood pressure reduction, and minimization of CBV by suppressing $CMRO_2$ with thiopental and promoting precapillary vasoconstriction with dihydroergotamine. Evidence in support of the Lund approach includes case series managed according to this protocol with good outcomes,[22] and cerebral microdialysis studies demonstrating that significant oxidative stress in the form of increased lactate/pyruvate ratios does not consistently occur until CPP falls below 50 mm Hg.[23]

It seems most likely that both the high- and low-CPP strategies described above are valid depending on the individual circumstances of the patient. In this view, no single approach should be generalized to all patients; instead, CPP should be optimized based on individualized physiologic monitoring. Advanced multimodality monitoring techniques such as brain tissue oxygen monitoring, jugular bulb oximetry, signal-processed electroencephalography (EEG), and microdialysis may eventually allow clinicians to fine tune CPP and MAP goals based on the specific physiologic circumstances in a particular patient at any given point in time during acute injury. This approach makes better physiologic sense and may eventually be the ultimate goal in the future.

Neurocritical Care Monitoring

Hyperventilation

Hyperventilation has long played a role in ICP therapy. A decrease in Pco_2 causes vasoconstriction, which lowers CBV and thus ICP. The effect is almost immediate, but often transient, with a steady loss of effect occurring within the first hour. In conditions characterized by excessive vasodilation and cerebral hyperemia, the effect of hyperventilation may be sustained for days. Intracranial pressure is directly related to CBV. Hyperventilation works by directly reducing CBF through vasoconstriction. A reduction of CBF could potentially limit blood flow to ischemic areas of the brain, with only a modest reduction in ICP through its indirect effects on CBV.

Studies have demonstrated a risk of exacerbation of cerebral ischemia with ongoing hyperventilation. As such, the use of hyperventilation should occur in the setting of ICP crisis and emergency as a transient method before other therapies are available. The routine application of extreme hyperventilation (less than 30 mm Hg) within the first few hours of TBI is generally considered harmful because of the risk of exacerbation of ischemia.[24] If necessary, jugular venous oxygen saturation or brain tissue oxygen monitoring can be used as a guide during hyperventilation to ensure adequate brain oxygen delivery.[25,26]

Osmotherapy

If CPP is optimized, the patient is sedated, and ICP remains elevated, osmotherapy should be initiated. Mannitol, given in a 20% solution at a dose of 0.25 to 1.5 g/kg, mediates an ICP-lowering effect through two mechanisms. First, it is an osmotic diuretic that creates a concentration gradient across the blood-brain barrier and extracts free water from the brain. This decreases brain volume and lowers ICP.[20] Also, mannitol increases CPP through plasma expansion, and promotes vasoconstriction and CBV reduction by decreasing blood viscosity and improving CBF.[27] Mannitol can lower ICP within minutes. It should be given in a single rapid bolus (0.25 to 1.5 g/kg), and may be repeated as frequently as once an hour when ICP is elevated. Complications of mannitol therapy include dehydration and renal failure. Hypertonic saline (2 to 5 mL/kg of 7.5% saline or 0.5 to 2.0 mL/kg of 23.4% saline over 30 minutes) is an alternative to mannitol for treating acutely elevated ICP. It has been shown to be at least as effective[28,29] for acutely lowering ICP, and has the advantage of boosting MAP, CPP, and intravascular volume when patients are dehydrated. The main complication specific to hypertonic saline therapy is congestive heart failure due to fluid overload. For this reason, the use of a continuous IV infusion of 3% hypertonic saline (at a certain rate: typically starting at 50 mL per hour, titrating up to the serum sodium target of about 150 mEq/L) may not be the best method if volume overload is a concern. In such a case, a bolus dosing may be preferred. Once patients are on a steady dose of continuous IV 3% saline with a serum sodium level approximately 150 mEq/L, it is advised that the hypertonic saline should be weaned very slowly (over several days), if deemed appropriate, as it is not uncommon to observe rebound intracranial hypertension upon abrupt cessation of the infusion (patients with space-occupying lesions may even herniate).

Currently, there are insufficient data to suggest one concentration or method (continuous or bolus) over another. Hypertonic saline bolus therapy does appear to be as effective as mannitol in reducing refractory elevated ICP and improving CPP transiently. However, many issues remain to be clarified, including the exact mechanism of action of hypertonic saline, the best mode of administration and concentration, and its risks and complications.

Pentobarbital

Failure of hyperventilation and osmotherapy to control ICP should prompt consideration of the initiation of pentobarbital infusion.[30] Consideration of pentobarbital in this setting should also trigger reconsideration of performing hemicraniectomy or the application of hypothermia. The mechanism of action of pentobarbital is a profound reduction of the cerebral metabolic rate. Pentobarbital can be given in repeated 5-mg/kg boluses every 15 to 30 minutes until the ICP is controlled (usually 10 to 20 mg/kg is required), and then continuously infused at 1 to 4 mg/kg per hour. An EEG should be continuously recorded, and the pentobarbital titrated to produce a burst-suppression pattern, with approximately 6- to 8-second interbursts, to avoid overmedication (although the goal is ICP control, not burst suppression on EEG, per se). The most common complication of pentobarbital therapy is hypotension owing to its cardiac suppression, and vasopressors and inotropes are often needed for hemodynamic support. Ileus may occur as well, and feeding may have to be given parenterally during treatment. Delayed, inadequate hemodynamic support may lead to acute kidney failure (and hence multiorgan failure) and severe acid-base imbalance, leading to a much more difficult situation.

Hypothermia

If all of the above therapies fail to control ICP, induced hypothermia to 32°C to 34°C can effectively lower otherwise refractory ICP. Hypothermia reduces ICP by lowering $CMRO_2$ requirements and thus CBV. The recommended temperature goal is 32°C to 34°C, which is considered mild-to-moderate hypothermia because there are fewer complications than at lower temperatures. Hypothermia can be achieved using various surface and endovascular cooling methods coupled to a rectal, esophageal, pulmonary artery, or bladder thermometer. Rapid infusion of large-volume cold fluids (30 mL/kg of 0.9% saline cooled to 4°C to 5°C) may be suitable for core cooling, especially as an effective, cost-effective method of administering a hypothermia-induction agent. Cold saline infusion should be used from the beginning while trying to set up a more controllable temperature-modulatory device. Therapeutic hypothermia has been clinically demonstrated to control ICP in a small series of patients refractory to pentobarbital,[31] but large controlled studies are lacking in this regard. Common potential complications of hypothermia include nosocomial infection, hypotension, cardiac arrhythmias, coagulopathy, shivering, hypokalemia, hyperglycemia, and ileus. Particular caution should be exercised when rewarming patients because rebound ICP readily occurs. Rewarming must be done slowly (0.10°C to 0.33°C per hour) and in a controlled fashion.

! CRITICAL CONSIDERATIONS

- The Monro-Kellie hypothesis states that the brain is encased in a confined space, and any space-occupying lesion or increased volume of intracranial constituents may lead to elevated ICP.
- ICP values should be considered along with CPP (therefore MAP), as it is important to understand that the ICP value alone as an absolute value may not carry any clinical significance. Evidence supports that an extremely low CPP (less than 50 mm Hg), especially in the setting of systemic hypotension, may lead to worse outcomes.
- The injured brain may not have adequate compliance, and therefore has a low threshold for a rapidly rising ICP. Any clinician dealing with an ICP crisis should be aware of pathologic waves and poorly compliant ICP waveforms.
- It is important to understand that a normal ICP value with poor compliance seen on the waveform may suggest that any minor change in patient's condition such as head position and pain/sedation status may trigger an ICP crisis.

- Understanding the compliance helps neurointensivists and surgeons make decision about the duration and magnitude of CSF diversion and ventricular drain management.
- Currently, optimizing CPP at this time is being done in an arbitrary fashion, but with continued data from multimodality monitoring, it may be possible to tailor individualized, goal-directed therapy for brain resuscitation in the future. It is important to remember that a higher CPP does not necessarily mean better perfusion.
- ICP management should be done in an organized, stepwise approach. Traditionally accepted medical therapy for ICP includes sedation, osmotherapy, and pentobarbital. There are multiple small series in the literature reporting hypothermia (target core body temperature of 32°C to 34°C) as an effective method of reducing an otherwise refractory ICP. While this needs to be studied with large prospective trials before recommending it as a routine therapy, it is not unreasonable to consider this therapy as one of the last resorts.

REFERENCES

1. Sorenson S, Krauss JF. Occurrence, severity, and outcomes of brain injury. *J Head Trauma Rehabil.* 1991;6:1-10.
2. Marshall LF, Gautille, T, Klauber MR, et al. The outcome of severe closed head injury. *J Neurosurg.* 1991;75:S28-S36.
3. Fishman RA. *Cerebrospinal Fluid in Diseases of the Nervous System.* Philidelphia, PA: WB Saunders; 1980:19-62, 93.
4. Strandgaard S, Paulson OB. Cerebral autoregulation. *Stroke.* 1984;15:413-416.
5. Shinnoj E, Strangaard S. Pathogenesis of hypertensive encephalopathy. *Lancet.* 1973;1:461-462.
6. Lassen NA, Agnoli A. The upper limit of autoregulation of cerebral blood flow on the pathogenesis of acute hypertensive encephalopathy. *Scand J Clin Lab Invest.* 1973;30:113-116.
7. Lundberg N. Continuous recording and control of ventricular fluid pressure in neurosurgical practice. *Acta Psychiatr Scand Suppl.* 1960;149:1-19.
8. Mayhall CG, Archer NH, Lamb VA, et al. Ventriculostomy related infections: a prospective epidemiologic study. *N Engl J Med.* 1984;310:553-559.
9. Lozier AP, Sciacca RR, Romagnoli MF, Connolly ES. Ventriculostomy-related infections: a critical review of the literature. *Neurosurgery.* 2002;51:170-182.
10. Durward QJ, Amacher AL, DelMaestro RF, et al. Cerebral and cardiovascular responses to head elevation in patients with intracranial hypertension. *J Neurosurg.* 1983;59:938-944.
11. Rossi S, Roncati Zanier E, Mauri I, Columbo A, Stocchetti N. Brain temperature, body core temperature, and intracranial pressure in acute cerebral damage. *J Neurol Neurosurg Psychiatry.* 2001;71:448-454.
12. Clifton GL, Miller ER, Sung CC, et al. Lack of effect of induction of hypothermia after acute brain injury. *N Engl J Med.* 2001;344:556-563.
13. Shackford SR. Fluid resuscitation in head injury. *J Intensive Care Med.* 1990;5:59-68.
14. Vahedi K, Hofmeijer J, Juettler E, et al. Early decompressive surgery in malignant infarction of the middle cerebral artery: a pooled analysis of three randomized controlled trials. *Lancet Neurol.* 2007;6:315-322.
15. Gupta R, Connolly ES, Mayer S, Elkind MS. Hemicraniectomy for massive middle cerebral artery territory infarction: a systematic review. *Stroke.* 2004;35:539-543.
16. Albanese J, Viviand X, Potie F, Rey M, Alliez B, Martin C. Sufentanil, fentanyl, and alfentanil in head trauma patients: a study on cerebral hemodynamics. *Crit Care Med.* 1999; 27:407-411.
17. Kelly DF, Goodale DB, Williams J, et al. Propofol in the treatment of moderate and severe head injury: A randomized, prospective double-blinded pilot trial. *J Neurosurg.* 1999:90;1042-1052.
18. Rosner MJ, Rosner SD, Johnson AH. Cerebral perfusion pressure: management protocol and clinical results. *J Neurosurg.* 1995;83:949-962.
19. Oertel M, Kelly DF, Lee JH, et al. Efficacy of hyperventilation, blood pressure elevation, and metabolic suppression therapy in controlling intracranial pressure after head injury. *J Neurosurg.* 2002;97:1045-1053.

20. Mayer SA, Chong J. Critical care management of increased intracranial pressure. *J Intensive Care Med.* 2002;17:55-67.

21. Contant CF, Valadka AB, Gopinath SP, et al. Adult respiratory distress syndrome: a complication of induced hypertension after severe head injury. *J Neurosurg.* 2001; 95:560-568.

22. Eker C, Asgiersson B, Grände PO, Schálen W, Nordström CH. Improved outcome after head injury with a therapy based on principles for brain volume regulation and improved microcirculation. *Crit Care Med.* 1998;26:1881-1886.

23. Nordström CH, Reinstrup P, Xu W, Gärdenfors A, Ungerstedt U. Assessment of the lower limit for cerebral perfusion pressure in severe head injuries by bedside monitoring of regional energy metabolism. *Anesthesiol.* 2003;98:809-814.

24. Muizelaar JP, Marmarou A, Ward JD, et al. Adverse effects of prolonged hyperventilation in patients with severe head injury: a randomized clinical trial. *J Neurosurg.* 1991;75:731-739.

25. Sheinberg M, Kaner MJ, Robertson CS, et al., Continuous monitoring of jugular venous oxygen saturation in head-injured patients. *J Neurosurg.* 1992;76:212-217.

26. Dings J, Meixensberger J, Amschler J, et al.: Continuous monitoring of brain tissue Po_2: a new tool to minimize the risk of ischemia caused by hyperventilation therapy. *Zentralbl Neurochir.* 1996:57:177-183.

27. Muizelaar JP, Wei EP, Kontos HA, et al. Mannitol causes compensatory cerebral vasoconstriction in response to blood viscosity changes. *J Neurosurg.* 1983;59:822-828.

28. Suarez JI, Qureshi AI, Bhardwaj A, et al. Treatment of refractory intracranial hypertension with 23.4% saline. *Crit Care Med.* 1998;26:1118-1122.

29. Qureshi AI, Wilson DA, Traystman RJ. Treatment of elevated intracranial pressure in experimental intracerebral hemorrhage: comparison between mannitol and hypertonic saline. *Neurosurgery.* 1999;44:1055-1063.

30. Eisenberg HM, Frankowski RF, Contant CF, et al. High-dose barbiturate control of elevated intracranial pressure in patients with severe head injury. *J Neurosurg.* 1988;69:15-23.

31. Shiozaki T, Sugimoto H, Taneda M, et al. Effect of mild hypothermia on uncontrollable intracranial hypertension after severe head injury. *J Neurosurg.* 1993;79:363-368.

Neurocritical Care Monitoring

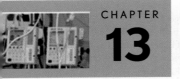

CHAPTER

13

Continuous Electroencephalogram Monitoring in the Intensive Care Unit

Santiago Ortega-Gutierrez, MD
Emily Gilmore, MD
Jan Claassen, MD, PhD

A 60-year-old man presented to the emergency department (ED) with progressive dysarthria and confusion over the prior 24 hours. In the last month, his wife states that her husband complained of episodic headaches that occasionally were associated with nausea. On examination, he was obtunded and moaning to painful stimulation. He had a left gaze preference, but localized equally with his arms and legs. The tone in his legs was increased with bilateral upgoing toes. His noncontrast head computed tomographic (CT) scan (Figure 13-1) performed in the ED revealed a left frontal lesion with mass effect and midline shift. He was admitted to the neurologic intensive care unit (NeuroICU, NICU) for further evaluation and management.

Does his head CT explain the mental status?

There is a mismatch between the neurologic examination and imaging findings; therefore, alternate causes for altered mental status must be explored. The frontal left hypodensity with a surrounding hyperdensity should not account for such a degree of obtundation. Depending on the clinical scenario, this may take the form of obtaining further history or diagnostic tests.

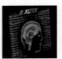

Upon further questioning, this patient's wife states that over the last 2 weeks he had been more forgetful, with fluctuating irritability that would last anywhere from minutes to hours. She denies any rhythmic jerking of his arms or legs or loss of consciousness. There had been no evidence of incontinence or tongue biting. Upon arrival in the NICU, a magnetic resonance image (MRI) with and without gadolinium was performed, and he was subsequently connected to continuous electroencephalographic (cEEG) monitoring (Figure 13-2).

When can cEEG monitoring be helpful in the ICU setting?

The goal of neuromonitoring is to identify secondary brain injury as early as possible and prevent permanent injury by triggering timely interventions. Ideally, such monitoring should

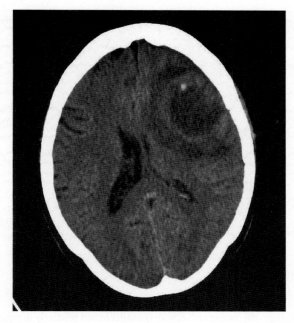

Figure 13-1. Noncontrast head CT with left frontal lesion with mass effect and midline shift.

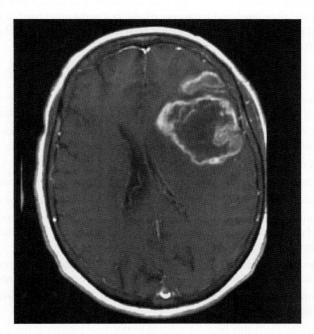

Figure 13-2. Magnetic resonance imaging showed a heterogeneously enhancing lesion in the left frontal lobe with mass effect. The diagnosis of high-grade glioma was suspected, steroids were started, and neurosurgery was consulted. Continued electroencephalographic monitoring was initiated, and a representative page is shown below.

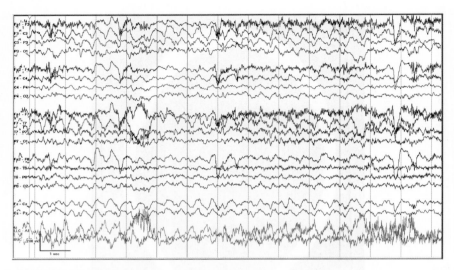

Figure 13-2. (*Continued*)

be highly sensitive and specific, noninvasive, widely available and relatively inexpensive, pose no risks to patients, have high inter- and intra-rater reliability, and have good temporal and spatial resolution. Limitations of cEEG monitoring include high cost, vulnerability to artifact and medications, poor spatial resolution, and poor inter- and intra-rater reliability. On the other hand, it is noninvasive (as long as it is limited to surface EEG monitoring), has great temporal resolution, and allows assessment of neuronal activity.

Applications of cEEG in the ICU

1. To rule out subclinical or nonconvulsive seizures in patients with:
   • Persistently impaired mental status after a convulsive seizure or convulsive status epilepticus (SE)
   • Ongoing or frequently recurring movements, including isolated eye movements, that may or may not represent seizures
   • Impaired mental status and a history of epilepsy
   • Unexplained impaired brain function after basic evaluation (labs and imaging)
   • Acute brain injury with stupor or coma, including post anoxic coma, and sepsis
   • Unexplained fluctuations in mental status, including those secondary to hypoxia and increased intracranial pressure (ie, hydrocephalus, intracranial hemorrhage, and intraventricular hemorrhage)
2. To characterize paroxysmal clinical events, including posturing, rigidity, tremors, chewing, or even autonomic spells such as sudden hypertension, tachycardia, bradycardia, or apnea
3. Epileptiform activity or periodic discharges on initial EEG (often performed for not more than 30 minutes)
4. To detect cerebral ischemia (ie, subarachnoid hemorrhage patients at risk for delayed cerebral ischemia)
5. To guide medication titration and quantify seizure frequency in patients with refractory status epilepticus (RSE)

Table 13-1. EEG and Neuronal injury Associated with Cerebral Blood Flow Changes

CBF level (mL/100 g/min)	EEG change	Degree of neuronal injury
35-70	Normal	No injury
25-35	Loss of fast beta frequencies	Reversible
18-25	Background slowing to theta frequencies (5-7 Hz)	Reversible
12-18	Background slowing to delta frequencies (1-4 Hz)	Reversible
< 8-10	Suppression of all frequencies	Neuronal death

Abbreviations: CBF, cerebral blood flow; EEG, electroencephalographic. *(Derived from Jordan KG. Emergency EEG and continuous EEG monitoring in acute ischemic stroke. J Clin Neurophysiol. 2004;21:341-52.)*

What finding on cEEG could explain the patient's intermittent deficits?

Nonconvulsive seizures (NCSs) and nonconvulsive status epilepticus (NCSE) are frequently seen in the ICU setting. These can present similar to the patient described in this case. Even in the medical ICU population after excluding all patients with any clinical suspicion of seizures, approximately 8% of comatose patients have electrographic seizures.[1,2] Electrographic seizures can be detected by cEEG in 20% to 48% and NCSE in 14% in the aftermath of clinically successfully treated convulsive SE.[3,4] In the acute brain injury setting, electrographic seizures are even more frequent but the incidence clearly depends on the underlying etiology. However, no population-based studies are available to date; thus, the real incidence is unknown. In the NICU setting, subclinical seizures were seen in 18% of a cohort of 570 consecutive patients who underwent cEEG for the detection of subclinical seizures or to evaluate an unexplained decrease in consciousness (Table 13-1). In this study, seizures were more frequently recorded in younger patients with a history of epilepsy, patients who had convulsive seizures prior to start of cEEG monitoring, and those who were comatose at the time cEEG was started. When stratified by etiology, either periodic epileptiform discharges (PEDs), NCSs, or NCSE can be seen in one-quarter to one-half of those undergoing monitoring (Table 13-2). While the majority of seizures will be recorded in the first 24 hours, frequently 48 hours or more of cEEG are needed to record the first seizure in comatose patients (Figure 13-3).[5]

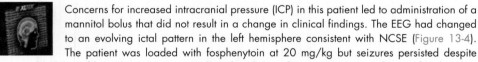

Concerns for increased intracranial pressure (ICP) in this patient led to administration of a mannitol bolus that did not result in a change in clinical findings. The EEG had changed to an evolving ictal pattern in the left hemisphere consistent with NCSE (Figure 13-4). The patient was loaded with fosphenytoin at 20 mg/kg but seizures persisted despite repeated boluses of lorazepam. He was intubated and started on a continuous infusion of midazolam (for details, refer to the status epilepticus protocol in Chapter 3).

How can quantitative EEG (qEEG) be helpful in the next 24 hours in the management of NCSE?

In addition to looking at the raw EEG data, the EEG recordings can be subjected to quantitative analysis. A number of different quantification methods are available with most commercially available EEG software. Quantification techniques include the calculation of power spectra by means of fast Fourier transform (FFT), which then can be used to calculate ratios of fast over slow activ-

Table 13-2. Prevalence of Abnormal Epileptiform Patterns Including Seizures With and Without Acute Brain Injury

Diagnosis	PEDs (N = 1071)	Surface EEG NCS (N = 570)	NCSE (N = 570)	TCME NCS (N = 40)
CNS infection	23%	9%	17%	NA
Toxic-metabolic encephalopathy	26%	13%	8%	NA
Epilepsy-related seizures	11%	11%	20%	75% (3/4)
Brain tumor	17%	11%	12%	NA
Postneurosurgery	13%	15%	8%	NA
SAH	16%	5%	13%	55% (11/20)
TBI	13%	10%	8%	50% (3/6)
ICH	17%	4%	9%	29% (2/7)
Unexplained decrease in LOC	10%	10%	5%	NA
AIS	16%	2%	7%	50% (1/2)

Abbreviations: AIS, acute ischemic stroke; ICH, intracranial hemorrhage; LOC, level of consciousness; NCSs, nonconvulsive seizures; NCSE, nonconvulsive status epilepticus; PEDs, periodic epileptiform discharges; SAH, subarachnoid hemorrhage; TBI, traumatic brain injury; TCME: transcortical minidepth electrode. *(Derived from Claassen J, Jetté N, Chum F, et al. Electrographic seizures and periodic discharges after intracerebral hemorrhage. Neurology 2007;69:1356-1365; Claassen J, Hirsch LJ, Frontera JA, et al. Prognostic significance of continuous EEG monitoring in patients with poor-grade subarachnoid hemorrhage. Neurocrit Care 2006;4:103-112; Claassen J, Mayer SA, Kowalski RG, Emerson RG, Hirsch LJ. Detection of electrographic seizures with continuous EEG monitoring in critically ill patients. Neurology 2004;62:1743-1749, and unpublished data.)*

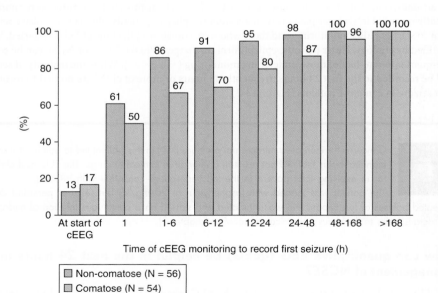

Figure 13-3. Time to detect the first seizure in 110 of 570 critically ill patients who had seizures recorded on continuous electroencephalography. *(From Claassen J, Mayer SA, Kowalski RG, et al. Detection of electrographic seizures with continuous EEG monitoring in critically ill patients. Neurology. 2004;62:1743-1748.)*

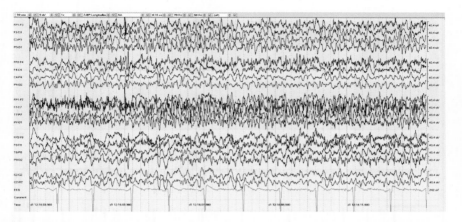

Figure 13-4. Continuous electroencephalograph revealing a left hemispheric seizure predominantly seen in the temporal leads.

ity or other parameters. These can be displayed as numbers or graphically as compressed spectral arrays (CSAs), histograms, or as staggered arrays, which have the potential to unmask subtle background changes when trended over time. The qEEG parameters may include total power, frequency activity totals (eg, total or percentage alpha power), spectral edge frequencies (eg, frequency below which 50% of the EEG resides), amplitude-integrated interval, frequency ratios (eg, alpha-to-delta ratio), and brain symmetry index.[6] Other more automated EEG data reduction display formats include the cerebral function monitor (CFAM), EEG density modulation, automated analysis of segmented EEG (AAS-EEG), and bispectral index (BIS) monitor.[7-11] However, qEEG should always be interpreted in the context of the raw EEG since artifacts, medications, and other clinical events may cause very similar findings to epileptiform findings (Figure 13-5). This is particularly true for software packages that display "user-friendly" composite scores, and any outputs that are based on unpublished algorithms ("proprietary information") should be viewed with great caution. The qEEG parameters are particularly useful for seizure quantification and to estimate effects of seizure treatment once the qEEG "footprint" of a seizure has been identified.

For continued NCSE in this patient, a midazolam drip was rapidly titrated up until seizures were controlled. The next morning he underwent tumor resection while on midazolam with no complications. Postoperatively, midazolam was weaned, and on postoperative day 2, he was transferred to the floor with signs of a mild residual neglect. Biopsy revealed glioblastoma multiforme.

What else may qEEG offer?

In addition to seizure quantification, qEEG is useful for trending patterns over time as the transitions may not be as evident on review of the raw data. The qEEG and raw EEG in Figure 13-6 illustrate resolution of NCSE over an extended period of time.

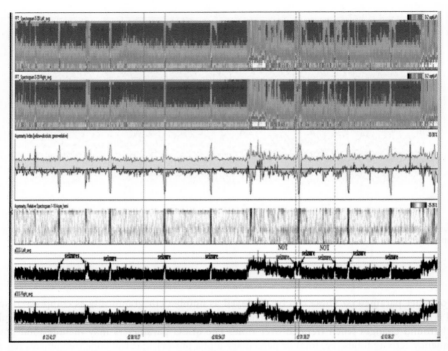

Figure 13-5. Note: This quantitative electroencephalogram (qEEG) was taken from a different patient than the one in the case presented here. A 4-hour qEEG recording with multiple nonconvulsive seizures (*labeled*) maximal on the left as evident on aEEG (higher amplitude on the left) and the relative asymmetry index, going sharply downward (more power in the left) with each seizure. The standard spectrogram and the asymmetry spectrogram both demonstrate involvement of all frequencies. Note the two episodes labeled as "no seizures" in which the amplitude-integrated EEG (aEEG) tracing jumps up in a manner almost identical to the prior and subsequent seizures. However, review of the raw EEG revealed muscle artifact. *(From Hirsch LJ, Brenner RP. Atlas of EEG in Critical Care. Hoboken, NJ: Wiley-Blackwell, 2010. Figure 13-7.10, page 238.)*

In addition to the quantitative measures described above, seizure detection programs using specialized EEG signal–processing software can be used for screening large cEEG datasets, allowing the reviewer to hone in on marked segments (Figure 13-7, top row). These programs may be based on a simple FFT-based frequency analysis, may recognize specific waveform patterns, or incorporate a complex learning algorithm that recognizes more combinations and sequential developments of typical waveforms. Based on the FFT analysis of EEG, CSA graphs can be generated to determine the occurrence of subclinical seizures once the "CSA signature" or footprint of a seizure in an individual patient has been determined.[12] This can be used to quickly screen a 24-hour recording and quantify the frequency of seizures.

Others have investigated the utility of the cerebral function analyzing monitor (CFAM) to detect seizures, but sensitivity was particularly low for partial seizures.[12] Algorithms were limited by a high false-positive rate with good sensitivity.[12] While promising, commercially available automated seizure-detection software has been developed for use in epilepsy-monitoring units and programmed to identify seizures from healthy patients. However, seizures in brain-injured and often medically sick comatose patients have rather different patterns, which are typically less organized, have a slower maximum frequency, and are longer in duration with unclear on and off settings. Thus, in order to

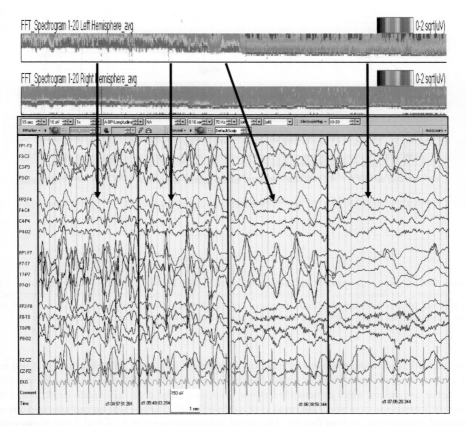

Figure 13-6. Resolution of partial nonconvulsive status epilepticus shown on compressed spectral array (CSA). CSA showing gradual resolution of nonconvulsive status epilepticus over a few hours. CSA is particularly useful for recognition of such long-term trends. Arrows indicate approximate time periods in the CSA from which the EEG samples are taken. Y-axis: frequency, 0 Hz at bottom, 60 Hz at top. X-axis: time (approximately 4 hours shown). Color scale (Z-axis) power of given frequency (scale in upper right; microvolts/Hz). Z-axis: voltage, measured in microvolts/Hz.

utilize seizure-detection programs in the NeuroICU, new software will need to be developed and programmed to more accurately identify complex ICU ictal patterns. Automated seizure-detection software based on multichannel, digitized real-time FFT (2 seconds per epoch, 2 minutes averaging) and trends of total EEG power has been used by some groups with reasonable success but has not been verified on an independent dataset.[11,12]

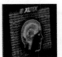

A 57-year-old woman was admitted to the NICU with aneurysmal subarachnoid hemorrhage (aSAH) from a right posterior communicating artery aneurysm (Hunt and Hess grade IV, Fisher 3, modified Fisher grade 3), which was clipped. Her postoperative noncontrast head CT that day did not reveal any infarcts. Her Glasgow Coma Scale (GCS) score was 14 and she was subsequently extubated. Transcranial Doppler flow velocities were mildly elevated on postbleed day 6 without any new neurologic findings. Hypervolemic hypertensive therapy was initiated with a target

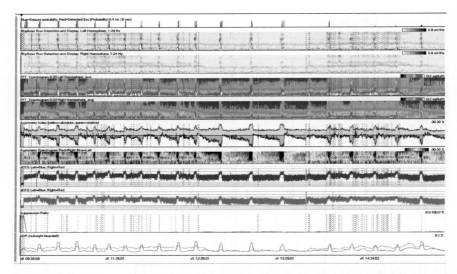

Figure 13-7. Different quantitative electroencephalographic (qEEG) tools including seizure probability (*top row*), rhythmic run detection (*second and third row from top*), CSA (*4th and 5th rows from top*), asymmetry indices (*6th and 7th rows from top*), amplitude-integrated EEG (*8th and 9th rows from top*), suppression rate (*10th row from top*), and alpha-to-delta ratio (*bottom row*), all clearly detecting frequent recurrent seizure activity.

systolic blood pressure greater than 180 mm Hg. On postbleed day 7, her GCS dropped to 12 and her CT scan revealed an acute stroke in the left internal capsule (Figure 13-8). She was taken for a digital subtraction angiogram, which demonstrated severe vasospasm in the distal right middle cerebral and left vertebral arteries. The tortuosity of the vessel precluded angioplasty, but she was treated with intra-arterial verapamil and papaverine. Later that day, her clinical status deteriorated to a GCS of 7 with a new onset of left hemiparesis. Unfortunately, her clinical status continued to deteriorate and she died on postbleed day 8 after CT showed widespread infarction.

Is there any role for cEEG monitoring in this patient?

Yes. Symptomatic vasospasm and the associated delayed cerebral ischemia (DCI) are common complications that occur in 20% to 40% of patients with SAH.[13] A number of treatments are available, but making the diagnosis of DCI can be challenging, particularly in those with a limited neurologic examination. Ideally, timely recognition of ischemia leads to interventions that prevent infarction. In addition to recording ictal activity, cEEG may detect decreased cerebral perfusion in the setting of vasospasm after SAH. EEG is very sensitive to ischemia and may reveal changes at a reversible stage of reduced cerebral blood flow (CBF) and neuronal dysfunction (25 to 30 mL/100 g per minute; Table 13-1). The raw EEG progresses through predictable stages with increasing degrees of hypoperfusion, including loss of fast activity, increased slowing, and background attenuation[14,15]

The patient was monitored with cEEG from post-bleed day 3 to 8 of her hospitalization. As seen below (Figure 13-9) the cEEG alpha/delta ratio (ADR) progressively decreased after day 6, particularly in the right anterior region, to settle into a steady trough level later that night reflective of decrease in faster frequencies and slowing over the right hemisphere.

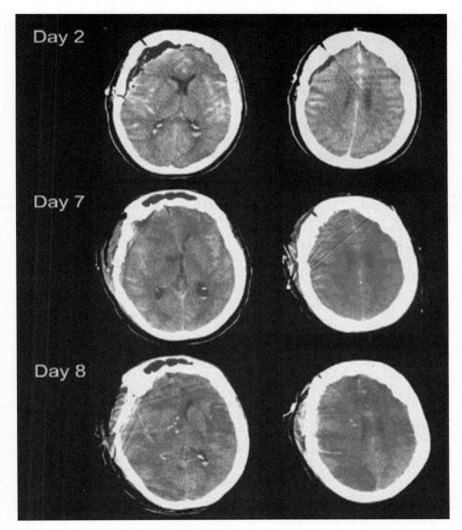

Figure 13-8. Computed tomographic (CT) scan of the head performed on subarachnoid hemorrhage days 2, 7, and 8. On day 2, thick subarachnoid blood is noted along with the site of the craniotomy after clipping. On day 7, a hypodensity in the right internal capsule is noted. On day 8, hypodensities are noted throughout the cerebral hemispheres affecting different vascular areas including the right and left middle cerebral arteries as well as the right posterior cerebral artery. *(With permission from Claassen J, Hirsch LJ, Kreiter KT, et al. Quantitative continuous EEG for detecting delayed cerebral ischemia in patients with poor grade subarachnoid hemorrhage. Clin Neurophysiol. 2004;115:2699-2710.)*

These changes occurred several hours before transcranial Doppler (TCD) velocities were obtained and clinical symptoms were noted. A transient increase of the right anterior and posterior ADRs were noted after the infusion of intra-arterial vasodilators during angiogram. However, the increase was transient and several hours later the ADR decreased again, reflecting progression of her vasospasm. Figure 13-10 shows a sample of the raw EEG on days 7 and 8, which demonstrates an increase in delta frequency activity and a decrease in faster frequency activity, more pronounced in the right hemisphere.

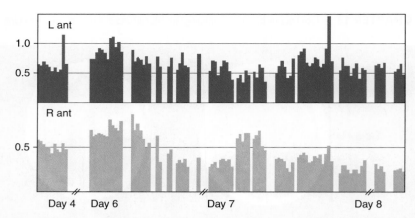

Figure 13-9. Alpha-to-delta ratio calculated from left and right anterior surface EEG leads. (*Modified from Claassen J, Hirsch LJ, Kreiter KT, et al. Quantitative continuous EEG for detecting delayed cerebral ischemia in patients with poor-grade subarachnoid hemorrhage. Clin Neurophysiol. 2004;115:2699-2710. Figure 13-2, page 2705.*)

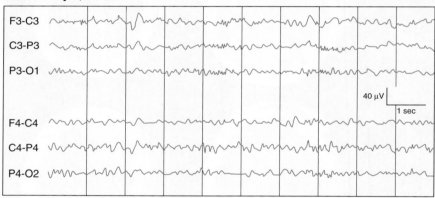

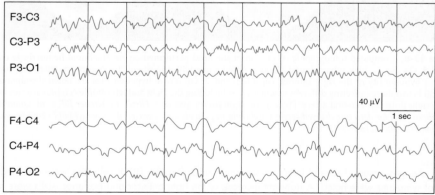

Figure 13-10. Surface electroencephalocardiogram on days 6 and 7 demonstrating new-onset right hemispheric slowing on day 7. (*From Claassen J, Hirsch LJ, Kreiter KT, et al. Quantitative continuous EEG for detecting delayed cerebral ischemia in patients with poor-grade subarachnoid hemorrhage. Clin Neurophysiol. 2004;115:2699-2710. Figure 13-4, page 2707.*)

In what scenario is cEEG most frequently used to detect ischemia?

EEG was first used to detect ischemia during carotid endarterectomy (CEA) and is still used to monitor for ischemia during cross-clamping (Figure 13-11). In acute ischemic stroke, reocclusion occurs in about 34% after successful recanalization with tissue plasminogen activator (tPA).[16] Quantitative EEG parameters

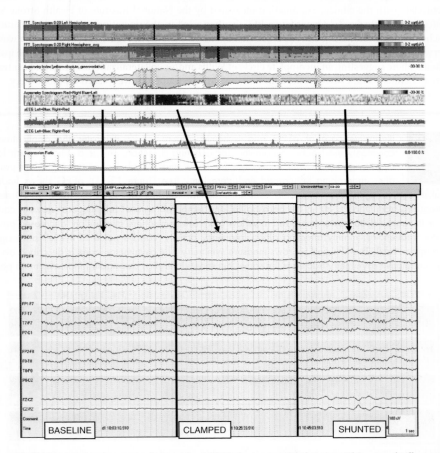

Figure 13-11. Continuous electroencephalography (qEEG) during carotid clamping. This example illustrates the rise in asymmetry after clamping of the carotid artery during endarterectomy. A right-sided attenuation after clamping was observed on raw EEG that is then restored with a common-carotid-to-internal-carotid shunt, which was placed for the duration of the procedure. Although the asymmetry was evident on the raw EEG, it was accentuated on the compressed spectral array (CSA). This is a two-hour epoch where the qEEG shows findings typical of cortical dysfunction frequently seen in ischemia. The first two rows depict spectrograms from 0 to 20 Hz in the bilateral hemispheres. Right hemisphere attenuation (decreased power) of faster frequencies, mainly affecting alpha frequency activity can be noted in the right hemisphere (*red box*). The third row measures symmetry. The asymmetry index shows total absolute asymmetry in *yellow*; this is calculated by comparing asymmetry at each pair of homologous electrodes. The absolute values are summed to give a total asymmetry score; this can only be positive and upward on this display and goes up with asymmetry at any frequency. The *green* relative asymmetry tracing is the same, but shows laterality: downgoing indicates more power on the left and upgoing on the right. The forth row in *red* and *blue* is the asymmetry spectrogram. It shows asymmetry at each frequency from 1 to 18 Hz averaged over the entire hemisphere. *Blue* means more power on the left in that frequency. Here, it shows increased frequency activity on the left correlating with the loss of all frequency of activity on the right. The fifth row is the suppression ratio (percentage of frequencies below 5 μV). During the periods of ischemia the suppression ratio increases over on the right. This technology is not only essential in the operating room, but can also be applied to the neuromonitoring setting in the ICU.

such as the brain symmetry index (BSI) and the acute delta change index correlate with the degree of cerebral perfusion after acute ischemic stroke (AIS) measures by diffusion and perfusion-weighted imaging MRI.[17] Some studies suggest that the qEEG parameter known as regional attenuation without delta (RAWOD) has a distinctive early pattern reflecting hemispheric infarction and may help to anticipate which patients might benefit from thrombolytic therapy.[18] Furthermore, EEG parameters such as BSI correlate with the clinical examination measured by the National Institute of Health Stroke Scale of outcome after stroke.[19,20] Quantitative EEG is often used in the operating room at our institution for ischemia detection during CEA as illustrated by the case shown in Figure 13-11 in which a woman underwent clamping of the internal carotid artery (ICA) and had pronounced attenuation of the ipsilateral hemisphere suggesting an incomplete circle of Willis and/or collateralization. To minimize intraoperative ischemia, a shunt between the common carotid artery and ICA was placed for the surgery.

Illustrative case of qEEG and ischemia. Figure 13-12 illustrates the application of commonly used qEEG parameters for ischemia detection. This is a 4-hour epoch for a middle-aged man with a negative head CT and MRI, but persistent right hemiparesis after undergoing left carotid endarterectomy (see Figure 13-11). qEEG shows findings typical of cortical dysfunction frequently seen in ischemia. The first four rows of Figure 13-10 depict spectrograms from 0 to 20 Hz in the parasagittal and temporal regions. Left temporal slowing can be seen as increased delta power (more red in yellow box). Left hemisphere attenuation (decreased power) of faster frequencies, mainly affecting alpha frequency activity, can be noted in the left parasagittal region (green box). The fifth and six rows measure symmetry. The asymmetry index is described above. The green relative asymmetry tracing is the same, but shows laterality: downgoing indicates more power

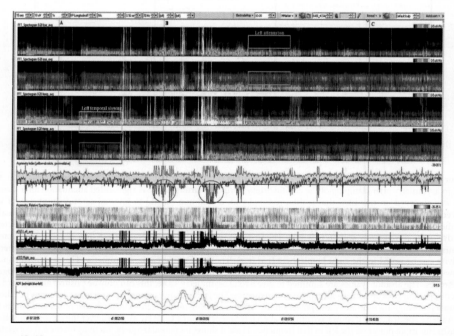

Figure 13-12. Illustration of the application of commonly used continuous electroencephalographic parameters for ischemia detection. See text. *(From Hirsch LJ, Brenner RP. Atlas of EEG in Critical Care. Hoboken, NJ: Wiley-Blackwell, 2010. Figure 13-7.6, page 228.)*

on the left, and upgoing on the right. The sixth row in red and blue is the asymmetry spectrogram. Again, it shows asymmetry at each frequency from 1 to 18 Hz averaged over the entire hemisphere. Here it shows that higher frequencies (greater than 6 Hz) are increased on the right and slower frequencies (less than 4 Hz) are increased on the left, which is characteristic of ischemia. The bottom row shows the alpha-to-delta ratio on each side (red = right and blue = left). Note that the ratio is persistently higher on the right, suggesting ischemia on the contralateral side.

A few investigations reported on the applicability of qEEG parameters for the detection of DCI and/or vasospasm after a SAH. While the ideal qEEG parameter for assessing ischemia is a matter of debate, most include some ratio of fast-to-slow activity.[21] Variability of relative alpha and post stimulation ADRs have been shown to correlate with DCI in good- and poor-grade SAH patients. Changes in relative alpha variability have been detected up to 2 days before the onset of clinical symptoms.[15] Among 34 patients with poor grade, a SAH monitored with cEEG, a single drop greater than 50% (sensitivity 89% and specificity 84%, PPV 67% and NPV 96%) and six consecutive recordings with 10% or more reduction in the baseline ADR (sensitivity 100%, specificity 76%, PPV 60% and NPV 100%) correlated well with the development of DCI.[21] Other qEEG methods to characterize ischemia include the compressed spectral array (CSA), suppression-burst ratio, amplitude-integrated EEG, or the asymmetry indices.[15]

This patient underwent cEEG monitoring and developed new-onset right hemispheric slowing on postbleed day 7. As seen in the figure (Figure 13-9), the cEEG ADR progressively decreased after day 6, particularly in the right anterior region, to settle into a steady trough level later that night, reflective of the decrease in faster frequencies and slowing over the right hemisphere (Figure 13-10). These changes occurred several hours before TCD velocities were obtained and clinical symptoms were noted. A transient increase of the right anterior and posterior ADRs were noted after the infusion of intra-arterial vasodilators during angiogram. However, the increase was transient and several hours later the ADR decreased again, reflecting progression of her vasospasm.

A 55-year-old man was admitted with an intraventricular hemorrhage in the setting of phencyclidine abuse. Several days into his hospitalization, he developed refractory hypotension that initially resulted in a drop in the mean arterial pressure (MAP) and cerebral perfusion (Figure 13-13, red and blue dotted line). A delayed increase in the intracranial pressure (ICP) was observed 30 minutes later (Figure 13-13, black dotted line). At that time, he showed clinical signs of herniation. Despite aggressive medical management, the herniation could not be reversed and he progressed to brain death.

What do you expect his qEEG parameters including CSA, amplitude integrated EEG, and suppression burst ratio will have shown?

A review of the quantitative and raw EEG with hemodynamic parameters is shown in Figure 13-13.

A 25-year-old black male was admitted to the NICU with a traumatic brain injury (TBI) after surviving a motor vehicle accident while driving under the influence of alcohol. He was intubated in the field, where his initial GCS was 5. Trauma workup revealed a hemorrhagic contusion in the right frontal and temporal lobes. Intraparenchymal ICP and tissue brain oxygenation monitors were placed. cEEG was connected and revealed diffuse

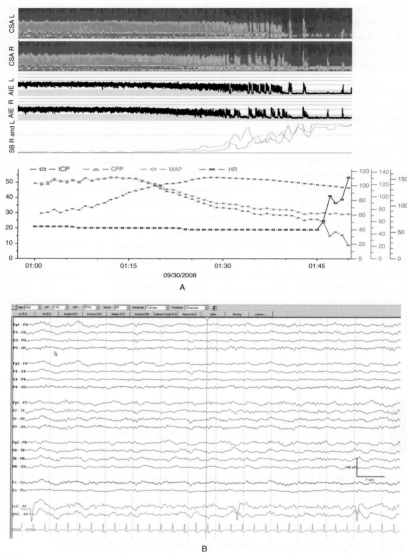

Figure 13-13. (A) 1-hour of quantitative electroencephalographic (qEEG) analysis demonstrates attenuation of all frequencies in the compressed spectral array (CSA), particularly on the right. The amplitude-integrated EEG reveals a drop in the maximum amplitude per epoch, and the suppression ratio (*red and blue lines*) depicts the increasingly suppressed EEG background. Interestingly, qEEG parameters changed gradually as the mean arterial pressure (MAP) and cerebral perfusion pressure (CPP) start to decrease, which is at least 15 minutes prior to the development of refractory intracranial pressure (ICP) crisis. Within an hour, the raw EEG changes from diffuse background with subtle attenuation on the right (**B**) to a severely suppressed background (**C**). *(From Kurtz P, Hanafy KA, Claassen J. Cur Opinion Crit Care 2009;15:99-109, Figure 13-2, page 101-102.)*

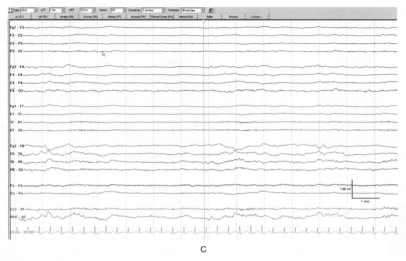

C

Figure 13-13. (*Continued*)

slowing, but no electrographic seizures. Despite increased sedation, several boluses of propofol, and osmotherapy agents, he continued to have refractory ICP elevations, leading to a pentobarbital bolus of 100 mg and the initiation of hypothermia. His cEEG before and after the pentobarbital bolus is shown in Figure 13-14.

Can cEEG be utilized to monitor response to therapy other than anti-epileptics?

EEG monitoring can be especially useful in evaluating the response to interventions that aim to depress neuronal activity and brain metabolism. As described in Chapter 12, cEEG is essential in guiding successful treatment of refractory status epilepticus. It gives clinicians an end point that allows adjustment of IV medications to maintain enough suppression of the EEG background while minimizing adverse effects. Pharmacologic coma remains a tool for the treatment of refractory ICP elevations,

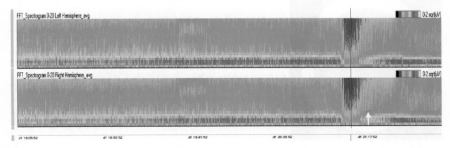

Figure 13-14. At baseline, the compressed spectral array (CSA) shows a mixture of theta and delta frequencies (*yellow and red*) and alpha and beta (*green*) electroencephalographic (EEG) power, with slightly higher delta and theta frequency power over the left hemisphere. After the pentobarbital bolus (*red arrow*), attenuation of faster frequencies (*loss of green bilaterally*) and increase in slower frequencies can be clearly seen in the CSA. As the medication wears off (*white arrow*), there is a gradual return of higher frequency power (*return of green*). This weaning off of the pentobarbital effect can be difficult to appreciate on review of the raw EEG.

especially when occurring acutely. Although effective in reducing ICP, its use is coupled with a high risk of systemic complications, including hypotension, renal failure, cardiac depression, and hepatic dysfunction. The goal is to use the minimum dose required to achieve the goals of ICP control and decrease metabolism.[22]

Continuous EEG may also provide information about the level of sedation in the critically ill, especially in the setting of neuromuscular blockade. A number of commercially available qEEG-based tools such as the Bispectral Index,[23] Patient State Index,[24] and Entropy Monitor and Narcotrend[25] have been used in operating rooms and ICUs for decades to monitor sedation levels. These single-purpose devices use proprietary algorithms and have been shown to be very inconsistent, particularly when confronted with EEGs showing seizures or ischemia. For the time being one can only ask for extreme caution when using these "black-box" analytical methods in the acute brain injury or ICU setting.

An obtunded 73-year-old man with a large right hemispheric infarct was admitted to the NICU for close monitoring with a particular concern for herniation. On hospital day 2, his mental status remained poor and hypothermia to 35°C was initiated along with invasive multimodality intracranial monitoring. As part of the invasive monitoring "bundle," an eight-contact miniature depth electrode was placed in the right frontal lobe in the area of presumed ischemic penumbra, along with an ICP monitor, a brain tissue oxygen tension monitor, and a cerebral microdialysis catheter. Scalp EEG leads were also in place (Figure 13-15).

What could be a benefit of depth electrode monitoring as a component of multimodality brain monitoring to complement scalp EEG?

Preliminary studies from our group have suggested that a small depth electrode inserted near the cortex in severely brain-injured patients (acute brain injury resulting in coma at risk for secondary brain injury) may improve the signal-to-noise ratio of EEG (ie, shivering obliterating surface recordings), clarify suspicious but not clearly epileptiform patterns (ie, rhythmic slowing without clear evolution), detect seizures not seen on the surface, and detect changes that indicate secondary complications

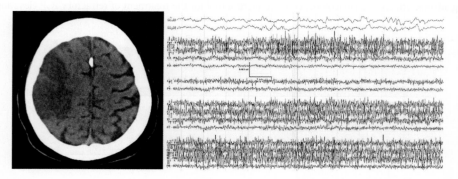

Figure 13-15. The image on the left shows the noncontrast head computerized tomographic scan with a well-demarcated hypodensity involving the right frontal and parietal lobes. Effacement of sulci and gyri is also noted. The image on the right shows the baseline electroencephalogram at 9:00 PM, which reveals a continuous mixture of alpha, delta, and theta frequencies in the depth electrode recording *(top two channels)*. The scalp recording is obscured by muscle artifact, likely from microshivering. *(From Hirsch LJ, Brenner RP. Atlas of EEG in Critical Care. Hoboken, NJ: Wiley-Blackwell; 2010. Figure 13-7.49, page 291.)*

(ie, ischemia).[25,26] The significance of depth-only findings is currently unclear and should not lead to management changes without any additional data to corroborate the impression.[27]

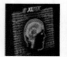 At 9:45 PM, this patient's EEG recorded from the depth electrode became discontinuous, with a suppression burst pattern predominating. The scalp EEG showed no significant changes. Around 4 AM the depth electrode became more suppressed, while the scalp EEG remained obscured by myogenic artifact. Subsequently, the depth EEG began to recover, with periodic delta waves by 6:20 AM and resumption of a continuous pattern by 7:25 AM (Figure 13-16). A concomitant review of the multimodality data revealed that after the prominent EEG change (Figure 13-16, red line) occurred there was a significant drop in brain tissue oxygen tension (slowly drifting to a critical level less than 15). The lactate-to-pyruvate ratio, measured by microdialysis (for details, see Chapter 14; normal less than 40), was markedly elevated during the entire time. A noncontrast head CT the next day revealed hemorrhagic transformation of the ischemic infarct (Figure 13-17).

In this case, the depth electrode showed the potential to improve the signal-to-noise ratio and identification of a secondary complication; that is, hemorrhagic transformation of an acute ischemic stroke. Additionally, depth electrode monitoring may allow clarification of unclear surface EEG patterns or show ictal patterns that are not evident on the scalp EEG recording (Figures 13-18 and 13-19).

What are high-frequency oscillations and what is cortical spreading depression?

A number of studies have observed high-frequency oscillations using intracortical EEG recordings in normal subjects and patients with epilepsy.[28-32] This phenomenon has also been termed *microseizures* and cannot be recorded by regular surface electrodes. Interestingly, these microseizures are more frequent in brain regions that generated seizures and also sporadically evolved into large-scale clinical seizures. The relationship to depth-only seizures in patients undergoing depth electrode monitoring, and if this is present in patients with acute brain injury, is currently unknown.

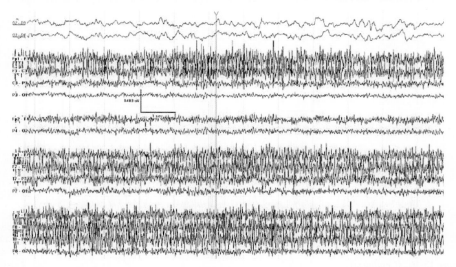

Figure 13-16. Sequence of changes in electroencephalography from the patient discussed in the text.

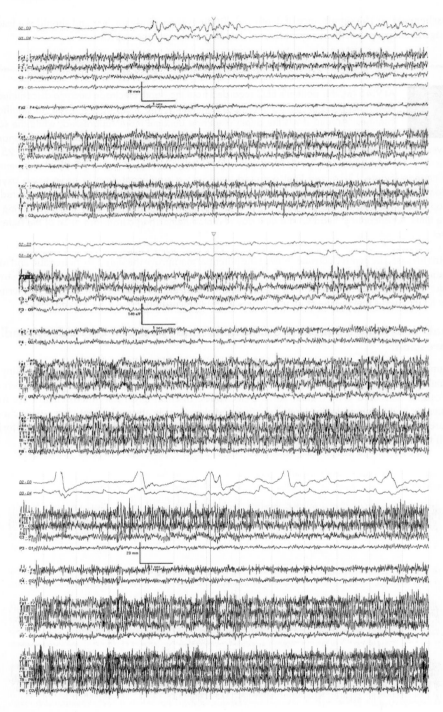

Figure 13-16. (*Continued*)

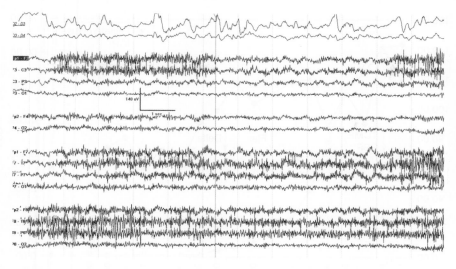

Figure 13-16. (*Continued*)

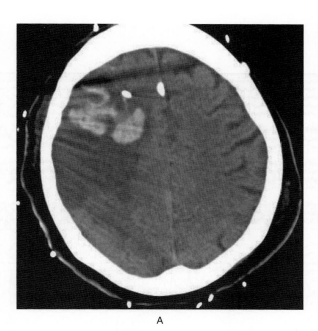

A

Figure 13-17. **A.** Computerized scan of head reveals hypodensity in the middle cerebral artery region with a hyperdensity that represents acute blood. **B.** Seventeen hours of multimodality monitoring data are displayed and discussed in the text. (*From Waziri A, Claassen J, Stuart RM, et al. Intracortical electroencephalography in acute brain injury. Ann Neurol. 2009;66:366-377. Figure 13-5, page 372.*)

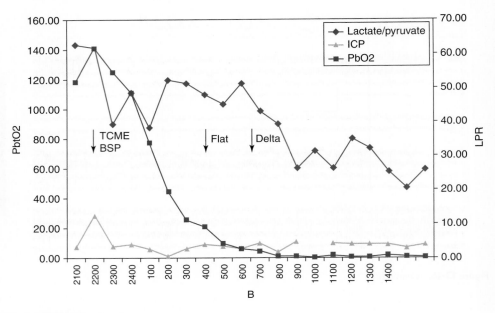

Figure 13-17. (*Continued*)

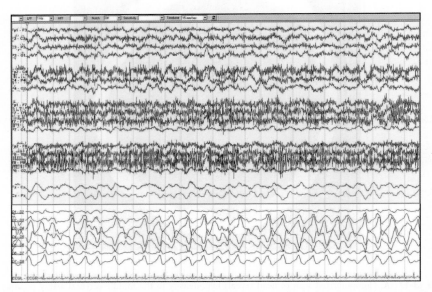

Figure 13-18. A 20-year-old woman admitted to the NeuroICU with a traumatic brain injury with hemorrhagic shear injury in the corpus callosum, right posterior pons, and left frontal lobe. Scalp electroencephalography and depth electrode recording is shown in this figure, conveying the improved signal-to-noise ratio in the depth recording.

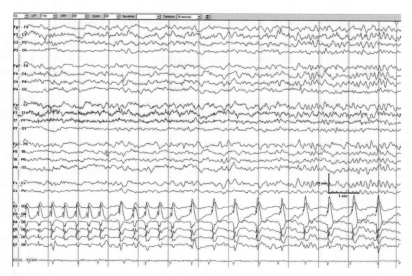

Figure 13-19. A 74-year-old woman with a Hunt and Hess grade III right anterior communicating artery subarachnoid hemorrhage who underwent clipping and postoperative scalp electroencephalography (EEG) and depth electrode monitoring. The scalp EEG showed a moderate degree of diffuse cerebral slowing, which was worse over the right hemisphere with evolving seizures in the depth recording, maximal at D4-D5. In the depth channels *(bottom 8 channels above)*, there is an evolving rhythmic 3-Hz spike and wave pattern that spreads in field, increases in amplitude, and then slows to 1 to 2 Hz at offset. These occurred every 2 to 3 minutes in a cyclic manner. There was no scalp EEG correlate despite good-quality EEG. There was no obvious change in the microdialysis biomarkers. *(From Waziri A, Claassen J, Stuart RM, et al. Intracortical electroencephalography in acute brain injury. Ann Neurol. 2009;66:366-377. Figure 13-5, page 372. Figure 13-4, page 371.)*

Cortical spreading depression as well as slow and prolonged peri-injury depolarizations lasting minutes have been reported in a number of recent studies in patients with acute brain injury.[33-36] Both patterns are thought to indicate compromised metabolism. Clinically, they may be used to detect infarct enlargement in patients with MCA infarction[35] and DCI after aSAH.[34]

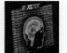

You are called to consult on a 69-year-old man in the surgical ICU who had a cardiopulmonary arrest after undergoing cardiothoracic surgery. The initial rhythm was asystole and his return of spontaneous circulation (ROSC) was 15 minutes. He was treated with hypothermia for 24 hours and slowly rewarmed over the subsequent 36 hours. At 72 hours, he remained in a coma despite being off sedation and paralytics. Neurology has been consulted for prognostication purposes.

Is there a role for cEEG?

Abnormal epileptiform EEG patterns with or without clinical correlates including periodic discharges and seizures can be frequently seen after cardiac arrest. Periodic epileptiform patterns, seizures, loss of reactivity and absence of normal sleep architecture, suppression burst, flat background[37-38] have been associated with poor outcome after cardiac arrest. In the era of induced hypothermia after cardiac arrest,[39] the prognostic implications of EEG findings have to be revisited, and anecdotally it is clear that good outcomes are possible even in patients with status epilepticus after cardiac arrest.

Does cEEG monitoring have a role outside of the NeuroICU?

Yes. Studies reporting the seizure frequencies in non-neurologic ICUs are limited. Over a 2-year period, 12.3% of 1758 admitted medical ICU patients experienced some type of neurologic complications. Among those, seizures (28%) were the second most common complication after metabolic encephalopathy and usually occurred in the context of metabolic disarrangement.[40] These include, but are not limited to, hyponatremia, hypo- or hyperglycemia, hypocalcemia, drug intoxication or withdrawal uremia, and hepatic failure and hypertensive encephalopathy.[41] Septic encephalopathy is the most common type of metabolic encephalopathy encountered in the medical ICU and is found in up to 70% of patients.[42,43] Recently, a review of 257 patients admitted to the medical ICU and submitted to cEEG monitoring found NCSs in 11% of the cohort of 19% of those with sepsis. In fact, sepsis was an independent predictor of NCS, and the presence of electrographic seizures was associated with poor outcome.[44,45] The true overlap between seizures and sepsis will need to be studied prospectively.

What are current limitations to implementing cEEG monitoring in the ICU setting?

Obstacles to more widespread use of this technique include expense of equipment and personnel, 24-hour availability of technicians to maintain high-quality recordings, and the presence of encephalographers available to review the studies in real time.[46] Few studies have investigated the clinical impact of cEEG-driven interventions and health care economics associated with cEEG monitoring. The key to developing an efficient and proficient cEEG service is being able to train nurses and medical staff to recognize both basic EEG patterns and their changes over time as well as common artifacts encountered in the ICU setting (Figure 13-20). Common artifacts may mimic seizures, including chest percussion, oscillating beds, ventilators, chewing, and rhythmic movements. Other artifacts in the ICU include electrical artifact (60 Hz) from dialysis, extracorporeal membrane oxygenation (ECMO), pumps/drips, heating/cooling devices, and electric beds. Identification of artifacts is greatly aided by use of video EEG. In the light of increased

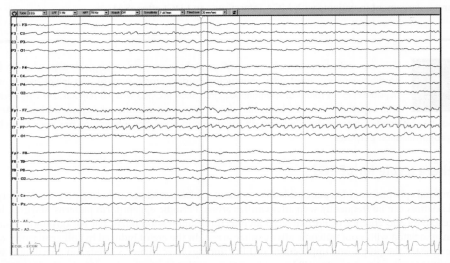

Figure 13-20. Common electroencephalographic artifacts seen in the ICU. Panels 1, 2, and 3 reflect chest percussion artifact; Panel 4 is respirator artifact; and Panel 5 is chewing artifact.

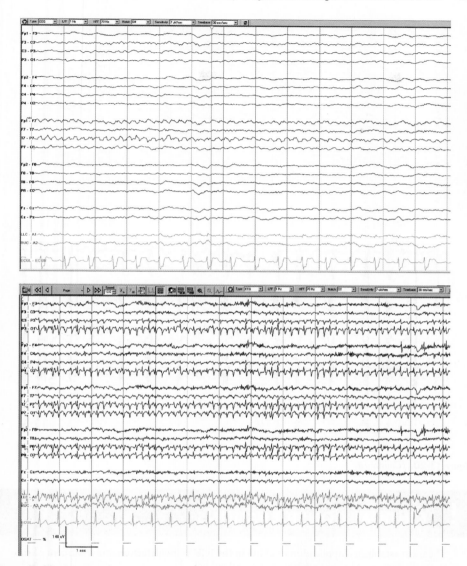

Figure 13-20. (*Continued*)

availability of CT- and MRI-compatible electrodes as well as prospective studies assessing the impact on outcomes, such monitoring is crucial and will help make cEEG a valuable tool in the armamentarium of neuromonitoring devices.[47]

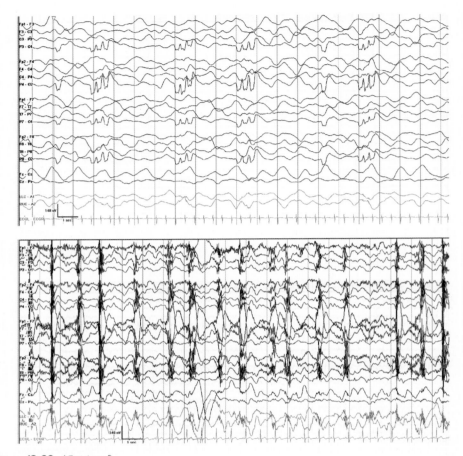

Figure 13-20. (*Continued*)

! CRITICAL CONSIDERATIONS

- The most established application of cEEG in the ICU is the detection and treatment of subclinical seizures and nonconvulsive status epilepticus.

- Quantification of seizure frequency and titration medications used to treat seizures can be facilitated using qEEG parameters.

- Ischemia can be detected using cEEG, and detection of DCI from vasospasm is one clinical application.

- Seizures are frequent in comatose patients in the medical ICU, particularly those with sepsis.

- The relationship between ICP and EEG patterns is poorly understood. It appears that EEG activity is not influenced by high ICP until cerebral perfusion pressure and cerebral blood flow are severely compromised.

- EEG may help guide sedation but is currently poorly studied in the ICU setting.
- The EEG may be used by the trained intensivist as an extension of the clinical examination. Phenomena like EEG reactivity to stimuli may serve as objective end points in clinical practice and potential clinical trials.
- Abnormal electrographic patterns frequently seen in the acute brain injury setting include depth seizures not seen on the surface, cortical spreading depression, and peri-infarct depolarization. All of these are poorly understood.

Neurocritical Care Monitoring

REFERENCES

1. Towne AR, Waterhouse EJ, Boggs JG, et al. Prevalence of nonconvulsive status epilepticus in comatose patients. *Neurology.* 2000;55:1421-1423.

2. Oddo M, Carrera E, Claassen J, et al. Continuous electroencephalography in the medical intensive care unit. *Crit Care Med.* 2009;37:2051-2056.

3. DeLorenzo RJ, Waterhouse EJ, Towne AR, et al. Persistent nonconvulsive status epilepticus after the control of convulsive status epilepticus. *Epilepsia.* 1998;39:833-840.

4. Treiman DM, Meyers PD, Walton NY, et al. A comparison of four treatments for generalized convulsive status epilepticus. Veterans Affairs Status Epilepticus Cooperative Study Group. *N Engl J Med.* 1998;339:792-798.

5. Claassen J, Mayer SA, Kowalski RG, et al. Detection of electrographic seizures with continuous EEG monitoring in critically ill patients. *Neurology.* 2004;62:1743-1748.

6. Suzuki A, Mori N, Hadeishi H. Computerized monitoring system in neurosurgical intensive care. *J Neurosci Methods.* 1988;26:133-139.

7. Bricolo A, Faccioli F, Grosslercher JC, et al. Electrophysiological monitoring in the intensive care unit. *Electroencephalogr Clin Neurophysiol Suppl.* 1987;39:255-263.

8. Chiappa KH, Ropper AH. Evoked potentials in clinical medicine (first of two parts). *N Engl J Med.* 1982;306(19):1140-1150.

9. Newton DE. Electrophysiological monitoring of general intensive care patients. *Intensive Care Med.* 1999;25:350-352.

10. Fleming RA, Smith NT. Density modulation—A technique for the display of three-variable data in patient monitoring. *Anesthesiology.* 1979;50:543-546.

11. Maynard DE, Jenkinson JL. The cerebral function analysing monitor. Initial clinical experience, application and further development. *Anaesthesia.* 1984;39:678-690.

12. Claassen J, Baeumer T, Hansen HC. Continuous EEG for monitoring on the neurological intensive care unit. New applications and uses for therapeutic decision making. *Nervenarzt.* 2000;71:813-821.

13. Frontera JA, Claassen J, Schmidt JM, et al. Prediction of symptomatic vasospasm after subarachnoid hemorrhage: The modified Fisher scale. *Neurosurgery.* 2006;59:21-27.

14. Claassen J, Hirsch LJ, Kreiter KT, et al. Quantitative continuous EEG for detecting delayed cerebral ischemia in patients with poor-grade subarachnoid hemorrhage. *Clin Neurophysiol.* 2004;115:2699-2710.

15. Vespa PM, Nuwer MR, Juhász C, et al. Early detection of vasospasm after acute subarachnoid hemorrhage using continuous EEG ICU monitoring. *Electroencephalogr Clin Neurophysiol.* 1997;103:607-615.

16. Alexandrov AV, Grotta JC. Arterial reocclusion in stroke patients treated with intravenous tissue plasminogen activator. *Neurology.* 2002;59:862-867.

17. Van Putten MJ, Tavy DL. Continuous quantitative EEG monitoring in hemispheric stroke patients using the brain symmetry index. *Stroke.* 2004;35:2489-2492.

18. Schneider AL, Jordan KG. Regional attenuation without delta (RAWOD): a distinctive EEG pattern that can aid in the diagnosis and management of severe acute ischemic stroke. *Am J Electroneurodiagnostic Technol.* 2005;45:102-117.

19. Finnigan SP, Rose SE, Walsh M, et al. Correlation of quantitative EEG in acute ischemic stroke with 30-day NIHSS score: comparison with diffusion and perfusion MRI. *Stroke.* 2004;35:899-903.

20. Rose SE, Janke AL, Griffin M, et al. Improved prediction of final infarct volume using bolus delay-corrected perfusion-weighted MRI: implications for the ischemic penumbra. *Stroke.* 2004;35:2466-2471.

21. Claassen J, Hirsch LJ, Kreiter KT, et al. Quantitative continuous EEG for detecting delayed cerebral ischemia in patients with poor-grade subarachnoid hemorrhage. *Clin Neurophysiol.* 2004;115: 2699-2710.

22. Vespa PM, Nenov V, Nuwer MR. Continuous EEG monitoring in the intensive care unit: early findings and clinical efficacy. *J Clin Neurophysiol.* 1999;16:1-13.

23. Simmons LE, Riker RR, Prato BS, et al. Assessing sedation during intensive care unit mechanical ventilation with the Bispectral Index and the Sedation-Agitation Scale. *Crit Care Med.* 1999;27: 1499-1504.

24. Prichep LS, Gugino LD, John ER, et al. The Patient State Index as an indicator of the level of hypnosis under general anaesthesia. *Br J Anaesth.* 2004;92:393-399.

25. Bauerle K, Greim CA, Schroth M, et al. Prediction of depth of sedation and anaesthesia by the Narcotrend EEG monitor. *Br J Anaesth.* 2004;92:841-845.

26. Waziri A, Claassen J, Stuart RM, et al. Intracortical electroencephalography in acute brain injury. *Ann Neurol.* 2009;66:366-377.

27. Stuart RM, Waziri A, Weintraub D, et al. Intracortical EEG for the detection of vasospasm in patients with poor-grade subarachnoid hemorrhage. *Neurocrit Care.* 2010;13:355-358.

28. Claassen J, Schmidt MJ, Tu B, et al. Seizures and ictal patterns on depth EEG monitoring after subarachnoid hemorrhage. *Epilepsia* [abstract]. In press.

29. Bragin A, Wilson CL, Staba RJ, et al. Interictal high-frequency oscillations (80-500 Hz) in the human epileptic brain: entorhinal cortex. *Ann Neurol.* 2002;52:407-415.

30. Schevon CA, Ng SK, Cappell J, et al. Microphysiology of epileptiform activity in human neocortex. *J Clin Neurophysiol.* 2008;25:321-330.

31. Worrell GA, Gardner AB, Stead SM, et al. High-frequency oscillations in human temporal lobe: simultaneous microwire and clinical macroelectrode recordings. *Brain.* 2008;131(Pt 4):928-937.

32. Schevon CA, Trevelyan AJ, Schroeder CE, et al. Spatial characterization of interictal high frequency oscillations in epileptic neocortex. *Brain.* 2009; 132(Pt 11):3047-3059.

33. Stead M, Bower M, Brinkmann BH, et al. Microseizures and the spatiotemporal scales of human partial epilepsy. *Brain.* 2010;133:2789-2797.

34. Dreier JP, Woitzik J, Fabricius M, et al. Delayed ischemic neurological deficits after subarachnoid hemorrhage are associated with clusters of spreading depolarizations. *Brain.* 2006;129(Pt 12):3224-3237.

35. Dohmen C, Sakowitz OW, Fabricius M, et al. Co-Operative Study of Brain Injury Depolarizations (COSBID). Spreading depolarizations occur in human ischemic stroke with high incidence. *Ann Neurol.* 2008;63:720-728.

36. Fabricius M, Fuhr S, Bhatia R, et al. Cortical spreading depression and peri-infarct depolarization in acutely injured human cerebral cortex. *Brain.* 2006;129(Pt 3):778-790.

37. Young GB, Doig G, Ragazzoni A. Anoxic-ischemic encephalopathy: clinical and electrophysiological associations with outcome. *Neurocrit Care.* 2005;2: 159-164.

38. Wijdicks EF, Hijdra A, Young GB, et al. Quality Standards Subcommittee of the American Academy of Neurology. Practice parameter: prediction of outcome in comatose survivors after cardiopulmonary resuscitation (an evidence-based review): Report of the Quality Standards Subcommittee of the American Academy of Neurology. *Neurology.* 2006;67:203-210.

39. Bernard SA, Gray TW, Buist MD, et al. Treatment of comatose survivors of out-of-hospital cardiac arrest with induced hypothermia. *N Engl J Med.* 2002;346: 557-563.

40. Bleck TP, Smith MC, Pierre-Louis SJ, et al. Neurologic complications of critical medical illnesses. *Crit Care Med.* 1993;21:98-103.

41. Abou Khaled KJ, Hirsch LJ. Advances in the management of seizures and status epilepticus in critically ill patients. *Crit Care Clin.* 2006;22:637-659.

42. Razvi SS, Bone I. Neurological consultations in the medical intensive care unit. *J Neurol Neurosurg Psychiatry.* 2003;74(suppl 3):16-23.

43. Barlas I, Oropello JM, Benjamin E. Neurologic complications in intensive care. *Curr Opin Crit Care.* 2001;7:68-73.

44. Jette N, Claassen J, Emerson RG, et al. Frequency and predictors of nonconvulsive seizures during continuous electroencephalographic monitoring in critically ill children. *Arch Neurol.* 2006;63:1750-1755.

45. Oddo M, Carrera E, Claassen J, et al. Continuous electroencephalography in the medical intensive care unit. *Crit Care Med.* 2009;37:2051-2056.

46. Young GB. Continuous EEG monitoring in the ICU. *Acta Neurol Scand.* 2006;114:67-68.

47. Kull LL, Emerson RG. Continuous EEG monitoring in the intensive care unit: Technical and staffing considerations. *J Clin Neurophysiol.* 2005;22:107-118.

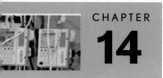

14

Multimodality Neuromonitoring

Raimund Helbok, MD
Pedro Kurtz, MD
Jan Claassen, MD, PhD

A 34-year-old right-handed woman with history of smoking presented with a sudden onset of severe occipital headache followed by loss of consciousness that started while cleaning her bathroom. In the emergency department, she was found to be arousable to deep stimulation, her pupils were very sluggish and almost nonreactive at 3-mm diameter, and she was withdrawing to painful stimulation bilaterally. When her mental status further declined, she was intubated for airway protection. Head computerized tomographic (CT) scanning (Figure 14-1) revealed subarachnoid hemorrhage (SAH) with thick blood filling the basal cisterns, hydrocephalus, and bilateral intraventricular hemorrhage (IVH). CT angiography revealed an aneurysm of the anterior communicating artery (ACoM). She was transferred to the nearest tertiary medical care center.

Cerebral angiography revealed an 8 cm × 4 cm ACoM aneurysm which was coiled on SAH day 1 (Figure 14-2). Additionally, angiography revealed severe, bilateral anterior cerebral artery vasospasm, which improved after treatment with 12 mg of intra-arterial (IA) verapamil. The postprocedural CT scan revealed global cerebral edema and worsening hydrocephalus. An external ventricular drainage catheter was placed. Postoperatively, the patient was found to be in coma with intact brainstem reflexes, bilateral posturing to painful stimulation, and bilateral positive Babinski signs. At that time, the treating physicians decided to place a multimodality neuromonitoring bundle through a right frontal burr hole consisting of a parenchymal intracranial pressure (ICP) monitor, a brain tissue oxygenation probe, and a microdialysis catheter.

What is the purpose of invasive neuromonitoring in comatose patients?

One of the most important goals of neurologic critical care is to detect secondary brain injury at a time when permanent damage can still be prevented. The clinical examination remains the gold standard for the assessment of patients with neurologic disease despite great advances in neuroimaging and other diagnostic tools. Furthermore, in medical intensive care unit (ICU) patients, daily interruption of sedation has been shown to decrease the duration of mechanical ventilation, shorten hospital stay, and, in combination with spontaneous breathing trials, lead to improved outcome.[1,2] There is some evidence suggesting that daily interruption of sedation is safe even in patients with brain injury,[3] but this remains controversial.[4] Clearly, there are a number of patients with acute brain injury in whom interruption of sedation is contraindicated such as those with ongoing status epilepticus, severe ICP crises, or respiratory failure requiring sedation. Comatose and sedated patients with brain injury are often compared to a "black box" when assessing the neurologic status.

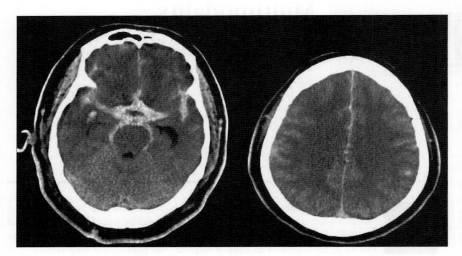

Figure 14-1. Selected cuts of the admission head computed tomography without contrast demonstrating diffuse filling of the basal cisterns (*left image*) and signs of diffuse global edema (*right image*).

Using clinical parameters alone, it may be difficult to differentiate changes in brain physiology that warrant interventions from medication effects. Clinical examinations lack sensitivity to detect some secondary complications such as nonconvulsive status epilepticus (NCSE)[5] or silent infarction.[6] Inter- and intra-rater reliability may be a factor to consider depending on the skill of the examiner.[7]

Commonly used clinical scales may be too crude to detect secondary complications. The most widely used clinical scale in the ICU environment is the Glasgow Coma Scale (GCS),[8] which was developed to facilitate rapid communication between first responders and specialized brain-injury units to triage traumatic brain injury (TBI) patients. This widely used scale does not reliably detect secondary complications and has been shown in some studies to have poor predictive power for outcome.[9] More recently, modifications such as the FOUR score have been proposed,[10] but likely these will not be adequate monitors to detect secondary injury in brain-injured patients.[11] Invasive monitoring of the brain has the advantage of allowing real-time continuous assessment of

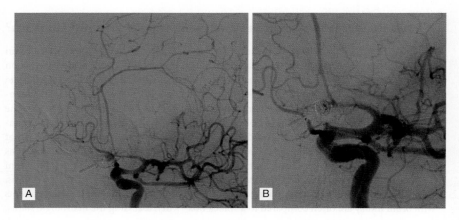

Figure 14-2. A. Cerebral angiography demonstrating an 8 cm × 4 cm anterior communicating artery aneurysm and severe vasospasm. **B.** The patient underwent coil embolization of the aneurysm.

brain physiology and has been shown to be safe.[12-14] Additionally, as outlined below, neuromonitoring may be used to quantify the effect of interventions and prognosticate the outcome.

Which monitoring devices should be placed in this patient?

The most established monitoring technique to assess ICP can be accomplished with probes placed in, for example, the ventricle, brain parenchyma, subarachnoid space, or subdural space. Most commonly, intraventricular or intraparenchymal monitoring probes are used because of safety and accuracy concerns. Measuring ICP allows calculation of cerebral perfusion pressure (CPP) using the simple formula: CPP = mean arterial pressure (MAP) − ICP. Importantly, the CPP reflects a global assessment of the pressure gradient that should not be confused with the amount of blood flow to the brain, called the cerebral blood flow (CBF), or an assessment of brain metabolism or oxygenation status ($Pbto_2$). Currently, no consensus exists regarding the selection of monitoring devices for specific patient groups. The selection of devices needs to be made based on the questions that the clinician wants to have answered for a specific patient and based on local experience with monitoring devices. An overview about existing monitoring devices separated by their spatial and temporal data resolution is displayed in Table 14-1. Findings from just one device may be more difficult to interpret than

Table 14-1. Choices of Neuromonitoring Devices

Monitored phenomenon or physiology	High spatial resolution[a]	High temporal resolution[a]
Intracranial pressure	NA	Pressure monitors inserted into the ventricle, brain parenchyma, subarachnoid or subdural space
Neuronal injury	Imaging techniques (ie, apparent diffusion coefficient or diffusion tensor imaging on MRI)	Microdialysis (ie, glycerol)
Large white matter tracts	MRI diffusion tensor imaging, evoked potentials	Continuous evoked potentials
Large blood vessels	Digital subtraction, MR or CT angiography, duplex	Continuous duplex
Flow velocity in blood vessels	TCD (large vessels)	Continuous TCD
Brain perfusion	MR or CT perfusion, arterial spin labeling, SPECT, PET	Thermal diffusion-based microcatheter, near-infrared spectroscopy
Neuronal activity and function	Functional MRI, resting state MRI	cEEG, intracortical EEG
Tissue oxygenation	PET	Clark electrode measuring partial brain tissue oxygenation, near-infrared spectroscopy
Cerebral metabolism	PET, MR spectroscopy, resting state MRI	Microdialysis, difference calculated between arterial and jugular venous oxygenation

Abbreviations: cEEG, continuous electroencephalography; CT, computed tomography; EEG, electroencephalography; MRI, magnetic resonance imaging; NA, not applicable; PET, positron emission tomography; SPECT, single-photon emission computed tomography; TCD, transcranial Doppler.

[a]Here, spatial resolution refers to the ability to visualize brain structure or function, whereas temporal resolution refers to the ability to monitor specific physiologic phenomena over time.

Neurocritical Care Monitoring

a more complete assessment that quantifies pressure, metabolism, and oxygenation status at the same time. Additionally, CBF monitors and intracranial electroencephalographic (EEG) monitoring are being used in some centers.[15,16] Bedside monitoring facilitates immediate detection of changing brain physiology and allows targeted treatment before obvious and often irreversible clinical deterioration occurs.[17] However, the use of invasive neuromonitoring remains controversial.[13,18-20]

In this patient, we selected ICP monitoring because of the high risk for intracranial hypertension (both with external ventricular drainage catheter [EVD] and parenchymal catheter). Additionally, we initiated brain oxygen tension (Pbto$_2$) and neurochemical monitoring (cerebral microdialysis) because of the high risk of secondary complications in this patient including ischemia from vasospasm.

Where should monitoring devices be placed?

All monitoring devices discussed above measure local brain physiology. Knowledge about catheter location is crucial for the treating neurointensivist in order to correctly interpret the collected data. Currently, no consensus exists regarding the desired placement of devices in relation to injured brain tissue. Generally, most practitioners recommend placement in tissue at highest risk for secondary complications. In patients with spontaneous SAH, the tissue at highest risk for vasospasm and delayed cerebral ischemia (DCI) are those in the area perfused by the ruptured artery.[21] However, vasospasm is a diffuse pathology and delayed ischemia may occur in a distant area. Therefore, local invasive neuromonitoring may miss the onset of DCI. In patients with focal brain injury such as intracranial hemorrhage (ICH), cerebral contusion, or a well-demarcated area of hypodensity in a vascular distribution consistent with an infarct, a perilesional placement is generally attempted. Currently used placement techniques at the bedside through a burr hole are not very accurate in reaching this goal. Placement of neuromonitoring devices inside the lesion, that is, within an infarct or hemorrhage, will not yield any meaningful data.[12] Using a CT-guided neuronavigated approach may allow for more accurate perilesional catheter placement. In patients with a diffuse or nonfocal injury (diffuse SAH, multifocal bilateral injuries, global cerebral edema, confined IVH), the neuromonitoring devices are generally placed in the frontal lobe of the nondominant hemisphere. A CT scan after neuromonitoring device placement is recommended to determine probe location and to detect procedure-related complications such as bleeding.

What are the complications of invasive neuromonitoring?

In the absence of large multicenter trials, no exact numbers are known but the most significant complications include intracerebral, subdural, or epidural bleeding; encephalitis or meningitis; and device malfunctioning or misplacement.[22,23] A major bleeding risk is higher in patients who receive an antiplatelet agent such as clopidogrel or aspirin. Caution is warranted in those receiving antiplatelet agents and those with a low platelet count or dysfunctional platelets (ie, during uremia). Most series report an infection risk of 5% or lower,[23,24] while antibiotic prophylaxis remains controversial.[23-25]

When should Pbto$_2$ be monitored?

Based on very little data, there are recommendations for Pbto$_2$ monitoring in patients with TBI. Guidelines from the Brain Trauma Foundation recommend monitoring of brain tissue oxygen tension (Pbto$_2$) or jugular venous oxygen saturation (Svjo$_2$) if hyperventilation is used (level III).[26] Further, it is advised to address brain tissue oxygen tension levels below 15 mm Hg with appropriate treatment strategies (level III).[27] For other diagnoses there are no recommendations to be found. SAH guidelines published in 2009 by the American Heart Association do not address the issue of Pbto$_2$ measurement.[28]

Pbto$_2$ is a marker of the balance between oxygen delivery and oxygen consumption in brain cells. Pbto$_2$ is assessed using a Clark electrode that samples the tension of oxygen in the extracellular fluid, reflecting a small volume of brain (17 mm^3) at the distal end of the probe. The health of the brain tissue that is monitored with the probe significantly correlates with the behavior of the brain oxygen measurements.[29,30] In healthy normal brain, $Pbto_2$ is 25 to 35 mm Hg at all times, and there is a good correlation between CPP and $Pbto_2$ when $Pbto_2$ is low, suggesting intact autoregulation. In dead brain tissue, $Pbto_2$ levels are generally less than 5 mm Hg and no correlation with CPP is observed. If the probe is placed in the penumbra, $Pbto_2$ may be low and there is a general correlation with CPP, suggesting disturbed autoregulation.[29,30]

A number of studies found a good correlation between a low $Pbto_2$ (less than 15 mm Hg) and poor outcome after SAH[31] and in TBI patients.[13,30,32-36] However, from these data, it is not clear if the low $Pbto_2$ is just a surrogate marker for the extent of brain injury. The idea behind cerebral oxygen monitoring is to address these changes to hypoxic values with appropriate treatment strategies. $Pbto_2$-guided therapy to prevent hypoxic brain injury has been associated with improved outcome in uncontrolled, single-center trials.[20,37,38] Based on this finding, a multicenter randomized controlled trial in patients with severe TBI (GCS 8 or less) is under way (National Institute of Neurological Disease and Stroke [NINDS]–funded phase II trial entitled Randomized Controlled Trial of Brain Tissue Oxygenation Monitoring).

 In our patient, the bundle was placed into the right frontal white matter. Biochemical analyses revealed lactate-to-pyruvate ratio (LPR) values ranging between 22 and 29 and brain glucose in the range of 0.8 to 1.2 mmol/L. $PbtO_2$ was 22 mm Hg. The patient developed ventilator-associated pneumonia, which was treated with aminopenicillin. Clinical examination showed improvement with normal brainstem reflexes and withdrawal responses to painful stimulation. Routine transcranial Doppler (TCD) sonography revealed normal velocity in anterior and posterior circulation. On day 5, $PbtO_2$ dropped to 10 mm Hg without a change in brain metabolism or the clinical examination.

What is the meaning of the decrease in $PbtO_2$ and how should the patient be treated?

What we measure with $Pbto_2$ is the balance between oxygen delivery and oxygen consumption in brain cells. $Pbto_2$ may be influenced by a whole host of different local factors including oxygen consumption of neurons and glia, oxygen diffusion conditions and gradients in the sampled brain tissue, the number of perfused capillaries per tissue volume, the length and diameter of perfused capillaries, the capillary perfusion rate and microflow pattern, and the hemoglobin oxygen release in the microcirculation. Systemic factors that may influence $Pbto_2$ measurements include arterial blood pressure, ICP, Pao_2, $Paco_2$, pH, temperature, the blood Hgb content, blood viscosity, and the hematocrit.

One study suggests that local brain tissue oxygen tension is more closely related to CBF and the diffusion of dissolved plasma oxygen rather than total oxygen delivery to the brain and oxygen metabolism of the brain cell.[39] Strategies to influence low $Pbto_2$ are multiple and should be decided on an individual basis (Figure 14-3). While $Pbto_2$ may increase in one patient after CPP optimization or improvement of cardiac function, other patients may benefit from an increase in oxygen transport capacity (blood transfusion). Additional monitoring devices (CBF, brain temperature, EEG) may be helpful for the clinician to narrow down the differential diagnosis of a low $Pbto_2$.

Low $Pbto_2$ values may be observed without changes in brain metabolism as this strongly depends on the duration of brain hypoxia. Basic strategies to minimize oxygen consumption of the brain include aggressive fever management, treatment of shivering,[40,41] management of pain and agitation (sedation and adequate analgesia), and optimization of positioning of the upper part of the body (30 degrees or more).

Basic principles

- Aggressive fever management
- Adequate sedation-analgesia to prevent pain and agitation
- Treatment of shivering
- Optimized body positioning (30°)
- Treatment of elevated ICP
- $CO_2 \geq 35$ mm Hg unless ICP >20 mm Hg
  → Individual cutoff based on correlation
  of CO_2/$Pbto_2$ and $Pbto_2$/CBF

↓

CPP optimization

1. **Intravascular volume status**
   SVV (< 10%)
   GEDI (600-800 mL/m^2)
   PAWP (10-14 mm Hg)
2. **Optimization of cardiac output**
   Preload (volume challenge, bolus)
   Inotropic agents (dobutamine 2-20 µg/kg/min)
3. **Titration of MAP to $Pbto_2$ > 20 mm Hg**
   Levophed (2-20 µg/min)
   Phenylephrine

↓

ICP < 20 mm Hg

- CSF diversion by EVD
- Sedation and analgesia
- Surgical decompression
- Short-term hyperventilation
- Osmotic agents
  - Mannitol (1-1.5 g/kg IV bag infused over 30 min, q6h;
    avoid serum Osm > 360 mOsm/L, Osm gap > 10)
  - Hypertonic saline 23.4% (30 mL over 5 min IV, q4-6h;
    avoid serum Na > 160 mg/dL)
- Therapeutic hypothermia
- EEG-guided barbiturate coma

↓

Blood transfusion

- Can be considered, specially in SAH patients with severe vasospasm
- Increase oxygen capacity to the brain and may increase $Pbto_2$
- No convincing effect on brain metabolism so far

Hyperoxia

- Increases brain tissue oxygen tension
- So far no convincing effect on brain metabolism

↓

Decreasing metabolic need of brain tissue

- Treatment of seizures
- Treatment of fever, maybe hypothermia
- Treatment of raised ICP

Figure 14-3. Treatment options to increase brain tissue oxygen tension ($Pbto_2$). CPP, cerebral perfusion pressure; CSF, cerebrospinal fluid; EEG, electroencephalography; EVD, extraventricular drainage; GEDI, global end-diastolic index; ICP, intracranial pressure; MAP, mean arterial pressure; PAWP, pulmonary capillary wedge pressure; SAH, subarachnoid hemorrhage; SVV, stroke volume variation.

The following text questions use a correlational data analysis approach to better understand brain physiology in the acute brain injury setting. This approach may help clinicians to understand complex physiologic relationships and identify optimal physiologic targets in real time. Additionally, the behavior of physiologic parameters in relation to interventions (eg, increasing MAP/CPP, optimizing cardiac output, decreasing ICP, blood transfusion, ventilator strategies) may identify individualized thresholds such as MAP goals and assess cerebral autoregulation.

What is the relationship between CO_2 and $PbtO_2$?

In general there is a close relationship between $PbtO_2$ and $PacO_2$ as well as end-tidal CO_2 (Figure 14-4). Hyperventilation leads to cerebral vasoconstriction and may cause infarction. In TBI patients, hyperventilation is only recommended as a temporizing measure for increased ICP (level III) and should not be used in the first 24 hours after head injury (Level III).[26] Prophylactic hyperventilation is not recommended (level II), and if hyperventilation is used, jugular venous oxygen saturation ($SvjO_2$) or brain tissue oxygen tension ($PbtO_2$) measurements are recommended to monitor oxygen delivery (level III).[26]

Neurocritical Care Monitoring

 In our patient, we chose a CO_2 target of 30 to 33 mm Hg using end-tidal CO_2 measurements.

How do you interpret Figure 14-5 and what are treatment options?

Figure 14-5 illustrates the tight correlation between CPP and $PbtO_2$ in our patient during a 24-hour monitoring period. Brain tissue hypoxia ($PbtO_2$ less than 15 mm Hg) is observed at CPP values of 90 mm Hg and

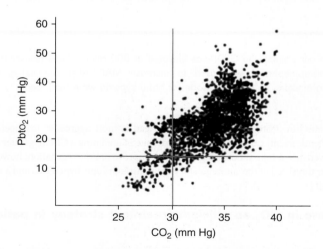

Figure 14-4. This figure illustrates the correlation between end-tidal CO_2 and $PbtO_2$ in our patient. Monitoring of CO_2 is crucial even in awake patients after severe brain injury. Despite these recommendations, a recent survey conducted in Europe showed that prophylactic hyperventilation (30-35 mm Hg) is still commonly used after severe traumatic brain injury.[42] Additionally, these investigators found that $PbtO_2$ or $SvjO_2$ monitoring is rarely implemented even if patients were hyperventilated to a level below 30 mm Hg. A low CO_2 level is associated with tissue hypoxia after severe head injury, and unintentional spontaneous hyperventilation may be a common and underrecognized cause of brain tissue hypoxia after severe brain injury.[43,44]

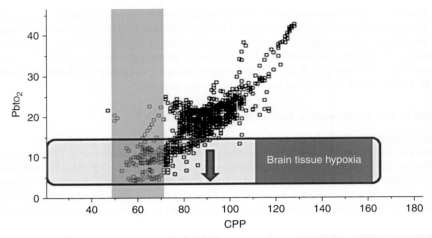

Figure 14-5. Correlation of cerebral perfusion pressure (CPP) and Pbto₂ over 24-hour time period. Every dot represents a specific time point during 24 hours of CPP and the corresponding Pbto₂ value.

lower. There are several treatment options to optimize CPP in this patient. As a first step, the intravascular volume status should be optimized, which may be estimated using a clinical assessment or monitored parameters such as the stroke volume variation, the global end-diastolic index (GEDI), or the pulmonary artery wedge pressure. If optimizing volume status does not result in improved CPP and Pbto₂ numbers, MAP may be titrated up to achieve Pbto₂ improvements greater than 20 mm Hg. Depending on cardiac performance (which can be estimated using the cardiac index or the ejection fraction), this can be achieved using pressors including norepinephrine, phenylephrine, milrinone, dobutamine, or dopamine.

In our patient, the GEDI was elevated at 800 after volume resuscitation and Levophed (norepinephrine) was used to increase MAP. After optimizing these physiologic parameters, no further episodes of brain hypoxia were seen. See Figure 14-6.

This case illustrates how Pbto₂-guided therapy may lead to more aggressive management. Additionally, hypoxic and ischemic events can also be observed despite maintaining a CPP of greater than 70 mm Hg in patients with severe brain injury. Lowering CPP may improve brain oxygenation; however, once the CPP reaches the lower threshold of the autoregulatory breakthrough zone, hyperemia and a secondary increase in ICP may result (Figure 14-7).[45]

Is an increase in FIO₂ an efficient treatment strategy in patients with low Pbto₂?

Increasing FIO₂ effectively increases local brain oxygen partial pressure. However, this does not necessarily lead to an improvement in brain metabolism. What has been described is a simultaneous decrease in lactate and pyruvate, leaving the lactate-to-pyruvate ratio overall unchanged. This would suggest that hyperoxia may lead to retardation of the metabolism rather than stimulation.[46] Another study showed that hyperoxia may decrease brain lactate levels.[47] Contrarily, hyperbaric hyperoxygenation may have a positive effect on Pbto₂ and brain metabolism.[48]

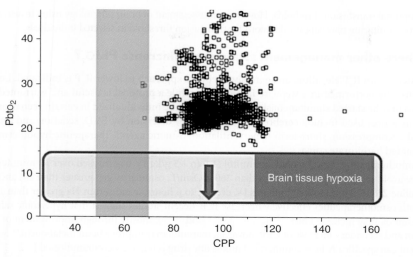

Figure 14-6. Correlation of CPP and Pbto$_2$ over 24-hour time period after fluid resuscitation with 1000 mL normal saline and initiation of vasopressor therapy using norepinephrine.

Our patient's hemoglobin was 8.5 mg/dL with a PbtO$_2$ level below 12 mm Hg. Should this patient be transfused?

Blood transfusions increase oxygen transport capacity to the brain and have been shown to increase Pbto$_2$ after severe head injury without improving brain metabolism.[49] In a randomized controlled trial, a transfusion threshold of less than 7 mg/dL was not associated with increased 30-day mortality rate in critically ill patients.[50] For neurologic ICU (NeuroICU, NICU) patients, there is conflicting evidence about the optimal transfusion threshold. Decisions regarding blood transfusions in patients with SAH must be individualized because optimal transfusion triggers are not known (level III).[51] Currently, there are a number of trials underway to compare different transfusion thresholds for SAH patients.[51-56] Subpopulations of SAH patients such as those with ongoing DCI from vasospasm may benefit from higher transfusion thresholds (ie, keeping hemoglobin greater than 10 mg/dL).[55,57] Patients with moderate-to-severe TBI do not benefit from a "liberal" transfusion strategy (level II).[51] Recent reports on multimodal neuromonitoring and hemoglobin suggest that low hemoglobin is associated with brain metabolic distress (LPR greater than 40) and low cerebral glucose concentration (less than 0.7 mmol/L).[49,58] Currently, data are too preliminary to

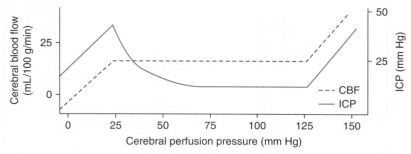

Figure 14-7. Idealized relationship between cerebral perfusion pressure and cerebral blood flow (CBF) with intact autoregulation. ICP, intracranial pressure. *(Modified from Mayer SA CJ. Critical care management of increased intracranial pressure. J Intensive Care Med. 2002;17:55-67.)*

define optimal transfusion thresholds. However, the assessment of brain physiology using invasive multi-modality monitoring may support decisions for transfusion threshold in selected individuals.

Are there other management strategies to increase PbtO$_2$?

For patients with ICP elevation, an aggressive stepwise approach to lower ICP is indicated. Lowering ICP is usually performed in a stepwise fashion, and while a protocol is useful and warranted, interventions may be started simultaneously and may need to be individualized in certain scenarios. Some of the measures used include cerebrospinal fluid (CSF) diversion by EVD, sedation and analgesia, surgical decompression, short-term hyperventilation, osmotic agents, therapeutic hypothermia, and EEG-guided barbiturate coma.

Osmotherapeutic agents include mannitol (1.0 to 1.5 g/kg IV bag infused over 30 minutes, every 6 hours; avoid serum osmolarity greater than 360 mOsm/L, osmolarity gap greater than 10) and hypertonic saline 23.4% (30 mL over 5 minutes IV, every 4 to 6 hours, avoid serum Na greater than 160 mg/dL). Both osmotherapeutics effectively decrease ICP. Recent studies suggest that hypertonic saline, but not mannitol, may increase PbtO$_2$[59,60] (Figures 14-8 and 14-9), mostly through improvement of cardiac function and secondary increase of CPP; however, mannitol may improve brain metabolism.[61] So far, no treatment can specifically be recommended unless one drug is relatively contraindicated (Figure 14-10).

Does optimization of cardiac performance in patients with normal ICP improve oxygenation status?

Yes, it may. As shown in Figure 14-11, cerebral oxygenation, as measured by PbtO$_2$, may improve with increased cardiac output. Carbon dioxide can be optimized with the use of inotropic agents in volume-resuscitated patients with inadequate cardiac output or through the infusion of fluids in preload-responsive patients. In patients with inadequate oxygen delivery to the brain despite normal ICP and CPP, the improvement in cardiac performance may further optimize cerebral blood flow and potentially improve aerobic metabolism.

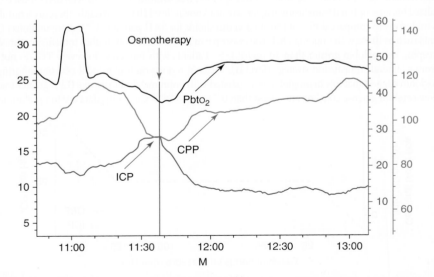

Figure 14-8. The *green arrow* in this graph indicates the time of administration of osmotherapy for the treatment of elevated intracranial pressure (ICP) (> 20 mm Hg). Following osmotherapy, ICP decreased and both cerebral perfusion pressure (CPP) and PbtO$_2$ improved. (Note: This graph is taken from a different patient from the one discussed in this case.)

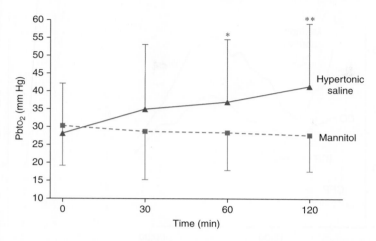

Figure 14-9. Line graph illustrating mean (SD) brain tissue oxygen pressure (Pbto$_2$) at baseline (time 0) and at 30, 60, and 120 minutes after hypertonic saline and mannitol bolus administration. *P = .05; **P = .01 for comparisons between the two treatments. *(From Oddo M, Levine JM, Frangos S, et al. Effect of mannitol and hypertonic saline on cerebral oxygenation in patients with severe traumatic brain injury and refractory intracranial hypertension. J Neurol Neurosurg Psychiatry. 2009;80:916-920.)*[59]

Can a correlational analysis of multimodality parameters be used to assess autoregulatory status?

Yes. It has been known for more than a decade that there is a relationship between the autoregulatory status of a patient and the arterial blood pressure (BP) versus ICP correlation.[62] This has been termed the pressure reactivity index (PRx) and is calculated as a moving correlation between BP and ICP.

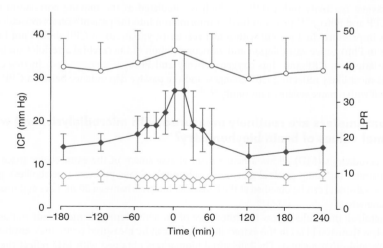

Figure 14-10. Line graph that shows the average time course of lactate-to-pyruvate ratio (LPR), intracranial pressure (ICP), and brain tissue oxygen pressure before (−180 min to 0), at (time = 0), and after (0-240 min) mannitol 20% infusion. LPR is calculated as a ratio between the lactate and the pyruvate and is discussed in Table 14-3. Error bars represent means and 1 standard error of n = 22 individual trials. *(From Helbok RKS, Schmidt JM, Kurtz P, et al. Effect of mannitol on brain metabolism and tissue oxygenation in severe hemorrhagic stroke. J Neurol Neurosurg Psychiatry. 2011;82:378-383.)*

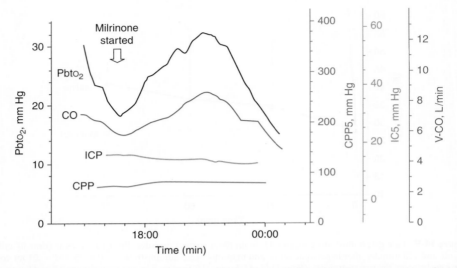

Figure 14-11. Multimodality parameters during a trial of milrinone with resultant improvement in cardiac output and improved $Pbto_2$ without changes in intracranial pressure (ICP) or cerebral perfusion pressure (CPP) in a woman with poor-grade subarachnoid hemorrhage and declining $Pbto_2$ levels despite normal cardiac output and CPP.

A negative correlation is seen in patients with vasoreactivity, whereas a positive correlation indicates a passive pressure response system and is seen in absent vasoreactivity (Figure 14-12).

Do any of the multimodality parameters allow further insight into the autoregulatory status?

Yes, the oxygen reactivity index (ORx), which is calculated as the moving correlation coefficient between CPP and $Pbto_2$,[63-65] provides further information into the patient's cerebrovascular response to changes in pressure. In a patient with intact reactivity, variations in CPP should not be reflected in changes in $Pbto_2$ since vasodilation and vasoconstriction of the cerebral arterioles should prevent passive variations in CBF and thus oxygen delivery and $Pbto_2$ (Figure 14-13). In this case, $Pbto_2$ variation is most likely reflecting CBF changes, and the passive dependence between CPP and $Pbto_2$ is associated with a more severe brain injury.[63-65]

Which parameters are routinely measured with microdialysis, and what are the normal values of brain biochemistry?

Cerebral microdialysis (MD) allows a neurochemical assessment of the extracellular space. Values of various substrates including cerebral glucose (= substrate), lactate, pyruvate (metabolites), glycerol, or glutamate (= substrate) can be obtained at the bedside at intervals between 20 minutes and usually 1 hour (routine parameters) (Figure 14-14).[66]

In general, all molecules below the cutoff size of the semipermeable membrane (either less than 20 kDa or less than 100 kDa) in the extracellular space can be measured (cytokines, antibiotics, anticonvulsants, and other agents). The interstitial biomarkers obtained with MD reflect the net effect of several processes: energy supply, diffusion, and consumption. A simplistic approach on changes in routine parameters obtained by cerebral MD is given in Table 14-2. A typical ischemic pattern includes a marked decrease in brain glucose, increase in LPR and LGR (lactate-to-glucose ratio), and a moderate increase in brain lactate and a decrease in brain pyruvate.[21]

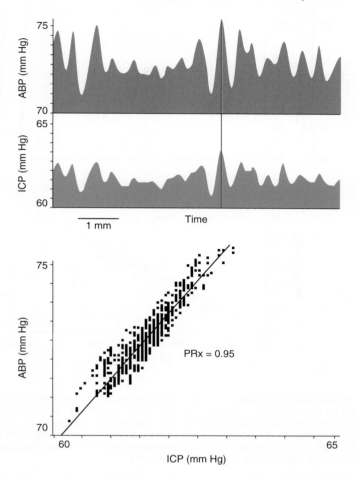

Figure 14-12. Pressure reactivity index calculated as the correlation coefficient between arterial and intracranial pressure in a patients with absent autoregulation. ABP, arterial blood pressure; ICP, intracranial pressure; PRx, pressure reactivity index. (*From Czosnyka M, Smielewski P, Kirkpatrick P, Laing RJ, Menon D, Pickard JD. Continuous assessment of the cerebral vasomotor reactivity in head injury. Neurosurgery. 1997;41:11-17; discussion 17-19.*)

Many other metabolites, including adenosine, inosine, hypoxanthine urate, glutathione, cysteine, glycine, and gamma-aminobutyric acid (GABA) have been studied and others such as taurine, interleukins, and a number of amino acids are under investigation.[21] The clinical role that these metabolites may play remains to be determined.

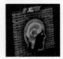 On day 6, our patient developed prolonged brain tissue hypoxia (PbtO$_2$) and worsening of brain metabolism with increasing LPR and decreasing brain glucose (Figure 14-15).

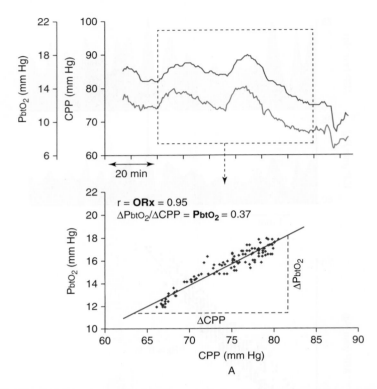

A

Figure 14-13. Moving correlation coefficient between cerebral perfusion pressure (CPP) and Pbto$_2$ variation. The panels on the left show a very close correlation between changes in CPP and Pbto$_2$ with an oxygen reactivity index (ORx) of 0.95, suggesting disturbed reactivity. The panels on the right show no correlation between CPP and Pbto$_2$ with an ORx of − 0.04, suggesting intact reactivity. *(From Jaeger M, Schuhmann MU, Soehle M, Meixensberger J. Continuous assessment of cerebrovascular autoregulation after traumatic brain injury using brain tissue oxygen pressure reactivity. Crit Care Med. 2006;34:1783-1788.)*

What is the relationship between PbtO$_2$ and brain metabolism, and what is the most likely cause for the increase in LPR and decreasing levels of brain glucose in this patient?

Prolonged episodes (more than 25 minutes) of profound brain tissue hypoxia (Pbto$_2$ less than 10 mm Hg) are associated with marked metabolic changes (including increasing MD-LPR and decreasing MD-glucose; see Figure 14-16).[67-69] MD-glucose, MD-lactate, MD-pyruvate, or lactate-to-pyruvate ratio may be indicators for the detection of secondary complications involving hypoxia or ischemia. Brain biochemistry may predict neurologic deterioration secondary to cerebral vasospasm even hours before the symptoms occur.[17] Poor outcome has been associated with elevated lactate, lactate-to-pyruvate ratio, and glutamate and low glucose in SAH [31,70-74] and TBI[75-77] patients.

The MD changes depicted in Figure 14-16 were observed on postbleed day 7, which was in the middle of the typical time period for the onset of vasospasm. Additionally, our patient was a high-risk patient, given that she had a high Hunt and Hess grade and a modified Fisher score of 4.[78] She also had already exhibited vasospasm on the admission

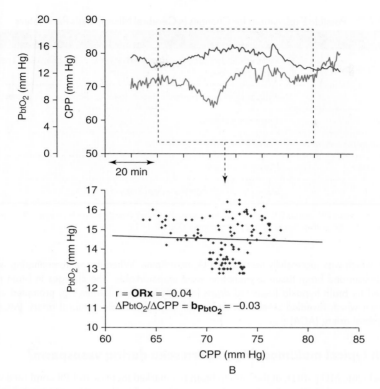

Figure 14-13. (*Continued.*)

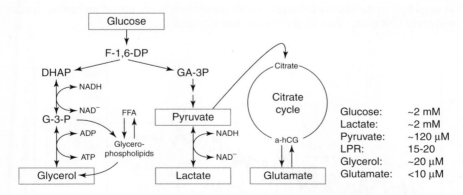

Glucose:	~2 mM
Lactate:	~2 mM
Pyruvate:	~120 µM
LPR:	15-20
Glycerol:	~20 µM
Glutamate:	<10 µM

Figure 14-14. The metabolites routinely measured at the bedside are shown in red boxes. The list on the right shows normal values of brain tissue metabolites in sedated patients (microdialysis membrane length: 10 mm; perfusion fluid rate 0.3 µL/min; membrane cutoff 20 kDa). ADP, adenosine diphosphate; ATP, adenosine triphosphate; DHAP, dihydroxyacetone phosphate; F-1,6-DP, fructose-1,6-diphosphatase; FFA, free fatty acid; G-3-P, glucose-3-phosphate; GA-3P, glyceraldehyde phosphate dehydrogenase; NAD, nicotinamide adenine dinucleotide; NADH, reduced nicotinamide adenine dinucleotide. (*From Hutchinson PJ, O'Connell MT, Al-Rawi PG, et al. Clinical cerebral microdialysis: A methodological study. J Neurosurg. 2000;93:37-43.*)

Table 14-2. Possible Explanations for Changes in Cerebral Microdialysis Parameters

Biomarker	Interpretation
↓ Glucose	Reduced capillary perfusion, decreased systemic supply, or increased cellular uptake of glucose
↑ Glucose	Hyperemia, increased systemic glucose levels, or decreased cellular metabolism
↑ Lactate	Anaerobic metabolism
↑ Lactate-to-pyruvate ratio	Marker of ischemia
↑ Glutamate	Marker of ischemia
↑ Glycerol	Destruction of cell membranes caused by energy failure

(From Hillered L, Vespa PM, Hovda DA. Translational neurochemical research in acute human brain injury: The current status and potential future for cerebral microdialysis. J Neurotrauma. 2005;22:3-41.)

angiogram, which was successfully treated with IA nicardipine. When the neuromonitoring was started, brain metabolism and brain tissue oxygenation were unremarkable. The changes in brain metabolism accompanied by brain hypoxia (repeated drops in PbtO$_2$ less than 10 mm Hg) prompted us to obtain an angiogram which revealed severe vasospasm of the right middle cerebral artery (MCA) and the anterior cerebral artery (ACA) (Figure 14-17).

What is a typical multimodality pattern seen during vasospasm?

A typical ischemic MD pattern of the human brain is a marked increase in LPR combined with a very low MD-glucose level.[79] Other biochemical changes observed in the setting of acutely brain-injured patients are summarized in Table 14-3, including the nonischemic glycolysis.[80]

Let us go back to the observed changes in brain metabolism in our patient prompting us to an angiogram: LPR greater than 40, glucose less than 0.7 mmol/L.

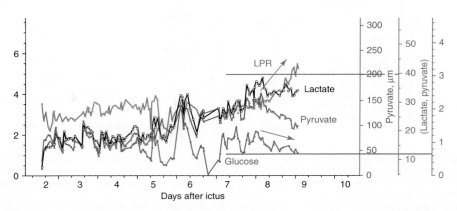

Figure 14-15. Microdialysis variables plotted over 10 days for our patient. Arrows demonstrate the change in LPR (*red arrow,* increase) and brain glucose (*green arrow,* decrease) to a level of lactate-pyruvate ratio (LPR) > 40 (*red line*) and brain glucose < 0.7 mmol/L (*green line*).

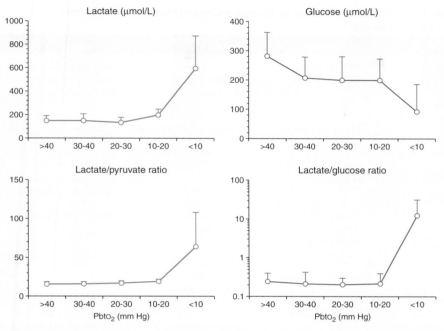

Figure 14-16. Lactate and lactate-to-pyruvate ratios rise and glucose drops with $Pbto_2$ levels < 10. *(From Hillered L, Vespa PM, Hovda DA. Translational neurochemical research in acute human brain injury: The current status and potential future for cerebral microdialysis. J Neurotrauma. 2005;22:3-41.)*

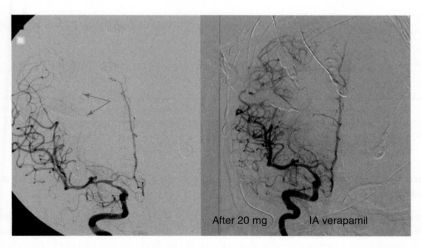

Figure 14-17. Cerebral angiography revealed severe vasospasm of the right middle cerebral artery and the anterior cerebral artery *(left image)*. Following administration of 20 mg of intra-arterial (IA) verapamil, radiographic improvement of cerebral vasospasm was documented *(right image)*. *Blue arrows* indicate the location of multimodal neuromonitoring probes.

Table 14-3. Possible Explanations for Changes in Cerebral Microdialysis Parameters and Treatment Options

Biomarker	Interpretation	Etiology	Intervention
↓ Glucose	Reduced capillary perfusion	Ischemia/hypoxia, vasospasm, edema, ICP crisis, hyperventilation	Increasing brain perfusion (address vasospasm, improve CPP, osmotherapy, normocapnia)
	Decreased systemic supply	Decreased or normal blood glucose	Adjustment of serum glucose
	Increased cellular uptake of glucose	Seizure, ICP crisis, shivering	Antiepileptic drugs, osmotherapy, antishivering management, sedation
↑ Glucose	Hyperemia, increased systemic supply, decreased cellular metabolism	Reperfusion, hyperglycemia, deep sedation	No specific intervention needed
↑ Lactate	Anaerobic metabolism	Ischemia/hypoxia, ICP crisis, hyperventilation	
↑ LPR and decreased pyruvate	Decreased oxygen delivery	Ischemia/hypoxia, vasospasm, edema, ICP crisis, hyperventilation	Improving brain perfusion, osmotherapy, blood transfusion (?), normocapnia
↑ LPR and normal or increased pyruvate	Increased oxygen consumption, mitochondrial dysfunction	Inflammation, fever, seizure	Fever control, temperature control, seizure control, sedation
↑ Glutamate	Excitotoxicity	Marker of ischemia (vasospasm, stroke, hyperventilation, ICP crisis), seizure	Improving brain perfusion, normocapnia, seizure control
↑ Glycerol	Destruction of cell membranes caused by energy failure	Ischemia/hypoxia (vasospasm, stroke), seizure	Improving brain perfusion, seizure control

Abbreviations: CPP, cerebral perfusion pressure; ICP, intracranial pressure; LPR, lactate-to-pyruvate ratio. (From Hillered L, Vespa PM, Hovda DA. Translational neurochemical research in acute human brain injury: The current status and potential future for cerebral microdialysis. J Neurotrauma. 2005;22:3-41.)

What are the definitions of metabolic distress and metabolic crisis (MC) and how do they affect outcome?

Metabolic distress is commonly defined as LPR greater than 40, whereas metabolic crisis comprises the combination of LPR greater than 40 and brain glucose less than 0.7 mmol/L.[21,79-81] Metabolic distress/crisis, therefore, is a composite value that reflects, in the direct measurement of brain glucose and its anaerobic and aerobic metabolites (lactate/pyruvate), the difference between energy supply and demand.[21,81] A reduction in energy supply can be caused by reduced CBF, which decreases the oxygen and glucose supply, resulting in a shift to anaerobic metabolism with increased brain lactate.[79] Alternatively, low glucose availability can lead to a decrease in brain pyruvate without an increase in lactate.[76,80] Elevated LPR with and without low MD-glucose, high brain-serum glucose variability, high MD-lactate, and high MD-glutamate concentration, measured in the interstitial space by MD, have been linked with poor outcome in patients with acute brain injury (including TBI and SAH patients).[70-76,82-84] The etiology of MC is diverse, including low CPP, elevated ICP, spreading depolarizations, and others.[83-86]

Our patient was treated with 20 mg IA verapamil. What are the expected hemodynamic changes and how may IA calcium channel blockers affect brain homeostasis?

IA calcium channel blockers are a treatment option in severe vasospasm (papaverine, verapamil, nicardipine, nimodipine).[87-93] Awareness of side effects, depending on the half-life of the drug, and the total dose given is warranted. Cerebral vasodilation may cause intracranial hypertension, which lasted for 3 hours after high-dose IA verapamil in a small series of SAH patients (Figure 14-18).[22,87,88,94] Furthermore, CPP may decrease secondary to a drop in MAP as a systemic side effect. Close hemodynamic monitoring up to 12 hours following treatment is necessary. Preliminary data suggest that brain metabolism is not affected by this intervention; however, an increased brain perfusion may result in increase of substrate delivery (glucose) to the brain.[94]

What is the relationship between serum glucose and brain glucose, and how should this patient be managed?

There is generally a close correlation between serum and brain glucose, which renders the central nervous system vulnerable to episodes of hypoglycemia (Figure 14-19). A critical threshold for MD-glucose is generally believed to be 0.7 mmol/L. Tight glucose control (4.4 to 6.2 mmol/L) with intravenous insulin was implemented in a large number of ICUs after 2001, when a randomized controlled trial showed the survival benefit of surgical ICU patients.[95] However, the results could not be replicated in mixed populations of critically ill patients, mostly because of hypoglycemic episodes in the tight glycemic controlled group,[96] and a recent study actually favored a more liberal glucose regimen (less than 180 mg/dL).[97] Multimodal neuromonitoring studies showed that tight glycemic control may be associated with MC in severely brain-injured patients (Figure 14-20).[98,99] Insulin therapy may decrease brain glucose despite serum normoglycemia.[99,100] As a treatment strategy, invasive monitoring can be used to ensure that the energy supply to the brain (serum glucose and oxygen) should be adjusted to meet the individual demand of the brain tissue to prevent cerebral hypoglycemic episodes.

Are there other factors besides serum glucose influencing brain tissue glucose levels?

Yes. A decrease in brain glucose concentration can be triggered by several primary and secondary complications in patients with severe brain injury such as ischemia, hypoxia, intracranial hypertension, seizures, vasospasm, and others.[101,102] Beyond delivery and consumption, impaired glucose transportation through GLUT-1 transporters may limit the passage of glucose through the blood-brain barrier and decrease its brain tissue concentration.[103,104] Thus, ineffective upregulation or dysfunction of GLUT-1 transporters can potentially limit glucose utilization by the neuron and astrocyte. In a high-energy-demand environment, this may lead to energy failure.[71,105] Another potential cause of low brain tissue glucose is the hyperglycolysis observed in the acute phase after severe brain injury (TBI and SAH). If the overstimulated glycolytic pathway is not supplied with enough substrate, tissue concentrations of glucose may be decreased. A recent study using ^{13}C-labeled acetate and lactate nuclear magnetic resonance (NMR) spectra of microdialysate fluid confirmed that we only have an incomplete understanding of brain metabolism in the acute brain injury state.[106] These investigators found that the brain may be able to utilize lactate as a fuel, and they proposed the mechanism shown in Figure 14-21.

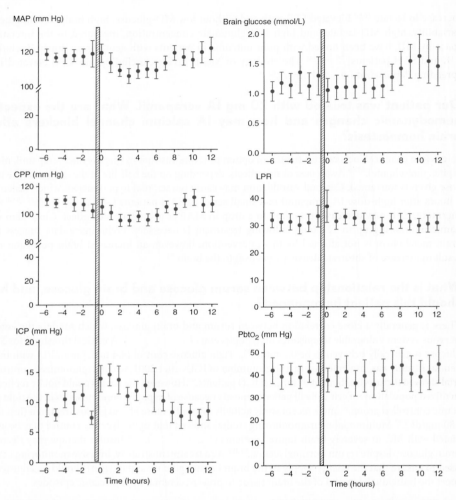

Figure 14-18. These graphs show the average time course of serum MAP, CPP, ICP, and brain glucose, LPR, and Pbto₂ before and after intra-arterial verapamil. Error bars represent means and 1 standard error of individual trials. X-axis represents hours before (−6 to −1), at (time = 0), and after therapy (1-12). The gray bar reflects the period of cerebral angiography. CPP, cerebral perfusion pressure; ICP, intracranial pressure; LPR, lactate-to-pyruvate ratio. *(From Stuart RM, Helbok R, Kurtz P, et al. High-dose intra-arterial verapamil for the treatment of cerebral vasospasm after subarachnoid hemorrhage: prolonged effects on hemodynamic parameters and brain metabolism. Neurosurgery. 2011;68:337-45).*

How should variations in lactate and pyruvate concentrations be interpreted when LPR is not affected?

Patients with severe brain injury will often present parallel fluctuations of lactate and pyruvate that do not affect LPR. Usually, increases in the concentrations of both metabolites reflect increased metabolic activity, such as that seen during rewarming from hypothermia (Figure 14-22). On the other hand, decreased metabolic activity, such as what is observed during sedation, is reflected by reductions of pyruvate and lactate tissue concentrations. If enough substrate delivery and oxygenation are

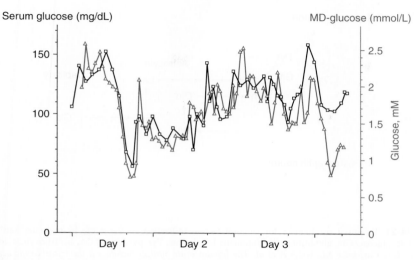

Figure 14-19. This graph shows serum glucose and brain glucose during 3 days of monitoring in our patient.

available, variations of metabolic activity should not lead to energy failure and increased LPR. However, if increased metabolic demand (eg, interruption of sedation, rewarming) leads to unbalanced delivery and consumption of substrate and oxygen, LPR will likely increase.

What information could be added by monitoring regional CBF (rCBF)?

Continuous monitoring of rCBF is possible through a thermal diffusion (TD) microprobe inserted into the brain parenchyma.[107] The microprobe consists of a thermistor in the distal tip and a temperature

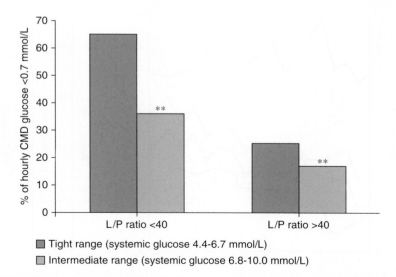

Figure 14-20. This graph shows that tight systemic glucose control is associated with brain energy crisis, which in turn is associated with increased mortality. CMD, cerebral microdialysis. L/P, lactate/pyruvate. (*From Oddo M, Schmidt JM, Carrera E, et al. Impact of tight glycemic control on cerebral glucose metabolism after severe brain injury: A microdialysis study. Crit Care Med. 2008;36:3233-3238.*)

Presynaptic neuron

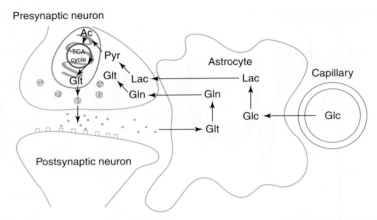

Figure 14-21. Proposed mechanism for cerebral lactate utilization in the acute brain injury setting. Ac, acetate; Glc, glucose; Gln, glutamine; Glt, glutamate; Lac, lactate; Pyr, pyruvate; TCA, tricarboxylic acid. *(From Gallagher CN, Carpenter KL, Grice P, et al. The human brain utilizes lactate via the tricarboxylic acid cycle: A ^{13}C-labelled microdialysis and high-resolution nuclear magnetic resonance study. Brain. 2009;132:2839-2849.)*

sensor 5 mm proximal. The thermistor is heated to 2°C above tissue temperature and rCBF is calculated by a mathematical model using the tissue's ability to transport heat, which depends on tissue perfusion.[108] The sample volume is approximately 27 mm³. The microprobe should be inserted in the vascular region of interest 20 to 25 mm deep, thus reflecting white matter perfusion, and secured with a metal bolt. TD-rCBF should be integrated into other modalities of neuromonitoring, such as MD and tissue oxygenation. Anaerobic metabolism and Pbto$_2$ reductions in patients with severe SAH, combined with dynamic changes in rCBF, clearly point to an ischemic injury due

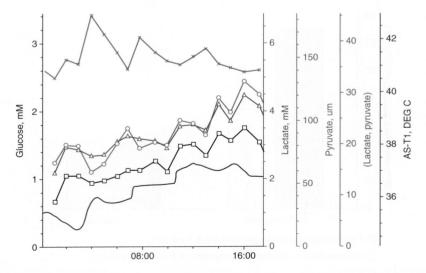

Figure 14-22. This graph demonstrates the rewarming phase of a 60-year-old male patient submitted to hypothermia after resuscitation from cardiac arrest. There is a rise of 2°C to 3°C with a corresponding elevation in the concentration of lactate, pyruvate, and glucose but no increase in the lactate-to-pyruvate ratio, suggesting a balanced increase in metabolism.

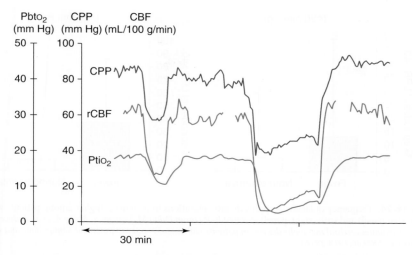

Figure 14-23. This graph demonstrates concomitant changes in regional cerebral blood flow (CBF) as measured by thermal diffusion and Pbto$_2$ and cerebral perfusion pressure (CPP). This suggests that reductions in cerebral oxygenation are due to reduced tissue perfusion that may resolve with CPP optimization. *(From Jaeger M, Soehle M, Schuhmann MU, Winkler D, Meixensberger J. Correlation of continuously monitored regional cerebral blood flow and brain tissue oxygen. Acta Neurochir (Wien). 2005;147:51-56; discussion 56).*

to vasospasm.[109-111] On the other hand, metabolic distress with stable rCBF may indicate hypoxic hypoxia or mitochondrial dysfunction. rCBF has been shown to correlate fairly with Pbto$_2$ and reflect perfusion changes due to systemic parameters such as CPP (Figure 14-23).[112] Thus, it can aid in goal-directed management of CPP and cardiac output management. Although it makes physiologic sense to incorporate rCBF to multimodality monitoring of patients with severe SAH and TBI, there are very little data to support its role in diagnosis and management of cerebral hypoperfusion.

Is jugular bulb oximetry monitoring indicated for patients with severe TBI and severe SAH?

Jugular venous oxygen saturation (Svjo$_2$) has been extensively used in patients with severe TBI and is currently included in the TBI management guidelines published by the Brain Trauma Foundation.[27] Measurement of Svjo$_2$ and the arterial-jugular difference of oxygen content (AJDo$_2$) offers a global estimate of the balance between oxygen delivery and extraction by the brain.[113,114] Both parameters have been associated with secondary brain injury and outcome after severe TBI.[113] Patients with low (less than 50% to 55%) and high (greater than 80%) Svjo$_2$ have worse outcomes than those with values in the middle range. Critically low values of Svjo$_2$ reflect cerebral hypoperfusion with increased oxygen extraction. Exhaustion of this compensatory mechanism results in secondary ischemic injury to the brain. After TBI, high Svjo$_2$ is usually associated with hyperemia, which may lead to intracranial hypertension. Patients with low AJDo$_2$ have also been shown to have worse outcomes than the ones with normal values. This may be the result of an inability to compensate for increased oxygen extraction in a context of high metabolic demand, reflecting more severe brain injury.[113]

There is a paucity of data on the use of Svjo$_2$ monitoring for patients with poor-grade SAH. A few small studies have shown that Svjo$_2$ decreases prior to the development of symptomatic vasospasm.[114] The physiologic rationale of Svjo$_2$ monitoring extensively applied to TBI patients (balance between oxygen delivery and consumption) should remain valid for patients with severe brain injury with other etiologies and justify its use in some selected patients.

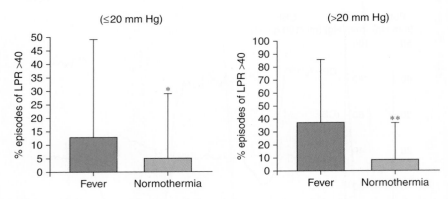

(≤20 mm Hg)　　　　　　　　　　　　　(>20 mm Hg)

Figure 14-24. Frequency of lactate-to-pyruvate ratio elevations in patients is higher among patients with fever without (left panel) and with (right panel) elevated ICP. *(From Oddo M, Frangos S, Milby A, et al. Induced normothermia attenuates cerebral metabolic distress in patients with aneurysmal subarachnoid hemorrhage and refractory fever. Stroke. 2009;40:1913-1916).*

What is the effect of fever on multimodality parameters?

Fever is common after subarachnoid hemorrhage[115] and can effectively be controlled by intravascular or surface-cooling devices.[116,117] Treatment of fever is nowadays routine in neurocritical care and may improve outcome.[116] Besides infections, fever has been linked to severity of injury, hemorrhage load, occurrence of vasospasm, and elevated ICP.[118-120] Recently, fever has been associated with high LPR[121] (Figure 14-24). These data furthermore suggest that fever control may improve brain metabolism. Although these results have to be confirmed in larger studies, beneficial effects of fever control on brain homeostasis may be explained by a reduction in ICP and a decrease in metabolic need.[120]

A 41-year-old woman presented with iatrogenic SAH from the left A2 callosomarginal artery aneurysm after sinus surgery. Course complicated by ICP crises, vasospasm, and ventriculitis. Her continuous EEG (cEEG) demonstrated periodic epileptiform discharges that occurred in runs (Figure 14-25).

Can multimodality monitoring help in the interpretation of questionable EEG findings?

The answer is not entirely clear, but multimodality monitoring may in select cases help clarify questionable EEG patterns.[122] At times that the patient's EEG had these ictal/interictal patterns she had a rise in LPR, glycerol, and glutamate (Figure 14-26). Her glucose initially rose and then dropped. This led to further investigation and she was found to have developed ACA strokes in the territory of the neuromonitoring bundle secondary to vasospasm.

A 70-year-old woman admitted with Hunt and Hess grade IV SAH, with hydrocephalus and medial right frontal ICH. She was found to have an anterior communicating artery aneurysm that became coiled. Multimodality monitoring including ICP and intracortical electroencephalography (ICE) were started (Figures 14-27 and 14-28).

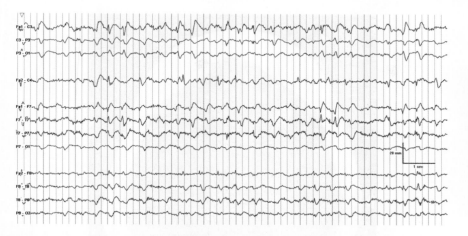

Figure 14-25. Surface electroencephalographic scan demonstrating runs of periodic epileptiform discharges originating primarily from the left hemisphere.

How do you interpret the EEG findings in Figure 14-28 (reference axes indicate 20-mm tracing height and a 1-second time interval. Filter settings are LFF 0.1 Hz, HFF 70 Hz, and notch 60 Hz)?

The scalp EEG demonstrates diffuse background slowing (top 12 tracings) and the depth EEG shows highly epileptiform discharges (bottom 4 tracings).

 The patient's course was complicated by vasospasm combined with sepsis and systemic hypotension refractory to medical intervention. Her corresponding EEG tracings, ICP and CPP curves, together with a compressed spectral array analysis of her surface and depth EEG recordings are shown in Figure 14-29.

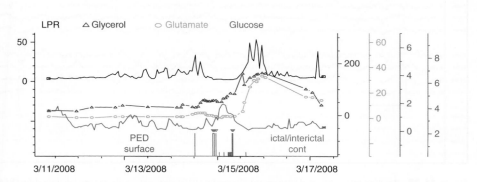

Figure 14-26. Following ictal/interictal patterns on depth recording (red triangles) and periodic epileptiform discharges with a frequency up to 2 Hz. Cerebral glucose is seen to rise, followed by glycerol and glutamate rises.

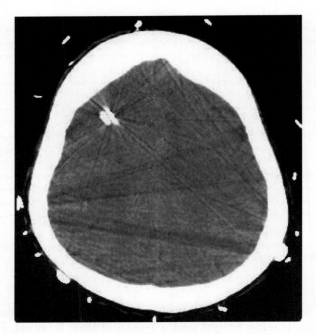

Figure 14-27. Computed tomography after monitoring bundle placement shows probe location in the right frontal lobe. *(From Waziri A, Claassen J, Stuart RM, et al. Intracortical electroencephalography in acute brain injury. Ann Neurol. 2009;66:366-377.)*

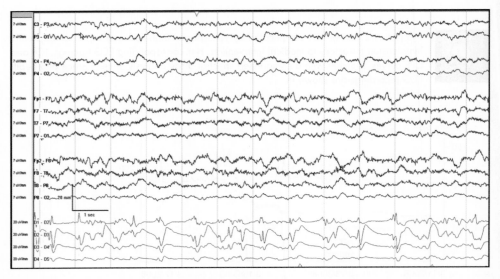

Figure 14-28. Baseline intracortical electroencephalography (ICE) and surface electroencephalography (EEG). *(From Waziri A, Claassen J, Stuart RM, et al. Intracortical electroencephalography in acute brain injury. Ann Neurol. 2009;66:366-377.)*

How do you interpret the monitoring findings?

The ICE shows an evolution from the highly epileptiform initial baseline EEG (see Figure 14-28) to a burst-suppression pattern and ultimately nearly complete attenuation, whereas the overlying scalp coverage did not demonstrate an obvious concerning change. Quantitative EEG analysis of a 6-hour period surrounding the identification of ICE-specific changes is shown. The top two rows are derived from scalp EEG, and the bottom two rows from the intracortical electrode. After a period of slow decrease, a significant and permanent decline in EEG total power was seen in isolation from the intracortical electrode (*arrow*) with a similarly obvious and dramatic change in the ICE spectrogram. A similar trend could not be appreciated from the scalp-derived quantitative EEG trends. This event was associated with a period of progressive decrease in CPP (*purple line*), as well as a delayed and significant increase in ICP (*blue line*); the corresponding time interval is marked with dotted lines.

What happened to the patient?

Owing to decreasing CPP, the patient developed diffuse widespread infarction of her brain (Figure 14-30).

What is spreading depolarization and how relevant is it for the acutely injured brain?

Cortical spreading depression (CSD) is a 1- to 5-mm per minute wave of depolarization in the gray matter. CSDs are recorded by subdural electrocorticography electrode strips and occur both in healthy cortical tissue (reversible) and the diseased brain[16] under conditions of energy compromise (ischemia, hypoxia, hypoglycemia). CSDs are associated with neuronal injury.[123] CSDs in the peri-ischemic brain

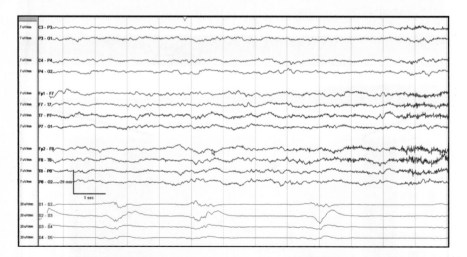

Figure 14-29. EEG, ICP, CPP, and qEEG tracings. The qEEG tracing depicts compressed spectral arrays (CSAs) and total power plots. Both are based on fast Fourier transformation of the raw EEG signal and plotted over time (x-axis). The CSA visualizes how much of the raw EEG is faster and how much is slower frequencies (color coded: from very little to a lot of dark blue – green – yellow – red – white; on y-axis, slow frequencies at the bottom and fast frequencies at the top). Histograms with total power plots have the power on the y-axis. In the above sample, the top two qEEG CSA plots are from the left and right hemisphere, respectively, and the bottom two ones are from the depth electrode (third from top CSA depth and bottom plot total power from depth). (for more details, see Chapter 13). CPP, cerebral perfusion pressure; EEG, electroencephalography; ICE, intracortical electroencephalography; IPP, intracranial pressure; qEEG, quantitative EEG. *(Waziri A, Claassen J, Stuart RM, et al. Intracortical electroencephalography in acute brain injury. Ann Neurol. 2009;66:366-377.)*

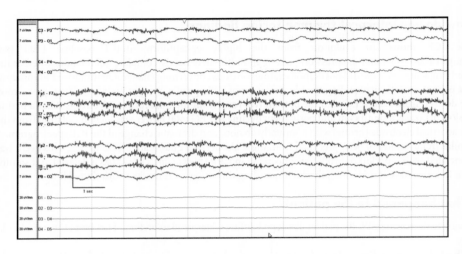

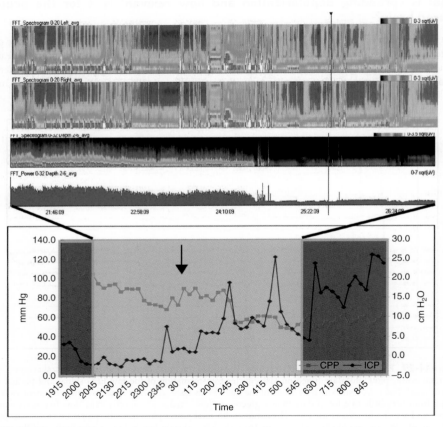

Figure 14-29. (*Continued.*)

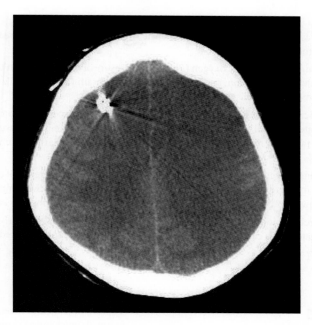

Figure 14-30. Computed tomographic imaging demonstrating infarction of bilateral anterior cerebral artery and left middle cerebral artery regions, likely secondary to hypoperfusion in the setting of preexisting vasospasm. *(Waziri A, Claassen J, Stuart RM, et al. Intracortical electroencephalography in acute brain injury. Ann Neurol. 2009;66:366-377.)*

tissue are referred as "peri-infarct depolarization" (PID).[124] CSDs and PID indicate compromised metabolism and are commonly observed after TBI, malignant MCA infarction, and SAH.[16,125-127] It has been suggested that the vasodilatory response of CSD indicates progressive ischemia, whereas the following vasoconstrictive response—also referred to as cortical spreading ischemia—may contribute to progression of ischemic lesions.[125] This novel technology may have potential to monitor for ongoing ischemia in severe brain injury.

Does neuromonitoring improve outcome?

This has not been adequately studied and all studies so far were underpowered to investigate this question. This may be the wrong question to ask. In patients with cEEG monitoring, this technique was helpful in decision making: "decisive" 54%, "contributing" 32%, "noncontributing" 14% (retrospective, depends on cooperation with ICU physicians).[128] Currently, clinical trials are under way to test if multimodality-targeted management strategies impact on outcome.

! CRITICAL CONSIDERATIONS

One of the most important goals of neurocritical care medicine is to detect secondary brain injury at a time when permanent damage can still be prevented. Thus, the main purpose of invasive neuromonitoring is to create this window of opportunity between the onset of functional disarray and neuronal injury. It is therefore, of fundamental importance for any unit that engages in invasive brain monitoring to have the infrastructure in place to react to detected changes in a timely fashion.

- Partial pressure of brain tissue oxygen ($Pbto_2$) is a measure of cerebral oxygen tension reflecting oxygen delivery, diffusion, and consumption in the brain tissue. Optimizing $Pbto_2$ may potentially improve aerobic metabolism.

- Cerebral microdialysis is a technique through which the concentrations of lactate, glucose, pyruvate, glycerol, and glutamate can be monitored in the brain tissue. Alterations in these metabolites may be early indications of metabolic disarray, such as anaerobic metabolism.

- Jugular venous oxygen saturation ($Svjo_2$) and the arterial-jugular difference of oxygen content ($AJDo_2$) are measures of global oxygen extraction by the brain. High $Svjo_2$ may reflect hyperemia and low $Svjo_2$ may reflect inadequate cerebral perfusion and possibly ischemia.

- Regional cerebral blood flow (rCBF) is a direct assessment of local brain tissue perfusion, and a surrogate of this can be obtained with a thermal diffusion probe inserted into the brain parenchyma.

REFERENCES

1. Kress JP, Pohlman AS, O'Connor MF, Hall JB. Daily interruption of sedative infusions in critically ill patients undergoing mechanical ventilation. *N Engl J Med.* 2000;342:1471-1477.

2. Girard TD, Kress JP, Fuchs BD, et al. Efficacy and safety of a paired sedation and ventilator weaning protocol for mechanically ventilated patients in intensive care (awakening and breathing controlled trial): a randomised controlled trial. *Lancet.* 2008;371:126-134.

3. Skoglund K, Enblad P, Marklund N. Effects of the neurological wake-up test on intracranial pressure and cerebral perfusion pressure in brain-injured patients. *Neurocrit Care.* 2009;11: 135-142.

4. Helbok R, Badjatia N. Is daily awakening always safe in severely brain injured patients? *Neurocrit Care.* 2009;11:133-134.

5. Claassen J, Mayer SA, Kowalski RG, Emerson RG, Hirsch LJ. Detection of electrographic seizures with continuous EEG monitoring in critically ill patients. *Neurology.* 2004;62:1743-1748.

6. Schmidt JM, Rincon F, Fernandez A, et al. Cerebral infarction associated with acute subarachnoid hemorrhage. *Neurocrit Care.* 2007;7:10-17.

7. Rowley G, Fielding K. Reliability and accuracy of the Glasgow Coma Scale with experienced and inexperienced users. *Lancet.* 1991;337: 535-538.

8. Teasdale G, Jennett B. Assessment of coma and impaired consciousness. A practical scale. *Lancet.* 1974;2:81-84.

9. Balestreri M, Czosnyka M, Chatfield DA, et al. Predictive value of Glasgow Coma Scale after brain trauma: change in trend over the past ten years. *J Neurol Neurosurg Psychiatry.* 2004;75: 161-162.

10. Wijdicks EF, Bamlet WR, Maramattom BV, Manno EM, McClelland RL. Validation of a new coma scale: the FOUR score. *Ann Neurol.* 2005;58:585-593.

11. Giacino JT, Schnakers C, Rodriguez-Moreno D, Kalmar K, Schiff N, Hirsch J. Behavioral assessment in patients with disorders of consciousness: gold standard or fool's gold? *Prog Brain Res.* 2009;177:33-48.

12. Carrera E, Schmidt JM, Fernandez L, et al. Spontaneous hyperventilation and brain tissue hypoxia in patients with severe brain injury. *J Neurol Neurosurg Psychiatry.*81:793-797.

13. Maloney-Wilensky E, Gracias V, Itkin A, et al. Brain tissue oxygen and outcome after severe traumatic brain injury: a systematic review. *Crit Care Med.* 2009;37:2057-2063.

14. Harris CH, Smith RS, Helmer SD, Gorecki JP, Rody RB. Placement of intracranial pressure monitors by non-neurosurgeons. *Am Surg.* 2002;68:787-790.

15. Waziri A, Claassen J, Stuart RM, et al. Intracortical electroencephalography in acute brain injury. *Ann Neurol.* 2009;66:366-377.

16. Dreier JP, Woitzik J, Fabricius M, et al. Delayed ischemic neurological deficits after subarachnoid hemorrhage are associated with clusters of spreading depolarizations. *Brain.* 2006;129: 3224-3237.

17. Sarrafzadeh AS, Sakowitz OW, Kiening KL, Benndorf G, Lanksch WR, Unterberg AW. Bedside microdialysis: a tool to monitor cerebral metabolism in subarachnoid hemorrhage patients? *Crit Care Med.* 2002;30:1062-1070.

18. Steiner LA, Coles JP, Czosnyka M, et al. Cerebrovascular pressure reactivity is related to global cerebral oxygen metabolism after head injury. *J Neurol Neurosurg Psychiatry.* 2003;74: 765-770.

19. Narotam PK, Burjonrappa SC, Raynor SC, Rao M, Taylon C. Cerebral oxygenation in major pediatric trauma: its relevance to trauma severity and outcome. *J Pediatr Surg.* 2006;41: 505-513.

20. Narotam PK, Morrison JF, Nathoo N. Brain tissue oxygen monitoring in traumatic brain injury and major trauma: outcome analysis of a brain tissue oxygen-directed therapy. *J Neurosurg.* 2009;111:672-682.

21. Hillered L, Vespa PM, Hovda DA. Translational neurochemical research in acute human brain injury: the current status and potential future for cerebral microdialysis. *J Neurotrauma.* 2005;22:3-41.

22. Stuart RM, Schmidt M, Kurtz P, et al. Intracranial multimodal monitoring for acute brain injury: a single institution review of current practices. *Neurocrit Care.*12:188-198.

23. Stuart RM, Schmidt M, Kurtz P, et al. Intracranial multimodal monitoring for acute brain injury: a single institution review of current practices. *Neurocrit Care.*

24. Dings J, Meixensberger J, Jager A, Roosen K. Clinical experience with 118 brain tissue oxygen partial pressure catheter probes. *Neurosurgery.* 1998;43:1082-1095.

25. Lozier AP, Sciacca RR, Romagnoli MF, Connolly ES Jr. Ventriculostomy-related infections: a critical review of the literature. *Neurosurgery.* 2008;62(suppl 2):688-700.

26. Bratton SL, Chestnut RM, Ghajar J, et al. Guidelines for the management of severe traumatic brain injury. XIV. Hyperventilation. *J Neurotrauma.* 2007;24(suppl 1):S87-S90.

27. Bratton SL, Chestnut RM, Ghajar J, et al. Guidelines for the management of severe traumatic brain injury. X. Brain oxygen monitoring and thresholds. *J Neurotrauma.* 2007;24(suppl 1):S65-S70.

28. Bederson JB, Connolly ES Jr, Batjer HH, et al. Guidelines for the management of aneurysmal subarachnoid hemorrhage: A statement for healthcare professionals from a special writing group of the stroke council, American Heart Association. *Stroke.* 2009;40:994-1025.

29. Sarrafzadeh AS, Kiening KL, Bardt TF, Schneider GH, Unterberg AW, Lanksch WR. Cerebral oxygenation in contusioned vs. nonlesioned brain tissue: monitoring of $Ptio_2$ with Licox and Paratrend. *Acta Neurochir Suppl.* 1998;71:186-189.

30. Kiening KL, Hartl R, Unterberg AW, Schneider GH, Bardt T, Lanksch WR. Brain tissue Po_2-monitoring in comatose patients: implications for therapy. *Neurol Res.* 1997;19:233-240.

31. Kett-White R, Hutchinson PJ, Al-Rawi PG, Gupta AK, Pickard JD, Kirkpatrick PJ. Adverse cerebral events detected after subarachnoid hemorrhage using brain oxygen and microdialysis probes. *Neurosurgery.* 2002;50:1213-1221; discussion 1221-1222.

32. Bardt TF, Unterberg AW, Hartl R, Kiening KL, Schneider GH, Lanksch WR. Monitoring of brain tissue Po_2 in traumatic brain injury: effect of cerebral hypoxia on outcome. *Acta Neurochir Suppl.* 1998;71:153-156.

33. van den Brink WA, van Santbrink H, Steyerberg EW, et al. Brain oxygen tension in severe head injury. *Neurosurgery.* 2000;46:868-876; discussion 876-878.

34. Valadka AB, Gopinath SP, Contant CF, Uzura M, Robertson CS. Relationship of brain tissue Po_2 to outcome after severe head injury. *Crit Care Med.* 1998;26:1576-1581.

35. Zauner A, Doppenberg EM, Woodward JJ, Choi SC, Young HF, Bullock R. Continuous monitoring of cerebral substrate delivery and clearance: Initial experience in 24 patients with severe acute brain injuries. *Neurosurgery.* 1997;41:1082-1091; discussion 1091-1093.

36. Tolias CM, Reinert M, Seiler R, Gilman C, Scharf A, Bullock MR. Normobaric hyperoxia—Induced improvement in cerebral metabolism and reduction in intracranial pressure in patients with severe head injury: a prospective historical cohort-matched study. *J Neurosurg.* 2004;101:435-444.

37. Meixensberger J, Jaeger M, Vath A, Dings J, Kunze E, Roosen K. Brain tissue oxygen guided treatment supplementing ICP/CPP therapy after traumatic brain injury. *J Neurol Neurosurg Psychiatry.* 2003;74:760-764.

38. McCarthy MC, Moncrief H, Sands JM, et al. Neurologic outcomes with cerebral oxygen monitoring in traumatic brain injury. *Surgery.* 2009;146:585-590; discussion 590-591.

Neurocritical Care Monitoring

39. Rosenthal G, Hemphill JC 3rd, Sorani M, et al. Brain tissue oxygen tension is more indicative of oxygen diffusion than oxygen delivery and metabolism in patients with traumatic brain injury. *Crit Care Med.* 2008;36:1917-1924.

40. Badjatia N, Strongilis E, Gordon E, et al. Metabolic impact of shivering during therapeutic temperature modulation: The Bedside Shivering Assessment Scale. *Stroke.* 2008;39:3242-3247.

41. Badjatia N, Strongilis E, Prescutti M, et al. Metabolic benefits of surface counter warming during therapeutic temperature modulation. *Crit Care Med.* 2009;37:1893-1897.

42. Neumann JO, Chambers IR, Citerio G, et al. The use of hyperventilation therapy after traumatic brain injury in Europe: an analysis of the BrainIT database. *Intensive Care Med.* 2008;34:1676-1682.

43. Coles JP, Minhas PS, Fryer TD, et al. Effect of hyperventilation on cerebral blood flow in traumatic head injury: clinical relevance and monitoring correlates. *Crit Care Med.* 2002;30:1950-1959.

44. Carrera E, Schmidt JM, Fernandez L, et al. Spontaneous hyperventilation and brain tissue hypoxia in patients with severe brain injury. *J Neurol Neurosurg Psychiatry.* 2010;81:793-797.

45. Mayer SA CJ. Critical care management of increased intracranial pressure. *J Intensive Care Med.* 2002;17:55-67.

46. Magnoni S, Ghisoni L, Locatelli M, et al. Lack of improvement in cerebral metabolism after hyperoxia in severe head injury: a microdialysis study. *J Neurosurg.* 2003;98:952-958.

47. Menzel M, Doppenberg EM, Zauner A, et al. Cerebral oxygenation in patients after severe head injury: monitoring and effects of arterial hyperoxia on cerebral blood flow, metabolism and intracranial pressure. *J Neurosurg Anesthesiol.* 1999;11:240-251.

48. Rockswold SB, Rockswold GL, Zaun DA, et al. A prospective, randomized clinical trial to compare the effect of hyperbaric to normobaric hyperoxia on cerebral metabolism, intracranial pressure, and oxygen toxicity in severe traumatic brain injury. *J Neurosurg.* 2010;112:1080-1090.

49. Oddo M, Milby A, Chen I, et al. Hemoglobin concentration and cerebral metabolism in patients with aneurysmal subarachnoid hemorrhage. *Stroke.* 2009;40:1275-1281.

50. Hebert PC, Wells G, Blajchman MA, et al. A multicenter, randomized, controlled clinical trial of transfusion requirements in critical care. Transfusion requirements in critical care investigators, Canadian Critical Care Trials Group. *N Engl J Med.* 1999;340:409-417.

51. Napolitano LM, Kurek S, Luchette FA, et al. Clinical practice guideline: red blood cell transfusion in adult trauma and critical care. *Crit Care Med.* 2009;37:3124-3157.

52. Kramer AH, Gurka MJ, Nathan B, Dumont AS, Kassell NF, Bleck TP. Complications associated with anemia and blood transfusion in patients with aneurysmal subarachnoid hemorrhage. *Crit Care Med.* 2008;36:2070-2075.

53. Kramer AH, Zygun DA. Anemia and red blood cell transfusion in neurocritical care. *Crit Care.* 2009;13:R89.

54. Zygun DA, Nortje J, Hutchinson PJ, Timofeev I, Menon DK, Gupta AK. The effect of red blood cell transfusion on cerebral oxygenation and metabolism after severe traumatic brain injury. *Crit Care Med.* 2009;37:1074-1078.

55. Naidech AM, Jovanovic B, Wartenberg KE, et al. Higher hemoglobin is associated with improved outcome after subarachnoid hemorrhage. *Crit Care Med.* 2007;35:2383-2389.

56. Dhar R, Zazulia AR, Videen TO, Zipfel GJ, Derdeyn CP, Diringer MN. Red blood cell transfusion increases cerebral oxygen delivery in anemic patients with subarachnoid hemorrhage. *Stroke.* 2009;40:3039-3044.

57. Naidech AM, Drescher J, Ault ML, Shaibani A, Batjer HH, Alberts MJ. Higher hemoglobin is associated with less cerebral infarction, poor outcome, and death after subarachnoid hemorrhage. *Neurosurgery.* 2006;59:775-779; discussion 779-780.

58. Kurtz P, Schmidt JM, Claassen J, et al. Anemia is associated with metabolic distress and brain tissue hypoxia after subarachnoid hemorrhage. *Neurocrit Care.* 2010;13:10-16.

59. Oddo M, Levine JM, Frangos S, et al. Effect of mannitol and hypertonic saline on cerebral oxygenation in patients with severe traumatic brain injury and refractory intracranial hypertension. *J Neurol Neurosurg Psychiatry.* 2009;80:916-920.

60. Rockswold GL, Solid CA, Paredes-Andrade E, Rockswold SB, Jancik JT, Quickel RR. Hypertonic saline and its effect on intracranial pressure, cerebral perfusion pressure, and brain tissue oxygen. *Neurosurgery.* 2009;65:1035-1041; discussion 1041-1042.

61. Helbok RKS, Schmidt JM, Kurtz P, et al. Effect of mannitol on brain metabolism and tissue oxygenation in severe hemorrhagic stroke. *J Neurol Neurosurg Psychiatry.* 2011;82:378-383.

62. Czosnyka M, Smielewski P, Kirkpatrick P, Laing RJ, Menon D, Pickard JD. Continuous assessment of the cerebral vasomotor reactivity in head injury. *Neurosurgery.* 1997;41:11-17; discussion 17-19.

63. Lang EW, Czosnyka M, Mehdorn HM. Tissue oxygen reactivity and cerebral autoregulation after severe traumatic brain injury. *Crit Care Med.* 2003;31:267-271.

64. Barth M, Woitzik J, Weiss C, et al. Correlation of clinical outcome with pressure-, oxygen-, and flow-related indices of cerebrovascular reactivity in patients following aneurysmal SAH. *Neurocrit Care.* 2010;12:234-243.

65. Jaeger M, Schuhmann MU, Soehle M, Meixensberger J. Continuous assessment of cerebrovascular autoregulation after traumatic brain injury using brain tissue oxygen pressure reactivity. *Crit Care Med.* 2006;34:1783-1788.

66. Hutchinson PJ, O'Connell MT, Al-Rawi PG, et al. Clinical cerebral microdialysis: a methodological study. *J Neurosurg.* 2000;93:37-43.

67. Hutchinson PJ, Al-Rawi PG, O'Connell MT, et al. Monitoring of brain metabolism during aneurysm surgery using microdialysis and brain multiparameter sensors. *Neurol Res.* 1999;21:352-358.

68. Kett-White R, Hutchinson PJ, Czosnyka M, et al. Effects of variation in cerebral haemodynamics during aneurysm surgery on brain tissue oxygen and metabolism. *Acta Neurochir Suppl.* 2002;81:327-329.

69. Kett-White R, Hutchinson PJ, Al-Rawi PG, et al. Cerebral oxygen and microdialysis monitoring during aneurysm surgery: effects of blood pressure, cerebrospinal fluid drainage, and temporary clipping on infarction. *J Neurosurg.* 2002;96:1013-1019.

70. Persson L, Valtysson J, Enblad P, et al. Neurochemical monitoring using intracerebral microdialysis in patients with subarachnoid hemorrhage. *J Neurosurg.* 1996;84:606-616.

71. Cesarini KG, Enblad P, Ronne-Engstrom E, et al. Early cerebral hyperglycolysis after subarachnoid hemorrhage correlates with favourable outcome. *Acta Neurochir (Wien).* 2002;144:1121-1131.

72. Staub F, Graf R, Gabel P, Kochling M, Klug N, Heiss WD. Multiple interstitial substances measured by microdialysis in patients with subarachnoid hemorrhage. *Neurosurgery.* 2000;47:1106-1115; discussion 1115-1116.

73. Sarrafzadeh A, Haux D, Kuchler I, Lanksch WR, Unterberg AW. Poor-grade aneurysmal subarachnoid hemorrhage: relationship of cerebral metabolism to outcome. *J Neurosurg.* 2004;100:400-406.

74. Helbok R, Schmidt JM, Kurtz P, et al. Systemic glucose and brain energy metabolism after subarachnoid hemorrhage. *Neurocrit Care.* 2010;12:317-323.

75. Goodman JC, Valadka AB, Gopinath SP, Uzura M, Robertson CS. Extracellular lactate and glucose alterations in the brain after head injury measured by microdialysis. *Crit Care Med.* 1999;27:1965-1973.

76. Vespa PM, McArthur D, O'Phelan K, et al. Persistently low extracellular glucose correlates with poor outcome 6 months after human traumatic brain injury despite a lack of increased lactate: a microdialysis study. *J Cereb Blood Flow Metab.* 2003;23:865-877.

77. Chamoun R, Suki D, Gopinath SP, Goodman JC, Robertson C. Role of extracellular glutamate measured by cerebral microdialysis in severe traumatic brain injury. *J Neurosurg.* 2010;113:564-570.

78. Claassen J, Bernardini GL, Kreiter K, et al. Effect of cisternal and ventricular blood on risk of delayed cerebral ischemia after subarachnoid hemorrhage: the Fisher Scale revisited. *Stroke.* 2001;32:2012-2020.

79. Hlatky R, Valadka AB, Goodman JC, Contant CF, Robertson CS. Patterns of energy substrates during ischemia measured in the brain by microdialysis. *J Neurotrauma.* 2004;21:894-906.

80. Vespa P, Bergsneider M, Hattori N, et al. Metabolic crisis without brain ischemia is common after traumatic brain injury: a combined microdialysis and positron emission tomography study. *J Cereb Blood Flow Metab.* 2005;25:763-774.

81. Bellander BM, Cantais E, Enblad P, et al. Consensus meeting on microdialysis in neurointensive care. *Intensive Care Med.* 2004;30:2166-2169.

82. Kurtz P, Schmidt J, Claassen J, et al. Serum glucose variability and brain-serum glucose ratio predict metabolic distress and mortality after severe brain injury. *Crit. Care* 2009;13.

83. Samuelsson C, Hillered L, Zetterling M, et al. Cerebral glutamine and glutamate levels in relation to compromised energy metabolism: a microdialysis study in subarachnoid hemorrhage patients. *J Cereb Blood Flow Metab.* 2007;27:1309-1317.

84. Schulz MK, Wang LP, Tange M, Bjerre P. Cerebral microdialysis monitoring: determination of normal and ischemic cerebral metabolisms in patients with aneurysmal subarachnoid hemorrhage. *J Neurosurg.* 2000;93:808-814.

Neurocritical Care Monitoring

85. Johnston AJ, Steiner LA, Coles JP, et al. Effect of cerebral perfusion pressure augmentation on regional oxygenation and metabolism after head injury. *Crit Care Med*. 2005;33:189-195; discussion 255-257.

86. Strong AJ. The management of plasma glucose in acute cerebral ischemia and traumatic brain injury: more research needed. *Intensive Care Med*. 2008;34:1169-1172.

87. Tejada JG, Taylor RA, Ugurel MS, Hayakawa M, Lee SK, Chaloupka JC. Safety and feasibility of intra-arterial nicardipine for the treatment of subarachnoid hemorrhage-associated vasospasm: initial clinical experience with high-dose infusions. *AJNR Am J Neuroradiol*. 2007;28: 844-848.

88. Keuskamp J, Murali R, Chao KH. High-dose intraarterial verapamil in the treatment of cerebral vasospasm after aneurysmal subarachnoid hemorrhage. *J Neurosurg*. 2008;108:458-463.

89. Elliott JP, Newell DW, Lam DJ, et al. Comparison of balloon angioplasty and papaverine infusion for the treatment of vasospasm following aneurysmal subarachnoid hemorrhage. *J Neurosurg*. 1998;88:277-284.

90. Feng L, Fitzsimmons BF, Young WL, et al. Intraarterially administered verapamil as adjunct therapy for cerebral vasospasm: safety and 2-year experience. *AJNR Am J Neuroradiol*. 2002;23:1284-1290.

91. Biondi A, Ricciardi GK, Puybasset L, et al. Intra-arterial nimodipine for the treatment of symptomatic cerebral vasospasm after aneurysmal subarachnoid hemorrhage: preliminary results. *AJNR Am J Neuroradiol*. 2004;25:1067-1076.

92. Badjatia N, Topcuoglu MA, Pryor JC, et al. Preliminary experience with intra-arterial nicardipine as a treatment for cerebral vasospasm. *AJNR Am J Neuroradiol*. 2004;25:819-826.

93. Allen GS, Ahn HS, Preziosi TJ, et al. Cerebral arterial spasm—a controlled trial of nimodipine in patients with subarachnoid hemorrhage. *N Engl J Med*. 1983;308:619-624.

94. Stuart RM HR, Kurtz P, Schmidt MJ, et al. High-dose intra-arterial verapamil for the treatment of cerebral vasospasm after subarachnoid hemorrhage: prolonged effects on hemodynamic parameters and brain metabolism. *Neurosurgery*. 2011;68:337-345; discussion 345.

95. van den Berghe G, Wouters P, Weekers F, et al. Intensive insulin therapy in the critically ill patients. *N Engl J Med*. 2001;345:1359-1367.

96. Brunkhorst FM, Engel C, Bloos F, et al. Intensive insulin therapy and pentastarch resuscitation in severe sepsis. *N Engl J Med*. 2008;358:125-139.

97. Finfer S, Chittock DR, Su SY, et al. Intensive versus conventional glucose control in critically ill patients. *N Engl J Med*. 2009;360: 1283-1297.

98. Oddo M, Schmidt JM, Carrera E, et al. Impact of tight glycemic control on cerebral glucose metabolism after severe brain injury: a microdialysis study. *Crit Care Med*. 2008;36:3233-3238.

99. Vespa P, Boonyaputthikul R, McArthur DL, et al. Intensive insulin therapy reduces microdialysis glucose values without altering glucose utilization or improving the lactate/pyruvate ratio after traumatic brain injury. *Crit Care Med*. 2006;34:850-856.

100. Schlenk F, Graetz D, Nagel A, Schmidt M, Sarrafzadeh AS. Insulin-related decrease in cerebral glucose despite normoglycemia in aneurysmal subarachnoid hemorrhage. *Crit Care*. 2008;12:R9.

101. Abi-Saab WM, Maggs DG, Jones T, et al. Striking differences in glucose and lactate levels between brain extracellular fluid and plasma in conscious human subjects: effects of hyperglycemia and hypoglycemia. *J Cereb Blood Flow Metab*. 2002;22:271-279.

102. Zazulia AR, Videen TO, Powers WJ. Transient focal increase in perihematomal glucose metabolism after acute human intracerebral hemorrhage. *Stroke*. 2009;40:1638-1643.

103. Gould GW, Holman GD. The glucose transporter family: structure, function and tissue-specific expression. *Biochem J*. 1993;295 (Pt 2):329-341.

104. Maher F, Vannucci SJ, Simpson IA. Glucose transporter proteins in brain. *FASEB J*. 1994;8: 1003-1011.

105. Bergsneider M, Hovda DA, Shalmon E, et al. Cerebral hyperglycolysis following severe traumatic brain injury in humans: a positron emission tomography study. *J Neurosurg*. 1997;86:241-251.

106. Gallagher CN, Carpenter KL, Grice P, et al. The human brain utilizes lactate via the tricarboxylic acid cycle: a 13C-labelled microdialysis and high-resolution nuclear magnetic resonance study. *Brain*. 2009;132:2839-2849.

107. Vajkoczy P, Roth H, Horn P, et al. Continuous monitoring of regional cerebral blood flow: experimental and clinical validation of a novel thermal diffusion microprobe. *J Neurosurg*. 2000;93: 265-274.

108. Lee SC, Chen JF, Lee ST. Continuous regional cerebral blood flow monitoring in the neurosurgical intensive care unit. *J Clin Neurosci*. 2005;12:520-523.

109. Vajkoczy P, Horn P, Bauhuf C, et al. Effect of intra-arterial papaverine on regional cerebral blood flow in hemodynamically relevant cerebral vasospasm. *Stroke.* 2001;32:498-505.

110. Thome C, Vajkoczy P, Horn P, Bauhuf C, Hubner U, Schmiedek P. Continuous monitoring of regional cerebral blood flow during temporary arterial occlusion in aneurysm surgery. *J Neurosurg.* 2001;95:402-411.

111. Vajkoczy P, Horn P, Thome C, Munch E, Schmiedek P. Regional cerebral blood flow monitoring in the diagnosis of delayed ischemia following aneurysmal subarachnoid hemorrhage. *J Neurosurg.* 2003;98:1227-1234.

112. Jaeger M, Soehle M, Schuhmann MU, Winkler D, Meixensberger J. Correlation of continuously monitored regional cerebral blood flow and brain tissue oxygen. *Acta Neurochir (Wien).* 2005;147:51-56; discussion 56.

113. Stocchetti N, Canavesi K, Magnoni S, et al. Arterio-jugular difference of oxygen content and outcome after head injury. *Anesth Analg.* 2004;99:230-234.

114. Heran NS, Hentschel SJ, Toyota BD. Jugular bulb oximetry for prediction of vasospasm following subarachnoid hemorrhage. *Can J Neurol Sci.* 2004;31:80-86.

115. Fernandez A, Schmidt JM, Claassen J, et al. Fever after subarachnoid hemorrhage: risk factors and impact on outcome. *Neurology.* 2007;68:1013-1019.

116. Badjatia N, Fernandez L, Schmidt JM, et al. Impact of induced normothermia on outcome after subarachnoid hemorrhage: a case-control study. *Neurosurgery.* 2010;66:696-700; discussion 700-701.

117. Broessner G, Beer R, Lackner P, et al. Prophylactic, endovascular based, long-term normothermia in ICU patients with severe cerebrovascular disease: bicenter prospective, randomized trial. *Stroke.* 2009;40:e657-665.

118. Oliveira-Filho J, Ezzeddine MA, Segal AZ, et al. Fever in subarachnoid hemorrhage: relationship to vasospasm and outcome. *Neurology.* 2001;56:1299-1304

119. Dorhout Mees SM, Luitse MJ, van den Bergh WM, Rinkel GJ. Fever after aneurysmal subarachnoid hemorrhage: relation with extent of hydrocephalus and amount of extravasated blood. *Stroke.* 2008;39:2141-2143.

120. Rossi S, Zanier ER, Mauri I, Columbo A, Stocchetti N. Brain temperature, body core temperature, and intracranial pressure in acute cerebral damage. *J Neurol Neurosurg Psychiatry.* 2001;71:448-454.

121. Oddo M, Frangos S, Milby A, et al. Induced normothermia attenuates cerebral metabolic distress in patients with aneurysmal subarachnoid hemorrhage and refractory fever. *Stroke.* 2009;40:1913-1916.

122. Claassen J. How I treat patients with EEG patterns on the ictal-interictal continuum in the neuro ICU. *Neurocrit Care.* 2009;11:437-444.

123. Iijima T, Mies G, Hossmann KA. Repeated negative dc deflections in rat cortex following middle cerebral artery occlusion are abolished by mk-801: effect on volume of ischemic injury. *J Cereb Blood Flow Metab.* 1992;12:727-733.

124. Hossmann KA. Periinfarct depolarizations. *Cerebrovasc Brain Metab Rev.* 1996;8:195-208.

125. Dreier JP, Major S, Manning A, et al. Cortical spreading ischaemia is a novel process involved in ischaemic damage in patients with aneurysmal subarachnoid hemorrhage. *Brain.* 2009;132:1866-1881.

126. Dohmen C, Sakowitz OW, Fabricius M, et al. Spreading depolarizations occur in human ischemic stroke with high incidence. *Ann Neurol.* 2008;63:720-728.

127. Hartings JA, Strong AJ, Fabricius M, et al. Spreading depolarizations and late secondary insults after traumatic brain injury. *J Neurotrauma.* 2009;26:1857-1866.

128. Jordan KG. Continuous EEG monitoring in the neuroscience intensive care unit and emergency department. *J Clin Neurophysiol.* 1999;16:14-39.

Neurocritical Care Monitoring

15 Advanced Hemodynamic Monitoring

Kiwon Lee, MD, FACP, FAHA, FCCM
Pedro Kurtz, MD

 A 57-year-old man with history of hypertension and gastric ulcer presents after a sudden onset of severe headache followed by nausea and vomiting. The patient arrived in the emergency department (ED) after becoming stuporous in the ambulance. On arrival at the ED, he was hemodynamically unstable—blood pressure (BP) 80/40 mm Hg—and was promptly intubated. He was given fluid resuscitation with the infusion of 2 L of crystalloids, with blood pressure recovering to 140/80 mm Hg. Computed tomography (CT) of the head revealed acute subarachnoid hemorrhage (SAH) filling the basal cistern, bilateral sylvian fissures with thick hemorrhages (modified Fischer grade 3), and early evidence of hydrocephalus (Figure 15-1). The patient was transferred to the neurologic intensive care unit (NeuroICU, NICU) where an external ventricular drain (EVD) was urgently placed and urgent angiography was planned. Even after EVD placement, the patient remained comatose, with intact brainstem reflexes. Vital signs were as follows: BP 150/70 mm Hg, HR 120 bpm in sinus rhythm, RR 22 breaths/min (mechanical ventilation at assist control–pressure-controlled mode), temperature 37°C.

Patients in the acute phase after aneurysmal SAH are at increased risk for rebleeding. The highest rates of rebleeding occur in the first 3 days after SAH, and therefore clipping or coiling of the ruptured aneurysm should be performed as soon as possible after admission. While the aneurysm is unsecured, systemic hypertension should be avoided but hemodynamic stability is crucial to avoid cerebral hypoperfusion, acute ictal infarcts, and cerebral circulatory arrest.[1]

Liberal fluid resuscitation with crystalloids is commonly necessary in poor-grade SAH patients before securing the aneurysm. Although frequently hypertensive, patients may present with relative intravascular volume depletion—due to natriuresis and to the systemic inflammatory response associated with severe brain injury—and this was why this patient responded appropriately to 2 L of normal saline, which was necessary to maintain end-organ perfusion. On arrival at the ICU, this patient should receive a central venous access and an arterial line. If a mean arterial pressure (MAP) goal of at least 60 to 70 mm Hg is not achieved, vasopressors and inotropic agents should be initiated. This patient's ruptured aneurysm has not been secured yet, therefore systemic hypertension and intracranial hypertension must be treated promptly. Typically, systolic blood pressure less than 140 to 160 mm Hg or MAP less than 100 mm Hg can be used to as a general target. At this point, urine output, central venous pressure (CVP), arterial lactate levels, and central venous oxygen saturation (ScvO$_2$) are assessed to refine the evaluation of hemodynamic stability. Urine output < 0.5 mL/kg/h, lactate levels above 2 mmol/L, and ScvO$_2$ below 65% generally represent systemic hypoperfusion and further fluid resuscitation should target CVP > 8 mm Hg, ScvO$_2$ > 70%, and the reduction of arterial lactate.[2]

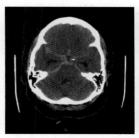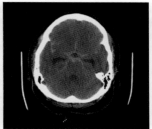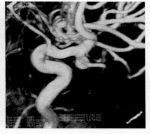

Figure 15-1. Poor-grade subarachnoid hemorrhage (SAH) with modified Fisher grade 3 caused by a right internal carotid artery aneurysm rupture.

The patient received a cerebral angiography that revealed an aneurysm in the intracranial part of the right internal carotid artery. Endovascular coiling was undertaken with successful occlusion of the aneurysm sac. When the patient returns to the ICU, which systemic and cerebral monitoring devices should be placed?

A comprehensive approach to goal-directed interventions requires that organ function is assessed to indicate the need and evaluate the response to specific treatments. The ideal monitoring tools in the ICU should be continuous, noninvasive (when possible), and accurate measurements of the end-organ function of interest. In order to monitor cerebral function parameters, there are no good substitutes to intracranial probes that measure intracranial pressure (ICP), brain tissue oxygen tension, and aerobic metabolic activity. Recently, advanced multimodal monitoring has been focused on systemic and cerebral parameters and the interrelation between them, as shown in Table 15-1.

Hemodynamic monitoring is a cornerstone of the management of critically ill neurologic patients. There are commercially available, minimally invasive, continuous cardiac output monitoring systems available in United States such as the Vigileo (Edwards Lifesciences, Irvine, CA) and PICCO (Phillips Healthcare, Andover, MA) devices, both of which monitor MAP and pulse contour analysis of the arterial waveform in order to generate continuous cardiac output measurements.[3-7] Both technologies also offer continuous measurement of stroke volume variation (SVV), which may be used as a surrogate for volume or fluid responsiveness in mechanically ventilated patients. As SSV may vary during different phases of respiration (due to preload variation during inspiration and expiration), SVV is considered more reliable in patients who are being sedated and mechanically ventilated on a set rate without any added spontaneous breaths. Arrhythmia also affects SVV data. The PICCO system further calculates extravascular lung water (EVLW) and global end-diastolic volumes based on a transpulmonary thermodilution curve.[7] Through a central venous line, preferably on the subclavian site, CVP and Scvo$_2$ are continuously monitored. Arterial-lactate and arterial-venous delta CO$_2$ (a-v Δco$_2$) allow estimation of tissue hypoperfusion and inadequate systemic CO$_2$ washout, an indication of inappropriate cardiac output.[2,8-11]

Multimodal monitoring parameters of brain function are shown in Table 15-1. It is composed of intracranial measurements of ICP, partial pressure of brain tissue oxygen (Pbto$_2$), microdialysis (MD), regional cerebral blood flow (rCBF: Hemedex, Inc, Cambridge, MA), and cortical depth continuous electroencephalography (cEEG).[12-19] In addition to the intracranial monitoring, surface cEEG and jugular bulb oximetry complete the armamentarium of tools available. The intracranial modalities are usually used as a bundle, inserted into a multilumen bolt, and/or tunneled in as necessary. Pbto$_2$ is a measure of tissue oxygen tension and is believed to reflect the balance between delivery, consumption, and tissue diffusion of oxygen.[20-23] Microdialysis allows measurement of glucose, lactate, and pyruvate in a small volume of tissue around the catheter. High lactate-to-pyruvate (L/P)

Table 15-1. Multimodal Monitoring—Systemic and Cerebral Parameters

Modality	Purpose and general goals	Description and comments
SYSTEMIC		
Continuous cardiac index (CI)	Above 2.5 L/min/m²	Body surface area (BSA) indexed cardiac output based on pulse contour analysis of arterial waveform
Mean arterial pressure (MAP)	Above 70 mm Hg	Invasive MAP through radial or femoral artery
Stroke volume variation (SVV)	Below 10%	Ventilation-induced variability of stroke volume
Global end-diastolic volume index (GEDVI)	Above 600 mL/m²	Estimated maximal volume of four heart chambers based on transpulmonary thermodilution curve
Central venous oxygen saturation (ScvO₂)	Above 70%	Blood oximetry measured by central venous catheter located at right atrium or superior vena cava
Central venous pressure (CVP)	Above 5 mm Hg	Intravascular pressure measured by central venous catheter located at right atrium or superior vena cava
Extravascular lung water index (ELWI)	Below 10 mL/kg	Estimate of the intrathoracic volume of water outside the blood vessels based on transpulmonary thermodilution
CEREBRAL		
Continuous electro-encephalography (cEEG)	Seizure and ischemia detection	Surface continuous EEG with quantitative parameters
Intracranial pressure (ICP)	Below 20 mm Hg	Intracranial parenchymal or ventricular pressure
Cerebral perfusion pressure (CPP)	Above 60 mm Hg	MAP-ICP
Brain tissue oxygen tension (PbtO₂)	Above 15 mm Hg	Partial pressure of oxygen measured at brain tissue level
Cerebral microdialysis	Lactate/pyruvate ratio < 40 and glucose > 0.7 mmol/L	Lactate, pyruvate, and glucose measured at brain tissue level
Brain tissue perfusion (rCBF)	Above 20 mL/100 g/min	Regional brain tissue perfusion based on thermodilution method
Depth continuous EEG	Seizure and ischemia detection	Subcortical continuous EEG
Jugular venous bulb oximetry (SjvO₂)	Above 65%	Blood oximetry measured at jugular venous bulb

ratios (LPRs) indicate anaerobic metabolism, and if associated with low brain glucose, suggest tissue metabolic crisis.[24,25] Tissue perfusion (rCBF) around the area of the probe is estimated through a thermodilution method between two thermistors along the probe (Hemedex).[18] For more clinically applicable information, see Chapter 14.

Multimodal cerebral monitoring was placed in the right hemisphere. It included a triple-lumen bolt with ICP, PbtO$_2$, and MD probes and a double-lumen bolt with a depth electroencephalographic (EEG) electrode and a rCBF probe. A PICCO catheter was placed in the femoral artery allowing for continuous monitoring of cardiac index (CI) and SVV, as well as intermittent assessment of global end-diastolic volume index (GEDVI) and EVLW. What should be the hemodynamic goals for this patient?

Systemic hemodynamic resuscitation should always precede brain-targeted interventions. Comatose patients with severe brain injury are likely to be mechanically ventilated and should be monitored with an invasive arterial line, a central venous catheter, and an ICP pressure probe. Semi-invasive continuous monitoring of cardiac output and SVV are possible through pulse contour analysis of the arterial waveform. GEDVI is used as a volumetric static measure of preload and EVLW measurements as an indicator of pulmonary edema. CVP and Scvo$_2$ complement this comprehensive list of hemodynamic monitoring parameters.

Markers of end-organ hypoperfusion, such as high lactate and low Scvo$_2$, indicate inadequate oxygen delivery and should prompt interventions in order to achieve optimal mean arterial pressure and cardiac output.[2,11,26] Assessment of fluid responsiveness should follow based on GEDVI and SVV. SVV greater than 10% and GEDVI less than 600 mL/m^2 generally indicate that the patient will respond to a fluid challenge with either 500 mL of crystalloid or 250 mL of colloid solution.[27] An increase in cardiac output confirms the response to the fluid challenge. After optimal preload is achieved, MAP should be maintained above 70 mm Hg, with norepinephrine and CI kept above 2.5 L/min/m^2 with dobutamine or milrinone if necessary.

After hemodynamic stabilization, end-organ perfusion parameters should be reassessed. Urine output greater than 0.5 mL/kg per hour, clearance of arterial lactate, Scvo$_2$ greater than 70%, and a-v Δco$_2$ less than 6 are good indicators of effective systemic resuscitation.

How should the optimal cerebral perfusion pressure (CPP) be defined, and what are the cerebral multimodal monitoring goals in this patient?

The goal of advanced neuromonitoring in patients with severe brain injury is to allow early detection of complications and ensure adequate delivery of oxygen and nutrients to the brain in order to avoid permanent damage. After the primary event, a number of processes can lead to secondary brain injury. Nonconvulsive seizures after traumatic brain injury, vasospasm after subarachnoid hemorrhage, expansion of the hematoma after intracerebral hemorrhage, and increased ICP after cardiac arrest are examples of detectable complications that progress in the ICU and can be discovered by comprehensive monitoring of brain function. Early detection and prompt intervention can potentially prevent irreversible damage.

Continuous multimodality neuromonitoring includes ICP, Pbto$_2$, MD, continuous EEG (cEEG) (surface and depth), and tissue perfusion. These probes are introduced at the bedside through a multilumen bolt and/or tunneled in subcutaneously. All the data are stored and continuously displayed at the bedside along with systemic monitoring parameters. An integrative approach to brain oxygenation, metabolism, electrical activity, and perfusion allows the clinician to understand the pathophysiology of events and to individualize clinical therapy. Small elevations in ICP below traditional thresholds may compromise perfusion and lead to brain tissue hypoxia and metabolic crisis. Early treatment to optimize perfusion may reverse these alterations and avoid a vasodilatory cascade that leads to refractory intracranial hypertension.[28] Similarly, a reduction in regional blood flow to ischemic levels may cause reduced alpha-to-delta ratios, elevated LPRs, and low $Pbto_2$.[21,25,29-32] Early CPP optimization and balloon angioplasty may also reverse ischemia and avoid permanent deficits.

CPP is the primary determinant of CBF and oxygen delivery to the brain.[33-35] It is thus a powerful and practical tool at the bedside to achieve adequate balance between oxygen and nutrient delivery and the brain's metabolic demand. Instead of relying on arbitrary thresholds to target CPP, functional assessment of the brain permits goal-directed management of cerebral hemodynamics and individualized targets of optimal CPP. The main goals used to optimize CPP are to maintain $Pbto_2$ greater than 15 to 20 mm Hg, $Sjvo_2$ greater than 65%, LPR less than 40, and rCBF greater than 20 mL/100 g per minute.[25,36] The first step is usually to optimize cardiac preload with fluids in patients who are fluid responsive. Once adequate preload and an SVV less than 10% are achieved, MAP and cardiac output can be improved with vasopressors and inotropes, respectively. CI and CPP should initially be kept above 2.5 L/min/m^2 and above 60 to 70 mm Hg, respectively.

CPP and cardiac output, though critically important, are only two pieces of the homeostatic puzzle where factors such as blood rheology, serum osmotic pressure, glucose, and arterial Po_2 influence ongoing neuronal injury. Taking into account the complexity and interactions between these variables, efforts should be made to adjust sedation, serum osmolarity, and blood glucose control and exclude surgical complications through neuroimaging while the hemodynamic status is optimized.

If brain physiologic targets are not yet achieved, further efforts to increment CPP and cardiac output should be undertaken. Supranormal levels are defined as optimal if they correlate with improvements in the cerebral oxygenation and metabolic profile.

On postbleed day 5, the patient shows a reduction in $PbtO_2$ from 25 to 16 mm Hg and an increase in MD-lactate, without critical values of LPR (LPR greater than 30). An echocardiogram performed 2 days earlier had revealed a moderate left ventricular (LV) dysfunction and maximum troponin level of 4 on postbleed day 2. What would be an appropriate approach to a patient with suspected vasospasm and myocardial dysfunction?

Vasospasm is a major concern after SAH, especially between days 4 and 14 after the initial hemorrhage. Up to 50% of patients develop varying degrees of symptomatic vasospasm after SAH. Patients with diffuse and thick cisternal clots are at increased risk for delayed cerebral infarcts due to vasospasm. There is increasing evidence that multimodality monitoring allows detection of cerebral ischemia due to vasospasm before clinical signs develop.[21,22,25,31,37] Integrating electrical activity monitoring through quantitative EEG, oxygenation with $Pbto_2$, and oxidative metabolism measured by MD may create a window of opportunity for intervention before clinical signs appear and permanent deficits take place. Recent evidence suggests this window may vary from hours to a few days (Figure 15-2).[24,38]

Although there is no level I type of evidence, dynamic changes in the alpha-to-delta ratio on EEG, a relative reduction in $Pbto_2$, or elevation in the LPR may be considered an alarming feature to alert the bedside nurse or clinician of potential ongoing ischemia. Repeated clinical and transcranial Doppler examinations should be performed daily, preferably multiple times each day. If significant vasospasm is suspected, especially in a comatose or sedated patient, in addition to CT angiography, a perfusion scan may be helpful to evaluate the extent of the perfusion deficit. At the same time, a trial of increased CPP and cardiac output may be considered with reversal of the altered parameters mentioned above as the goal. A positive response to improved CBF is seen within minutes for the continuously measured $Pbto_2$ and quantitative EEG (qEEG) parameters and is reflected in the next 1 to 2 hours of MD-measured lactate and pyruvate. If a positive response is achieved, these supranormal levels of cardiac output and CPP may be defined as optimal for that particular patient. In patients with stunned myocardium and left ventricular (LV) dysfunction, caution is advised since excessive MAP and CPP (especially those patients who are on vasopressors without any inotropic property) may result in increased left

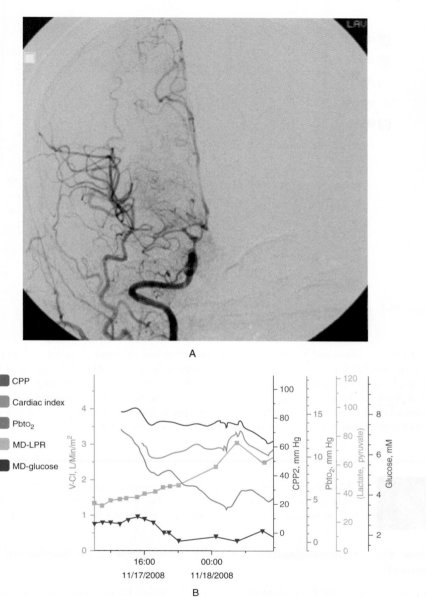

A

B

Figure 15-2. A. Cerebral angiography shows vasospasm of the right middle cerebral and anterior cerebral arteries. **B.** Multimodality panel demonstrates a steep reduction of Pbto$_2$ along with an increase in the lactate-to-pyruvate ratio (LPR) with normal levels of cerebral perfusion pressure (CPP) and cardiac index (CI). **C.** After initiation of milrinone and norepinephrine, increases in CI and CPP improve cerebral oxygenation and metabolism.

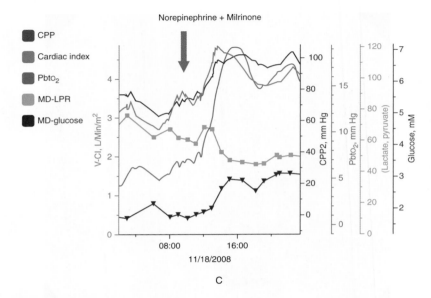

Figure 15-2. (*Continued.*)

ventricular afterload and lead to reduced cardiac output and pulmonary congestion.[39] In the setting of myocardial dysfunction, a combination of norepinephrine with either dobutamine or milrinone should be utilized to achieve hyperdynamic/hypertensive therapy while providing some contractility support for the myocardium. Hypertensive/hyperdynamic therapy (plus euvolemic, not hypervolemic) is often not sufficient to treat severe vasospasm, and intra-arterial vasodilators and balloon angioplasty are often necessary for refractory symptomatic vasospasm.[35,40]

A 63-year-old patient admitted with severe traumatic brain injury (TBI) after a motor vehicle accident presents on posttrauma day 4 with ventilator-associated pneumonia (VAP), worsening pulmonary gas exchange, and severe sepsis (Figure 15-3).

How should hemodynamic and CPP management be conducted in this patient?

A recent update of the Brain Trauma Foundation Guidelines for the management of patients with severe TBI addresses the evidence available on CPP management, including the role of brain tissue oxygenation and metabolism.[36] It suggests that there is a clinical threshold of CPP, between 50 and 60 mm Hg, below which CBF is compromised and poor outcome is more likely. Studies have shown that CPP values below 60 mm Hg are associated with low $Pbto_2$ and $Sjvo_2$ and that these findings are related to poor outcome. MD studies have also suggested that ischemia, as measured by altered LPRs, is more frequent when CPP trends below 50 mm Hg.

The guidelines' update also emphasizes recent evidence from a randomized clinical trial comparing treatment based on CPP and ICP goals. CPP was kept above 70 mm Hg in one group, while the

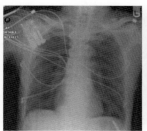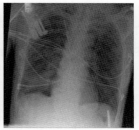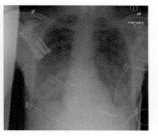

Figure 15-3. Chest radiography on posttrauma days 1, 4, and 5 (*above*). The second radiograph demonstrates a new right lower lobe infiltrate that evolved into a ventilator-associated pneumonia. After 1 day, the patient presented with bilateral pulmonary infiltrates and a Pao_2/Fio_2 (P/F) ratio of 180, confirming acute respiratory distress syndrome (ARDS).

other group was treated to maintain ICP below 20 to 25 mm Hg and avoid CPP less than 50 mm Hg. There was no difference in outcome between the two groups, and the CPP-based management group (CPP greater than 70 mm Hg) had a fivefold increased incidence of acute respiratory distress syndrome (ARDS).[41] Similar results were found in a retrospective analysis of a randomized clinical trial (RCT) where CPP-targeted therapy was associated with ARDS and this complication was strongly related to vasopressor administration.[42]

The body of evidence available suggests that finding an optimal CPP is crucial to the management of patients with TBI.[36] The optimal level should be individualized after assessing cerebral autoregulation, oxygenation, metabolic and electrical profiles, and their responses to changes in CPP. It may be useful to assess autoregulation in the acute phase after severe TBI through the moving correlations between MAP and ICP (pressure reactivity index)[43,44] and CPP and $Pbto_2$ (oxygen reactivity index).[45] Impaired autoregulation indicates that CBF is dependent on CPP and that unnecessarily high CPP levels may lead to increased cerebral blood volume and ICP. It is wise to avoid CPP levels below 60 mm Hg. ICP levels above 25 mm Hg would need to be treated with sedatives/analgesics and osmolar therapy followed by barbiturates and hypothermia in refractory cases.[36] Concomitantly, optimal CPP can be pursued based on pressure and oxygen reactivity index analysis.

Cardiac preload assessment always precedes efforts to increase systemic vascular resistance with vasopressors and myocardial contractility with inotropes. The goal is to avoid *consistently* low CVP less than 5 mm Hg, keep GEDVI greater than 600 mL/m², and maintain stroke volume or pulse pressure variation below 10%. Extreme caution to avoid unnecessary fluid overloading is warranted during the course of fluid resuscitation. It might be useful to use fluid boluses of crystalloid as needed instead of continuous infusion of large volumes of fluid. After every fluid challenge, cardiac output improvement needs to be assessed. Ineffective fluid challenges would fail to increase cardiac output and CBF, and only contribute to pulmonary edema. While high extravascular lung water measurements are not necessarily a contraindication to fluid administration, special caution is needed in patients with values above 10 to 15 mL/kg.[7,46]

Vasopressors and inotropes should be initiated for patients who fail to maintain minimum values of CPP (greater than 50 to 60 mm Hg) and cardiac index (greater than 2.5 L/min/m²) after fluid resuscitation. The next step is to titrate CPP and CI to meet individual needs based on physiologic information from multimodality monitoring (Figure 15-4). In patients who present with reduced $Pbto_2$ and elevated LPR—less than 15 to 20 mm Hg and above 40, respectively—one may consider doing a trial of increased CPP and/or cardiac output in order to further improve brain oxygenation.[47,48] Dynamic improvement of oxygenation and metabolism suggest that the supranormal values achieved are necessary to maintain brain homeostasis and avoid secondary injury.

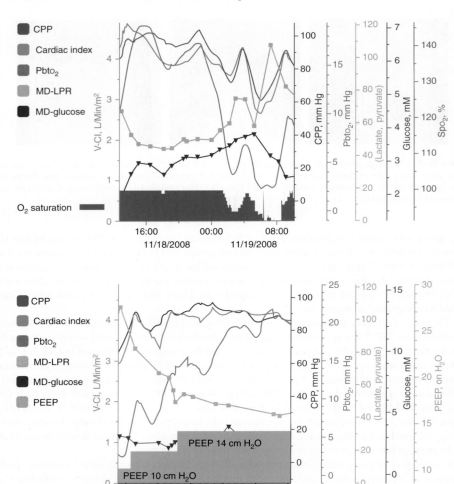

Figure 15-4. The top multimodality panel shows a reduction in Pbto$_2$ and increase in the lactate-to-pyruvate ratio (LPR) along with peripheral oxygen desaturation during worsening pulmonary gas exchange (*top panel*). Cerebral oxygenation and metabolism later improved with lung recruitment and optimal positive end-expiratory pressure (PEEP) levels (*middle panel*). After 1 day of negative fluid balance and improved gas exchange, PEEP was reduced from 14 to 10 cm H$_2$O without worsening of Pbto$_2$ or LPR.

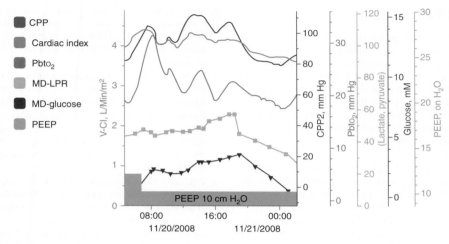

Figure 15-4. (*Continued.*)

! CRITICAL CONSIDERATIONS

- Hemodynamic monitoring is a cornerstone of the management of critically ill neurologic patients.
- While brain resuscitation is critical in the early phase of brain injury, adequate brain resuscitation cannot be done efficiently without addressing the hemodynamic status.
- Euvolemic therapy is critical for all brain injury patients—as adequate hemodynamic status is the key for delivery of oxygen and cerebral metabolic rate of oxygen consumption need for the injured brain.
- Although there is no level I type of evidence, dynamic changes in the alpha-to-delta ratio on EEG, a relative reduction in $Pbto_2$, or elevation in the LPR may be considered an alarming feature to alert the bedside nurse or clinician of potential ongoing ischemia.
- Markers of end-organ hypoperfusion, such as high lactate and low $Scvo_2$, indicate inadequate oxygen delivery and should prompt interventions in order to achieve optimal MAP and cardiac output.
- Assessment of fluid responsiveness may be possible by following GEDVI, SVV, and pulse pressure variation. CVP is a poor indicator for fluid responsiveness or intravascular volume status. SVV greater than 10% and GEDVI less the 600 mL/m² generally indicate that the patient will respond to a fluid challenge with either 500 mL of crystalloid or 250 mL of colloid solution.
- The main goals used to optimize CPP are to maintain $Pbto_2$ greater than 15 to 20 mm Hg, $Sjvo_2$ greater than 65%, LPR less than 40, and rCBF greater than 20 mL/100 g per minute. The first step is usually to optimize cardiac preload with fluids in patients who are fluid responsive. Once adequate preload and an SVV less than 10% are achieved, MAP and cardiac output can be improved with vasopressors and inotropes, respectively. CI and CPP should initially be kept above 2.5 L/min/m² and above 60 to 70 mm Hg, respectively.

REFERENCES

1. Bederson JB, Connolly ES Jr, Batjer HH, et al. Guidelines for the management of aneurysmal subarachnoid hemorrhage: a statement for healthcare professionals from a special writing group of the Stroke Council, American Heart Association. *Stroke.* 2009;40:994-1025.

2. Rivers E, Nguyen B, Havstad S, et al. Early goal-directed therapy in the treatment of severe sepsis and septic shock. *N Engl J Med.* 8 2001;345:1368-1377.

3. Ostergaard M, Nielsen J, Rasmussen JP, Berthelsen PG. Cardiac output—Pulse contour analysis vs. pulmonary artery thermodilution. *Acta Anaesthesiol Scand.* 2006;50:1044-1049.

4. de Waal EE, Kalkman CJ, Rex S, Buhre WF. Validation of a new arterial pulse contour-based cardiac output device. *Crit Care Med.* 2007;35:1904-1909.

5. Mayer J, Boldt J, Schollhorn T, Rohm KD, Mengistu AM, Suttner S. Semi-invasive monitoring of cardiac output by a new device using arterial pressure waveform analysis: a comparison with intermittent pulmonary artery thermodilution in patients undergoing cardiac surgery. *Br J Anaesth.* 2007;98:176-182.

6. Mayer J, Boldt J, Wolf MW, Lang J, Suttner S. Cardiac output derived from arterial pressure waveform analysis in patients undergoing cardiac surgery: validity of a second generation device. *Anesth Analg.* 2008;106:867-872.

7. Berkowitz DM, Danai PA, Eaton S, Moss M, Martin GS. Accurate characterization of extravascular lung water in acute respiratory distress syndrome. *Crit Care Med.* 2008;36:1803-1809.

8. Vallee F, Vallet B, Mathe O, et al. Central venous-to-arterial carbon dioxide difference: an additional target for goal-directed therapy in septic shock? *Intensive Care Med.* 2008;34:2218-2225.

9. Bakker J, Vincent JL, Gris P, Leon M, Coffernils M, Kahn RJ. Veno-arterial carbon dioxide gradient in human septic shock. *Chest.* 1992;101:509-515.

10. Cuschieri J, Rivers EP, Donnino MW, et al. Central venous-arterial carbon dioxide difference as an indicator of cardiac index. *Intensive Care Med.* 2005;31:818-822.

11. Otero RM, Nguyen HB, Huang DT, et al. Early goal-directed therapy in severe sepsis and septic shock revisited: concepts, controversies, and contemporary findings. *Chest.* 2006;130:1579-1595.

12. Waziri A, Arif H, Oddo M, et al. Early experience with a cortical depth electrode for ICU neurophysiological monitoring. *Epilepsia.* 2007;48(suppl 6):208-209.

13. Jaeger M, Soehle M, Schuhmann MU, Winkler D, Meixensberger J. Correlation of continuously monitored regional cerebral blood flow and brain tissue oxygen. *Acta Neurochir (Wien).* 2005;147:51-56; discussion 56.

14. Lee SC, Chen JF, Lee ST. Continuous regional cerebral blood flow monitoring in the neurosurgical intensive care unit. *J Clin Neurosci.* 2005;12:520-523.

15. Thome C, Vajkoczy P, Horn P, Bauhuf C, Hubner U, Schmiedek P. Continuous monitoring of regional cerebral blood flow during temporary arterial occlusion in aneurysm surgery. *J Neurosurg.* 2001;95:402-411.

16. Vajkoczy P, Horn P, Bauhuf C, et al. Effect of intra-arterial papaverine on regional cerebral blood flow in hemodynamically relevant cerebral vasospasm. *Stroke.* 2001;32:498-505.

17. Vajkoczy P, Horn P, Thome C, Munch E, Schmiedek P. Regional cerebral blood flow monitoring in the diagnosis of delayed ischemia following aneurysmal subarachnoid hemorrhage. *J Neurosurg.* 2003;98:1227-1234.

18. Vajkoczy P, Roth H, Horn P, et al. Continuous monitoring of regional cerebral blood flow: experimental and clinical validation of a novel thermal diffusion microprobe. *J Neurosurg.* 2000;93:265-274.

19. Stuart RM, Schmidt M, Kurtz P, et al. Intracranial Multimodal Monitoring for Acute Brain Injury: a Single Institution Review of Current Practices. *Neurocrit Care.* 2010;12:188-198.

20. Stewart C, Haitsma I, Zador Z, et al. The new Licox combined brain tissue oxygen and brain temperature monitor: assessment of in vitro accuracy and clinical experience in severe traumatic brain injury. *Neurosurgery.* 2008;63:1159-1164; discussion 1164-1165.

21. Rose JC, Neill TA, Hemphill JC 3rd. Continuous monitoring of the microcirculation in neurocritical care: an update on brain tissue oxygenation. *Curr Opin Crit Care.* 2006;12:97-102.

22. Rosenthal G, Hemphill JC 3rd, Sorani M, et al. Brain tissue oxygen tension is more indicative of oxygen diffusion than oxygen delivery and metabolism in patients with traumatic brain injury. *Crit Care Med.* 2008;36:1917-1924.

23. Rosenthal G, Hemphill JC, Sorani M, et al. The role of lung function in brain tissue oxygenation following traumatic brain injury. *J Neurosurg.* 2008;108:59-65.

24. Hillered L, Vespa PM, Hovda DA. Translational neurochemical research in acute human brain injury: the current status and potential future for cerebral microdialysis. *J Neurotrauma.* 2005;22:3-41.

25. Bellander BM, Cantais E, Enblad P, et al. Consensus meeting on microdialysis in neurointensive care. *Intensive Care Med.* 2004;30:2166-2169.

26. Nguyen HB, Rivers EP, Knoblich BP, et al. Early lactate clearance is associated with improved outcome in severe sepsis and septic shock. *Crit Care Med.* 2004;32:1637-1642.

27. Michard F, Teboul JL. Predicting fluid responsiveness in ICU patients: a critical analysis of the evidence. *Chest.* 2002;121:2000-2008.

28. Lescot T, Abdennour L, Boch AL, Puybasset L. Treatment of intracranial hypertension. *Curr Opin Crit Care.* 2008;14:129-134.

29. Helbok R, Schmidt JM, Kurtz P, et al. Systemic glucose and brain energy metabolism after subarachnoid hemorrhage. *Neurocrit Care.* 2010;12:317-323.

30. Oddo M, Schmidt JM, Carrera E, et al. Impact of tight glycemic control on cerebral glucose metabolism after severe brain injury: a microdialysis study. *Crit Care Med.* 2008;36:3233-3238.

31. Claassen J, Hirsch LJ, Kreiter KT, et al. Quantitative continuous EEG for detecting delayed cerebral ischemia in patients with poor-grade subarachnoid hemorrhage. *Clin Neurophysiol.* 2004;115:2699-2710.

32. Carrera E, Schmidt JM, Fernandez L, et al. Spontaneous hyperventilation and brain tissue hypoxia in patients with severe brain injury. *J Neurol Neurosurg Psychiatry.* 2010;81:793-797.

33. Johnston AJ, Steiner LA, Coles JP, et al. Effect of cerebral perfusion pressure augmentation on regional oxygenation and metabolism after head injury. *Crit Care Med.* 2005;33:189-195; discussion 255-257.

34. White H, Venkatesh B. Cerebral perfusion pressure in neurotrauma: a review. *Anesth Analg.* 2008;107:979-988.

35. Diringer MN, Axelrod Y. Hemodynamic manipulation in the neuro-intensive care unit: cerebral perfusion pressure therapy in head injury and hemodynamic augmentation for cerebral vasospasm. *Curr Opin Crit Care.* 2007;13:156-162.

36. Bratton SL, Chestnut RM, Ghajar J, et al. Guidelines for the management of severe traumatic brain injury. X. Brain oxygen monitoring and thresholds. *J Neurotrauma.* 2007;24(suppl 1):S65-S70.

37. Claassen J, Mayer SA, Hirsch LJ. Continuous EEG monitoring in patients with subarachnoid hemorrhage. *J Clin Neurophysiol.* 2005;22:92-98.

38. Belli A, Sen J, Petzold A, Russo S, Kitchen N, Smith M. Metabolic failure precedes intracranial pressure rises in traumatic brain injury: a microdialysis study. *Acta Neurochir (Wien).* 2008;150:461-469; discussion 470.

39. Naidech AM, Kreiter KT, Janjua N, et al. Cardiac troponin elevation, cardiovascular morbidity, and outcome after subarachnoid hemorrhage. *Circulation.* 2005;112:2851-2856.

40. Diringer MN. Management of aneurysmal subarachnoid hemorrhage. *Crit Care Med.* 2009;37:432-440.

41. Robertson CS, Valadka AB, Hannay HJ, et al. Prevention of secondary ischemic insults after severe head injury. *Crit Care Med.* 1999;27:2086-2095.

42. Contant CF, Valadka AB, Gopinath SP, Hannay HJ, Robertson CS. Adult respiratory distress syndrome: a complication of induced hypertension after severe head injury. *J Neurosurg.* 2001;95:560-568.

43. Steiner LA, Coles JP, Johnston AJ, et al. Assessment of cerebrovascular autoregulation in head-injured patients: a validation study. *Stroke.* 2003;34:2404-2409.

44. Steiner LA, Coles JP, Czosnyka M, et al. Cerebrovascular pressure reactivity is related to global cerebral oxygen metabolism after head injury. *J Neurol Neurosurg Psychiatry.* 2003;74:765-770.

45. Jaeger M, Schuhmann MU, Soehle M, Meixensberger J. Continuous assessment of cerebrovascular autoregulation after traumatic brain injury using brain tissue oxygen pressure reactivity. *Crit Care Med.* 2006;34:1783-1788.

46. Huber W, Umgelter A, Reindl W, et al. Volume assessment in patients with necrotizing pancreatitis: a comparison of intrathoracic blood volume index, central venous pressure, and hematocrit, and their correlation to cardiac index and extravascular lung water index. *Crit Care Med.* 2008;36:2348-2354.

47. Joseph M, Ziadi S, Nates J, Dannenbaum M, Malkoff M. Increases in cardiac output can reverse flow deficits from vasospasm independent of blood pressure: a study using xenon computed tomographic measurement of cerebral blood flow. *Neurosurgery.* 2003;53:1044-1051; discussion 1051-1052.

48. Muench E, Horn P, Bauhuf C, et al. Effects of hypervolemia and hypertension on regional cerebral blood flow, intracranial pressure, and brain tissue oxygenation after subarachnoid hemorrhage. *Crit Care Med.* 2007;35:1844-1851; quiz 1852.

Neurocritical Care Monitoring

Evoked Potentials in the Operating Room and ICU

Errol Gordon, MD
Jan Claassen, MD

Evoked potentials are well established as diagnostic and monitoring tools in the operating room (OR) as well as the intensive care unit (ICU) setting. They may help clinicians to detect injury to peripheral nerves and the spinal cord during surgery, and help prognosticate outcome after traumatic brain injury (TBI) and cardiac arrest.

 A 55-year-old woman complained for several years of neck stiffness and pain for which she was medicating herself with nonsteroidal anti-inflammatory drugs. Over the past several months, she noted having more difficulty getting around and increasing clumsiness. She denied any bowel or bladder symptoms. Her examination revealed increased tone in all of her extremities with bilateral positive Babinski signs and sustained ankle clonus. Strength was full power on confrontation testing throughout. No sensory level was appreciated. Her primary care physician sent her for a computerized tomographic (CT) scan of the cervical spine, which revealed significant spondylosis and canal stenosis that was worse at C5-C6 and C6-C7, with posteriorly displaced discs. A cervical magnetic resonance image (MRI) revealed cord compression with cord signal changes at C5-C6. After getting these results, the primary care physician referred her to a local orthopedic surgeon who recommended decompression of C5-C6 and C6-C7. He mentioned that he will be using intraoperative neurophysiologic monitoring during the case.

What is the role of intraoperative neurophysiologic monitoring?

During operative procedures requiring anesthesia resulting in depressed consciousness surgeons have limited means to assess the integrity of the nervous system using clinical examination techniques alone. Monitoring techniques during surgery or interventions (such as interventional neuroradiologic procedures) may allow documentation of acute, but still reversible, changes in neurologic function. Additionally, these techniques can be used intraoperatively to assist in identifying important neural structures. Techniques commonly used for intraoperative monitoring include electroencephalography (EEG) and evoked potentials; the later will be discussed in this chapter. Evoked potentials include somatosensory evoked potentials (SSEPs), brainstem auditory evoked potentials (BAEPs), visual evoked potentials (VEPs), and motor evoked potentials (MEPs). Each of these specifically assesses different sensory or motor pathways and can be selected based on the individual clinical scenario. Wiedemayer et al 2002[1] reported that of 423 operations with intraoperative monitoring, surgical decisions were successfully modified in 5.2%. Using both SSEP and BAEP monitoring, the rates were: true-positive findings with intervention, 42 cases (9.9%); true-positive findings without intervention, 42 cases (9.9%), false-positive findings, 9 cases (2.1%), false-negative findings, 16 cases (3.8%), and true-negative findings, 314 cases (74.2%).

What are evoked potentials?

Evoked potentials (EPs) are electric potentials recorded from the nervous system following presentation of a stimulus, which can be auditory, visual, or *electrical*. EPs are orders of magnitude smaller in amplitude than EEG signals and require signal averaging and precise localization of the recording electrode to measure a response.[2] The recorded potential is time-locked to the stimulus and most of the noise occurs randomly, allowing the noise to be averaged out by collecting repeated responses. EPs can be recorded from cerebral cortex, brainstem, spinal cord, and peripheral nerves. Usually, the term *evoked potential* is reserved for responses involving either recordings from, or stimulation of, central nervous system structures. Thus, evoked compound motor action potentials (CMAPs) or sensory nerve action potentials (SNAPs) as used in nerve conduction studies (NCS) are generally not thought of as evoked potentials, although they do meet the above definition. Clinically, the recorded electric potentials are evaluated for morphology, latency, and amplitude. These values may then be compared to laboratory-established norms or compared to the contralateral side, in which case patients may serve as their own control.

What are visual, somatosensory, and motor evoked potentials and how are they generated?

Visual Evoked Potentials (VEPs)

These are generated by placing a recording electrode over or near to the visual cortex and applying visual stimuli such as a flashing light or a flickering checkerboard.[3] Measured from the primary recording electrodes over the primary visual cortex, these stimuli typically produced a negative deflection at approximately 75 milliseconds (N75) and a positive deflection at approximately 100 milliseconds (P100).

Somatosensory Evoked Potentials (SSEPs)

This test assesses the integrity of the dorsal column-lemniscal system.[4] This pathway projects via the dorsal column of the spinal cord to the cuneate nucleus in the lower brainstem, to the ventroposterior lateral thalamus, to the primary somatosensory cortex, and then to a wide network of cortical areas involved in somatosensory processing. Median and tibial nerves are most often stimulated in SSEP testing, although others (eg, ulnar, peroneal) may be used when appropriate.

The stimulus for SSEPs is a brief electric pulse delivered by a pair of electrodes placed on the skin above the nerve. To minimize artifact produced by electric stimulation, a ground electrode is placed between the stimulation site and the recording site. Both standard surface disc electrodes and needle electrodes can be used as recording electrodes. For upper limb SSEP recording, electrodes are placed at the clavicle between the heads of the sternocleidomastoid muscles (Erb point) and on the skin overlying cervical bodies 6-7. On the scalp, electrodes are placed at CP3 and CP4 of the International 10-20 System. For tibial SSEPs, electrodes are placed in the popliteal fossa and over the lumbar vertebra. At least two bipolar channels (eg, CPz-Fpz and CP3-CP4) should be used to record the cortical component. The SSEP waveform is obtained by averaging typically from 500 to 2000 stimuli; it is necessary to repeat at least two independent averages to demonstrate reproducibility. SSEPs are recorded using a broad bandpass filter with high-pass and low-pass filters set typically to 30 and 2000 Hz, respectively. Notch filters to eliminate power line noise (50 or 60 Hz) should be used with caution because of their tendency to create "ringing" oscillatory artifacts.

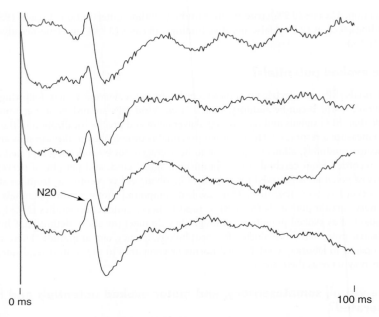

Figure 16-1. Normal median somatosensory evoked potential (SSEP) in a 65-year-old woman undergoing a lumbar laminectomy.

A normal median SSEP waveform is shown in Figure 16-1 and normal values in Table 16-1.[5] The purpose of obtaining peripheral potentials (ie, N9, Erb point) is to differentiate peripheral causes of conduction delays as seen in peripheral neuropathy from central ones. The P14 is generated in the caudal medial lemniscus within the lower medulla and the N20 reflects activation

Table 16-1. Normal Values for Evoked Potentials from Healthy Volunteers

	Recording site	Latency, mean (ms)	Latency, upper limit (ms)
Median SSEP			
N9	Erb point	9.8	11.5
N13	Cervical spine (C7)	13.3	14.5
N20	Contralateral cortex (CP3 or CP4)	19.8	23.0
Intervals median			
CCT (P14-N20)	-	5.6	6.6
Tibial SSEP			
N8	Popliteal fossa	8.5	10.5
N22	Lumbar spine (L1)	21.8	25.2
P30	Fz-Cv7	29.2	34.7
P39	Cz-Fz	38.0	43.9
Intervals tibial			
N22-P30	-	7.4	10.2
P30-P39	-	8.7	13.4

(Carrera ER, Claassen J. Brainstem auditory evoked potentials and somatosensory evoked potentials. In: LeRoux PD, Levine JM, Kofke WA eds. Monitoring in Neurocritical Care. Philadelphia: Elsevier; 2010.)

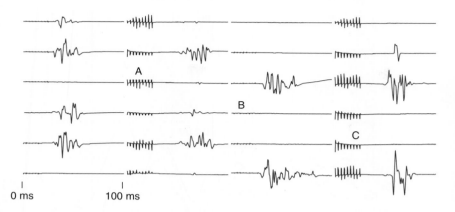

Figure 16-2. Normal motor evoked potential (MEP) in the patient seen in Figure 16-1. Columns A and C represent the left and right abductor pollicis, respectively. Columns B and D represent the left and right flexor hallucis longus, respectively.

of the primary somatosensory receiving area, located in the posterior bank of the rolandic fissure in Brodmann area 3b. Middle and late latency potentials are less frequently used. A delayed or absent signal at the Erb point may suggest a brachial plexus injury. A delayed or absent potential at the base of the brain may suggest pathology in the upper cervical cord or brainstem. If the typical brainstem potentials (ie, N14) are present, but cortical potentials like the N20 are not seen, this suggests disruption to the thalamicocortical projections, which may be related to pathology such as tumors, anoxic injury, or ischemia.

Motor Evoked Potentials (MEPs)

Other evoked potentials typically used in the operating room are MEPs (Figure 16-2). These EPs are generated using magnetic stimulation at or close to the primary motor cortex and have the recording electrode placed in the relevant muscle.

A 42-year-old man presented with several months of persistent headaches and decreased hearing on the right. Examination by his primary physician revealed an otherwise normal neurologic examination. The headaches were not controlled with pain medication and were progressively becoming more severe. An MRI was ordered and he was found to have a 3 cm × 2.5 cm pontomedullary mass. He was referred to a neurosurgeon for further evaluation. The neurosurgeon planned to surgically remove the tumor using intraoperative monitoring with brainstem auditory evoked potentials (BAEPs).

Describe BAEPs

BAEPs are produced by an audible clicking stimulus. The first 10 milliseconds on the response elicited from the audio stimulus represents the electric transmission of that signal through the brainstem and thus is known as the BAEPs.[3] Recording electrodes are between the Cz (according to the international 10-20 system) and the ipsilateral ear. The normal BAEP typically shows five to six peaks labeled with corresponding Roman numerals (Figure 16-3). Although generators of individual peaks are still somewhat controversial, commonly identified generators include the distal auditory

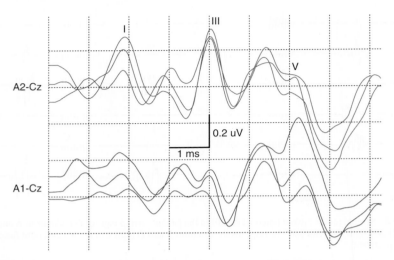

Figure 16-3. A 49-year-old woman found to have a right frontal brain tumor with normal brainstem auditory evoked potential (BAEP) bilaterally (click 90 db, noise 60 db; recorded from the right ear).

nerve (wave I), auditory nerve as it exits the porus acoustics or the cochlear nucleus (wave II), the cochlear nucleus or ipsilateral superior olivary nucleus (wave III), the superior olive or nucleus or axons of the lateral lemniscus (wave IV), and the inferior colliculus and ventral lateral lemniscus (wave V). As waves II and IV are less reliably recorded across individuals, clinical interpretation is based primarily on assessment of waves I, III, and V.

How can BAEPs be interpreted?

Absence or delays in wave V with a normal wave I latency can be seen with conduction abnormalities central to the distal portion of cranial nerve VIII, while absence of wave I with preserved wave V may reflect a problem with the peripheral hearing apparatus or with the auditory nerve, but commonly reflects technical difficulty of recording wave I. Functional disruption of the brainstem may cause loss of waves II to V with preseveration of wave I. Unilaterally abnormal BAEPs most often reflect ipsilateral brainstem damage. More rostral structures, including generators within the primary auditory cortex and surrounding areas, are responsible for longer latency components[6]; however, similar to other EPs, the later components of the BAEPs are substantially affected by arousal state and are less commonly used in the OR or ICU setting.[7]

Practical use of EPs in the OR

In the OR, EPs are used for two related purposes: (1) to minimize postoperative injury and (2) to guide treatment. Monitoring may detect functional impairment of neuronal function before permanent deficits occur. Intraoperatively, neuronal function is at risk from a number of mechanisms, including direct surgical transection, transmission of heat from surgical devices, stress, compression, and compromise of blood supply. In addition to EPs, recording needles may be placed in muscles of pertinent myotomes to look for spontaneous electromyographic (EMG) activity caused by stimulation of the relevant nerve. The surgeon may also have a specialized dissecting device that also serves as a stimulating electrode. EMG activity in the muscles of the face may, for example, signal the surgeon that he/she is dissecting too close to the facial nerve while trying to remove a pontomedullary tumor.

A surgeon may also apply an electric stimulus to a screw placed during back surgery. The corresponding EMG activity detected in the relevant muscle may give the surgeon an idea of how close the screw is to the nerve root.

What specific considerations pertain to using EPs in the OR?

ORs are electrically noisy environments with abundant artifacts from use of surgical equipment such as a Bovie device and also ungrounded electric equipment. Consideration must also be given to the type of stimulation and recording electrodes that are used. It is also important to note the placement of the ground electrode on the patient. Stray current from various surgical devices may travel along the surface of the skin and cause burns at the site of electrodes. Specific consideration should be given to the type of electrodes used. Surface electrodes are appropriate for awake patients, but they may be easily dislodged and replacement may be very challenging in a prepped and draped patient. Needle electrodes are less likely to be dislodged and have a very low infection risk. Neurologic injury may occur from positioning and baseline studies, post-induction but prior to the final positioning, and may be helpful to differentiate EP changes present at baseline from those due to positioning or the surgical intervention.

Do medications commonly used in the OR or the ICU affect EPs?

Subcortical components (ie, waves I to V of the BAEP) are relatively unaffected by most medications commonly used in the OR and the ICU, whereas cortical ones are more susceptible to medication effects, especially at high doses. Sedative medications, including benzodiazepines, propofol, barbiturates, nitrous oxide, and halogenated inhalational agents, all depress the cortical components of evoked potentials in a dose-related manner.[8-10] Interpeak changes may be more stable (ie, I to V interpeak latencies for BAEPs) and comparing left- and right-sided recordings may be useful, particularly for SSEPs. Neuromuscular blockade should not affect SSEP,[2] but will affect MEPs.

 A 62-year-old man was witnessed passing out at his gym after leaving the treadmill. Bystanders found him to be unresponsive and without a pulse, and immediately started cardiopulmonary resuscitation (CPR). An automated external defibrillator (AED) was placed and the patient was defibrillated twice. Emergency medical services (EMS) arrived 10 minutes after the collapse and found him in ventricular fibrillation. After two rounds of electric cardioversion, he went into sinus rhythm. He was intubated in the field and brought to the closest emergency department. Total time from collapse to return of spontaneous circulation was estimated to be 25 minutes. On arrival at the hospital, the patient had a blood pressure of 90/60 mm Hg, not requiring blood pressure support, a heart rate of 98, and a temperature of 36.6°C. An electrocardiogram (ECG) revealed inferior lateral ST depression and T-wave inversion with a troponin I level of 1.2 (peaked the next day at 3.6). On neurologic examination, he was noted to have pupils of 5 mm and nonreactive to light, intact corneal reflexes bilaterally, and absent gag or cough reflexes. The patient did not have any spontaneous breathing, and no motor responses were elicited to painful stimuli in all extremities.

SSEP for prognostication after cardiac arrest

EPs and particularly SSEPs are frequently used to predict outcome after cardiac arrest and have been recommended for prognostication. These recommendations are based on one prospective and a number of retrospective studies.[11-20] The prospective study of 407 cardiac arrest patients showed that bilaterally absent N20s were seen in 45% of patients who were comatose at 72 hours, and all of these had poor outcome.[20] In a meta-analysis of 4500 postanoxic patients, bilaterally absent N20s within the first week had a 100% specificity to predict poor outcome.[19] Combining SSEPs with other predictors of outcome after cardiac arrest such as EEG or serum markers of neuronal injury improves prognostic accuracy.[16-18] While some predictions can be made for poor recovery, it is much more difficult to predict good outcome.

 This patient underwent 24 hours of induced hypothermia (goal temperature 33°C) followed by slow rewarming (0.1°C per hour). After rewarming, the neurologic examination revealed no spontaneous eye opening; pupils unreactive bilaterally to light; intact corneal, gag, and cough reflexes; and extensor posturing bilaterally with both upper extremities to pain.

Does therapeutic hypothermia have an effect on the utility of SSEPs in post-cardiac arrest patients?

Two randomized control studies have shown that therapeutic hypothermia post–cardiac arrest related to ventricular fibrillation and ventricular tachycardia improves both survival[21] and neurologic outcome.[21,22] In a prospective study of 111 cardiac arrest patients who underwent therapeutic hypothermia,[23] none of the patients who had absent SSEPs 24 hours after weaning of sedation had a favorable neurologic outcome. Another study,[24] which was retrospective, looked at 185 therapeutic hypothermia patients post–cardiac arrest. This study found that of the 36 patients who had bilaterally absent SSEPs, only one patient had a good recovery. The mean time to SSEP study was 3 days. In a small control study by Tiainen et al[25] of 60 cardiac arrest patients, 30 of whom underwent therapeutic hypothermia, no patient in either the hypothermia group or the normothermia group with absent SSEPs awoke. These SSEPs were preformed 24 hours post–cardiac arrest, and so the patients in the hypothermia group had a mean temperature of 33°C. Despite these studies, larger prospective studies need to be performed to determine the utility of SSEPs in prognosticating after cardiac arrest.

Do BAEPs have any utility in prognostication after cardiac arrest?

BAEPs have rarely been studied systematically in cardiac arrest patients. In a small cohort of 13 patients, middle latency auditory evoked responses (MLAEPs) were absent in all patients who died or remained in a persistent vegetative state.[14] In the study by Tiainen et al[25] mentioned above, BAEPs were found not to be useful for prognostication after cardiac arrest.

What is the significance of the EP grading system and neurologic injury?

One study[14] examined the value of using median nerve SSEP, BAEP, and MLAEP in 131 ICU patients who were comatose as a result of anoxic ischemic injury, TBI, complication of neurosurgery, or encephalitis. These investigators used a grading system to categorize electrophysiologic studies and test the accuracy to prognosticate outcome (Table 16-2). This grading system is not widely used clinically.

Electrophysiologic studies were preformed between days 1 and 46 after onset of coma.[14] Among patients with anoxic brain injury, 38% recovered with SSEP grade 1 classification. No patient recovered from coma with grade 2 or 3 in the anoxic ischemic group. In the TBI patients, 81% with grade 1 median SSEP recovered from coma, whereas 86% recovered with a grade 2 SSEP. No one in the TBI

Table 16-2. Grading System for Reporting Evoked Potentials

Grading	SSEP	BEAR	MLAEP
1	Normal SSEP at least on one side	Normal	Normal
2	Bilateral amplitude reduction	Increase in I-V interval without amplitude change	Isolated delay in Pa (Pa > 31.6) latency without Na-Pa amplitude reduction
3	Bilateral absent cortical responses	Amplitude ratio of V/I < 0.5	Na-Pa amplitude < 0.3 μV
4	NA	No detectable wave IV or V	No Pa detected
5	NA	Only wave I present	NA

(From Logi F, Fischer C, Murri L, Mauguière F. The prognostic value of evoked responses from primary somatosensory and auditory cortex in comatose patients. Clin Neurophysiol. 2003;114:1615-1627.)

group recovered with grade 3. In the poststroke group, 60% recovered from coma with grade 1 median SSEP, 69% recovered with grade 2, and again no one recovered from coma with grade 4 SSEP. Of note, no patient in the anoxic group with an N20-P24 amplitude of less than 1.2 μV recovered. This was not noted in the TBI patients or the poststroke patients. In summary, absent primary cortical median nerve SSEP responses were very accurate in predicting poor outcome after anoxic brain injury.[14] Many studies have not taken dynamic changes of the EP findings into account, but some evidence suggests that secondary loss of initially present cortical responses carries a poor prognosis.[14]

What are event-related potentials (ERPs) and are they useful in predicting recovery from coma?

ERPs are long-latency potentials also visualized through signal-averaging techniques of the EEG[26] and are thought to reflect more complex cognitive processing of stimuli. Examples of ERPs include P300, N100, and MMN (mismatch negativity). The N100 is thought to represent attention,[27] the P300 is elicited by a rare task related stimulus,[26] while the MMN is elicited by an "oddball" sound in a sequence of sounds.[26] A meta-analysis compared the predictive ability of late-stage EPs for awakening from coma due to ischemia, hemorrhage, trauma, anoxic injury, metabolic etiologies, and postoperative causes (Table 16-3).[28] The presence of a N100 had a sensitivity of 71% (CI 66-76) and specificity of 57% (CI 51-63) for good outcome across the several studies. The MMN had a sensitivity of 38% (CI 32-43) and specificity of 91% (CI 85-95). The P300 had a sensitivity 62% (CI 53-69) and specificity of 77% (CI 70-82).

MMN showed a relatively high specificity for recovery of wakefulness, particularly in anoxic injury.[29] Fischer et al found the MMN to be the most powerful prognostic indicator for awakening from a coma and used it as the initial criterion to prepare a decision tree that they proposed for post–cardiac arrest prognostication.[29] This is not widely used.

Can temperature affect the EP?

The bulk of our experience of using EP in the hypothermic patient stems from intraoperative cases, particularly during cardiac and neurovascular surgery, but this needs to be considered for ICU patients given the increasingly widespread use of therapeutic hypothermia. In a cohort of nine aortic surgery patients, subcortical SSEP components (P13 and N14) became more consistently recognized at profound hypothermia (less than 20°C) when compared to normothermia; however, cortical components disappeared.[30] A linear correlation between decreasing temperature

Neurocritical Care Monitoring

Table 16-3. Sensitivity and Specificity of the Presence of Late-Stage Evoked Potentials for Awakening (Glasgow Outcome Score > 2) in Comatose Patients from Various Etiologies

ERP	Etiology	Sensitivity	Specificity
		% (CI)	% (CI)
N100	Stroke and hemorrhage	73 (64-80)	43 (32-55)
	Anoxic brain injury	83 (64-94)	61 (51-71)
	Traumatic brain injury	64 (54-72)	48 (29-68)
	Encephalopathy	85 (54-97)	28 (10-54)
MMN	Stroke and hemorrhage	41 (31-52)	86 (74-94)
	Anoxic brain injury	50 (30-70)	94 (84-98)
	Traumatic brain injury	34 (26-43)	90 (72-97)
	Encephalopathy	37 (10-74)	86 (42-99)
P300	Stroke and hemorrhage	86 (56-97)	63 (45-78)
	Anoxic brain injury	52 (32-70)	85 (76-91)
	Traumatic brain injury	76 (65-85)	80 (62-91)
	Encephalopathy	86 (42-99)	56 (30-79)

(From Daltrozzo J, Wioland N, Mutschler V, Koychoubey B. Predicting coma and other low responsive patients outcome using event-related brain potentials: a meta-analysis. Clin Neurophysiol. 2007;118:606-614.)

and increasing cortical and peripheral SSEP latencies (N10, P14, and N19) was seen in another cohort of cardiac surgery patients,[31] while the amplitude was poorly correlated with the temperature. Whereas cortical potentials disappeared between 20°C and 25°C, peripheral components remained stable.

There is a linear increase of BAEP latencies and interpeak intervals by approximately 7% per drop of each degree celsius.[32] At 26°C, BAEP normal values are approximately doubled. Longer latency components may disappear with moderate degrees of hypothermia, but ultimately all components will disappear below temperatures of 14°C or 20°C.[33,34]

In a recent study of patients with cardiac arrest undergoing therapeutic hypothermia (goal 33°C), SSEPs and BAEPs were used to study patients between 24 and 28 hours after the arrest.[25] The investigators confirmed previously established EP prognosticators (ie, poor outcome with bilaterally absent N20 in the SSEP) in the setting of induced hypothermia. BAEPs had no additional value in outcome prediction.

A 14-year-old boy was admitted in a deep coma (Glasgow Coma Scale [GCS] score 3) with suspected severe diffuse axonal injury and had elevated intracranial pressure (ICP). Median nerve SSEPs (Figure 16-4), absent left cortical responses, and prolongation with a severely decreased amplitude right cortical responses.

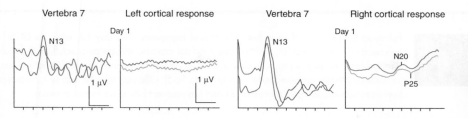

Figure 16-4. Refer to text for explanation. *(From Claassen J, Hansen HC. Early recovery after closed traumatic head injury: Somatosensory evoked potentials and clinical findings. Crit Care Med. 2001;29:494-502.)*

How can EPs after TBI be used and what is the significance of the above SSEP?

Many studies have investigated the utility of EPs after TBI and demonstrated the ability to predict short-term mortality rate and long-term outcome. Most studies agree that bilaterally absent cortical SSEP responses in the setting of intact peripheral and spinal potentials universally indicate poor outcome.[35-38] Those with normal SSEPs (N = 553) have a favorable outcome (normal or moderate disability; Figure 16-5) in 71% of cases compared to unfavorable outcome (severe disability, vegetative state, or death) in 99% of those with bilaterally absent SSEPs (N = 777).[39] The positive predictive value and sensitivity are 71% and 59%, respectively, for normal SSEP, predicting favorable outcome; and 99% and 46.2%, respectively, for bilaterally absent SSEP, predicting unfavorable outcome. SSEPs perform favorably when compared to other predictors of outcome after severe TBI, including the GCS, pupillary or motor responses, CT, and EEG.[40] The predictive accuracy of abnormal, but present, cortical responses such as in our patient or unilateral abnormalities is more ambiguous.

Can serial SSEPs offer additional information?

Serial EPs may detect recovery[41,42] (see Figure 16-5) or secondary injury (ie, blossoming hemorrhages or ICP crises) after TBI.

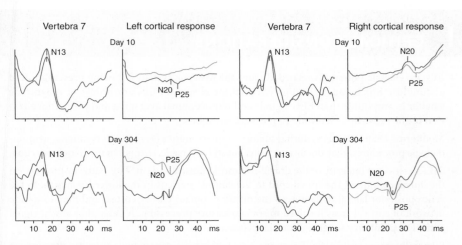

Figure 16-5. Follow-up somatosensory evoked potentials (SSEPs) after traumatic brain injury. *(From Claassen J, Hansen HC. Early recovery after closed traumatic head injury: somatosensory evoked potentials and clinical findings. Crit Care Med. 2001;29:494-502.)*

Neurocritical Care Monitoring

Follow-up SSEPs revealed some first indication of improvement on day 10, while his GCS first improved on day 13 post-TBI, and the patient did not move his left side purposefully until day 26. Twenty-three days after injury, latencies of the right cortical projection were within normal limits, whereas amplitudes remained reduced (see Figure 16-5). One year after the accident, he suffered from minimal residual speech impairment and has returned fully to his former activities.

Can EPs other than SSEPs be useful after TBI?

BAEP abnormalities are more frequently seen in TBI patients with poor outcome.[43,44] Applying the above introduced grading system[44] to TBI patients, 75% of those with grade 1 or 2 BAEPs recovered from coma compared to 50% of those with grade 3 or 4. MLAEPs performed similarly.

What role do EPs play in managing patients with intracranial hemorrhage (ICH), acute ischemic stroke (AIS), or subarachnoid hemorrhage (SAH)?

SSEPs do not provide the same predictive accuracy of poor outcome in coma from other neurologic injuries and are currently not widely used for these patients. However, BAEP and SSEP abnormalities are seen in SAH with poor functional outcome.[45,46] Bilaterally absent cortical potentials carry a similarly dismal prognosis as in other etiologies discussed above.[45]

EPs in determining brain death

Many practice parameter guidelines accept EPs as one option of a confirmatory test.[47] The American Academy of Neurology (AAN) recently updated guidelines on the determination of brain death.[48] SSEPs were not noted to be one of the typical ancillary tests that are used. Patients evolving to brain death will lose subcortical SSEPs and all BAEP responses when investigated with serial examinations.[49,50] Loss of the median nerve SSEP noncephalic P14 and of its cephalic referenced reflection N14 as well as the N18 is seen in brain death.[50,51]

! CRITICAL CONSIDERATIONS

- EPs are electric potentials recorded from the nervous system following presentation of a stimulus, which can be auditory, visual, or electrical. EPs are orders of magnitude smaller in amplitude than EEG signals and require signal averaging and precise localization of the recording electrode to measure a response.

- Monitoring techniques used during surgery or interventions (such as interventional neuroradiologic procedures) may document acute, but still reversible, changes in neurologic function.

- SSEPs assess the integrity of the dorsal column-lemniscal system. This pathway projects via the dorsal column of the spinal cord to the cuneate nucleus in the lower brainstem, to the ventroposterior lateral thalamus, to the primary somatosensory cortex, and then to a wide network of cortical areas involved in somatosensory processing. A delayed or absent signal at the Erb point may suggest a brachial plexus injury.

- Bilaterally absent cortical SSEP responses are highly predictive of poor outcome after cardiac arrest and traumatic brain injury.

- Subcortical components of the BAEP are relatively unaffected by most medications commonly used in the OR and the ICU, whereas cortical ones are more susceptible to medication effects, especially at high doses.
- Sedative medications including benzodiazepines, propofol, barbiturates, nitrous oxide, and halogenated inhalational agents all depress the cortical components of EPs in a dose-related manner.
- Interpeak changes may be more stable (ie, I to V interpeak latencies for BAEPs) and comparing left- and right-sided recordings may be useful, particularly for SSEPs.
- Neuromuscular blockade should not affect SSEP, but will affect MEPs.

REFERENCES

1. Wiedemayer H, Fauser B, Sandalcioglu IE, Schafer H, Stolke D. The impact of neurophysiological intraoperative monitoring on surgical decisions: a critical analysis of 423 cases. *J Neurosurg.* 2002; 96:255262.

2. Freye E. Cerebral monitoring in the operating room and the intensive care unit—An introductory for the clinician and a guide for the novice wanting to open a window to the brain. Part II: sensory-evoked potentials (SSEP, AEP, VEP). *J Clin Monit Comput.* 2005;19:77-168.

3. Moller AR. *Intraoperative Neurophysiological Monitoring.* 2nd ed. Totowa, NJ: Humana Press; 2006.

4. Cruccu G, Aminoff MJ, Curio G, et al. Recommendations for the clinical use of somatosensory-evoked potentials. *Clin Neurophysiol.* 2008;119:1705-1719.

5. Carrera ER, Claassen J. Brainstem auditory evoked potentials and somatosensory evoked potentials. In: LeRoux PD, Levine JM, Kofke WA, eds. *Monitoring in Neurocritical Care.* Philadelphia: Elsevier; 2010.

6. Yvert B, Crouzeix A, Bertrand O, Seither-Preisler A, Pantev C. Multiple supratemporal sources of magnetic and electric auditory evoked middle latency components in humans. *Cereb Cortex.* 2001;11:411-423.

7. Linden DE. The P300: where in the brain is it produced and what does it tell us? *Neuroscientist.* 2005;11:563-576.

8. Legatt AD. BAEPs in surgery. In: Marc RN, ed. *Handbook of Clinical Neurophysiology.* St. Louis, MO: Elsevier; 2008:334-349.

9. Drummond J, Todd MM, Schubert A, Sang H. Effect of the acute administration of high dose pentobarbital on human brain stem auditory and median nerve somatosensory evoked responses. . *Neurosurgery.* 1987;20:830-835.

10. Liu E, Wong HK, Chia CP, Lim HJ, Chen ZY, Lee TL. Effects of isoflurane and propofol on cortical somatosensory evoked potentials during comparable depth of anaesthesia as guided by bispectral index. *Br J Anaesth.* 2005;94:193-197.

11. Zandbergen EG, Koelman JH, de Haan RJ, Hijdra A. SSEPs and prognosis in postanoxic coma: only short or also long latency responses? *Neurology.* 2006;67:583-586.

12. Madl C, Kramer L, Domanovits H, et al. Improved outcome prediction in unconscious cardiac arrest survivors with sensory evoked potentials compared with clinical assessment. *Crit Care Med.* 2000;28:721-726.

13. Gendo A, Kramer L, Hafner M, et al. Time-dependency of sensory evoked potentials in comatose cardiac arrest survivors. *Intensive Care Med.* 2001;27: 1305-1311.

14. Logi F, Fischer C, Murri L, Mauguiere F. The prognostic value of evoked responses from primary somatosensory and auditory cortex in comatose patients. *Clin Neurophysiol.* 2003;114:1615-1627.

15. Berek K, Lechleitner P, Luef G, et al. Early determination of neurological outcome after prehospital cardiopulmonary resuscitation. *Stroke.* 1995;26: 543-549.

16. Young GB, Doig G, Ragazzoni A. Anoxic-ischemic encephalopathy: clinical and electrophysiological associations with outcome. *Neurocrit Care.* 2005;2:159-164.

17. Chen R, Bolton CF, Young B. Prediction of outcome in patients with anoxic coma: a clinical and electrophysiologic study. *Crit Care Med.* 1996;24:672-678.

18. Bassetti C, Bomio F, Mathis J, Hess CW. Early prognosis in coma after cardiac arrest: a prospective clinical, electrophysiological, and biochemical study of 60 patients. *J Neurol Neurosurg Psychiatry.* 1996;61:610-615.

19. Zandbergen EG, de Haan RJ, Stoutenbeek CP, Koelman JH, Hijdra A. Systematic review of early

prediction of poor outcome in anoxic-ischaemic coma. *Lancet.* 1998;352:1808-1812.

20. Zandbergen EG, Hijdra A, Koelman JH, et al. Prediction of poor outcome within the first 3 days of postanoxic coma. *Neurology.* 2006;66:62-68.

21. Hypothermia after Cardiac Arrest Study Group. Mild therapeutic hypothermia to improve the neurologic outcome after cardiac arrest. *N Engl J Med.* 2002;346:549-556.

22. Bernard SA, Gray TW, Buist MD, et al. Treatment of comatose survivors of out-of-hospital cardiac arrest with induced hypothermia. *N Engl J Med.* 2002;346:557-563.

23. Rossetti AO, Oddo M, Logroscino G, Kaplan PW. Prognostication after cardiac arrest and hypothermia: a prospective study. *Ann Neurol.* 2010;67:301-307.

24. Leithner C, Ploner CJ, Hasper D, Storm C. Does hypothermia influence the predictive value of bilateral absent N20 after cardiac arrest? *Neurology.* 2010;74:965-969.

25. Tiainen M, Kovala TT, Takkunen OS, Roine RO. Somatosensory and brainstem auditory evoked potentials in cardiac arrest patients treated with hypothermia. *Crit Care Med.* 2005;33:1736-1740.

26. Duncan CC, Barry RJ, Connolly JF, et al. Event-related potentials in clinical research: guidelines for eliciting, recording, and quantifying mismatch negativity, P300, and N400. *Clin Neurophysiol.* 2009;120:1883-1908.

27. Papageorgiou C, Giannakakis GA, Nikita KS, Anagnostopoulos D, Papadimitriou GN, Rabavilas A. Abnormal auditory ERP N100 in children with dyslexia: comparison with their control siblings. *Behav Brain Funct.* 2009;5:26.

28. Daltrozzo J, Wioland N, Mutschler V, Kotchoubey B. Predicting coma and other low responsive patients outcome using event-related brain potentials: a meta-analysis. *Clin Neurophysiol.* 2007;118:606-614.

29. Fischer C, Luaute J, Nemoz C, Morlet D, Kirkorian G, Mauguiere F. Improved prediction of awakening or nonawakening from severe anoxic coma using tree-based classification analysis. *Crit Care Med.* 2006;34:1520-1524.

30. Guerit JM, Soveges L, Baele P, Dion R. Median nerve somatosensory evoked potentials in profound hypothermia for ascending aorta repair. *Electroencephalogr Clin Neurophysiol.* 1990;77:163-173.

31. Markand ON, Warren C, Mallik GS, King RD, Brown JW, Mahomed Y. Effects of hypothermia on short latency somatosensory evoked potentials in humans. *Electroencephalogr Clin Neurophysiol.* 1990;77:416-424.

32. Markand ON, Lee BI, Warren C. et al. Effects of hypothermia on brainstem auditory evoked potentials in humans. *Ann Neurol.* 1987;22:507-513.

33. Kusakari J, Inamura N, Sakurai T, Kawamoto K. Effect of hypothermia upon the electrocochleogram and auditory evoked brainstem response. *Tohoku J Exp Med.* 1984;143:351-359.

34. Rosenblum SM, Ruth RA, Gal TJ. Brain stem auditory evoked potential monitoring during profound hypothermia and circulatory arrest. *Ann Otol Rhinol Laryngol.* 1985;94:281-283.

35. Rumpl E, Prugger M, Battista HJ, Badry F, Gerstenbrand F, Dienstl F. Short latency somatosensory evoked potentials and brain-stem auditory evoked potentials in coma due to CNS depressant drug poisoning. Preliminary observations. *Electroencephalogr Clin Neurophysiol.* 1988;70:482-489.

36. Sleigh JW, Havill JH, Frith R, Kersel D, Marsh N, Ulyatt D. Somatosensory evoked potentials in severe traumatic brain injury: a blinded study. *J Neurosurg.* 1999;91:577-580.

37. Procaccio F, Polo A, Lanteri P, Sala F. Electrophysiologic monitoring in neurointensive care. *Curr Opin Crit Care.* 2001;7:74-80.

38. Chiappa KH, Hoch DB. Electrophysiologic monitoring. In: Roper AH, ed. *Neurological and Neurosurgical intensive Care.* New York: Raven Press; 1993:147-183.

39. Carter BG, Butt W. Review of the use of somatosensory evoked potentials in the prediction of outcome after severe brain injury. *Crit Care Med.* 2001;29:178-186.

40. Carter BG, Butt W. Are somatosensory evoked potentials the best predictor of outcome after severe brain injury? A systematic review. *Intensive Care Med.* 2005;31:765-775.

41. Fossi S, Amantini A, Grippo A, et al. Continuous EEG-SEP monitoring of severely brain injured patients in NICU: methods and feasibility. *Neurophysiol Clin.* 2006;36:195-205.

42. Claassen J, Hansen HC. Early recovery after closed traumatic head injury: somatosensory evoked potentials and clinical findings. *Crit Care Med.* 2001;29:494-502.

43. Rappaport M, Hemmerle AV, Rappaport ML. Short and long latency auditory evoked potentials in traumatic brain injury patients. *Clin Electroencephalogr.* 1991;22:199-202.

44. Cant BR, Hume AL, Judson JA, Shaw, NA. The assessment of severe head injury by short-latency somatosensory and brain-stem auditory evoked potentials. *Electroencephalogr Clin Neurophysiol.* 1986;65:188-195.

45. Ritz R, Schwerdtfeger K, Strowitzki M, Donauer E, Koenig J, Steudel WI. Prognostic value of SSEP in early aneurysm surgery after SAH in poor-grade patients. *Neurol Res.* 2002;24:756-764.

46. Schick U, Dohnert J, Meyer JJ, Vitzthum HE. Prognostic significance of SSEP, BAEP and serum S-100B monitoring after aneurysm surgery. *Acta Neurol Scand.* 2003;108:161-169.

47. Wijdicks EF. Brain death worldwide: accepted fact but no global consensus in diagnostic criteria. *Neurology.* 2002;58:20-25.

48. Wijdicks EF, Varelas PN, Gronseth GS, Greer DM. Evidence-based guideline update: determining brain death in adults: report of the Quality Standards Subcommittee of the American Academy of Neurology. *Neurology.* 2010;74:1911-1918.

49. Starr A. Auditory brain-stem responses in brain death. *Brain.* 1976;99:543-554.

50. Buchner H, Ferbert A, Hacke W. Serial recording of median nerve stimulated subcortical somatosensory evoked potentials (SEPs) in developing brain death. *Electroencephalogr Clin Neurophysiol.* 1988;69:14-23.

51. Sonoo M, Tsai-Shozawa Y, Aoki M, et al. N18 in median somatosensory evoked potentials: a new indicator of medullary function useful for the diagnosis of brain death. *J Neurol Neurosurg Psychiatry.* 1999;67:374-378.

Neurocritical Care Monitoring

17 Neurophysiologic Decision Support Systems

Michael J. Schmidt, PhD, MSc

The field of biomedical informatics can be defined as the scientific discipline that deals with biomedical information, data, and knowledge including their storage, retrieval, and optimal use for problem solving and decision making.[1] The fields of bioinformatics, imaging informatics, clinical informatics, and public health informatics are all grouped under this larger umbrella.[1,2] Most relevant to this chapter, clinical informatics is motivated by applied problems in clinical care encompassing both patient-specific information and knowledge-based information. The electronic medical record is an application based on patient-specific information, whereas MEDLINE, which is provided by the National Library of Medicine, is a key resource for health-related knowledge retrieval.[2] A clinical decision support system (CDSS) is a computer program designed to help clinicians make diagnoses or management decisions[3] and often relies on both patient-specific and knowledge-based information.[2]

The goal of invasive neuromonitoring, or multimodality monitoring, is to provide neurophysiologic decision support at the bedside. Advanced monitoring techniques can provide real-time information regarding the relative health or distress of the brain. This information can be used to set physiologic end points to guide goal-directed therapy and thereby create and maintain an optimal physiologic environment for the comatose injured brain to heal.[4] From a critical standpoint, multimodality monitoring as a clinical decision support system is still in its infancy. Patient-specific information from patient monitors and devices are not easy to obtain, manipulate, or visualize, and knowledge-based information is largely dependent on what is known by the clinician looking at the data. That said, the field is now starting to evolve rapidly and the realization of the potential benefits of multimodality monitoring, and CDSSs in general, is only going to increase. This chapter is designed to help you implement neurophysiologic decision support systems in your intensive care unit (ICU).

Are neurophysiologic decision support systems really needed in the ICU?

It is true that there is a paucity of CDSSs of any type operating in the ICU,[5] and yet it may be the clinical setting in greatest need for such systems. Clinicians may be confronted with more than 200 variables[6] during morning rounds, and yet people are not able to judge the degree of relatedness between more than two variables.[7] Our ability to collect patient data far exceeds our intellectual capacity to understand it unassisted[5] and greatly contributes to conditions of constant information overload that can lead to preventable medical errors.[7,8] Implementation of CDSSs to help us understand the clinical meaning of patient data is essential.[9,10]

Why are ICU CDSSs not already widely available?

Generally speaking, there is a lack of clinical informatics infrastructure to support these systems. Adoption of electronic health record (EHR) systems is being promoted by the Department of Health and Human Services through the office of National Coordinator for

Health Information Technology by means of forums and regulations. The American Recovery and Reinvestment Act of 2009 (ARRA) has also authorized centers for Medicare and Medicaid Services (CMS) to provide reimbursement incentives up to $44,000 for each eligible health care professional who uses a certified EHR in a meaningful manner. Starting in 2015, financial penalties will be levied until EHRs are utilized according to the meaningful use of the terms.[11-13] ICUs have been migrating from paper-based to computerized charting systems for over a decade.[14] Despite all of these efforts, as of 2009, it is estimated that hospitals only have an EHR adoption rate of about 12%.[12]

How can CDSSs based on patient monitoring information be used to improve ICU care, or asked another way, how can I justify the need for neurophysiologic decision support systems to hospital administrators?

At a minimum you should have two goals. First, you should have tools to evaluate the effectiveness of treatments that are initiated to modify physiologic end points or improve clinical conditions. If you drill a hole into a patient's head and place an intracranial pressure (ICP) microprobe into the patient's brain, you should be able to easily monitor the effectiveness of your treatment decisions. I have yet to meet a hospital administrator or information technologist who has disagreed with this point. For instance, clinicians should be able to easily answer these questions:

- How fast does ICP drop after mannitol administration?
- Are repeated mannitol doses just as effective as earlier doses, or are more frequent doses now required?
- Is it safe to continue to give mannitol? What is the osmolar gap?
- Does increasing blood pressure increase or decrease ICP?
- Does adding sedation or reducing temperature provide additional ICP reduction?
- Has medical management failed; is it time to consider a surgical option?

These basic questions are difficult to answer in the absence of neurophysiologic decision support tools.

Second, neurophysiologic decision support systems should elucidate the physiologic status of the patient and how such physiology impacts other metrics of brain health like brain oxygenation and/or cerebral metabolism. An application of this (discussed in Chapter 15) is the assessment of cerebral autoregulation status. Often understanding patient physiologic status provides a context for treatment interventions rather than leading to a specific intervention. For example, if a patient with a subarachnoid hemorrhage has elevated ICP in the context of disturbed autoregulation, increasing blood pressure to increase cerebral perfusion (eg, to counteract cerebral vasospasm) may risk further ICP elevations, thereby increasing the risk of tissue compression or cerebral herniation. In this context, knowledge of cerebral autoregulation status helps the clinician weigh the risk/reward profile of different treatment options rather than directly evaluating the effectiveness of a specific treatment.

There are other potential benefits that can be realized by CDSS if patient-specific data can be collected and provided to support these systems.[15,16] These include automatic early detection of secondary complications before clinical symptoms occur (eg, sepsis detection[17]), computerized implementation of clinical protocols (eg, administration of insulin[18]), and general support of clinical decision making (eg, clinical dashboard[19]). As ICU clinical information infrastructure improves, the potential benefits provided by CDSS will only increase in the future.

How does the Food and Drug Administration (FDA) regulate CDSSs?

The FDA does regulate medical software as a device. One category of medical software is "software accessories," which is actively regulated by the FDA. Software accessories are attached to (or used with) other medical devices such as a patient physiologic monitor. For example, systems for digital analysis and graphical representation of electroencephalographic (EEG) data connected to EEG acquisition systems are FDA regulated. In contrast, it has been unclear how, or to what extent (if at all), stand-alone software should be regulated by the FDA.[20] With respect to neurophysiologic decision support systems, in general, all-in-one monitoring solutions connect directly with patient monitoring devices and, therefore, fall into the regulated FDA category of software accessory. In contrast, ICU-wide solutions often start by collecting data from patient monitors and storing it in a database. In a second separate step, data analysis and visualization software query data from the database, thereby being classified as stand-alone software that has not been regulated. There is the potential for causing harm when using CDSS,[21] and issues regarding liability and negligence with CDSS use are not currently clear.[20] Two independent organizations have been focusing on these issues,[22,23] and in 2011 the FDA announced Class I requirements (ie, requiring general controls) for 'Medical Device Data Systems' and Class I, II, or III requirements for 'Mobile Medical Applications' depending on what the application does. An application that allows a user to input patient-specific information and - using formulae or processing algorithms - output a patient-specific result, diagnosis, or treatment recommendation to be used in clinical practice constitutes a regulated software application. Discuss these new regulations with vendors and if you plan to create applications to help analyze patient data call the FDA and find out if there are regulatory requirements that must be met.

What kind of data do I need to collect in order to realize any or all of the benefits of neurophysiologic decision support systems?

High-resolution physiologic data from the patient monitor and tertiary patient monitoring devices are the most fundamental data that are required to support neurophysiologic decision support systems. Real-time information from infusion pumps about treatments and other intervention information is the second most critical patient-specific data that you need. These two types of data together will enable you to evaluate the physiologic effect of treatment interventions and to make determinations about a patient's physiologic status. Your understanding of the patient can be enhanced if you can integrate these data with laboratory, clinical examination, nutrition, and any other information that is captured digitally.

What about EEG data?

I have already implied that EEG monitoring systems are FDA regulated, and indeed they are. Historically, EEG monitoring and neurophysiologic decision support systems have been separated with little integration. This is beginning to change. EEG systems are starting to integrate patient monitoring data into its system or making quantitative EEG parameters available for export into neurophysiologic decision support systems. EEG vendors will be able to tell you specifics for their systems, and options in this regard increase every year. Kull and Emerson[24] cover in detail considerations related to EEG monitoring in the ICU.

The hospital is planning to implement an EHR system in our ICU. Will the hospital plan cover everything I need?

The most likely answer is no. The hospital plan will probably focus on complying with "meaningful use" standards including electronic prescribing, health information exchange among clinicians and hospitals, and automated reporting of quality performance.[11] The benefit to the hospital is that electronic data collection is in principle more efficient, helps reduce medical errors and resulting lawsuits, improves medical device management, reduces costs,[9,25,26] and will provide the maximum financial incentives for EHR adoption.[12] This will almost certainly cover laboratory, clinical examination, and other tertiary data normally documented on paper charts, including intervention information. All of these data can be helpful to incorporate into a neurophysiologic decision support system. However, high-resolution patient monitoring data—the essential ingredient to any type of neurophysiologic decision support system—will probably not be considered a priority. Traditionally, EHR systems are not designed to capture and store high-resolution physiologic data, although some EHR systems specifically designed for the critical care settings do attempt to address this (eg, MetaVision for ICUs,[27] iMD*soft*, Needham, MA).

Still it is unlikely that even critical care EHR systems will come preconfigured to collect data from neuromonitoring devices that do not plug into the monitor. A customized solution, or more likely, an entirely separate data acquisition plan will be needed for this purpose (and for EEG monitoring as well).

What is the best plan for creating a neurophysiologic decision support system?

There is no right answer to this question and typically the "right" solution will be different depending on the particular situation of your institution. There are many choices to consider that fundamentally revolve around the three critical areas including:

1. Collection and storage of high-resolution data from the patient monitor and secondary monitoring devices that do not plug into the patient monitor.

2. Integration of patient monitoring data with other types of patient information, such as medication infusion information.

3. Analyzing, visualizing, and otherwise synthesizing patient data converting it into useful clinical information that supports diagnosis and management decisions.

Specifically, the first and biggest choice you need to consider is whether you plan to monitor a small number of patients using a portable monitoring solution that can be moved from room-to-room, or if you plan on creating an ICU-wide solution. Small-scale solutions are akin to purchasing a medical device that takes data directly from the patient monitor and peripheral devices in order to display the data on its screen. This choice offers a convenient all-in-one solution that includes equipment for data acquisition and software for analysis and visualization in one package. Cart-based portable solutions often can include EEG monitoring with trending of patient vital signs from the patient monitor. These systems tend to be easy to use by staff, easy to maintain, and purchasing one is likely the quickest path to implementing a live system in the ICU (Figure 17-1). Cart-based neuromonitoring solutions are

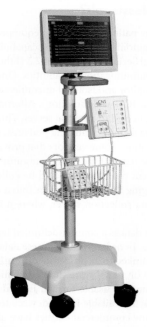

Figure 17-1. All-in-one electroencephalographic and neuromonitoring solutions by Component Neuromonitoring System (CNS) technology.

Neurocritical Care Monitoring

usually FDA approved and, therefore, are priced similar to an expensive medical device—a cost benefit is not necessarily realized with this option. These CDSS devices also have some of the other drawbacks of any medical device, including difficulty integrating it with other hospital clinical information systems, options to use the collected data for CDSS outside the all-in-one system is extremely limited, and archiving the data for clinical research purposes is often cumbersome and may not lend itself to group analysis. Finally, analysis and visualization options are fixed unless your system exports real-time data to another source that allows you to manipulate and visualize it how you choose.

In contrast, ICU-wide solutions are more complicated to initiate and expensive to maintain, but usually offer greater short- and long-term flexibility. Data from all the patient monitors and peripheral devices in the ICU are collected simultaneously and stored on an enterprise level central server.[25,28] A server is simply a class of computers with large computational and storage capacities that manage, store, and retrieve data for other computers or devices.[29] This central server will need to be operated and maintained over time, most often by hospital information technology, which is an expense that must be budgeted for. You will need to assess the extent to which hospital administrators and information technology (IT) understand and are committed to neurophysiologic decision support in the ICU. I recommend this as an essential prerequisite before seriously considering ICU-wide solutions. Ideally, patient data are stored in a nonproprietary Open Database Connectivity (ODBC) database like the Microsoft SQL Server. In this format, patient data can be queried for use by any number of CDSS programs in the future. CDSS programs that query data from a database, as opposed to directly from the monitor, fall into the category of stand-alone software and are not generally regulated by the FDA at this time. Data in an ODBC database will also better facilitate clinical research. Unlike the all-in-one solution, you may need additional software systems to analyze and/or view the data (Figure 17-2).

What do I need to know about collecting high-resolution patient monitoring data in order to communicate effectively with commercial vendors, hospital administrators, and IT professionals?

Most bedside devices including the patient monitor are equipped with RS-232 (digital) and analog (waveform) data output ports for automatic data output capabilities. Some newer models to output data from devices include Universal Serial Bus (USB), 802.3 (Ethernet), IEEE 11073, or even wireless (eg, 802.11b/g, Bluetooth) data communication capabilities. One strategy is to collect data by connecting directly to each patient monitor and isolated unconnected medical devices. This is typically the strategy for all-in-one and some ICU-wide solutions. Alternatively, most patient monitors operate on a closed intranet and are connected to a central server. This facilitates providing data from the patient monitor to a central nursing station or nursing pod area, or perhaps transferring hourly data to an EHR system for nurse verification. Some vendors that provide an ICU-wide solution to patient data collection do so by pulling the data off the patient monitor central server. However, data from devices not connected to the patient monitor must still be collected from each individual device. This can be accomplished by plugging individual devices into a communication hub that transmits the data from the device to the data collection server, where it is integrated with data pulled from the monitor.

Medical devices usually output data as a comma-delimited text string (eg, 16, 24.5, HIGH, 53.76, 2, 11, and so on) every few seconds. In order to collect these data, this text string must be converted into individual data points that are linked to its proper identification label. This translation is referred to as a device interface, or a small bit of software that automatically converts data outputted from the device into understandable data in a usable format. Each device has its own specifications for data communication, which usually is available in the device's technical manual or can be obtained from the device manufacturer. Many commercial entities have already written device interfaces for cardiopulmonary and neuromonitoring devices. Make a list of devices that you want and make sure

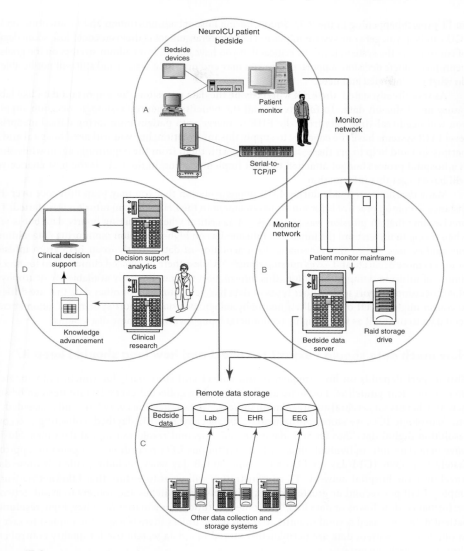

Figure 17-2. ICU-wide solution for neurophysiologic decision support illustration.

your vendor of choice supports them. Also, consider purchasing data interfaces for future, but as of yet unknown, devices.

Should I coordinate efforts to create a neurophysiologic decision support system in the ICU with that of ICU EHR implementation by the hospital?

Yes, and I would strongly encourage it, especially if you plan to implement an ICU-wide monitoring solution. First, you will need capital funds to purchase equipment and long-term operating funds to support your monitoring program over time. Connecting neurophysiologic decision support to the budget for EHR implementation could be helpful. Even if these budgets remain separate, the best time to get a neurophysiologic decision system implemented is when the hospital already has an IT project happening in the ICU. Simply having hospital administration and IT attention on the ICU can help you get your system in place. The counterargument is that you could lose some degree of control over the system. It will be critical that you have buy-in from administrators on the goals of neurophysiologic decision support, or else you may end up with a system and still will not be able to do what you intended and need.

As was already stated, the EHR will likely be the data repository for important data like laboratory and infusion data. To fully realize all the benefits of neurophysiologic decision support you will need real-time data from the EHR to merge with patient monitoring data. Enterprise-level EHR systems have the capacity to supply this information, but you will need hospital and IT permission and help to get these data. Working with them from the beginning, again while there is a hospital project budget attached to EHR implementation in the ICU, is the best chance you will have to get this information.

Many decisions are made during EHR implementation that you may want influence over. For instance, common practice is for nurses to document in the EHR when an infusion was started. The precise time that an infusion was started is not as critical when evaluating hourly data but is vital when trying to understand the impact an infusion has on high-resolution monitoring data. Numerous studies have shown that automatic documentation of data directly to an EHR from infusion pumps is more accurate and saves nursing time.[30-32] Unless there is a voiced clinical need for precise timing of infusion pump information, this information will not be easily available for neurophysiologic decision support tools. Other types of data like ventilator data or other data that are difficult to collect might be left out. Ideally, a neurophysiologic decision support system can automatically send data to the EHR as well. I highly recommend being involved in these discussions.

How much data should I expect to collect and how long should I keep it?

This in part depends on how frequently you collect and store data, for which, unfortunately, there is no clear guideline. For some applications, data collected every 10 minutes can be sufficient, whereas for cerebral autoregulation indices,[33] data collection every 5 seconds is needed. In our neurologic ICU, we store approximately 200 megabytes (MB)/day/bed, collecting 5-second resolution digital data into an SQL database and 2-second resolution digital data plus 240-Hz waveform data into individual binary files. Continuous EEG recordings can generate approximately 1 gigabyte (GB)/day for EEG alone, and 20 GB/day when including video. If these data travel over the hospital network, IT administrators will want to ensure that Ethernet networks employ 1 GB per second or greater connections between switches and routers to avoid network performance slowdowns or data loss.[34] In some institutions, as a matter of policy, high-resolution patient data are erased several months after discharge unless there is a specific request to save it. In our ICU, all patient data are permanently stored in a data warehouse for quality control and clinical research purposes.

What is a data warehouse?

A data warehouse is a collection of decision support technologies to enable better and faster decisions,[35] and is composed of multiple servers and networked data storage to support clinical decision making and research. A data warehouse, then, is where laboratory, imaging, intervention, physiologic, and all other patient databases reside. Traditional data warehouses are set up to bring several different kinds of data (eg, laboratory and physiologic) together into a unified database to be utilized by clinical support software tools. According to the National Institutes of Health (NIH) road map, the goal of translational research is to translate scientific discovery that typically begins at "the bench" into practical applications that progress to the clinical level, or the patient's "bedside."[36] A data warehouse is a critical component for clinical informatics translational research, whereby new uses of patient information can be researched and then brought to the bedside for clinical use through the implementation of a CDSS.

How can I create a clinical research database without a lot of experience?

Clinical research has yielded an understanding of many physiologic patterns that should be acted on when observed at the patient bedside. Continued clinical research is vital to advancing the field of neurophysiologic decision support systems. Dr. Urban Ungerstedt from the Karolinska Institute, Stockholm, Sweden, is most widely known for his work in cerebral microdialysis (eg, see references 37 and 38). Dr. Ungerstedt has recently initiated a collaborative project with support of the Karolinska Institute and the Neurocritical Care Society to provide free software support for research multimodal data acquisition.[39] This organization is also committed to connecting researchers together for collaboration on multimodal monitoring projects. This is a good place to start.

Data about the clinical course of patients will also need to be collected. The desire to document and time stamp the entire clinical course of a patient must be balanced with limited resources to do so. Try to capture too many variables and the quality and accuracy of data can go down, whereas not capturing enough information results in not being able to meaningfully address research questions. *How to Research* [40] is a good reference on conducting research that covers the entire research process from formulating a question to writing a manuscript for publication. I strongly encourage you to take advantage of collaboration opportunities through *www.multimodalmonitoring.org* and connect with investigators already conducting research in your area of interest.

What commercial options are available for neurophysiologic decision support systems?

The field is expanding and more systems and configurations emerge each year. The systems listed below are ones that I am familiar with, but undoubtedly there are other viable options in the marketplace. Features are added to these systems frequently. Contact system vendors for current lists of capabilities, and absolutely search on your own because new systems seem to appear annually. Online search term suggestions include ICU information systems, ICU data acquisition systems, NeuroICU monitoring, critical care information system, and critical care information management.

Be very clear about what you want to be able to do with the data, both now and for the future, and what data you need to have. You can always delete or thin data; be biased toward collecting too much data too frequently. If you purchase a solution that stores data in an ODBC database like the Microsoft SQL server, know that you can use standard data mining packages like IBM SPSS Modeler Professional[41] or Statistica Data Miner,[42] and/or other standard data visualization packages like MATLAB[43] and R.[44] Working with hospital IT to help you evaluate all your options is highly recommended.

Cart-based all-in-one systems:

- Component Neuromonitoring System[45] (CNS Technology, Ambler, PA)
- Eclipse Neurologic Workstation[46] (Axon Systems, Hauppauge, NY)
- Neuro Workbench[47] (Nihon Kohden, Foothill Ranch, CA)

ICU-wide enterprise systems:

- Bedmaster EX[48] (Excel Medical, Jupiter, FL)
- Patient Monitoring Solutions[49] (General Electric, Waukesha, WI)
- Healthcare Informatics and Patient Monitoring[50] (Philips Healthcare, Andover, MA)

Hybrid systems (can be configured for portable use or for the entire ICU):

- ICM+[51] (University of Cambridge, Cambridge, UK)
- ICU Pilot[52] (CMA Microdialysis, Holliston, MA)
- Customized solutions[45] (CNS Technology, Ambler, PA)

Dashboard systems:

- Clinical Command and Control[53] (Global Care Quest, El Segundo, CA)
- CareAware Critical Care[54] (Cerner Corporation, Kansas City, MO)

REFERENCES

1. Shortliffe E, Blois M. The computer meets medicine and biology: emergence of a discipline. *Biomed Inform.* 2006:3-45.
2. Hersh W. Medical informatics: Improving health care through information. *JAMA.* 2002;288:1955.
3. Musen M, Shahar Y, Shortliffe E. Clinical decision-support systems. *Biomed Inform.* 2006:698-736.
4. Wartenberg KE, Schmidt JM, Mayer SA. Multimodality monitoring in neurocritical care. *Crit Care Clin.* 2007;23:507-538.
5. De Turck F, Decruyenaere J, Thysebaert P, et al. Design of a flexible platform for execution of medical decision support agents in the intensive care unit. *Comput Biol Med.* 2007;37:97-112.
6. Morris G, Gardner R. Computer Applications. In: Hall J, Schmidt G, Wood L, eds. *Principles of Critical Care.* New York: McGraw-Hill; 1992: 500-514.
7. Imhoff M. Detecting relationships between physiological variables using graphical modeling. In: *Annual Symposium.* Proc AMIA; 2002:340-344.
8. Jennings D, Amabile T, Ross L. Informal assessments: data-based versus theory-based judgments. In: Kahnemann D, Slovic P, Tversky A, eds. *Judgments Under Uncertainity: Heuristics Biases.* Cambridge, UK: Cambridge University Press; 1982:211-230.
9. Adhikari N, Lapinsky S. Medical informatics in the intensive care unit: overview of technology assessment. *J Crit Care.* 2003;18:41-47.
10. Martich GD, Waldmann CS, Imhoff M. Clinical informatics in critical care. *J Intensive Care Med.* 2004;19:154-163.
11. Jha A. Meaningful use of electronic health records. *JAMA.* 2010;304:1709.
12. Jha A, DesRoches C, Kralovec P, Joshi M. A progress report on electronic health records in US hospitals. *Health Affairs.* 2010;29:1951.
13. Blumenthal D. Launching HITECH. *N Engl J Med.* 2010;362:382-385.
14. Donati A, Gabbanelli V, Pantanetti S, et al. The impact of a clinical information system in an intensive care unit. *J Clin Monit Comput.* 2008;22:31-36.
15. Custer J, Spaeder M, Fackler J. Critical care decision support. *Contemp Crit Care.* 2008;6.
16. Mann E, Salinas J. The use of computer decision support systems for the critical care environment. *AACN Adv Crit Care.* 2009;20:216.
17. Hooper M, Martin J, Weavind L, et al. Automated surveillance of modified SIRS criteria is an effective tool for detection of sepsis in the medical intensive care unit. *Am J Respir Crit Care.* 2010;181:A6137.
18. Campion T, Waitman L, May A, Ozdas A, Lorenzi N, Gadd C. Social, organizational, and contextual characteristics of clinical decision support systems for intensive insulin therapy: a literature review and case study. *Int J Med Inform.* 2009;18:115-119.
19. Sloane E, Rosow E, Adam J, Shine D. Clinical engineering department strategic graphical dashboard to enhance maintenance planning and asset management. *Conf Proc IEEE Eng Med Biol Soc.* 2005;7:7107-7110.
20. Goodman K. Ethical and legal issues in decision support. *Clin Decision Support Systems.* 2007:126-139.
21. Tsai TL, Fridsma DB, Gatti G. Computer decision support as a source of interpretation error: the case of electrocardiograms. *J Am Med Inform Assoc* 2003;10:478-483.
22. Haitsma IK, Maas AI. Advanced monitoring in the intensive care unit: brain tissue oxygen tension. *Curr Opin Crit Care.* 2002;8:115-120.
23. Johnston AJ, Gupta AK. Advanced monitoring in the neurology intensive care unit: microdialysis. *Curr Opin Crit Care,* 2002;8:121-127.
24. Kull LL, Emerson RG. Continuous EEG monitoring in the intensive care unit: technical and staffing considerations. *J Clin Neurophysiol.* 2005;22:107-118.
25. Martich G, Waldmann C, Imhoff M. Clinical informatics in critical care. *J Intensive Care Med.* 2004;19:154.
26. Clemmer TP. Computers in the ICU: where we started and where we are now. *J Crit Care.* 2004;19:201-207.
27. Metavision for ICUs. (Accessed 2010, at http://www.imd-soft.com/metavision-for-icus)
28. Chelico JD, Wilcox A, Wajngurt D. Architectural design of a data warehouse to support operational and analytical queries across disparate clinical databases. Paper presented at the American Medical Informatics Association, Chicago, IL.
29. Chou D, Sengupta S. *Infrastructure and Security.* New York, NY: Academic Press; 2008.

30. Sapo M, Wu S, Asgari S, et al. A comparison of vital signs charted by nurses with automated acquired values using waveform quality indices. *J Clin Monit Comput*. 2009;23:263-271.

31. Vawdrey D, Gardner R, Evans R, et al. Assessing data quality in manual entry of ventilator settings. *J Am Med Inform Assoc*. 2007;14:295-303.

32. Dalto JD, Johnson KV, Gardner RM, Spuhler VJ, Egbert L. Medical Information Bus usage for automated IV pump data acquisition: evaluation of usage patterns. *Int J Clin Monit Comput*. 1997;14:151-154.

33. Steiner LA, Czosnyka M, Piechnik SK, et al. Continuous monitoring of cerebrovascular pressure reactivity allows determination of optimal cerebral perfusion pressure in patients with traumatic brain injury. *Crit Care Med*. 2002;30:733-738.

34. Kull L, Emerson R. Continuous EEG monitoring in the intensive care unit: technical and staffing considerations. *J Clin Neurophysiol*. 2005;22:107-118.

35. Chaudhuri S, Dayal U. An overview of data warehousing and OLAP technology. *ACM Sigmod Rec*. 1997;26:65-74.

36. Re-engineering the Clinical Research Enterprise. 2009. (Accessed at http://nihroadmap.nih.gov/clinicalresearch/overview-translational.asp)

37. Ungerstedt U. Microdialysis—Principles and applications for studies in animals and man. *J Intern Med*. 1991;230:365-373.

38. Ungerstedt U, Rostami E. Microdialysis in neurointensive care. *Curr Pharm Des*. 2004;10:2145-2152.

39. Multimodal Monitoring. (Accessed 2010, at http://www.multimodal.org)

40. Blaxter L, Hughes C, Tight M. *How to Research*. 3rd ed. Buckingham, GBR: Open University Press; 2006.

41. IBM SPSS Modeler Professional. (Accessed 2010, at http://www.spss.com/software/modeling/modeler-pro/)

42. Statistica Data Miner. (Accessed 2010, at http://www.statsoft.com/products/data-mining-solutions/)

43. MATLAB - The Language of Technical Computing. (Accessed 2010, at http://www.mathworks.com/products/matlab/)

44. The R Project for Statistical Computing. (Accessed 2010, at http://www.r-project.org/)

45. Component Neuromonitoring System ™. (Accessed 2010, at http://www.cnstechnology.com/index.php)

46. Eclipse Neurological Workstations. (Accessed 2010, at http://www.axonsystems.com/eclipse.htm)

47. Neuro Workbench ™. (Accessed 2010, at http://www.nkusa.com/neurology_cardiology/#aa.)

48. Bedmaster EX. (Accessed 2010, at http://www.excel-medical.com/)

49. Patient Monitoring Solutions. (Accessed 2010, at http://www.gehealthcare.com/euen/patient_monitoring/products/iconnect/index.html)

50. Healthcare Informatics and Patient Monitoring. (Accessed 2010, at http://www.healthcare.philips.com/main/products/hi_pm/products/index.wpd)

51. ICM+. (Accessed 2010, at http://www.neurosurg.cam.ac.uk/icmplus/about.html)

52. ICU Pilot. (Accessed 2010, at http://www.microdialysis.se/software/icupilot-software?stat=)

53. Clinical Command and Control (Accessed 2010, at http://www.globalcarequest.com/surgeonconnect.html)

54. CareAware™ Critical Care. (Accessed 2010, at https://store.cerner.com/hospitals_and_health_systems/critical_care)

Neurocritical Care Intervention

Section Editor: Stephan A. Mayer, MD, FCCM

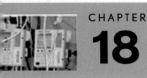

CHAPTER

18

Sedation

Amy L. Dzierba, PharmD, BCPS
Vivek K. Moitra, MD
Robert N. Sladen, MBChB, MRCP, FRCP

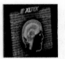

A 66-year-old man with a history of coronary artery disease, chronic renal insufficiency, alcoholic cirrhosis, hypertension, and anxiety is brought to the emergency department after a motor vehicle accident. He has traumatic brain injury and rib fractures. After tracheal intubation, he is transferred to the intensive care unit (ICU) for further management. The patient appears agitated and uncomfortable. He is tachycardic, with a heart rate of 120 bpm; hypertensive with a blood pressure of 188/72 mm Hg; and tachypneic, breathing 38 breaths/min. His home medications include aspirin and clopidogrel.

What is the difference between sedation and analgesia?

It is useful to consider sedation as having three components: anxiolysis (which is indicated for every ICU patient), hypnosis (ie, the induction of sleep, which may be indicated in sicker patients), and amnesia (loss or lack of recall). Sedation is distinct from analgesia, the relief of pain; and sedative agents such as propofol and the benzodiazepines (lorazepam and midazolam) have no analgesic effects. Sedating a patient for agitation induced by pain may further disinhibit their control functions and lead to a paradoxical increase in agitation (see below). Also, although amnesia is essential during general anesthesia in the operating room, the potent anterograde amnesia induced by benzodiazepines—even at subhypnotic doses—

results in confusion and disorientation on awakening, and may predispose toward ICU delirium. In contrast, propofol provides amnesia only during sleep, so emergence is smoother.

What is the first step in managing this patient's sedation and analgesia?

The neurointensivist should adopt an "analgesia first" or "A-1" approach to relieve the patient's pain before administration of sedation.[1] This will avoid disinhibiting a patient whose agitation is due to pain, as discussed above. There is evidence that an A-1 approach decreases sedation requirements and time on the ventilator.[2-6] ICU patients experience pain and discomfort with procedures such as tracheal intubation, endotracheal tube suctioning, and repositioning. Failure to treat pain exacerbates endogenous catecholamine activity, which predisposes to myocardial ischemia, hypercoagulability, hypermetabolic states, sleep deprivation, and delirium.[7,8]

Opioids are the mainstay of pain management in the ICU. Synthetic analgesics such as fentanyl and remifentanil are commonly used. These agents are administered as a bolus or as an infusion to manage pain and facilitate synchronous mechanical ventilation. Fentanyl, a short-acting opioid, has an intravenous onset time of less than 1 minute and duration of action of ½ to 1 hour. Duration of analgesia increases with prolonged infusions or repeated dosing. Fentanyl does not have an active metabolite and its pharmacokinetics is not altered by renal failure. However, uremia potentiates its pharmacodynamic effect, and sensitivity to sedation and respiratory depression is increased. Fentanyl has a high hepatic extraction ratio and its metabolism is slowed in patients with liver disease (eg, cirrhosis) or hepatic dysfunction (eg, congestive heart failure, shock).[9]

Remifentanil is an ultrashort-acting opioid and as such may be preferred for patients who require frequent neurologic evaluations. It is metabolized directly in the blood by plasma esterases and has an elimination half-life of 8 to 9 minutes. Described as a "forgiving opioid," remifentanil is characterized by a rapid onset and offset of action that is independent of liver or renal function.[10,11] Infusion of remifentanil has an onset of action of 1 minute[10] and rapidly achieves steady-state plasma levels. Its analgesic and sedative effects dissipate within 3 to 10 minutes of discontinuation of an infusion. Abrupt discontinuation of an infusion (eg, disconnect, empty bag) can precipitate the sudden return of severe pain and discomfort with hypertension and tachycardia.

In a randomized controlled trial comparing remifentanil infusion (0.15 mcg/kg per minute) with morphine, the duration of mechanical ventilation, time to tracheal extubation, and the interval between tracheal extubation and ICU discharge were significantly shorter with remifentanil.[3] Nonetheless, because of its high cost and the risk of sudden discontinuation (see above), remifentanil is not widely used in the ICU in the United States.

Bradycardia, hypotension, respiratory depression, nausea, and skeletal muscle rigidity are potential adverse effects of opioids. Given this patient's chronic renal insufficiency, morphine and meperidine should not be prescribed because they have active metabolites that are eliminated by the kidneys. Although it does not accumulate in renal failure, hydromorphone has a half-life of 2 to 3 hours, which makes it difficult to titrate for frequent neurologic assessment.

Epidural analgesia effectively prevents chest wall splinting after rib fractures, but placement of an epidural catheter is contraindicated in patients who have received a dose of clopidogrel within 7 days.

Are the goals for sedation and analgesia different in the neurologically compromised patient?

In addition to decreasing anxiety, pain, and discomfort, sedatives and analgesics can also be used to treat neurologic dysfunction directly (Table 18-1). These drugs manage intracranial hypertension, reduce seizure activity, and decrease cerebral metabolic rate of oxygen ($CMRO_2$). Indeed, inadequate sedation and analgesia may allow intracranial pressure (ICP) to increase in patients with impaired cerebral autoregulation after brain injury. It is important to recognize the interdependence between therapeutic sedation and analgesia, the harmful consequences of inadequate sedation and analgesia,

Table 18-1. Intravenous Analgesics and Sedatives

Medication	Intermittent (Bolus) dose	Infusion dose	Onset of action	Half-life	Active metabolites	ICP effect	Seizure effect	$CMRO_2$	Unique adverse effects
Fentanyl[a]	25-50 mcg	10-400 mcg/hr	2 min	1.5-6 h	No	Minimal change	None	Minimal change to decrease	Accumulation of parent compound
Remifentanil	Not recommended	0.05-0.2 mcg/kg/min	3-10 min	No		Minimal change	None	Minimal change to decrease	Hyperalgesia
Hydromorphone[a]	0.25-0.5 mg	0.5-1 mg/hr	15 min	2-3 h	No	Minimal change	None	Minimal change to decrease	
Morphine[a]	0.5-10 mg	1-10 mg/h	15 min	3-7 h	Yes	Increase	None	Minimal change to decrease	Histamine release Accumulation of metabolite in renal failure
Midazolam[a]	1-2 mg	1-10 mg/h	2-5 min	3-11 h	Yes	Minimal change	Attenuates seizures	Minimal change to decrease	Accumulation of parent compound Accumulation of metabolite in renal failure
Lorazepam	0.5-1 mg	1-10 mg/h	5-20 min	8-15 h	No	Minimal change	Attenuates seizures	Minimal change to decrease	High-dose PG–related acidosis or renal failure
Propofol[a]	Not recommended	5-70 mcg/kg/min	Immediate	26-32 h	No	Decrease	Attenuates seizures	Decrease	PRIS, infection risk Elevated triglycerides
Dexmedetomidine[a]	Not recommended	0.2-1.5 mcg/kg/h	30 min	2-5 h	No	No change	None	Decrease	Bradycardia

Abbreviation: $CMRO_2$, cerebral metabolic rate of oxygen; ICP, intracranial pressure; PG, propylene glycol; mcg, micrograms; mg, milligrams; PRIS, propofol infusion syndrome.

[a]Dose adjustment recommended with hypothermia.

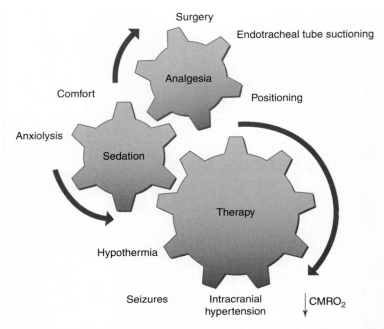

Figure 18-1. Interdependence between sedation and analgesia and treatment of neurologic conditions. CMRO$_2$, cerebral metabolic rate of oxygen.

and neurologic outcomes (Figure 18-1). In addition, when choosing sedatives and analgesics, shorter-acting drugs are usually preferred for the ease of following patients' neurologic examinations.

How do commonly used sedatives and analgesics affect ICP, seizure threshold, and cerebral metabolic rate (CMR)?

Table 18-1 outlines the neurologic effects of commonly used sedative and analgesic agents. Propofol suppresses electroencephalogram (EEG) activity and decreases seizure activity at high doses.[12] Although propofol manages refractory status epilepticus, investigators also report proconvulsant activity with its use.[13-17] Like barbiturates, propofol decreases the CMR and the cerebral blood flow (CBF) to decrease ICP. Hypotension, from propofol-induced vasodilation, may decrease cerebral perfusion pressure (CPP). Benzodiazepines are potent anticonvulsants that inhibit seizure activity when seizures are provoked via antagonism of the γ-aminobutyric acid (GABA) receptor. Benzodiazepines minimally affect ICP and CBF. Dexmedetomidine does not decrease ICP or affect seizure threshold. With the exception of morphine, opioids do not affect ICP or CBF independent of carbon dioxide arterial tension. Cautious use of sedatives is advised in patients whose lungs are not mechanically ventilated. Sedatives and analgesics can depress the respiratory rate and cause hypercarbia, which increases ICP via cerebral vasodilation. The benefits of sedative therapy to manage ICP, the CMR, and seizure threshold cannot be realized without intensive management of ventilation and avoidance of hypercarbia.

Is ketamine contraindicated in patients with traumatic brain injury?

A little over 40 years ago during the Vietnam War, ketamine, a nonbarbiturate phencyclidine derivative,[18] was considered an ideal "battlefield anesthetic."[19] Like the fixed combination preparation of fentanyl and droperidol (Innovar), ketamine became popular for neuroleptanesthesia, a state of dissociative anesthesia in which the patient appears to be calm and nonreactive to pain, with maintained airway reflexes. However, its popularity waned because of an undesirable side-effect profile: hallucinations, delirium, lacrimation, tachycardia, and potential for an increase in ICP and coronary ischemia. Concerns about its psychotropic effects limited its use as a sedative in the ICU. Recent research, however, suggests that with lower doses (60-120 mcg/kg per hour), ketamine may not be associated with untoward effects and may improve outcomes. Ketamine sedation may benefit patients who are critically ill. It prevents opioid-induced hyperalgesia, decreases inflammation, and reduces bronchoconstriction.[20-23]

Concerns about using ketamine in the ICU stem from its mind-altering effects, which include hallucinations and unpleasant emergence recall. When sedatives such as propofol and midazolam were prescribed with ketamine, psychiatric effects were attenuated.[24-27] Analgesic effects were found at plasma concentrations lower than plasma concentrations that produced psychotomimetic effects.[24,28-30]

Clinicians have avoided ketamine in patients at risk for elevated ICP, which also may increase in patients receiving ketamine who are breathing spontaneously. Some studies have shown, however, that ketamine does not increase CBF or ICP if CO_2 levels are controlled.[31,32] In children with intracranial hypertension whose lungs were mechanically ventilated, ketamine decreased ICP and increased CPP.[33] In combination with benzodiazepines, ketamine prevented fluctuations in ICP.[34-36] Hemodynamic variables appear to be preserved with ketamine in patients with brain or spinal cord injuries.[37] These results suggest that the adequacy of sedation is more important than the choice of sedative in the management of ICP.

The potential for neuroprotection against ischemic damage with ketamine is intriguing. Ketamine binds N-methyl-D-aspartate (NMDA) and sigma opioid receptors to produce intense analgesia. It crosses the blood-brain barrier rapidly and reaches maximal effect in 1 minute. During neuronal injury, the NMDA receptor is activated to release Ca^{2+} and glutamate by ischemic neurons, which initiates cell necrosis and apoptosis.[38] Blockade of NMDA receptors may be therapeutic.[39,40]

Supplemental sedation with ketamine can decrease opioid requirements and their adverse effects. In critically ill patients, there are two potential pathways to develop allodynia (ie, the sensation of pain from a stimulus that does not normally produce pain), hyperalgesia, and eventually chronic pain syndromes. Surgical and trauma patients and patients who undergo painful procedures in the ICU experience prolonged noxious stimuli, which can cause central sensitization and lead to a chronic pain syndrome.[41-43] Opioids themselves can induce hyperalgesia. Ketamine antagonizes the NMDA receptor to block these responses, reducing windup pain and central hyperexcitability. Several studies report that ketamine decreases opioid-induced hyperalgesia.[23,44]

How should sedation and analgesia be assessed?

A sedation scale should have well-defined criteria for each level of sedation. It should be easy to administer, demonstrate reliability and validity, and provide clear goals for sedation end points.[45,46] A sedation scale can facilitate the appropriate level of sedation to promote comfort, facilitate mechanical ventilation, prevent hypotension, or avoid decreases in CPP.

Two commonly used sedation scales are listed in Table 18-2. The Ramsay Sedation Scale is a simple 6-point scale that has been in regular use since it was first described in 1974.[47] It incorporates four levels of increasing sedation but only one level of agitation, and for this reason has been criticized for being imbalanced. The Richmond Agitation-Sedation Scale (RASS) has achieved prominence recently because it is more balanced across levels of sedation and agitation, correlates better with electroencephalographic (EEG) assessment, and has been integrated with an assessment of delirium called the Confusion Assessment Method for the ICU (CAM-ICU).[48,49] Several other instruments for

Neurocritical Care Intervention

Table 18-2. Sedation Scales

Modified Ramsay Sedation Scale		
1	Awake	Anxious, agitated, restless
2	Awake	Cooperative, orientated, serene
3	Awake	Responding only to commands
4	Asleep	Brisk response to stimulation*
5	Asleep	Sluggish response to stimulation*
6	Asleep	No response to stimulation*

Richmond Agitation-Sedation Scale (RASS)		
Score	Assessment	Description
+4	Combative	Overtly combative, violent, danger to staff with observation
+3	Very agitated	Pulls or removes tube(s) or catheters, aggressive with observation
+2	Agitated	Frequent nonpurposeful movement with observation or dyssynchrony with ventilator
+1	Restless	Anxious, apprehensive, but not aggressive
0		Alert and calm upon observation
−1	Drowsy	With loud speaking voice awakens > 10 s, not fully alert
−2	Light sedation	With loud speaking voice briefly awakens to voice < 10 s
−3	Moderate sedation	With loud speaking voice has movement or eye opening without eye contact
−4	Deep sedation	Movement to physical stimulation
−5	Unarousable	No response to physical stimulation

*stimulation = glabellar tap or loud noise

assessment of sedation focus on agitation and physiologic parameters. The Riker Sedation-Agitation Scale (SAS), the Motor-Activity Assessment Scale (MAAS), the Adaptation to the Intensive Care Environment (ATICE), and the AVRIPAS scale, which incorporates heart rate and respiration, have all been utilized to guide sedation.[50-54]

It is important to note that these scales assess the level of sedation only, and not pain, anxiety, or level of cognition; they cannot be used in the presence of neuromuscular blockade; and none of them has been exclusively validated in patients with neurologic injury.

If the patient is able to cooperate, pain can be assessed using a verbal or visual analog scale (VAS). In a nonintubated patient, the patient is simply asked to rate his/her own pain, with "0" for no pain and "10" for the worst pain imaginable. Although pain is subjective, the patient is his/her own control, and the change in VAS in response to a therapeutic intervention may be quite helpful. In patients who are too sedated to respond, signs of pain are manifest by increased sympathetic activity, which includes tachycardia (and even ectopic rhythms), hypertension, lacrimation, sweating, and papillary dilation. These are the same signs the anesthesiologist looks for to detect inadequate anesthesia in the operating room.

On ICU day 3, the patient's ICP is elevated; he has fever and worsening neurologic function. His heart rate is 68 bpm; his blood pressure is 140/70 mm Hg. His kidney injury is
acute with a creatinine clearance of 30 mL/min. He is treated for ventilator-associated
pneumonia with linezolid, piperacillin, and tazobactam. Therapeutic hypothermia is initiated. After he has been cooled to a temperature of 36.5°C, the patient begins to shiver. A dexmedetomidine infusion is initiated and the patient's heart rate decreases to 50 bpm. The patient continues
to shiver.

How are sedative doses adjusted in patients who undergo therapeutic hypo-thermia?

It is important to recognize that the hypothalamic threshold for the onset of shivering is directly regulated by feedback from cutaneous temperature receptors. The warmer the skin, the lower the central
temperature declines before the onset of shivering, and vice versa. Therefore, the most effective non-
pharmacologic means of suppressing shivering is skin warming. This may be impracticable during
surface cooling but can be very effective during central (intravascular) cooling and avoids excessive
use of antishivering drugs, which engender the caveats described below.

Drugs commonly used to suppress shivering during therapeutic hypothermia are listed in
Figure 18-2. Of all the opioids, meperidine has the most potent antishivering effect, but high doses

Neurocritical Care Intervention

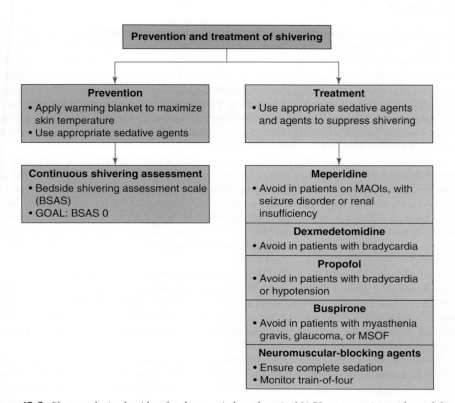

Figure 18-2. Pharmacologic algorithm for therapeutic hypothermia. MAOIs, monoamine oxidase inhibitors;
MSOF, multisystem organ failure.

are associated with respiratory depression, hypotension, and tachycardia. Dexmedetomidine is an α_2 agonist that is quite effective in suppressing shivering,[55-59] but it also decreases catecholamine levels and may provoke bradycardia and hypotension in susceptible patients. Its sister compound, clonidine, is equally effective but long-acting and much more difficult to titrate. Buspirone is a mild anxiolytic agent that has central antiserotonin effects and has been shown to have synergistic effects on shivering suppression with both meperidine and dexmedetomidine.[55,60] Magnesium infusions are also used but are not very effective in suppressing shivering. Propofol is a potent sedative that suppresses the shivering threshold in a dose-dependent manner, but it induces vasodilation and hypotension at higher doses. Neuromuscular blockade should be used as a last resort, and only when it is assured that the patient is completely sedated (Ramsay level 6 or RASS level −5).

Drug metabolism and clearance are closely related to the overall metabolic rate and decrease during hypothermia.[61-63] Most medications used to control shivering undergo biotransformation in the liver. With decreased hepatic blood flow and an altered cytochrome P450 (CYP450) enzyme system, medications or their active metabolites may accumulate and the risk of drug toxicity is magnified. Hypothermia also affects drug distribution and response.[64] It is prudent to make empiric dose adjustments for medications such as fentanyl, meperidine, midazolam, propofol, and dexmedetomidine. The Bedside Shivering Assessment Scale (BSAS), a method to quantify shivering, also serves as a convenient tool to assess responsiveness to medications used to suppress shivering [65] (see Figure 18-2).

What are the neurologic consequences of sedating this patient with dexmedetomidine?

Dexmedetomidine is a highly selective agonist at the α_2 adrenoreceptor, which is a subgroup of noradrenergic receptors (α_{2A}, α_{2B}, α_{2C}) distributed throughout the body in the central, peripheral, and autonomic nervous systems. Stimulation of presynaptic receptors in the sympathetic nervous system inhibits norepinephrine release. Simultaneously, activation of central postsynaptic receptors hyperpolarizes neurons. The end result is diminished sympathetic activity through a negative feedback loop as norepinephrine output is decreased. The resulting sympatholysis is characterized by bradycardia, low blood pressure, anxiolysis, and sedation. Dexmedetomidine also acts at spinal receptors to modulate analgesia and has an opioid-sparing effect. And, as indicated previously, it is effective in suppressing shivering in patients during therapeutic hypothermia.[55-59]

In contrast to GABA agonists, dexmedetomidine sedates without changes in the respiratory rate, oxygen saturation, or arterial carbon dioxide tension.[66] Unlike benzodiazepines, clinical doses of dexmedetomidine are not associated with anterograde amnesia; patients are easily arousable from light levels of sedation and emerge without confusion or disorientation. When left undisturbed, they go back to their previous level of sedation. Thus, dexmedetomidine produces interactive or cooperative sedation and facilitates neurologic examination.[67-69] Although dexmedetomidine may decrease the incidence of delirium in the ICU, this effect has not been extensively studied in neurointensive care patients.[70,71]

Dexmedetomidine decreases CBF, which could be deleterious in patients who are at risk for neuronal injury.[72,73] Animal studies suggest that dexmedetomidine prevents a reduction in the CMR when CBF is compromised, resulting in an imbalance of oxygen supply and demand.[74,75] A recent study in healthy human volunteers confirmed the decrease in CBF but also showed that the CBF-to-CMR ratio is preserved.[76] Dexmedetomidine may impair autoregulation of cerebral vasculature in patients with sepsis who become hypercapnic.[77]

The locus ceruleus, a blue-staining medullary nucleus that contains many noradrenergic neurons, mediates transmission of sympathetic nervous system impulses from the cortex to the brainstem. It is thought to modulate arousal, vigilance, sleep, and the sleep-wake cycle.[67] Dexmedetomidine acts on the α_{2A} receptors in the locus ceruleus to decrease transmission of noradrenergic output and consequently produces anxiolysis and sedation. In contrast, drugs such as propofol or midazolam that act directly at the GABA receptor do not suppress norepinephrine transmission, which may explain why they are more likely to be associated with delirium.[71] This difference may also explain why dexmedetomidine is associated with meaningful interaction without cognitive compromise.[69] Unlike other sedatives, α_2 agonists appear to promote sleep through nonrapid eye movement pathways.[67]

In addition to its sedative and analgesic properties, dexmedetomidine may have other clinical applications in intensive care. It not only facilitates weaning from mechanical ventilation by decreasing the need for opioids or benzodiazepines that might depress respiration, but also allows continuation of anxiolysis and analgesia after tracheal extubation.[78-89] It is very helpful in the management of withdrawal syndromes and other hyperadrenergic states. In neurointensive care, dexmedetomidine can prevent or treat paroxysmal autonomic instability with dystonia (PAID).[90]

In a patient with bradycardia, should dexmedetomidine be discontinued?

The decision to discontinue dexmedetomidine really depends on the severity of bradycardia (eg, < 40 bpm) and whether it is associated with hemodynamic instability. Bradycardia induced by α_2-adenergic agonists is a consequence of the suppression of norepinephrine output from the locus ceruleus. It is exacerbated by concomitant vagal stimulation (visceral stretch, endoscopy), antiarrhythmic drugs such as β blockers or amiodarone, or drugs with vagotonic or sympatholytic effects such as neostigmine or fentanyl. Avoidance of these factors will minimize the incidence of bradycardia with dexmedetomidine. In the treatment of shivering, combination therapy with meperidine and/or buspirone decreases dexmedetomidine dose requirements and, therefore, the risk of unintended bradycardia.[59]

Should this patient's shivering be treated with meperidine?

Meperidine is singular among the opioids through its ability to suppress shivering at the mu, kappa, and α_{2B} adenoreceptors.[59,91] However, meperidine has an active metabolite, normeperidine, which possesses neuroexcitatory effects and is cleared by the kidney.[45] In patients with renal insufficiency, accumulation of normeperidine may cause seizures. Meperidine may precipitate a serotonin syndrome in patients treated with linezolid, a weak monoamine oxidase inhibitor (MAOI).

 After initiation of skin counterwarming, dexmedetomidine sedation, and buspirone and magnesium infusion, the patient continues to shiver. A propofol infusion is started.

What changes are initially expected with propofol therapy?

Propofol may be rapidly titrated to reduce the vasoconstriction and shivering threshold.[92] Reductions in CBF and CMR have also been observed.[93,94] As a result of its short half-life, this agent may be preferred for patients in whom rapid awakening is important.[45,92] Nonetheless, there are several caveats with its use.

Propofol is a potent sedative that decreases catecholamine levels, induces vasodilation, and limits baroreflex cardiovascular responses. Thus, although propofol sedation or anesthesia may promptly lower ICP,[95-97] it may (especially in volume-depleted patients) also induce hypotension and thus decrease CPP.[96,98]

Although propofol has been used to treat status epilepticus, a seizure-like phenomenon has been reported during induction and emergence from propofol anesthesia.[13-17,99] Because propofol is so highly lipid soluble, it is suspended in a 20% fat emulsion, which may predispose to infection (so the drug must be handled aseptically), hypertriglyceridemia, and pancreatitis.[100-104] High-dose propofol (> 50 mcg/kg/min) infusions in the setting of shock, or high endogenous or exogenous catecholamines, and corticosteroids may rarely be associated with a potentially fatal syndrome that appears to result from an intracellular block in fat oxidation resulting in intractable lactate acidosis, myocardial depression and death, the so-called propofol infusion syndrome (PRIS).[105]

When should neuromuscular-blocking agents be initiated?

Muscle paralysis with neuromuscular blockers should be considered only if the patient is completely sedated (Ramsay level 6 or RASS level −5) and all physical and pharmacologic maneuvers have failed to control shivering. Neuromuscular blockers abolish the muscular activity associated with shivering—they do not affect centrally mediated thermoregulatory control.

There are many caveats with the use of neuromuscular blockers. The worst outcome is to have a patient awake and paralyzed! Clinicians have to be careful not to treat the patient as an inanimate object. Complete immobilization increases the risk of pressure injury, deep vein thrombosis, and critical illness polyneuropathy.

For all these reasons, limitation of neuromuscular blockade to the induction and rewarming phase is preferable. The depth of block should always be monitored by a twitch monitor to ensure that at least one twitch in a train-of-four is preserved; this is the best means to avoid overdose and delayed reversal. *cis*-Atracurium is preferred as a neuromuscular-blocking agent because it undergoes spontaneous (Hoffmann) dissociation in the blood and its elimination is independent of liver or kidney function.

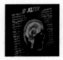

Neuromuscular blockade is initiated with an infusion of *cis*-Atracurium to manage the patient's shivering. His ICP remains elevated.

Should the bispectral index monitor (BIS) be used to evaluate the depth of sedation?

Assessment of sedation and analgesia is semiquantitative at best, and it is impossible to ensure the adequacy of amnesia or analgesia in a patient who is paralyzed. Oversedation may prolong mechanical ventilation and length of patient stay. Undersedation may result in patient discomfort, hemodynamic instability, and increased oxygen consumption.

The BIS monitor is a neurophysiologic monitor that uses Fourier transform analysis to process EEG signals via proprietary software to generate a value ranging from 0 to 100. In general, a score less than 60 may be associated with inhibition of memory formation under general surgical anesthesia. The BIS monitor is well established (although not completely without controversy) in the operating room, where its use has been associated with decreased sedative requirements and faster recovery from anesthesia.[106,107]

Several ICU studies suggest that there is a correlation between the BIS score and sedation scales.[108-110] A small study of neurologic patients suggests that BIS may decrease sedative requirements compared to assessment using the Ramsay Scale.[111] However, BIS values may be confounded by catecholamine levels, electrical equipment such as electrocardiographic (ECG) leads, grimacing, shivering, temperature fluctuation, and increased muscle tone. Although consensus guidelines recommend against the routine use of BIS monitoring to replace clinical assessments of the patient,[45] it seems logical to monitor the patient undergoing neuromuscular blockade to ensure adequate sedation.

Should sedation be interrupted daily in a patient with intracranial hypertension?

In the general ICU population, there is evidence that daily interruption of sedative medications and daily breathing trials decrease the duration of mechanical ventilation, shorten ICU length of stay, and minimize exposure to sedative medications.[112,113] Interruption also appears to minimize the adverse events associated with prolonged tracheal intubation.[114-116] However, the pros and cons of this practice have not been formulated for patients with neurologic injury.

One randomized, controlled trial showed no difference in the duration of mechanical ventilation or ICU length of stay in a subgroup of head-injured patients who received sedative interruption.[117] In patients with severe traumatic brain injury or subarachnoid hemorrhage in whom direct monitoring was used to study the effects of sedative interruption on ICP and CPP, a different picture emerged.[118] The mean ICP almost doubled, and in nearly 40% of patients, this increase in ICP was associated with a decrease in CPP.

Abrupt discontinuation of long-term, high-dose sedatives and analgesics may precipitate a hyperadrenergic withdrawal syndrome that may dramatically increase $CMRO_2$ and precipitate seizures in vulnerable patients. Continuous EEG monitoring may be helpful in assessing the response to sedation titration. The most appropriate time to taper or discontinue sedation in the neurologically injured patient is still unknown. Although daily sedation interruption is advocated by many for the general ICU population, it is inappropriate to withdraw sedation in patients with elevated ICP and unconscionable in patients on neuromuscular blockade.

The patient develops status epilepticus and is sedated with high doses of lorazepam and propofol, as well as fentanyl. After 7 days, the patient becomes tachypneic and develops an anion-gap acidosis. To assess his neurologic function, lorazepam is discontinued, yet the patient remains unresponsive to painful stimuli. The patient has not had a bowel movement for 7 days.

What laboratory test should be ordered in the context of sedative therapy?

High doses of sedative medications are administered to manage patients with seizures and intracranial hypertension. Benzodiazepines such as midazolam and lorazepam are lipid soluble and accumulate in fat stores, so prolonged infusions result in markedly delayed emergence. Lorazepam is diluted in propylene glycol, which has been associated with acute kidney injury and metabolic acidosis. The osmolar gap should be calculated in patients receiving lorazepam doses greater than 1 mg/kg per day.

As previously mentioned, high-dose propofol (> 50 mcg/kg/min) infusions in the setting of shock, high endogenous or exogenous catecholamines, and corticosteroids may rarely be associated with the so-called propofol infusion syndrome (PRIS). A recent case series noted three cases of PRIS in 50 neurologic ICU (NICU) patients on vasopressor therapy.[119] All patients were treated with escalating doses of propofol to manage intracranial hypertension. The pathogenesis of PRIS appears to involve mitochondrial dysfunction, impaired fatty acid oxidation, and metabolite accumulation. Characteristic findings include progressive lactic acidosis (an important warning sign), triglyceride elevations, and arrhythmias; death is usually due to intractable cardiac failure.

After discontinuation of lorazepam, the patient remains unresponsive. Should flumazenil be administered?

Flumazenil is a selective, competitive inhibitor of benzodiazepines at the GABA receptor; it antagonizes their pharmacologic effects in a dose-dependent fashion.[120] Flumazenil undergoes extensive first-pass

Neurocritical Care Intervention

hepatic metabolism and its duration of action is less than 30 minutes. Patients quickly return to the level of sedation they were at prior to its administration. To achieve a longer effect, repeated doses or continuous infusion is usually necessary. However, it is more prudent to restrict the use of flumazenil to confirming a diagnosis of lorazepam overdose and then supporting the patient to allow ultimate elimination of the benzodiazepine. Ultimately the decision to administer flumazenil should be tempered by the knowledge that abrupt reversal of benzodiazepine sedation and its anticonvulsant effects may lead to an undesirable increase in ICP, precipitate seizures, and provoke a withdrawal syndrome.[121]

Should methylnaltrexone be administered?

Opioids remain the primary source of analgesia in the ICU, and may be infused for many days in critically ill patients. Among the common undesired side effects are nausea, vomiting, pruritus, urinary retention, delayed gastric emptying, suppression of bowel motility, constipation, and ileus.

Methylnaltrexone and alvimopan are members of a new class of drug: peripherally acting mu-opioid-receptor antagonists (PAMORAs). In contrast to naloxone, these medications do not cross the blood-brain barrier and, therefore, do not antagonize the central (analgesic) effects of opioids. They act on peripheral receptors only, blocking side effects such as constipation and ileus, while preserving analgesia. The Food and Drug Administration (FDA) has approved subcutaneous methylnaltrexone for the relief of opioid-induced constipation and oral alvimopan to facilitate the return of gut dysfunction after anastomotic bowel surgery.

To treat this patient's constipation, a multimodal approach is warranted that includes careful tapering of opioid doses, subcutaneous methylnaltrexone, and a bowel regimen.

! CRITICAL CONSIDERATIONS

- Analgesia should be provided prior to institution of sedation.
- Sedatives should be used cautiously in nonintubated patients with neurologic compromise. Sedatives that depress respiratory function can increase arterial carbon dioxide tension and increase ICP.
- Ketamine may be used safely in brain-injured patients whose lungs are mechanically ventilated and who are receiving a GABA antagonist.
- Dexmedetomidine has several unique roles in the neurologic ICU including "cooperative sedation" and the treatment and prevention of shivering with hypothermia.
- Propofol decreases ICP but may also decrease CPP in volume-depleted patients.
- Prolonged infusions of propofol and lorazepam may cause a metabolic acidosis.

REFERENCES

1. Riker RR, Fraser GL. Altering intensive care sedation paradigms to improve patient outcomes. *Crit Care Clin.* 2009;25:527-538, viii-ix.
2. Breen D, Karabinis A, Malbrain M, Morais R, et al. Decreased duration of mechanical ventilation when comparing analgesia-based sedation using remifentanil with standard hypnotic-based sedation for up to 10 days in intensive care unit patients: a randomised trial [ISRCTN47583497]. *Crit Care.* 2005;9:R200-210.
3. Dahaba AA, Grabner T, Rehak PH, List WF, Metzler H. Remifentanil versus morphine analgesia and sedation for mechanically ventilated critically ill patients: a randomized double blind study. *Anesthesiology.* 2004;101:640-646.
4. Muellejans B, Lopez A, Cross MH, Bonome C, Morrison L, Kirkham AJ. Remifentanil versus fentanyl for analgesia based sedation to

provide patient comfort in the intensive care unit: a randomized, double-blind controlled trial [ISRCTN43755713]. *Crit Care.* 2004;8:R1-R11.

5. Muellejans B, Matthey T, Scholpp J, Schill M. Sedation in the intensive care unit with remifentanil/propofol versus midazolam/fentanyl: a randomised, open-label, pharmacoeconomic trial. *Crit Care.* 2006;10:R91.

6. Rozendaal FW, Spronk PE, Snellen FF, et al. Remifentanil-propofol analgo-sedation shortens duration of ventilation and length of ICU stay compared to a conventional regimen: a centre randomised, cross-over, open-label study in the Netherlands. *Intensive Care Med.* 2009;35:291-298.

7. Hall LG, Oyen LJ, Murray MJ. Analgesic agents. Pharmacology and application in critical care. *Crit Care Clin.* 2001;17:899-923, viii.

8. Lewis KS, Whipple JK, Michael KA, Quebbeman EJ. Effect of analgesic treatment on the physiological consequences of acute pain. *Am J Hosp Pharm.* 1994;51:1539-1554.

9. Devlin JW, Roberts RJ. Pharmacology of commonly used analgesics and sedatives in the ICU: benzodiazepines, propofol, and opioids. *Crit Care Clin.* 2009;25:431-449, vii.

10. Egan TD, Lemmens HJ, Fiset P, et al. The pharmacokinetics of the new short-acting opioid remifentanil (GI87084B) in healthy adult male volunteers. *Anesthesiology.* 1993;79:881-892.

11. Rosow C. Remifentanil: a unique opioid analgesic. *Anesthesiology.* 1993;79:875-876.

12. Mirski MA, Hemstreet MK. Critical care sedation for neuroscience patients. *J Neurol Sci.* 2007;261:16-34.

13. Herrema IH. A 10-second convulsion during propofol injection? *Anaesthesia.* 1989;44:700.

14. Wood PR, Browne GP, Pugh S. Propofol infusion for the treatment of status epilepticus. *Lancet.* 1988;1:480-481.

15. Victory RA, Magee D. A case of convulsion after propofol anaesthesia. *Anaesthesia.* 1988;43:904.

16. Serrano-Pozo A, Lopez-Munoz MM, Franco-Macias E, Boza-Garcia F, Chaparro-Hernandez P. [Generalised clonic tonic seizures triggered by anaesthesia with propofol and sevoflurane]. *Rev Neurol.* 2004;39:693-694.

17. Walder B, Tramer MR, Seeck M. Seizure-like phenomena and propofol: a systematic review. *Neurology.* 2002;58:1327-1332.

18. Domino EF, Chodoff P, Corssen G. Pharmacologic effects of Ci-581, a new dissociative anesthetic, in man. *Clin Pharmacol Ther.* 1965;6:279-291.

19. Malchow RJ, Black IH. The evolution of pain management in the critically ill trauma patient: emerging concepts from the global war on terrorism. *Crit Care Med.* 2008;36:S346-S357.

20. Angst MS, Clark JD. Opioid-induced hyperalgesia: a qualitative systematic review. *Anesthesiology.* 2006;104:570-587.

21. De Kock M, Lavand'homme P, Waterloos H. 'Balanced analgesia' in the perioperative period: is there a place for ketamine? *Pain.* 2001;92:373-380.

22. Lois F, De Kock M. Something new about ketamine for pediatric anesthesia? *Curr Opin Anaesthesiol.* 2008;21:340-344.

23. Joly V, Richebe P, Guignard B, et al. Remifentanil-induced postoperative hyperalgesia and its prevention with small-dose ketamine. *Anesthesiology.* 2005;103:147-155..

24. Himmelseher S, Durieux ME. Ketamine for perioperative pain management. *Anesthesiology.* 2005;102:211-220.

25. Badrinath S, Avramov MN, Shadrick M, Witt TR, Ivankovich AD. The use of a ketamine-propofol combination during monitored anesthesia care. *Anesth Analg.* 2000;90:858-862.

26. Friedberg BL. Propofol-ketamine technique: dissociative anesthesia for office surgery (a 5-year review of 1264 cases). *Aesthetic Plast Surg.* 1999;23:70-75.

27. Morse Z, Sano K, Kanri T. Effects of a midazolam-ketamine admixture in human volunteers. *Anesth Prog.* 2004;51:76-79.

28. Bowdle TA, Radant AD, Cowley DS, Kharasch ED, Strassman RJ, Roy-Byrne PP. Psychedelic effects of ketamine in healthy volunteers: relationship to steady-state plasma concentrations. *Anesthesiology.* 1998;88:82-88.

29. Hartvig P, Valtysson J, Lindner KJ, et al. Central nervous system effects of subdissociative doses of (S)-ketamine are related to plasma and brain concentrations measured with positron emission tomography in healthy volunteers. *Clin Pharmacol Ther.* 1995;58:165-173.

30. Tucker AP, Kim YI, Nadeson R, Goodchild CS. Investigation of the potentiation of the analgesic effects of fentanyl by ketamine in humans: a double-blinded, randomised, placebo controlled, crossover study of experimental pain[ISRCTN83088383]. *BMC Anesthesiol.* 2005;5:2.

31. Pfenninger E, Grunert A, Bowdler I, Kilian J. The effect of ketamine on intracranial pressure during haemorrhagic shock under the conditions of both spontaneous breathing and controlled ventilation. *Acta Neurochir (Wien).* 1985;78:113-118.

32. Schwedler M, Miletich DJ, Albrecht RF. Cerebral blood flow and metabolism following ketamine administration. *Can Anaesth Soc J.* 1982;29: 222-226.

33. Bar-Joseph G, Guilburd Y, Tamir A, Guilburd JN. Effectiveness of ketamine in decreasing intracranial pressure in children with intracranial hypertension. *J Neurosurg Pediatr.* 2009;4:40-46.

34. Himmelseher S, Durieux ME. Revising a dogma: ketamine for patients with neurological injury? *Anesth Analg.* 2005;101:524-534, table of contents.

35. Strebel S, Kaufmann M, Maitre L, Schaefer HG. Effects of ketamine on cerebral blood flow velocity in humans. Influence of pretreatment with midazolam or esmolol. *Anaesthesia.* 1995;50: 223-228.

36. Albanese J, Arnaud S, Rey M, Thomachot L, Alliez B, Martin C. Ketamine decreases intracranial pressure and electroencephalographic activity in traumatic brain injury patients during propofol sedation. *Anesthesiology.* 1997;87: 1328-1334.

37. Hijazi Y, Bodonian C, Bolon M, Salord F, Boulieu R. Pharmacokinetics and haemodynamics of ketamine in intensive care patients with brain or spinal cord injury. *Br J Anaesth.* 2003;90:155-160.

38. Meldrum BS. Glutamate as a neurotransmitter in the brain: review of physiology and pathology. *J Nutr.* 2000;130:1007S-1015S.

39. Prass K, Dirnagl U. Glutamate antagonists in therapy of stroke. *Restor Neurol Neurosci.* 1998;13:3-10.

40. Himmelseher S, Pfenninger E, Georgieff M. The effects of ketamine-isomers on neuronal injury and regeneration in rat hippocampal neurons. *Anesth Analg.* 1996;83:505-512.

41. Li J, Simone DA, Larson AA. Windup leads to characteristics of central sensitization. *Pain.* 1999;79:75-82.

42. Oye I. Ketamine analgesia, NMDA receptors and the gates of perception. *Acta Anaesthesiol Scand.* 1998;42:747-749.

43. Mao J, Price DD, Mayer DJ. Mechanisms of hyperalgesia and morphine tolerance: a current view of their possible interactions. *Pain.* 1995;62: 259-274.

44. Stubhaug A, Breivik H, Eide PK, Kreunen M, Foss A. Mapping of punctuate hyperalgesia around a surgical incision demonstrates that ketamine is a powerful suppressor of central sensitization to pain following surgery. *Acta Anaesthesiol Scand.* 1997;41:1124-1132.

45. Jacobi J, Fraser GL, Coursin DB, et al. Clinical practice guidelines for the sustained use of sedatives and analgesics in the critically ill adult. *Crit Care Med.* 2002;30:119-141.

46. Sessler CN, Grap MJ, Brophy GM. Multidisciplinary management of sedation and analgesia in critical care. *Semin Respir Crit Care Med.* 2001;22:211-226.

47. Ramsay MA, Savege TM, Simpson BR, Goodwin R. Controlled sedation with alphaxalone-alphadolone. *BMJ* 1974;2:656-659.

48. Ely EW, Truman B, Shintani A, et al. Monitoring sedation status over time in ICU patients: reliability and validity of the Richmond Agitation-Sedation Scale (RASS). *JAMA.* 2003;289: 2983-2991.

49. Sessler CN, Grap MJ, Ramsay MA. Evaluating and monitoring analgesia and sedation in the intensive care unit. *Crit Care.* 2008;12(suppl 3):S2.

50. Sessler CN, Gosnell MS, Grap MJ, et al. The Richmond Agitation-Sedation Scale: validity and reliability in adult intensive care unit patients. *Am J Respir Crit Care Med.* 2002;166:1338-1344.

51. Riker RR, Picard JT, Fraser GL. Prospective evaluation of the Sedation-Agitation Scale for adult critically ill patients. *Crit Care Med.* 1999;27:1325-1329.

52. Hogg LH, Bobek MB, Mion LC, et al. Interrater reliability of 2 sedation scales in a medical intensive care unit: a preliminary report. *Am J Crit Care.* 2001;10:79-83.

53. De Jonghe B, Cook D, Griffith L, et al. Adaptation to the Intensive Care Environment (ATICE): development and validation of a new sedation assessment instrument. *Crit Care Med.* 2003;31:2344-2354.

54. Avripas MB, Smythe MA, Carr A, Begle RL, Johnson MH, Erb DR. Development of an intensive care unit bedside sedation scale. *Ann Pharmacother.* 2001;35:262-263.

55. Lenhardt R, Orhan-Sungur M, Komatsu R, et al. Suppression of shivering during hypothermia using a novel drug combination in healthy volunteers. *Anesthesiology.* 2009;111:110-115.

56. Nicolaou G, Chen AA, Johnston CE, Kenny GP, Bristow GK, Giesbrecht GG. Clonidine decreases vasoconstriction and shivering thresholds, without affecting the sweating threshold. *Can J Anaesth.* 1997;44:636-642.

57. Delaunay L, Bonnet F, Liu N, Beydon L, Catoire P, Sessler DI. Clonidine comparably decreases the thermoregulatory thresholds for vasoconstriction and shivering in humans. *Anesthesiology.* 1993;79:470-474.

58. Talke P, Tayefeh F, Sessler DI, Jeffrey R, Noursalehi M, Richardson C. Dexmedetomidine does not

alter the sweating threshold, but comparably and linearly decreases the vasoconstriction and shivering thresholds. *Anesthesiology.* 1997;87:835-841.

59. Doufas AG, Lin CM, Suleman MI, et al. Dexmedetomidine and meperidine additively reduce the shivering threshold in humans. *Stroke.* 2003;34:1218-1223.

60. Mokhtarani M, Mahgoub AN, Morioka N, et al. Buspirone and meperidine synergistically reduce the shivering threshold. *Anesth Analg.* 2001;93:1233-1239.

61. Fukuoka N, Aibiki M, Tsukamoto T, Seki K, Morita S. Biphasic concentration change during continuous midazolam administration in brain-injured patients undergoing therapeutic moderate hypothermia. *Resuscitation.* 2004;60:225-230.

62. Koska AJ 3rd, Romagnoli A, Kramer WG. Pharmacodynamics of fentanyl citrate in patients undergoing aortocoronary bypass. *Cardiovasc Dis.* 1981;8:405-412.

63. Leslie K, Sessler DI, Bjorksten AR, Moayeri A. Mild hypothermia alters propofol pharmacokinetics and increases the duration of action of atracurium. *Anesth Analg.* 1995;80:1007-1014.

64. Puig MM, Warner W, Tang CK, Laorden ML, Turndorf H. Effects of temperature on the interaction of morphine with opioid receptors. *Br J Anaesth.* 1987;59:1459-1464.

65. Badjatia N, Strongilis E, Gordon E, et al. Metabolic impact of shivering during therapeutic temperature modulation: the Bedside Shivering Assessment Scale. *Stroke.* 2008;39:3242-3247.

66. Venn RM, Hell J, Grounds RM. Respiratory effects of dexmedetomidine in the surgical patient requiring intensive care. *Crit Care.* 2000;4:302-308.

67. Nelson LE, Lu J, Guo T, Saper CB, Franks NP, Maze M. The alpha2-adrenoceptor agonist dexmedetomidine converges on an endogenous sleep-promoting pathway to exert its sedative effects. *Anesthesiology.* 2003;98:428-436.

68. Shelly MP. Dexmedetomidine: a real innovation or more of the same? *Br J Anaesth.* 2001;87:677-678.

69. Venn RM, Grounds RM. Comparison between dexmedetomidine and propofol for sedation in the intensive care unit: patient and clinician perceptions. *Br J Anaesth.* 2001;87:684-690.

70. Riker RR, Shehabi Y, Bokesch PM, et al. Dexmedetomidine vs midazolam for sedation of critically ill patients: a randomized trial. *JAMA.* 2009;301:489-499.

71. Pandharipande PP, Pun BT, Herr DL, et al. Effect of sedation with dexmedetomidine vs lorazepam on acute brain dysfunction in mechanically ventilated patients: the MENDS randomized controlled trial. *JAMA.* 2007;298:2644-2653.

72. Prielipp RC, Wall MH, Tobin JR, et al. Dexmedetomidine-induced sedation in volunteers decreases regional and global cerebral blood flow. *Anesth Analg.* 2002;95:1052-1059.

73. Zornow MH, Maze M, Dyck JB, Shafer SL. Dexmedetomidine decreases cerebral blood flow velocity in humans. *J Cereb Blood Flow Metab.* 1993;13:350-353.

74. Zornow MH, Fleischer JE, Scheller MS, Nakakimura K, Drummond JC. Dexmedetomidine, an alpha 2-adrenergic agonist, decreases cerebral blood flow in the isoflurane-anesthetized dog. *Anesth Analg.* 1990;70:624-630.

75. Karlsson BR, Forsman M, Roald OK, Heier MS, Steen PA. Effect of dexmedetomidine, a selective and potent alpha 2-agonist, on cerebral blood flow and oxygen consumption during halothane anesthesia in dogs. *Anesth Analg.* 1990;71:125-129.

76. Drummond JC, Dao AV, Roth DM, et al. Effect of dexmedetomidine on cerebral blood flow velocity, cerebral metabolic rate, and carbon dioxide response in normal humans. *Anesthesiology.* 2008;108:225-232.

77. Kadoi Y, Saito S, Kawauchi C, Hinohara H, Kunimoto F. Comparative effects of propofol vs dexmedetomidine on cerebrovascular carbon dioxide reactivity in patients with septic shock. *Br J Anaesth.* 2008;100:224-229.

78. Maccioli GA. Dexmedetomidine to facilitate drug withdrawal. *Anesthesiology.* 2003;98:575-577.

79. Multz AS. Prolonged dexmedetomidine infusion as an adjunct in treating sedation-induced withdrawal. *Anesth Analg.* 2003;96:1054-1055.

80. Baddigam K, Russo P, Russo J, Tobias JD. Dexmedetomidine in the treatment of withdrawal syndromes in cardiothoracic surgery patients. *J Intensive Care Med.* 2005;20:118-123.

81. Kent CD, Kaufman BS, Lowy J. Dexmedetomidine facilitates the withdrawal of ventilatory support in palliative care. *Anesthesiology.* 2005;103:439-441.

82. Farag E, Chahlavi A, Argalious M, et al. Using dexmedetomidine to manage patients with cocaine and opioid withdrawal, who are undergoing cerebral angioplasty for cerebral vasospasm. *Anesth Analg.* 2006;103:1618-1620.

83. Rovasalo A, Tohmo H, Aantaa R, Kettunen E, Palojoki R. Dexmedetomidine as an adjuvant in the treatment of alcohol withdrawal delirium: a case report. *Gen Hosp Psychiatry.* 2006;28:362-363.

Neurocritical Care Intervention

84. Stemp LI, Karras GE Jr. Dexmedetomidine facilitates withdrawal of ventilatory support. *Anesthesiology.* 2006;104:890; author reply 890.

85. Darrouj J, Puri N, Prince E, Lomonaco A, Spevetz A, Gerber DR. Dexmedetomidine infusion as adjunctive therapy to benzodiazepines for acute alcohol withdrawal. *Ann Pharmacother.* 2008;42:1703-1705.

86. Tobias JD. Dexmedetomidine to treat opioid withdrawal in infants following prolonged sedation in the pediatric ICU. *J Opioid Manag.* 2006;2:201-205.

87. Tobias JD. Subcutaneous dexmedetomidine infusions to treat or prevent drug withdrawal in infants and children. *J Opioid Manag.* 2008;4:187-191.

88. Siobal MS, Kallet RH, Kivett VA, Tang JF. Use of dexmedetomidine to facilitate extubation in surgical intensive-care-unit patients who failed previous weaning attempts following prolonged mechanical ventilation: a pilot study. *Respir Care.* 2006;51:492-496.

89. Arpino PA, Kalafatas K, Thompson BT. Feasibility of dexmedetomidine in facilitating extubation in the intensive care unit. *J Clin Pharm Ther.* 2008;33:25-30.

90. Goddeau RP, Jr., Silverman SB, Sims JR. Dexmedetomidine for the treatment of paroxysmal autonomic instability with dystonia. *Neurocrit Care.* 2007;7:217-220.

91. De Witte J, Sessler DI. Perioperative shivering: physiology and pharmacology. *Anesthesiology.* 2002;96:467-484.

92. Matsukawa T, Kurz A, Sessler DI, Bjorksten AR, Merrifield B, Cheng C. Propofol linearly reduces the vasoconstriction and shivering thresholds. *Anesthesiology.* 1995;82:1169-1180.

93. Van Hemelrijck J, Fitch W, Mattheussen M, Van Aken H, Plets C, Lauwers T. Effect of propofol on cerebral circulation and autoregulation in the baboon. *Anesth Analg.* 1990;71:49-54.

94. Stephan H, Sonntag H, Schenk HD, Kohlhausen S. [Effect of Disoprivan (propofol) on the circulation and oxygen consumption of the brain and CO_2 reactivity of brain vessels in the human]. *Anaesthesist.* 1987;36:60-65.

95. Kelly DF, Goodale DB, Williams J, et al. Propofol in the treatment of moderate and severe head injury: a randomized, prospective double-blinded pilot trial. *J Neurosurg.* 1999;90:1042-1052.

96. Pinaud M, Lelausque JN, Chetanneau A, Fauchoux N, Menegalli D, Souron R. Effects of propofol on cerebral hemodynamics and metabolism in patients with brain trauma. *Anesthesiology.* 1990;73:404-409.

97. Hartung HJ. [Intracranial pressure in patients with craniocerebral trauma after administration of propofol and thiopental]. *Anaesthesist.* 1987;36:285-287.

98. Hutchens MP, Memtsoudis S, Sadovnikoff N. Propofol for sedation in neuro-intensive care. *Neurocrit Care.* 2006;4:54-62.

99. Fukushima H, Ishiyama T, Oguchi T, Masui K, Matsukawa T, Kumazawa T. [Refractory generalized convulsions in a patient undergoing brain tumor resection during propofol anesthesia]. *Masui.* 2004;53:691-692.

100. Bennett SN, McNeil MM, Bland LA, et al. Postoperative infections traced to contamination of an intravenous anesthetic, propofol. *N Engl J Med.* 1995;333:147-154.

101. Henry B, Plante-Jenkins C, Ostrowska K. An outbreak of *Serratia marcescens* associated with the anesthetic agent propofol. *Am J Infect Control.* 2001;29:312-315.

102. Eddleston JM, Shelly MP. The effect on serum lipid concentrations of a prolonged infusion of propofol—Hypertriglyceridaemia associated with propofol administration. *Intensive Care Med.* 1991;17:424-426.

103. Leisure GS, O'Flaherty J, Green L, Jones DR. Propofol and postoperative pancreatitis. *Anesthesiology.* 1996;84:224-227.

104. Casserly B, O'Mahony E, Timm EG, Haqqie S, Eisele G, Urizar R. Propofol infusion syndrome: an unusual cause of renal failure. *Am J Kidney Dis.* 2004;44:e98-e101.

105. Vasile B, Rasulo F, Candiani A, Latronico N. The pathophysiology of propofol infusion syndrome: a simple name for a complex syndrome. *Intensive Care Med.* 2003;29:1417-1425.

106. Forestier F, Hirschi M, Rouget P, et al. Propofol and sufentanil titration with the bispectral index to provide anesthesia for coronary artery surgery. *Anesthesiology.* 2003;99:334-346.

107. Gan TJ, Glass PS, Windsor A, et al. Bispectral index monitoring allows faster emergence and improved recovery from propofol, alfentanil, and nitrous oxide anesthesia. BIS Utility Study Group. *Anesthesiology.* 1997;87:808-815.

108. Deogaonkar A, Gupta R, DeGeorgia M, et al. Bispectral Index monitoring correlates with sedation scales in brain-injured patients. *Crit Care Med.* 2004;32:2403-2406.

109. Turkmen A, Altan A, Turgut N, Vatansever S, Gokkaya S. The correlation between the Richmond agitation-sedation scale and bispectral index during dexmedetomidine sedation. *Eur J Anaesthesiol.* 2006;23:300-304.

110. Riker RR, Fraser GL, Simmons LE, Wilkins ML. Validating the Sedation-Agitation Scale with the Bispectral Index and Visual Analog Scale in adult ICU patients after cardiac surgery. *Intensive Care Med.* 2001;27:853-858.

111. Olson DM, Thoyre SM, Peterson ED, Graffagnino C. A randomized evaluation of bispectral index-augmented sedation assessment in neurological patients. *Neurocrit Care.* 2009;11:. 20-27.

112. Kress JP, Pohlman AS, O'Connor MF, Hall JB. Daily interruption of sedative infusions in critically ill patients undergoing mechanical ventilation. *N Engl J Med.* 2000;342:1471-1477.

113. Girard TD, Kress JP, Fuchs BD, et al. Efficacy and safety of a paired sedation and ventilator weaning protocol for mechanically ventilated patients in intensive care (Awakening and Breathing Controlled Trial): a randomised controlled trial. *Lancet.* 2008;371:126-134.

114. Schweickert WD, Gehlbach BK, Pohlman AS, Hall JB, Kress JP. Daily interruption of sedative infusions and complications of critical illness in mechanically ventilated patients. *Crit Care Med.* 2004;32:1272-1276.

115. Kress JP, Gehlbach B, Lacy M, Pliskin N, Pohlman AS, Hall JB. The long-term psychological effects of daily sedative interruption on critically ill patients. *Am J Respir Crit Care Med.* 2003;168:1457-1461.

116. Kress JP, Vinayak AG, Levitt J, et al. Daily sedative interruption in mechanically ventilated patients at risk for coronary artery disease. *Crit Care Med.* 2007;35:365-371.

117. Anifantaki S, Prinianakis G, Vitsaksaki E, et al. Daily interruption of sedative infusions in an adult medical-surgical intensive care unit: randomized controlled trial. *J Adv Nurs.* 2009;65:1054-1060.

118. Skoglund K, Enblad P, Marklund N. Effects of the neurological wake-up test on intracranial pressure and cerebral perfusion pressure in brain-injured patients. *Neurocrit Care.* 2009;11:135-142.

119. Smith H, Sinson G, Varelas P. Vasopressors and propofol infusion syndrome in severe head trauma. *Neurocrit Care.* 2009;10:166-172.

120. Schulte am Esch J, Kochs E. Midazolam and flumazenil in neuroanaesthesia. *Acta Anaesthesiol Scand Suppl.* 1990;92:96-102.

121. Spivey WH. Flumazenil and seizures: analysis of 43 cases. *Clin Ther.* 1992;14: 292-305.

Neurocritical Care Intervention

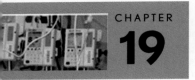

Fever and Temperature Modulation

Neeraj Badjatia, MD, MSc, FCCM

A 46-year-old woman was brought back to the neurologic intensive care unit after undergoing coiling of a right middle cerebral artery aneurysm that had ruptured the previous day. On examination, she required mild sternal rub to remain awake, and was able to follow simple, one-step commands. There were cranial nerve abnormalities, but a mild left pronation drift was noted. Overall, an unchanged examination from presentation. While in the operating room, a left subclavian central line and radial arterial line were placed along with a right external ventricular drain. On posthemorrhage day 5 (postoperative day 4), she developed a fever with a temperature of 39°C.

Why is controlling fever after brain injury important?

Fever after brain injury independently worsens outcome. One of the important mechanisms is by exacerbating inflammatory cascades. Postinjury elevations in temperature have been shown to increase inflammatory processes, including elevations in proinflammatory cytokines, the increased accumulation of polymorphonuclear leukocytes in injured tissue.[1] The hypothalamus is a key center for thermoregulation and damage to this structure can result in hyperthermia. Vascular and inflammatory cascades appear to be extremely sensitive to mild elevations in temperature following CNS injury.

Several studies also suggest that one of the key impacts of fever is an increase in neuronal excitotoxicity. Elevations in temperature have been reported to increase neurotransmitter release, accelerate free-radical production, increase intracellular glutamate concentrations, and potentiate the sensitivity of neurons to excitotoxic injury.[1] In an experimental microdialysis study of focal ischemia, glutamate release was significantly higher in hyperthermic than normothermic rats, indicating the importance of focal brain temperature on neurotransmitter release.[2] Other investigators have observed increases in cellular depolarization in the ischemic penumbra surrounding damaged neuronal tissue, increased neural intracellular acidosis, and inhibition of enzymatic protein kinases, which are responsible for synaptic transmission and cytoskeletal function in relation to elevations in core body temperature.[3] At the molecular level, elevations in temperature have been shown to enhance the expression of heat-shock proteins, as well as receptor expression associated with glutamate neurotransmission.[4]

Experimental and clinical studies have suggested that fever can also directly induce nervous system injury.[5] In these circumstances, it is usually a temperature higher than 40°C for extended periods that produces abnormalities in the blood-brain barrier, as well as profound cardiovascular, metabolic, and hemodynamic dysfunction. Thus, mechanisms underlying hyperthermia-induced pathophysiology and secondary hyperthermia following central nervous system (CNS) injury are similar.

A recent meta-analysis of all brain injury types found that fever is related to morbidity and mortality.[6] However, several important questions regarding the impact timing and duration of fever on outcome remain unanswered. Is it the fever seen within the first 24 hours or within the first 10 days the most influential on outcome? Which is more important in influencing outcome: the number of febrile episodes or the overall burden of temperatures above 37°C in the first week? Both clinical and experimental evidence indicate that each type of injury may have an optimal time window for fever control.

What are the initial management steps for fever in this patient?

The new onset of fever should trigger a careful diagnostic evaluation to find a source of infection. It is important to be familiar with the patient's history, with particular attention being paid to predisposing causes of fever. For example, patients presenting in coma who require emergent endotracheal intubation are likely at a higher risk for developing pneumonia from aspiration. In addition to auscultation of the lung fields and careful abdominal examination, particular attention should be paid to any surgical wounds or skin ulcerations as well as for cerebrospinal fluid (CSF) leaks (otorrhea or rhinorrhea) in patients who underwent a craniotomy. Review of chest radiographs should focus on any evidence of new infiltrates or effusions. Initial laboratory tests should focus on peripheral white blood cells (WBCs) and cultures of blood, urine, sputum, and CSF in patients with an external ventricular or lumbar drain. If the patient is endotracheally intubated or has a tracheotomy, obtain a sample of sputum for Gram stain either by blind suctioning or bronchoalveolar lavage. Central venous catheters that have been in place for longer than 96 hours should be removed, and the tip should be submitted for semiquantitative microbiology. In patients receiving antibiotics for more than 3 days, a stool sample should be analyzed for the presence of *Clostridium difficile* toxin (Figure 19-1).

What methods can be utilized for controlling fever in this patient?

Pharmacologic Interventions

Endogenous pyrogens released by leukocytes in response to infection, drugs, blood products, or other stimuli cause fever by stimulating cerebral prostaglandin E synthesis and as a result raise the hypothalamic temperature set point.[7] Antipyretic agents including acetaminophen, aspirin, and other nonsteroidal anti-inflammatory drugs (NSAIDs) are believed to block this process by inhibiting cyclooxygenase-mediated prostaglandin synthesis in the brain, resulting in a lowering of the hypothalamic set point. This activates the body's two principal mechanisms for heat dissipation: vasodilation and sweating.[7] The effectiveness of antipyretic agents is tightly linked to conditions where thermoregulation is intact. Therefore, they are more likely to be ineffective in brain-injured patients with impaired thermoregulatory mechanisms. Corticosteroids also have antipyretic properties but are not used clinically to treat fever because of their side effects.

Whether acetaminophen alone is more effective than placebo for treating fever in adult ICU patients is still unclear. The majority of studies have been conducted in the pediatric population, where weight-adjusted doses have been shown to be effective in reducing fever. In the adult neurocritical care population, acetaminophen has been most widely studied in an attempt to maintain normothermia in patients with acute stroke. Koennecke and Leistner[8] showed that treatment with acetaminophen in a daily dose of 4000 mg resulted in a substantial reduction of the proportion of patients with body temperatures over 37.5°C (the amount of temperature reduction was not reported). Kasner et al[9] observed a difference of 0.2°C in body temperature in favor of treatment with acetaminophen (approximately 4 g per day) as compared to placebo in patients with hemorrhagic or ischemic stroke, although not statistically significant. Two recent phase II studies have demonstrated that perhaps a higher dose of acetaminophen (6000 mg per day) is more effective in

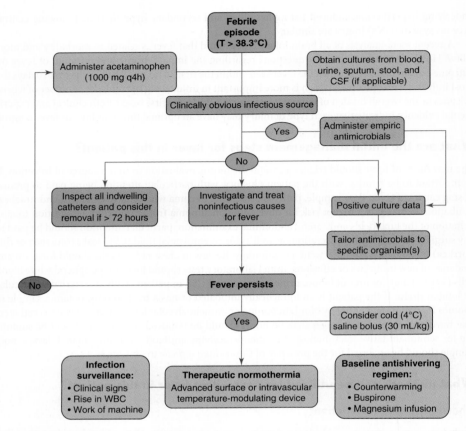

Figure 19-1. Approach toward febrile patient in the neurologic intensive care unit. CSF, cerebrospinal fluid; WBCs, white blood cells.

maintaining normothermia/preventing fever. Based on the results from these studies, a large phase III study assessing the ability to maintain normothermia after acute ischemic stroke is under way.[10]

Ibuprofen has been widely studied in the pediatric population, with equivalent or superior efficacy as compared to acetaminophen. However, only one randomized, controlled study has been conducted in adult patients with brain injury, which demonstrated that ibuprofen (2400 mg per day) was not shown to be better than acetaminophen or placebo in maintaining normothermia after ischemic stroke.[10] A recent small randomized study of a continuous infusion of diclofenac sodium (0.04 mg/kg per hour) was found to be effective in reducing the burden of fever and number of febrile events in critically injured traumatic brain injury (TBI) and subarachnoid hemorrhage (SAH) patients.[11] Although no adverse effects related to increasing hemorrhage rates were reported, larger studies are needed before this therapy can be widely utilized.

Nonpharmacologic Interventions

External cooling

External cooling reduces body temperature by promoting heat loss without affecting the hypothalamic set point. Four modes of heat transfer constitute the basis of interventions to promote heat loss: (1) evaporation (eg, water sprays or sponge baths); (2) conduction (eg, ice packs, water-circulating cooling blankets, immersion); (3) convection (eg, fans, air-circulating cooling blankets); and (4) radiation (ie, exposure of the skin).[12] In patients with temperature elevations caused by impaired thermoregulation, such as what occurs after brain injury, antipyretic agents are usually ineffective, and temperature reduction may only be achieved by external cooling. However, external cooling can result in reflex shivering and vasoconstriction as the body attempts to generate heat and counteract the cooling process.

Few controlled studies have evaluated the efficacy of external cooling interventions for lowering body temperature in humans. Previous experimental studies have shown that the combination of evaporative and convection cooling, with water sprays or sponging and forced airflow, is more effective than conduction cooling or either method alone for reducing temperature in non–brain-injured patients with hyperthermia.[13] In a study of febrile neurocritical care patients treated with acetaminophen, air-blanket cooling had a small benefit that did not reach statistical significance.[14]

Water-circulating cooling blankets, a form of conductive cooling, are the most commonly used treatment for acetaminophen-refractory fever in critically ill adults. However, there are few data regarding their efficacy. Two small controlled studies have evaluated external cooling in adult ICU patients. One study compared the use of acetaminophen alone with tepid water sponging or with a water-circulating cooling blanket in febrile neurologic patients and found no difference between the three treatments.[15] Another study of febrile patients under sedation, analgesia, and mechanical ventilation found that ice-water sponging was superior to two IV NSAIDs[16] in a nonrandomized crossover study. A large observational study found no difference in the mean cooling rate in febrile ICU patients treated with or without water-circulating cooling blankets.[17] A feature commonly found with water circulating blankets is the wide fluctuations in temperature that occur, with temperature overshoot being very common.

Recent engineering advancements have introduced a new set of surface-cooling blankets that are much more efficient at achieving and maintaining normothermia (Figure 19-2). Each system works by utilizing tightly wrapped pads that circulate cold water to promote conductive heat loss. In a randomized controlled trial of 53 neurologically injured patients that had a fever (temperature ≥ 38.3°C) for at least 2 hours after the administration of 650 mg of acetaminophen were randomized to treatment with an advanced cooling blanket system or a conventional water-circulating cooling blanket. Despite having a slightly higher baseline mean temperature, patients treated with the advanced system experienced a 75% reduction in fever burden and became normothermic faster than the control group, despite a significantly higher rate of shivering.[18]

Intravascular cooling

Over the past few years, a number of intravascular devices have become available to lower body temperature (Figure 19-2). They all work to control fever by directly lowering the blood temperature with cooled saline, which circulates through balloons or channels around an intravascular catheter. While there is no direct contact with the blood, the cold saline solution extracts heat from the blood, thus lowering body temperature.[13]

Infusion of 4°C normal saline is an appealing option because it is inexpensive and easy to administer in the critical care setting. The use of cold saline boluses has recently been studied and advocated for the induction of hypothermia in cardiac arrest patients.[19] A small case series also found the rapid infusion of large-volume cold saline to be a safe and effective method to achieve normothermia in select brain-injured patients.[20] In addition to its rapid onset, the large volume of infusion can help offset the fluid imbalance that may be observed during the induction of hypothermia. Therefore, the administration of large-volume cold saline could be considered during the induction phase of fever control.

Neurocritical Care Intervention

The nurse administers 1000 mg of acetaminophen through the patient's nasogastric tube. Cultures from blood, urine, sputum, and CSF were sent to the laboratory. All the lines were inspected and were noted not to appear infected. A decision is made to initiate aggressive fever control to maintain normothermia with an advanced temperature-modulating device.

What is the evidence for aggressive fever control after brain injury?

Clinical Evidence

Subarachnoid hemorrhage

Fever after SAH occurs in up to 70% of all patients in the first 10 days after SAH. In addition to disease severity and the amount of SAH present, the presence of intraventricular hemorrhage is a strong risk factor for the development of fever.[21] Experimental models have demonstrated that the presence of even the smallest amount of blood within the CSF can induce fever.[22]

(A) Gaymar

(surface-cooling device using wrap-around pads)

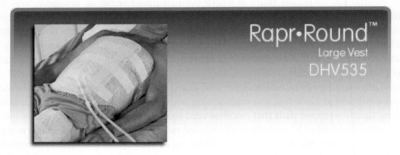

Gaymar's Rapr-Round large vest DHV535

Gaymar's Medi-Therm MTA7900 system for temperature modulation

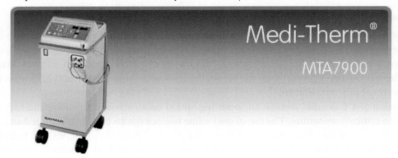

Figure 19-2. Food and Drug Administration–approved temperature-modulation devices. **A.** Gaymar surface-cooling device using wrap-around pads. **B.** Cincinnati Sub-Zero surface-cooling device using a cool blanket. **C.** Medivance Arctic Sun, surface temperature modulation using conductive gel pads. **D.** Philips InnerCool RTx endovascular system using a conductive metal catheter. **E.** Zoll intravascular temperature management system using balloon catheters.

(B) Cincinnati Sub-Zero
   (surface-cooling device using a cool blanket)

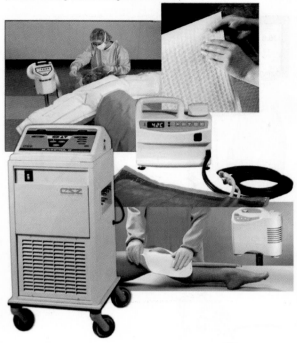

(C) Medivance Arctic Sun
   (surface temperature modulation using conductive gel pads)

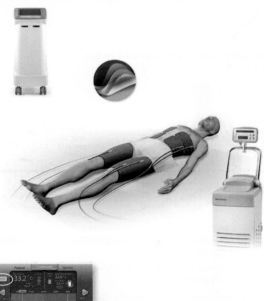

Figure 19-2. (*Continued.*)

(D) Philips InnerCool RTx endovascular system
(using conductive metal catheter)

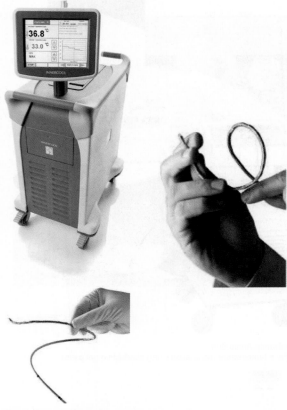

(E) Zoll intravascular temperature management system
(using balloon catheters)

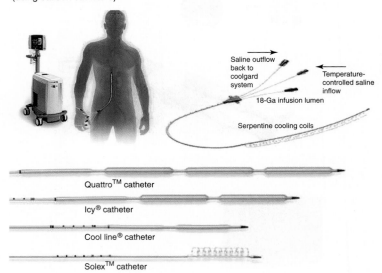

Saline outflow back to coolgard system

Temperature-controlled saline inflow

18-Ga infusion lumen

Serpentine cooling coils

Quattro™ catheter

Icy® catheter

Cool line® catheter

Solex™ catheter

Figure 19-2. (*Continued.*)

Clinically, the febrile response has been implicated in the development of cerebrovascular vaso-spasm after SAH.[23] Numerous recent studies have found that after controlling for baseline predictors of poor outcome, fever is associated with an increased risk of death or severe disability, loss of inde-pendence in instrumental activities of daily living (IADL), and cognitive impairment.[6] A recent case-control study that matched SAH patients by age, severity of injury, and amount of blood on initial computed tomographic (CT) scan found that the application of therapeutic normothermia for the first 2 weeks after hemorrhage was associated with an improvement in 12-month outcomes. This study also found a higher rate of pneumonia and longer ICU length of stay in the therapeutic normo-thermia group.[24] These preliminary findings point to the fine balance between infectious risks and benefit of prolonged fever control.

Cardiac arrest

Recent reports have demonstrated the benefit of therapeutic hypothermia for the first 12 to 24 hours after cardiac arrest,[25,26] and hypothermia has been adopted as the standard of care for survivors of cardiac arrest by the American Heart Association.[27] However, the ongoing importance of con-trolling temperature and preventing fever after the initial 24 hours has not been well studied. Previously published studies indicated that the occurrence of fever in the first 72 hours after cardiac arrest was very common and was independently associated with poor outcome.[28,29] It is not known whether there is still a high incidence of fever in the 48 hours after hypothermia, nor what the influence of applying hypothermia in the first 24 hours may have on the impact of subsequent fever. It may be reasonable to conclude, however, that ongoing maintenance of fever control (therapeutic normothermia) is beneficial for at least 48 hours after 24 hours of therapeutic hypothermia.

Spinal cord injury

Fever is a common complication in patients with spinal cord injury (SCI), with the most common cause being infections, especially pneumonia and urinary tract infections.[1] However, similar to brain-injured patients, this population also has a high incidence of thermoregulatory problems, deep venous thrombosis, and fever of unknown etiology.[30] Experimental studies have shown that inducing hyperthermia immediately after cord injury is associated with increased tissue damage and worse outcomes in behavioral and histopathologic measures as compared to normothermic conditions.[1] No clinical studies to date have looked at fever after spinal cord injury, limiting the support for aggressive maintenance of normothermia in this patient population beyond the initial resuscitation phase and into the ICU setting.

Stroke

Decades of experimental research have consistently pointed to the negative influence of fever at the time of ischemia. Maintaining normothermia acutely after ischemia stabilizes the blood-brain barrier, reduces cerebral metabolism, ischemic depolarizations, and free-radical production.[3] Clinical studies have dem-onstrated the strong independent association between fever and stroke severity as well as outcome both at admission and in the first 24 hours after ischemic stroke[6]; however, the impact fever has beyond 24 hours has not been well studied. Mechanisms that influence secondary injury in ischemic stroke remain active for several days, and, clinically, the period for peak cerebral edema occurs within the first 3 to 5 days postinjury. Aggressive control of temperature during this time period may be warranted.

The clinical and experimental evidence for the impact of fever after intracerebral hemorrhage (ICH) is much more limited but comes to the same essential conclusion that fever in the acute stage after ICH is detrimental. Schwarz et al demonstrated that the development of fever within the first 72 hours after injury was associated with outcome on discharge, even after accounting for measures of injury severity.[31] While clinical data are lacking with regard to the importance of fever beyond 72 hours, cerebral edema in ICH is known to persist for longer periods than seen in ischemic stroke and, therefore, these patients may require a longer period of fever control.

Traumatic brain injury

Fever early after TBI is associated with a poor Glasgow Coma Scale on presentation, the presence of diffuse axonal injury, cerebral edema on the initial head CT scan, systolic hypotension, hyperglycemia, and leukocytosis.[32] Like all other brain injuries, fever after TBI is likely related to both the development of infection and degree of hypothalamic dysfunction from injury. Observational studies have found that the occurrence of fever in the first week after injury is associated with increased intracranial pressure (ICP), neurologic impairment, and prolonged ICU stay.[33] The largest cohort study is by Jiang et al, who reported a strong relationship between fever and outcome in a study of 846 TBI patients.[34] Taken together, these studies indicate that fever at any time in the first week after injury is associated with intermediate decline and long-term poor outcome and should be treated aggressively.

In order to initiate normothermia with an advanced temperature-modulating device, the nurse informs the ICU team that a continuous measure of core temperature is necessary.

Where is the ideal location for core temperature monitoring during therapeutic normothermia?

While most of the literature reports fever in relation to core body temperature, it is important to note that brain temperature is often higher than core body temperature. Rossi et al found that the incidence of temperature measurements exceeding 38°C in the brain was 15% higher as compared to simultaneously measured core body temperature from the pulmonary artery.[35] The difference between brain and core temperatures has been found to range up to 2°C depending on the characteristics of the patient, the probe placement, and interactions with other physiologic variables.[35,36] As patients become febrile, the gap between brain and core temperatures increases, which may indicate that the true incidence of febrile temperatures in the brain may be even higher than reported in large observational studies that have only measured core body temperature.

However, brain temperature monitoring requires specialized invasive intracranial monitoring, which is not indicated in the majority of brain-injured patients, and current practice is to target core body temperature. The most accurate measure of core body temperature is obtained from a pulmonary artery catheter, which faces the same limitation of the invasive intracranial monitoring. As a result, the two most common modes of obtaining a continuous core temperature reading is via either a bladder temperature probe or an esophageal temperature probe. A bladder temperature probe has the advantage of being attached to a Foley catheter and, therefore, can serve dual purposes. Accurate bladder temperatures rely on normal urinary flow such that both polyuria and oliguria can result in wide fluctuations in temperature readings and render a bladder monitor inaccurate. This is a significant and common limitation that should be considered when using bladder temperatures during normothermia or hypothermia therapy. Esophageal temperature monitors are often isolated probes that serve only to measure temperature, although there are some probes available that are intertwined into an existing nasogastric tube. The great advantage of esophageal temperature as the measure of body temperature is its close correspondence to temperature in the pulmonary artery. However, some means of ensuring that the temperature probe is placed in the lower esophagus is necessary (eg, verification by chest radiography) since catheters may tend to form into a "U" shape in swallowing so that the tip is high in the esophagus even though a sufficient length of catheter has been swallowed.

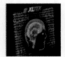

On the postbleed day 8, the patient is noted to have persistent episodes of shivering accompanied by an increase in the workload of the temperature-modulating device. The WBC count is noted to be 11.4×10^9 cells/L (previous day 10.2×10^9 cells/L), and the chest radiograph shows a possible retrocardiac infiltrate. However, the core body temperature remains less than 38°C and all preliminary cultures are negative.

How does one track the development of infection during therapeutic normothermia?

Fever is not only a cardinal sign of infection, it is also an adaptive response that enhances the ability to fight infection, and by inducing normothermia, this adaptive response may be impaired. A prospective, randomized clinical trial demonstrated that treatment of septic patients with intravenous ibuprofen for 48 hours improved physiologic end points but did not decrease the incidence of organ failure or 30-day mortality.[37] These studies suggest that the febrile response may have beneficial effects. This should always be weighed against the lack of evidence for the routine use of therapeutic normothermia in brain-injured patients.

Should the risk of ongoing secondary injury of fever be deemed to be greater than the risk of eliminating fever, routine infection surveillance is important. Unfortunately, no standard approach on the best way to do this surveillance currently exists. One large randomized controlled study of therapeutic normothermia using an intravascular cooling device obtained cultures and a chest radiograph if the WBC count rose by 20% or temperature exceeded 38°C. Others have advocated obtaining cultures when the water temperature in water-circulating blankets dips below 10°C even though this may not be directly related to the development of infection. The inability to accurately detect infection during therapeutic normothermia can result in antibiotic misuse and selection of resistant organisms.

The NeuroICU teams decided not to start antibiotics, but rather they performed a fiberoptic bronchoscopy in order to obtain a quantitative bronchiolar lavage (BAL) sample in addition to searching for additional causes of fever.

What additional tests should be performed to assess for additional causes of fever?

More extensive diagnostic evaluation should be considered in a graded fashion based on history, physical examination findings, laboratory results, persistence of fever despite presumably appropriate antimicrobial chemotherapy, or clinical instability. These additional tests and procedures include diagnostic thoracentesis, paracentesis, and lumbar puncture. Imaging studies should be considered, including abdominal or cardiac ultrasonography and head, chest, or abdominal CT.

Although fever in the ICU is most commonly due to infection, myriad noninfectious causes of systemic inflammation can also result in hyperthermia. Important noninfectious causes of fever in ICU patients are listed in Table 19-1. Although it is believed that fever from noninfectious causes

Neurocritical Care Intervention

Table 19-1. Common Noninfectious Causes of Fever

Cardiovascular
  Myocardial infarction
  Pericarditis
  Deep venous thrombosis
Pulmonary
  Atelectasis
  Pulmonary embolism
Hepatobiliary/Gastrointestinal
  Acalculous cholecystitis
  Acute pancreatitis
  Toxic megacolon
  Noninfectious hepatitis
Endocrine
  Hyperthyroidism
  Adrenal insufficiency
  Pheochromocytoma
Other
  Drug reactions ("drug fever")
  Transfusion reactions
  Tumors
  Malignant hyperthermia
  Neuroleptic malignant syndrome
  Serotonin syndrome
  Drug withdrawal

rarely results in a high core temperature, data in support of this view are lacking. As well, infections are rarely, if ever, associated with core temperatures greater than 40°C. When the core temperature is this high, the clinician should also suspect malignant hyperthermia or neuroleptic malignant syndrome.

The BAL sample demonstrates gram-negative rods (greater than 10,000 colony-forming units [CFU]) and appropriate empiric antibiotics are initiated. However, the ICU nursing staff reports that the patient continues to shiver.

What is the importance of the shivering response?

The shivering/vasoconstriction response is dependent on a temperature set point mediated via the preoptic nucleus of the anterior hypothalamus. The thermoregulatory system utilizes a series of positive- and negative-feedback loops to minimize fluctuations, maintaining core body temperature within 0.1°C to 0.2°C. The overall goal of such tight control is to reduce oxygen utilization and caloric expenditure to maximize metabolic efficiency as well as protect crucial enzymatic function.

In normal conditions, the hypothalamus coordinates a response to maintain core body temperature at normothermia (37°C), and the shivering/vasoconstriction response begins once temperatures fall below 36°C. In brain-injured patients, the set point is believed to be elevated, and as a result, the thermoregulatory response can be seen when lowering body temperatures to normothermic levels. In fact, the incidence of shivering has been reported to occur in up to 40% of patients undergoing therapeutic normothermia.

The metabolic consequences of this response can be extensive. An important and consistent consequence is a dramatic increase in resting energy expenditure (REE), carbon dioxide production (Vco_2), and oxygen consumption (Vo_2). By affecting several muscular groups for prolonged periods, shivering triggers an increase in metabolic demand, which translates into higher Vo_2 combined with increased respiration.[38] The clinical consequences include increased tissue ischemia, which has been associated with increased morbidity rate in postoperative cardiac surgery patients.[39] The increase of Vo_2 linked to shivering is proportional to the affected muscular mass and can increase the basal rate of oxygen consumption by two- to threefold.[38] Factors associated with an increased response include young age, higher muscle mass, and low serum magnesium.[40] The increased metabolic demand of uncontrolled shivering can lead to a dramatic change in the utilization of carbohydrates, lipids, and protein, promoting catabolism in critically ill patients.[41] For all these reasons, uncontrolled shivering can eliminate any benefit of fever control, making combating and preventing shivering crucial when inducing and maintaining normothermia.

How should shivering be treated?

The ability to differentiate the graded metabolic response to shivering is important during therapeutic normothermia, particularly as an end point for antishiver interventions. Previous measures of shivering in the postoperative setting provided qualitative assessments that may not have translated to the brain-injured patient.[42] More recently, a simple grading scale, the Bedside Shivering Assessment Scale (BSAS),[43] was developed by assessing the correlation of bedside shivering assessments with systemic metabolic stress quantified by indirect calorimetry (Table 19-2).

By clinically assessing the muscular involvement in the trunk and limbs, the BSAS provides an accurate representation of the metabolic impact of shivering. The ability to accurately identify the intensity of shivering has distinct advantages when developing a rationale approach toward treating shivering without oversedation.

When adopting a stepwise approach toward shiver control that coincides with the initiation of therapeutic normothermia, less sedating options (eg, surface counterwarming) are preferred as the initial interventions (Table 19-3). Cheng et al[44] have shown that a linear relationship exists between core temperature and the average skin temperature for the appearance of shivering in the nonanesthetized patient. The threshold temperature for shivering is equal to the sum of 20% of the mean skin temperature and 80% of the core temperature. Therefore, to inhibit shivering, the average skin temperature must be raised by at least 4°C to be as efficient as a 1°C increase in core temperature. Radiant heat systems first applied in the recovery room proved to be an efficient way of preventing postanaesthetic shivering[45] or rapidly inhibiting it when it occurs. A recent prospective study demonstrated that

Neurocritical Care Intervention

Table 19-2. The Bedside Shivering Assessment Scale (BSAS)

Score	Term	Description
0	No	Absence of shivering on palpation of neck or pectoralis muscles
1	Mild	Localized to the neck and/or thorax; may be present only on palpation
2	Moderate	Involvement of the upper extremities ± neck or pectoralis muscles
3	Severe	Generalized, whole body involvement

Table 19-3. Stepwise Protocol for Shivering Control for Induced Normothermia

Indication	Intervention	Application	Rationale
Standing	Acetaminophen	1000 mg orally every 4 h	Minimizes the pyrogenic response
	Buspirone	30 mg orally every 8 h	Works synergistically with opioids to lower the shivering threshold
	Skin counterwarming	Forced-air convection warming blanket (Bair Hugger[a]) at 43°C	Temperature receptors on the skin surface send impulses to the brain, partially inhibiting shivering response
	Magnesium	Bolus with 4 g intravenously, infuse 1 g/h and titrate to serum magnesium of 3-4 mg/dL	Magnesium sulfate results in cutaneous vasodilation, increases skin temperature, and improves comfort
Step 1 (if BSAS > 1)	Meperidine	25-75 mg intravenous bolus Alternatively, 0.5-1.0 mg/kg/h infusion	Meperidine decreases the shivering threshold
	Dexmedetomidine	Loading dose 1 μg/kg followed by an infusion of 0.3-1.5 μg/kg/h	Reduces the shivering threshold in humans Synergistic with meperidine
Step 2[b] (if BSAS > 1)	Propofol[c]	30-100 μg/kg/min	No specific antishivering properties

Abbreviation: BSAS, bedside shivering assessment scale.

[a]Manufactured by Arizant Inc, Eden Prairie, MN.

[b]Discontinuation of therapeutic normothermia should be strongly considered if patients are shivering refractory to measures outlined in Step 1.

[c]Requires mechanical ventilation.

the application of a forced-air warming blanket set at 43°C can effectively limit the metabolic impact of shivering in brain-injured patients. Surface counterwarming is a safe, effective, cheap, and nonsedating antishivering intervention that should be applied in all patients.

Pharmacologic interventions without significant sedating effects include buspirone and magnesium. Buspirone is a serotonin 1A (5-HT$_{1A}$) partial agonist that has shown special antishivering activity by activating hypothalamic heat-loss mechanisms. It is only mildly sedating and provides a good synergistic effect when combined with other antishivering interventions. The main disadvantage of buspirone is that it is administered orally and, therefore, may not be reliably absorbed in critically ill patients.[46] The intravenous administration of magnesium promotes both cutaneous vasodilation and muscle mild relaxation. Magnesium may also confer some protection from tissue ischemia, although recent studies of its neuroprotective properties have not been conclusive. Regardless, low serum magnesium levels have been shown to be a risk factor in the development of shivering, and all efforts should be made to maintain serum levels between 3 and 4 mg/dL. Levels higher than this may be associated with depressed sensorium and respiratory effort.

When these initial measures are not effective, pharmacologic agents that are more effective, but also more sedating, medications are utilized. Dexmedetomidine is a centrally acting α agonist that has distinct advantages of being an infusion with a short half-life. In tests with healthy volunteers, it is very effective in lowering the shivering threshold, and it has a synergistic impact when combined with buspirone.[46] The main limitations of the use of dexmedetomidine are bradycardia and hypotension which can be encountered at the higher doses necessary to achieve shiver control.

The most effective antishivering pharmacologic agent is meperidine.[46] It is the only opiate to have special "antishiver" properties owing to its κ-receptor activity (in addition to μ-receptor activity). It may also have central $α_2$-agonist activity. Given the short half-life of its antishivering properties, multiple dosing is required to achieve sustained shiver control, which often results in prolonged sedation. Lowering of the seizure threshold, especially in the setting of renal insufficiency, also limits its long-term utilization.

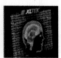
A surface counterwarming device is placed and magnesium and buspirone initiated. The patient's BSAS score is maintained at 1 or less with intermittent use of dexmedetomidine. On postbleed day 14, the NeuroICU team decides to discontinue therapeutic normothermia. Over the next 4 hours, the patient's temperature is noted to rise to 39°C and is accompanied by a decline in arousal, although the ICP remains unchanged. This prompts reinitiation of normothermia, at which point the patient's examination returns to its previous baseline.

Neurocritical Care Intervention

How does one determine the timing for discontinuing therapeutic normothermia?

There is currently no clinical evidence for the duration that fever impacts outcome after each form of brain injury. Without such information it is impossible to understand what the optimal duration should be for therapeutic normothermia. Most studies have observed that the fever burden in the first week after injury is important in determining outcome. SAH studies have extended the duration of importance out to the first 14 days after injury. Therefore, it would be reasonable to maintain normothermia for at least the first week after injury (2 weeks for SAH patients). Additional issues, such as the impact of ongoing fever on ICP, may be factored into a continued need for fever control beyond this time frame. As well, a decline in mental status is occasionally observed with the rebound fever that occurs with discontinuation of a temperature-modulating device. It is reasonable to reinstitute normothermia and attempt discontinuation at a later time. The phenomenon of rebound fever with discontinuation of a device is nearly universal and may have to do with the impact of these powerful devices on the hypothalamic thermoregulatory feedback loops, although the exact mechanisms are not known.

! CRITICAL CONSIDERATIONS

- Fever after brain injury is a very common occurrence.
- Fever may lead to worse outcomes after brain injuries.
- Although aggressive fever management and maintenance of normothermia are logical therapeutic interventions, one must keep in mind that there is no level 1 evidence to support this approach.

- When advanced temperature-modulation devices are utilized for normothermia, the management should be accompanied by a stepwise antishivering regimen. Such an approach should target the metabolic impact of shivering and minimize the use of long-acting sedatives.
- The utility of normothermia will depend on future research that will aim to identify the timing and target temperature that will optimize long-term recovery.

REFERENCES

1. Dietrich WD, Bramlett HM. Hyperthermia and central nervous system injury. *Prog Brain Res.* 2007;162:201-217.

2. Takagi K, Ginsberg MD, Globus MY, Martinez E, Busto R. Effect of hyperthermia on glutamate release in ischemic penumbra after middle cerebral artery occlusion in rats. *Am J Physiol.* 1994;267(Pt 2): H1770-1776.

3. Ginsberg MD, Busto R. Combating hyperthermia in acute stroke: a significant clinical concern.[see comment]. *Stroke.* 1998;29:529-534.

4. Kim Y, Truettner J, Zhao W, Busto R, Ginsberg MD. The influence of delayed postischemic hyperthermia following transient focal ischemia: alterations of gene expression. *J Neurol Sci.* 1998;159:1-10.

5. Sharma HS, Hoopes PJ. Hyperthermia induced pathophysiology of the central nervous system. *Int J Hyperthermia.* 2003;19:325-354.

6. Greer DM, Funk SE, Reaven NL, Ouzounelli M, Uman GC. Impact of fever on outcome in patients with stroke and neurologic injury: a comprehensive meta-analysis. *Stroke.* 2008;39:3029-3035.

7. Mackowiak PA. Concepts of fever. *Arch Intern Med.* 1998;158:1870-1881.

8. Koennecke HC, Leistner S. Prophylactic antipyretic treatment with acetaminophen in acute ischemic stroke: a pilot study. *Neurology.* 2001;57:2301-2303.

9. Kasner SE, Wein T, Piriyawat P, et al. Acetaminophen for altering body temperature in acute stroke: a randomized clinical trial [see comment]. *Stroke.* 2002;33:130-134.

10. Dippel DW, van Breda EJ, van der Worp HB, et al. Effect of paracetamol (acetaminophen) and ibuprofen on body temperature in acute ischemic stroke PISA, a phase II double-blind, randomized, placebo-controlled trial [ISRCTN98608690]. *BMC Cardiovasc Disord.* 2003;3:2.

11. Cormio M, Citerio G. Continuous low dose diclofenac sodium infusion to control fever in neurosurgical critical care [see comment]. *Neurocrit Care.* 2007;6:82-89.

12. Polderman KH. Application of therapeutic hypothermia in the ICU: opportunities and pitfalls of a promising treatment modality. Part 1: indications and evidence [see comment]. *Intensive Care Med.* 2004;30:556-575.

13. Badjatia N. Therapeutic temperature modulation in neurocritical care. *Curr Neurol Neurosci Rep.* 2006;6:509-517.

14. Mayer S, Commichau C, Scarmeas N, Presciutti M, Bates J, Copeland D. Clinical trial of an air-circulating cooling blanket for fever control in critically ill neurologic patients [see comment]. *Neurology.* 2001;56:292-298.

15. Morgan SP. A comparison of three methods of managing fever in the neurologic patient. *J Neurosci Nurs.* 1990;22:19-24.

16. Poblete B, Romand JA, Pichard C, Konig P, Suter PM. Metabolic effects of i.v. propacetamol, metamizol or external cooling in critically ill febrile sedated patients [see comment]. *Br J Anaesth.* 1997;78:123-127.

17. O'Donnell J, Axelrod P, Fisher C, Lorber B. Use and effectiveness of hypothermia blankets for febrile patients in the intensive care unit [see comment]. *Clin Infect Dis.* 1997;24:1208-1213.

18. Mayer SA, Kowalski RG, Presciutti M, et al. Clinical trial of a novel surface cooling system for fever control in neurocritical care patients [see comment]. *Crit Care Med.* 2004;32:2508-2515.

19. Bernard S, Buist M, Monteiro O, Smith K. Induced hypothermia using large volume, ice-cold intravenous fluid in comatose survivors of out-of-hospital cardiac arrest: a preliminary report. *Resuscitation.* 2003;56:9-13.

20. Badjatia N, Bodock M, Guanci M, Rordorf GA. Rapid infusion of cold saline (4°C) as adjunctive treatment of fever in patients with brain injury. *Neurology.* 2006;66:1739-1741.

21. Commichau C, Scarmeas N, Mayer SA. Risk factors for fever in the neurologic intensive care unit. *Neurology.* 2003;60:837-841.

22. Frosini M, Sesti C, Valoti M, et al. Rectal temperature and prostaglandin E2 increase in cerebrospinal fluid of conscious rabbits after intracerebroventricular injection of hemoglobin. *Exp Brain Res.* 1999;126:252-258.

23. Oliveira-Filho J, Ezzeddine MA, Segal AZ, et al. Fever in subarachnoid hemorrhage: relationship to vasospasm and outcome. *Neurology.* 2001;56:1299-1304.

24. Badjatia N, Fernandez L, Fernandez A, et al. Impact of therapeutic normothermia on outcome after subarachnoid hemorrhage. 60th Annual Meeting of the American Academy of Neurology. Chicago, IL, 2007.

25. Hypothermia after Cardiac Arrest Study Guide. Mild therapeutic hypothermia to improve the neurologic outcome after cardiac arrest [see comment] [erratum appears in *N Engl J Med* 2002;346:1756]. *N Engl J Med.* 2002;346:549-556.

26. Bernard SA, Gray TW, Buist MD, et al. Treatment of comatose survivors of out-of-hospital cardiac arrest with induced hypothermia [see comment]. *N Engl J Med.* 2002;346:557-563.

27. 2005 American Heart Association (AHA) guidelines for cardiopulmonary resuscitation (CPR) and emergency cardiovascular care (ECC) of pediatric and neonatal patients: pediatric basic life support [reprint of *Circulation.* 2005;112(24 suppl):IV1-203; PMID: 16314375]. *Pediatrics.* 2006;117:e989-e1004.

28. Takasu A, Saitoh D, Kaneko N, Sakamoto T, Okada Y. Hyperthermia: is it an ominous sign after cardiac arrest? *Resuscitation.* 2001;49:273-277.

29. Zeiner A, Holzer M, Sterz F, et al. Hyperthermia after cardiac arrest is associated with an unfavorable neurologic outcome. *Arch Intern Med.* 2001;161:2007-2012.

30. Beraldo PS, Neves EG, Alves CM, Khan P, Cirilo AC, Alencar MR. Pyrexia in hospitalised spinal cord injury patients. *Paraplegia.* 1993;31:186-191.

31. Schwarz S, Hafner K, Aschoff A, Schwab S. Incidence and prognostic significance of fever following intracerebral hemorrhage. *Neurology.* 2000;54:354-361.

32. Cairns CJ, Andrews PJ. Management of hyperthermia in traumatic brain injury. *Curr Opin Crit Care.* 2002;8:106-110.

33. Jones PA, Andrews PJ, Midgley S, et al. Measuring the burden of secondary insults in head-injured patients during intensive care. *J Neurosurg Anesthesiol.* 1994;6:4-14.

34. Jiang JY, Gao GY, Li WP, Yu MK, Zhu C. Early indicators of prognosis in 846 cases of severe traumatic brain injury. *J Neurotrauma.* 2002;19:869-874.

35. Rossi S, Zanier ER, Mauri I, Columbo A, Stocchetti N. Brain temperature, body core temperature, and intracranial pressure in acute cerebral damage. *J Neurol Neurosur Psychiatry.* 2001;71:448-454.

36. Henker RA, Brown SD, Marion DW. Comparison of brain temperature with bladder and rectal temperatures in adults with severe head injury. *Neurosurgery.* 1998;42:1071-1075.

37. Bernard GR, Wheeler AP, Russell JA, et al. The effects of ibuprofen on the physiology and survival of patients with sepsis. The Ibuprofen in Sepsis Study Group [see comment]. *N Engl J Med.* 1997;336(13):912-918.

38. Alfonsi P. Postanaesthetic shivering: Epidemiology, pathophysiology, and approaches to prevention and management. *Drugs.* 2001;61:2193-2205.

39. Ralley FE, Wynands JE, Ramsay JG, Carli F, MacSullivan R. The effects of shivering on oxygen consumption and carbon dioxide production in patients rewarming from hypothermic cardiopulmonary bypass. *Can J Anaesth.* 1988;35:332-337.

40. Ciofolo MJ, Clergue F, Devilliers C, Ben Ammar M, Viars P. Changes in ventilation, oxygen uptake, and carbon dioxide output during recovery from isoflurane anesthesia. *Anesthesiology.* 1989;70:737-741.

41. Haman F, Legault SR, Rakobowchuk M, Ducharme MB, Weber JM. Effects of carbohydrate availability on sustained shivering. II: Relating muscle recruitment to fuel selection [erratum appears in *J Appl Physiol.* 2004;96:1576]. *J Appl Physiol.* 2004;96:41-49.

42. Holtzclaw BJ. Postoperative shivering after cardiac surgery: a review. *Heart Lung.* 1986;15:292-302.

43. Badjatia N, Strongilis E, Gordon E, et al. Metabolic impact of shivering during therapeutic temperature modulation: the Bedside Shivering Assessment Scale. *Stroke.* 2008;39:3242-3247.

44. Cheng C, Matsukawa T, Sessler DI, et al. Increasing mean skin temperature linearly reduces the core-temperature thresholds for vasoconstriction and shivering in humans. *Anesthesiology.* 1995;82:1160-1168.

45. Weyland W, Weyland A, Hellige G, et al. Efficiency of a new radiant heater for postoperative rewarming. *Acta Anaesthesiol Scand.* 1994;38:601-606.

46. De Witte J, Sessler DI. Perioperative shivering: physiology and pharmacology. *Anesthesiology.* 2002;96:467-484.

CHAPTER

20

Endovascular Surgical Neuroradiology

Raqeeb Haque, MD
Celina Crisman, BS
Brian Hwang, MD
E. Sander Connolly, MD
Philip M. Meyers, MD

A 45-year-old man with a history of hypertension and tobacco abuse presents to the emergency department following the onset of a severe holocranial headache. He denies nausea, vomiting, head trauma, and previous headaches. His temperature is 38°C, heart rate 110 bpm, blood pressure 150/87 mm Hg. His left pupil is dilated and nonreactive to light. A computed tomographic (CT) brain scan shows diffuse subarachnoid hemorrhage. Catheter cerebral arteriography demonstrates a posterior communicating artery aneurysm (Figure 20-1).

What are the morbidity and mortality rates accompanying aneurysmal subarachnoid hemorrhage (SAH)?

Spontaneous rupture of a cerebral aneurysm causing SAH is a life-threatening condition and carries an immediate mortality rate of 10% to 20%.[1] Survival through the initial incident provides no guarantee, however; 12% to 30% of patients fail to recover neurologically, and by 6 months mortality may increase to 50%. Furthermore, as many as one-third of survivors remain dependent following aneurysmal hemorrhage.[2]

How effective is endovascular therapy in the treatment of ruptured aneurysms?

Following initial stabilization and diagnosis, attention necessarily turns toward the prevention of recurrent hemorrhage and vasospasm, both causes of significant morbidity and mortality after the initial hemorrhage.[1] Endovascular therapy is able to address both concerns, and now has an established role in treatment of ruptured cerebral aneurysms. Generally, this is accomplished by endovascular occlusion of the aneurysm with microcoils.

Since the 1960s, it has been known that surgically clipping ruptured aneurysms to prevent recurrent hemorrhage produced results superior to those associated with nonsurgical management. Endovascular coil occlusion of a cerebral aneurysm has been shown to accomplish the same goal: prevention of recurrent hemorrhage. Since its approval in 1991, endovascular coil occlusion of ruptured aneurysms has steadfastly garnered acceptance and has become the treatment modality of choice in patients with SAH due to ruptured aneurysms. Advantages of endovascular treatment include femoral access without a craniotomy and access to midline aneurysms without brain retraction.

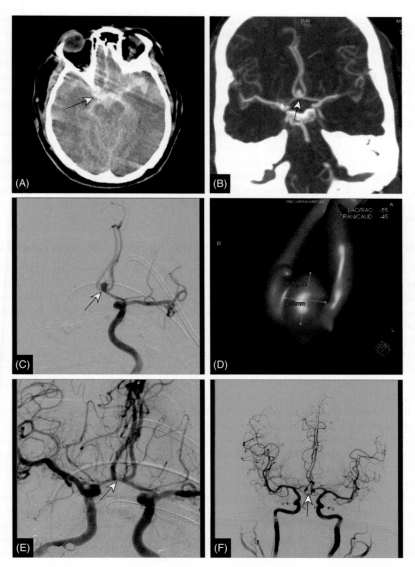

Figure 20-1. A 48-year-old man with headache and vomiting. **A.** Nonenhanced computed tomographic (CT) brain scan reveals subarachnoid hemorrhage into the basilar cisterns (*arrow*). **B.** CT angiography with coronal reconstructions demonstrates an aneurysm of the anterior communicating artery (AComA) (*arrow*). **C** and **D.** Catheter angiography of left internal carotid artery in a frontal oblique projection during the arterial phase with 3-dimensional reconstructions confirms the presence of a 6.4 mm × 4.8 mm AcomA aneurysm (*arrow*). **E** and **F.** Angiography post–coil embolization demonstrates no flow into the AComA aneurysm (*arrow*).

The effectiveness of endovascular intervention was directly compared to that of surgical clipping in the International Subarachnoid Aneurysm Trial (ISAT). This trial randomized 2143 patients presenting with SAH attributable to aneurysm rupture and deemed suitable for endovascular treatment or surgical clipping. Patients randomized to endovascular intervention experienced significantly better outcomes. Death or dependence at 1 year in the endovascular group was 23.7% compared with 30.6% in the surgical group. The absolute risk reduction in dependence or death associated with endovascular treatment was 6.9%. After 5 years of follow-up, the dependence rates did not vary significantly between groups; yet, survival in the endovascular group, even after 7 years of follow-up, remained significantly higher. In addition to decreased mortality, endovascular patients also experienced substantially fewer seizures despite a slightly greater incidence of recurrent SAH. After 3258 patient-years of follow-up, there were seven repeat hemorrhages in the endovascular group compared with two rebleeds in 3107 patient-years in the surgical group. This may be related in part to the durability of aneurysm occlusion: Sixty-six percent of follow-up angiograms in the endovascular group demonstrated complete aneurysm occlusion compared with 82% of surgically clipped aneurysms. Meanwhile, 8% of angiograms from endovascularly treated patients demonstrated incomplete occlusion with aneurysm refilling compared with 6% of angiograms of clipped aneurysms.[3,4] Despite lower rates of complete vascular occlusion, endovascular treatment represents a clinically effective treatment for many cases of ruptured aneurysms and is well supported by clinical outcomes as an acceptable treatment method in appropriately selected patients with SAH.

Which patients should undergo endovascular treatment for aneurysmal SAH?

The effectiveness and safety of endovascular intervention was initially demonstrated in 1990 when patients deemed unacceptable surgical candidates were treated with GDC (Guglielmi Detachable Coil, Target Therapeutics, Inc, Fremont, CA) occlusion of their aneurysms.[5] At that time, reasons to forgo surgical treatment included poor neurologic or medical status, anticipated surgical difficulty, failed surgery, or patient refusal to undergo surgery. Complete aneurysm occlusion was accomplished in 70.8% of small aneurysms with a small neck, 35% of large aneurysms, and 50% of giant aneurysms.[6,7] As a result of procedural complications, 1.74% of patients died, and 4.47% of them died because of the severity of the initial hemorrhage. The GDC procedure received Food and Drug Administration (FDA) approval in 1991, and the use of endovascular coil treatment has increased since that time.

Patients with severe medical comorbidities that could affect their likelihood of withstanding prolonged intracranial surgery are prime candidates for endovascular treatment. Patients with a coagulopathy or those who require chronic anticoagulation are also frequently considered for endovascular over conventional surgery. Evidence derived from multiple retrospective studies has established the safety of endovascular intervention in patients over the age of 70 years with ruptured aneurysms; in such patients, endovascular treatment is generally preferred to surgical clipping.[8]

Clinical grade has a bearing in determining the appropriate intervention. High-grade SAH patients (Hunt and Hess or World Federation of Neurologic Surgeons [WFNS] grades IV and V) present greater surgical challenges, as an edematous or ischemic brain in the setting of increased intracranial pressure (ICP) often responds poorly to surgical manipulation. However, endovascular therapies are less hindered by conditions such as swelling.[9] A study of endovascular treatment in patients with high-grade SAH due to aneurysm rupture resulted in a favorable outcome in 62% of grade IV and 25% of grade V patients, or in 52.5% of total included patients.[10] A study combining endovascular treatment with aggressive medical management, including hypervolemic hemodilution and hypertensive treatment, in WFNS grade V patients produced encouraging results. A majority of patients (55%) experienced a favorable outcome, while the mortality rate was 18%.[11] Thus, there exists growing support for endovascular intervention in patients with high-grade SAH, particularly when coupled with aggressive medical management.

Several specific complications may affect the decision to proceed with surgical or endovascular intervention. The development of an intracerebral hematoma (ICH) following aneurysmal rupture is associated with increased morbidity and mortality compared with SAH alone. The condition may require surgery owing to the need for hematoma evacuation and decompression. Clipping of the ruptured aneurysm may be undertaken simultaneously. Despite evacuation of the hemorrhage, particularly in WFNS grades IV and V, mortality in ICH patients remains high, ranging from 21% to 85%.[12,13]

For this reason, a sequential approach involving endovascular aneurysm occlusion followed quickly by surgical evacuation of the hematoma was proposed. One series using this approach in patients with WFNS grade IV or V SAH and ICH due to aneurysm rupture demonstrated favorable outcomes in 48% of patients, with death occurring in 21%.[14] This strategy may be particularly useful when ICH develops opposite to the side of the ruptured aneurysm. Chung et al reported a series of ruptured anterior communicating artery (AComA) aneurysms complicated by significant ICH, making the ICH difficult to evacuate from the optimal site for aneurysm access. These investigators treated AComA aneurysms using endovascular coil occlusion, then evacuated the ICH through a burr hole craniotomy. They observed no rebleed during follow-up and reported that more than half of the patients experienced moderate to good recovery.[15] Thus, evidence suggests that the occlusion of ruptured aneurysms associated with ICH via endovascular means followed by surgical evacuation is a safe and effective approach to a common situation traditionally associated with very high mortality.

Finally, the location and morphology of the aneurysm determine suitability for endovascular treatment. Aneurysms occurring in the posterior circulation are typically better candidates for endovascular treatment based on anatomic considerations. The relationship of these aneurysms to important perforator arteries and cranial nerves creates a great risk of surgical morbidity. Patients with multiple aneurysms in different vascular distributions and SAH of uncertain origin are also well served by endovascular treatment. However, aneurysms with tortuous proximal vessels, severe vasospasm, vessels affected by atherosclerosis, or those that are very distally located may present challenges to endovascular access.[16]

It is widely accepted that aneurysms with small necks, or inflow regions, relative to fundus size, are particularly amenable to endovascular therapy, while giant and fusiform aneurysms are not without the use of adjunctive devices. This is largely due to the tendency of endovascularly placed coils to herniate into the parent vessel. However, stent-assisted techniques as well as balloon-assisted techniques, which will be discussed in greater detail, help to reduce the failure rate of endovascular treatment in aneurysms with a low dome-to-neck ratio. The relative dimensions of an aneurysm no longer pose an absolute contraindication to endovascular management.

Middle cerebral artery (MCA) aneurysms represent one of the most common sites of intracranial aneurysms, accounting for roughly 20%, and are often managed surgically rather than endovascularly for several reasons. These aneurysms are easily accessible via craniotomy with little brain retraction. Furthermore, MCA aneurysms pose challenges to endovascular treatment, given that they often have wide necks and involve branch vessels. When 53 patients with 58 bifurcation or trifurcation aneurysms of the MCA were evaluated, 88% had a dome-to-neck ratio under 2%, and in 40% branch vessels were incorporated into the aneurysm sac.[17] However, endovascular therapy, while not generally the preferred option, is not precluded in the case of MCA aneurysms. Indeed, a recent study of 16 patients with wide-necked MCA aneurysms, including 10 acutely ruptured aneurysms, treated with stent-assisted embolization found no recurrence, rebleeding, or neurologic deterioration following an average of 20 months of follow-up.[18]

How does timing of endovascular treatment affect its success?

Intervention in the care of patients with aneurysmal SAH is primarily undertaken to prevent rebleeding, an event that increases mortality to 70% to 90%.[19,20] The risk of rebleed is greatest in the first 24 hours, reaching 19%, and by 4 weeks the cumulative risk reaches 40%.[1,19] Notably, the risk of rebleeding is greatest in those patients with high clinical grades.[1] Generally, every effort is made to secure the aneurysm as rapidly as possible as soon as the patient is medically stable.

Surgical series have yielded conflicting timing of aneurysm clipping, with some studies demonstrating higher rates of vasospasm and concordant morbidity in patients receiving early surgery, while others demonstrated a benefit associated with very early surgery (0 to 3 days following rupture). Most studies, however, yielded similar results with regard to the generally poorer outcome associated with surgical intervention when the risk of vasospasm is greatest; generally 6 to 10 days postrupture.[21]

Endovascular treatment itself has not been associated with increased vasospasm, and endovascular treatment of vasospasm can be undertaken at the time of aneurysm treatment if necessary. For these reasons, the timing issues involved in conventional surgery do not apparently hold true for endovascular intervention.[22] A retrospective study divided patients into three groups depending on when they underwent endovascular coil embolization following the development of aneurysmal SAH: within 48 hours, 3 to 10 days, or 11 to 30 days. Statistically, there was no difference in the percentage of patients experiencing favorable outcomes within each group. There was additionally no difference in the percentage of patients within each group who experienced an improvement in their clinical grade over the course of follow-up.[23] These results suggest that the amount of time elapsed between the rupture and the endovascular intervention has little bearing on the clinical result; nonetheless, treating as soon as possible is recommended given the risk of rerupture.

Should patients be maintained on anticoagulants during endovascular treatment?

Endovascular treatment involves placement of prosthetic materials (generally platinum-based coils) within a patient's vasculature to induce thrombosis of the ruptured aneurysm. Excessive thrombus formation could result in vessel occlusion and stroke. Excessive clotting is avoided by the routine use of intravenous heparin to maintain an activated clotting time (ACT) during treatment only. Although there is not universal agreement, many operators aim for an ACT two and a half to three times the baseline value. Following the procedure, the heparin effect can be reversed with protamine sulfate. Patients with small intraparenchymal hematomas have been heparinized safely; furthermore, prior placement of a ventriculostomy is not an absolute contraindication to heparin administration at the time of aneurysm treatment.[16] Patients with experimental use of intra-arterial stents in the presence of SAH, however, may require chronic antiplatelet therapy, a relative contraindication to their use.[16]

Seven days following presentation, the patient exhibited agitation and a reduced level of consciousness, mild aphasia, and left hemiparesis. The patient spontaneously became hypertensive. CT scan demonstrated no recurrent hemorrhage, hydrocephalus, or confluent areas of infarction. What was the likely etiology and role for endovascular treatment?

The patient was likely experiencing cerebral vasospasm, which follows aneurysmal SAH in up to 70% of patients, with 20% to 30% becoming symptomatic and experiencing a delayed ischemic neurologic deficit (DIND).[24] This condition remains one of the most challenging events following SAH, with death or permanent neurologic deficits occurring in as many as 20% of symptomatic patients, and generally presents between days 6 and 8.[25] Digital subtraction angiography continues to represent the gold standard for diagnosis; however, transcranial Doppler (TCD), CT, magnetic resonance (MR) angiography, and perfusion studies are often used for diagnosis and to guide treatment.[24] The medical management of cerebral vasospasm consists of the "triple H": hemodilution, hypertension, and volume expansion. Hypertensive therapy and adequate hydration are now considered the most important components. However, endovascular modalities provide additional options for management of medically refractory vasospasm.

Current endovascular treatment paradigms use intra-arterial administration of potent vasodilators directly into the cerebral arteries and balloon dilatation of narrowed arteries. Although vasospasm is primarily a disease of cerebral arterioles, transluminal balloon angioplasty (TBA) using microballoons mounted on microcatheters can be used to dilate the largest cerebral arteries at the skull base. The procedure, which is usually under heparin anticoagulation and often combined with intra-arterial infusion of vasodilators (IAVIs), has been supported by a number of studies that demonstrated clinical improvement in 31% to 80% of patients.[26-29] A meta-analysis evaluating combined TBA and IAVI demonstrated clinical improvement in 62%.[30] The procedure has shown benefit whether performed immediately or more than 24 hours following the onset of symptoms; however, evidence associated earlier intervention with better results to prevent extensive cerebral infarction.[27,31,32] Probably the most compelling evidence for the role of endovascular therapy was reported in a large population study by Johnston: At 70 university medical centers offering endovascular therapy, including balloon angioplasty for vasospasm, there was a 16% overall improvement in patient survival.[33] TBA may potentially reduce the risk of vasospasm when applied prophylactically, and in a recent multicenter clinical trial TBA significantly reduced the incidence of DIND; however, benefits must be weighed against the risk of vessel rupture inherent to the procedure, which occurred in 4 of 85 patients undergoing prophylactic TBA in this multicenter trial.[34] For this reason, prophylactic therapy is generally not recommended.

If the aneurysm had been discovered incidentally, would intervention be warranted?

Intracranial aneurysms occur in approximately 0.2% to 9.9% of the general population, as determined by autopsy studies.[35] Aneurysm rupture is uncommon, yet represents the most devastating sequela of intracranial aneurysms. Other manifestations and symptoms of intracranial aneurysms potentially include severe headaches, mass effect with focal neurologic deficits and cranial nerve palsies. The onset of a third-nerve palsy in association with a growing posterior communicating artery heralds impending rupture. An increasing number of patients are diagnosed with asymptomatic intracranial aneurysms following imaging studies, such as MR imaging (MRI). Indeed, a recent study on incidental findings accompanying MRI found asymptomatic intracranial aneurysms in 1.8% of patients undergoing MRI evaluation.[36]

Each intracranial aneurysm carries a risk of spontaneous rupture, which is thought to be decreased following endovascular occlusion, although this specific assertion remains unproven. Each intervention carries its own risks, ranging from iatrogenic rupture and intracranial bleeding to thrombosis and resultant stroke.

The International Study of Unruptured Intracranial Aneurysms prospectively followed patients with unruptured aneurysms and found an overall rupture rate of 3%, with 65% mortality in those experiencing hemorrhage; however, the study also established that the rate of rupture varies with size and location. Over a follow-up period extending 5 years, patients with no history of aneurysm rupture and with anterior circulation aneurysms under 7 mm, 7 to 12 mm, 13 to 24 mm, and greater than 25 mm experienced rupture rates of 0%, 2.6%, 14.5%, and 40%, respectively. Patients with a similar background, but aneurysms found in the posterior circulation or the posterior communicating artery, had different rates of rupture: a rate of 2.5% for those smaller than 7 mm, 14.5% for 7 to 12 mm, 18.4% for 13 to 24 mm, and 50% for those larger than 25 mm.[37] In addition, those patients who had suffered a ruptured aneurysm in the past proved more likely to suffer rupture of a previously unruptured aneurysm than their counterparts with no history of rupture.[38] Additional factors increasing the risk of rupture include severe headaches, tobacco use, and a family history of aneurysmal SAH. Age alone did not have a significant effect, even though cerebral aneurysms are more common with advancing age.[16]

The International Study of Unruptured Intracranial Aneurysms followed groups of patients undergoing surgical or endovascular intervention, and facilitated comparisons between the possible approaches to unruptured aneurysms, even though the numbers were too small to achieve statistical significance. Groups undergoing intervention generally contained proportionally more patients with larger aneurysms; however, the endovascular group included a greater proportion of older patients, larger aneurysms (>25 mm), and aneurysms of the posterior circulation as compared with the surgical cohort. The overall morbidity and mortality rate observed 1 year following endovascular surgery was 9.5%, which was slightly less than the 12.15% observed in the surgical group. The study demonstrated that factors, including large aneurysm size and location within the posterior circulation, associated with a greater risk of rupture in the absence of intervention also increased the risk of morbidity and mortality in the groups receiving surgical or endovascular treatment. While age was associated with a poorer prognosis in the surgical groups, it had a less notable impact on the prognosis of those patients treated endovascularly. The study concluded that patients with aneurysms under 7 mm and no history of aneurysm rupture had the lowest risk of rupture, whereas patients with anterior circulation aneurysms under 25 mm experienced the lowest rate of morbidity and mortality associated with interventions.[37] Current practice varies widely. Treatment, often in the form of coil embolization, is offered to patients with aneurysms 7 mm or larger. Decisions must be made on a case-by-case basis, however, and treatment for a smaller aneurysm may be appropriate for patients incurring an increased risk of rupture, such as those who smoke, have a family history of aneurysmal SAH, or who have an aneurysm that is symptomatic or demonstrates growth on serial imaging.[16] Patients with a history of SAH and coexisting aneurysms should be considered for treatment regardless of size. In those patients opting to forgo treatment or those with small aneurysms, periodic follow-up with MRI/magnetic resonance angiography (MRA) or CT/computed tomographic angiography (CTA) is advised.[39]

What techniques are used to treat intracranial aneurysms and what are the indications for each?

Endovascular intervention was originally applied to intracranial aneurysms through the use of detachable coils. There are currently six vendors of endovascular microcoils for aneurysm treatment, and each boasts specific proprietary advantages, although none has been proven to be superior over others. After careful angiographic assessment of the aneurysm, a microcatheter is advanced into the aneurysm lumen under fluoroscopic guidance. Subsequently, coils are introduced into the lumen, with the morphology and size of the initial coil selected to match the aneurysm lumen size and to span the aneurysm neck. Aneurysm occlusion is deemed optimal when there is no contrast opacification of the aneurysm lumen. Incomplete aneurysm occlusion may be accepted if there is concern that the placement of additional coils would lead to aneurysm rupture or cause obstruction of the parent artery. Surveillance evaluation after endovascular aneurysm occlusion is commonly performed to assess the durability of treatment. Catheter angiography or MRI/MRA performed at intervals for approximately 18 months is most commonly performed for follow-up.[16]

Coil embolization is appropriate for most aneurysms, particularly those with a lumen-to-neck ratio equal to or greater than 2, but is not ideal for fusiform aneurysms, those with vessels originating from the aneurysm, and those with a very large neck relative to parent artery lumen.[16] In a recent study on aneurysms of the posterior circulation, coil embolization succeeded in completely occluding the aneurysm in 80% of cases, while 20% remained incompletely occluded. Complications occurred in 6% and were limited to thromboembolic events causing transient symptoms. Intraprocedural aneurysm rupture represents a serious complication, which is fortunately infrequent, and was found in a retrospective review of 7 years of endovascular intervention to affect approximately 1% of procedures. There is additionally the risk of aneurysm regrowth or recanalization with the need for additional treatment, which affected 7% of patients in that study.[16]

Balloon-assisted coiling, which enhances conformation of the coil mass to the shape of the aneurysm, represents an option for wide-neck aneurysms. A temporary balloon is inflated in the parent artery to occlude the neck of the aneurysm while a microcatheter placed into the lumen of the aneurysm is used for coil deposition. The balloon provides a temporary barrier until the aggregate coil mass develops a stable configuration in the aneurysm sac. The technique is associated with occlusion rates of up to 83%, and a series studying its application in wide-necked aneurysms demonstrated a complete occlusion rate of 26% with subtotal occlusion in 53% in difficult aneurysms with wide necks.[40] However, the procedure is more technically demanding and carries an increased risk of rupture, which may be twice as great as that associated with unassisted coil embolization.[41]

Endovascular treatment of wide-neck aneurysms may not be possible even using balloon-remodeling technique. Coronary stents were initially applied off-label in the late 1990s to augment endovascular occlusion of wide-neck cerebral aneurysms. In 2002, the first dedicated neurovascular stent was approved for endovascular occlusion of cerebral aneurysms. Since 2002, several additional devices are now available to treat cerebral aneurysm either by providing a permanent barrier to coil occlusion of cerebral aneurysms or flow remodeling to channel cerebral blood flow away from the aneurysm to induce aneurysm thrombosis and healing. Vascular thrombosis causing stroke remains a major concern following stent placement.[42] Antithrombotic therapy, usually including use of aspirin and clopidogrel, is used to control the risk of thromboembolism until a neointimal layer covers the prosthetic devices.

Ethylene vinyl copolymer (Onyx, eV3, Inc, Maple Grove, MN) is delivered as a liquid suspension in organic solvent through a microcatheter into an aneurysm but rapidly precipitates to form a solid upon contact with blood. With a balloon inflated over the neck of the aneurysm to prevent extension of the polymer into the lumen of the parent vessel, Onyx is slowly injected to fill the aneurysm. The procedure has been studied in patients deemed poor candidates for coil embolization, as well as in those with aneurysms that recurred or failed to respond to endovascular coil embolization or surgical clipping. Investigators achieved complete occlusion in 79% of aneurysms and subtotal occlusion in 13%. However, there was a risk of delayed occlusion of the parent vessel, which affected 9 of 119 patients.[43]

Arteriovenous malformations (AVMs) can cause nontraumatic cerebral hemorrhage. What is the prevalence and typical presentation of an AVM?

AVMs represent aberrant development of the cerebral vasculature. As early as the perinatal period, AVMs may first be recognized as abnormal rests of irregular vessels, or nidi, replacing normal brain. The diagnostic hallmark of an AVM is rapid flow of arterial blood directly into venous structures, bypassing the usual capillary network on a catheter arteriogram. This produces a low-resistance, high-flow system placing high stress on the involved vessels. Consequently, AVMs may be associated with aneurysms along the cerebral blood vessels supplying or draining the AVM. Aneurysms may also occur within the nidi and may be responsible for hemorrhage in some individuals.

The prevalence of AVMs is not known with certainty. An early autopsy study located 30 AVMs among 5754 consecutively performed autopsies, and estimated prevalence at 0.52%.[44,45] However, estimates of prevalence vary, and a subsequent, retrospective, population-based study supported 10.3 per 100,000 as the prevalence of detected intracranial AVMs.[46,47] The New York Islands Arteriovenous Malformation Study was a population study that prospectively followed over 9 million people in the New York metropolitan area and showed an incidence of 1.34 per 100,000 person-years.[48] While a relatively rare disease, AVMs can cause significant neurologic morbidity and mortality.

AVMs often present with headaches and seizures, occurring in as many as a third of cases, and focal neurologic deficits. Such presentations are theoretically associated with hypoperfusion of the normal brain parenchyma surrounding the AVM as blood flows preferentially through the lower resistance pathways of the AVM called "steal phenomenon"; however, this phenomenon has not been definitively demonstrated in conjunction with symptomatic AVMs. Headaches alone may be experienced by patients with AVMs; however, it should be noted that workups initiated because of the sole symptom of headache yield a diagnosis of AVM in only approximately 0.2% of cases. Furthermore, headaches occurring in the absence of other neurologic symptoms constitute only approximately 0.3% of AVM presentations.[49] Up to 15% of AVMs are discovered incidentally while asymptomatic; usually during MRI or CT scanning for other reasons.[45] The most devastating and also one of the most common presentations, in more than 50% of AVMs, involves intracerebral hemorrhage.[50,51]

Neurocritical Care Intervention

How are AVMs diagnosed and which imaging modalities are used in their assessment (Figure 20-2)?

A variety of conventional imaging modalities are useful in the assessment of brain AVMs and may also lead to the diagnosis of asymptomatic AVMs. As mentioned previously, cross-sectional imaging studies such as CT and MRI are most often acquired first. Catheter angiography permits more accurate assessment of the underlying vascular anatomy of an AVM, including the anatomy of arterial supply and venous drainage, as well as the vascular nidus itself. Conventional MRI and complete catheter angiography provide important information for treatment planning.[51,52]

The role of additional assessment tools like functional MRI (fMRI) during treatment planning remains to be determined. fMRI helps to localize the malformation in relation to eloquent parts of the brain. fMRI may be particularly valuable for treatment planning because AVMs appear to cause reorganization of brain function. Likely a developmental process, AVMs may displace functional areas of cortex such that functional centers do not appear in the standard locations.[53]

What is the incidence of hemorrhage associated with AVMs, and what increases the risk of hemorrhage?

The risk of hemorrhage incurred by patients with diagnosed AVMs has been estimated by several studies. Among 139 patients presenting to Columbia University with no history of hemorrhage, the annual risk of hemorrhage was 2.2%.[54] An annual risk of 2% to 4% for patients with no history of hemorrhage is widely accepted based on the results of several studies following patients not receiving intervention or treatment.[54-56] Notably, the risk profile differs for patients having experienced a previous AVM hemorrhage, as demonstrated by a prospective study with approximately 380 patient-years of follow-up. Within the first year there is a risk of 15.42%; however, this risk decreases to 5.32% over the next 4 years, eventually reaching a plateau at 1.72% after 5 years.[55] These findings are supported by other studies of AVM populations.[57,58]

Factors associated with an increased risk of hemorrhage include infratentorial location (relative risk of 2.65) and deep venous drainage (relative risk 2.50). Young age at presentation (less than 30 years) has also been associated with increased risk, but not at statistically significant levels. Finally, intranidal aneurysms and high intranidal pressures also increase risk. Pressure measurement in feeding arteries of small AVMs demonstrated significantly higher pressures than those of large aneurysms.[59] In effect, smaller AVMs (diameter ≤ 3 cm) are associated with hemorrhage at presentation significantly more often than larger AVMs.

How are AVMs categorized and when is treatment appropriate?

The Spetzler and Martin (SM) grading scale is a commonly used descriptor and reflects surgical outcomes based on size, location, and venous drainage pattern. This grading scale (Table 20-1) correlates with surgical morbidity and mortality.[52]

The surgical morbidity for grade I, II, and III lesions is in the range of 1% to 3%. Thus, surgical intervention is recommended for all grade I and II lesions. A case-by-case approach is recommended for grade III AVMs. In grade IV lesions, surgery was associated with 31% morbidity, and the risk climbs to 50% when grade V lesions were operated.[60] Accordingly, no generalized recommendations were issued regarding grade IV or V AVMs, and it is necessary to individualize the treatment approach. Currently, AVMs are often managed using some combination of endovascular embolization, radiosurgery, and surgery for resection. Treatment resulted in deterioration in 19% of grade I and II patients, 35% of grade III patients, and 42% of patients with either grade IV or V AVMs.[51, 59]

The association between treatment risk and SM grading is more tenuous when considering endovascular treatment. Following 545 endovascular procedures, 14% of patients experienced new neurologic deficits, 2% of which proved persistent and disabling. Investigators found that the risk of

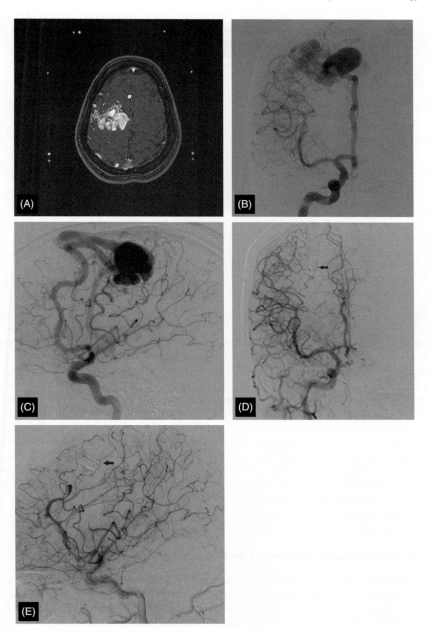

Figure 20-2. A 26-year-old woman presented with left hand paresthesias. **A.** Magnetic resonance imaging brain scan. Gradient echo image for stereotactic radiosurgery shows a pial arteriovenous malformation (AVM) in the right frontal lobe. **B** and **C.** Catheter angiography of the right internal carotid artery in frontal (B) and lateral (C) projections during the arterial phase demonstrates rapid arteriovenous shunting with hypertrophy of the intracranial right internal carotid artery and branches of the anterior and middle cerebral arteries supplying the AVM. **D** and **E.** Following endovascular embolization, final angiographic sequences show substantial reduction in arteriovenous shunting prior to surgical resection. When carefully performed, preoperative embolization of AVMs augments the safety of surgical resection.

Table 20-1. Spetzler and Martin Grading System

Category	No. Points
AVM Size	
Small (< 3 cm)	1
Medium (3-6 cm)	2
Large (> 6 cm)	3
Localization	
Noneloquent	0
Eloquent	1
Venous drainage	
Superficial only	0
Deep	1

Abbreviation: AVM, arteriovenous malformation.

neurologic deterioration following endovascular intervention did not correlate with SM grading, any of the components of the grading system, infratentorial location, the presence of aneurysms, or mode of presentation. Of the variables assessed, only age, lack of neurologic deficit at presentation, and number of embolizations significantly increased treatment risk.[61]

A subsequent study based on 295 embolization procedures and reporting good outcomes in 90.5% of patients evaluated outcomes based on the Glasgow Outcome Scale (GOS) and found that those with SM grades III through V, deep venous drainage, and periprocedural hemorrhage had a significantly increased risk of poor outcome.[62] Similarly, Starke et al defined the correlation of AVM features with endovascular treatment risk in a comprehensive treatment paradigm.[63] The resulting AVM Embolization Prognostic Risk Score assigned 1 point for a treatment plan requiring more than one embolization, 1 point for a small-diameter AVM (less than 3 cm), 1 point for eloquent location, 1 point for deep venous drainage, and 3 points for large size (greater than 6 cm). Among 222 patients undergoing embolization prior to microsurgery or radiotherapy, no patients with a score of 0 experienced postprocedural deficits. There was a new deficit rate of 6% associated with a score of 1, a 15% new deficit rate associated with a score of 2, a 21% rate associated with a score of 3, and a new deficit rate of 50% in patients with a score of 5.[63]

When is endovascular treatment undertaken for an AVM?

Endovascular embolization of brain AVMs is classically described as an adjunct to surgical resection. In fact, the two liquid embolic agents used to treat cerebral AVMs are specifically approved by the FDA for preoperative embolization. With that said, endovascular embolization of AVMs can be performed using a variety of substances. Embolic agents, including liquids, such as N-butyl-cyanoacrylate (NBCA; Trufill, Cordis Neurovascular, Inc, Miami Lakes, FL), ethylene vinyl copolymer (Onyx, ev3 Neurovascular, Irvine, CA), and undiluted ethanol; as well as particulates, polyvinyl alcohol (Contour, Boston Scientific, Natick, MA), and gelatin spheres (Embospheres, Merit Medical Systems Inc., South Jordan, Utah); and coils from a variety of manufacturers, may be used to occlude an AVM. Each agent has unique advantages and disadvantages. NBCA has received FDA approval and polymerizes to form a solid shortly after exposure to blood. An admixture consisting of NBCA and oil, with the ratio determining the rate of polymerization, is radiopaque and a permanent embolic agent upon polymerization. Furthermore, it causes an inflammatory response in occluded vessels, enhancing its permanence. Particles, often composed of polyvinyl alcohol, are radiolucent and must often be used in conjunction with a radiopaque contrast to provide an indication of placement. Furthermore, recanalization is more common with these particulates than with liquid agents, and the migration of embolic materials into the venous drainage is a theoretical possibility that must be avoided.[51,52]

Endovascular embolization can decrease the flow through the AVM nidus and thus reduce the risk of potentially catastrophic intraoperative hemorrhage. Its advantages include reduced surgical time and operative blood loss, and since embolized vessels are easily visualized, preoperative embolization may help with intraoperative navigation. Precise placement of the embolic agents is crucial to prevent stroke or hemorrhage. Embolization of normal arterial branches with a liquid embolic agent risks symptomatic neurologic deficits, which embolization of the venous drainage of an active AVM can create a surgical emergency with hyperpressurization of the nidus and hemorrhage. While feeding artery embolization may be performed with a relatively low risk of complications, embolization of proximal feeder vessels tends to encourage the growth of en passage collateral channels to the nidus, which may complicate surgery with additional bleeding from these friable white matter collaterals.

Preoperative embolization is useful in the treatment of deep-seated lesions. It is used to occlude feeding arteries with associated aneurysms; it can be used as an adjunct to radiosurgery to occlude high-risk features following hemorrhage; and it is often performed in the management of large AVMs (SM grades III to V) with the aim of decreasing surgical risk.[64] The strategy has proven effectiveness in reducing the size of the nidus. In a recent study using Onyx to preoperatively treat patients with SM grade I to IV AVMs, investigators achieved a mean nidus reduction of 84%. They achieved complete AVM resection with surgery in 98%, with no recurrence after follow-up. Following this combined treatment approach, 38% had a nondisabling neurologic deficit, whereas 7% had a disabling deficit.[65] In 202 patients who underwent endovascular embolization of AVMs prior to definitive treatment using either surgical resection or radiosurgery at a major academic medical center, Starke et al described a 2.5% risk of morbidity and no mortality.[63]

Radiotherapy for the treatment of AVMs applies highly focused radiation to the AVM nidus, causing progressive inflammation and vascular sclerosis with resultant thrombosis of the nidus. The advantages of radiotherapy for AVM include its low rate of complications and suitability for patients who are poor candidates for surgical therapy. It is relatively safe for AVMs proximal to eloquent cortex and is most effective for small (3 cm or smaller) AVMs. However, its effects are not immediate and patients remain with a risk of hemorrhage until obliteration of the lesion, which occurs in approximately 80% and is a process that generally takes 2 to 3 years.[51] There are three potential goals of embolization prior to radiosurgery: (1) decreasing the diameter of the nidus to less than 3 cm; (2) eradicating risk factors for hemorrhage such as intranidal and venous aneurysms; and (3) reducing arterial inflow in patients with symptoms, likely due to venous hypertension.[51] Many investigators recommend the use of a relatively permanent embolic agent, such as NBCA or ethylene vinyl copolymer, since less permanent agents such as particulate agents have been associated with higher recanalization rates.[51,52,66] A study utilizing NBCA to preoperatively embolize AVMs in 125 patients, including grades II through VI, determined that embolization produced total occlusion in 11.2% of AVMs and reduced the volume of 76% of AVMs enough to permit radiosurgery, which then produced total occlusion in 65% of partially embolized AVMs. During the latent phase of radiosurgery, partially embolized patients experienced a hemorrhage rate of 3% per year, arguably comparable to the natural history of unruptured AVMs. After 1 year of follow-up, investigators found an 11.8% recanalization rate.[67] A recent study compared outcomes in patients treated with embolization followed by radiosurgery to those treated with radiosurgery alone. The groups were matched such that postembolization volume was comparable to the volume of unembolized AVMs in the radiosurgery-only group. AVM location and marginal dose of radiation were also equal between the groups. This study showed that patients undergoing radiation alone had a significantly higher likelihood of AVM obliteration (70% compared with 47%). Such patients also experienced better clinical outcomes (64% versus 47%); yet, these differences were not statistically significant.[68] Although preradiosurgical embolization for the reduction of nidus size did not render the embolized AVM comparable to a naturally smaller

AMV, embolization followed by radiosurgery should not be interpreted as an ineffective treatment paradigm. There remains a role for combined therapy to treat larger aneurysms or those that are deep seated and adjacent to eloquent cortex.

Curative embolization of AVMs, defined as the cessation of blood flow through the AVM on catheter angiography, may be achieved through the use of embolization alone. Historically, nidus size has limited the effectiveness of embolization to cure AVMs. In an early study, 71% of AVMs less than 4 mL were fully occluded following endovascular treatment with NBCA, whereas similar results were accomplished in only 15% of AVMs between 4 and 8 mL.[69] A subsequent study suggested that successful complete occlusion hinged more on the identification of favorable angiographic features, such as a fistulous nidus and a limited number of dominant feeding arteries, than on size. This series reported cure in 74% of favorable AVMs, with an overall cure rate of 40%.[70] Thus, endovascular cure rates are limited and highly dependent on anatomic features of the AVM.

In selected circumstances, generally where surgical intervention is inappropriate and radiosurgery is not feasible and symptoms, such as seizures, are present, palliative embolization may be cautiously undertaken. In an early study involving 10 patients with AVMs deemed unresectable, 7 of 10 patients improved in terms of seizure reduction and mental status following partial nidal obliteration.[71] Partial obliteration has also improved limb function in lesions proximal to the rolandic cortex.[72] Any benefits of palliative embolization generally result from the reduction of the vascular steal phenomenon. Steal phenomenon defines the low-resistance blood flow through the AVM that impairs arterial flow to the surrounding normal brain or causes venous hypertension. However, owing to the rapid development of collaterals, clinical improvement stemming from palliative embolization may be transient, and this strategy may ultimately potentially worsen the long-term clinical course by increasing the risk of intracerebral hemorrhage.[73]

How are dural arteriovenous fistulas (dAVFs) distinguished from AVMs?

Classically, dAVFs constitute approximately 10% to 15% of all intracranial AVMs. We now recognize that dural fistulas are an etiologically distinct entity. They are different from pial (ie, brain) AVMs in their involvement of the intracranial dural sinuses or cortical veins. There is often no defined core, or nidus, and dAVFs are generally thought to be acquired, rather than congenital, following skull fractures or a thrombotic event in a venous sinus or cortical vein.[74] The gold standard for visualization of dAVFs remains catheter angiography, although lesions may also be identified through the use of MRI/ MRA, contrast-enhanced CT, or CTA. Table 20-2 presents a classification system for dAVFs based upon venous drainage and the amount of shunting, which roughly predict clinical course.[75]

Type I lesions exhibit a benign clinical course. In a clinical series, 0% of type I lesions presented with intracerebral hemorrhage, whereas 2% presented with nonhemorrhagic neurologic deficits. Type II lesions display a more aggressive course, presenting with hemorrhage in 11% and deficit in 39%. The higher likelihood of an aggressive course leads to a recommendation for treatment in most type II dAVFs. Hemorrhagic presentations occurred in 48% of type III lesions, with deficits in 79%.[75] Again, treatment is recommended for these lesions. Considering all types of dAVFs as a whole, the annual risk of intracranial hemorrhage is approximately 1.5%. This risk increases to 7.4% in patients who have previously experienced intracerebral hemorrhage.[76] Tentorial, middle cranial fossa, and orbital

Table 20-2. Dural Arteriovenous Fistula Classification

Type I	Shunting directly into a dural venous sinus or meningeal vein; anterograde flow only
Type II	Shunting into a dural venous sinus or meningeal vein; there is retrograde flow into subarachnoid veins
Type III	Direct shunting into subarachnoid veins

lesions are associated with more aggressive clinical courses, as are those with cortical or retrograde venous drainage.[77] Notably, the neurologic symptoms associated with dAVFs depend on the location of the lesion, with cranial nerve syndromes, aphasia, weakness, dysesthesia, dementia, exophthalmos, and visual impairment all within the realm of possibilities.

How are dural AVMs managed endovascularly?

Current endovascular strategies for the treatment of dAVFs largely resemble the procedures used for AVMs. As is the case for AVMs, only a minority of dAVFs are cured through transarterial embolization. The combination of radiosurgery followed by transarterial embolization, often within 48 hours, yields more promising results. A study involving 105 patients treated in this manner found that at an average of 14 months following the intervention, 68% of patients had fully obliterated dAVFs, whereas 14% had near-total obliteration and demonstrated no cortical venous drainage.[77] The most significant distinction between the management of dAVFs and AVMs is the option of curative transvenous embolization. Transvenous embolization requires endovascular access to the segment of venous sinus receiving the entire drainage of the fistula. Furthermore, the targeted vasculature must be separate from venous pathways necessary for the drainage of normal brain. If full occlusion of the draining segment is not carefully performed, redirection of venous drainage to delicate cortical veins may further exacerbate the shunt pathophysiology, an event likely to lead to acute hemorrhage.[74,77] Transvenous embolization has demonstrated effectivity in treating the transverse, sigmoid, or cavernous sinuses. In a series of patients treated for dAVFs, all eight patients undergoing transvenous embolization experienced complete occlusion, as compared with five of nine receiving transarterial treatment.[78] In a large retrospective study of 135 patients with carotid cavernous fistulas spanning 15 years, 76% were treated with transvenous embolization, which came into favor over the course of the study. After an average follow-up of 56 months, 90% of patients were considered clinically cured.[79] Thus, it is a singularly effective strategy, which must nonetheless be applied cautiously.

If a 68-year-old woman with a history of poorly managed hypertension presents to the emergency department with hemiparesis present for the past 8 hours and vital signs that are currently stable, what are the next steps in management?

Given this patient's presentation, acute stroke is an important consideration. Over 750,000 strokes occur each year; 80% of these are ischemic, while the remainder prove to be hemorrhagic, a distinction that can often be made with the aid of CT scanning.[80] Specialized imaging modalities, including diffusion/perfusion MRI and multimodal CT, assist in the definition of viable ischemic tissue, although such information does not generally form the basis of treatment decisions (Figure 20-3).

Treatment options pertinent to ischemic stroke include intravenous thrombolytics, intra-arterial thrombolytics, and mechanical embolectomy. Notably, these strategies are contraindicated in the patient with hemorrhagic stroke, in whom they exacerbate hemorrhage and cause clinical deterioration. Currently, intravenous administration of alteplase within 3 hours of stroke onset is the only FDA-approved treatment for acute ischemic stroke. The National Institute of Neurological Disorders and Stroke (NINDS) stroke trial found that significantly more patients (38%) randomized to treatment with intravenous alteplase experienced a complete, or near-complete, recovery after 3 months of follow-up compared with those treated with placebo (21%). While patients treated with alteplase experienced a higher risk of hemorrhage (6.4% versus 0.6%), there was no significant mortality difference between the groups at 3 months.[81] Features such as smaller clot size and more distal location of the clot increase the likelihood of a favorable outcome following fibrinolysis with intravenous alteplase.[81] Owing to this short time window, only 1% to 3% of otherwise eligible patients receive treatment with IV thrombolytics.[82,83]

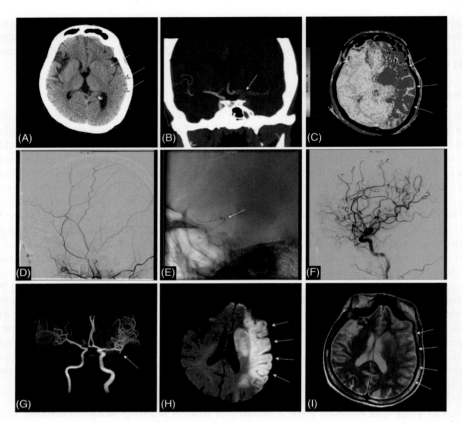

Figure 20-3. A 45-year-old woman with sudden global aphasia and hemiplegia. **A.** Computed tomographic (CT) brain scan shows indistinct basal ganglion structures, loss of the insular ribbon, gray-white junction, and sulcation in the middle cerebral distribution of the left hemisphere (*arrows*). **B.** CT angiography with coronal reconstructions reveal the absence of contrast opacification in the intracranial left internal carotid, proximal, and middle cerebral artery (MCA) branches. **C.** CT perfusion study depicting mean transi time (MTT) shows dramatically increased transient time throughout the left MCA distribution. **D.** Catheter angiography of the left common carotid artery in the lateral projection during the arterial phase shows opacification in external artery branches alone. There is no contrast filling of the cerebral arteries. **E.** Fluororadiograph of the cranium in the lateral projection during endovascular stroke treatment shows a Penumbra suction thrombectomy catheter in the left internal carotid and middle cerebral arteries (*arrow*). **F.** Catheter arteriography of the left common carotid artery after successful mechanical thrombectomy shows restoration of blood flow to the majority of the left cerebral hemisphere; TIMI 3 recanalization. **G.** Magnetic resonance (MR) angiography following endovascular revascularization using the Penumbra suction thrombectomy system and intra-arterial fibrinolysis; TIMI 3 recanalization is maintained. **H.** Diffusion-weighted MRI. **I.** T2 MRI. Despite a successful revascularization procedure within the conventional time period for acute stroke intervention (less than 8 hours of stroke onset), imaging shows extensive ischemic infarction in the MCA region comparable to that depicted by the CT perfusion study on admission. Despite best efforts, not all strokes can be successfully treated.

Intra-arterial (IA) fibrinolysis remains unproven, yet it has become the community standard and part of the standard approach to acute ischemic stroke. It has been shown to have a higher recanalization rate, at 63.2%, than intravenous thrombolysis, at 46.2%.[84] The procedure is performed based on the angiographic visualization of a large cerebral artery occlusion and under fluoroscopic guidance, thus only the amount of thrombolytic agent needed to achieve apparent restoration of flow is used. In the Prolysis in Acute Cerebral Thromboembolism (PROACT II) study, intra-arterial fibrinolysis was tested in a 3- to 6-hour time period from stroke onset. Thus, it is most often used for patients ineligible for IV thrombolysis owing to presentation outside the 3-hour window or for those who fail to respond to intravenous fibrinolysis as determined by the treating physician. Particularly favorable outcomes have followed intra-arterial thrombolysis of occlusions in the internal carotid artery, middle cerebral artery, and basilar artery, whereas thrombi in these locations are generally too large for effective treatment with IV thrombolytics.[85] A recent meta-analysis demonstrated a significant reduction in the odds of dependency or death associated with IA thrombolysis. Similarly, the randomized, controlled trial known as PROACT II demonstrated increased rates of recanalization and functional independence following intra-arterial administration of recombinant prourokinase compared with that of heparin alone.[86,87] Although patients who received IA prourokinase showed a significantly greater risk of intracranial hemorrhage within the first 24 hours, the clinical outcomes in the treatment group were superior to treatment with heparin alone.[88]

Currently, endovascular treatment using various mechanical means to restore cerebral blood flow following acute ischemic stroke is undergoing testing. Embolectomy with or without IA or intravenous fibrinolysis provides an additional option for acute ischemic stroke patients. Recent studies have extended the treatment window to 8 hours. The MERCI Retriever (Concentric Medical, Inc, Mountain View, CA), which has obtained FDA approval, is designed to trap thrombi through inflation of a small balloon distal to thrombus. The device then directs the thrombus into a microcatheter, which is subsequently withdrawn from the patient's body. The MERCI trial demonstrated that mechanical embolectomy significantly increased the portion of patients (48%) experiencing recanalization as compared with historical controls (18%), while demonstrating an association between recanalization and favorable outcome as well as decreased mortality, at least among patients undergoing treatment.[89] The Multi-MERCI trial introduced a device designed to better trap small thrombi breaking off from the original thrombus, and also included patients not achieving recanalization following attempted IV thrombolysis. Recanalization followed deployment of the device in 55%, while clinically significant procedure-related complications occurred in 5.5% of patients.[90] Outcome correlated with thrombus location, with the highest rates of recanalization being attained in the posterior circulation and the lowest in the M1 branch of the middle cerebral artery. The procedure appeared safe in patients recently exposed to IV thrombolytics as these patients experienced no statistically significant increase in rates of intracerebral hemorrhage or procedure-related complications. The mortality rate was higher in patients undergoing mechanical embolectomy as compared with control patients in the PROACT II study for IA thrombolysis. However, once only patients satisfying the eligibility criteria of the PROACT II study were considered, the difference ceases to be significant.[90,91]

The Penumbra System(Penumbra, Inc, Alameda, CA) represents a newer generation of neuro-thrombectomy devices designed to remove thrombi causing ischemic stroke from intracranial vessels. It received FDA approval for commercial use based on favorable results in a multicenter study including 125 patients with neurologic defects, who presented within 8 hours of symptom onset and had an angiographic occlusion (TIMI grade 0 or 1).[92] (TIMI refers to the Thrombolysis in Myocardial Infarction grading system, which was applied to stroke in the PROACT II trial. A score of 0 describes complete occlusion, while a score of 3 refers to complete recanalization.) Postprocedure, 81.6% of patients were revascularized to TIMI scores of 2 (48%) or 3 (52%). Procedural events occurred in 16 (12.8%) and were considered serious in 3 (2.4%). Adverse events, however, were not uniformly attributable to the use of the device. In 35 (28%) patients, intracranial hemorrhage (ICH) was detected on 24-hour CT, but 14 (11.2%) proved to be symptomatic. Although nine patients with detected ICH had received intravenous lytic therapy and three received IA lytic therapy, the investigators did not deem either form of lytic therapy a safety hazard when used with the Penumbra System. Good clinical outcome, defined as improvement by 4 or more points on the National Institute of Health Stroke Scale (NIHSS) score by discharge or a 30-day modified Rankin score (mRS) equal to or less than 2, was achieved by 41.6% of patients. At 90 days of follow-up, 25% of patients achieved an mRS equal to or less than 2; all-cause mortality at this time was 32.8%.[92] The effectiveness of the device was further supported by a retrospective study of 139 patients meeting device-approval criteria following its release. While 96% of target vessels had TIMI scores of 2 or 3, 84% had scores of 2 or 3 following thrombectomy with the Penumbra System. ICH at 24 hours occurred in 18 patients (13%), and was symptomatic in 10 patients (7.2%). Fifty six percent of patients improved by at least 4 points on the NIHSS. Such results support mechanical embolectomy as a promising treatment modality for ischemic stroke patients.

A 60-year-old patient has a history of past stroke and intracranial atherosclerosis (Figure 20-4). How may endovascular procedures, including angioplasty and stenting, improve this patient's prognosis?

Intracranial atherosclerotic disease (ICAD) carries a significant risk and has been recognized as the cause of 8% to 10% of ischemic strokes by population-based and hospital patient–based studies.[93-95]

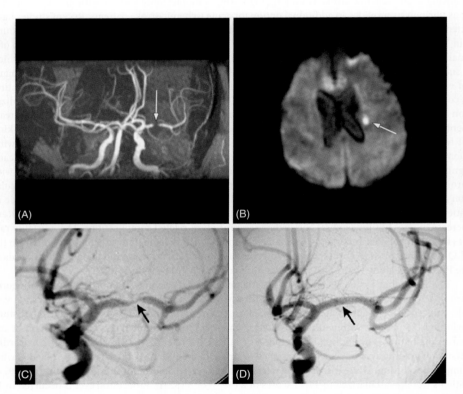

Figure 20-4. A 60-year-old woman with transient speech arrest and a small acute left frontal stroke. **A.** Magnetic resonance angiography of the circle of Willis demonstrates a flow gap (*arrow*) in the M1 segment of the middle cerebral artery indicating severe stenosis. **B.** Magnetic resonance imaging brain scan with diffusion-weighted sequence demonstrates an acute infarct in the paraventricular left frontal lobe (*arrow*) likely due to arterial-to-arterial embolization. **C.** Catheter angiography of the left internal carotid artery in the frontal projection during the arterial phase reveals severe (80%-90%) stenosis of the M1 segment of the left middle cerebral artery (*arrow*). **D.** Endovascular revascularization with stent-supported angioplasty using a 2.4 mm × 9.0 mm Wingspan stent resulted in restoration of the vessel lumen and cessation of further embolization (*arrow*). The patient has been monitored periodically using transcranial Doppler ultrasonography for evidence of restenosis but has maintained normal Doppler velocities and no further strokes or transient ishemic attacks.

Table 20-3. Hemodynamic Effects of Intracranial Atherosclerotic Disease

Stage 0	Normal cerebral hemodynamics
Stage 1	Reflex vasodilation with increased cerebral blood volume and prolonged mean transit time; preserved cerebral blood flow and normal oxygen extraction coefficient
Stage 2	Misery perfusion with falling cerebral blood flow and increased oxygen extraction coefficient

(From Derdeyn CP, Grubb RL Jr, Powers WJ. Cerebral hemodynamic impairment: Methods of measurement and association with stroke risk. Neurology. 1999;53:251-259.)

When transient ischemic attacks are considered in addition to ischemic stroke, approximately 100,000 people in the United States experience ischemic events due to ICAD each year. ICAD is associated with diabetes mellitus, smoking, hypertension, and hypercholesterolemia, and can lead to hemodynamic compromise by producing local thrombosis, occluding perforator arteries, or otherwise causing perfusion failure.[96] It is this hemodynamic compromise, which may be divided into three categories, that ultimately increases the risk of ipsilateral stroke (Table 20-3[97]).

Numerous studies have associated symptomatic intracranial atherosclerosis with a high risk of stroke or death. Patients with symptomatic ICAD, followed in the Warfarin Versus Aspirin Symptomatic Intracranial Disease Study for Stroke (WASID), experienced a 9% to 12% annual risk of ischemic stroke, with 77% of strokes occurring within the first year of follow-up despite optimal medical management and either systemic anticoagulation or antiplatelet therapy. Stenosis of at least 70% increased this risk; such lesions carried a 19% annual risk of stroke in the symptomatic territory.[98] Similarly, the EC/IC (extracranial/intracranial) Bypass Trial demonstrated that patients treated medically, with management of stroke risk factors and 1300 mg per day of aspirin, for symptomatic ICAD experienced an annual mortality and stroke rate of 8% to 10%.[99] Annual rates of stroke or death attributable to vascular causes are even higher in those failing antithrombotic therapy, and have been shown to approach 56%.[100]

Given the risk associated with symptomatic intracranial atherosclerosis, the failure of medical management to sufficiently mitigate that risk, and lack of a demonstrable decreased risk of recurrent ischemic events following extracranial/intracranial bypass procedures, interventions including angioplasty and stenting have been pursued. Initial procedures were largely corollaries of established techniques in interventional cardiology, utilizing percutaneous coronary intervention balloons to dilate intracranial vessels. However, cerebral arteries differ from their coronary counterparts on several grounds, generally exhibiting smaller diameters, a well-developed tunica media, and a relatively scarce tunica adventitia.[96] Accordingly, they are more prone to vasospasm and also more likely to rupture at lower forces than are coronary arteries. Furthermore, intracranial vessels may be exceedingly tortuous. Endovascular catheter technology has since progressed, making it an increasingly viable and accepted intervention for patients with ICAD. Currently, patients most likely to undergo endovascular treatment for ICAD remain symptomatic despite optimal medical management with stenosis greater than 50%.[96] However, decisions regarding individual patients must be made on an individual basis.

Balloon angioplasty has been performed with successful results reported in several case studies. A recent large study followed 120 patients with 124 symptomatic intracranial stenoses treated with angioplasty. Pretreatment stenoses averaged 82.2%, and ranged from 50% to 95%; angioplastic intervention reduced the average to 36%, with a range from 0% to 90%. The investigators observed a combined periprocedural stroke and death rate of 5.8%; after an average of 42.3 months of follow-up, the overall rate of stroke or death was 4.4% annually.[101] As expected with any procedure, certain atherosclerotic lesions are more amenable to angioplastic manipulation.

Table 20-4. Angiographic Features of Hemodynamically Significant Intracranial Stenoses

Type A	Short (< 5 mm in length); concentric or moderately eccentric; nonocclusive
Type B	Tubular (5-10 mm in length); extremely eccentric or fully occluded, moderately angulated, < 3 months old
Type C	Diffuse (more than 10 mm in length); extremely angulated (> 90°); very tortuous proximal segment or total occlusion; ≥ 3 months

Mori and colleagues correlated angiographic features of hemodynamically significant intracranial stenoses with clinical success of intracranial percutaneous transluminal cerebral balloon angioplasty (PTCBA).[96,102]

Clinical success rates for types A, B, and C (as described in Table 20-4) were 92%, 86%, and 33%, respectively. Type C lesions were most likely to undergo restenosis, with 100% demonstrating restenosis after 1 year; conversely, no type A lesions restenosed. Risk of fatal or nonfatal ischemic stroke or ipsilateral bypass surgery similarly related to type, with cumulative risks of 8%, 26%, and 87% observed in types A, B, and C, respectively. [102] Thus, the success of angioplasty depends strongly on the characteristics of the lesion.

Despite the general success of balloon angioplasty, certain complications associated with the procedure, such as elastic recoil and intimal dissection, are averted through stent-supported angioplasty. The Stenting of Symptomatic Atherosclerotic Lesions in the Vertebral or Intracranial Arteries (SSYLVIA) trial introduced the Neurolink stent (Guidant Corporation; Menlo Park, CA), a balloon expandable intracranial stent composed of interconnected bare stainless steel rings and specifically designed to be flexible enough to navigate the tortuous intracranial vessels without causing injury. The multicenter, prospective feasibility study involved patients with symptoms attributable to a single lesion with greater than 50% stenosis. The majority of patients, 43 of 61 (70.5%) had intracranial stenosis, while all others had extracranial vertebral artery stenosis. In 95% of cases the stent was successfully placed, such that less than 30% residual stenosis remained. Within the first 30 days, 6.6% of patients had nonfatal strokes; 7.3% of patients suffered strokes between 30 days and 1 year following stent placement. Restenosis greater than 50% occurred in 32.4% of patients with intracranial lesions; however, 61% of all patients demonstrating restenosis remained asymptomatic, with no strokes or transient ischemic attacks (TIAs).[103] Although the manufacturers of Neurolink received a humanitarian device exemption (HDE) from the FDA to treat patients with significant atherosclerotic disease, the device is not currently available for commercial use.

The Wingspan stent (Boston Scientific SMART; San Leandro, CA) has also received an HDE and is available to treat patients refractory to medical therapy with symptomatic intracranial stenosis greater than 50%.[96] It combines balloon dilatation with the subsequent placement of a self-expanding microstent. The study underlying the HDE involved 45 patients with symptomatic intracranial stenosis greater than 50% in a vessel 2.5 to 4.5 mm in diameter, who had been proven to be refractory to medical therapy.[104] Angioplasty and stent deployment was successful in 98% of patients. The 30-day postintervention combined ipsilateral stroke and death rate was 4.5%, whereas the 6-month ipsilateral stroke and death rate was 7.1%. The 6-month rate of all strokes was 9.7%, and all-cause mortality at the same time point was 2.3%. Patients averaged a 74.9% degree stenosis at baseline, which decreased to 31.9% after stenting. At the 6-month follow-up, the average degree of stenosis was 28%. Three patients, however, lost lumen diameter and restenosed to greater than 50% by 6 months of follow-up but were not symptomatic.[104]

Since intimal hyperplasia and vascular remodeling theoretically lead to restenosis, stents secreting antiproliferative drugs have been studied as a means of preventing restenosis. Recently, 18 patients were treated with either sirolimus- or paclitaxel-eluting stents.[105] All patients had symptomatic intracranial stenosis greater than 50% despite medical treatment. Within the first month, one major stroke and no deaths occurred; there were no additional such events at the 6-month time point. One of seven patients undergoing follow-up angiography at 6 months had developed restenosis greater than 50%.[105] A larger study also investigating drug-eluting stents detected 1 restenosis from 26 treated intracranial lesions (5%).[106]

There exists debate concerning whether angioplasty alone or angioplasty followed by stent placement provides better results. A recent multicenter study compared 95 primary angioplasty procedures against 98 intracranial stent placements.[107] There were no significant differences between the groups in terms of age, gender, or medical history, including hypertension, diabetes, and previous stroke or TIA. Preprocedure stenosis averaged 89.2% and 90.1% in patients undergoing primary angioplasty and those undergoing stent placement, respectively. However, residual stenosis greater than 50% was significantly more common in the angioplasty-treated group, at 15% of patients compared with 4%. The angioplasty-treated group had one periprocedural death and seven periprocedural strokes, whereas the stent-treated group had two periprocedural deaths and seven strokes. These differences as well as differences in terms of stroke- and death-free survival at 2 years were not significant. Similarly, where follow-up data were available, there was no significant difference in the occurrence of restentosis at follow-up: 25 of 66 (38.9%) in the angioplasty-treated group versus 23 of 68 (34%) in the stent-treated group. The investigators concluded that stent placement conferred no significant benefit over angioplasty alone except in the reduction of residual stenosis.

A meta-analysis conducted by Siddiq et al again compared angioplasty and stent placement in patients with symptomatic ICAD.[108] In pooling selected publications, the investigators established a significantly lower rate of death or stroke at 1 year in patients treated with stent placement (14.2%) as opposed to those undergoing primary angioplasty (19.7%). However, periprocedural death and stroke did not differ significantly between the groups. Stent placement was also associated with a lower percentage of restenosis at 11.1% compared with angioplasty alone at 14.2%.[108] These findings indicate that angioplasty followed by stenting may provide benefits over angioplasty alone; however, treatment decisions must be made by experienced interventionalists on a case-by-case basis.

How does a history of ischemia affect the use of contrast during angiography?

The ischemic brain has increased sensitivity to iodinated contrast. Use of nonionic, iso-osmolar contrast should be limited to 6 mg/kg total, even in patients with good renal function.[96]

How should patients be managed to reduce both the risk of hemorrhage and that of thrombosis?

In order to prevent reperfusion hemorrhage, a complication that occurs in up to 5% of otherwise successful procedures, mean arterial blood pressure should be lowered by 25% to 30%. Antihypertensive agents that reduce both pressure and pulsatility through α- and β-receptor blockade are ideal unless contraindicated for cardiopulmonary causes. Heparin may be discontinued postoperatively; however, clopidogrel at a dose of 75 mg daily for at least 6 weeks and indefinite aspirin therapy is recommended.[96]

How often should angiographic follow-up be provided?

Angiographic follow-up is recommended beginning at 3 months, given the occurrence of 100% restenosis by 3 months in type C lesions observed in a retrospective study.[96,109] Further follow-up should be arranged on a case-by-case basis.

! CRITICAL CONSIDERATIONS

Endovascular treatment for aneurysms

- Endovascular therapy is currently the first-line intervention for a ruptured aneurysm in selected cases.
- Candidates for endovascular aneurysm occlusion include the following:
  - Otherwise healthy patients, elderly patients, patients with medical comorbidities, patients on chronic anticoagulation, patients with a small or noncompressive intracranial hematoma, patients with poor-grade aneurysmal SAH
- Relative contraindications to endovascular aneurysm treatment may include the following considerations:
  - Patients with very tortuous vessels and some fusiform or wide-neck aneurysms
- Following acute SAH, coil embolization should be performed as soon as possible to prevent recurrent hemorrhage; however, the procedure has provided benefit as many as 30 days following known aneurysm rupture.
- Coil embolization with stent placement is useful for treatment of wide-neck aneurysms but requires antithrombotic therapy, generally with aspirin, clopidogrel, or other antiplatelet agent, and is not well tested in the treatment of acute aneurysmal SAH.
- Balloon-assisted coil occlusion of cerebral aneurysms can achieve better occlusion and may be useful in the management of wide-neck aneurysms.
- Vasospasm often follows aneurysmal SAH by 3 to 8 days, is associated with increased mortality, and may be treated with transluminal balloon angioplasty and IA vasodilator administration.
- Patients treated with endovascular coil occlusion of cerebral aneurysms should be monitored with catheter angiography or MRI/MRA at regular intervals for at least 18 months. Interval surveillance thereafter may be useful to monitor for development of additional aneurysms.[110]
- Endovascular aneurysm treatment may be considered for patients with incidentally discovered aneurysms generally greater than 7 mm in diameter, in symptomatic patients, those with a family history of SAH or a history of smoking, or prior treatment of ruptured aneurysm(s).

Endovascular treatment for AVMs

- The reported prevalence of brain AVMs is as high as 10.3 per 100,000.
- The annual risk of hemorrhage for patients with known intracranial AVMs may be as high as 2% to 4% and is increased for 5 years following a recent bleed, with exclusive deep venous drainage and an infratentorial location.
- Surgical prognosis is most commonly assessed according to the SM Scale, which takes into account size, localization, and venous drainage.
- Endovascular intervention is undertaken with one of several goals:
  - Prior to surgery: While this strategy does reduce the size of the nidus, it is associated with morbidity and mortality risks, particularly in patients with deep venous drainage or localization proximal to eloquent cortex.

- Prior to radiosurgery: This strategy is useful for large or deep-seated AVMs and reduces the size of the nidus, but not such that a diminished nidus assumes the risk/benefit profile of a similarly sized natural AVM.
- Endovascular "cure": Complete obliteration is uncommon following embolization alone, but may be achieved, especially in smaller AVMs.
- Palliation: Endovascular treatment may reduce symptoms associated with the vascular steal phenomenon.

Endovascular management of dAVFs

- Dural fistulas are a heterogeneous group of arteriovenous shunt lesions and constitute 10% to 15% of intracranial AVMs.
- Dural fistulas predominantly involve intracranial dural sinuses or cortical veins.
- Dural fistulas are often graded according to patterns of venous drainage: type I has a benign course, whereas grades II and III are more aggressive, with increasing symptoms and risk of bleed, and often require intervention.
- Endovascular transarterial embolization may be palliative but is most often not curative.
- Radiosurgery followed by transarterial embolization is effective in some lesions.
- dAVFs are often amenable to curative transvenous embolization in appropriately selected cases.

Endovascular therapy for acute ischemic stroke

- Intravenous fibrinolysis is FDA approved for treatment of acute ischemic stroke and has been proven effective in multiple controlled trials. Intravenous fibrinolysis is generally considered for treatment of patients presenting within 3 hours of stroke onset. Based upon data from the European Cooperative Acute Stroke Study (ECASS) III trial, many physicians now extend the treatment window to 4.5 hours from stroke onset.
- IA fibrinolysis is not an FDA-approved application of fibrinolytic agents but is often considered the community standard for treatment of ischemic stroke patients ineligible for intravenous fibrinolysis up to 6 hours after symptom onset.
- Mechanical revascularization significantly increases recanalization in acute ischemic stroke owing to large artery occlusion. While still unproven, recanalization is associated with an increased likelihood of a favorable outcome and decreased risk of death.

Endovascular procedures for stroke prevention

- Intracranial atherosclerotic disease causes 8% to 10% of ischemic strokes.
- Patients with symptomatic intracranial stenosis are at an increased risk of ipsilateral stroke despite medical therapy.
- Angioplasty alone or followed by stent placement improves prognosis.
- Angioplasty followed by stent placement may provide superior results to angioplasty alone; however, treatment decisions must be made on an individual basis.

Neurocritical Care Intervention

REFERENCES

1. Rosenorn J, Eskesen V, Schmidt K, Ronde F. The risk of rebleeding from ruptured intracranial aneurysms. *J Neurosurg.* 1987;67:329-332.

2. Hop JW, Rinkel GJ, Algra A, van Gijn J. Case-fatality rates and functional outcome after subarachnoid hemorrhage: a systematic review. *Stroke* 1997;28:660-664.

3. Molyneux A, Kerr R, Stratton I, et al. International Subarachnoid Aneurysm Trial (ISAT) of neurosurgical clipping versus endovascular coiling in 2143 patients with ruptured intracranial aneurysms: a randomised trial. *Lancet.* 2002;360:1267-1274.

4. Molyneux AJ, Kerr RS, Yu LM, et al. International subarachnoid aneurysm trial (ISAT) of neurosurgical clipping versus endovascular coiling in 2143 patients with ruptured intracranial aneurysms: a randomised comparison of effects on survival, dependency, seizures, rebleeding, subgroups, and aneurysm occlusion. *Lancet.* 2005;366:809-817.

5. Koebbe CJ, Veznedaroglu E, Jabbour P, Rosenwasser RH. Endovascular management of intracranial aneurysms: current experience and future advances. *Neurosurgery.* 2006;59(suppl 3):S93-S102; discussion S103-S113.

6. Vinuela F, Duckwiler G, Mawad M. Guglielmi detachable coil embolization of acute intracranial aneurysm: perioperative anatomical and clinical outcome in 403 patients. *J Neurosurg.* 1997;86:475-482.

7. Vinuela F, Duckwiler G, Mawad M. Guglielmi detachable coil embolization of acute intracranial aneurysm: perioperative anatomical and clinical outcome in 403 patients. 1997. *J Neurosurg.* 2008;108:832-839.

8. Bradac GB, Bergui M, Fontanella M. Endovascular treatment of cerebral aneurysms in elderly patients. *Neuroradiology.* 2005;47:938-941.

9. Johnston SC, Higashida RT, Barrow DL, et al. Recommendations for the endovascular treatment of intracranial aneurysms: a statement for healthcare professionals from the Committee on Cerebrovascular Imaging of the American Heart Association Council on Cardiovascular Radiology. *Stroke.* 2002;33:2536-2544.

10. Bracard S, Lebedinsky A, Anxionnat R, et al. Endovascular treatment of Hunt and Hess grade IV and V aneurysms. *AJNR Am J Neuroradiol.* 2002;23:953-957.

11. van Loon J, Waerzeggers Y, Wilms G, Van Calenbergh F, Goffin J, Plets C. Early endovascular treatment of ruptured cerebral aneurysms in patients in very poor neurological condition. *Neurosurgery.* 2002;50:457-464; discussion 464-465.

12. Jeong JH, Koh JS, Kim EJ. A less invasive approach for ruptured aneurysm with intracranial hematoma: Coil embolization followed by clot evacuation. *Korean J Radiol.* 2007;8:2-8.

13. Nowak G, Schwachenwald D, Schwachenwald R, Kehler U, Muller H, Arnold H. Intracerebral hematomas caused by aneurysm rupture. Experience with 67 cases. *Neurosurg Rev.* 1998;21:5-9.

14. Niemann DB, Wills AD, Maartens NF, Kerr RS, Byrne JV, Molyneux AJ. Treatment of intracerebral hematomas caused by aneurysm rupture: coil placement followed by clot evacuation. *J Neurosurg.* 2003;99:843-847.

15. Chung J, Kim BM, Shin YS, Lim YC, Park SK. Treatment of ruptured anterior communicating artery aneurysm accompanying intracerebral hematomas: endovascular coiling followed by hematoma evacuation with burr hole trephination and catheterization. *Acta Neurochir (Wien).* 2009;151:917-923; discussion 923.

16. Jabbour PM, Tjoumakaris SI, Rosenwasser RH. Endovascular management of intracranial aneurysms. *Neurosurg Clin North Am.* 2009;20:383-398.

17. Jayaraman MV, Do HM, Versnick EJ, Steinberg GK, Marks MP. Morphologic assessment of middle cerebral artery aneurysms for endovascular treatment. *J Stroke Cerebrovasc Dis.* 2007;16:52-56.

18. Yang P, Liu J, Huang Q, et al. Endovascular treatment of wide-neck middle cerebral artery aneurysms with stents: a review of 16 cases. *AJNR Am J Neuroradiol.* 2010;31:940-946.

19. Inagawa T, Kamiya K, Ogasawara H, Yano T. Rebleeding of ruptured intracranial aneurysms in the acute stage. *Surg Neurol.* 1987;28:93-99.

20. van Gijn J, Kerr RS, Rinkel GJ. Subarachnoid haemorrhage. *Lancet.* 2007;369:306-318.

21. Taylor B, Harries P, Bullock R. Factors affecting outcome after surgery for intracranial aneurysm in Glasgow. *Br J Neurosurg.* 1991;5:591-600.

22. Yalamanchili K, Rosenwasser RH, Thomas JE, Liebman K, McMorrow C, Gannon P. Frequency of cerebral vasospasm in patients treated with endovascular occlusion of intracranial aneurysms. *AJNR Am J Neuroradiol.* 1998;19:553-558.

23. Baltsavias GS, Byrne JV, Halsey J, Coley SC, Sohn MJ, Molyneux AJ. Effects of timing of coil embolization after aneurysmal subarachnoid hemorrhage on procedural morbidity and outcomes. *Neurosurgery.* 2000;47:1320-1329; discussion 1329-1331.

24. Haque R, Kellner CP, Komotar RJ, et al. Mechanical treatment of vasospasm. *Neurol Res.* 2009;31:638-643.

25. Komotar RJ, Zacharia BE, Otten ML, Mocco J, Lavine SD. Controversies in the endovascular management of cerebral vasospasm after intracranial aneurysm rupture and future directions for therapeutic approaches. *Neurosurgery.* 2008;62:897-905; discussion 905-897.

26. Coyne TJ, Montanera WJ, Macdonald RL, Wallace MC. Percutaneous transluminal angioplasty for cerebral vasospasm after subarachnoid hemorrhage. *Can J Surg.* 1994;37:391-396.

27. Eskridge JM, McAuliffe W, Song JK, et al. Balloon angioplasty for the treatment of vasospasm: results of first 50 cases. *Neurosurgery.* 1998;42:510-516; discussion 516-517.

28. Fujii Y, Takahashi A, Yoshimoto T. Effect of balloon angioplasty on high grade symptomatic vasospasm after subarachnoid hemorrhage. *Neurosurg Rev.* 1995;18:7-13.

29. Firlik AD, Kaufmann AM, Jungreis CA, Yonas H. Effect of transluminal angioplasty on cerebral blood flow in the management of symptomatic vasospasm following aneurysmal subarachnoid hemorrhage. *J Neurosurg.* 1997;86:830-839.

30. Hoh BL, Ogilvy CS. Endovascular treatment of cerebral vasospasm: transluminal balloon angioplasty, intra-arterial papaverine, and intra-arterial nicardipine. *Neurosurg Clin North Am.* 2005;16:501-516, vi.

31. Bejjani GK, Bank WO, Olan WJ, Sekhar LN. The efficacy and safety of angioplasty for cerebral vasospasm after subarachnoid hemorrhage. *Neurosurgery.* 1998;42:979-986; discussion 986-987.

32. Rosenwasser RH, Armonda RA, Thomas JE, Benitez RP, Gannon PM, Harrop J. Therapeutic modalities for the management of cerebral vasospasm: timing of endovascular options. *Neurosurgery.* 1999;44:975-979; discussion 979-980.

33. Johnston SC. Effect of endovascular services and hospital volume on cerebral aneurysm treatment outcomes. *Stroke.* 2000;31:111-117.

34. Zwienenberg-Lee M, Hartman J, Rudisill N, et al. Effect of prophylactic transluminal balloon angioplasty on cerebral vasospasm and outcome in patients with Fisher grade III subarachnoid hemorrhage: results of a phase II multicenter, randomized, clinical trial. *Stroke.* 2008;39:1759-1765.

35. Wiebers DO. Unruptured intracranial aneurysms: natural history and clinical management. Update on the international study of unruptured intracranial aneurysms. *Neuroimaging Clin North Am.* 2006;16:383-390, vii.

36. Vernooij MW, Ikram MA, Tanghe HL, et al. Incidental findings on brain MRI in the general population. *N Engl J Med.* 2007;357:1821-1828.

37. Wiebers DO, Whisnant JP, Huston J 3rd, et al. Unruptured intracranial aneurysms: natural history, clinical outcome, and risks of surgical and endovascular treatment. *Lancet.* 2003;362:103-110.

38. International Study of Unruptured Intracranial Aneurysms Investigators. Unruptured intracranial aneurysms—risk of rupture and risks of surgical intervention. *N Engl J Med.* 1998;339:1725-1733.

39. Bederson JB, Awad IA, Wiebers DO, et al. Recommendations for the management of patients with unruptured intracranial aneurysms: a Statement for healthcare professionals from the Stroke Council of the American Heart Association. *Stroke.* 2000;31:2742-2750.

40. Akiba Y, Murayama Y, Vinuela F, Lefkowitz MA, Duckwiler GR, Gobin YP. Balloon-assisted Guglielmi detachable coiling of wide-necked aneurysms: Part I—experimental evaluation. *Neurosurgery.* 1999;45:519-527; discussion 527-530.

41. Moret J, Cognard C, Weill A, Castaings L, Rey A. [Reconstruction technic in the treatment of wide-neck intracranial aneurysms. Long-term angiographic and clinical results. Apropos of 56 cases.] *J Neuroradiol.* 1997;24:30-44.

42. Jabbour P, Koebbe C, Veznedaroglu E, Benitez RP, Rosenwasser R. Stent-assisted coil placement for unruptured cerebral aneurysms. *Neurosurg Focus.* 2004;17:E10.

43. Molyneux AJ, Cekirge S, Saatci I, Gal G. Cerebral Aneurysm Multicenter European Onyx (CAMEO) trial: results of a prospective observational study in 20 European centers. *AJNR Am J Neuroradiol.* 2004;25:39-51.

44. McCormick WF. The pathology of vascular ("arteriovenous") malformations. *J Neurosurg.* 1966;24:807-816.

45. Zhao J, Wang S, Li J, Qi W, Sui D, Zhao Y. Clinical characteristics and surgical results of patients with cerebral arteriovenous malformations. *Surg Neurol.* 2005;63:156-161; discussion 161.

46. Brown RD, Jr., Wiebers DO, Torner JC, O'Fallon WM. Incidence and prevalence of intracranial vascular malformations in Olmsted County, Minnesota, 1965 to 1992. *Neurology.* 1996;46:949-952.

47. Berman MF, Sciacca RR, Pile-Spellman J, et al. The epidemiology of brain arteriovenous

malformations. *Neurosurgery.* 2000;47:389-396; discussion 397.

48. Stapf C, Mast H, Sciacca RR, et al. The New York Islands AVM Study: design, study progress, and initial results. *Stroke.* 2003;34:e29-33.

49. Al-Shahi R, Warlow C. A systematic review of the frequency and prognosis of arteriovenous malformations of the brain in adults. *Brain.* 2001;124(Pt 10):1900-1926.

50. Brown RD, Jr., Wiebers DO, Torner JC, O'Fallon WM. Frequency of intracranial hemorrhage as a presenting symptom and subtype analysis: a population-based study of intracranial vascular malformations in Olmsted County, Minnesota. *J Neurosurg.* 1996;85:29-32.

51. Ogilvy CS, Stieg PE, Awad I, et al. Recommendations for the management of intracranial arteriovenous malformations: a statement for healthcare professionals from a special writing group of the Stroke Council, American Stroke Association. *Circulation.* 2001;103:2644-2657.

52. Strozyk D, Nogueira RG, Lavine SD. Endovascular treatment of intracranial arteriovenous malformation. *Neurosurg Clin North Am.* 2009;20:399-418.

53. Latchaw RE, Hu X, Ugurbil K, Hall WA, Madison MT, Heros RC. Functional magnetic resonance imaging as a management tool for cerebral arteriovenous malformations. *Neurosurgery.* 1995;37:619-625; discussion 625-626.

54. Mast H, Young WL, Koennecke HC, et al. Risk of spontaneous haemorrhage after diagnosis of cerebral arteriovenous malformation. *Lancet.* 1997;350:1065-1068.

55. Yamada S, Takagi Y, Nozaki K, Kikuta K, Hashimoto N. Risk factors for subsequent hemorrhage in patients with cerebral arteriovenous malformations. *J Neurosurg.* 2007;107:965-972.

56. Hernesniemi JA, Dashti R, Juvela S, Vaart K, Niemela M, Laakso A. Natural history of brain arteriovenous malformations: a long-term follow-up study of risk of hemorrhage in 238 patients. *Neurosurgery.* 2008;63:823-829; discussion 829-831.

57. Jane JA, Kassell NF, Torner JC, Winn HR. The natural history of aneurysms and arteriovenous malformations. *J Neurosurg.* 1985;62:321-323.

58. Itoyama Y, Uemura S, Ushio Y, et al. Natural course of unoperated intracranial arteriovenous malformations: study of 50 cases. *J Neurosurg.* 1989;71:805-809.

59. Spetzler RF, Hargraves RW, McCormick PW, Zabramski JM, Flom RA, Zimmerman RS. Relationship of perfusion pressure and size to risk of hemorrhage from arteriovenous malformations. *J Neurosurg.* 1992;76:918-923.

60. Hamilton MG, Spetzler RF. The prospective application of a grading system for arteriovenous malformations. *Neurosurgery.* 1994;34:2-6; discussion 6-7.

61. Hartmann A, Pile-Spellman J, Stapf C, et al. Risk of endovascular treatment of brain arteriovenous malformations. *Stroke.* 2002;33:1816-1820.

62. Ledezma CJ, Hoh BL, Carter BS, Pryor JC, Putman CM, Ogilvy CS. Complications of cerebral arteriovenous malformation embolization: multivariate analysis of predictive factors. *Neurosurgery.* 2006;58:602-611; discussion 602-611.

63. Starke RM, Komotar RJ, Otten ML, et al. Adjuvant embolization with *N*-butyl cyanoacrylate in the treatment of cerebral arteriovenous malformations: outcomes, complications, and predictors of neurologic deficits. *Stroke.* 2009;40:2783-2790.

64. Ezura M, Takahashi A, Jokura H, Shirane R, Yoshimoto T. Endovascular treatment of aneurysms associated with cerebral arteriovenous malformations: experiences after the introduction of Guglielmi detachable coils. *J Clin Neurosci.* 2000;7(suppl 1):14-18.

65. Weber W, Kis B, Siekmann R, Jans P, Laumer R, Kuhne D. Preoperative embolization of intracranial arteriovenous malformations with Onyx. *Neurosurgery.* 2007;61:244-252; discussion 252-244.

66. Pollock BE, Kondziolka D, Lunsford LD, Bissonette D, Flickinger JC. Repeat stereotactic radiosurgery of arteriovenous malformations: factors associated with incomplete obliteration. *Neurosurgery.* 1996;38:318-324.

67. Gobin YP, Laurent A, Merienne L, et al. Treatment of brain arteriovenous malformations by embolization and radiosurgery. *J Neurosurg.* 1996;85:19-28.

68. Andrade-Souza YM, Ramani M, Scora D, Tsao MN, terBrugge K, Schwartz ML. Embolization before radiosurgery reduces the obliteration rate of arteriovenous malformations. *Neurosurgery.* 2007;60:443-451; discussion 451-452.

69. Wikholm G, Lundqvist C, Svendsen P. Embolization of cerebral arteriovenous malformations: Part I—Technique, morphology, and complications. *Neurosurgery.* 1996;39:448-457; discussion 457-459.

70. Valavanis A, Yasargil MG. The endovascular treatment of brain arteriovenous malformations. *Adv Tech Stand Neurosurg.* 1998;24:131-214.

71. Kusske JA, Kelly WA. Embolization and reduction of the "steal" syndrome in cerebral

arteriovenous malformations. *J Neurosurg.* 1974; 40:313-321.

72. Fox AJ, Girvin JP, Vinuela F, Drake CG. Rolandic arteriovenous malformations: improvement in limb function by IBC embolization. *AJNR Am J Neuroradiol.* 1985;6:575-582.

73. Kwon OK, Han DH, Han MH, Chung YS. Palliatively treated cerebral arteriovenous malformations: follow-up results. *J Clin Neurosci.* 2000;7(suppl) 1:69-72.

74. McConnell KA, Tjoumakaris SI, Allen J, et al. Neuroendovascular management of dural arteriovenous malformations. *Neurosurg Clin North Am.*2009;20:431-439.

75. Davies MA, TerBrugge K, Willinsky R, Coyne T, Saleh J, Wallace MC. The validity of classification for the clinical presentation of intracranial dural arteriovenous fistulas. *J Neurosurg.* 1996;85: 830-837.

76. Soderman M, Pavic L, Edner G, Holmin S, Andersson T. Natural history of dural arteriovenous shunts. *Stroke.* 2008;39:1735-1739.

77. Brown RD Jr, Flemming KD, Meyer FB, Cloft HJ, Pollock BE, Link ML. Natural history, evaluation, and management of intracranial vascular malformations. *Mayo Clin Proc.* 2005;80:269-281.

78. Dawson RC, 3rd, Joseph GJ, Owens DS, Barrow DL. Transvenous embolization as the primary therapy for arteriovenous fistulas of the lateral and sigmoid sinuses. *AJNR Am J Neuroradiol.* 1998;19:571-576.

79. Meyers PM, Halbach VV, Dowd CF, et al. Dural carotid cavernous fistula: definitive endovascular management and long-term follow-up. *Am J Ophthalmol.* 2002;134:85-92.

80. Cloft HJ, Rabinstein A, Lanzino G, Kallmes DF. Intra-arterial stroke therapy: an assessment of demand and available work force. *AJNR Am J Neuroradiol.*2009;30:453-458.

81. The National Institute of Neurological Disorders and Stroke rt-PA Stroke Study Group. Tissue plasminogen activator for acute ischemic stroke. *N Engl J Med.* 1995;333:1581-1587.

82. Kim D, Jahan R, Starkman S, et al. Endovascular mechanical clot retrieval in a broad ischemic stroke cohort. *AJNR Am J Neuroradiol.* 2006;27:2048-2052.

83. Furlan AJ. CVA: reducing the risk of a confused vascular analysis. The Feinberg Lecture. *Stroke.* 2000;31:1451-1456.

84. Rha JH, Saver JL. The impact of recanalization on ischemic stroke outcome: a meta-analysis. *Stroke.* 2007;38:967-973.

85. Gonner F, Remonda L, Mattle H, et al. Local intra-arterial thrombolysis in acute ischemic stroke. *Stroke.* 1998;29:1894-1900.

86. Saver JL. Intra-arterial fibrinolysis for acute ischemic stroke: the message of melt. *Stroke.* 2007;38:2627-2628.

87. Furlan A, Higashida R, Wechsler L, et al. Intra-arterial prourokinase for acute ischemic stroke. The PROACT II study: a randomized controlled trial. Prolyse in Acute Cerebral Thromboembolism. *JAMA.* 1999;282:2003-2011.

88. Kase CS, Furlan AJ, Wechsler LR, et al. Cerebral hemorrhage after intra-arterial thrombolysis for ischemic stroke: the PROACT II trial. *Neurology.* 2001;57:1603-1610.

89. Smith WS, Sung G, Starkman S, et al. Safety and efficacy of mechanical embolectomy in acute ischemic stroke: results of the MERCI trial. *Stroke.* 2005;36:1432-1438.

90. Smith WS, Sung G, Saver J, et al. Mechanical thrombectomy for acute ischemic stroke: final results of the Multi MERCI trial. *Stroke.* 2008;39:1205-1212.

91. Josephson SA, Saver JL, Smith WS. Comparison of mechanical embolectomy and intraarterial thrombolysis in acute ischemic stroke within the MCA: MERCI and Multi MERCI compared to PROACT II. *Neurocrit Care.* 2009;10:43-49.

92. The Penumbra Pivotal Stroke Trial: Safety and effectiveness of a new generation of mechanical devices for clot removal in intracranial large vessel occlusive disease. *Stroke.* 2009;40:2761-2768.

93. Sacco RL, Kargman DE, Gu Q, Zamanillo MC. Race-ethnicity and determinants of intracranial atherosclerotic cerebral infarction. The Northern Manhattan Stroke Study. *Stroke.* 1995;26:14-20.

94. Segura T, Serena J, Castellanos M, Teruel J, Vilar C, Davalos A. Embolism in acute middle cerebral artery stenosis. *Neurology.* 2001;56:497-501.

95. Wityk RJ, Lehman D, Klag M, Coresh J, Ahn H, Litt B. Race and sex differences in the distribution of cerebral atherosclerosis. *Stroke.* 1996;27:1974-1980.

96. Meyers PM, Schumacher HC, Tanji K, Higashida RT, Caplan LR. Use of stents to treat intracranial cerebrovascular disease. *Annu Rev Med.* 2007;58:107-122.

97. Derdeyn CP, Grubb RL Jr, Powers WJ. Cerebral hemodynamic impairment: methods of measurement and association with stroke risk. *Neurology.* 1999;53:251-259.

98. Chimowitz MI, Lynn MJ, Howlett-Smith H, et al. Comparison of warfarin and aspirin for

Neurocritical Care Intervention

symptomatic intracranial arterial stenosis. *N Engl J Med.* 2005;352:1305-1316.

99. The EC/IC Bypass Study Group. Failure of extracranial-intracranial arterial bypass to reduce the risk of ischemic stroke. Results of an international randomized trial. *N Engl J Med.* 1985;313:1191-1200.

100. Thijs VN, Albers GW. Symptomatic intracranial atherosclerosis: outcome of patients who fail antithrombotic therapy. *Neurology.* 2000;55:490-497.

101. Marks MP, Wojak JC, Al-Ali F, et al. Angioplasty for symptomatic intracranial stenosis: clinical outcome. *Stroke.* 2006;37:1016-1020.

102. Mori T, Fukuoka M, Kazita K, Mori K. Follow-up study after intracranial percutaneous transluminal cerebral balloon angioplasty. *AJNR Am J Neuroradiol.* 1998;19:1525-1533.

103. Stenting of Symptomatic Atherosclerotic Lesions in the Vertebral or Intracranial Arteries (SSYLVIA): study results. *Stroke.* 2004;35:1388-1392.

104. Bose A, Hartmann M, Henkes H, et al. A novel, self-expanding, nitinol stent in medically refractory intracranial atherosclerotic stenoses: the Wingspan study. *Stroke.* 2007;38:1531-1537.

105. Qureshi AI, Kirmani JF, Hussein HM, et al. Early and intermediate-term outcomes with drug-eluting stents in high-risk patients with symptomatic intracranial stenosis. *Neurosurgery.* 2006;59:1044-1051; discussion 1051.

106. Gupta R, Al-Ali F, Thomas AJ, et al. Safety, feasibility, and short-term follow-up of drug-eluting stent placement in the intracranial and extracranial circulation. *Stroke.* 2006;37:2562-2566.

107. Siddiq F, Vazquez G, Memon MZ, et al. Comparison of primary angioplasty with stent placement for treating symptomatic intracranial atherosclerotic diseases: a multicenter study. *Stroke.* 2008;39:2505-2510.

108. Siddiq F, Memon MZ, Vazquez G, Safdar A, Qureshi AI. Comparison between primary angioplasty and stent placement for symptomatic intracranial atherosclerotic disease: meta-analysis of case series. *Neurosurgery.* 2009;65:1024-1033; discussion 1033-1034.

109. Mori T, Fukuoka M, Kazita K, Mori K. Follow-up study after percutaneous transluminal cerebral angioplasty. *Eur Radiol.* 1998;8:403-408.

110. Juvela S, Porras M, Heiskanen O. Natural history of unruptured intracranial aneurysms: a long-term follow-up study. *J Neurosurg.* 1993;79:174-182.

Perioperative Surgical Care

Section Editor: E. Sander Connolly, MD

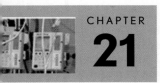

CHAPTER
21
Brain Aneurysm and Arteriovenous Malformation Surgery

Raqeeb Haque, MD
Ivan S. Kotchetkov, BA
Brian Y. Hwang, MD
E. Sander Connolly, MD

Ruptured intracranial aneurysms. A 56-year-old man is admitted to the neurologic intensive care unit (NICU, NeuroICU) after he develops a nonradiating frontal headache associated with photophobia, nausea, and one episode of nonbilious, nonbloody vomiting 30 minutes prior to his arrival at the emergency department. Noncontrast head computed tomography (CT) is consistent with acute subarachnoid hemorrhage—Blood is seen in the middle cerebral artery cisterns extending into the sylvian fissures bilaterally (Figure 21-1).

What are your initial management considerations for this patient?

In order to make an appropriate treatment decision for this patient, etiology of the subarachnoid hemorrhage (SAH), whether aneurysmal or traumatic, must first be determined. Most frequently, intracranial aneurysms present to clinical attention with symptoms of major aneurysmal rupture and, therefore, constitute a distinct clinical entity in the setting

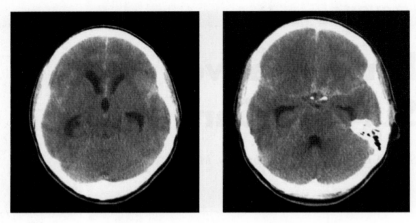

Figure 21-1. Noncontrast computed tomographic scan demonstrating subarachnoid hemorrhage.

of SAH. Although rupture nearly always results in SAH, it may also be accompanied by intracerebral hemorrhage (ICH), intraventricular hemorrhage (IVH), and, less often, subdural hemorrhage. This chapter discusses neurologic intensive care specific to surgical interventions for both ruptured and unruptured aneurysms. For NICU management of SAH and its related complications, see Chapter 1.

Symptoms that support a diagnosis of acute SAH due to aneurysmal rupture include:

- Worst headache of life, often with vomiting.
- Unilateral third cranial nerve palsy.
- Sixth nerve palsy.
- In the setting of concomitant ICH: hemiparesis, aphasia, amnesia, deterioration due to cerebral edema.
- In many cases, patients may present with sudden severe headache, but without any focal neurologic symptoms.

What diagnostic studies should be performed before deciding on a definitive treatment strategy and what medications should he be started on in the meantime?

If an aneurysmal rupture is suspected, a noncontrast head CT scan must be performed immediately to assess for subarachnoid blood. In the first 12 hours after the initial bleed, noncontrast head CT has a 98% to 100% sensitivity for SAH, which decreases to 93% at 24 hours[1-5] and to 57% to 85% after 6 days.[6,7] If the head CT does not reveal SAH, a mass lesion, or hydrocephalus, a lumbar puncture with analysis of the cerebrospinal fluid for xanthochromia should be performed.[8]

The gold standard for evaluation of cerebral aneurysms remains digital subtraction angiography (DSA), which demonstrates the source of SAH in approximately 85% of patients. Two less invasive modalities are increasingly being used, magnetic resonance angiography (MRA) and CT angiography. Three-dimensional time-of-flight MRA has a sensitivity to detect cerebral aneurysms between 55% and 93%.[9-12] Dichotomizing by size, the sensitivity is 85% to 100% for aneurysms 5 mm or greater, but only 56% for those less than 5 mm in size.[11,13,14] CT angiography, however, is the more frequently used noninvasive modality, as it is faster and more readily available. In addition, it has sensitivity for aneurysms between 77% and 100% and specificity between 79% and 100%.[15-21]

Recommended initial therapy includes:

1. Cefazolin sodium injection 1 g IV q8h
2. Nimodipine oral 60 mg PO q4h
3. Levetiracetam injection 1000 mg IVPB q12h
4. Dexamethasone oral 10 mg PO q6h
5. Esomeprazole oral 40 mg PO daily
6. Acetaminophen oral 650 mg PO q4h
7. Ondansetron injection 4 mg IV q3h

DSA demonstrates a 4 mm × 3 mm aneurysm extending medially from the internal carotid artery at the level of the posterior communicating artery (Figure 21-2). Three hours later, the patient develops a third nerve palsy. How do you interpret this finding?

Newly diagnosed cranial nerve (CN) III involvement in the setting of a posterior communicating artery aneurysm implies expansion of the vascular lesion with impending risk of rebleeding. Rebleeding is the major cause of death in patients who survive the initial hemorrhage but do not undergo surgical intervention.[22-24] Table 21-1 demonstrates common interpretations of emerging neurologic signs with regard to location of an expanding aneurysm.

The progression of neurologic deficits in the setting of aneurysmal rupture plays an integral role in deciding on surgical management of the aneurysm. The grading scale proposed by Hunt and Hess[25] (see Chapter 1) is a useful tool, but does not replace a comprehensive neurologic examination that can

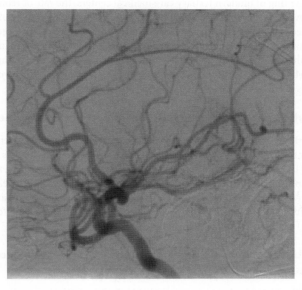

Figure 21-2. Digital subtraction angiographic scan demonstrating a 4 mm × 3 mm posterior communicating artery aneurysm.

Table 21-1. Neurologic Signs and Common Interpretations of Aneurysm Location and Expansion

Sign	Location/Interpretation
CN III palsy	Rapid aneurysmal expansion or small focal hemorrhage
CN III palsy accompanied by mydriasis, absent light reflex, and focal eye pain	Aneurysm at posterior communicating artery and internal carotid junction
CN VI palsy	Cavernous sinus aneurysm
Visual field deficit	Supraclinoid carotid aneurysm
Occipital and posterior cervical pain	Posterior inferior cerebellar artery or anterior inferior cerebellar artery aneurysm
Pain in or behind the eye and in low temple	Middle cerebral artery aneurysm

Abbreviation: CN, cranial nerve. *(From Ropper AH. Neurological and Neurosurgical Intensive Care. 4th ed. Philadelphia, PA: Lippincott Williams & Wilkins; 2004.)*

give an accurate and even quantitative assessment of neurologic deterioration as well as its underlying pathophysiology. Therefore, a careful neurologic examination at admission and subsequent points during the hospital stay is an important tool for assessing the outcomes of surgery and identifying, treating, and preventing postoperative complications.

What are the patient's risks of rebleeding?

In untreated SAH, the greatest risk of rebleeding occurs on the first day (4%), with a daily frequency of 1.5% until 13 days. By 2 weeks' post-ictus, the rebleed rate is 15% to 20%, and up to 50% by 6 months.[24] In the setting of modern tertiary care medical centers, the rate of rebleeding is nearly 7% when prehospital events are excluded,[26] although a number of studies refer to a 10% to 20% incidence of "ultraearly" rebleeds by taking into account events that occur before patients receive neurosurgical attention.[27-30] Overall, rebleed events in the first day are associated with a drastically reduced chance of survival, with functional independence at 3 months (modified Rankin score [mRS], ≤ 4; OR, 0.08; 95% CI, 0.02 to 0.34).[26] The goal of surgical and endovascular treatment is to prevent this occurrence, and since the 1980s there has been a shift toward early intervention.[31]

Is antifibrinolytic therapy appropriate for prevention of rebleeding?

The use of antifibrinolytic therapy for the prevention of rebleeding is controversial, as it has been shown to significantly decrease the incidence of rebleeding by 40% to 60%, but has also been shown to increase the risk of ischemic neurologic deficits by a similar margin.[32,33] However, recent evidence has shown that when antifibrinolytic therapy is prophylactically administered before early surgery, preoperative rebleeding rates can be reduced effectively and ischemic complications can be minimized by postsurgical discontinuation of antifibrinolytics.[28,34] ε-Aminocaproic acid (36 g/day) or tranexamic acid (6 to 12 g/day) can be used for these purposes.[35]

Should the patient receive surgical clipping of his posterior communicating artery aneurysm?

Interventions that directly address the aneurysm that caused the initial hemorrhage must be carefully considered alongside supportive and prophylactic therapies that treat the primary brain injury and prevent cerebral vasospasm, delayed ischemia, and hydrocephalus. Surgical treatment of an aneurysm is accomplished through craniotomy and aneurysm neck clipping to definitively exclude it from the circulation, thereby removing the risk of rebleeding.

At admission, large amounts of subarachnoid blood visible on CT, which are related to the development and severity of symptomatic vasospasm,[36] make early surgery a strong consideration. In fact, the use of hyperdynamic therapy for the treatment of vasospasm becomes a much safer option once an aneurysm has been secured with surgical clipping. Any conditions that contribute to instability of the aneurysm, including seizures and abrupt changes in blood pressure, may also make early intervention beneficial. However, if a patient has active vasospasm or severe cerebral edema at the time of evaluation, then surgery should be delayed.

If hemorrhage happened on the same day as your evaluation, when should microsurgical clipping be attempted?

The timing of intervention is still a source of debate,[37] but there are substantial efforts to carry out early management protocols[31] on account of broad-based support for their implementation garnered through favorable outcome data.[37-40] There is a widely recognized trade-off between early surgical risk of operative mortality and the benefits it confers in terms of rebleeding prevention. In 1990, the International Cooperative Study on the Timing of Aneurysm Surgery, which prospectively followed 3521 patients, reported no difference in outcome between intervention at 0 to 3 days after the original bleed versus 11 to 14 days, but outcomes were definitively worse in the 7- to 10-day interval.[39] No subsequent randomized controlled trials have been performed, but more recent observational studies and meta-analyses have argued that the benefits derived from reduction of rebleeding appear to outweigh the risks of early intervention.[35,37,38,40]

At our institution, we favor early surgery to prevent rebleeding. Early intervention is strongly indicated in cases where rebleeding has already occurred at least once. Likewise, any indications of an impending rebleed, such as an increase in aneurysm size on serial angiography or new neurologic deficits, including third nerve palsy in the setting of a posterior communicating artery aneurysm,[41] should prompt the clinician to consider surgical intervention. It is important to note that hyperdynamic therapy and bed rest do not prevent rebleeding.[42] This patient should receive immediate surgical intervention.

Before you can proceed with surgery, the patient's mental status deteriorates. He is stuporous and has minimal withdrawal response to painful stimuli. What are his options for surgical management given his current status?

This patient has a Hunt and Hess grade IV SAH. Although good medical and neurologic conditions (Hunt and Hess grade < 4) encourage favorable outcomes,[43,44] surgery also remains an appropriate option for patients in poor neurologic condition, as up to 40% of Hunt and Hess grade IV and V patients have been shown to have a good outcome (modified Rankin score 0 to 3) following surgical intervention.[45,46]

Perioperative Surgical Care

A 41-year-old woman with a history of asthma, methadone use, and IV drug use, including heroin and cocaine, was injecting these drugs when she had sudden onset of headache and witnessed loss of consciousness. Noncontrast head CT showed diffuse SAH with clot in the anterior suprasellar region. DSA showed a 6- to 7-mm anterior communicating artery aneurysm (Figure 21-3). While awaiting surgery, the patient's baseline blood pressure of 145/90 increased to 205/152 mm Hg.

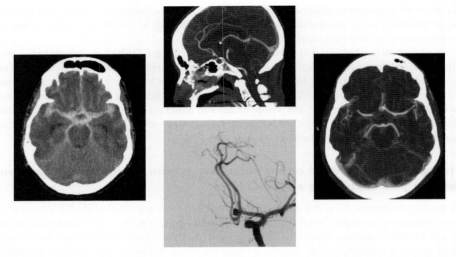

Figure 21-3. Computed tomographic, computed angiographic, and digital subtraction angiographic scans demonstrating subarachnoid hemorrhage from a 6- to 7-mm anterior communicating artery aneurysm.

How should this patient be treated?

While the aneurysm remains unsecured, careful blood pressure and volume management must be performed. As a general guideline, this involves maintenance of a target systolic pressure of less than 180 mm Hg and a target mean arterial pressure between 100 and 120 mm Hg, but a definitive target must be established by taking the patient's baseline blood pressure into account.[47] Some studies have found that rebleeding is more common when systolic blood pressure is above 150 mm Hg[27] or 160 mm Hg,[29] while others have found no relationship between blood pressure and rebleed rates.[26] Differences among these studies are related to the variable use of antihypertensive medications and inconsistent observation times.[48] At our center, we aim for blood pressure control with short-acting continuous infusion agents that can be delivered safely and with a reliable dose-response profile, such as nicardipine, labetalol, and esmolol. For specific protocols on blood pressure management, refer to Chapter 24.

In anticipation of aneurysmal clipping, what medications should be started preoperatively?

Upon admission, patients should be started on prophylactic anticonvulsants because of increased seizure incidence in the setting of aneurysmal rupture, as nearly 8% of patients experience seizures at SAH onset and more than 20% of patients experience them after initial hemorrhage.[49,50] Meperidine (Demerol) should be avoided for analgesia because it can lower the seizure threshold, and fentanyl should be used for pain relief instead of morphine to avoid histamine release. Dexamethasone (Decadron) can be given to relieve headache and neck pain and should be started preoperatively when preparing for craniotomy.

When anticipating early surgery, patients should be held NPO (nothing by mouth), and the clinical team must evaluate platelet count, bleeding time, and clotting parameters. Hematocrit levels above 40% significantly increase serum viscosity, as do levels of serum fibrinogen greater than 250 mg/dL. Serum viscosity may play an important role in the setting of vasospasm prevention and treatment, but this assertion has not been definitively evaluated.[51] A hematocrit above 40% at admission can be corrected with delivery of 5% IV colloids or hypertonic saline.[52,53] A hematocrit between 28% and 32% is considered ideal by many clinicians.[54] Patients with large hemorrhages may be in a state of catecholamine excess due to hypothalamic dysfunction. Myofibrillar necrosis may occur as a result of prolonged myocardial fiber contraction stimulated by high levels of catecholamines, and therefore serum levels of troponin and creatine kinase must be obtained to evaluate for the possibility of myocardial ischemia.

The patient undergoes successful clipping of her aneurysm, which is confirmed by intraoperative CT angiography. Neurologic deterioration is noted on the first day of recovery and head CT demonstrates ventriculomegaly (Figure 21-4). Routine labs are significant for hyponatremia.

How do you proceed?

Hydrocephalus is common in the setting of aneurysmal rupture, occurring in 20% to 30% of cases.[35] It should be promptly treated by placement of an external ventricular drain (EVD), as there is class I evidence to demonstrate that ventriculostomy improves neurologic status in patients who are symptomatic.[55-57] Fluid therapy with normal saline and 20 mEq KCl/L at 2 mL/kg per hour should be given to prevent hyponatremia caused by cerebral salt wasting because volume contraction has been shown to be correlated with the incidence of symptomatic vasospasm.[58] Fludrocortisone[59] and hypertonic saline[60] can also be used to improve sodium balance. Management of hypovolemia and hyponatremia in connection with cerebral salt wasting and hypervolemia secondary to the syndrome of inappropriate secretion of antidiuretic hormone (SIADH) are discussed in Chapter 1.

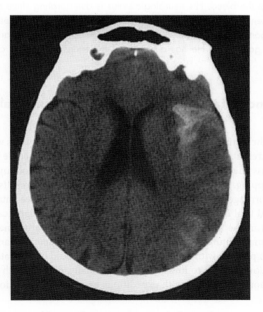

Figure 21-4. Computed tomographic scan demonstrating ventriculomegaly.

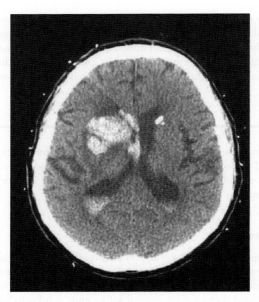

Figure 21-5. Computed tomographic scan demonstrating the presence of intracranial hemorrhage in patient with subarachnoid hemorrhage.

  You admit a 77-year-old man with a large right frontotemporal SAH and ICH (Figure 21-5). Angiography demonstrates a right middle cerebral artery aneurysm as the source of the bleed. His neurologic status is deteriorating since arrival at the emergency department. Currently, he is nonresponsive to voice and produces only minimal movement on the right side in response to painful stimulation with no eye opening. Pupils are small and nonreactive. He has no corneal or gag reflex. He has a history of hypertension and his current blood pressure is 260/165 mm Hg.

How does the concomitant presence of ICH affect surgical considerations in this patient?

When ICH occurs in the setting of aneurysmal rupture, radiographic studies will often reveal a hematoma at the middle cerebral artery bifurcation extending down to the circle of Willis. The presence of major ICH with mass effect and focal neurologic deficits favors craniotomy for hematoma evacuation and aneurysm clipping.[47] Notable in this context, however, are the results from the Surgical Trial in Intracerebral Hemorrhage (STICH), which was based on prospective data of 1033 patients. This randomized controlled trial demonstrated that ICH patients do not significantly benefit from early hematoma evacuation in the first 72 hours compared with conservative management of ICH.[61] In the setting of aneurysmal rupture, craniotomy with hematoma evacuation and duraplasty should be considered carefully in patients with ICH, and intervention should be indicated for large hematomas producing rapid deterioration due to mass effect. Additionally, patients with a > 3-cm diameter cerebellar hemorrhage should be treated with expeditious hematoma evacuation as the procedure can be lifesaving.[62]

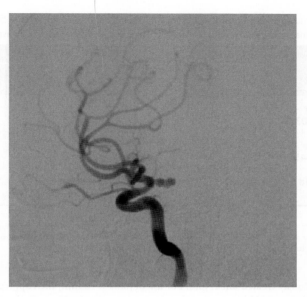

Figure 21-6. Digital subtraction angiographic scan demonstrating a 3 mm × 6 mm unruptured lobulated posterior communicating artery aneurysm.

Unruptured intracranial aneurysms. A 50-year-old woman with a prior history of SAH presents with 2 days of progressive decrease in eye movements and ptosis of her left eye. She also describes a new-onset migraine-like headache, which started approximately 2 weeks ago, but presently denies photophobia and neck stiffness. Angiography reveals a new 3 mm × 6 mm lobulated unruptured aneurysm that projects posteriorly from the left posterior communicating artery (Figure 21-6).

What is the main management consideration for this patient?

Surgical management of unruptured intracranial aneurysms (UIAs) centers on identifying those patients for whom the risk of aneurysmal rupture and consequent SAH exceeds the risks of procedural intervention. Almost 80% of nontraumatic SAH is due to aneurysmal rupture,[63] and the 30-day fatality rate of SAH is estimated to be near 15%.[64] Therefore, the risk of rupture must be taken very seriously. Unfortunately, management of UIAs continues to be fraught with controversy that is in large part due to a lack of definitive data on the natural history of UIAs.

What is this patient's risk of rupture?

Although UIAs are common, with an estimated prevalence in the general population of 2%,[65] their average annual rupture rate is considered to be relatively low, ranging from 0.3% to 0.7%.[66,67] However, the risk of rupture is heavily influenced by aneurysm size, location, and history of prior SAH from a separate but successfully treated aneurysm. In the retrospective arm of the International Study of Unruptured Intracranial Aneurysms (ISUIA), UIAs that were < 10 mm in diameter had a rupture rate of 0.05% per year, but this rate increased to 0.5% for patients who had a history of

Table 21-2. Cumulative Rupture Rates for Unruptured Intracranial Aneurysms at 5 Years: Results from the International Study of Unruptured Intracranial Aneurysms, Prospective Phase

Location	Size				
	< 7 mm no SAH (%)	< 7 mm with SAH (%)	7-12 mm (%)	13-24 mm (%)	≥ 25 mm (%)
A-comm/anterior circulation (n = 1037)	0	1.5	2.6	14.5	40
P-comm/posterior circulation (n = 445)	2.5	3.4	14.5	18.4	50
Cavernous carotid artery (n = 210)	0	0	0	3.0	6.4

Abbreviations: A-comm, anterior communicating artery; P-comm, posterior communicating artery; SAH, subarachnoid hemorrhage. No SAH, no prior history of SAH; with SAH, prior history of SAH from another surgically treated aneurysm. (Adapted from Wiebers DO, Whisnant JP, Huston J 3rd, et al. Unruptured intracranial aneurysms: Natural history, clinical outcome, and risks of surgical and endovascular treatment. Lancet. 2003;62:103-110.)

SAH from a previously treated aneurysm. For aneurysms > 10 mm, the rupture rate was near 1% per year irrespective of SAH history, but for giant aneurysms (> 25 mm), the rate was 6% in the first year.[66]

More recently, the prospective arm of the ISUIA, which followed 1692 patients, reported a cumulative rupture rate of 0%, 2.6%, 14.5%, and 40.0% over 5 years for anterior circulation aneurysms that were < 7 mm, 7 to 12 mm, 13 to 24 mm, and ≥ 25 mm in diameter, respectively. For posterior circulation aneurysms, the rates were 2.5%, 14.0%, 18.4%, and 50.0% over the same 5-year period (Table 21-2).[67] In summary, larger aneurysms and those located in the vertebrobasilar circulation or the posterior communicating artery are at significantly higher risk of rupture than other aneurysms. Small aneurysms (< 7 mm in the ISUIA) have a very low risk of rupture 5 years from diagnosis unless the patient has a history of SAH.[67] Other comorbidities, such as history of hypertension, abuse of alcohol or tobacco, and family history of aneurysms and SAH, should be taken into account as they may increase the risk of rupture.[68]

What type of management is most appropriate for this patient?

The risk of aneurysmal rupture must be weighed against the risks of morbidity and mortality associated with surgical intervention. In a meta-analysis of 61 studies with 2460 total patients, Raaymakers et al found that surgical clipping of UIAs was associated with a 10.9% morbidity and 2.6% mortality rate.[69] In this cohort, 54% of the aneurysms were in the anterior circulation and 30% were > 10 mm in diameter.[69] Conversely, in a meta-analysis that solely included asymptomatic UIAs, morbidity and mortality rates were 4.1% and 1.0%, respectively, but 94% of aneurysms were located in the anterior circulation and 28% were greater than 10 mm, likely favoring better outcomes.[70]

Given these statistics on surgical morbidity and mortality, patients with UIAs must be recommended for surgery only when the risk of rupture under conservative management is high. Age plays a central role in this decision making since rupture risk is significantly higher for younger patients owing to accumulation over a greater number of years. Younger patients are also less prone to suffer adverse effects from surgery and thus may benefit most from surgical clipping. The patients for whom management recommendations are most difficult to make include those with (1) UIAs in the anterior circulation 5 to 10 mm in diameter, (2) UIAs in the posterior circulation 3 to 10 mm in diameter, and (3) any UIAs 3 to 10 mm in diameter when there is a history of SAH. This is because the natural history of these lesions and their surgical risks are similar.[68] Randomized clinical trials comparing conservative management and surgical intervention will be necessary to define appropriate management guidelines in these situations.

A 34-year-old man presents with severe intractable headaches, but no other significant medical history. Diagnostic studies reveal a 6-mm unruptured aneurysm in the anterior communicating artery.

How does this patient's presentation affect management?

UIAs may present symptomatically when they exert pressure on nearby brain parenchyma or cranial nerves. Mass effect from giant aneurysms can involve brainstem compression resulting in hemiparesis and cranial neuropathies. CN III involvement is the most common cranial neuropathy found with an expanding aneurysm, and Table 21-1 reviews typical neurologic deficits associated with expansion at specific aneurysmal locations. In 2% to 3% of cases, UIAs may manifest as ischemic strokes downstream from the aneurysmal sac.[71,72] Seizures may be coincident with UIAs, but most often arise from localized gliosis rather than aneurysmal expansion per se.[72] Headaches are a common manifestation of UIAs, and the "worst headache of my life" description can also apply to cases that do not rupture. In cases where the disruption caused by symptoms outweighs the risks of surgical treatment, the UIA should be recommended for surgical clipping.

Currently, the guidelines of the Stroke Council of the American Heart Association, which were issued in 2000, before the results from the prospective phase of the ISUIA, remain applicable to management decisions[73]:

- The treatment of small incidental intracavernous aneurysms is not generally indicated. For large symptomatic intracavernous aneurysms, treatment decisions should be individualized on the basis of patient age, severity and progression of symptoms, and treatment alternatives. The higher risk of treatment and shorter life expectancy in older individuals must be considered in all patients and favors observation in older patients with asymptomatic aneurysms.

- Symptomatic intradural aneurysms of all sizes should be considered for treatment, with relative urgency for the treatment of acutely symptomatic aneurysms. Symptomatic large or giant aneurysms carry higher surgical risks that require a careful analysis of individualized patient and aneurysmal risks and surgeon and center expertise.

- Coexisting or remaining aneurysms of all sizes in patients with SAH due to another treated aneurysm carry a higher risk for future hemorrhage than do similar-sized aneurysms without a prior SAH history and warrant consideration for treatment. Aneurysms located at the basilar apex carry a relatively high risk of rupture. Treatment decisions must take into account the patient's age, existing medical and neurologic conditions, and relative risks of repair. If a decision is made for observation, reevaluation on a periodic basis with CT/MRA or selective contrast angiography should be considered, with changes in aneurysmal size sought, although careful attention to technical factors will be required to optimize the reliability of these measures.

- In consideration of the apparent low risk of hemorrhage from incidental small (<10 mm) aneurysms in patients without previous SAH, treatment rather than observation cannot be generally advocated. However, special consideration for treatment should be given to young patients in this group. Likewise, small aneurysms approaching the 10-mm diameter size, those with daughter sac formation and other unique hemodynamic features, and patients with a positive family history for aneurysms or aneurysmal SAH deserve special consideration for treatment. In those managed conservatively, periodic follow-up imaging evaluation should be considered and is necessary if a specific symptom should arise. If changes in aneurysmal size or configuration are observed, this should lead to special consideration for treatment.

• Asymptomatic aneurysms of ≥ 10 mm in diameter warrant strong consideration for treatment, taking into account patient age, existing medical and neurologic conditions, and relative risks for treatment.

This patient will undergo surgical clipping of his aneurysm. What type of preoperative management is indicated in his situation?

A thorough radiologic workup is necessary to develop an appropriate surgical strategy. DSA with selective cerebral arterial injection is the gold standard for the imaging of UIAs, but head CT and MRI can also be useful in providing information on these lesions, particularly when calcification or thrombosis is present, which cannot be detected by DSA.[74] Multislice CT angiography is often used instead of DSA because of its quicker image acquisition, lower cost, and minimal invasiveness, but it is less sensitive and specific than DSA.[75] Likewise, MRA is a minimally invasive procedure, but its sensitivity for detection significantly decreases at aneurysm sizes below 6 mm.[74]

In addition to a general medical examination and routine preoperative laboratory studies, the importance of a careful neurologic examination, as discussed in the section on aneurysmal rupture above, cannot be emphasized enough for its role in identifying postoperative improvement or morbidity.

During surgery, the most dreaded complication is intraoperative rupture of the aneurysm. High-quality preoperative angiography is absolutely essential to give a detailed understanding of the aneurysm's position and all sources of collateral circulation in case temporary clips need to be applied to trap the aneurysm in the event of rupture or difficult neck dissection.

As prophylaxis against possible intraoperative aneurysm rupture and adverse effects of vascular manipulation during the procedure, patients should receive anticonvulsants (phenytoin [Dilantin] IV loading dose 15 mg/kg), corticosteroids, and calcium channel blockers (nimodipine 60 mg PO q4h). Prophylaxis with H_2 blockers (eg, cimetidine) or proton pump inhibitors (eg, omeprazole) is common against gastrointestinal complications from steroids.

The patient is rebleeding from what was thought to be a well-clipped aneurysm. What must be done?

The most important complications after aneurysm surgery that differ from routine craniotomies are rebleeding from an incompletely clipped aneurysm, hydrocephalus secondary to SAH, and delayed cerebral ischemia due to vasospasm or perforator occlusion. The major complications after aneurysm surgery are presented in Table 21-3.

Incomplete occlusion must be followed with serial angiography, and reoperation is necessary in the setting of aneurysmal expansion and rebleeding. Prevention of rebleeding is accomplished through careful surgical clipping and verification with immediate postoperative angiography. Postoperative angiography can reveal the presence of an aneurysmal rest, indicating that the neck is not fully occluded by the surgical clip, unintentional vessel occlusion, or another unclipped aneurysm, all of which may be indications for a secondary procedure for clip adjustment.

The patient develops hydrocephalus. How should the patient be managed?

Hydrocephalus may often present asymptomatically, but a CT scan should be performed in the presence of even subtle cognitive alterations to assess the role of ventriculomegaly in neurologic deterioration. Little reservation should be given to placement of an EVD if indicated by CT and neurologic deficits. Ventriculoperitoneal shunt placement should also be considered after EVD placement when chronic cerebrospinal fluid (CSF) diversion is necessary.

Table 21-3. Major Complications of Aneurysm Surgery

Timing and type	Complication	Management
Immediate postoperative neurologic deficit	Deterioration due to ischemia from intraoperative perforator occlusion	Use intraoperative angiography to check for perforator occlusion and return patient to operating suite to adjust clip placement
Delayed neurologic deficit	Subdural, epidural, or intracerebral hemorrhage	When profuse hemorrhage seen on CT with rapid neurologic deterioration, proceed with immediate surgical evacuation
	Stroke	Immediate CT or MR diffusion-weighted imaging to rule out acute infarct
	Hydrocephalus	If symptomatic, use EVD placement or ventriculoperitoneal shunting
	Vasospasm	Ischemic areas on CT or increased cerebral blood flow on TCD should prompt hyperdynamic therapy if the aneurysm is secured, mannitol administration, and/or balloon angioplasty
	Seizures	Constant EEG monitoring is necessary in the postoperative period, along with anticonvulsant administration, beginning even before the operation for prophylactic purposes
	Electrolyte imbalance	Monitor serum electrolytes and initiate appropriate fluid treatment when necessary
	Meningitis	Use antibiotics if indicated by CSF analysis from lumbar puncture
Systemic medical problems	Myocardial infarction	If indicated by ECG and troponin or creatine kinase levels, use appropriate medical treatment
	Deep vein thrombosis	IVC filter in early postoperative period or anticoagulation medications can be used starting at 6 days' postoperative
	Pulmonary embolism	IVC filter in early postoperative period or anticoagulation medications can be used starting at 6 days' postoperative
	Respiratory failure	Intubation
	Urinary tract infection	Antibiotic treatment
	Pulmonary infection	Antibiotic treatment

Abbreviations: CSF, cerebrospinal fluid; CT, computed tomography; ECG, electrocardiography; EEG, electroencephalography; EVD, external ventricular drain; IVC, inferior vena cava; MR, magnetic resonance; TCD, transcranial Doppler.

Perioperative Surgical Care

What type of monitoring must be conducted on this patient postoperatively? What are the most important diagnostic modalities in the NICU setting s/p UIA clipping?

The most important monitoring is timely and consistent neurologic examination of the patient. Whenever neurologic deterioration occurs, CT scanning is a valuable diagnostic tool. Delayed neurologic deterioration occurring secondary to vasospasm is suspected when the CT is negative for hydrocephalus and hematoma and transcranial Doppler (TCD) monitoring reveals high flow velocities. Vasospasm can be treated with calcium channel blockers, balloon angioplasty, and hyperdynamic therapy, and is reviewed thoroughly in Chapter 1.

CT scans can be used to detect a developing subdural, epidural, or intracerebral hemorrhage. Reexploration is necessary to remove large hematomas. In some cases, meningitis may cause neurologic deterioration, and lumbar puncture is necessary to evaluate CSF for the presence of neutrophils, low glucose, or high protein concentration. Furthermore, electrolyte imbalances from diabetes insipidus or cerebral salt wasting should be monitored by routine laboratory studies and treated with fluid therapy as discussed in Chapter 1.

Electrophysiologic monitoring in the first 48 to 72 hours after surgery must be performed to assess for seizure activity. Therapeutic levels of anticonvulsant drugs should only be withdrawn after patients are definitively seizure-free.

The patient develops nonspecific T wave and ST changes. His peak troponin level is 8.4. What should be done?

Medically, myocardial infarction may be caused by catecholamine excess and is suspected in the face of unexplained changes in vital signs, a high troponin or creatine kinase level, and electrocardiographic (ECG) abnormalities. Use of 12-lead ECG monitoring in the recovery room, nitrate administration, and avoidance of hypertension are indicated in this setting.

Other medical complications may also occur. Deep venous thrombosis (DVT) may occur in the lower extremity, necessitating Doppler monitoring of this region. Thigh-high compression stockings should be used to avoid DVT complications. An inferior vena cava filter can be used in the acute postoperative setting to prevent pulmonary embolism in the presence of DVT, but heparin and warfarin can be initiated 5 days after surgery. Pulmonary embolism can be suspected from worsening arterial blood-gas and ECG abnormalities, but a pulmonary angiogram is required to definitively confirm the diagnosis.

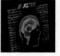

Arteriovenous malformations. A 46-year-old man previously in excellent general health experiences sudden onset of the worst headache of his life. He has the headache for 3 days and then decides to seek medical attention. A CT scan shows no obvious hemorrhage; however, it reveals abnormal calcifications in the right occipital region (Figure 21-7). He is suspected to have an arteriovenous malformation (AVM) in that area.

While you await an MRI study, what is your major management consideration if this patient has an AVM?

One of the greatest challenges of microsurgical management of AVMs lies in balancing the risk of surgery against the probability of hemorrhage, neurologic deficit, or seizure from the lesion. Microsurgery is not appropriate for all AVM patients, and a thorough understanding of the natural history of AVMs is important in making clinical decisions regarding possible interventions.

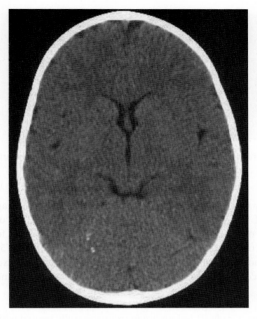

Figure 21-7. Computed tomographic scan demonstrating right occipital calcifications.

What are the risks of hemorrhage for this patient if the AVM is left untreated?

In general, AVMs carry a 2% to 4% annual risk of hemorrhage, which rises to 6% to 18% in the first year after an initial hemorrhage. Over a patient's lifetime, this translates into a 17% to 90% risk of rehemorrhage.[76-81] Multivariate modeling has demonstrated that young[82] or old[83] age may increase hemorrhage risk, but results regarding patient sex have been in disagreement.[82,84] Aneurysms are often found to be associated with AVMs in roughly 7% to 41% of cases. These may form inside or near the AVM nidus, in arterial feeders, or at a distance from the AVM. Potential rupture of such aneurysms increases the risk of AVM hemorrhage and, therefore, must be monitored radiographically.[81,85] The goal of microsurgical intervention for AVMs is complete obliteration of the AVM nidus and to eliminate the risk of hemorrhage.

MRI confirms the presence of an AVM, and DSA demonstrates a right occipital AVM with an associated early draining vein and blush, fed by posterior, lateral, and medial choroidal as well as the three branches of the inferior division of the posterior carotid artery (PCA) (Figure 21-8).

How do you proceed in evaluating this case?

Most commonly, operative risk is assessed using the Spetzler and Martin (SM) grading system for AVMs, which has been widely validated for outcome prediction following microsurgery.[76, 86–89] SM grading factors in such AVM characteristics as location, size, and venous drainage pattern provide a basis for exploring AVM management decisions (Table 21-4). Grade I and II lesions are often treated with

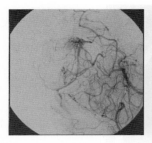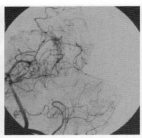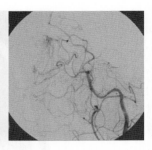

Figure 21-8. Digital subtraction angiographic scan demonstrating right occipital arteriovenous malformation and feeders.

microsurgery, especially when the AVM presents with a history of hemorrhage. Favorable outcomes following microsurgical intervention have been observed in 92% to 100% of patients with grade I lesions and 94% to 95% of patients with grade II lesions.[86,87,89] Microsurgery for grade III AVMs produces excellent or good outcomes in 68% to 96% of cases[86,87] and in 71% to 75% of cases for grade IV AVMs.[76,86,89] Finally, grade V AVMs have been reported to have a good or excellent outcome in only 50% to 70% of cases, accompanied by a 14% to 25% rate of poor outcome and a 0% to 5% mortality rate.[76,86,87,90]

Given these figures, microsurgery with adjunctive endovascular therapy is often recommended for grade I and II patients. Grade III lesions are more successfully treated with endovascular therapy followed by microsurgery if they are greater than 6 cm in size (grade IIIA), or with endovascular therapy followed by radiosurgery if they have deep venous drainage and/or are localized to eloquent areas (cortical M1, S1, or V1 regions, which are areas responsible for speech, hypothalamus, thalamus, internal capsule, brainstem, or cerebellar peduncles or nuclei) of the brain (grade IIIB).[90] Generally, grade IV and V patients are recommended for observation or, in some cases, multimodality treatment. Figure 21-9 summarizes this approach.[81] In the case above, the patient's lesion would be classified as SM grade IIIA, and therefore should be treated with endovascular embolization followed by microsurgery for definitive resection.

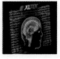
A 64-year-old man with a past history of hypertension presents with the worst headache of his life followed by witnessed loss of consciousness. A noncontrast head CT scan reveals a severe posterior fossa hemorrhage secondary to a cerebellar AVM (Figure 21-10).

Table 21-4. Spetzler and Martin Grading System for Arteriovenous Malformations

Characteristic	Classification	Points assigned
Eloquent location	No	0
	Yes	1
Venous drainage	Superficial	0
	Deep	1
Size	Small (< 3 cm)	1
	Medium (3-6 cm)	2
	Large (> 6 cm)	3

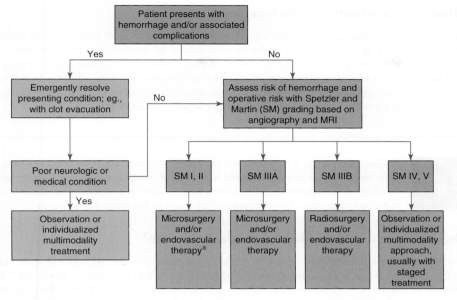

Figure 21-9. Management of cerebral arteriovenous malformations. [a]Radiosurgery is an option, especially in unruptured cases.

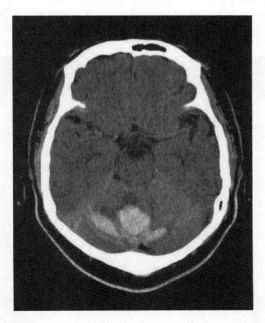

Figure 21-10. Computed tomographic scan demonstrating cerebellar arteriovenous malformation with hemorrhage.

What are the priorities for his treatment?

Generally, AVM microsurgery is an elective procedure except in emergent cases in which patients present with ICH or life-threatening hydrocephalus caused by hemorrhage. In these cases, clot removal constitutes the primary objective of surgical intervention and resection is only performed after the hematoma-related complications are resolved and the anatomy of the AVM can be carefully elucidated with angiography. If the AVM is readily visualized during clot removal, such as with superficial AVMs, microsurgical resection can be performed together with clot removal.

A 46-year-old woman is diagnosed with seizures. Fifteen years ago, while being evaluated for scalp melanoma, head scans revealed a small AVM overlying an area of cystic encephalomalacia, indicating that she had a previous hemorrhage from the AVM that had tracked down to the ventricular cavity. On reevaluation, DSA shows an SM grade II AVM (Figure 21-11).

Should she be recommended for surgical resection?

The presence of focal neurologic symptoms, including seizures, precipitated by AVM are considered to be a factor that favors surgery since AVM excision can lead to symptom resolution.[85] For instance, in a series of surgically treated AVMs that included 102 patients at 2 year follow-up, 82% were symptom-free 2 years after microsurgery and almost half improved enough so as to discontinue anticonvulsants.[91] Although good seizure control often results from microsurgery, it is affected by duration of seizures, age at onset, and seizure location. Studies with longer-term follow-up are needed to investigate the continuing effects of microsurgery on seizures secondary to AVMs.[81,92]

Overall, the best candidates for microsurgical resection are those with an absence of significant medical comorbidities, with a good life expectancy, and with AVMs < 6 cm in size that are located in noneloquent brain areas. A higher risk of hemorrhage, such as seen with AVMs that have associated aneurysms or obstruction of venous outflow, serves as another indication for microsurgical resection.

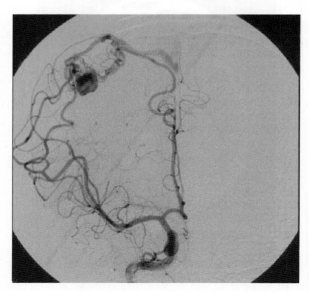

Figure 21-11. Digital subtraction angiographic scan demonstrating Spetzler and Martin grade II arteriovenous malformation.

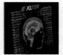 A 41-year-old woman in generally good medical condition has a minor head injury from a motor vehicle accident, and she is sent for a CT scan that demonstrates an incidental 2.5-cm left frontal arteriovenous malformation. The patient is completely asymptomatic from this malformation. The malformation is on the orbital frontal cortex fed mostly by middle cerebral branches and some anterior cerebral branches with superficial venous drainage.

How should she be managed?

Management of patients who are asymptomatic, however, remains controversial. In a recent prospective, population-based study of 114 patients with unruptured AVMs, there was no difference in long-term outcome between patients receiving microsurgery and those undergoing conservative management for their AVM, suggesting that monitoring of such lesions may be the best option if there is no history of hemorrhage.[93] However, if nonconservative management is attempted with this patient, then embolization followed by definitive resection of the malformation are recommended as treatment.

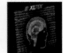 A 46-year-old male who is suffering severe headaches that are more severe when being exposed to paint and similar chemicals receives a CT scan that reveals a massive AVM in the right parieto-occipitotemporal region with evidence of large venous draining varices. DSA shows that a prominent right middle meningeal artery and right medial tentorial arteries provide its arterial blood supply (Figure 21-12).

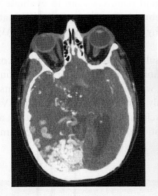
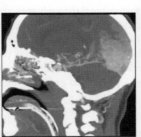
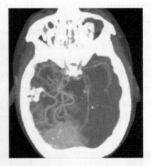

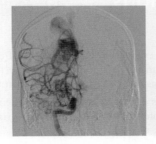
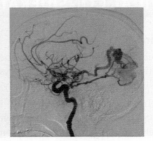

Figure 21-12. Computed tomographic scan and digital subtraction angiographic scan demonstrating large arteriovenous malformation indicated for staged treatment.

How do you plan for surgical management in this patient?

AVMs are thought to decrease blood flow to the rest of the brain through vascular steal, thereby compromising autoregulatory function of the cerebral vasculature and producing a state of chronic vasodilation. After AVM resection, blood flow to the rest of the brain increases significantly above normal and can lead to severe edema and hemorrhage. First described by Spetzler et al,[94] the development of malignant cerebral edema or hemorrhage due to normal perfusion pressure breakthrough is the most important complication following AVM surgery.

When surgical intervention is indicated for a large AVM with a high degree of direct arteriovenous shunting, staged treatment of the lesion is recommended for a more gradual reduction in lesion size. This can be accomplished with staged endovascular embolization of arterial feeders before complete surgical resection, thereby minimizing complications associated with normal perfusion pressure breakthrough.[95]

The patient undergoes surgical intervention for his AVM. Despite the best efforts of the neurovascular team at staged treatment, he develops severe cerebral edema after final resection. How do you approach postoperative management of normal perfusion pressure breakthrough?

Postoperative NICU care of AVM patients consists of strict blood pressure control and careful maintenance of euvolemia.[96] Using an arterial catheter, the systolic blood pressure should be maintained at the patient's baseline blood pressure, and parenteral antihypertensives may be used to lower the systolic pressure to < 110 mm Hg in healthy young patients. An indwelling catheter should be used to control urine output. Normotension should be maintained for at least 24 to 48 hours postoperatively. Neurologic status must be constantly monitored, and any observed changes should immediately be followed by an urgent head CT scan to evaluate for the presence of cerebral hemorrhage or hydrocephalus. Cerebral infarctions can be evaluated on diffusion-weighted imaging with MRI. Antiseizure prophylaxis is also needed after AVM surgery.

Although normal pressure perfusion breakthrough may result in hemorrhage, the most common cause of postoperative hemorrhage remains subtotal resection of the AVM. For this reason, it is imperative to perform an angiogram postoperatively to assess whether there are any remnants of the AVM at the site of surgery. When an angiogram reveals only partial obliteration of the AVM, the patient should return to the operating suite until complete excision is attained. Additionally, any complication in the postoperative period warrants prompt evaluation of the patient by angiogram to help in the diagnosis and treatment intervention.

! CRITICAL CONSIDERATIONS

Ruptured Intracranial Aneurysms

- Subarachnoid hemorrhage (SAH) should be evaluated with noncontrast CT or lumbar puncture for xanthochromia. In cases of aneurysmal SAH, the aneurysm(s) must be additionally evaluated using DSA or CTA to adequately assess size and location for treatment planning.
- Rebleeding from a ruptured aneurysm(s) is of paramount concern in the management of aneurysmal SAH, and the aim of surgical intervention is to eliminate the risk of rebleeding by definitively excluding the aneurysm from the circulation.

- Patients with ruptured aneurysms should be considered for early surgery, especially when there are signs of aneurysm expansion, impending rebleeding, or in the context of multiple rebleeds. Antifibrinolytic therapy can be used before early surgery in order to reduce the incidence of rebleeding, but should be discontinued immediately after surgery because of the risk of ischemic neurologic deficits.

- Early surgery for ruptured aneurysm is also favored when there is a large amount of subarachnoid blood on CT, which significantly increases the risk of vasospasm. Surgery should not be performed in patients with active vasospasm. Patients in poor neurologic condition (Hunt and Hess grades IV and V) still stand to benefit from surgery.

- Control of blood pressure near the patient's baseline or below 150 to 160 mm Hg is recommended before and after surgery for ruptured aneurysm. Prophylactic treatment with anticonvulsant therapy is essential in the perioperative period.

- Postoperatively after surgery for ruptured aneurysm, hydrocephalus should be promptly managed with EVD placement, and patients should be treated with appropriate IV fluids if they develop hypervolemia/hypovolemia and hypernatremia/hyponatremia.

Unruptured Intracranial Aneurysms

- Surgical management of UIAs centers around balancing the natural history of the lesion with regard to the possibility of rupture and hemorrhage against the risks of surgical morbidity and mortality.

- While the natural history of UIAs remains controversial, a number of studies have identified characteristics that significantly increase rupture risk and, therefore, favor surgical intervention. These include larger aneurysm size, location in the posterior circulation, and prior history of SAH from another surgically treated aneurysm (see Table 21-2). Moreover, patient age is an important factor, given the higher cumulative rupture risk of younger patients. The presence of symptoms related to the aneurysm, including seizures or intractable headaches, also makes surgical clipping a reasonable option as they may be relieved or resolved after the procedure.

- The most important postoperative complications after surgery for UIAs are development of delayed neurologic deficits due to vasospasm, stroke, hydrocephalus, seizures, and electrolyte imbalances. Any neurologic deterioration should prompt immediate radiologic evaluation for rehemorrhage, acute infarct, or ventriculomegaly.

- Prophylactic treatment with the calcium channel blocker nimodipine is a cornerstone of vasospasm management after surgery for UIAs, and active spasm deserves consideration for balloon angioplasty. Routine blood work and ECG tracings should be monitored for the development of acute myocardial infarction that may be precipitated by excess catecholamine. Other complications should be managed as in the setting of aneurysmal SAH and are detailed in Table 21-3.

Arteriovenous Malformations

- In the management of AVMs, the probability of hemorrhage, neurologic deficits, or seizures arising from the vascular lesion should be carefully weighed against the risks of surgery.

- Spetzler and Martin grading (see Table 21-4) provides a useful framework for evaluating the surgical risks of the patient with regard to size, location, and venous drainage of the AVM and can be used to select the most appropriate candidates for surgery. Each patient should

Perioperative Surgical Care

be evaluated individually by a multidisciplinary team, and endovascular or radiosurgical therapy serves as a useful adjunct to surgical resection in many cases.

- In general, SM grade I and II AVMs have the best outcomes following surgical resection. Grade III AVMs may have beneficial results from surgery when they are greater than 6 cm in size, but are not located in an eloquent area of the brain with deep venous drainage. Grade IV and V AVMs are recommended for observation or a multimodality approach with staged treatment.

- AVM resection is normally an elective procedure unless the patient presents with emergent hemorrhage. In such situations, resolution of hemorrhage with decompression and clot evacuation is the highest priority. Surgical resection should only be attempted after high-quality diagnostic studies have been performed to elucidate the precise anatomy of the AVM.

- Asymptomatic AVMs with low risk of bleeding should be managed conservatively, as the benefit of microsurgery has not been demonstrated in such cases.

- Staged treatment is a crucial aspect of intervention for large AVMs that have multiple arterial feeders that attract significant amounts of cerebral blood flow. For these lesions, multiple endovascular embolizations are required to reduce the risk of normal perfusion pressure breakthrough.

- Normal perfusion pressure breakthrough may result in hemorrhage and malignant cerebral edema and, therefore, presents the most significant management consideration after AVM surgery outside of complications of routine craniotomies. NICU care should center on strict blood pressure control (<110 mm Hg systolic in healthy young patients) and maintenance of euvolemia.

- Perioperative antiseizure prophylaxis, prompt treatment of hydrocephalus, and close neurologic monitoring should also be performed.

REFERENCES

1. Morgenstern L, Luna-Gonzales H, Huber J, et al. Worst headache and subarachnoid hemorrhage: prospective, modern computed tomography and spinal fluid analysis. *Ann Emerg Med.* 1998;32:297-304.

2. Sames T, Storrow A, Finkelstein J, Magoon M. Sensitivity of new-generation computed tomography in subarachnoid hemorrhage. *Acad Emerg Med.* 1996;3:16-20.

3. Sidman R, Connolly E, Lemke T. Subarachnoid hemorrhage diagnosis: lumbar puncture is still needed when the computed tomography scan is normal. *Acad Emerg Med.* 1996;3:827-831.

4. Tomasello F, d'Avela D, de Divitiis O. Does lamina terminalis fenestration reduce the incidence of chronic hydrocephalus after subarachnoid hemorrhage? *Neurosurgery.* 1999;45:827-831.

5. van der Wee N, Rinkel GJ, Hasan D, van Gijn J. Detection of subarachnoid haemorrhage on early CT: is lumbar puncture still needed after a negative scan? *J Neurol Neurosurg Psychiatry.*1995; 58:357-359.

6. Edlow J. Diagnosis of subarachnoid hemorrhage. *Neurocrit Care.* 2005;2:99-109.

7. van Gijn J, van Dongen K. The time course of aneurysmal haemorrhage on computed tomograms. *Neuroradiology.* 1982;23:153-156.

8. Cruickshank A, Auld P, Beetham R, et al. Revised national guidelines for analysis of cerebrospinal fluid for bilirubin in suspected subarachnoid haemorrhage. *Ann Clin Biochem.* 2008;45:238-244.

9. Anzalone N, Triulzi F, Scotti G. Acute subarachnoid haemorrhage: 3D time-of-flight MR angiography versus intra-arterial digital angiography. *Neuroradiology.* 1995;37:257-261.

10. Horikoshi T, Fukamachi A, Nishi H, Fukasawa I. Detection of intracranial aneurysms by three-dimensional time-of-flight magnetic resonance angiography. *Neuroradiology.* 1994;36:203-207.

11. Huston J, Nichols D, Luetmer P, et al. Blinded prospective evaluation of sensitivity of MR

angiography to known intracranial aneurysms: Importance of aneurysm size. *Am J Neuroradiol.* 1994;15:1607-1614.

12. Schuierer G, Huk W, Laub G. Magnetic resonance angiography of intracranial aneurysms: comparison with intra-arterial digital subtraction angiography. *Neuroradiology.* 1992;5:50-54.

13. Atlas S. Magnetic resonance imaging of intracranial aneurysms. *Neuroimaging Clin N Am.* 1997; 7:709-720.

14. Wilcock D, Jaspan T, Holland I, Cherryman G, Worthington B. Comparison of magnetic resonance angiography with conventional angiography in the detection of intracranial aneurysms in patients presenting with subarachnoid haemorrhage. *Clin Radiol.* 1996;51:330-334.

15. Alberico RA, Patel M, Casey S, Jacobs B, Maguire W, Decker R. Evaluation of the circle of Willis with three-dimensional CT angiography in patients with suspected intracranial aneurysms. *AJNR Am J Neuroradiol.* 1995;16:1571-1578.

16. Hope JK, Wilson JL, Thomson FJ. Three-dimensional CT angiography in the detection and characterization of intracranial berry aneurysms. *Am J Neuroradiol.* 1996;17:439-445.

17. Korogi Y, Takahashi M, Katada K, et al. Intracranial aneurysms: detection with three-dimensional CT angiography with volume rendering—comparison with conventional angiographic and surgical findings. *Radiology.* 1999;211:497-506.

18. Liang EY, Chan M, Hsiang JH, et al. Detection and assessment of intracranial aneurysms: value of CT angiography with shaded-surface display. *Am J Roentgenol.* 1995;165:1497-1502.

19. Ogawa T, Okudera T, Noguchi K, et al. Cerebral aneurysms: evaluation with three-dimensional CT angiography. *AJNR Am J Neuroradiol.* 1996;17:447-454.

20. Vieco P, Shuman W, Alsofrom G, Gross C. Detection of circle of Willis aneurysms in patients with acute subarachnoid hemorrhage: a comparison of CT angiography and digital subtraction angiography. *AJR Am J Roentgenol.* 1995;165:425-430.

21. Wilms G, Guffens M, Gryspeerdt S, et al. Spiral CT of intracranial aneurysms: correlation with digital subtraction and magnetic resonance angiography. *Neuroradiology.* 1996;38:S20-S25.

22. Broderick J, Brott T, Tomsick T, Miller R, Huster G. Intracerebral hemorrhage more than twice as common as subarachnoid hemorrhage. *J Neurosurg.* 1993;8:188-191.

23. Kassell NF, Torner JC. Aneurysmal rebleeding: a preliminary report from the Cooperative Aneurysm Study. *Neurosurgery.* 1983;13:479-481.

24. Winn HR, Richardson AE, Jane JA. The long-term prognosis in untreated cerebral aneurysms: I. The incidence of late hemorrhage in cerebral aneurysm: a 10-year evaluation of 364 patients. *Ann Neurol.* 1977;1:358-370.

25. Hunt WE, Hess RM. Surgical risk as related to time of intervention in the repair of intracranial aneurysms. *J Neurosurg.* 1968; 28:14-20.

26. Naidech AM, Janjua N, Kreiter KT, et al. Predictors and impact of aneurysm rebleeding after subarachnoid hemorrhage. *Arch Neurol.* 2005;62:410-416.

27. Fujii Y, Takeuchi S, Sasaki O, Minakawa T, Koike T, Tanaka R. Ultra-early rebleeding in spontaneous subarachnoid hemorrhage. *J Neurosurg.* 1996;84:35-42.

28. Hillman J, Fridriksson S, Nilsson O, Yu Z, Saveland H, Jakobsson KE. Immediate administration of tranexamic acid and reduced incidence of early rebleeding after aneurysmal subarachnoid hemorrhage: a prospective randomized study. *J Neurosurg.* 2002;97:771-778.

29. Ohkuma H, Tsurutani H, Suzuki S. Incidence and significance of early aneurysmal rebleeding before neurosurgical or neurological management. *Stroke.* 2001;32:1176-1180.

30. Sorteberg W, Slettebo H, Eide PK, Stubhaug A, Sorteberg A. Surgical treatment of aneurysmal subarachnoid haemorrhage in the presence of 24-h endovascular availability: management and results. *Br J Neurosurg.* 2008;22:53-62.

31. Komotar RJ, Schmidt JM, Starke RM, et al. Resuscitation and critical care of poor-grade subarachnoid hemorrhage. *Neurosurgery.* 2009;64:397-410; discussion 410-411.

32. Kassell NF, Torner JC, Adams HP Jr. Antifibrinolytic therapy in the acute period following aneurysmal subarachnoid hemorrhage. Preliminary observations from the Cooperative Aneurysm Study. *J Neurosurg.* 1984;61:225-230.

32. Torner JC, Kassell NF, Wallace RB, Adams HP Jr. Preoperative prognostic factors for rebleeding and survival in aneurysm patients receiving antifibrinolytic therapy: report of the Cooperative Aneurysm Study. *Neurosurgery.* 1981;9:506-513.

34. Starke RM, Kim GH, Fernandez A, et al. Impact of a protocol for acute antifibrinolytic therapy on aneurysm rebleeding after subarachnoid hemorrhage. *Stroke.* 2008;39:2617-2621.

35. Bederson JB, Connolly ES Jr, Batjer HH, et al. Guidelines for the management of aneurysmal subarachnoid hemorrhage: a statement for healthcare professionals from a special writing group of the Stroke Council, American Heart Association. *Stroke.* 2009;40:994-1025.

Perioperative Surgical Care

36. Fisher CM, Kistler JP, Davis JM. Relation of cerebral vasospasm to subarachnoid hemorrhage visualized by computerized tomographic scanning. *Neurosurgery.* 1980;6:1-9.

37. van der Jagt M, Hasan D, Dippel DW, van Dijk EJ, Avezaat CJ, Koudstaal PJ. Impact of early surgery after aneurysmal subarachnoid haemorrhage. *Acta Neurol Scand.* 2009;119:100-106.

38. de Gans K, Nieuwkamp DJ, Rinkel GJ, Algra A. Timing of aneurysm surgery in subarachnoid hemorrhage: a systematic review of the literature. *Neurosurgery.* 2002;50:336-340; discussion 340-342.

39. Kassell NF, Torner JC, Jane JA, Haley EC Jr, Adams HP. The International Cooperative Study on the Timing of Aneurysm Surgery. Part 2: Surgical results. *J Neurosurg.* 1990;73:37-47.

40. Milhorat TH, Krautheim M. Results of early and delayed operations for ruptured intracranial aneurysms in two series of 100 consecutive patients. *Surg Neurol.* 1986;26:123-128.

41. Soni SR. Aneurysms of the posterior communicating artery and oculomotor paresis. *J Neurol Neurosurg Psychiatry.* 1974;37:475-484.

42. Biller J, Godersky JC, Adams HP Jr. Management of aneurysmal subarachnoid hemorrhage. *Stroke.*1988;19:1300-1305.

43. Ogilvy CS, Cheung AC, Mitha AP, Hoh BL, Carter BS. Outcomes for surgical and endovascular management of intracranial aneurysms using a comprehensive grading system. *Neurosurgery.* 2006;59:1037-1042; discussion 1043.

44. Proust F, Hannequin D, Langlois O, Freger P, Creissard P. Causes of morbidity and mortality after ruptured aneurysm surgery in a series of 230 patients. The importance of control angiography. *Stroke.* 1995;26:1553-1557.

45. Le Roux PD, Elliott JP, Newell DW, Grady MS, Winn HR. Predicting outcome in poor-grade patients with subarachnoid hemorrhage: a retrospective review of 159 aggressively managed cases. *J Neurosurg.* 1996;85:39-49.

46. Mocco J, Ransom ER, Komotar RJ, et al. Preoperative prediction of long-term outcome in poor-grade aneurysmal subarachnoid hemorrhage. *Neurosurgery.* 2006;59:529-538; discussion 529-538.

47. Wijdicks EF, Kallmes DF, Manno EM, et al. Subarachnoid hemorrhage: neurointensive care and aneurysm repair. *Mayo Clin Proc.* 2005;0:550-559.

48. Rose JC, Mayer SA. Optimizing blood pressure in neurological emergencies. *Neurocrit Care.* 2004;1:287-299.

49. Baker CJ, Prestigiacomo CJ, Solomon RA. Short-term perioperative anticonvulsant prophylaxis for the surgical treatment of low-risk patients with intracranial aneurysms. *Neurosurgery.* 1995;37:863-870; discussion 870-861.

50. Lin CL, Dumont AS, Lieu AS, et al. Characterization of perioperative seizures and epilepsy following aneurysmal subarachnoid hemorrhage. *J Neurosurg.* 2003;99:978-985.

51. Ropper AH. *Neurological and Neurosurgical Intensive Care.* 4th ed. Philadelphia, PA: Lippincott Williams & Wilkins; 2004.

52. Perel P, Roberts I. Colloids versus crystalloids for fluid resuscitation in critically ill patients. *Cochrane Database Syst Rev,* 2007;CD000567.

53. Vermeulen LC Jr, Ratko TA, Erstad BL, Brecher ME, Matuszewski KA. A paradigm for consensus. The University Hospital Consortium guidelines for the use of albumin, nonprotein colloid, and crystalloid solutions. *Arch Intern Med.* 1995;155:373-379.

54. Solomon RA, Fink ME, Lennihan L. Early aneurysm surgery and prophylactic hypervolemic hypertensive therapy for the treatment of aneurysmal subarachnoid hemorrhage. *Neurosurgery.* 1988;23:699-704.

55. Hasan D, Vermeulen M, Wijdicks EF, Hijdra A, van Gijn J. Management problems in acute hydrocephalus after subarachnoid hemorrhage. *Stroke.* 1989;20:747-753.

56. Milhorat TH. Acute hydrocephalus after aneurysmal subarachnoid hemorrhage. *Neurosurgery.* 1987;20:15-20.

57. Rajshekhar V, Harbaugh RE. Results of routine ventriculostomy with external ventricular drainage for acute hydrocephalus following subarachnoid haemorrhage. *Acta Neurochir (Wien).* 1992;115:8-14.

58. Solomon RA, Post KD, McMurtry JG 3rd. Depression of circulating blood volume in patients after subarachnoid hemorrhage: implications for the management of symptomatic vasospasm. *Neurosurgery.* 1984;15:354-361.

59. Mori T, Katayama Y, Kawamata T, Hirayama T. Improved efficiency of hypervolemic therapy with inhibition of natriuresis by fludrocortisone in patients with aneurysmal subarachnoid hemorrhage. *J Neurosurg.* 1999;91:947-952.

60. Suarez JI, Qureshi AI, Parekh PD, et al. Administration of hypertonic (3%) sodium chloride/acetate in hyponatremic patients with symptomatic vasospasm following subarachnoid hemorrhage. *J Neurosurg Anesthesiol.* 1999;11:178-184.

61. Mendelow AD, Gregson BA, Fernandes HM, et al. Early surgery versus initial conservative treatment in patients with spontaneous supratentorial intracerebral haematomas in the International Surgical

Trial in Intracerebral Haemorrhage (STICH): a randomised trial. *Lancet.* 2005;365:387-397.

62. Ott KH, Kase CS, Ojemann RG, Mohr JP. Cerebellar hemorrhage: diagnosis and treatment. A review of 56 cases. *Arch Neurol.* 1974;31:160-167.

63. van Gijn J, Rinkel GJ. Subarachnoid haemorrhage: diagnosis, causes and management. *Brain.* 2001;124:249-278.

64. Kleindorfer D, Broderick J, Khoury J, et al. The unchanging incidence and case-fatality of stroke in the 1990s: a population-based study. *Stroke.* 2006; 37:2473-2478.

65. Rinkel GJ, Djibuti M, Algra A, van Gijn J. Prevalence and risk of rupture of intracranial aneurysms: a systematic review. *Stroke.* 1998;29:251-256.

66. International Study of Unruptured Intracranial Aneurysms Investigators. Unruptured intracranial aneurysms—Risk of rupture and risks of surgical intervention. *N Engl J Med.* 1998;339: 1725-1733.

67. Wiebers DO, Whisnant JP, Huston J 3rd, et al. Unruptured intracranial aneurysms: natural history, clinical outcome, and risks of surgical and endovascular treatment. *Lancet.* 2003;62: 103-110.

68. Burns JD, Brown RD, Jr. Treatment of unruptured intracranial aneurysms: surgery, coiling, or nothing? *Curr Neurol Neurosci Rep.* 2009; 9:6-12.

69. Raaymakers TW, Rinkel GJ, Limburg M, Algra A. Mortality and morbidity of surgery for unruptured intracranial aneurysms: a meta-analysis. *Stroke.* 1998;29:1531-1538.

70. King JT Jr, Berlin JA, Flamm ES. Morbidity and mortality from elective surgery for asymptomatic, unruptured, intracranial aneurysms: a meta-analysis. *J Neurosurg.* 1994;81:837-842.

71. Bhardwaj A, Mirski MAZ, Ulatowski JA. *Handbook of Neurocritical Care.* Totowa, NJ: Humana Press, 2004.

72. Raps EC, Rogers JD, Galetta SL, et al. The clinical spectrum of unruptured intracranial aneurysms. *Arch Neurol.* 1993;50:265-268.

73. Bederson JB, Awad IA, Wiebers DO, et al. Recommendations for the management of patients with unruptured intracranial aneurysms: a statement for healthcare professionals from the Stroke Council of the American Heart Association. *Stroke.* 2000;31:2742-2750.

74. Adams WM, Laitt RD, Jackson A. The role of MR angiography in the pretreatment assessment of intracranial aneurysms: a comparative study. *AJNR Am J Neuroradiol.* 2000;21:1618-1628.

75. Chappell ET, Moure FC, Good MC. Comparison of computed tomographic angiography with digital subtraction angiography in the diagnosis of cerebral aneurysms: a meta-analysis. *Neurosurgery.* 2003;52:624-631; discussion 630-662.

76. Hartmann A, Mast H, Mohr JP, et al. Morbidity of intracranial hemorrhage in patients with cerebral arteriovenous malformation. *Stroke.* 1998;29: 931-934.

77. Hamilton MG, Spetzler RF. The prospective application of a grading system for arteriovenous malformations. *Neurosurgery.* 1994;34:2-6; discussion 6-7.

78. Hernesniemi JA, Dashti R, Juvela S, Vaart K, Niemela M, Laakso A. Natural history of brain arteriovenous malformations: a long-term follow-up study of risk of hemorrhage in 238 patients. *Neurosurgery.* 2008;63:823-829; discussion 829-831.

79. Kondziolka D, McLaughlin MR, Kestle JR. Simple risk predictions for arteriovenous malformation hemorrhage. *Neurosurgery.* 1995;37:851-855.

80. Ondra SL, Troupp H, George ED, Schwab K. The natural history of symptomatic arteriovenous malformations of the brain: A 24-year follow-up assessment. *J Neurosurg.* 1990;73:387-391.

81. Starke RM, Komotar RJ, Hwang BY, et al. Treatment guidelines for cerebral arteriovenous malformation microsurgery. *Br J Neurosurg.* 2009;23:376-386.

82. Yamada S, Takagi Y, Nozaki K, Kikuta K, Hashimoto N. Risk factors for subsequent hemorrhage in patients with cerebral arteriovenous malformations. *J Neurosurg.* 2007;107:965-972.

83. Stapf C, Mast H, Sciacca RR, et al. Predictors of hemorrhage in patients with untreated brain arteriovenous malformation. *Neurology.* 2006;66:1350-1355.

84. Mast H, Young WL, Koennecke HC, et al. Risk of spontaneous haemorrhage after diagnosis of cerebral arteriovenous malformation. *Lancet.* 1997;350:1065-1068.

85. Nakaji P, Spetzler RF. Indications for surgical treatment of arteriovenous malformations. *Neurosurg Clin N Am.* 2005;16:365-366, x.

86. Hartmann A, Stapf C, Hofmeister C, et al. Determinants of neurological outcome after surgery for brain arteriovenous malformation. *Stroke.* 2000;31:2361-2364.

87. Heros RC, Korosue K, Diebold PM. Surgical excision of cerebral arteriovenous malformations: late results. *Neurosurgery.* 1990;26:570-577; discussion 577-578.

88. Pik JH, Morgan MK. Microsurgery for small arteriovenous malformations of the brain: results in 110 consecutive patients. *Neurosurgery.* 2000;47:571-575; discussion 575-577.

89. Spetzler RF, Martin NA. A proposed grading system for arteriovenous malformations. 1986. *J Neurosurg.* 2008;108:186-193.

90. de Oliveira E, Tedeschi H, Raso J. Multidisciplinary approach to arteriovenous malformations. *Neurol Med Chir (Tokyo).* 1998;38(suppl):177-185.

91. Piepgras DG, Sundt TM Jr, Ragoowansi AT, Stevens L. Seizure outcome in patients with surgically treated cerebral arteriovenous malformations. *J Neurosurg.* 1993;78:5-11.

92. Yeh HS, Tew JM Jr, Gartner M. Seizure control after surgery on cerebral arteriovenous malformations. *J Neurosurg.* 1993;78:12-18.

93. Wedderburn CJ, van Beijnum J, Bhattacharya JJ, V, et al. Outcome after interventional or conservative management of unruptured brain arteriovenous malformations: a prospective, population-based cohort study. *Lancet Neurol.* 2008;7:223-230.

94. Spetzler RF, Wilson CB, Weinstein P, Mehdorn M, Townsend J, Telles D. Normal perfusion pressure breakthrough theory. *Clin Neurosurg.* 1978;25:651-672.

95. Tarr RW, Johnson DW, Horton JA, et al. Impaired cerebral vasoreactivity after embolization of arteriovenous malformations: assessment with serial acetazolamide challenge xenon CT. *AJNR Am J Neuroradiol.* 1991;12:417-423.

96. Ogilvy CS, Stieg PE, Awad I, et al. AHA Scientific Statement: recommendations for the management of intracranial arteriovenous malformations: a statement for healthcare professionals from a special writing group of the Stroke Council, American Stroke Association. *Stroke.* 2001;32:1458-1471.

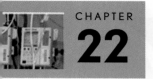
External Ventricular Drain Management and Ventriculoperitoneal Shunt

Paul R. Gigante, MD

Brian Y. Hwang, MD

E. Sander Connolly, MD

A 56-year-old woman with history of hypertension and hyperlipidemia presented with a sudden onset of severe headache followed by nausea and vomiting. She was taken by ambulance to the nearby emergency department (ED).
In the ED, the patient was alert and oriented to person, place, and time but was lethargic and uncooperative, without focal neurologic deficit. Noncontrast head computed tomographic (CT) scan demonstrated thick hyperdensity in the sylvian and interhemispheric fissures, as well as in the basilar cisterns. Her third and lateral ventricles were notably dilated. She was diagnosed with subarachnoid hemorrhage (SAH) with evidence of early hydrocephalus, and was urgently transferred to the neurologic intensive care unit (NICU, NeuroICU) for further management.

On arrival to the NICU she was lethargic, mumbling incoherently, not following commands, pupils were symmetrically reactive, and she moved all extremities with good strength. Vital signs: heart rate 88 bpm, respiratory rate 16 breaths/min, temperature 37.4°C (99.4°F), blood pressure 110/60 mm Hg. See Figure 22-1.

Does this patient need an external ventricular drain (EVD)? What are the indications for EVD placement?

This patient's presentation is consistent with Hunt and Hess (HH) grade III and Fisher grade 3 SAH (see Chapter 1 for information on SAH grading). Radiographic evidence of acute hydrocephalus along with neurologic decline (failure to follow commands) call for emergent placement of an external ventricular drain (EVD) to alleviate intracranial hypertension. EVDs serve three primary functions in SAH: to monitor intracranial pressure (ICP), to drain cerebrospinal fluid (CSF) for treatment of hydrocephalus, and/or to acutely reduce ICP. EVD placement is therefore indicated when a patient is thought to have symptomatic hydrocephalus and/or elevated ICP, based on neurologic examination and radiographic findings.

Ventriculostomy is considered standard-of-care for treating SAH-associated hydrocephalus and has been shown to improve both short- and long-term outcomes.[1] However, there is no standard, evidence-based guideline for EVD placement in SAH patients. Although the Glasgow Coma Scale (GCS) score (eg, 12 or less)[2] and HH grade (eg, III or

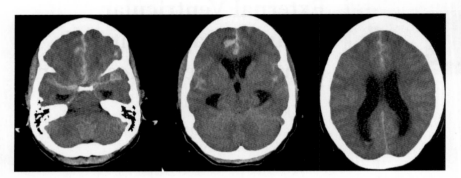

Figure 22-1.

greater)[3] have been used to establish an objective threshold for ventriculostomy, the procedure should be generally considered in patients who demonstrate clinical or radiologic deterioration or have an unreliable neurologic examination. Patients who present comatose or severely lethargic are almost universally considered for emergent ventriculostomy.[4] At our institution, all SAH patients not following commands are strong candidates for EVD insertion (Figure 22-2). Minimal improvement in neurologic status despite normalization of the ICP in these patients may point to other etiologies such as seizure, medication effect, or metabolic derangement and prompts immediate investigation. As for those with fluctuating levels of consciousness, the impact of ventriculostomy on outcome remains unclear and, therefore, careful risk-benefit analysis is warranted.[2] Figure 22-3 outlines our ICP management protocol for patients admitted to our NICU with aneurysmal SAH (aSAH).

Similarly, EVD placement is recommended in a variety of other neurologic conditions causing symptomatic acute hydrocephalus related to either noncommunicating or communicating hydrocephalus or evidence of elevated ICP.[1] Common causes of obstructive or noncommunicating hydrocephalus include posterior fossa tumors, intraventricular hemorrhage, and intraventricular cysts or tumors; communicating hydrocephalus may be caused by SAH, intraventricular hemorrhage, and meningitis; elevated ICP without significant hydrocephalus is commonly caused by closed-head trauma.[5] Normalization of ICP with EVDs can prevent secondary cortical injury, improve neurologic status,

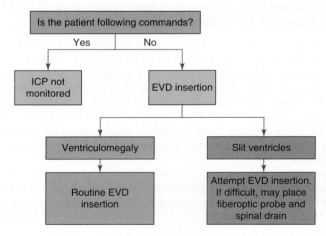

Figure 22-2. Algorithm for the decision to place an external ventricular drain in the setting of subarachnoid hemorrhage.

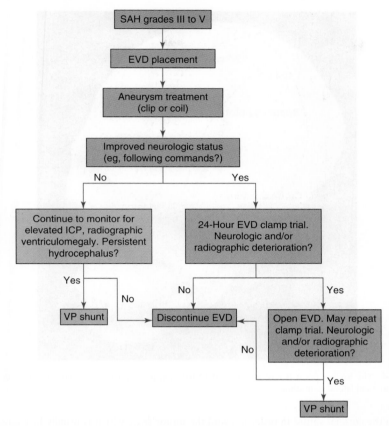

Figure 22-3. Algorithm for the management of subarachnoid hemorrhage–associated hydrocephalus. External ventricular drain (EVD) challenge is generally initiated within 1 week of EVD placement. Ventriculoperitoneal (VP) shunting is appropriate for patients with persistent hydrocephalus. ICP, intracranial pressure; SAH, subarachnoid hemorrhage.

and enhance operative exposure during surgery.[6-9] Of note, normal ICP ranges for adults and young children are considered less than 10 to 15 and 3 to 7, respectively.[5]

Another indication for EVD placement is to aid wound healing in the postoperative neurosurgical patient. Those who undergo operations of the posterior fossa, for example, via a suboccipital or a far lateral approach, are at particularly high risk for a postoperative CSF leak through their incision. Therefore, the neurosurgeon often leaves an EVD in the patient for a few days postoperatively, which allows for drainage of CSF through the EVD and alleviation of CSF pressure on the fresh incision. Once the incision has begun to heal and there is no evidence of CSF leak, the EVD can be removed.[5]

How is an EVD placed?

The EVD is placed by making a frontal incision and single burr hole in the skull, so that the catheter can be passed through the frontal lobe and into the lateral ventricle, with the goal of placing the catheter tip at the foramen of Monro. The nondominant frontal lobe is preferred as an entry point because it minimizes the risk of significant neurologic deficit in the event of a procedural complication such as subdural, epidural, or intraparenchymal hemorrhage.[5] The burr hole entry point should be lateral to midline (in the mid-pupillary line) to avoid the sagittal sinus and its tributaries, and

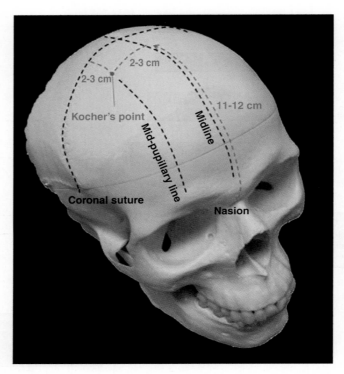

Figure 22-4. The Kocher point is typically located 12 to13 cm posterior to the nasion in the anteroposterior direction and 3 cm lateral to midline.

anterior to the coronal suture in order to avoid the motor strip, which is usually located 4 to 5 cm behind the coronal suture. This well-known entry point is called the Kocher point, and is typically located 12 to 13 cm posterior to the nasion in the anteroposterior (A-P) direction, and 3 cm lateral to midline (Figure 22-4). These measurements should always be correlated with anatomic landmarks by palpating the coronal suture through the scalp and ensuring the entry point is anterior, as well as visually ensuring the entry point lies in the mid-pupillary line. Although a right-sided (nondominant frontal lobe) placement is preferred, the EVD may be placed through the left side if the surgeon needs to avoid a lesion or hemorrhage in the right frontal lobe or lateral ventricle. In trauma patients, the surgeon may prefer to pass the EVD through whichever frontal lobe has already been injured in order to minimize risk to the remaining normal parenchyma. When the Kocher point is used as an entry point, the trajectory of the EVD pass through the parenchyma should be aimed at the medial canthus in a medial-lateral direction and the tragus in an A-P direction. This trajectory is usually achieved if the EVD is aimed exactly perpendicular to the skull surrounding the burr hole. Depending on the size of the lateral ventricles, the surgeon may pass the catheter 4 to 5 cm into the parenchyma before feeling a "pop" sound indicating entry into the lateral ventricle, with CSF return through the catheter. In order to advance the catheter tip to the foramen of Monro, the EVD is usually "soft passed" (advancing the catheter without the stylet) to a total of 6.5 to 7.0 cm from the outer table of the skull. The catheter is then tunneled a short distance under the scalp, in a direction that avoids a potential future shunt pathway.

The rate of EVD catheter misplacement can be as high as 60%, morbidity rate as high as 28%, and hemorrhagic complications 17.5%.[8,10] Therefore, a routine postplacement CT scan is recommended to ensure correct placement and rule out hemorrhagic complications.

Does it matter who places the EVD and where it is placed?

EVDs can be placed either in the operating room (OR) or at the bedside using local anesthesia.[11,12] The OR provides a more sterile, controlled environment where acute complications can be efficiently managed. However, waiting for an OR room may delay treatment when emergent EVD is needed, and transporting critically ill patients leaves physicians without resources during transport. Although EVD placement in an ICU setting may increase the risk of severe infection, there are no conclusive data to determine how the environment of EVD placement affects the overall complication rate and outcome.[11,13]

EVDs have traditionally been placed by neurosurgeons to ensure that the person who places the device can also manage procedure-associated complications, such as subdural or intracerebral hemorrhage. Recently, an increasing number of EVDs and ICP monitors have been placed by nonneurosurgeons, including neurointensivists, nurse practitioners, physician assistants, trauma surgeons, and general surgery residents.[14] The impact of EVD placement by nonneurosurgeons on procedural success, complication rates, and outcomes is yet to be determined. Nevertheless, the increasing trend toward nonneurosurgeon EVD and ICP monitor placement, if proven equally safe and effective, may provide patients with more expeditious care in select environments.

Although an EVD is thought to offer the most accurate ICP measurements, the surgeon may be unable to place an EVD in patients with collapsed ventricles, slit ventricles, or significant mass effect.[5] In such cases, ICP can be monitored via placement of a fiberoptic parenchymal ICP bolt, which is a small fiberoptic cable passed through a burr hole and into the parenchymal edge, usually at the Kocher point. If an ICP bolt is placed and the team believes intracranial CSF volume is contributing to critically elevated ICP, a spinal drain can be placed in patients with communicating hydrocephalus. Just like an EVD, the spinal drain allows for lowering of ICP and treatment of hydrocephalus through CSF drainage. In effect, a parenchymal ICP bolt in conjunction with a spinal drain can serve the same functions as an EVD.[15] Although intraparenchymal monitors are easily placed and can be disconnected during patient transport without the need for recalibration, they cannot accurately detect pressure alterations in deeper parts of the brain.[15,16] The devices are also associated with mechanical failure, fragility, and monitor malfunction. Table 22-1 describes advantages and disadvantages of ICP-monitoring devices.

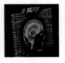 Prior to receiving an external ventriculostomy, the 56-year-old patient presented above undergoes CT angiography, which reveals a 10 mm × 8 mm × 6 mm pericallosal aneurysm. See Figure 22-5.

Will EVD placement increase this patient's risk of rebleeding?

EVD placement has been suggested to increase the risk of rebleeding in aSAH patients.[2,17,18] An abrupt drop in ICP and resultant increase in the transmural pressure on the aneurysm are thought to cause the rebleeding.[19] However, elevated risk of rebleeding in aSAH patients after EVD placement remains controversial, and no study to date has conclusively established a causal relationship.[20,21] Of note, patients requiring an EVD tend to present with worse HH grade, which in turn is associated with independent risk factors for rebleeding, such as larger aneurysm and dense SAH. Furthermore, conflicting results may be attributed to the failure to account for the following confounding variables: clinical grade, aneurysm treatment timing, duration of EVD placement during which the aneurysm remained untreated, and the interval between onset of SAH and EVD placement.[21,22] In the absence of conclusive data, the presence of an aneurysm should not be a contraindication for EVD placement in the setting of SAH-associated hydrocephalus. Nevertheless, ICP should be normalized gradually to minimize the theoretical risk of rebleeding.

Perioperative Surgical Care

Table 22-1. Characteristics of Intracranial Pressure (ICP)-Monitoring Devices

Device	Advantages	Disadvantages
Intraventricular catheter	Gold standard of accuracy	Most invasive
	Allows cerebrospinal fluid (CSF) drainage and sampling	Sometimes difficult to place in ventricle
	Allows ICP control	Cathether can become occluded by blood or tissue
	Inexpensive	Needs repositioning of transducer level with change in head position
		Potential infection
Fiberoptic probe	Can be placed in the subdural, subarachnoid, intraventricular, intraparenchymal spaces	Cannot be calibrated after placement
	Minimal artifact and drift	Breakage of the fiberoptic cable
	High resolution of waveform	Higher cost
	Less risk of infection	
	No need to adjust for patient position	
Subdural, epidural catheter/sensor	Least invasive	Increasing baseline drift over time, accuracy, reliability sometimes questionable
	Easily and quickly placed	Does not provide CSF sampling

(Adapted from Zhong J, Dujovny M, Park HK, Perez E, Perlin AR, Diaz FG. Advances in ICP monitoring techniques. Neurol Res. 2003;25:339-350.)

The patient's EVD is successfully placed. How should it be set and managed?

After the EVD is placed, the patient's head is elevated 30 degrees to reduce ICP and increase venous return. The drainage bag is fixed to a pole next to the bed, with "0" set exactly at the level of the external auditory meatus, which is approximately at the level of the foramen of Monro and, thus,

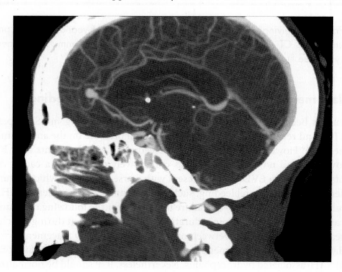

Figure 22-5.

the intraventricular catheter tip[5] (Figure 22-6). The drainage port can then be set at a certain level above or below this reference point ("0") with the valve open. Whenever the intraventricular pressure exceeds the level of the open drainage port, CSF should drain. For example, if the drainage port is set at 15 cm H_2O (15 cm above the "0" reference point), CSF should only drain when the intraventricular pressure exceeds 15 cm H_2O. The level of the drain can be titrated to the desired spillover pressure.

At our institution, we set the EVD open at 20 cm H_2O immediately after placement in SAH patients whose aneurysms remain unprotected to prevent overdrainage and the aforementioned theoretical

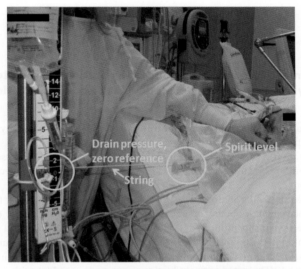

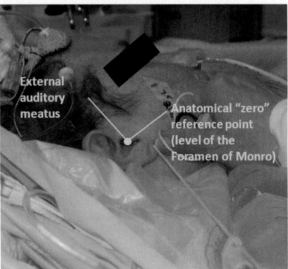

Figure 22-6. Proper EVD setup is demonstrated, with alignment of the "0" at the external auditory meatus.

creation of a transmural pressure gradient across the aneurysm wall. Postoperatively, once the aneurysm has been protected with clipping or coiling, we may lower the EVD to 5, 10, or 15 cm H_2O, depending on the patient's clinical status and degree of radiographic hydrocephalus. The lower the EVD is set, the more CSF is drained. An alternative approach is to drain off a fixed amount of CSF per unit of time up to a maximum of 20 mL per hour, which is roughly the rate of normal CSF production.[5] Overdrainage should be avoided as it can lead to acute subdural hemorrhage or even theoretical herniation.

In the setting of a posterior fossa tumor, EVDs are often placed intra-operatively.[5] CSF can be drained prior to opening the dura to relax the brain away from the dura. During the postoperative period, the EVD is usually set at a low height (eg, 10 mm H_2O) for 24 hours, and is progressively elevated over a 48-hour period and discontinued by 72 hours. Of note, both mm Hg and mm H_2O are commonly used for pressure measurements. Conversion factors between the two units are as following:

$$1 \text{ mm Hg} = 1.35 \text{ cm } H_2O$$

$$1 \text{ cm } H_2O = 0.735 \text{ mm Hg}$$

What are the most common infectious complications associated with EVDs? Should prophylactic antibiotic be used? What about antibiotic-coated catheters?

Soft tissue infection and ventriculitis are the most common ventriculostomy-related infections (VRI).[23,24] Less common are intraparenchymal abscesses, subdural empyema, and osteomyelitis. Steroid use and duration of catheter placement are known risk factors for EVD-associated infection,[25] and there have been no conclusive studies regarding the effects of systemic infection on the risk of neurologic infection.

While surgeons universally give one dose of antibiotic (ie, Ancef [cefazolin] 1 to 2 g) prior to skin incision for EVD placement, as in any operation, prophylactic antibiotic use for the entire duration the EVD is in place remains institution- and physician-dependent. As presented in Table 22-2, data for prophylactic antibiotic use remain conflicting and inconclusive. There is currently an ongoing clinical trial comparing perioperative prophylactic systemic antibiotics (PSA) (ampicillin/sulbactam and ceftriaxone) with EVDs coated with antibiotics versus prolonged PSA with a standard EVD. An interim report including analysis of 110 patients reported no viral respiratory infections.

How should an EVD be managed? How often should ICP be checked on the pressure transducer? What should the waveforms look like?

Once an EVD is placed, it should be checked regularly (eg, 2 to 4 hours) to ensure that it is functioning properly. The system should be assessed for patency, position, and reliability of ICP measurements. Any changes in ICP and neurologic examination also warrant close examination of the system. The drip chamber should be emptied into the drainage bag on a regular basis to keep the chamber from becoming full. Drain position should also be checked to make sure that it is at the prescribed level. Whenever the level of a patient's head is changed in relation to the drip chamber, the stopcock should be closed to drainage until the prescribed level is reestablished. Patients undergoing magnetic resonance imaging (MRI) or CT scan should have the stopcock closed for the duration of the scan because the drainage system generally cannot be set up on a pole at the appropriate level during a scan. Otherwise, if the physician intends for the EVD to be open and continuously draining CSF, it should only be clamped when measuring ICP, obtaining CSF samples, or following administration of intrathecal medications. Efforts should be made to minimize clamping time in EVD-dependent patients. If the physician suspects the monitor does not accurately reflect the ICP, he or she can test for a change in ICP by lowering the head of the bed or applying gentle pressure on the jugular veins bilaterally; either of these procedures should increase ICP.

ICP waveforms reflect transmission of systemic blood pressure to the intracranial compartment.[5] The waveforms consist of the arterial systolic pressure waves and the central venous A waves, which

Table 22-2. Clinical Trials that Evaluate the Effects of Prophylactic Antibiotics on the Incidence of External Ventricular Drain (EVD)–Associated Infection Rate

Reference No. (year)	Study type	No. of patients	Design	Duration	Infection rate (%)	P value
Blomstedt [26] (1985)	Retrospective	122	Placebo vs prolonged trimethoprim-sulfamethoxazole	Drainage duration	6.5 vs 23.3	< 0.001
Poon et al[27] (1998)	Retrospective	228	Perioperative ampicillin + sulbactam vs prolonged ampicillin, sulbactam, aztreonam	Perioperative vs drainage duration	3 vs 11	0.01
Zabramski et al[28] (2003)	Prospective, randomized, controlled	288	Standard EVD vs EVD coated with minocycline, rifampin	Drainage duration	36.7 vs 17.9	< 0.0012
Arabi et al[23] (2005)	Retrospective	99	No antibiotics vs prolonged cefazolin, ceftriaxone, cefuroxime	Drainage duration	29.3 vs 12.1	0.03
Lackner et al[29] (2008)	Retrospective	40	Standard EVD vs EVD coated with silver nanoparticles	Drainage duration	0 vs 25	< 0.05
Tamburrini et al[30] (2008)	Prospective, randomized, controlled	47	Standard EVD vs EVD coated with clindamycin, rifampicin	Drainage duration	31.8 vs 2.1	0.003

are, in turn, superimposed on slower respiratory variations.[5] ICP rises during cardiac systole due to distention of the intracranial arteriolar vasculatures, and during expiration because the concomitant pressure elevation in the superior vena cava reduces venous outflow from the cranium.[5,31]

Under normal circumstances, ICP elevation plateaus at a level at which further increase in the intracranial volume is balanced by CSF absorption. However, volume expansion beyond a critical point leads to a rapid and persistent increase in the ICP along with decreasing cerebral compliance.[32] In a normal, compliant brain, the first peak (P1 or the percussive wave), which represents the arterial pressure, is taller than the second peak (P2 or the tidal wave) which reflects brain rigidity. As the ICP rises to the level of arterial pressure, the waveforms demonstrate prominent arterial pressure waves, with the tidal wave becoming taller than the percussive wave as the brain loses compliance.[5,33]

In 1960, Lundberg described the three ICP wave patterns outlined in Table 22-3. Like ICP measurements, assessment of the waveforms should be evaluated with the stopcock turned off to the drain but open to the pressure transducer.

The nursing staff reports that CSF has not drained in the past 2 hours and the EVD system appears to be blocked. What should be done?

If the EVD is open to drainage, the nursing staff should monitor and record CSF output every 1 to 2 hours. The amount of CSF drained in a day is typically about 250 mL, and although uncommon, can reach up to 450 to 700 mL if the patient fails to absorb any CSF.[5]

If no CSF has drained, the waveform is dampened or lost, or blockage is suspected, one should consider the algorithm in Figure 22-7.

Perioperative Surgical Care

Table 22-3. Characteristics of Lundberg Waves

	Description/Significance
Lundberg A (plateau) waves	Mean wave > 50 mm Hg. Entire wave lasts 5-20 min, then returns to slightly elevated baseline. Always considered pathologic. Occurs when ICP exceeds the limits of cerebral compliance; reflects ischemia.
Lundberg B waves (pressure pulses)	Mean wave > 20-50 mm Hg. The wave oscillates at a frequency of 0.5-2.0 waves/min and the entire wave lasts up to 3 min. May be due to respiratory changes and variations in cerebral blood flow. Can be seen in sleep. Suggests that Lundberg A waves may form.
Lundberg C waves (preterminal wave)	Mean wave < 20 mm Hg. The wave oscillates at a frequency of 4-8 waves/min. Have been seen in healthy subjects and may represent transmission of cyclic variation in systemic blood pressure to ICP. High amplitude may be preterminal.

Abbreviation: ICP, intracranial pressure. *(Adapted from Siddiqi J. Neurosurgical Intensive Care. New York, NY: Thieme; 2008.)*

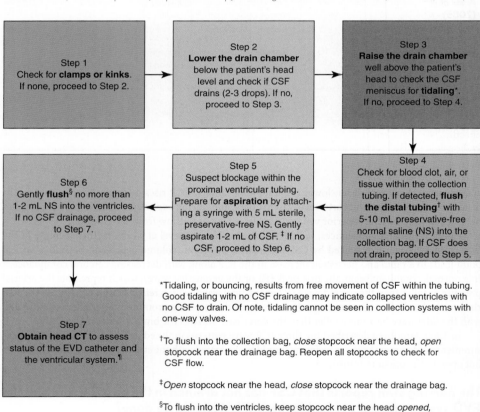

Step 1
Check for **clamps or kinks**. If none, proceed to Step 2.

Step 2
Lower the drain chamber below the patient's head level and check if CSF drains (2-3 drops). If no, proceed to Step 3.

Step 3
Raise the drain chamber well above the patient's head to check the CSF meniscus for **tidaling***. If no, proceed to Step 4.

Step 6
Gently **flush**§ no more than 1-2 mL NS into the ventricles. If no CSF drainage, proceed to Step 7.

Step 5
Suspect blockage within the proximal ventricular tubing. Prepare for **aspiration** by attaching a syringe with 5 mL sterile, preservative-free NS. Gently aspirate 1-2 mL of CSF. ‡ If no CSF, proceed to Step 6.

Step 4
Check for blood clot, air, or tissue within the collection tubing. If detected, **flush the distal tubing**† with 5-10 mL preservative-free normal saline (NS) into the collection bag. If CSF does not drain, proceed to Step 5.

Step 7
Obtain head CT to assess status of the EVD catheter and the ventricular system.¶

*Tidaling, or bouncing, results from free movement of CSF within the tubing. Good tidaling with no CSF drainage may indicate collapsed ventricles with no CSF to drain. Of note, tidaling cannot be seen in collection systems with one-way valves.

†To flush into the collection bag, *close* stopcock near the head, *open* stopcock near the drainage bag. Reopen all stopcocks to check for CSF flow.

‡*Open* stopcock near the head, *close* stopcock near the drainage bag.

§To flush into the ventricles, keep stopcock near the head *opened*, stopcock near the drainage bag *closed*.

¶Sterility is critical to minimize the risk of ventriculitis.

Figure 22-7. Algorithm for troubleshooting external ventricular drain (EVD) blockage. CSF, cerebrospinal fluid; CT, computed tomography; EVD, external ventricular drain.

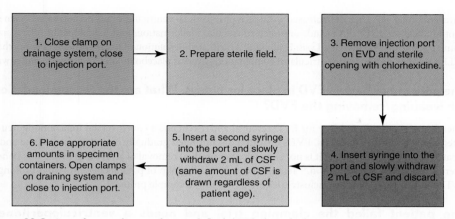

Figure 22-8. Steps for sampling cerebrospinal fluid (CSF) through the external ventricular drain (EVD) injection port.

How should CSF be drawn from the EVD access ports? How often?

CSF should be drawn to screen for infection in a febrile patient, to assess CSF protein level prior to ventriculoperitoneal shunt placement, to measure CSF levels of intraventricularly administered antibiotics (every 24 hours), and to check antibiotic response in patients with CSF infection (every 24 hours).

Generally, routine prospective sampling of CSF is not advised as it can increase the risk of infection.[25] Routine analysis of CSF may not predict EVD-associated infection, and no specific or reproducible changes in CSF parameters, including leukocytes, pleocytosis, and protein/glucose levels, are definitively predictive of infection.[34] Thus, CSF analysis should be performed only when there is a clinical suspicion of infection.[35] Figure 22-8 outlines how to sample CSF using EVD.

What are the indications for intraventricular administration of medications?

As for intraventricular antibiotic administration, no randomized controlled trial has been performed to determine its efficacy in treating central nervous system (CNS) device–associated infection. Owing to potential toxicity and difficult delivery, intraventricular administration of antibiotics is generally considered when conventional intravenous therapy has failed to sterilize the CSF, infection is caused by highly resistant organisms that are only sensitive to antibiotics with poor CSF penetration, and the device cannot be removed.[36,37]

No antibiotic has been approved by the Food and Drug Administration (FDA) for intraventricular use. The use of vancomycin and gentamicin has been reported more than any other antibiotic in the literature, and others are mostly limited to case reports.[38-40] Cephalosporins and penicillins should not be given intraventricularly because of significant neurotoxicity.[36,41] Intraventricular antibiotic dosing has not been standardized, and dosing has been guided by calculation of the "inhibitory quotient," which can be determined by dividing the trough CSF antibiotic concentration by the minimum inhibitory concentration (MIC) of the drug for the isolate; it should not exceed 10 to 20.[42]

Administration of intraventricular thrombolysis using tissue plasminogen activator (tPA), for example, is considered in patients with a significant amount of intraventricular hemorrhage (IVH) that will either clot the EVD repeatedly or impair the patient's own CSF outflow for a prolonged period.[43] Although unproven by any well-designed study, more rapid resolution of IVH through thrombolytic administration should theoretically reduce the complications associated with prolonged EVD usage in the ICU and aim to reduce the incidence of shunt-requiring hydrocephalus.[43] However, theoretical risks associated with

Perioperative Surgical Care

intraventricular tPA include increased incidence of infectious ventriculitis and hemorrhage.[44] General contraindications to IV tPA include unprotected vascular malformations and coagulopathy. A large, randomized controlled study, Clot Lysis: Evaluating Accelerated Resolution of Intraventricular Hemorrhage (CLEAR-IVH), testing intraventricular recombinant tPA versus placebo in IVH, is currently under way.

The patient has had an EVD in place for 6 days. What are the recommendations for weaning/removing the EVD?

There is no standard guideline for EVD removal and it remains a controversial topic among neurointensivists and neurosurgeons. EVDs are often discontinued gradually over days toward the end of a patient's ICU stay. However, it is not clear whether gradual removal of an EVD provides any benefit over more rapid discontinuation.[45] In addition, which subgroup of patients benefits from prolonged EVD placement remains inconclusive. Figure 22-9 shows a sample protocol.

The patient failed the clamping trial and needs a ventriculoperitoneal shunt (VPS). What are the known risk factors for shunt dependency following aneurysmal SAH? Does EVD increase one's risk of becoming shunt dependent? When is it not ideal to convert an EVD to a VPS?

Aneurysmal SAH (aSAH) is the leading cause of chronic hydrocephalus requiring VPS placement in adults, affecting approximately 35% of all cases.[46] Approximately 10% to 20% of these patients will require permanent CSF diversion with a shunt.[47,48] Obstruction of the arachnoid granulations by blood products, fibrosis of the leptomeninges and arachnoid granulations, adhesion formation within the ventricular system, and resulting alterations of CSF dynamics have all been suggested as possible mechanisms. Factors associated with the development of chronic hydrocephalus following aSAH include old age, high HH grade, female sex, acute hydrocephalus, posterior circulation aneurysm, and aneurysm size greater than 2.5 cm.[46,49,50] A high CSF protein level and large third ventricle diameter at EVD challenge may also predict challenge failure.[51] A number of retrospective studies

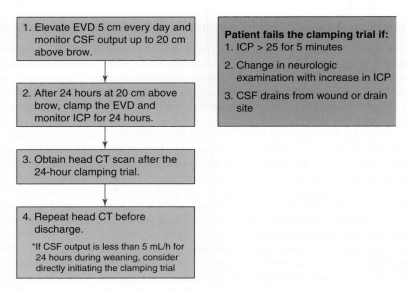

1. Elevate EVD 5 cm every day and monitor CSF output up to 20 cm above brow.

↓

2. After 24 hours at 20 cm above brow, clamp the EVD and monitor ICP for 24 hours.

↓

3. Obtain head CT scan after the 24-hour clamping trial.

↓

4. Repeat head CT before discharge.

*If CSF output is less than 5 mL/h for 24 hours during weaning, consider directly initiating the clamping trial

Patient fails the clamping trial if:
1. ICP > 25 for 5 minutes
2. Change in neurologic examination with increase in ICP
3. CSF drains from wound or drain site

Figure 22-9. Guideline for evaluating patients for external ventricular drain (EVD) removal; CSF, cerebrospinal fluid; CT, computed tomography; ICP, intracranial hemorrhage.

reported that prolonged or continuous CSF drainage is associated with an increased risk of chronic hydrocephalus.[52,53] However, causality of the association remains inconclusive.

EVD to VPS conversion is generally not performed in the presence of signs of infection (ie, fever), at the peak of vasospasm or elevated transcranial Doppler readings, and on the same day as percutaneous endoscopic gastrostomy (PEG) tube placement. Significantly increased CSF protein (greater than 200) and red blood cell (RBC) counts are thought to increase CSF viscosity and thus the likelihood of shunt blockage and malfunction.[51,52] However, proteinaceous and hemorrhagic CSF are common among SAH, IVH, and trauma patients requiring a VPS, and the decision to convert a temporary EVD to permanent VPS is left to the discretion of the neurointensivist and neurosurgeon.

Can the EVD site be used for VPS placement?

There are no clear guidelines on technique and placement site when converting an EVD to a permanent shunt in aSAH patients. A new site is routinely established for shunt placement in order to avoid the theoretical risk of infection from the previous incision and EVD. Although further investigation is warranted, there are data to suggest an EVD can be safely converted to a permanent shunt using the existing EVD site, particularly with the use of prophylactic antibiotics and antibiotic-coated catheters.[52]

! CRITICAL CONSIDERATIONS

- EVDs provide an accurate and reliable means to continuously or intermittently monitor and control ICP. EVDs are used in a variety of conditions associated with hydrocephalus and elevated ICP, such as SAH, posterior fossa or ventricular tumors, intraventricular or posterior fossa hemorrhages, trauma, meningitis, subdural hematoma, and ventricular cysts.
- EVD placement should be generally considered in aSAH patients who demonstrate clinical or radiologic deterioration or have an unreliable neurologic examination. Patients who present comatose or severely lethargic are almost universally considered for emergent ventriculostomy. Minimal improvement in neurologic status despite normalization of the ICP in these patients may point to other etiologies such as seizure, medication effect, or metabolic derangement and prompts immediate investigation.
- Although an EVD is thought to offer the most accurate ICP measurement, it may be difficult to place in the setting of significant mass effect or narrow/collapsed ventricles. In such cases, an ICP parenchymal bolt can be used to measure ICP, and spinal CSF drainage can be used to remove CSF and decrease ICP in patients with communicating hydrocephalus.
- EVD placement has been suggested to increase the risk of rebleeding in aSAH patients. However, an elevated risk of rebleeding in aSAH patients after EVD placement remains controversial and no study to date has conclusively established their causal relationship.
- Although one dose of preincision antibiotic is almost universally given prior to EVD or ICP monitor placement, the utility of prophylactic antibiotics for the duration the device is in place remains controversial. Therefore, prophylactic antibiotic use is at the treating physician's discretion.
- Generally, routine prospective sampling of CSF is not advised as it can increase the risk of infection. Routine analysis of CSF may not predict EVD-associated infection, and no specific or reproducible changes in CSF parameters, including leukocytes, pleocytosis, and protein/glucose levels, are predictive of infection. Thus, CSF analysis should be performed only when there is a clinical suspicion of infection.

Perioperative Surgical Care

- EVDs are often discontinued gradually after serial elevation of the drain level and a 24-hour "clamping trial." However, there is no clear evidence to suggest that gradual removal of EVD provides any benefit over more rapid discontinuation, or vice versa.
- EVD to VPS conversion is generally not performed in the presence of signs of infection (ie, fever), at the peak of vasospasm or elevated transcranial Doppler readings, and on the same day as PEG tube placement. Significantly elevated CSF protein and RBC counts may also influence the decision to convert to permanent VPS.

REFERENCES

1. Kusske JA, Turner PT, Ojemann GA, Harris AB. Ventriculostomy for the treatment of acute hydrocephalus following subarachnoid hemorrhage. *J Neurosurg.* 1973;38:591-595.
2. Hasan D, Vermeulen M, Wijdicks EF, Hijdra A, van Gijn J. Management problems in acute hydrocephalus after subarachnoid hemorrhage. *Stroke.* 1989;20:747-753.
3. Corsten L, Raja A, Guppy K, et al. Contemporary management of subarachnoid hemorrhage and vasospasm: the UIC experience. *Surg Neurol.* 2001;56:140-148; discussion 148-150.
4. Bederson JB, Connolly ES, Jr, Batjer HH, et al. Guidelines for the management of aneurysmal subarachnoid hemorrhage: a statement for healthcare professionals from a special writing group of the Stroke Council, American Heart Association. *Stroke.* 2009;40:994-1025.
5. Greenberg MS, Arredondo N. *Handbook of Neurosurgery.* 6th ed. New York, NY: Thieme; 2006.
6. Mack WJ, King RG, Ducruet AF, et al. Intracranial pressure following aneurysmal subarachnoid hemorrhage: monitoring practices and outcome data. *Neurosurg Focus.* 2003;14:e3.
7. Steinke D, Weir B, Disney L. Hydrocephalus following aneurysmal subarachnoid haemorrhage. *Neurol Res.* 1987;9:3-9.
8. Tomei G, Gaini SM, Giovanelli M, Rampini P, Granata G, Villani R. Intracranial pressure in subarachnoid hemorrhage. Preliminary report in 36 cases. *J Neurosurg Sci.* 1981;25:57-66.
9. Gambardella G, De Blasi F, Caruso G, Zema A, Turiano F, Collufio D. Intracranial pressure, cerebral perfusion pressure, and SPECT in the management of patients with SAH Hunt and Hess grades I-II. *Acta Neurochir Suppl.* 1998;71:215-218.
10. O'Neill BR, Velez DA, Braxton EE, Whiting D, Oh MY. A survey of ventriculostomy and intracranial pressure monitor placement practices. *Surg Neurol.* 2008;70:268-273; discussion 273.
11. Bekar A, Dogan S, Abas F, et al. Risk factors and complications of intracranial pressure monitoring with a fiberoptic device. *J Clin Neurosci.* 2009;16:236-240.
12. Gardner PA, Engh J, Atteberry D, Moossy JJ. Hemorrhage rates after external ventricular drain placement. *J Neurosurg.* 2009;110:1021-1025.
13. Clark WC, Muhlbauer MS, Lowrey R, Hartman M, Ray MW, Watridge CB. Complications of intracranial pressure monitoring in trauma patients. *Neurosurgery.* 1989;25:20-24.
14. Ehtisham A, Taylor S, Bayless L, Klein MW, Janzen JM. Placement of external ventricular drains and intracranial pressure monitors by neurointensivists. *Neurocrit Care.* 2009;10:241-247.
15. Zhong J, Dujovny M, Park HK, Perez E, Perlin AR, Diaz FG. Advances in ICP monitoring techniques. *Neurol Res.* 2003;25:339-350.
16. Mollman HD, Rockswold GL, Ford SE. A clinical comparison of subarachnoid catheters to ventriculostomy and subarachnoid bolts: a prospective study. *J Neurosurg.* 1988;68:737-741.
17. Pare L, Delfino R, Leblanc R. The relationship of ventricular drainage to aneurysmal rebleeding. *J Neurosurg.* 1992;76:422-427.
18. van Gijn J, Hijdra A, Wijdicks EF, Vermeulen M, van Crevel H. Acute hydrocephalus after aneurysmal subarachnoid hemorrhage. *J Neurosurg.* 1985;63:355-362.
19. Hasan D, Lindsay KW, Vermeulen M. Treatment of acute hydrocephalus after subarachnoid hemorrhage with serial lumbar puncture. *Stroke.* 1991;22:190-194.
20. Roitberg BZ, Khan N, Alp MS, Hersonskey T, Charbel FT, Ausman JI. Bedside external ventricular drain placement for the treatment of acute hydrocephalus. *Br J Neurosurg.* 2001;15:324-327.
21. Hellingman CA, van den Bergh WM, Beijer IS, et al. Risk of rebleeding after treatment of acute hydrocephalus in patients with aneurysmal subarachnoid hemorrhage. *Stroke.* 2007;38:96-99.

22. Fountas KN, Kapsalaki EZ, Machinis T, Karampelas I, Smisson HF, Robinson JS. Review of the literature regarding the relationship of rebleeding and external ventricular drainage in patients with subarachnoid hemorrhage of aneurysmal origin. *Neurosurg Rev.* 2006;29:14-18; discussion 19-20.

23. Arabi Y, Memish ZA, Balkhy HH, et al. Ventriculostomy-associated infections: incidence and risk factors. *Am J Infect Control.* 2005;33:137-143.

24. Dettenkofer M, Ebner W, Els T, et al. Surveillance of nosocomial infections in a neurology intensive care unit. *J Neurol.* 2001;248:959-964.

25. Hoefnagel D, Dammers R, Ter Laak-Poort MP, Avezaat CJ. Risk factors for infections related to external ventricular drainage. *Acta Neurochir (Wien).* 2008;150:209-214; discussion 214.

26. Blomstedt GC. Results of trimethoprim-sulfamethoxazole prophylaxis in ventriculostomy and shunting procedures. A double-blind randomized trial. *J Neurosurg.* 1985;62:694-697.

27. Poon WS, Ng S, Wai S. CSF antibiotic prophylaxis for neurosurgical patients with ventriculostomy: a randomised study. *Acta Neurochir Suppl.* 1998;71:146-148.

28. Zabramski JM, Whiting D, Darouiche RO, et al. Efficacy of antimicrobial-impregnated external ventricular drain catheters: a prospective, randomized, controlled trial. *J Neurosurg.* 2003;98:725-730.

29. Lackner P, Beer R, Broessner G, et al. Efficacy of silver nanoparticles-impregnated external ventricular drain catheters in patients with acute occlusive hydrocephalus. *Neurocrit Care.* 2008;8:360-365.

30. Tamburrini G, Massimi L, Caldarelli M, Di Rocco C. Antibiotic-impregnated external ventricular drainage and third ventriculostomy in the management of hydrocephalus associated with posterior cranial fossa tumours. *Acta Neurochir (Wien).* 2008;150:1049-1055; discussion 1055-1056.

31. Foltz EL, Blanks JP, Yonemura K. CSF pulsatility in hydrocephalus: respiratory effect on pulse wave slope as an indicator of intracranial compliance. *Neurol Res.* 1990;12:67-74.

32. Czosnyka M, Czosnyka Z, Momjian S, Pickard JD. Cerebrospinal fluid dynamics. *Physiol Meas.* 2004;25:R51-R76.

33. Siddiqi J. *Neurosurgical Intensive Care.* New York, NY: Thieme; 2008.

34. Beer R, Lackner P, Pfausler B, Schmutzhard E. Nosocomial ventriculitis and meningitis in neurocritical care patients. *J Neurol.* 2008;255(11):1617-1624.

35. Hader WJ, Steinbok P. The value of routine cultures of the cerebrospinal fluid in patients with external ventricular drains. *Neurosurgery.* 2000;46:1149-1153; discussion 1153-1155.

36. Wen DY, Bottini AG, Hall WA, Haines SJ. Infections in neurologic surgery. The intraventricular use of antibiotics. *Neurosurg Clin N Am.* 1992;3:343-354.

37. Sutherland GE, Palitang EG, Marr JJ, Luedke SL. Sterilization of Ommaya reservoir by instillation of vancomycin. *Am J Med.* 1981;71:1068-1070.

38. Segal-Maurer S, Mariano N, Qavi A, Urban C, Rahal JJ Jr. Successful treatment of ceftazidime-resistant *Klebsiella pneumoniae* ventriculitis with intravenous meropenem and intraventricular polymyxin B: case report and review. *Clin Infect Dis.* 1999;28:1134-1138.

39. Swayne R, Rampling A, Newsom SW. Intraventricular vancomycin for treatment of shunt-associated ventriculitis. *J Antimicrob Chemother.* 1987;19:249-253.

40. Cruciani M, Navarra A, Di Perri G, et al. Evaluation of intraventricular teicoplanin for the treatment of neurosurgical shunt infections. *Clin Infect Dis.* 1992;15:285-289.

41. Manzella JP, Paul RL, Butler IL. CNS toxicity associated with intraventricular injection of cefazolin. Report of three cases. *J Neurosurg.* 1988;68:970-971.

42. Tunkel AR, Hartman BJ, Kaplan SL, et al. Practice guidelines for the management of bacterial meningitis. *Clin Infect Dis.* 2004;39:1267-1284.

43. Nyquist P, LeDroux S, Geocadin R. Thrombolytics in intraventricular hemorrhage. *Curr Neurol Neurosci Rep.* 2007;7:522-528.

44. Lapointe M, Haines S. Fibrinolytic therapy for intraventricular hemorrhage in adults. *Cochrane Database Syst Rev.* 2002:CD003692.

45. Klopfenstein JD, Kim LJ, Feiz-Erfan I, et al. Comparison of rapid and gradual weaning from external ventricular drainage in patients with aneurysmal subarachnoid hemorrhage: a prospective randomized trial. *J Neurosurg.* 2004;100:225-229.

46. Komotar RJ, Hahn DK, Kim GH, et al. The impact of microsurgical fenestration of the lamina terminalis on shunt-dependent hydrocephalus and vasospasm after aneurysmal subarachnoid hemorrhage. *Neurosurgery.* 2008;62:123-132; discussion 132-134.

47. Auer LM, Mokry M. Disturbed cerebrospinal fluid circulation after subarachnoid hemorrhage and acute aneurysm surgery. *Neurosurgery.* 1990;26:804-808; discussion 808-809.

48. Joakimsen O, Mathiesen EB, Monstad P, Selseth B. CSF hydrodynamics after subarachnoid hemorrhage. *Acta Neurol Scand.* 1987;75:319-327.

49. Rincon F, Gordon E, Starke RM, et al. Predictors of long-term shunt-dependent hydrocephalus after aneurysmal subarachnoid hemorrhage. *J Neurosurg.* 2010;113:774-780.

50. Dorai Z, Hynan LS, Kopitnik TA, Samson D. Factors related to hydrocephalus after aneurysmal subarachnoid hemorrhage. *Neurosurgery.* 2003;52: 763-769; discussion 769-771.

51. Chan M, Alaraj A, Calderon M, et al. Prediction of ventriculoperitoneal shunt dependency in patients with aneurysmal subarachnoid hemorrhage. *J Neurosurg.* 2009;110:44-49.

52. Rammos S, Klopfenstein J, Augspurger L, et al. Conversion of external ventricular drains to ventriculoperitoneal shunts after aneurysmal subarachnoid hemorrhage: effects of site and protein/red blood cell counts on shunt infection and malfunction. *J Neurosurg.* 2008;109:1001-1004.

53. Hirashima Y, Kurimoto M, Hayashi N, et al. Duration of cerebrospinal fluid drainage in patients with aneurysmal subarachnoid hemorrhage for prevention of symptomatic vasospasm and late hydrocephalus. *Neurol Med Chir (Tokyo).* 2005;45:177-182; discussion 182-183.

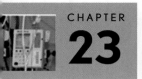

CHAPTER

23

Carotid Revascularization and EC-IC Bypass

Christopher Kellner, MD
Matthew Piazza, BA
Geoffrey Appelboom, MD
E. Sander Connolly, MD

The patient is an 83-year-old, right-handed woman with a past history of type 2 diabetes, hypertension, hyperlipidemia, and asthma who presents 10 days after experiencing an episode of right eye visual loss and left-sided hemiplegia lasting approximately 5 minutes, with spontaneous resolution. Given the transient nature of her symptoms, the patient did not seek medical care, but saw her primary care physician several days later, who subsequently ordered a magnetic resonance image/magnetic resonance angiogram (MRI/MRA) for further evaluation. She was sent to the emergency department (ED) when the scan was notable for subacute infarct in the right frontal cortex (Figure 23-1) and an absence of flow-related signal in the right common carotid bifurcation, highly suggestive of carotid stenosis (Figure 23-1). In the ED, the patient was in no acute distress, her vitals were stable, and her physical examination was notable for mild left facial asymmetry but an otherwise benign neurologic examination.

What is the next step in the management and workup of this patient?

The patient's imaging and physical examination findings are highly suggestive of an ischemic stroke in the right frontal cortex secondary to thromboembolism from a right carotid stenotic atherosclerotic lesion (while this patient's MRA is highly suspicious for carotid stenosis as the cause of the ischemic stroke, an electrocardiogram [ECG] and transesophageal echocardiogram should be ordered to rule out cardiac causes as well). Since this patient is well outside the time window for intravenous thrombolysis, she should be started on acetylsalicylic acid (ASA) 325 mg tid for secondary prevention of stroke and should receive further diagnostics for her suspected carotid artery disease.

Extracranial, large-vessel stenosis should be evaluated by at least two of the following three noninvasive modalities to determine the extent and degree of stenosis: MRA, computed tomographic angiography (CTA), and carotid Doppler ultrasound. Carotid Doppler ultrasound is a quick, inexpensive, and portable modality that is easily performed at the bedside and assesses stenosis via focal measurements of flow velocity; however, the quality of the study is highly dependent on the physician/technician. MRA, which can be performed with or without contrast, does not expose patients to radiation and has demonstrated greater discriminatory power than ultrasound in assessing high-grade stenosis.[1] CTA, while an excellent modality for identifying carotid occlusion, has less discriminatory power in identifying high-grade stenosis.[2] If stenting is considered as a possible treatment

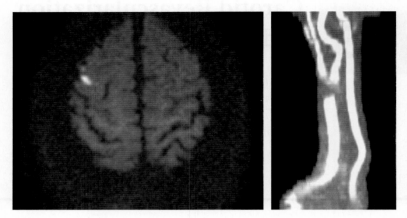

Figure 23-1. Magnetic resonance imaging/magnetic resonance angiography of patient demonstrating cortical infarct in frontal lobe (*left*) and loss of signal at the level of right carotid bifurcation (*right*).

modality, the patient can be evaluated with angiography, the gold standard for evaluating carotid disease, for possible intervention. However, it is a costly and an invasive procedure and is associated with risk of contrast nephropathy, especially in patients with underlying renal disease. This patient underwent carotid ultrasound, which demonstrated 80% to 90% stenosis of the right internal carotid artery (ICA) bifurcation, with confirmatory CTA showing severe atherosclerotic disease of the right carotid artery at the level of the bifurcation and a patent right ICA with 70% stenosis (Figure 23-2). Given this patient has symptomatic, high-grade stenosis 70% or greater present on at least two imaging modalities, neurosurgical intervention is indicated.[3]

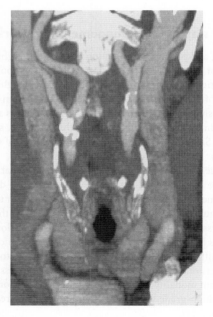

Figure 23-2. Computed tomographic angiography of patient showing significant calcification and high-grade stenosis of the right carotid bifurcation.

What intervention is most appropriate in this patient, carotid endarterectomy or endovascular stenting?

Carotid atherosclerotic disease can be treated surgically with carotid endarterectomy (CEA) or with carotid angioplasty and stenting (CAS). The evidence from randomized clinical trials comparing CEA with best medical management in both symptomatic and asymptomatic patients is substantial. The North American Symptomatic Carotid Endarterectomy Trial (NASCET) for surgical intervention found that CEA significantly reduced the risk of further stroke (17% at 2 years) and death (7% at 2 years) for patients with stenosis at or greater than 70%.[3] The Asymptomatic Carotid Artery Stenosis Trial (ACAS) found that patients with greater than 60% stenosis had a 6% reduction in risk of stroke or death at 5 years.[4] Since the results of these major trials, carotid stenting has surfaced as an alternative to surgery, especially in those patients who are poor surgical candidates.

The recent results from the Carotid Revascularization Endarterectomy versus Stenting Trial (CREST)[5] compared endovascular and surgical techniques in both symptomatic and asymptomatic patients and found comparable rates of the primary outcome measure of death, stroke, or myocardial infarction in the perioperative period and any ipsilateral stroke at 4 years, although perioperative stroke and myocardial infarction occurred more frequently in the stenting and CEA groups, respectively. However, the results of this trial should be interpreted with caution. The perioperative stroke but not myocardial infarction was associated with worse health status at 1 year in quality of life assessment, suggesting that the primary end point may have not been appropriately weighted to account for the greater morbidity rate associated with perioperative stroke and may have biased results in favor of stenting. Moreover, while rigorous credentialing of endovascular surgeons in this study is certainly a major strength of the design, such high standards may be possible only at highly specialized institutions. Hence, while carotid stenting is a suitable alternative in patients who are poor operative candidates, CEA remains the gold standard treatment for high-grade stenosis.

This patient has a number of cardiovascular risk factors and a possible history of angina, potentially placing her at high risk for surgery. However, carotid stenting may be difficult to accomplish safely and effectively in this patient for the following reasons. First, CTA demonstrates a significant amount of calcification at the bifurcation, which makes both the degree of stenosis and the anatomic margins difficult to evaluate. Second, the lesion of the location involves the bifurcation, which will complicate balloon positioning and inflation as well as stent deployment. Third, the proximal ICA has a tortuous appearance, which combined with the significant calcification creates a technically challenging situation for the endovascular surgeon and increases the risk of arterial trauma/dissection and thromboembolism. Hence, CEA is the best intervention for this patient, pending, of course, medical clearance by a cardiologist. She should also be continued on ASA up until surgery.[6]

Perioperative Surgical Care

This patient was subsequently seen by the cardiology service, who found no evidence for coronary artery disease based on history and physical examination and deemed her suitable for surgery. The patient remained on ASA 325 mg tid for 2 days and then proceeded to the operating room for CEA. The patient was placed under general anesthesia, intubated, and her neck was prepped and draped in the sterile fashion. A linear incision was made along the anterior border of the sternocleidomastoid muscle, and the usual neck dissection resulted in identification of the right common, external, and internal carotid arteries. The patient was heparinized and her blood pressure was elevated greater than 200 mm Hg. The segments of the carotid were cross-clamped, an arteriotomy was performed; the atherosclerotic plaque was identified and dissected from the intima, with copious irrigation with heparinized saline throughout the process. The arteriotomy was closed uneventfully, the arteries were unclamped, the systolic blood pressure (SBP) was lowered to 150s, and Doppler confirmed patency of the vessel. Of note, no electrocardiographic (EEG) changes were observed throughout the operation. The skin was closed, the patient was extubated and returned to the neurologic intensive care unit (NICU) for further management.

How should the patient be managed in the ICU postoperatively?

Management during the postoperative period after endarterectomy should focus on blood pressure control and early detection and management of complications of endarterectomy. Table 23-1 lists rates of complications after CEA. In the postoperative period after endarterectomy, blood pressure may be especially labile during the first 24 hours owing to changes in flow and pressure at the carotid sinus. Such variation in blood pressure can result in undesirable stress on the myocardium, especially in patients with multiple cardiovascular risk factors and underlying coronary artery disease, hence the importance of an appropriate preoperative workup. Even in the absence of blood pressure instability, it is our routine to monitor patients with serial troponin assessments for the first 24 hours together with continuous ECG and an arterial line. In the absence of other concerns, we aim to keep the blood pressure about 10 points below the baseline mean arterial pressure (MAP) as long as the ECG and troponin levels are normal. The other reason to maintain blood pressure in this range is to guard against hyperperfusion syndrome. This generally occurs in patients with impaired autoregulation and very tight stenosis with poor collaterals. It may present with headache, mental status change, seizures, or, in the worst case, hemorrhage. Patients at high risk for hyperperfusion syndrome or with early signs can be evaluated with transcranial doppler (TCD), MR perfusion, or CT perfusion to aid in diagnosis and management. Avoiding postoperative hypertension may also prevent untoward disruption of the arteriotomy site, especially in the case of patched repairs,

Table 23-1. Rates of Complications After Carotid Endarterectomy (CEA)

Type of complication	Frequency (%)	Pathophysiology
Acute coronary syndrome	0.5-2.3[3,5,7]	Hemodynamic disturbances following CEA in the setting of preexisting coronary atherosclerotic disease
Ischemic stroke	2.1-5.5[3,5,7]	Thromboembolism, carotid occlusion, hemodynamic disturbances
Seizure	0.8[8]	Hyperperfusion syndrome, emboli, intracerebral hemorrhage
Intracerebral hemorrhage	0.1-0.8[9,10]	Hyperperfusion syndrome in previously ischemic regions
Nerve injury	5.1 (0.5 at 4-month follow-up)[11]	Compression from retraction or direct injury; hypoglossal nerve injury the most common (1.6%) followed by marginal mandibular (1.0%) and recurrent laryngeal (1.0%)
Neck hematoma	1.7-1.9 requiring surgical intervention[12,13]	Postoperative bleeding; give protamine to reduce bleeding complications

and may play a role in preventing expanding neck hematoma, which rarely requires reoperation. In those patients without contraindications (eg, asthma, chronic obstructive pulmonary disease [COPD]), intravenous β blockers are an excellent first-line approach, but calcium channel blockers may also be used. In contrast, relative hypotension is to be particularly avoided in patients with preexisting microangiopathy such as those with severe long-standing hypertension and/or diabetes mellitus. In terms of agents of choice, phenylephrine may be used as a first-line therapy for relative hypotension and nitroprusside or dopamine added as needed.

In addition to careful management of blood pressure, repeated focused neurologic examinations should be frequent following endarterectomy for early detection of cerebral ischemia/stroke in addition to other surgery-related complications. In particular, expected deficits in the distribution of the ICA operated on are of importance (loss of vision in ipsilateral eye, contralateral motor/sensory disturbances, speech disturbances if operated artery supplies dominant hemisphere). Signs of injury to cranial nerves encountered during surgery should also be monitored: deviation of tongue to ipsilateral side for hypoglossal nerve injury; hoarseness for recurrent laryngeal nerve; lip asymmetry from mandibular nerve injury. The operative site should be examined frequently for neck hematoma. Antiplatelet agents, usually aspirin 325 mg, should be resumed immediately the morning following surgery.[14] Dipyridamole can also be given instead of aspirin, although the combination of medications has not proved beneficial in reducing the rate of restenosis after endarterectomy.[15]

 The patient is a 58-year-old, right-handed man with a past history of hypertension and hyperlipidemia who presents after several episodes of left-sided weakness that completely resolve after several minutes. Doppler ultrasound of the carotid arteries reveal 80% stenosis of the right ICA just distal to the bifurcation and 30% stenosis of the left ICA at the level of the bifurcation. MRA confirmed stenosis of the right ICA between 70% and 80%. The patient was subsequently scheduled for CEA. The surgery was uneventful; however, prior to extubation, the patient was noted to have a dense hemiplegia on the left side.

What is the next best course of action?

This patient underwent an uneventful CEA on the right side without any obvious intraoperative EEG changes and confirmed patency of arteriotomy site by Doppler ultrasound just prior to skin closure. Upon emergence from anesthesia, however, the patient developed a new neurologic deficit consistent with the distribution of the right ICA. The differential diagnosis for this patient's new left hemiplegia includes thromboembolism from the endarterectomized surface to a distal vessel, ischemia from prolonged cross-clamping, or in situ thrombosis at the surgical site; rarely, hyperperfusion may be a cause of neurologic symptoms in the immediate postoperative period. In this patient, given the absence of concerning EEG changes throughout the operation, ischemia secondary to hypoperfusion from cross-clamping is unlikely. Postoperative thrombosis of the endarterectomy site is the most common cause of major postoperative transient ischemic attack (TIA)/stroke[14] and should be emergently investigated using intraoperative angiography if readily available, although if suspicion is high for occlusion, reexploration should not be delayed. In addition, the patient should be given pressors (phenylephrine) to elevate blood pressure (preferably SBP in approximately 180-200 mm Hg range) as well as ample fluids to assist in the latter and to reduce blood viscosity. Heparinization and potentially long-term anticoagulation may be considered to prevent further thrombosis, although further studies are needed to evaluate the role of anticoagulation after postoperative thrombosis.

Angiography demonstrated complete occlusion of the right ICA. The patient was immediately prepped, draped, and dosed with heparin, blood pressure was elevated, and the skin incision and arteriotomy site were promptly reopened to reveal a large thrombus in the lumen. The thrombus was removed, and the arteriotomy was once again closed. Repeat angiography demonstrated successful revascularization; the patient was dosed again with heparin and started on a heparin drip. Upon emergence from anesthesia, the patient was noted to have resistance to gravity on the left side, was subsequently extubated without incident, and sent to the NICU. Postoperatively, the patient experienced significant blood pressure lability, with several episodes of prolonged hypertension that proved difficult to control. On postoperative day 1, the patient complained of dizziness and stridor; upon examination, he was noted to have a pulsatile mass deep to the incision site.

What is the diagnosis and what is the next step in management?

This patient is on a heparin drip following perioperative occlusion of the endarterectomy site and had multiple episodes of sustained hypertension during the early postoperative period, increasing risk for bleeding from both the arteriotomy site and the associated soft tissues of the neck. The new-onset stridor and pulsatile neck mass are concerning for ruptured arteriotomy closure. The stridorous breathing suggests compression of the trachea, and the first priority should be establishing a safe airway. Awake, fiberoptic intubation should be attempted by anesthesia. If this cannot be accomplished, the wound may have to be opened and the clot evacuated. This should be done in the OR if time permits. Once the clot is cleared and the bleeding has been controlled, the patient should be intubated and prepped for formal exploration of the wound. Emergent tracheostomy should be a last resort in a patient on heparin with a deviated trachea as this could lead to complete loss of the airway, especially in inexperienced hands.

The patient is a 62-year-old, right-handed woman, with a past history of chronic, poorly controlled hypertension and atrial fibrillation on warfarin (Coumadin), who presents 6 days following an uneventful endarterectomy of the right carotid artery for which she was discharged 4 days ago on ASA 325 mg tid. The patient felt well until the morning of admission when she complained to her husband of headache and nausea; in the early afternoon she developed weakness on her left side. Her husband brought her to the ED, where her vitals on admission were T 37.3°C (99.1°F), HR 67 bpm, BP 170/90 mm Hg, RR 13 breaths/min. On physical examination, the patient was alert and oriented twice and she demonstrated three-fifths strength on the left upper and lower extremities.

What is the most likely diagnosis?

This patient is most likely suffering from cerebral hyperperfusion syndrome (CHS) after CEA. Clinical CHS, which characteristically occurs several days after endarterectomy, results from an increase in cerebral blood flow from baseline in an area of the brain that has lost its autoregulatory capacity after chronic hypoperfusion from high-grade carotid stenosis.[16] This uncontrolled increase in cerebral blood flow leads to transudation of fluid into the brain parenchyma and cerebral edema formation. Reported rates after CEA range from 0.2% to 18.9%, depending on the clinical severity, and patients will typically present with headache, orbital pain, change in level of consciousness, and focal neurologic deficits. Rarely, CHS may lead to intracerebral hemorrhage (ICH). Hemorrhage is thought to be due to the existence of areas of ischemia secondary to perioperative emboli that in turn undergo hemorrhagic transformation when confronted with increases in cerebral blood flow. Patients typically present several days to weeks after surgery (peak incidence at postoperative day 6) with headache, focal neurologic signs, altered sensorium, and/or seizure. Patients with CHS complicated by ICH may additionally present with nausea and vomiting from rapid increase in intracranial pressure (ICP). Patients at greatest risk are those with advanced age, diabetes, high-grade stenosis, cerebrovascular atherosclerotic disease elsewhere, evidence of perioperative or intraoperative cerebral ischemia, sustained increases in cerebral blood flow as detected by TCD, uncontrolled hypertension in the postoperative period, and a preoperative decrease in cerebrovascular reactivity as detected by acetazolamide challenge.[16]

What is the next best step in management for this patient?

Patients experiencing headache without focal neurologic signs within the first week or 2 following surgery should undergo TCD; if a greater than 100% increase in perfusion is detected, patients should have aggressive blood pressure management, discontinuation of anticoagulants if they are on them (for atrial fibrillation), and possible administration of mannitol to reduce ICP and cerebral edema and antiepileptics for seizure prophylaxis.[17] Patients with severe headache or those patients who have focal neurologic signs should undergo emergent CT scan to rule out ICH, which may require surgical evacuation in a minority of cases. Negative CT scan warrants MRI/MR perfusion for evaluation of infarct, as new neurologic deficits may reflect cerebral infarcts from embolic clots; new infarcts should be further investigated using carotid Doppler ultrasound to evaluate for thrombosis at the endarterectomy site and TCD for HITs (high-intensity transients). In addition to the above steps, this patient should be monitored in an ICU with an arterial line and should have strict blood pressure management, as this is the key to preventing the potentially devastating consequences of CHS.

While the patient is being transported to the NICU she vomits twice and becomes stuporous. Her left-sided weakness progresses to dense hemiplegia and she has decreased pupillary reactivity. She vomits a third time and loses consciousness. What is most likely going on in this patient? What is the next best step in management for this patient?

The patient most likely has developed an ICH secondary to CHS. However, before any intervention, the patient should be assessed for ABCs (airway, breathing, circulation)! Ensure the airway is secure—This patient requires intubation as she is comatose and she cannot protect her airway. Once the patient's ABCs are secured, emergency CT scan is warranted to investigate the possibility of hemorrhage. While en route, if possible, intra-arterial and intravenous access should be promptly obtained, coagulation studies should be drawn, mannitol/hypertonic saline should be administered preemptively given the signs of increased ICP, and prophylactic antiepileptics should be administered.

CT scan of this patient's head demonstrated right putamenal hemorrhage with significant associated mass effect and intraventricular extension, compression of the third ventricle, and significant dilation of the lateral ventricles. Coagulation studies came back with an INR (international normalized ratio) greater than 4. What is the next best step in management?

In addition to the above measures, the patient has a coagulopathy that should be promptly corrected. Patients with therapeutic INRs (2 to 3 in most cases) should be treated with 2 to 3 units of fresh-frozen plasma, although this patient's supratherapeutic levels warrant 6 units.[14] Prothrombin complex concentrates may also be used for reversal of warfarin-induced anticoagulation. The patient may also benefit from external ventricular drainage to relieve increased ICP from hematoma compression and ventricular hemorrhage. Surgical hematoma evacuation may be useful in patients who have lobar or cerebellar hemorrhages, but such efforts in basal ganglia hemorrhage have been proved futile.[18] In cases that ventriculostomy is not effective in reducing regional ICP, hemicraniectomy can be considered without clot evacuation, but the data on its effectiveness are only anecdotal. Blood pressure (BP) should be monitored through a dedicated arterial line; while the most appropriate target for blood pressure after ICH is controversial, a target of 140/90 mm Hg is reasonable, although hypotension should be avoided to maintain adequate cerebral perfusion. Slightly higher BP may be allowed for chronic hypertensives. Normoglycemia[19] and normothermia[20] are also appropriate goals in this patient. See Chapter 2 for further details regarding management of ICH.

 The patient is a 59-year-old, right-handed man with a history of occlusion of the left ICA secondary to dissection, with residual right-sided weakness and dysphagia (Figure 23-3). Owing to the fact that he was experiencing frequent life-altering exercise-induced TIAs, he was admitted for direct revascularization and underwent an uncomplicated extracranial-intracranial (EC-IC) bypass. While the data from the EC-IC bypass study and the yet-to-be released, but halted, Carotid Occlusion Surgery Study (COSS) seem to question the utility of this procedure in preventing stroke in unselected patients, even with positron emission tomography (PET)–defined misery perfusion, some individual patients can experience a reduction in the frequency of their TIAs, which improves their quality of life. Moreover, the effects of bypass on cognition remain to be seen. No blood products were administered, and the patient emerged from anesthesia with no new neurologic deficits. He was transferred to the NICU for further management.

How should this patient be managed in the postoperative period?

Tight blood pressure control is crucial in this patient, preferably with systolic BP in the range of 130 to 160 mm Hg in the early postoperative period. Hypertension may cause bleeding both from

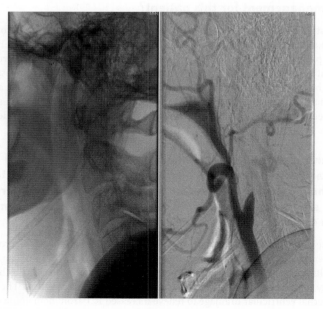

Figure 23-3. Cerebral angiography of patient demonstrating left internal carotid artery occlusion.

the anastomotic site, the open dural edges, or hemorrhage in reperfused areas, while hypotension may result in cerebral hypoperfusion and/or graft occlusion. The patient's BP should be monitored in the NICU with an arterial line, and short-acting pressors or vasodilators should be given as needed for BP control. Adequate intravenous fluids will also protect against hypotension. Frequent neurologic checks are necessary to monitor for new ischemic events, either from embolism or graft occlusion. Perioperative seizures can occur in this population as well, and perioperative antiepileptic drugs (AEDs) are generally felt to be of value. Frequent TCDs may be used to monitor graft patency, although some centers advocate MRA or CTA on the first postoperative day to evaluate the graft. Any new neurologic signs should be promptly investigated with CTA/CT or MRI/angiography, with the latter being more sensitive. Patients are generally operated on aspirin 81 mg daily without perioperative discontinuation. Perioperative dexamethasone is generally not indicated.

On postoperative day 1, this patient develops new-onset dysarthria and worsening of baseline right-sided weakness. What is the differential diagnosis and what is the next step in management?

The new onset of neurologic symptoms referable to the left hemisphere in this patient may represent ischemia secondary to either (1) occlusion of the graft, (2) thromboembolism from the right carotid artery, (3) hyperperfusion, or (4) subdural hematoma.

Graft patency may become compromised secondary to hypotensive episodes, inadequate IV hydration, surgical technique, quality of donor and recipient vessels, or excessively tight head dressing impairing flow through the donor vessel. TCDs may be used to quickly assess graft patency. If patency of the graft is in question, intravenous dextran may be administered to inhibit platelet function,[21] or a return to the operating room for graft revision may be necessary. CT should be ordered to rule out ICH due to hyperperfusion or epidural/subdural hematoma from graft/dural leakage. In these cases, surgical decompression and/or hematoma evacuation may be warranted and underscores the importance of prompt investigation of neurologic deterioration. It should be noted, however, that epidural hematoma formation secondary to oozing can be prevented intraoperatively using 50% protamine for heparin reversal or completely avoiding the use of heparin.[22] Arterial blowout at the anastomosis site may also occur leading to epidural or subdural hematoma, although this is quite rare with superficial temporal artery/middle cerebral artery (STA-MCA) bypass as this is a low-flow conduit.[22] Any patient with a hemorrhagic complication should have coagulation labs drawn and reversal of any underlying coagulopathy. MRI will be useful in identifying the presence of new infarcts, although intravenous tissue plasminogen activator (tPA) in these patients would be contraindicated given the close proximity of surgery. Additionally, seizure may be the cause of neurologic deficits in patients who are not placed on antiepileptic treatments.

Perioperative Surgical Care

! CRITICAL CONSIDERATIONS

- The evidence preferring surgery compared to medical management is substantial. The North American Symptomatic Carotid Endarterectomy Trial for surgical intervention found that CEA significantly reduced the risk of further stroke (17% at 2 years) and death (7% at 2 years) for patients with stenosis at or greater than 70%. The Asymptomatic Carotid Artery Stenosis Trial found that patients with greater than 60% stenosis had a 6% reduction in risk of stroke or death at 5 years.

- The recent results from the Carotid Revascularization Endarterectomy versus Stenting Trial (CREST)[5] compared endovascular and surgical techniques in both symptomatic and asymptomatic patients and found comparable rates of the primary outcome measure of death, stroke, or myocardial infarction in the perioperative period and any ipsilateral stroke at 4 years, although perioperative stroke and myocardial infarction occurred more frequently in the stenting and CEA groups, respectively.

- Clinical CHS, which characteristically occurs several days after endarterectomy, results from an increase in cerebral blood flow from baseline in an area of the brain that has lost its autoregulatory capacity after chronic hypoperfusion from high-grade carotid stenosis.

- While the data from the previous bypass study and the yet-to-be released, but halted, COSS, seem to question the utility of the EC-IC bypass surgery procedure in preventing stroke in unselected patients, even with PET-defined misery perfusion, some individual patients can experience a reduction in the frequency of their TIAs, which improves their quality of life. Also, the effects of bypass on cognitive function remain to be seen.

- Any new onset of neurologic symptoms referable to the ipsilateral cerebral hemisphere after EC-IC bypass may represent ischemia secondary to most likely one or a combination of the following: (1) occlusion of the graft, (2) thromboembolism from right carotid artery, (3) hyperperfusion, or (4) subdural hematoma.

REFERENCES

1. Nederkoorn PJ, van der Graaf Y, Hunink MGM. Duplex ultrasound and magnetic resonance angiography compared with digital subtraction angiography in carotid artery stenosis: a systematic review. *Stroke.* 2003;34:1324-1332.

2. Anderson GB, Ashforth R, Steinke DE, Ferdinandy R, Findlay JM. CT angiography for the detection and characterization of carotid artery bifurcation disease. *Stroke.* 2000;31:2168-2174.

3. North American Symptomatic Carotid Endarterectomy Trial Collaborators. Beneficial effect of carotid endarterectomy in symptomatic patients with high-grade carotid stenosis. *N Engl J Med.* 1991;325:445-453.

4. Executive Committee for the Asymptomatic Carotid Atherosclerosis Study. Endarterectomy for asymptomatic carotid artery stenosis. *JAMA.* 1995;273:1421-1428.

5. Brott TG, Hobson RW, Howard G, et al. Stenting versus endarterectomy for treatment of carotid-artery stenosis. *N Engl J Med.* 2010;363:11-23.

6. Carotid Endarterectomy Study Group. Results of a randomized controlled trial of carotid endarterectomy for asymptomatic carotid stenosis. *Mayo Clin Proc.* 1992;67:513-518.

7. Young B, Moore WS, Robertson JT, et al. An analysis of perioperative surgical mortality and morbidity in the asymptomatic carotid atherosclerosis study. ACAS Investigators. Asymptomatic Carotid Atherosclerosis Study. *Stroke.* 1996;27:2216-2224.

8. Naylor AR, Evans J, Thompson MM, et al. Seizures after carotid endarterectomy: hyperperfusion, dysautoregulation or hypertensive encephalopathy? *Eur J Vasc Endovasc Surg.* 2003;26:39-44.

9. Henderson RD, Phan TG, Piepgras DG, Wijdicks EF. Mechanisms of intracerebral hemorrhage after carotid endarterectomy. *J Neurosurg.* 2001;95:964-969.

10. Karapanayiotides T, Meuli R, Devuyst G, et al. Postcarotid endarterectomy hyperperfusion or reperfusion syndrome. *Stroke.* 2005;36: 21-26.

11. Cunningham EJ, Bond R, Mayberg MR, Warlow CP, Rothwell PM. Risk of persistent cranial nerve injury after carotid endarterectomy. *J Neurosurg.* 2004;101:445-448.

12. Stone DH, Nolan BW, Schanzer A, et al. Protamine reduces bleeding complications associated with carotid endarterectomy without increasing the risk of stroke. *J Vasc Surg.* 2010;51:559-564, 564.e1.

13. Welling RE, Ramadas HS, Gansmuller KJ. Cervical wound hematoma after carotid endarterectomy. *Ann Vasc Surg.* 1989;3:229-231.

14. Greenberg M. *Handbook of Neurosurgery.* New York, NY: Thieme; 2006.

15. Harker LA, Bernstein EF, Dilley RB, et al. Failure of aspirin plus dipyridamole to prevent restenosis

after carotid endarterectomy. *Ann Intern Med.* 1992;116:731-736.

16. van Mook WNKA, Rennenberg RJMW, Schurink GW, et al. Cerebral hyperperfusion syndrome. *Lancet Neurol.* 2005;4:877-888.

17. Moulakakis KG, Mylonas SN, Sfyroeras GS, Andrikopoulos V. Hyperperfusion syndrome after carotid revascularization. *J Vasc Surg.* 2009;49: 1060-1068.

18. Batjer HH, Reisch JS, Allen BC, Plaizier LJ, Su CJ. Failure of surgery to improve outcome in hypertensive putaminal hemorrhage. A prospective randomized trial. *Arch Neurol.* 1990;47: 1103-1106.

19. Passero S, Ciacci G, Ulivelli M. The influence of diabetes and hyperglycemia on clinical course after intracerebral hemorrhage. *Neurology.* 2003;61: 1351-1356.

20. Schwarz S, Hafner K, Aschoff A, Schwab S. Incidence and prognostic significance of fever following intracerebral hemorrhage. *Neurology.* 2000;54: 354-361.

21. Newell D, Vilela M. Superficial temporal artery to middle cerebral artery bypass. *Neurosurgery.* 2004; 54:1441-1448.

22. Sekhar LN, Kalavakonda C. Cerebral revascularization for aneurysms and tumors. *Neurosurgery.* 2002;50:321-331.

Postcraniotomy Complication Management

Raqeeb Haque, MD
Teresa J. Wojtasiewicz, BA
Brian Y. Hwang, MD
E. Sander Connolly, MD

 A 38-year-old woman with a history of medically refractory epilepsy since childhood underwent frontoparietal temporal craniotomy for implantation of subdural electrode array. Seven days after the initial craniotomy, the patient returned to the operating room (OR) for reelevation of her prior craniotomy site, removal of her electrode strip, and multiple pial transections. The area of epileptiform discharge was ablated and her intraoperative course was benign. Upon transfer to the neurologic intensive care unit (NICU, NeuroICU), the patient was unable to move her right arm and was sent for an urgent computed tomographic (CT) scan. The CT scan revealed no abnormalities and the patient recovered four-fifths motor function in her arm upon completion of the CT scan.

What complications are expected in this patient and what are her risk factors?

Given her history, this patient is at high risk for postoperative seizure. Therefore, her postoperative monitoring should include electroencephalographic (EEG) monitoring and seizure prophylaxis. Her focal neurologic deficit quickly resolved, which is not unusual in the immediate postoperative setting. Her team elected for CT to rule out an urgent cerebrovascular complication, such as a subdural hematoma, which may present acutely in the postoperative period.

Postoperative patients represent a large fraction of cases seen in the NICU. Many neurosurgical procedures involve a craniotomy (removal of a section of the cranium that is replaced). Procedures that may require craniotomy include:

- Brain tumor resection
- Aneurysmectomy
- Epilepsy grid placement
- Hematoma evacuation
- Brain abscess removal
- Implantation of a deep brain stimulator
- Insertion of a monitoring probe
- Ventriculostomy

The range of postoperative complications depends on the location of the operative site, length of operation, and patient characteristics.[1,2] Adverse postoperative events (eg, neoplasm, cerebrovascular insult, high intracranial pressure [ICP]) are associated with, and often directly result from, the disease process. In a small subset of patients, craniotomy itself can lead to unintended postoperative complications. The most common postcraniotomy complications are:

General medical complications:

- Hypotension/hypertension
- Nausea
- Infections
- Deep vein thrombosis
- Pulmonary embolism
- Pneumonia

Neurologic complications:

- Cerebrovascular complications
- Cerebrospinal fluid (CSF) leaks
- Hydrocephalus
- Edema and increased ICP
- Seizures

Medical complications are common in the NICU and affect more than 50% of neurosurgical patients.[3] History of psychiatric illness, asthma, carotid stenosis, and male sex are associated with increased risk of medical complications.[4] Neurologic complications are more commonly seen in patients with carotid stenosis and preexisting mental illness.[4] Infratentorial meningioma and craniopharyngioma are also associated with particularly high rates of neurologic and general medical complication rates.[3,4] Rates of postcraniotomy complications vary widely by procedure (Table 24-1).[2]

Potentially fatal complications can be managed appropriately to decrease mortality rate. Some of the most serious and potentially fatal complications include:

- Abscess formation (either subdural or intracerebral)
- Brain edema
- Hemorrhage

Table 24-1. Rates of Complications of Procedures Requiring Craniotomy

	Nonfatal complications (%)	Fatal complications (%)
Supratentorial tumor resection	7-30	1.7-5.0
Unruptured intracranial aneurysm	12-15	0-4
Ruptured intracranial aneurysm	25-70	7-30
Posterior fossa surgery	Varies by pathology and location: Overall 31.9[5]	0.3-2.5

(From Stevens RD. Postoperative care. In: Bhardwaj A, Mirski MAZ, Ulatowski JA, eds. Handbook of Neurocritical Care. Totowa, NJ: Humana Press; 2004.)

Table 24-2. Common Postoperative Complications in Various Stages of Postoperative Care[6]

Operation	Immediate complication	24–48 h	>48 h
Craniotomy/tumor	Cerebral edema Cerebral hemorrhage Subdural hemorrhage	Cerebrospinal fluid leak Vasospasm	Seizure
Surgical aneurysm repair	Stroke	Vasospasm Cerebral edema	Seizure
Arteriovenous malformation	Hemorrhage	Cerebral edema	Seizure
Cerebellopontine angle tumor	Epidural hematoma	Hydrocephalus	Seizure

(From Ropper AH, Gress DR, Dringer MN Green DM, Mayer SA, Bleck TP. Postoperative neurosurgical care. In: Neurological and Neurosurgical Intensive Care. Philadelphia, PA: Lippincott Williams & Wilkins; 2004:169-176.)

Different complications tend to present at different points in the postoperative course. Infections tend to present far later, while cerebrovascular events are more common during the early postoperative period. Table 24-2 presents a general perspective of the most common complications during various postoperative periods.[6] It is not a definitive summary of all possible complications of any surgery.

What kind of postoperative monitoring should be considered in postcraniotomy patients?

Appropriate postoperative monitoring is critical for the detection and management of postoperative complications. In the patient described above, EEG monitoring was especially important as the patient was at high risk for seizure activity. ICP and cerebral blood flow (CBF) monitors are excellent for detecting pressure changes signaling brain edema or hemorrhage, but are associated with a risk of infection.[7] EEG monitors for seizure activity are recommended, and adequate screening for postoperative seizures may require 24 hours or more of continuous EEG monitoring.[8] Detailed neurophysiologic monitoring modalities are discussed in Section 2 of this book. Complications most commonly occur within the first 24 to 48 hours after surgery, and early intervention is critical in improving the clinical course and outcome.[9] Generally, postoperative monitoring in the NICU includes a neurologic examination and blood pressure monitoring.

Neurologic Examination

Although intensive monitoring is readily available, especially in advanced NICUs, neurologic examination may be the earliest sign of postoperative deterioration.[10] Multiple scales can be used in clinical examination of postoperative patients—the widely accepted Glasgow Coma Scale (GCS) (Table 24-3) and the newer full outline of unresponsiveness (FOUR score)[11] (Table 24-4). Although the GCS is a validated measure of neurologic function,[12,13] the FOUR score, a new neurologic function score, offers more subtle discrimination of neurologic function, especially in patients who are deeply comatose or on a ventilator; has a high concordance between examiners; is easy to use, even by inexperienced staff; and can predict hospital mortality or decline to the Rankin score of 3 to 6.[11,14,15]

After surgery, ensure that the effects of anesthetics have sufficiently worn off. All patients should be monitored for sudden postoperative neurologic status. Perform baseline neurologic examination every hour. If this is not feasible, do it every 2 to 4 hours. If a patient's neurologic status changes (ie, GCS drop > 2), a CT scan should be ordered to rule out hemorrhage, CSF leak, edema, or infection. Common normal postoperative examination findings (often related to anesthetic side effects) and

Table 24-3. Glasgow Coma Scale [11]

Eye response
  4 = eyes open spontaneously
  3 = eye opening to verbal command
  2 = eye opening to pain
  1 = no eye opening

Motor response
  6 = obeys commands
  5 = localizing pain
  4 = withdrawal from pain
  3 = flexion response to pain
  2 = extension response to pain
  1 = no motor response

Verbal response
  5 = oriented
  4 = confused
  3 = inappropriate words
  2 = incomprehensible sounds
  1 = no verbal response

(From Wijdicks EFM, Bamlet WR, Maramattom BV, Manno EM, McClelland RL. Validation of a new coma scale: the FOUR score. Ann of Neurol. 2005;58:585-593.)

Table 24-4. FOUR Score

Eye response
  4 = eyelids open or opened, tracking, or blinking to command
  3 = eyelids open but not tracking
  2 = eyelids closed but open to loud voice
  1 = eyelids closed but open to pain
  0 = eyelids remain closed with pain

Motor response
  4 = thumbs-up, fist, or peace sign
  3 = localizing to pain
  2 = flexion response to pain
  1 = extension response to pain
  0 = no response to pain or generalized myoclonus status

Brainstem reflexes
  4 = pupil and corneal reflexes present
  3 = one pupil wide and fixed
  2 = pupil or corneal reflexes absent
  1 = pupil and corneal reflexes absent
  0 = absent pupil, corneal, and cough reflex

Respiration
  4 = not intubated, regular breathing pattern
  3 = not intubated, Cheyne-Stokes breathing pattern
  2 = not intubated, irregular breathing
  1 = breathes above ventilator rate
  0 = breathes at ventilator rate or apnea

(From Wijdicks EFM, Bamlet WR, Maramattom BV, Manno EM, McClelland RL. Validation of a new coma scale: The FOUR score. Ann of Neurol. 2005;58:585-593.)

Table 24-5. A Comparison of Common Normal and Abnormal Neurologic Findings After Craniotomy

Common postoperative neurologic findings	Concerning postoperative neurologic findings
Upturned Babinski reflex up to 2 h postoperatively	Vertigo
Unilateral pupillary dilation in awake patients	Pupillary changes in a fully awake patient
Eccentric pupil	New hemiparesis
Mild exacerbation of previous hemiparesis for up to 2 h postoperatively	New or worsened paresthesias
	Progressive drowsiness
Dysarthria	Rapidly increasing headache (especially with vomiting)
Asterixis	Facial paresis[a]
Transient headache	

[a]Some posterior fossa masses, especially acoustic neuromas, may impact the facial nerve and facial nerve weakness is a common postoperative finding.

abnormal findings should be differentiated[6] (Table 24-5). Causes of abnormal findings on postoperative examination include intracerebral hemorrhage, epidural hemorrhage, subdural hemorrhage, and brain edema.

Blood Pressure Monitoring

Postoperative hypertension

The incidence of postoperative hypertension is relatively high (30% to 80% depending on definition of hypertension[2]). A sudden increase in blood pressure may raise suspicion of a cerebrovascular event. Hypertension increases the risk of postoperative complications, including myocardial infarction, stroke, and cerebral hemorrhage.[16,17] It is important to discriminate postoperative hypertension from the Cushing reflexive hypertension secondary to elevated ICP. Treatment of hypertension must avoid decreasing cerebral hemodynamic parameters (cerebral blood flow, ICP, cerebral metabolic rate of oxygen) as it can lead to cerebral hypoperfusion.[2,18]

First-line agents: Intravenous β-adrenergic antagonists provide adequate blood pressure control[2]:

- Labetalol
- Metoprolol
- Esmolol

Second-line agents: With refractory hypertension or marked bradycardia where β-adrenergic antagonists are unsuitable, angiotensin-converting enzyme (ACE) inhibitors and vasodilators are options—Blood pressure control outweighs the risks.[2,18]

Blood pressure management (Figure 24-1) should be combined with appropriate pain management, as undercontrolled pain may increase blood pressure. Morphine or other opioids have sedative effects that make neurologic function more difficult to assess. Nonsteroidal anti-inflammatory drugs (NSAIDs) are favorable agents, but may need to be combined with opioid analgesics for adequate pain control.[19] Abrupt administration of an antihypertensive agent may lead to a sudden decrease in cerebral blood flow—Patients should be carefully monitored when receiving an intravenous (IV) bolus of antihypertensive medication.[18]

Postoperative hypotension

Postoperative hypotension is not as common as hypertension (2% to 5%), but can impact recovery and is associated with adverse events such as hemorrhage.[2] Neurogenic and septic shock should both also be considered in cases of hypotension.

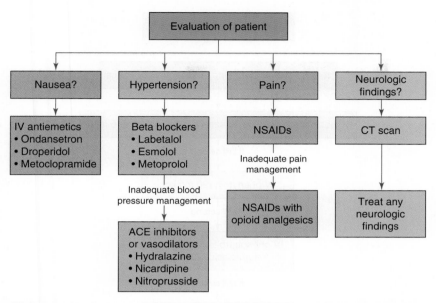

Figure 24-1. Algorithm for the clinical postoperative management of nausea, hypertension and pain. ACE, angiotensin-converting enzyme; CT, computed tomography; NSAIDs, nonsteroidal anti-inflammatory drugs.

Nausea

Neurosurgical patients are at high risk of postoperative nausea (over 30% to 50%).[2] This may lead to volume abnormalities, including elevated ICP and blood pressure. Treat nausea with one of the following:

- IV ondansetron (4 to 8 mg)
- IV droperidol (0.625 to 1.25 mg)
- IV metoclopramide (5 to 10 mg)

If vomiting does not stop and remains severe, intracranial hypertension may be suspected, and if neurologic function deteriorates, hemorrhage is a possibility—This necessitates a CT scan (Figure 24-1).

How should postoperative seizures be managed?

Postoperative seizures are common. They occur within a week of surgery in anywhere from 4% to 19% of patients.[20] Surgery for brain tumors, brain abscesses, arteriovenous malformations (AVMs), and aneurysms have all been associated with postoperative seizures.[20] Patients with a preexisting seizure disorder or metabolic abnormalities are also at increased risk for seizures. Although generalized tonic-clonic seizures are the most common seizure observed in the NICU, some patients will present with neurologic deterioration and decreased level of consciousness rather than convulsions.[21] Without EEG monitoring, comatose patients may have unrecognized status epilepticus.[22] Continuous EEG monitoring is critical for detecting these less common, nonconvulsive seizures. Preoperative prophylaxis with phenytoin and continuation of therapy reduce the incidence of seizures, but inadequate dosing (10 to 20 μg/dL is ideal) is common.[23,24] Seizures may be a manifestation of other pathologic processes, such as cerebral edema, intracranial hemorrhage, meningitis, or infection. Epilepsy management is discussed in detail in Chapter 3.

Perioperative
Surgical Care

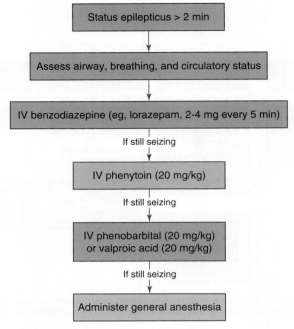

Figure 24-2. Seizure management protocol.

Patients with a single focal seizure lasting less than 2 minutes should be monitored carefully and considered for anticonvulsants.[25] Generalized seizures lasting more than 1 to 2 minutes should be aggressively treated (Figure 24-2).[26]

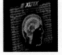 A 64-year-old man with a history of hypertension and coronary artery disease collapsed while walking his dog. In the emergency department, his blood pressure was measured at 240/150 mm Hg and a CT scan revealed intraventricular hemorrhage secondary to a right middle cerebral artery stroke. Angiography revealed extensive atherosclerosis with no aneurysms. Initially, he was following commands with a GCS of 13. Despite maximal medical therapy, his neurologic examination worsened to a GCS of 10, with signs of early herniation. Six days after admission, he underwent decompressive craniectomy. His neurologic function failed to improve, and a CT scan revealed a subgaleal hematoma (Figure 24-3), which was evacuated emergently.

What can be done to prevent postoperative hemorrhage?

This patient initially presented with massive intraventricular hemorrhage (IVH) and uncontrolled hypertension, cardiac disease, and atherosclerosis. He was at high risk for hemorrhagic stroke in the postoperative period. Unfortunately, despite aggressive monitoring and prompt recognition of his hematoma, this patient had a very poor neurologic outcome, as is likely with severe IVH. Postoperative hemorrhage, which commonly includes intracerebral, subdural, epidural, and subgaleal

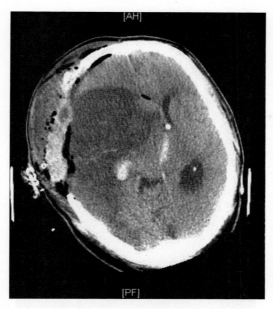

Figure 24-3. Computed tomographic scan revealing a subgaleal hematoma.

hemorrhages, is one of the most serious complications of neurologic surgery. Improved surgical technique has reduced the incidence of postoperative hemorrhage significantly—Postcraniotomy hemorrhage occurs in approximately 1% of patients.[27] The most common risks for postoperative bleeding include hypertension, administration of antiplatelet agents, and other clotting abnormalities.[27,28] These are often correctable—Preoperative evaluation is critical in reducing the incidence of postoperative hemorrhage. Neurologic deterioration, especially an altered level of consciousness, in the immediate postoperative period should be followed with CT and potentially magnetic resonance imaging (MRI) with diffusion to ensure appropriate detection of hemorrhage.[9] Urgent surgical decompression is required for many postoperative hemorrhages. Outcomes following hemorrhage are grim (80% of patients experience some permanent neurologic deficit).[27]

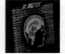 A 78-year-old man with a history of poorly controlled diabetes, hypertension, and ischemic stroke presented after falling in the shower. His wife brought him to the emergency department where CT showed a subdural hematoma (SDH) with overlying skull fracture. A craniotomy was performed immediately to evacuate the hematoma. Five days after the operation, the patient appeared agitated and had a fever of 102.3°F. His fever persisted for 12 hours despite an extensive fever workup, with negative blood cultures. Six days after his operation, a CT scan revealed subdural empyema (Figure 24-4).

What antibiotic prophylaxis is indicated to prevent infection? What kinds of infections are most common in the postoperative period?

This patient's unexplained fever prompted a fever workup and his injury, with skull fracture, predisposed him to bacterial infections. Prophylaxis and preoperative prevention are key in preventing

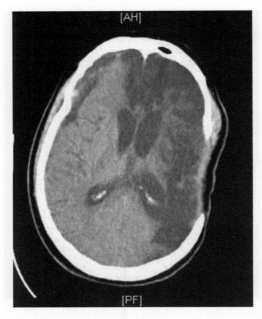

Figure 24-4. Computed tomographic scan revealing a subdural empyema.

postoperative infection.[29,30] Although the rates of infection are fairly low in neurosurgery, surgical techniques for minimizing infection should be used and patients should be given antibiotics with gram-positive and gram-negative coverage in the brief preoperative, intraoperative, and postoperative periods to minimize risk of infection.[29] Skin flora are the most common culprits in postoperative infections. A suitable regimen for broad-spectrum prophylactic operative coverage is:

- For "clean" operations: Cefazolin and cefoperazone/sulbactam have been shown to be equally effective for preoperative prophlaxis.[31]
- For "dirty" operations: Vancomycin 1.5 g/day and ceftazidime 6 g/day for 72 hours after the operation.[30]

Patients with an external ventricular drain (EVD) or other invasive devices, especially if the device remains for an extended period of time, may contribute to a higher risk of infection—EVD management is covered in Chapter 22 of this textbook.[32-34] In addition, neurosurgical patients should be monitored for nonoperative infections, including urinary tract infections, pneumonia, and infections of various catheters.[25] (See Section 10 of this book for detailed nonoperative infection management.) Although neurosurgery is generally associated with low rates of postoperative infection, the following complications are possible:

- Surgical site infection
- Meningitis
- Subdural empyema
- Brain abscess
- Catheter infection, especially CSF shunts.

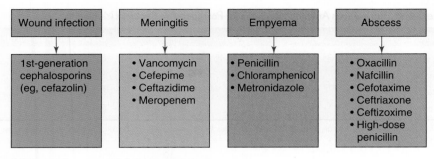

Wound infection	Meningitis	Empyema	Abscess
1st-generation cephalosporins (eg, cefazolin)	• Vancomycin • Cefepime • Ceftazidime • Meropenem	• Penicillin • Chloramphenicol • Metronidazole	• Oxacillin • Nafcillin • Cefotaxime • Ceftriaxone • Ceftizoxime • High-dose penicillin

Figure 24-5. Broad-spectrum infection management.

Management of each infection should begin with a broad-spectrum regimen (Figure 24-5), and once the organism has been identified, an antibiotic regimen should be tailored accordingly.

Surgical Site Infection

Wound infections occur in an estimate of 0% to 5.8% of cases.[29,31] Clinical symptoms including swelling and tenderness at the surgical site take at least 48 hours, possibly many days or weeks, to develop.[35] Once detected, wound infections should be treated immediately to prevent cranial osteomyelitis or meningitis, which can result from unrecognized and untreated wound infections.[36] Skull films, or CT with bony windows, may be helpful for comparison with later films in case osteomyelitis develops. Culture of the wound site will determine the specific antibiotic regimen needed. Because gram-positive cocci are the most common causes of wound infection (Figure 24-6), first-generation cephalosporins, such as cefazolin, are a good choice for initial broad-spectrum therapy.

Osteomyelitis

If repeat skull films or CT scans reveal spread to the underlying bone, excision of the infected bone flap or plate, with antibiotic treatment and drainage of the area, is critical.

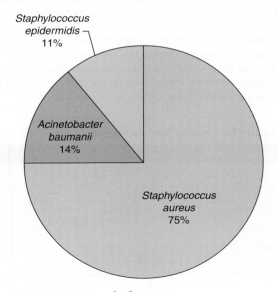

Figure 24-6. Most common organisms in wound infections.

Table 24-6. Intravenous Antibiotic Regimen for Postoperative Bacterial Meningitis [39]

Antibiotic	Dose	Duration of treatment (d)
Use vancomycin and one of the following:	30-45 mg/kg	8-12
Cefepime	6 g	8
Ceftazidime	6 g	8
Meropenem	6 g	8

(From Tunkel AR, Hartman BJ, Kaplan SL, et al. Practice Guidelines for the management of bacterial meningitis. Clin Infect Dis. 2004;9:1267-1284.)

Meningitis

Nosocomial meningitis may be very difficult to detect and often presents differently than community-acquired meningitis. The most common symptoms are fever and an altered level of consciousness, but these are nonspecific and easily mistaken for normal postoperative recovery.[36] Meningismus may be present in less than 50% of patients.[37] Lumbar puncture with analysis of the cell count, protein, glucose, Gram stain, and culture of the CSF are critical. However, Gram stain and cell count have low sensitivity in neurosurgical patients, and cell count may have low sensitivity, especially in patients who have had intracerebral hemorrhage.[37] In cases of diagnostic uncertainty, lactate levels of the CSF may prove helpful. A lactate level of over 4 mmol/L in the CSF has a high sensitivity and specificity for bacterial meningitis.[38] Patients should be treated with the antibiotics listed in Table 24-6.[39]

Aseptic meningitis from surgical trauma or immune reaction to blood in the central nervous system may account for up to 70% of postoperative meningitic findings. If repeated CSF analysis yields negative findings and the patient is determined to have aseptic meningitis, antibiotics can be safely discontinued.[40]

Subdural empyema

Subdural empyema (SDE) is fortunately a rare complication of craniotomy, but it is a surgical emergency and must be detected and treated immediately. Patients with subdural bacterial collections may present with fever, headache, seizures, periorbital edema, and various focal neurologic deficits.[41] As with postoperative bacterial meningitis, patients with postoperative SDE tend to present with more subtle symptoms and a more insidious onset than typical SDE patients.[42] An urgent CT scan in a patient with postoperative SDE may reveal a hypodense or isodense subdural collection with rim enhancement.[41]

Surgical evacuation of the abscess is critical and removal of the underlying bone flap may be necessary. Patients should be treated with postoperative medications listed in Table 24-7.[41]

Table 24-7. Postoperative Medication for Subdural Empyema

Antibiotics: 2 wk IV, then 4 wk oral of either	
Penicillin	100,000 units/kg/6 h
Chloramphenicol	15 mg/kg/6 h
Metronidazole	7.5 mg/kg/8 h
Prophylactic antiepileptic:	
Phenytoin, phenobarbitone, etc.	

(From Nathoo NFCS, Nadvi SSFCS, van Dellen JRP, Gouws EB. Intracranial subdural empyemas in the era of computed tomography: A review of 699 cases. Neurosurgery. 1999;44:529-535.)

Table 24-8. Postoperative Medication for Brain Abscess [43]

Antibiotics: 4–6 wk, followed by prolonged oral therapy
Antistaphylococcal penicillin → oxacillin, nafcillin
Third-generation cephalosporin → cefotaxime, ceftriaxone, ceftizoxime
High-dose penicillin
For patients with sinusitis or chronic lung infections (risk of *Bacteroides* species) → metronidazole

(From Leedom JH, Holtom PD. Infectious complications. In: Apuzzo MLJ, ed. Brain Surgery: Complication Avoidance and Management. New York, NY: Churchill Livingstone; 1993.)

Brain abscess

A brain abscess, like subdural empyema, is a life-threatening, rare complication that requires immediate attention. The time course of a bacterial abscess is similar to that of SDE. Symptoms may be subtle. The most common symptoms are headache and alteration in mental status.[43] CT has 95% to 99% sensitivity in detecting brain abscess.[44] However, the ring-enhancing lesion can be easily mistaken for other pathologic processes, including malignancy, infarction, and hematoma.[43] Upon diagnosis of an abscess, broad-spectrum antibiotic therapy should be as shown in Table 24-8.[43]

Brain abscesses must be either surgically aspirated or resected, and the organism detected will determine the antibiotic therapy that is required.

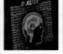

A 59-year-old woman with a history of well-controlled type II diabetes mellitus underwent an elective surgery to remove a 2.5-cm acoustic neuroma. A retrosigmoid craniotomy was performed and her tumor was more than 95% resected. The patient's intraoperative course was uneventful and she was transferred to the neurologic intensive care unit (NICU, Neuro-ICU) for postoperative management. Her neurologic status remained excellent. Two days after her operation, clear drainage from the wound site was noted, with no warmth or erythema. The drainage was monitored, with the presumptive diagnosis of cerebrospinal fluid (CSF) leak for 6 days, when a spinal drain was put in. Eight days after her operation, fluid drainage persisted. Two weeks after the operation, the patient returned to the OR for repair of her CSF leak. The deficit was repaired and she had an uneventful recovery.

When should this patient's CSF leak be repaired?

This patient presented with clear fluid and no pain or swelling at her surgical site, indicating no infection. Most CSF leaks resolve within a week without intervention, but some, like this patient, may require surgical repair.[1] Although CSF leaks are relatively rare, patients who have undergone posterior fossa surgery are at higher risk for CSF leaks (up to 13% of posterior fossa surgeries may result in this complication, but there is much variation based on the specific surgical approach).[5] Presentation of CSF leak may include:

- Direct drainage through the wound
- Otorrhea
- Rhinorrhea

Otorrhea and rhinorrhea CSF leaks are more commonly seen in more aggressive operative approaches, but intraoperative packing with bone wax has helped reduce the incidence of these complications.[45] Diagnosing a CSF leak can be challenging, as not all patients present with substantive fluid drainage. Fluid may be expressed when the patient stands or changes positions. Elevation of the patient's head may also be helpful in finding fluid.[46] If clear, nonbloody fluid can be collected, inspection can verify the identity of the drainage. If confirmation is needed, a β_2-transferrin assay is sensitive, as is glucose testing of nonbloody fluid (CSF glucose should be approximately 60% of serum glucose) to verify its identity.[46]

Treatment

CSF wound leakage can be handled conservatively—Most patients will resolve within 5 to 7 days without intervention.[5] Patients that do not resolve within this time can be treated with lumbar puncture and continuous spinal drainage—CSF should be drained at a rate of 5 to 15 mL/h.[25] Surgical packing for closure of the CSF fistula may rarely be required if these measures are ineffective (Figure 24-7).[1] Although meningitis and infection are potential sequelae of a CSF leak, antimicrobial prophylaxis is not indicated.[47]

How should hydrocephalus be recognized and managed in postoperative patients?

Hydrocephalus is particularly common after posterior fossa surgeries, ranging from 4.6% to 30.0% of operations.[5,48] It is unclear if the etiology of the hydrocephalus is related to the tumor or the surgery. The most common presenting symptom in patients with hydrocephalus is decreased level of consciousness, which is a relatively late finding. Earlier signs of hydrocephalus include headache, nausea/vomiting, gait disturbance, or abducens nerve palsy.[5,9] Hydrocephalus can also present with a CSF leak.[5] Sudden changes in systolic blood pressure or breathing can signal an acute, potentially life-threatening change in the pressure in the posterior fossa. CT scans compared with baseline CT scans from the preoperative or immediate postoperative period can establish a diagnosis of hydrocephalus. Hydrocephalus as a result of obstruction of the ventricular drainage system can be confused with hydrocephalus as a result of generalized cerebral edema.[9] Management is markedly different in these etiologies—CSF drainage through a ventriculostomy is indicated for obstructive hydrocephalus, but one should proceed with extreme caution in brain edema to avoid herniation.[9]

As mentioned before, brain edema can be confused with obstructive hydrocephalus. Brain edema can occur as a result of tissue manipulation during surgery, often developing 48–72 hours after the craniotomy.[9] CT should reveal hypodense areas consistent with cerebral edema. The treatment of cerebral edema consists of:

1. ICP monitoring: A monitor of intracranial pressure provides critical information of the course of postoperative edema and is a critical tool. Maintaining a cerebral perfusion pressure of at least 60 mm Hg is imperative to prevent brain injury. Chapter 12 of this book provides more details.

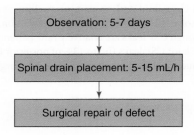

Figure 24-7. Cerebrospinal fluid leak management.

2. Hyperventilation: Immediate intubation and hyperventilation is critical in patients with severe, acute edema, especially patients showing evidence of brainstem dysfunction. Patients should be hyperventilated to achieve a P_{CO_2} of 30-35 mm Hg.[25]

3. Osmotic agents: Mannitol and hypertonic saline both have been shown to lower ICP.[49-52] There is controversy over which is preferred, but currently both are suitable options for managing brain edema. The target serum osmolarity of treatment is 300–310 mEq/L.[25]

4. Steroids: Steroids are very effective for treating edema after tumor surgery, but not as helpful in other postoperative situations.[2,25] Steroids should be administered to patients who have had a tumor removed (10 mg of dexamethasone every 4 hrs).

! CRITICAL CONSIDERATIONS

- Postoperative neurologic monitoring is critical for detecting complications of craniotomy.
- Analysis of metabolic function, clotting ability, and prophylactic antibiotics and anticonvulsants can reduce the incidence of postoperative complications.
- Emergent CT scanning can reveal pathologic processes, including abscess, brain edema, hydrocephalus, and hemorrhage.
- Treatment of bacterial infections should begin with a broad-spectrum regimen with good central nervous system permeability and follow with specific therapy.
- CSF leaks usually resolve on their own, but may require shunting or surgical revision.
- In suspected hydrocephalus, rule out brain edema before proceeding to ventriculostomy.
- Postoperative seizure management should focus on stopping the patient from seizing, then provide a bolus of anticonvulsant to prevent future seizures.
- Surgical treatment may be required for subdural empyema, brain abscess, hemorrhage, and rare CSF leaks.

Perioperative Surgical Care

REFERENCES

1. Post KD, Friedman ED, McCormick P. *Postoperative Complications in Intracranial Neurosurgery.* New York, NY: Thieme; 1993:241.
2. Stevens RD. Postoperative care. In: Bhardwaj A, Mirski MAZ, Ulatowski JA, eds. *Handbook of Neurocritical Care.* Totowa, NJ: Humana Press; 2004:91-122.
3. Manninen PH, Raman SK, Boyle K, el-Beheiry H. Early postoperative complications following neurosurgical procedures. *Can J Anaesth.* 1999;46:7-14.
4. Beauregard CL, Friedman WA. Routine use of postoperative ICU care for elective craniotomy: a cost-benefit analysis. *Surg Neurol.* 2003;60:483-489.
5. Dubey A, Sung WS, Shaya M, et al. Complications of posterior cranial fossa surgery—an institutional experience of 500 patients. *Surg Neurol.* 2009;72:369-375.
6. Ropper AH, Gress DR, Diringer MN, Green DM, Mayer SA, Bleck TP. Postoperative neurosurgical care. In: *Neurological and Neurosurgical Intensive Care.* Philadelphia, PA: Lippincott Williams & Wilkins; 2004:169-176.
7. Steiner LA, Andrews PJD. Monitoring the injured brain: ICP and CBF. *Br J Anaesth.* 2006;97:26-38.
8. Pfister D, Strebel SP, Steiner LA. Postoperative management of adult central neurosurgical patients: systemic and neuro-monitoring. *Best Pract Res Clin Anaesthesiol.* 2007;21:449-463.
9. Redmond AJ, Chiang VL. Postoperative management in the neurosurgical critical care unit. In: Torbey MT, ed. *Neurocritical Care.* New York, NY: Cambridge University Press; 2010:425.
10. Bullock R, Hannemann CO, Murray L, Teasdale GM. Recurrent hematomas following craniotomy for traumatic intracranial mass. *J Neurosurg.* 1990;72:9-14.

11. Wijdicks EFM, Bamlet WR, Maramattom BV, Manno EM, McClelland RL. Validation of a new coma scale: the FOUR score. *Ann Neurol.* 2005;58:585-593.

12. Teasdale G, Jennett B. Assessment of coma and impaired consciousness. A practical scale. *Lancet.* 1974;2:81-84.

13. Namen AM, Ely EW, Tatter SB, et al. Predictors of successful extubation in neurosurgical patients. *Am J Respir Crit Care Med.* 2001;163:658-664.

14. Iyer VN, Mandrekar JN, Danielson RD, Zubkov AY, Elmer JL, Wijdicks EF. Validity of the FOUR score coma scale in the medical intensive care unit. *Mayo Clin Proc.* 2009;84:694-701.

15. Wolf CA, Wijdicks EF, Bamlet WR, McClelland RL. Further validation of the FOUR score coma scale by intensive care nurses. *Mayo Clin Proc.* 2007;82:435-438.

16. Rose DK, Cohen MM, DeBoer DP. Cardiovascular events in the postanesthesia care unit: Contribution of risk factors. *Anesthesiology.* 1996;4:772-781.

17. Basali A, Mascha EJ, Kalfas I, Schubert A. Relation between perioperative hypertension and intracranial hemorrhage after craniotomy. *Anesthesiology.* 2000;93:48-54.

18. Varon J, Marik PE. Perioperative hypertension management. *Vasc Health Risk Manag.* 2008;4:615-627.

19. Cousins MJ, Umedaly HS. Postoperative pain management in the neurosurgical patient. *Int Anesthesiol Clin.* 1996;34:179-193.

20. Krauss WE, Post KD. General complications in neurological surgery. In: Post KD, Friedman E, McCormick P, eds. *Postoperative Complications in Intracranial Neurosurgery.* New York, NY: Thieme; 1993:241.

21. Varelas PN, Mirski MA. Seizures in the adult intensive care unit. *J Neurosurg Anesthesiol.* 2001;13:163-175.

22. Towne, ARM, Waterhouse EJM, Boggs JGM, et al. Prevalence of nonconvulsive status epilepticus in comatose patients. *Neurology.* 2000;54:340.

23. Kvam, DA, Loftus CM, Copeland B, Quest DO. Seizures during the immediate postoperative period. *Neurosurgery.* 1983;12:14-17.

24. Yeh JS, Dhir JS, Green AL, Bodiwala D, Brydon HL. Changes in plasma phenytoin level following craniotomy. *Br J Neurosurg.* 2006;20:403-406.

25. Rodrigue T, Selman WR. Postoperative management in the neurosciences critical care unit. In: Suarez JI, ed. *Critical Care Neurology and Neurosurgery.* Totowa, NJ: Humana Press; 2004:433-448.

26. Working Group on Status Epilepticus. Treatment of convulsive status epilepticus: recommendations of the epilepsy foundation of America's working group on status epilepticus. *JAMA.* 1993;270:854-859.

27. Kalfas IH, Little JR. Postoperative hemorrhage: a survey of 4992 intracranial procedures. *Neurosurgery.* 1988;23:343-347.

28. Palmer JD, Sparrow OC, Iannotti F. Postoperative hematoma: a 5-year survey and identification of avoidable risk factors. *Neurosurgery.* 1994;35:1061-1064; discussion 1064-1065.

29. Dempsey R, Rapp RP, Young B, Johnston S, Tibbs P. Prophylactic parenteral antibiotics in clean neurosurgical procedures: A review. *J Neurosurg.* 1988;69:52-57.

30. Cacciola F, Cioffi F, Anichini P, Di Lorenzo N. Antibiotic prophylaxis in clean neurosurgery. *J Chemother.* 2001;13:119-122.

31. Erman TMD, Yilmaz DMMD, Demirhindi HMD, et al. Postsurgical infection: comparative efficacy of intravenous cefoperazone/sulbactam and cefazoline in preventing surgical site infection after neurosurgery. *Neurosurg Q.* 2007;17:166-169.

32. Dasic D, Hanna SJ, Bojanic S, Kerr RS. External ventricular drain infection: the effect of a strict protocol on infection rates and a review of the literature. *Br J Neurosurg.* 2006;20:296-300.

33. Beer R, Lackner P, Pfausler B, Schmutzhard E. Nosocomial ventriculitis and meningitis in neurocritical care patients. *J Neurol.* 2008;255:1617-1624.

34. Hoefnagel D, Dammers R, Ter Laak-Poort MP, Avezaat CJ. Risk factors for infections related to external ventricular drainage. *Acta Neurochir (Wien).* 2008;150:209-214; discussion 214.

35. Hoff JT, Clarke HB. Adverse postoperative events. In: Apuzzo MLJ, ed. *Brain Surgery: Complication Avoidance and Management.* New York, NY: Churchill Livingstone; 1993:99-126.

36. Riechers RGI, Jarell AD, Ling GFS. Infections of the central nervous system. In: Suarez JI, ed. *Critical Care Neurology and Neurosurgery.* Totowa, NJ: Humana Press; 2004:515-532.

37. van de Beek D, Drake JM, Tunkel AR. Nosocomial bacterial meningitis. *N Engl J Med.* 362:146-154.

38. Leib SL, Boscacci R, Gratzl O, Zimmerli W. Predictive value of cerebrospinal fluid (CSF) lactate level versus CSF/blood glucose ratio for the diagnosis of bacterial meningitis following neurosurgery. *Clin Infect Dis.* 1999;29:69-74.

39. Tunkel AR, Hartman BJ, Kaplan SL, et al. Practice guidelines for the management of bacterial meningitis. *Clin Infect Dis.* 2004;9:1267-1284.

40. Zarrouk V, Vassor I, Bert F, et al. Evaluation of the management of postoperative aseptic meningitis. *Clin Infect Dis.* 2007;4:1555-1559.

41. Nathoo NFCS, Nadvi SSFCS, van Dellen JRP, Gouws EB. Intracranial subdural empyemas in the era of computed tomography: a review of 699 cases. *Neurosurgery.* 1999;44:529-535.

42. Post EM, Modesti LM. "Subacute" postoperative subdural empyema. *J Neurosurg.* 1981;55: 761-765.

43. Leedom JH, Holtom PD. Infectious complications. In: Apuzzo MLJ, ed. *Brain Surgery: Complication Avoidance and Management.* New York, NY: Churchill Livingstone; 1993:127-144.

44. Nielsen H, Gyldensted C. Computed tomography in the diagnosis of cerebral abscess. *Neuroradiology.* 1977;12:207-217.

45. Samii M, Matthies C. Management of 1000 vestibular schwannomas (acoustic neuromas): surgical management and results with an emphasis on complications and how to avoid them. *Neurosurgery.* 1997;40:11-21; discussion 21-23.

46. Sen CN, Sekhar LN. Complications of cranial base surgery. In: Post KD, Friedman E, McCormick P, eds. *Postoperative Complications in Intracranial Neurosurgery.* New York, NY: Thieme; 1993:111-133.

47. Klastersky J, Sadeghi M, Brihaye J. Antimicrobial prophylaxis in patients with rhinorrhea or otorrhea: a double-blind study. *Surg Neurol.* 1976;6: 111-114.

48. Duong DH, O'Malley S, Sekhar LN, Wright DG. Postoperative hydrocephalus in cranial base surgery. *Skull Base Surg.* 2000;10:197-200.

49. Infanti JL. Challenging the gold standard: Should mannitol remain our first-line defense against intracranial hypertension? *J Neurosci Nurs.* 2008;40:362-368.

50. Berger S, Schurer L, Hartl R, et al. 7.2% NaCl/10% dextran 60 versus 20% mannitol for treatment of intracranial hypertension. *Acta Neurochir Suppl (Wien).* 1994;60:494-498.

51. Himmelseher S. Hypertonic saline solutions for treatment of intracranial hypertension. *Curr Opin Anaesthesiol.* 2007;20:414-426.

52. Castillo LB, Bugedo GA, Paranhos JL. Mannitol or hypertonic saline for intracranial hypertension? A point of view. *Crit Care Resusc.* 2009;11:151-154.

Perioperative Surgical Care

Trauma and Surgical Intensive Care

Section Editors: Joseph Meltzer, MD
Vivek K. Moitra, MD

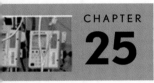

CHAPTER
25

Thoracic Trauma and Cardiothoracic Intensive Care Unit Management

Steven Miller, MD
Vivek K. Moitra, MD

Thoracic trauma. A 38-year-old woman is brought to the emergency department after exposure to an explosion. The patient is confused but able to answer questions, is short of breath and complaining of pain over her left chest with respiration, and opens her eyes to verbal command. She is tachycardic with a heart rate of 112 bpm; hypotensive with a blood pressure of 92/54 mm Hg; tachypneic, breathing 28 breaths/min; and has an oxygen saturation of 98% on 2 L of oxygen via nasal cannula. The physical examination is notable for decreased breath sounds over the right lung field and carbonaceous material in her nares.

What thoracic injuries should be considered immediately in this patient?

Patients who experience thoracic trauma may present with life-threatening injuries such as a pneumothorax, hemothorax, traumatic air embolism, cardiac tamponade, major airway injury, aortic rupture, myocardial rupture, and flail chest (Figure 25-1).[1-7]

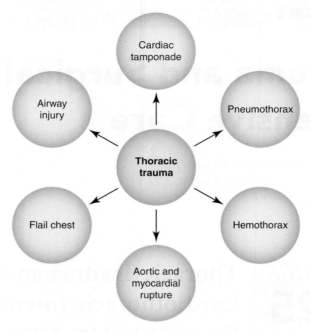

Figure 25-1. Life-threatening complications of thoracic trauma.

A pneumothorax occurs from an injury to the chest wall or lung. As the patient inspires, gas enters the pleural space, where it is trapped. When a one-way valve mechanism occurs at the site of injury, intrapleural pressure increases with each respiratory cycle. Eventually, the ipsilateral lung is compressed and displaced to the opposite side causing a tension pneumothorax. In a tension pneumothorax, kinking of the major vessels entering the heart, decreased venous return, and hypotension occur.[8] A hemothorax also occurs after blunt or penetrating thoracic trauma. The diagnosis is confirmed by placement of a chest tube and drainage of blood from the thoracic cavity. A double-lumen tube can be used for lung isolation to prevent further hypoxia (Figure 25-2).

There is paradoxical motion of the chest wall in patients with a flail chest. After rib injury, free-floating segments of a loose chest wall move in response to pleural pressure instead of the mechanical

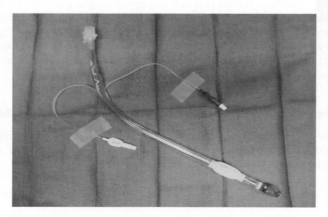

Figure 25-2. Double-lumen endotracheal tube.

positions of the rest of the chest wall. Compromised lung mechanics make inspiration difficult and lead to a pulmonary contusion as a loose chest wall collides with underlying lung tissue.

In patients who present with stridor or subcutaneous emphysema, major airway injury should be considered.[9] There should be a low threshold to intubate patients with suspected injury of the airway. Endotracheal intubation can be difficult when there are changes in the anatomy of the airway. Damage to the bronchial tree can lead to the development of a bronchovenous fistula resulting in a massive air embolus. The presentation of this process may be delayed and unmasked by positive-pressure ventilation.

Almost all patients with an aortic or myocardial rupture die prior to transfer to the intensive care unit (ICU).[3,10]

What is the clinical significance of singed hair and carbonaceous sputum in this patient's nares?

Multiple mechanisms contribute to respiratory failure after a burn injury. Most commonly, toxins contained in smoke injure and inflame the airway. Upper airway edema may completely obstruct the airway, and lower airway edema may close small airways and lead to pneumonia. Patients at risk may have stridor, wheezing, hoarseness, facial burns, or carbonaceous sputum, but these signs are not always present. In many cases, fiberoptic bronchoscopy may be necessary to reveal inhalation injury. If inhalation injury is suspected, the airway should be secured promptly by endotracheal intubation, as the progress of edema is unpredictable and may worsen with fluid resuscitation.

Should this patient be intubated?

Intubation is considered in trauma patients who present with diminished mental status and the inability to maintain an airway or clear secretions. Patients with a Glasgow Coma Scale (GCS) score equal to or less than 8 may be intubated to prevent secondary cerebral injury from hypoxemia or hypercapnia.[11] Additional indications for tracheal intubation after trauma include cardiopulmonary arrest, elevated intracranial pressure, acute hypoxemia, and transport to a less monitored situation.

Chest radiography shows two fractured ribs and the presence of a left-sided pneumothorax (Figure 25-3). A thoracostomy tube is inserted. The patient's tachypnea resolves, her heart rate decreases to 94 bpm, and her blood pressure increases to 120/70 mm Hg. The patient complains of left-sided chest pain and is unable to take deep breaths. Patient-controlled analgesia with morphine sulfate is administered. She continues to complain of pain with inspiration. Her oxygen saturation is 95% on 4 L of oxygen via nasal cannula. What can be done to manage this patient's pain?

Inadequate analgesia causes splinting and respiratory compromise and may lead to mechanical ventilation of the patient's lungs. Cautious use of opioid analgesics is advised in patients whose lungs are not mechanically ventilated. Thoracic epidural analgesia with continuous infusion of local anesthesia in the epidural space effectively prevents pulmonary splinting from rib fractures.[12,13] Placement of an epidural catheter is contraindicated in patients who are coagulopathic or suffer from head injury. An anesthesiologist should be consulted to place a thoracic epidural catheter. Repeated intercostal nerve blockade (Figure 25-4) anesthetizes the nerves of the chest wall without sedation. Disadvantages of this technique include the need for repeat injections and the risk of local anesthetic toxicity from intravascular uptake of medications.

Computerized tomographic (CT) scan of her head, abdomen, and pelvis are negative for additional pathology. On ICU day 2, the patient's oxygenation and tachypnea worsen, crackles are auscultated over her left lung field, and

Trauma and Surgical Intensive Care

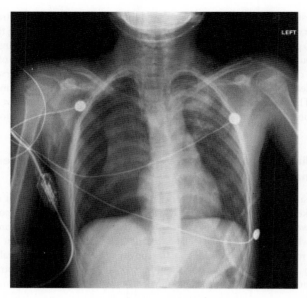

Figure 25-3. Chest radiography demonstrating two fractured ribs and a tension pneumothorax.

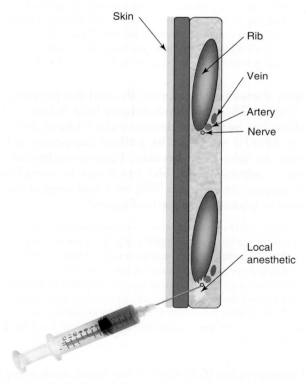

Figure 25-4. Illustration of an intercostal nerve block.

egophony is present over the left chest wall. Her heart rate is 112 bpm, blood pressure is 145/73 mm Hg, respiratory rate is 30 breaths/min, and oxygen saturation is 91% on 10 L of oxygen flow via a simple face mask. What is the differential diagnosis of this patient's respiratory failure?

The differential diagnosis for respiratory failure 2 days after thoracic injury includes pleural effusion; pulmonary contusion; pneumonia; recurrent pneumothorax from a dislodged thoracostomy tube; splinting with atelectasis; pericardial effusion with tamponade, cardiac contusion, and myocardial stunning; and congestive heart failure in the setting of fluid mobilization after trauma. Her unilateral findings of decreased breath sounds and egophony suggest pulmonary contusion and pneumonia.

What is a pulmonary contusion?

Twenty-five percent of patients who suffer from blunt force thoracic trauma are diagnosed with a pulmonary contusion.[14] Contusions develop over 24 to 48 hours, worsen with time, and resolve within 2 weeks. Initial chest radiography may be unremarkable or show unilateral infiltrates from capillary leak and edema (Figure 25-5). Compared to chest radiography, CT scans have a higher sensitivity (Figure 25-6).[15]

What are the complications of a pulmonary contusion?

Complications of pulmonary contusions are common. Pulmonary contusion may progress to parenchymal lung injury or noncardiogenic pulmonary edema (Figure 25-7). Noncardiogenic pulmonary edema results from increased permeability of the alveolar capillary membrane, creating a capillary leak syndrome with exudation of water and protein into the alveolar space. In its most dramatic form, it presents as the acute onset of a massive outpouring of proteinaceous fluid from the endotracheal tube. Noncardiogenic pulmonary edema is distinguished from cardiac failure by the finding of normal or low left atrial or pulmonary artery wedge pressures and a high protein concentration in the edema fluid (albumin concentration 90% or greater than that of serum albumin).

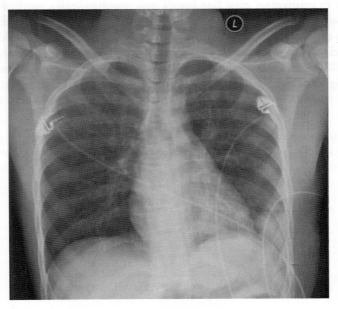

Figure 25-5. Chest radiograph of a patient with a pulmonary contusion.

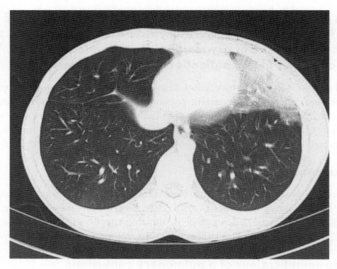

Figure 25-6. Computed tomographic scan showing a pulmonary contusion in the same patient as in Figure 25-5.

Pneumonia occurs after airway edema obstructs the airway. Chest radiography may not be diagnostic in the setting of a preexisting opacification from the pulmonary contusion. Prophylactic antibiotics are not recommended in the treatment of pulmonary contusions, but aggressive treatment of pneumonia after presumptive diagnosis is warranted since it is a prime cause of increased morbidity and mortality.

The patient is intubated and her lungs are mechanically ventilated. For the first 24 hours after intubation, the patient's oxygenation and ventilation deteriorate on assist control–volume control ventilation despite high levels of positive end-expiratory pressure (PEEP). Chest radiography shows diffuse air space–filling disease consistent with acute respiratory distress syndrome (ARDS) (Figure 25-8). Her arterial blood gas is notable for a PaO$_2$ of 45 mm Hg. Should this patient be placed on extracorporeal membrane oxygenation (ECMO)?

ECMO is a device therapy which circulates blood extracorporeally through an oxygenator, ie, "an artificial lung" that removes carbon dioxide, and returns blood to the body via venous or arterial cannulas. Cannulation can occur centrally or peripherally (Figure 25-9).[16] ECMO therapy is used for both

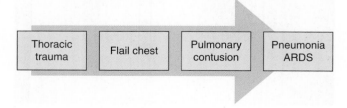

Figure 25-7. Complications of thoracic trauma. ARDS, acute respiratory distress syndrome.

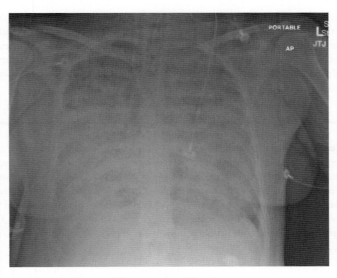

Figure 25-8. Chest radiograph showing diffuse air space–filling disease.

respiratory (ie, ARDS/acute lung injury [ALI],[17,18] pulmonary hemorrhage, ischemia reperfusion injury, or primary graft failure after lung transplant[19]) and hemodynamic support (ie, severe congestive heart failure with cardiogenic shock, failure to wean off of cardiopulmonary bypass during cardiac surgery, acute pulmonary embolus[20]). In venovenous ECMO (VV-ECMO), blood is returned to the circulation via a venous cannula to provide respiratory support. In veno-arterial ECMO (VA-ECMO),

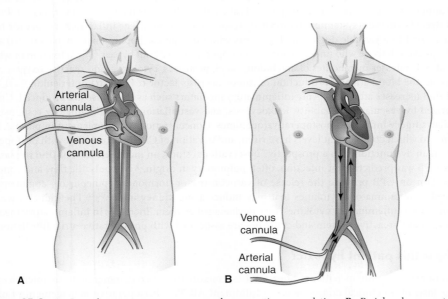

Figure 25-9. A. Central venovenous extracorporeal oxygenation cannulation. **B.** Peripheral veno-arterial extracorporeal oxygenation cannulation. *(From Marasco SF, Lukas G, McDonald M, McMillan J, Ihle B. Review of ECMO (extra corporeal membrane oxygenation) support in critically ill adult patients. Heart Lung Circ. 2008;17(suppl 4):S41-S47.)*

Trauma and Surgical Intensive Care

blood is returned to the circulation via an arterial cannula to provide respiratory and cardiac support. During ECMO therapy, consumption of clotting factors, contact activation, and platelet dysfunction cause coagulopathy and bleeding. At the same time microthrombi form, and low doses of heparinization are required to prevent clotting of the cannula and oxygenator.[16] In this trauma patient with single-organ failure and ARDS, VV-ECMO therapy should be considered if conventional mechanical ventilation is unsuccessful and the patient is not actively bleeding.

 Cardiothoracic intensive care. A 41-year-old woman is diagnosed with new mitral regurgitation. She undergoes a mitral valve repair under cardiopulmonary bypass for 3 hours. During the operation, she receives 6 units of packed red blood cells, 6 units of fresh-frozen plasma, and a 6-pack of platelets. In the ICU, her lungs are mechanically ventilated; she requires 12 µg per minute of norepinephrine to achieve a mean arterial blood pressure of 90/40 mm Hg; her oxygen saturation is 91% with a fractional inspired concentration of oxygen of 1 and her urine output is 10 mL per hour. Her laboratory values show a blood glucose level of 300 mg/dL, white blood cell count of 20,000 cells, and a creatinine of 2.4 mg/dL.

The patient has leukocytosis and hypotension. Should antibiotics be started for an infection?

During cardiac surgery, the metabolic and endocrine function of patients can range from mild hyperglycemia of no clinical consequence to the altered neuroendocrine responses of chronic critical illness. The postoperative management of metabolic derangements can be challenging because multiple factors compromise neuroendocrine function, including the inflammatory response to cardiac surgery and cardiac bypass. Cardiac surgery and cardiopulmonary bypass provoke acute inflammation. A cascade of stress responses is elicited, mediated by the release of various cytokines and stress hormones (systemic inflammatory response syndrome). The inflammatory cascade may be activated to a variable degree in all patients who undergo cardiopulmonary bypass (CPB) and perhaps even in those who undergo other major operations without bypass.[21-23] Activation of white blood cells releases metabolites of arachidonic acid, proteases, cytokines, and reactive oxygen species into the blood stream. Production of tumor necrosis factor α (TNF-α), interleukin 6 (IL-6), and IL-8 increases after CPB. Anti-inflammatory mediators such as IL-10 also are produced. Characterized by vascular permeability, leukocytosis, and vasodilation, the inflammatory response to cardiac surgery influences postoperative outcomes. Concentrations of complement in plasma, the degree to which complement levels have risen, and duration of CPB are correlated with postoperative organ dysfunction.[24] In a prospective observational study, an increased level of IL-6 in plasma after CPB was predictive for infection, often pulmonary in origin.[25] Nonpulsatile flow and contact activation on CPB provoke the release of vasoconstrictor hormones (epinephrine, angiotensin) as well as inflammatory cytokines that may induce acute kidney injury.[21,22] The kidneys, which sequester proinflammatory cytokines, may be damaged by them. Increases in inflammatory mediators such as C-reactive protein and cytokines are associated with postoperative atrial fibrillation.

Why is this patient hypoxic?

Pulmonary function in patients after CPB is consistently altered, ranging from microscopic atelectasis of no clinical consequence to fulminant ARDS.[13] Perioperative management of oxygenation and ventilation can be challenging because multiple factors compromise pulmonary function, including atelectasis, pleural disruption, impaired lung compliance, and the systemic inflammatory response to extracorporeal circulation. CPB represents a particular challenge to the patient with limited pulmonary reserve, who has a particularly high risk of postoperative pulmonary complications. Recruitment maneuvers and lung-protective ventilation should be performed in hypoxic patients with lung injury after cardiopulmonary bypass.

This patient's blood glucose is 300 mg/dL. Is the patient a poorly controlled patient with diabetes who forgot to take her insulin on the morning of surgery?

Hyperglycemia is a ubiquitous phenomenon after cardiac surgery. The metabolic consequences of cardiac surgery and cardiopulmonary bypass, characterized by elevations in circulating catecholamines, growth hormone, glucagon, and cortisol levels with a concomitant depression in insulin levels, promote hepatic glycogenolysis and gluconeogenesis. Hyperglycemia and insulin resistance marks this metabolic profile. Impaired skeletal muscle utilization of glucose (secondary to increased insulin resistance) and decreased entry into the liver reduce glucose clearance.[26,27]

The degree of postoperative hyperglycemia may be dependent on the duration of surgery, intraoperative medications (eg, steroids, epinephrine, or IV fluids containing dextrose), anesthetic agents, and dextrose in pump prime fluid.[28-32] Patients who undergo cardiac surgery with CPB under deep hypothermic circulatory arrest frequently develop hyperglycemia.[33] This is due to the profound inflammatory and stress response of CPB and/or hypothermia, which decreases insulin secretion and further augments insulin resistance.[29] Hyperglycemia after CPB may also reflect an increased reabsorption of glucose in the renal tubules.[34]

Significant insulin resistance develops intraoperatively during cardiac surgery and continues in the postoperative period.[35] This resistance is mediated by proinflammatory molecules, free fatty acids, and counterregulatory hormones.[36] In patients who develop postoperative infections, endotoxin potentiates hyperglycemia by stimulating the adrenergic system and increasing the levels of cytokines that cause insulin resistance.[37]

Intensive insulin therapy is controversial. Should an insulin infusion be initiated in this patient?

Varying recommendations have been proposed by professional organizations (American College of Endocrinology, Canadian Diabetes Association, American Diabetes Association, and the Society of Thoracic Surgeons).[38-41] A general theme of these guidelines is to maintain glucose levels <180 mg/dL perioperatively and between 140 and 180 mg/dL postoperatively. Although the Society of Thoracic Surgeons recommends to maintain a glucose level of <150 mg/dL in cardiac surgery patients with a complicated ICU course, it should be recognized that the recommendation is not based on a high level of evidence.[41] Maintaining glucose levels to < 180 mg/dL is a reasonable goal in most situations. Insulin should be administered preferably by IV infusion, and glucose should be monitored consistently by established monitors.[42]

Two hours after arrival at the ICU, the patient becomes more hypotensive. Her temperature is 37.5°C, and breath sounds are decreased over the right lung field. Her oxygen saturation decreases to 85%. Her central venous pressure increases from 8 mm Hg to 22 mm Hg over 10 minutes. ST-segment elevations are noted in the precordial leads. Does this patient have a pneumothorax?

Immediately after cardiac surgery, patients have chest tubes. Chest tubes are connected to pleurovacs, which are connected to wall suction. Occasionally, these connections become loose or suction is not applied. Large clots can form in the chest tube preventing drainage of blood or air from the patient's chest. The result is a hemothorax or pneumothorax causing hypoxia from atelectasis and shunt physiology.

This patient's central venous pressure is 22 mg Hg. Is she hypervolemic?

No! An acute increase in central venous pressure (CVP) after cardiac surgery is cardiac tamponade until proven otherwise. The cardiac surgeon should immediately open the chest to decrease extracardiac pressure in unstable patients. Acute increases in CVP also occur with right ventricular infarction or pulmonary hypertensive crisis. Echocardiography is useful to determine the etiology of the patient's changing hemodynamics. Sudden increases in CVP impair venous return and increase intracranial pressure and cerebral edema in patients with cerebral injury.

The patient's chest is opened at the bedside and her hemodynamics improve. On the morning after surgery, the patient receives 100 mg of furosemide for low urine output. Her CVP has increased gradually to 18 mm Hg. Her cardiac index is 1.3 L/min per square meter. Her mixed venous oxygen saturation is 55%. Why is this patient's urine output low?

The development of acute kidney injury (AKI) is a major cause of increased morbidity and mortality rates after cardiac surgery. AKI after cardiac surgery is associated with the initiation of renal replacement therapy and an increased incidence of gastrointestinal bleeding, respiratory infections, and sepsis.[43,44] In this setting, postoperative AKI leads to increased intensive care and hospital length of stay. Preventative strategies focus on preoperative optimization of renal function, judicious perioperative fluid balance, and "renoprotective" pharmacologic agents. These strategies appear to have only limited benefit because the incidence of postoperative renal failure has remained constant over the last two decades. Nevertheless, considerable research has been marshaled to protect the kidneys during the high-risk perioperative period when the kidney is placed at risk through preexisting impairment, nephrotoxins, renal ischemia, and the inflammatory process.

Several patient-specific risk factors are associated with the development of renal dysfunction after cardiac surgery: female gender, age, hypertension, diabetes mellitus, ventricular dysfunction, left main coronary artery disease, chronic obstructive pulmonary disease, sepsis, hepatic failure, and chronic kidney disease (CKD).[45] Because CKD also has various definitions, the association between preoperative CKD and postoperative renal injury is difficult to quantify accurately. Nevertheless, there is no doubt that the correlation is strong.[46-48] Recently, pulse pressure hypertension has been shown to precipitate worsening renal function in the setting of cardiac surgery.[49] Interestingly, there appears to be a complex relationship between apolipoprotein E (ApoE) and postoperative AKI. ApoE polymorphisms, although associated with atherosclerotic disease, may confer a degree of renal protection.[50,51]

Controversial procedure-related risk factors associated with kidney injury in the setting of cardiac surgery include length of CPB, cross-clamp time, off-pump versus on-pump, nonpulsatile flow, hemolysis, and hemodilution.[45] The occurrence, alone or in combination, of compromised hemodynamics, surgery, nephrotoxins, or an inflammatory process from CPB may precipitate perioperative AKI, particularly in the patient predisposed by preexisting renal insufficiency or a genetic predisposition. Although the renal medulla receives the minority of renal blood flow, the medullary process of urinary concentration has a high metabolic requirement. Any compromise to renal blood flow increases the regional perfusion imbalance and renders the medulla ischemic. Compromise may result from aortic occlusion, atheromatous embolism, hypotension, low blood flow states, and hypovolemia. Ultimately the pathophysiologic lesion characterizing the AKI of the perioperative cardiac period may be acute tubular necrosis.[45]

CPB and the interaction between blood components and the extracorporeal circuit can diminish renal blood flow through the release of vasoconstrictive compounds. It is important to note, however, that the development of AKI after cardiac surgery appears to vary with the type of surgery. Patients undergoing coronary artery bypass grafting (CABG) have the lowest incidence of injury followed by those undergoing valvular surgery. The highest incidence of renal dysfunction occurs in patients undergoing combined CABG and valvular surgery.[45,52]

Should continuous renal replacement therapy be initiated?

This patient's clinical picture is consistent with a low cardiac output. An elevation in CVP is concerning for a decrease in right ventricular cardiac output. Continuous renal replacement therapy (CRRT) is used in patients who are critically ill, unstable, and unable to tolerate the blood pressure variations of intermittent hemodialysis. Traditionally, renal replacement therapy is considered for patients with uremia, electrolyte abnormalities, acidosis, intoxication, and volume overload. After cardiac surgery, CRRT decreases myocardial edema, removes myocardial depressants, and optimizes the Starling relationship. In patients with evidence of right ventricular pressure overload who do not respond to diuretic therapy, removing intravascular volume via CRRT can improve blood pressure and cardiac output.

! CRITICAL CONSIDERATIONS

- Intubation is considered in trauma patients who present with diminished mental status and the inability to maintain an airway or clear secretions. Patients with a GCS score of 8 or less may be intubated to prevent secondary cerebral injury from hypoxemia or hypercapnia.
- The differential diagnosis for respiratory failure 2 days after thoracic injury includes pleural effusion; pulmonary contusion; pneumonia; recurrent pneumothorax from a dislodged thoracostomy tube; splinting with atelectasis, pericardial effusion with tamponade, cardiac contusion, and myocardial stunning; and congestive heart failure in the setting of fluid mobilization after trauma. In this patient, unilateral findings of decreased breath sounds and egophony suggest pulmonary contusion and pneumonia.
- ECMO therapy is used for both respiratory (ARDS/ALI, pulmonary hemorrhage, ischemia, reperfusion injury, or primary graft failure after lung transplant) and hemodynamic support (severe congestive heart failure with cardiogenic shock, failure to wean off of CPB during cardiac surgery, and acute severe pulmonary embolus).
- An acute increase in CVP after cardiac surgery is cardiac tamponade until proven otherwise. The cardiac surgeon should immediately open the chest to decrease extracardiac pressure in unstable patients. Acute increases in CVP also occur with right ventricular infarction or pulmonary hypertensive crisis. Echocardiography is useful to determine the etiology of the patient's changing hemodynamics.
- Sudden increases in CVP impair venous return and increase intracranial pressure and cerebral edema in patients with cerebral injury.

REFERENCES

1. Liman ST, Kuzucu A, Tastepe AI, Ulasan GN, Topcu S. Chest injury due to blunt trauma. *Eur J Cardiothorac Surg*. 2003;23:374-378.
2. Arthurs ZM, Starnes BW, Sohn VY, Singh N, Martin MJ, Andersen CA. Functional and survival outcomes in traumatic blunt thoracic aortic injuries: an analysis of the National Trauma Databank. *J Vasc Surg*. 2009;49:988-994.
3. Fitzgerald M, Spencer J, Johnson F, Marasco S, Atkin C, Kossmann T. Definitive management of acute cardiac tamponade secondary to blunt trauma. *Emerg Med Australas*. 2005;17:494-499.
4. Ball CG, Kirkpatrick AW, Laupland KB, et al. Incidence, risk factors, and outcomes for occult pneumothoraces in victims of major trauma. *J Trauma*. 2005;59:917-924;discussion 924-925.
5. O'Connor JV, Kufera JA, Kerns TJ, et al. Crash and occupant predictors of pulmonary contusion. *J Trauma*. 2009;66:1091-1095.
6. Budd JS. Effect of seat belt legislation on the incidence of sternal fractures seen in the accident department. *Br Med J (Clin Res Ed)*. 1985;291:785.

Trauma and Surgical
Intensive Care

7. Arajarvi E, Santavirta S. Chest injuries sustained in severe traffic accidents by seatbelt wearers. *J Trauma.* 1989;29:37-41.

8. Kulshrestha P, Munshi I, Wait R. Profile of chest trauma in a level I trauma center. *J Trauma.* 2004;57:576-581.

9. Cassada DC, Munyikwa MP, Moniz MP, Dieter RA Jr, Schuchmann GF, Enderson BL. Acute injuries of the trachea and major bronchi: importance of early diagnosis. *Ann Thorac Surg.* 2000;69:1563-1567.

10. Fulda G, Brathwaite CE, Rodriguez A, Turney SZ, Dunham CM, Cowley RA. Blunt traumatic rupture of the heart and pericardium: a ten-year experience (1979-1989). *J Trauma.* 1991;31:167-172;discussion 172-173.

11. Teasdale G, Jennett B. Assessment of coma and impaired consciousness. A practical scale. *Lancet.* 1974;2:81-84.

12. Luchette FA, Radafshar SM, Kaiser R, Flynn W, Hassett JM. Prospective evaluation of epidural versus intrapleural catheters for analgesia in chest wall trauma. *J Trauma.* 1994;36:865-869;discussion 869-870.

13. Bulger EM, Edwards T, Klotz P, Jurkovich GJ. Epidural analgesia improves outcome after multiple rib fractures. *Surgery.* 2004;136:426-430.

14. Richardson JD, Adams L, Flint LM. Selective management of flail chest and pulmonary contusion. *Ann Surg.* 1982;196:481-487.

15. Schild HH, Strunk H, Weber W, et al. Pulmonary contusion: CT vs plain radiograms. *J Comput Assist Tomogr.* 1989;13:417-420.

16. Marasco SF, Lukas G, McDonald M, McMillan J, Ihle B. Review of ECMO (extra corporeal membrane oxygenation) support in critically ill adult patients. *Heart Lung Circ.* 2008;17(suppl 4):S41-S47.

17. Linden VB, Lidegran MK, Frisen G, Dahlgren P, Frenckner BP, Larsen F. ECMO in ARDS: a long-term follow-up study regarding pulmonary morphology and function and health-related quality of life. *Acta Anaesthesiol Scand.* 2009;53:489-495.

18. Kuroda H, Masuda Y, Imaizumi H, Kozuka Y, Asai Y, Namiki A. Successful extracorporeal membranous oxygenation for a patient with life-threatening transfusion-related acute lung injury. *J Anesth.* 2009;23:424-426.

19. Bermudez CA, Adusumilli PS, McCurry KR, et al. Extracorporeal membrane oxygenation for primary graft dysfunction after lung transplantation: long-term survival. *Ann Thorac Surg.* 2009;87:854-860.

20. Kawahito K, Murata S, Adachi H, Ino T, Fuse K. Resuscitation and circulatory support using extracorporeal membrane oxygenation for fulminant pulmonary embolism. *Artif Organs.* 2000;24:427-430.

21. Gu YJ, Mariani MA, Boonstra PW, Grandjean JG, van Oeveren W. Complement activation in coronary artery bypass grafting patients without cardiopulmonary bypass: the role of tissue injury by surgical incision. *Chest.* 1999;116:892-898.

22. Wan S, LeClerc JL, Vincent JL. Inflammatory response to cardiopulmonary bypass: mechanisms involved and possible therapeutic strategies. *Chest.* 1997;112:676-692.

23. Warren OJ, Smith AJ, Alexiou C, et al. The inflammatory response to cardiopulmonary bypass: Part 1—Mechanisms of pathogenesis. *J Cardiothorac Vasc Anesth.* 2009;23:223-231.

24. Chenoweth DE, Cooper SW, Hugli TE, Stewart RW, Blackstone EH, Kirklin JW. Complement activation during cardiopulmonary bypass: evidence for generation of C3a and C5a anaphylatoxins. *N Engl J Med.* 1981;304:497-503.

25. Sander M, von Heymann C, von Dossow V, et al. Increased interleukin-6 after cardiac surgery predicts infection. *Anesth Analg.* 2006;102:1623-1629.

26. Bagry HS, Raghavendran S, Carli F. Metabolic syndrome and insulin resistance: perioperative considerations. *Anesthesiology.* 2008;108:506-523.

27. Schricker T, Lattermann R, Schrieiber M, Geisser W, Georgieff M, Radermacher P. The hyperglycemic response to surgery: pathophysiology, clinical implications and modification by the anaesthetic technique. *Clin Intensive Care.* 1998;9:118-128.

28. Kuntschen FR, Galletti PM, Hahn C. Glucose-insulin interactions during cardiopulmonary bypass. Hypothermia versus normothermia. *J Thorac Cardiovasc Surg.* 1986;91:451-459.

29. Rassias AJ. Intraoperative management of hyperglycemia in the cardiac surgical patient. *Semin Thorac Cardiovasc Surg.* 2006;18:330-338.

30. Lukins MB, Manninen PH. Hyperglycemia in patients administered dexamethasone for craniotomy. *Anesth Analg.* 2005;100:1129-1133.

31. Sebel PS, Bovill JG, Schellekens AP, Hawker CD. Hormonal responses to high-dose fentanyl anaesthesia. A study in patients undergoing cardiac surgery. *Br J Anaesth.* 1981;53:941-948.

32. Schricker T, Carli F, Schreiber M, et al. Propofol/sufentanil anesthesia suppresses the metabolic and endocrine response during, not after, lower abdominal surgery. *Anesth Analg.* 2000;90:450-455.

33. Lehot JJ, Piriz H, Villard J, Cohen R, Guidollet J. Glucose homeostasis. Comparison between hypothermic and normothermic cardiopulmonary bypass. *Chest.* 1992;102:106-111.

34. Braden H, Cheema-Dhadli S, Mazer CD, McKnight DJ, Singer W, Halperin ML. Hyperglycemia during normothermic cardiopulmonary bypass: the role of the kidney. *Ann Thorac Surg.* 1998;65:1588-1593.

35. Schricker T, Lattermann R, Fiset P, Wykes L, Carli F. Integrated analysis of protein and glucose metabolism during surgery: effects of anesthesia. *J Appl Physiol.* 2001;91:2523-2530.

36. Ljungqvist O, Nygren J, Thorell A. Insulin resistance and elective surgery. *Surgery.* 2000;128:757-760.

37. McGuinness OP. Defective glucose homeostasis during infection. *Annu Rev Nutr.* 2005;25:9-35.

38. Canadian Diabetes Association. 2008 Clinical Practice Guidelines for the Prevention and Management of Diabetes in Canada. *Can J Diabetes.* 2008;32:S72-S73.

39. American Diabetes Association. Standards of medical care in diabetes—2008. *Diabetes Care.* 2008;31(suppl 1):S12-S54.

40. Rodbard HW, Blonde L, Braithwaite SS, et al. American Association of Clinical Endocrinologists medical guidelines for clinical practice for the management of diabetes mellitus. *Endocr Pract.* 2007;13(suppl 1):S1-S68.

41. Lazar HL, McDonnell M, Chipkin SR, et al. The Society of Thoracic Surgeons practice guideline series: blood glucose management during adult cardiac surgery. *Ann Thorac Surg.* 2009;87:663-669.

42. Wahl HG. How accurately do we measure blood glucose levels in intensive care unit (ICU) patients? *Best Pract Res Clin Anaesthesiol.* 2009;23:387-400.

43. Ryckwaert F, Boccara G, Frappier JM, Colson PH. Incidence, risk factors, and prognosis of a moderate increase in plasma creatinine early after cardiac surgery. *Crit Care Med.* 2002;30:1495-1498.

44. Anderson RJ, O'Brien M, MaWhinney S, et al. Renal failure predisposes patients to adverse outcome after coronary artery bypass surgery. VA Cooperative Study #5. *Kidney Int.* 1999;55:1057-1062.

45. Rosner MH, Okusa MD. Acute kidney injury associated with cardiac surgery. *Clin J Am Soc Nephrol.* 2006;1:19-32.

46. Vossler MR, Ni H, Toy W, Hershberger RE. Preoperative renal function predicts development of chronic renal insufficiency after orthotopic heart transplantation. *J Heart Lung Transplant.* 2002;21:874-881.

47. Conlon PJ, Stafford-Smith M, White WD, et al. Acute renal failure following cardiac surgery. *Nephrol Dial Transplant.* 1999;14:1158-1162.

48. Chertow GM, Lazarus JM, Christiansen CL, et al. Preoperative renal risk stratification. *Circulation.* 1997;95:878-884.

49. Aronson S, Fontes ML, Miao Y, Mangano DT. Risk index for perioperative renal dysfunction/failure: critical dependence on pulse pressure hypertension. *Circulation.* 2007;115:733-742.

50. Chew ST, Newman MF, White WD, et al. Preliminary report on the association of apolipoprotein E polymorphisms, with postoperative peak serum creatinine concentrations in cardiac surgical patients. *Anesthesiology.* 2000;93:325-331.

51. Strittmatter WJ, Bova Hill C. Molecular biology of apolipoprotein E. *Curr Opin Lipidol.* 2002;13:119-123.

52. Grayson AD, Khater M, Jackson M, Fox MA. Valvular heart operation is an independent risk factor for acute renal failure. *Ann Thorac Surg.* 2003;75:1829-1835.

Abdominal Trauma

Brian Woods, MD

Emergency medical services (EMS) calls into the community hospital where you are working to alert the staff that they are bringing in by ambulance a 34-year-old male driver who survived a head-on automobile collision. Initial details over the radio inform you that he was found conscious in the car. An IV was started while he was placed in a cervical collar and on a trauma board for transport. He is currently lucid and conversant with EMS staff. His vitals are BP 100/70 mm Hg, pulse 100 bpm, respiratory rate 18 breaths/min, and pulse oximetry 99% on nasal cannula. He denies pain, but the EMS staff can smell alcohol. Initial field physical examination revealed head lacerations with some bleeding, but he is moving all extremities and he has no gross deformities.

What other information would you seek to elicit from the EMS staff? What instructions would you convey?

Initial reports from the field tend to be brief and consist of bare essentials to alert the receiving facility. The field staff focus on major presenting signs and symptoms that can be managed or temporized while preparing for and implementing transport to the hospital. Interventions such as splinting, intubation, IV placement, and, in some communities, drug administration are performed. Review and advice from the receiving physician or facility is often sought. The current paradigm emphasizes "scoop and run," or rapid transport to a definitive facility rather than aggressive and prolonged management in the field.[1] Some would even advocate against placement of IVs prior to beginning transport in urban areas, since the time to place IVs may be equivalent to the time of transport. Location and time of transport probably have a major effect on level and outcomes of care. Advanced life support (ALS) providers are more prevalent in the urban than the rural setting, which is probably the opposite of what is required. Interestingly, however, ALS has not been shown to provide benefit in the EMS setting, and the use of EMS causes delays in time of transport owing to advanced interventions for severe trauma. More concerning, ALS measures, particularly endotracheal intubation, worsened outcomes for patients with initial Glasgow Coma Scale (GCS) scores of less than 9.[2,3]

Estimated time of arrival (ETA) and information about the nature of the injury and patient help the receiving facility prepare personnel and resources appropriately. Further exchange of information might consist of requests for guidance from the receiving physician; otherwise, the EMS staff will focus on transport and patient stability. Transport, IV placement, and directly applied pressure to the head wounds along with vital signs and basic patient observation are the key at this time, which is known as the *prehospital phase*.

The patient is en route to your facility, which is a 50-bed rural hospital with a surgeon on home beeper call. ETA is 15 minutes. You are the

only physician covering the emergency department (ED). What preparations would you make?

This patient may arrive in stable condition with minor injuries that you can easily manage, or could decompensate at any point from overt or occult causes. A room or area should be set aside for this patient, with space for equipment and personnel. Nursing and support staff, including radiology, should be on standby. Endotracheal intubation equipment (laryngoscopes and endotracheal tubes of different sizes, a bag-mask device, end-tidal CO_2 confirmation device, oral or nasal airways, and suction at a minimum) should be prepared and checked. Warm IV fluid sets should be prepared. Standard monitors including noninvasive blood pressure, pulse oximetry, and continuous electrocardiography (ECG) must be present. The blood bank should be informed and asked to have un–cross-matched type O blood available if needed. Universal precautions must be observed; therefore, gowns, gloves, and eye/face protection should be donned. The surgeon should be called in. Arrangements for possible transfer to a higher level care facility should be initiated.

The patient arrives at your facility. EMS informs you that he remained stable during transport. He is moved to a hospital stretcher, still in the c-collar and on the trauma board. The bandages on his head are soaked with blood, and he is looking around and following commands. What do you do next?

You can begin a simple initial assessment as the patient rolls in. Is the patient conscious? Is he in distress? Does he have any gross injuries? Is your team assembled and prepared? EMS will give you a brief but fuller summary than performed over the radio. Details such as mechanism of injury, restrained versus unrestrained, time of extraction, and events during transport provide insight into likely sites and severity of injuries.

A simple and systematic approach is emphasized by the advanced trauma life support (ATLS) guidelines. Many of the steps can be performed in parallel by the team. Coordination by a team leader is essential, along with communication among team members.

A rapid primary survey is followed by treatment of abnormal vital functions. A secondary survey follows, and then definitive care.

ATLS guidelines reduce initial trauma management to ABCDE:

1. Airway maintenance with cervical spine protection
2. Breathing and ventilation
3. Circulation with hemorrhage control
4. Disability: neurologic status
5. Exposure/environmental control: completely undress the patient but prevent hypothermia[4]

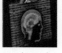 EMS confirms that he was an unrestrained driver who hit a roadside tree. There were skid marks leading up to the tree. He was found conscious, and extraction time was minimal. There was major impact damage to the front of the car, with "starring" of the windshield. The steering wheel was cracked. No air bag was deployed. EMS placed a 16-gauge IV en route. He denied significant medical history or allergies. EMS held pressure on bleeding anterior head lacerations. You begin your initial assessment. He is breathing comfortably with good chest rise and appears awake. The ER tech places a pulse oximeter probe and noninvasive blood pressure (NIBP) monitor along with ECG leads on the patient. BP is 90/65 mm Hg with a pulse of 120 bpm and SpO_2 of 99%. No significant ECG abnormalities are apparent on the monitor in leads II and V_5 other than the sinus tachycardia. Head-to-toe primary survey shows two approximately 8-cm lacerations on top of the head with some minor degloving. There is ongoing dark, venous-appearing blood loss here. No other head injury is apparent, and the ear

canals are clear. He is already moving his eyes and head to follow movement around him in the ED, and appears to do so comfortably. In fact, he is asking you, "Am I going to be OK, Doc?" You can smell alcohol on his breath. You do not see any blood or injured teeth on mouth inspection, and his airway is Mallampati 3. The face is uninjured. You take off the c-collar and have an assistant hold his head. There is no apparent neck injury and he has good carotid pulses. You replace the collar. Your team has already warmed the room, removed his clothing and placed him under warm blankets. You inspect the chest, abdomen, pelvis, and lower extremities visually and by palpation. He has some bruising of the lower chest, consistent with steering wheel impact. Otherwise you see nothing remarkable. The lungs are clear. His abdomen is flat but mildly tender in the upper region; there are no masses. Your team performs a logroll with neck stabilization and you inspect the back, which has no abnormalities. The perineal region and rectal examination are unremarkable. He has good strength and sensation in all his extremities to a brief examination.

Is this patient doing well? What are your next interventions?

You should be concerned about this patient. He suffered a high-energy impact without restraint and has a head injury along with signs of chest or abdominal injury. Table 26-1 outlines typical

Table 26-1. Mechanisms of Injury and Suspected Injury Patterns

Mechanism of injury	Suspected injury patterns
Frontal impact automobile collision	Cervical spine fracture
Bent steering wheel	Anterior flail chest
Knee imprint on dashboard	Myocardial contusion
Bull's-eye fracture of the windshield	Pneumothorax
	Traumatic aortic disruption
	Fractured spleen or liver
	Posterior fracture/dislocation of hip or knee
Side impact automobile collision	Contralateral neck sprain
	Cervical spine fracture
	Lateral flail chest
	Pneumothorax
	Traumatic aortic disruption
	Diaphragmatic rupture
	Fractured spleen/liver/kidney
	Fractured pelvis or acetabulum
Rear impact automobile collision	Cervical spine injury
	Soft tissue injury to neck
Ejection from vehicle	Precludes meaningful prediction of injury patterns, but increases risk of all injuries
Pedestrian struck by motor vehicle	Head injury
	Traumatic aortic disruption
	Abdominal visceral injuries
	Fractured lower extremities/pelvis

(From Fildes J, Brasel K, Burris DG, et al. Advanced Trauma Life Support Student Course Manual. 8th ed. Chicago, IL: American College of Surgeons; 2008:13.)

patterns of injury based on injury mechanism. The lack of severe abdominal pain and relative lack of physical findings can be masked by altered mental status. Furthermore, patients, particularly the young, can compensate for initial injury for some time before abruptly deteriorating. Significant injuries can remain relatively occult, dictating continued patient reassessment. The relative blood pressure stability provides no reassurance; hypotension is a late sign of decompensation.[5] The tachycardia is nonspecific but may portend ongoing blood loss or impending hemodynamic compromise.

You have performed a rapid primary survey and should now address vital functions while beginning a secondary survey. Fluid administration is indicated. The tachycardia could be due to pain, anxiety, or more likely ongoing blood loss. There is little or no disadvantage to a fluid bolus at this point. One to 2 L of normal saline or Ringer's lactate, warmed, should be given rapidly. A nasogastric tube (since there is no facial or skull base injury, the nasal route is appropriate) for lavage and a urinary catheter are important. You should also address the most obvious injury and source of blood loss; that is, the scalp lacerations. Scalp wounds can cause significant blood loss. The wound should be inspected gently but not probed. Depressed skull fracture or foreign material should be identified if possible. Leakage of clear fluid indicates cerebrospinal fluid (CSF) leak. Staples or sutures can quickly stop blood loss; since the scalp is highly vascular, infection is unlikely.

The patient's pulse reduces to 95 bpm after the fluid administration. His blood pressure remains the same. You perform another abdominal examination with similar results. A plain film of the chest is unremarkable, and laboratory studies are pending. It has been 25 minutes since his arrival. Nasogastric (NG) lavage and the urine are clear of blood. The nurse asks if you want to perform a FAST examination. What is the FAST examination? How is it performed? Who can perform it?

Current practice has incorporated the FAST (Focused Assessment with Sonography in Trauma) examination into trauma care worldwide. The basic premise of FAST is to identify fluid in the pericardium or peritoneum. An extended FAST (eFAST) examination is used at some centers; this protocol uses ultrasound to look for pathologic fluid or air in the thorax.

The FAST examination has four views (Figure 26-1); eFAST adds thoracic views.[6] The examination is usually performed initially with the patient supine. The patient can be moved, if clinically appropriate, to improve sonographic windows; for example, to the right lateral position to demonstrate fluid in the right upper quadrant. There is no established, widely accepted certification in FAST; however, United States surgical and emergency medicine residencies now promote training in this technique.

What are the FAST examination's test characteristics? What other diagnostic tools are at your disposal to evaluate this patient's abdominal trauma?

Evidence supports the widespread adoption of FAST. Ultrasound in abdominal trauma has been shown to improve patient outcomes, reduce the use of diagnostic peritoneal lavage (DPL) and computed tomography (CT), and shorten time to the operating room (OR).[7] Cost savings are significant; more than enough to pay for the cost of the ultrasound machine.[8] Scoring based on fluid depth in the abdomen correlates with need for laparotomy.[9] FAST can detect as little as 250 mL of free fluid in the abdomen, with an average positive FAST at 619 mL.[10]

Classic diagnostic tools for abdominal trauma are the DPL and the CT scan. DPL is sensitive for blood in the abdomen but is somewhat time consuming; requires operator experience; has reduced effectiveness or application in the pregnant, obese, or postsurgical patient; and is invasive. Use of the DPL has decreased with the advent of FAST. CT scan is sensitive not only for free fluid but also for solid

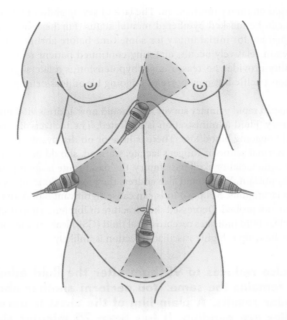

Figure 26-1. Focused assessment with sonography for trauma (FAST). Views are clockwise starting from top: pericardial, left upper quadrant, pouch of Douglas/retrovesicular space, right upper quadrant. *(From Sisley AC, Rozycki GS, Ballard RB, Namias N, Salomone JP, Feliciano DV. Rapid detection of traumatic effusion using surgeon-performed ultrasonography. J Trauma. 1998;44:291-296.)*

organ injury and free air, and is now widely available. However, it is costly and time consuming, as well as requiring transport of a potentially unstable patient out of a highly monitored setting (Table 26-2).[11]

FAST equipment is small and portable. It can be performed at the bedside by a member of the trauma team while initial review and resuscitation efforts are under way. ATLS guidelines recommend a repeat FAST examination 30 minutes after the first scan to demonstrate developing hemoperitoneum in slowly bleeding patients or patients close to the time of injury.[4]

How would you perform a DPL?

DPL is 98% sensitive for intraperitoneal bleeding but does not detect pericardial pathology. It is best performed by an experienced operator. The open or closed infraumbilical approach can be used. After NG tube and urinary catheter placement, the lower abdominal surface is made sterile. In the open technique, the infraumbilical area is locally anesthetized if indicated, a vertical incision is made, and then the soft tissue is dissected at the midline down to the peritoneum. The peritoneum is punctured and a peritoneal dialysis catheter or other appropriate tube is passed into the peritoneal cavity. The closed technique employs a catheter passed over a needle that is inserted into the peritoneum over a wire—essentially a Seldinger technique. If initial aspiration is negative for blood, gastrointestinal (GI) contents, or other foreign material, 1 L of warmed crystalloid is instilled. The fluid is distributed throughout the abdomen by gentle manipulation of the patient. The fluid should remain for a few minutes if conditions allow. The fluid is then drained. More than 30% return is adequate. The fluid should be sent for Gram stain, red blood cell (RBC) and white blood cell (WBC) counts. More than 100,000 RBCs/cc, more than 500 WBCs/cc, or positive Gram stain for bacteria or food fibers indicates the need for laparotomy. Note that the DPL does not detect retroperitoneal injury or diaphragmatic tears. The pregnant patient or prior surgical patient may require a supraumbilical approach. Potential

Table 26-2. Comparison of Focused Assessment with Sonography in Trauma (FAST), Diagnostic Peritoneal Lavage (DPL), and Computed Tomography (CT) in Abdominal Trauma

	FAST	DPL	CT
Advantages	Rapid	Rapid	Highly specific and sensitive for particular organ injury and intraperitoneal blood. Can be extended to include head, thorax, pelvis, extremities
	Good sensitivity and specificity for intra-abdominal fluid	98% sensitive for intraperitoneal bleeding	
	Noninvasive		
	Low cost		Noninvasive
	Available bedside		
Disadvantages	Operator experience-dependent	Invasive	Time consuming/transport delay
		Requires training	
	Limited by obesity, subcutaneous air, previous surgeries	Complicated by obesity, pregnancy, cirrhosis, coagulopathy, or preexisting surgery	Costly
			Requires cooperative patient
Contraindications	Lack of operator experience	Existing indication for laparotomy	Hemodynamic instability
			Allergy to contrast
Notes	Scan should be repeated to assess for slow bleeding	Open or Seldinger infraumbilical approach preferred	Gastrointestinal, diaphragmatic, and pancreatic injuries can be missed
	Can be used to assess pericardial fluid and cardiac function	Positive test is by gross aspiration, or > 100,000 RBC/mm^3, 500 WBC/mm^3, positive Gram stain	Patient must be monitored during transport and scan

(From Fildes J, Brasel K, Burris DG, et al. Advanced Trauma Life Support Student Course Manual. 8th ed. Chicago, IL: American College of Surgeons; 2008:117-118.)

complications of the DPL include bleeding, peritonitis from enteric perforation, urinary bladder injury, solid organ injury, and wound infection.[4]

What factors would lead you to employ one diagnostic test over another?

FAST, DPL, and CT are not mutually exclusive tests and can be used to complement management. There is no absolute standard of care when choosing among these tests, but clearly their availability and timing must be considered. An initial FAST examination for every trauma patient is standard at many centers.

Describe the basic anatomy assessed in the FAST examination

The right upper quadrant view looks at the Morrison pouch and thus for fluid in the right paracolic gutter between the liver and right kidney. The left upper quadrant view examines the space between the spleen and the left kidney; that is, the left paracolic gutter. Notably, the right paracolic gutter is longer than the left and tends to have more fluid in it during pathologic states since the phrenocolic ligament on the left side diverts fluid to the right. The rectovesical pouch in males or the pouch of Douglas in females is the most dependent intrapelvic space in the supine patient, and is thus the target of the FAST pelvic view. The pericardium, typically through the subxiphoid or subcostal view, is seen on the fourth view. Assessment of the diaphragms and pleural spaces bilaterally is performed in the eFAST.[11] Figure 26-2 is a sample left upper quadrant FAST view.

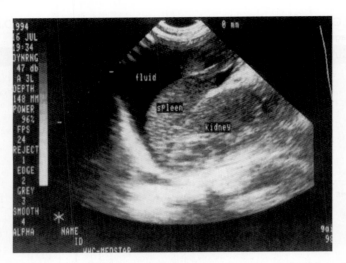

Figure 26-2. Positive left upper quadrant FAST examination view. *(From Rozycki GS, Ochsner MG, Schmidt JA, et al. A prospective study of surgeon-performed ultrasound as the primary adjuvant modality for injured patient assessment. J Trauma. 1995;39:492-498.)*

You find free fluid in the right upper quadrant view on your repeat FAST examination, but the other views are normal. The patient's pulse has increased again to the 120s, without change in the mean arterial pressure. He still has abdominal pain. Laboratory studies are unremarkable except for an elevated blood ethanol level. What is your interpretation of these findings?

Recurrent tachycardia after resolution with fluid along with developing FAST findings suggests intra-peritoneal bleeding. The lack of change in physical examination and lack of acute anemia should not reassure you. Circulating hemoglobin concentration does not change acutely with rapid hemorrhage.

The on-call surgeon arrives, reviews your findings, and recommends laparotomy. However, the OR staff are still en route and the OR will not be set up for some time. What do you do in the meantime?

ATLS guidelines recommend a low threshold for transfer of trauma patients to higher levels of care. You have stabilized and already begun resuscitation of this patient; further management requires the OR. At this point, you must decide between transfer to another, higher level of care facility or await arrival of your OR staff. This choice must be made using your knowledge of the resources at hand and time of transport to the next facility, as well as the patient's stability. You have already initiated arrangements with a team at a trauma center 40 minutes away by ground, which has 24-hour OR readiness. You and the surgeon decide that transfer is best for this patient (Table 26-3).

You confirm transfer with the trauma center's receiving physician, who requests a CT of the head, chest, abdomen, and pelvis prior to transfer to identify other potential injuries and define the abdominal process. What do you say?

Further studies will delay transfer and definitive care for this patient. While other pathology might be revealed by the scan, you have already identified his most threatening problem—hemoperitoneum—and its treatment—laparotomy. Further studies are not indicated pending resolution of his primary problem, and could worsen his condition. Even the entirely stable patient's transfer should not be delayed. This particular patient, however, is not stable and needs laparotomy as soon as possible (Table 26-4).

Table 26-3. Indications for Transfer to Higher Level of Care

Central nervous system	Head injury:
	    Penetrating injury or depressed skull fracture
	    Open injury with or without cerebrospinal fluid leak
	    Glasgow Coma Scale score < 15 or neurologically abnormal
	    Lateralizing signs
	Spinal cord injury or major vertebral injury

Chest	Widened mediastinum or signs suggesting great vessel injury Major chest wall injury or pulmonary contusion Cardiac injury Patients who may require prolonged intubation
Pelvis/abdomen	Unstable pelvic-ring disruption Pelvic-ring disruption with shock and continued hemorrhage Open pelvic injury Solid organ injury
Extremities	Severe open fractures Traumatic amputation with potential for reimplantation Complex articular fractures Major crush injury Ischemia
Multisystem injuries	Head injury with face, chest, abdominal, or pelvic injury Injury to more than two body organs Major burns or burns with associated injuries Multiple proximal long-bone fractures
Comorbid factors	Age > 55 y Age < 5 y Cardiac or respiratory disease Insulin-dependent diabetes Morbid obesity Pregnancy Immunosuppression
Secondary deterioration	Mechanical ventilation Sepsis Single- or multiple-organ failure Major tissue necrosis

(From Fildes J, Brasel K, Burris DG, et al. Advanced Trauma Life Support Student Course Manual. 8th ed. Chicago, IL: American College of Surgeons; 2008:272.)

Trauma and Surgical Intensive Care

You are on the trauma service at a tertiary care center. EMS calls in to say they are bringing in a 66-year-old woman who was assaulted and robbed. She was able to call 911 after the attack. EMS found her confused, tachycardic to the 130s, with a systolic BP of 80 mm Hg. She had clothing tears consistent with stab wounds, and there was blood on the ground. ETA is 20 minutes.

Table 26-4. Goals of Patient Transfer to Higher Level of Care

Goal	Notes
Timelines	Time between injury and appropriate care has direct effect on patient outcome
	Intervention prior to transfer should be weighed against need for timely higher level of care
Patient and facility factors	Physiologic instability that cannot be treated at presenting center indicates need for transfer
	Pain control and sedation can worsen patient status but may be necessary for safe transfer
	Receiving facility must be equipped to handle patient needs based on the trauma and initial survey
Transport mode	Depends on location, availability, and speed of transport
	Patient transport itself affects level of care to the patient and should be planned and accomplished quickly
Communication	Referring physician must initiate transfer, mode of transport, and must consult with receiving physician; appropriate documentation should be sent with or prior to patient; patient should be stabilized within capabilities of referring facility
	Receiving physician ensures receiving facility has capabilities appropriate to the patient, as well as to facilitate transport

(From Fildes J, Brasel K, Burris DG, et al. Advanced Trauma Life Support Student Course Manual. 8th ed. Chicago, IL: American College of Surgeons; 2008;270-273.)

What goals do you have for management of this patient?

ABCDE (see above), the treatment of abnormal vitals, and repeated assessment of traumatized patients.

The patient arrives. EMS had to intubate her en route for airway protection because of worsening mental status. Vecuronium was used to facilitate airway management. She has a 14-gauge IV and has normal saline running in; her second liter of IV fluid. She appears age appropriate, pale, and she is not moving. Her clothes, prior to removal, are covered in blood over the abdomen. You begin a primary survey. Notable findings are two stab wounds, one under the left breast and one just right of the umbilicus. Vital signs show a BP of 96/66 mm Hg and a pulse of 110 bpm. What should you do next?

This patient needs to be in a c-collar since we do not know if she suffered another injury, and she likely is unresponsive because of medications used to intubate, if not from injury. She needs a complete *primary* survey, which includes looking at the back, perineum, and rectum. Endotracheal tube position should be confirmed by breath sounds and end-tidal carbon dioxide ($ETCO_2$) concentration. A FAST examination can be done after she is turned. The room should be warmed and fluids made warm. Blood should be available, and labs sent. An oral gastric tube for lavage and a urinary catheter should be placed.

 You find another stab wound in the lower right back. It is bleeding slowly. The other wounds are not bleeding, and there is no sucking sound from the chest wound. You apply pressure dressings to all these wounds. Drainage from the stomach and urinary bladder are clear. Her abdomen is firm and you cannot assess if it is tender, but she is beginning to move her extremities and her head. FAST examination shows no fluid in the abdomen or pericardium. Her pulse rises to the 130s and her systolic pressure decreases to the 70s. Her labs return just as the chest plain film is obtained. Her hemoglobin is 8 g/dL.

What interventions would you make now?

She is bleeding somewhere and needs resuscitation with fluid and probably blood. If cross-matched blood is available, give several units in anticipation of ongoing blood loss; otherwise, you must use un–cross-matched but typed blood if she is already typed, or type O blood if you do not know the blood type. Since she is female, she may have been exposed to Rh antigens during pregnancy and, therefore, you should not use O+ blood if at all possible. Fresh-frozen plasma (FFP) should be given as well; recent trauma literature supports use of FFP to blood in a 1:1 ratio, although this is not a universal standard.[12] Another large-bore IV would prove to be useful.

Would you repeat the FAST examination, perform a DPL, or perform a CT?

Not if she fails to respond to fluids and blood. She would need to go directly to the OR for laparotomy. In fact, some experts would take any patient with penetrating wounds to the abdomen and hemodynamic instability to the OR immediately. A secondary survey should be repeated. Points of interest would be the chest, looking for pneumothorax, hemopneumothorax or a pericardial effusion, all of which can cause tachycardia, hypotension, and acute anemia. The left anterior chest wound, since it is below the nipple, could have caused an intra-abdominal injury. If she responds to the fluid and blood products, then a judgment can be made about conservative, expectant management (observation and studies) versus immediate laparotomy.

If this patient's injuries were gunshot wounds rather than stabs, how would this change your approach?

Gunshot wounds are high energy; stab wounds are low energy. Gunshot wounds to the abdomen typically mandate exploratory laparotomy since significant intraperitoneal injury will reach nearly 90%. Gunshots can also fragment or ricochet off bony structures, worsening injury. Small bowel, colon, liver, and vascular structures are the more common injured organs. Stab wounds to the abdomen are less likely to require exploratory laparotomy and, if the patient is stable, can be explored at the bedside. Organs injured by stab wounds are typically the liver, small bowel, diaphragm, and colon.[4] Indications for exploratory laparotomy in abdominal trauma are listed in Table 26-5. Gunshot wounds can vary widely depending on site of entry, type of bullet, and victim position. Entry and exit sites are not always identifiable. The projectile path within the body is not necessarily linear as the bullet can tumble prior to stopping, and it can subsequently migrate. CT scan, while highly useful in the stable patient with penetrating abdominal injury, does not obviate the need for serial observation or exploratory laparotomy.[13]

Your patient goes to the OR for an exploratory laparotomy. The surgeon performs a splenectomy for a large laceration. Two enterotomies (small bowel injuries) are discovered and repaired. A left colon perforation is also discovered and repaired. Frank spillage of stool into the peritoneum was discovered on opening. The back wound is explored in the OR and is washed out and closed primarily from the outside since it does not penetrate deeper than muscle. She does fairly well hemodynamically in the OR, receiving several liters of crystalloid and colloid along with a few units of red cells and FFP. The OR team places a central line. She remains intubated and is brought to your ICU. As the day progresses she becomes increasingly tachycardic and hypotensive, requiring

Table 26-5. Some Indications for Exploratory Laparotomy in Abdominal Trauma

Blunt abdominal trauma with positive FAST or other evidence of intraperitoneal bleeding
Hypotension with penetrating abdominal wound
Gunshot wound traversing peritoneal cavity, viscera, vascular structure, or retroperitoneum
Evisceration
Bleeding from the stomach, rectum, or genitourinary tract from penetrating trauma
Peritonitis
Free air, retroperitoneal air, or rupture of the hemidiaphragm after blunt trauma
Ruptured gastrointestinal tract, intraperitoneal bladder injury, renal pedicle injury, or severe visceral parenchymal injury demonstrated on computed tomographic scan

(From Fildes J, Brasel K, Burris DG, et al. Advanced Trauma Life Support Student Course Manual. 8th ed. Chicago, IL: American College of Surgeons; 2008:120.)

vasopressor support and ongoing fluid resuscitation. These interventions do not seem to help. The nurse calls you to report a decreasing urine output despite an elevated central venous pressure (CVP).

What is your diagnosis, and what do you do about it?

This patient is probably developing intra-abdominal hypertension (IAH) with signs of abdominal compartment syndrome in the setting of fecal peritonitis, bowel injury, and large fluid resuscitation. You should check a bladder pressure, and while that is obtained, call the surgeon, who will likely elect to open the abdomen. See Chapter 28 for more details regarding assessment and management of IAH. The CVP is elevated because of transmission of the high intra-abdominal pressures to the inferior vena cava (IVC). Similarly, catheter-measured cardiac filling pressures would be elevated, with a low cardiac output and stroke volume. This patient requires the fluid for resuscitation; the bowel edema is part of the natural history of her disease process and will have to be managed conservatively until resolution.

At what point would you start this patient on antibiotics? What antibiotics would you choose?

There is no evidence supporting antibiotic use in the patient with penetrating abdominal trauma sensu stricto.[14] However, patients undergoing exploratory laparotomy should receive one dose of antibiotic with gram-positive and gram-negative coverage prior to incision. Patients with evident hollow viscus injury should receive at least 1 day of such antibiotic. Our patient, who has fecal peritonitis, is more complex and will require several days of antibiotic treatment for gram-positives, gram-negatives, anaerobes, and possibly fungal pathogens as well since the patient is critically ill. The Infectious Disease Society of America/Surgical Infection Society guidelines recommend 4 to 7 days of treatment for complicated intra-abdominal infections; less than 24 hours of antibiotic are required for simple perforated bowel cases. These guidelines also detail antibiotic regimens.[15]

What other interventions should you perform for the abdominal trauma patient in your ICU?

The tertiary survey should be performed. This is essentially the final phase of the evaluation that began in the trauma bay. The patient's injuries and status should be reviewed literally from head to toe. A physical examination should be performed and a history elicited from the patient if possible. Laboratory and radiologic studies should be thoroughly reviewed. In this way, missed injuries or trauma sequelae can be identified. The tertiary survey typically takes place 24 hours after admission, and some centers repeat the tertiary survey prior to discharge.[16,17]

What are management options for the patient with liver injury?

Hepatic injury manifests as hypovolemic shock. Hemorrhage can be rapid enough that anemia is not seen on initial laboratory investigation. CT is sensitive for liver injury and can provide the basis for triage, but these images have not been found to correlate well with intraoperative findings. FAST is typically not useful for defining liver parenchymal injury. Surgical management can include direct ligation of vessels, debridement, or partial resection if indicated. Packing is performed for hard to control bleeding. Identification and control of bleeding can be challenging since the liver has three sources of blood: the hepatic artery, portal vein, and back bleeding from the hepatic veins. Injury at the hepatic veins or hepatic IVC can be especially hard to manage.[18] A common grading system for hepatic injury is given in Table 26-6. Traumatic hepatic injury even with high-grade liver laceration can be managed conservatively without operation with close observation, having cross-matched blood available, and fluid restriction with the aim of a low CVP to reduce venous bleeding.

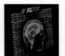 You admit a patient with polytrauma from a fall to your ICU. He is a 45-year-old construction worker who fell 30 ft, face-first, onto cement bags. He is intubated for a declining GCS score, is in a c-collar, and has multiple extremity injuries. CT scan results are consistent with head injury, lower thoracic spine injury, and multiple extremity fractures. He is hemodynamically stable and the initial plan is for stabilization of his spine fracture. Over the course of the day, however, a rising amylase level is noted.

Table 26-6. Liver Injury Scale.*

I	Hematoma	Subcapsular, < 10% surface area
	Laceration	Capsular tear, < 1 cm parenchymal depth
II	Hematoma	Subcapsular, nonexpanding, 10%-50% surface area; intraparenchymal, < 10 cm in diameter
	Laceration	1-3 cm parenchymal depth, < 10 cm long
III	Hematoma	Subcapsular, > 50% surface area or expanding; ruptured subcapsular or parenchymal hematoma; intraparenchymal hematoma > 10 cm or expanding
	Laceration	> 3 cm parenchymal depth
IV	Laceration	Parenchymal disruption involving 25%-75% of hepatic lobe or 1-3 segments within a single lobe
V	Laceration	Parenchymal disruption involving > 75% of hepatic lobe or > 3 segments within a single lobe
	Vascular	Juxtahepatic venous injuries
VI	Vascular	Hepatic avulsion

*Advance one grade for multiple injuries, up to grade III. (From Moore EE, Cogbill TH, Jurkovich GJ, Shackford SR, Malangoni MA, Champion HR. Organ injury scaling: Spleen and liver (1994 revision). J Trauma. 1995;38:Table 2.)

Trauma and Surgical Intensive Care

What do you suspect?

Pancreatic injury. This patient suffered blunt trauma to the epigastric area, energetic enough to cause thoracic spine fracture. Absence of hyperamylasemia on initial presentation does not rule out traumatic pancreatitis; conversely, not all elevations of amylase in trauma patients are caused by pancreatitis, a finding that is not well understood but may be due to translocation into the bloodstream.[19] In any case, traumatic pancreatitis must be assessed by serial CT if necessary. Management can range from observation to debridement, depending on CT findings and patient condition.

 A survivor of a side-on car collision is admitted to your ICU for stabilization. He was a restrained driver whose car was struck on its side by another vehicle. The door was crushed into the passenger compartment, and the extrication time was prolonged. Among other data, initial review in the trauma bay that included plain films showed significant pelvic fractures. Serial FAST examinations were negative. He received fluid and blood in the trauma bay prior to transfer to the ICU. The ICU nurse pages you, indicating that the patient's heart rate is now in the 120s and his systolic blood pressure has decreased since admission.

What do you ask the nurse to do?

Transfuse blood products—The patient likely has ongoing blood loss.

You examine the patient and find flank hematomas with a firm distended abdomen. You deliberately avoid manipulating the pelvis to assess instability, given the history and plain films available. What is your diagnosis?

Retroperitoneal bleed from the pelvic fracture should be uppermost. These can be quite difficult to control, but there are several interventions to stabilize the bleeding. In the first place, do no harm. Do not worsen the fracture and potentially the bleeding by rocking the pelvis to determine stability. Instead, if retroperitoneal hemorrhage from pelvic fracture is suspected, the pelvic bone should be stabilized with a commercial purpose-built device or by cinching a sheet around the patient's hips. Management can be expectant or can involve interventional radiology for embolization versus intraoperative management. The latter can lead to worse blood loss since the bleeding source can be difficult to identify and control in the OR. In such cases, packing and stabilization of the bony structures, then embolization, can be done.[20] Retroperitoneal hemorrhage can occur with both blunt and penetrating abdominal injuries, with or without bony involvement. Other concerns in the differential are pulmonary embolus (fat, air, or thrombotic), pericardial tamponade, pneumothorax, or great vessel injury. Neurogenic shock from a high spinal injury is less likely, given the tachycardia. Ongoing assessment of vital signs, imaging, or surgical exploration is indicated.

! CRITICAL CONSIDERATIONS

- ATLS guidelines provide an excellent basis for initial and ongoing management of abdominal trauma.
- Understanding the mechanism and probable resulting patterns of injury are important for effective treatment.

- Repeated surveys of the patient by examination and studies must be performed, and a high index of suspicion for occult injury maintained.
- Investigation of related injuries outside of the abdomen, particularly in the chest, must be considered.
- Early transfer to a definitive facility is a cornerstone of trauma management. Preparation and teamwork are paramount.
- Understanding the relative strengths and weaknesses of the FAST, DPL, and CT scan improve care.
- ICU management of the abdominal trauma patient should be viewed in continuum with the prehospital, trauma bay, and OR phases.
- Injuries not apparent during initial stages of treatment may manifest in the ICU or floor setting, particularly as patient time in the initial stages decreases.

REFERENCES

1. Smith RM, Conn AK. Prehospital care—Scoop and run or stay and play? *Injury.* 2009;40(suppl 4):S23-S26.

2. Cornwell EE 3rd, Belzberg H, Hennigan K, et al. Emergency medical services (EMS) vs non-EMS transport of critically injured patients: a prospective evaluation. *Arch Surg.* 2000;135:315-319.

3. Stiell IG, Nesbitt LP, Pickett W, et al. The OPALS Major Trauma Study: impact of advanced life-support on survival and morbidity. *CMAJ.* 2008;178:1141-1152.

4. Fildes J, Brasel K, Burris DG, et al. *Advanced Trauma Life Support Student Course Manual.* 8th ed. Chicago, IL: American College of Surgeons; 2008.

5. Baskett PJ. ABC of major trauma. Management of hypovolaemic shock. *BMJ.* 1990;300:1453-1457.

6. Sisley AC, Rozycki GS, Ballard RB, Namias N, Salomone JP, Feliciano DV. Rapid detection of traumatic effusion using surgeon-performed ultrasonography. *J Trauma.* 1998;44:291-296; discussion 6-7.

7. Melniker LA, Leibner E, McKenney MG, Lopez P, Briggs WM, Mancuso CA. Randomized controlled clinical trial of point-of-care, limited ultrasonography for trauma in the emergency department: the first sonography outcomes assessment program trial. *Ann Emerg Med.* 20 06;48:227-235.

8. Branney SW, Moore EE, Cantrill SV, Burch JM, Terry SJ. Ultrasound based key clinical pathway reduces the use of hospital resources for the evaluation of blunt abdominal trauma. *J Trauma.* 1997;42:1086-1090.

9. McKenney KL, McKenney MG, Cohn SM, et al. Hemoperitoneum score helps determine need for therapeutic laparotomy. *J Trauma.* 2001;50:650-654; discussion 4-6.

10. Branney SW, Wolfe RE, Moore EE, et al. Quantitative sensitivity of ultrasound in detecting free intraperitoneal fluid. *J Trauma.* 1995;39:375-380.

11. Noble VE, Nelson B, Sutingco AN. *Manual of Emergency and Critical Care Ultrasound.* New York, NY: Cambridge University Press; 2007.

12. Ho AM, Dion PW, Yeung JH, et al. Fresh-frozen plasma transfusion strategy in trauma with massive and ongoing bleeding. Common (sense) and sensibility. *Resuscitation.* 2010;81:1079-1081.

13. Goodman CS, Hur JY, Adajar MA, Coulam CH. How well does CT predict the need for laparotomy in hemodynamically stable patients with penetrating abdominal injury? A review and meta-analysis. *Am J Roentgenol.* 2009;193:432-437.

14. Brand M, Goosen J, Grieve A. Prophylactic antibiotics for penetrating abdominal trauma. *Cochrane Database Syst Rev.* 2009:CD007370.

15. Solomkin JS, Mazuski JE, Bradley JS, et al. Diagnosis and management of complicated intra-abdominal infection in adults and children: guidelines by the Surgical Infection Society and the Infectious Diseases Society of America. *Clin Infect Dis.* 2010;50:133-164.

16. Biffl WL, Harrington DT, Cioffi WG. Implementation of a tertiary trauma survey decreases missed injuries. *J Trauma.* 2003;54:38-43; discussion 43-44.

17. Trauma Tertiary Surveys. 2010. (Accessed 2/12/2010, at http://www.trauma.org/archive/nurse/tertiarysurvey.html)

18. Jarnagin WR. Liver and portal venous system. In: Doherty GM, ed. *Current Diagnosis and Treatment: Surgery.* 13th ed. New York, NY: McGraw-Hill; 2010;509-543.

19. Malinoski DJ, Hadjizacharia P, Salim A, et al. Elevated serum pancreatic enzyme levels after hemorrhagic shock predict organ failure and death. *J Trauma.* 2009;67:445-449.

20. Dyer GS, Vrahas MS. Review of the pathophysiology and acute management of haemorrhage in pelvic fracture. *Injury.* 2006;37:602-613.

Trauma and Surgical Intensive Care

Traumatic Vascular Injuries

27

Shahzad Shaefi, MD
Joseph Meltzer, MD

A 48-year-old female restrained car driver is involved in a motor vehicle accident. Her car slid off the road into a tree when it was traveling at 50 mph with air bag deployment. She did not lose consciousness. After a short extrication time, she is brought to the emergency department (ED). The patient is awake and alert, although somewhat confused. Her vital signs include a BP of 80/40 mm Hg, HR 120 bpm, sats 94% on an FIO$_2$ of 100% via nonrebreather face mask.

What are the immediate goals for this patient?

In the ED, many things need to be coordinated at once. Primary survey of airway, breathing, and circulation according to advanced trauma life support (ATLS) algorithms should be the immediate priority.[1] Establishment of adequate intravenous access, the collection of laboratory studies, and recognition of life-threatening injuries are paramount.

The primary survey reveals a patent airway but minimal breath sounds over the right hemithorax, with ecchymosis and crepitus on the right chest wall. She has a tense abdomen and pain upon palpation of her pelvis. A right open tibial fracture is noted. Plain chest radiography demonstrates an effusion in the right hemithorax. A tube thoracostomy is performed on the right, with return of air and 800 cc of bloody fluid without significant improvement in hemodynamics. Pelvic films show fractures of the pelvic ring and a right acetabular fracture. The pelvis is temporarily stabilized with a bedsheet. A FAST (focused assessment with sonography in trauma) examination shows free fluid in the abdomen, and the patient is taken to the operating room (OR) for an exploratory laparotomy. A splenectomy and hepatic debridement and surgical packing are performed, as well as external fixation of her tibial fracture. The abdomen is left open. After the OR, the patient is taken to the Interventional Radiology Suite, and two pelvic arterial injuries are coiled with hemodynamic stabilization. The patient is taken to the ICU sedated, endotracheally intubated, and mechanically ventilated.

What are the goals of care of this patient in the operating room?

The pendulum has shifted from surgical correction of all injuries fully to "damage control" of those immediate life-threatening injuries.[2-4] The rapid control of hemorrhage and prevention of coagulopathy, hypothermia, and acidosis are the perioperative goals. This is achieved via limiting the operative time as much possible with rapid transport to the intensive care unit (ICU) for further optimization. Damage-control surgery is the mainstay of acute surgical trauma care.[5,6] Polytrauma patients will often require multiple operations to deal with problems stemming from the initial traumatic insult.

Traumatic injury represents the leading cause of death nationally in those under 45 years of age and the fifth most common cause of death overall.[7] In the multiple trauma patients, the leading cause of death is catastrophic brain injury. Hemorrhage is the second most common cause of mortality.[8] Major vascular and severe neurologic injuries often occur together in the polytrauma victim.

What are the mechanisms of vascular and solid organ injuries?

The vascular tree and viscera can be affected by direct or indirect insult from blunt or penetrating trauma. Vessels can be injured by transection, rupture, or contusion. These injuries must be recognized rapidly and managed aggressively. Other vascular injuries such as dissection, true and pseudo-aneurysm formation, and embolism may develop immediately or in a delayed fashion.

Blunt Trauma

The mechanism of damage to the thoracic aorta following blunt trauma often reveals a consistent pattern of injury that is discrete from that of penetrating injury owing to physical forces and inherent points of aortic weakness. The thoracic aorta is relatively fixed at three points: the aortic valve, the ligamentum arteriosum, and the diaphragm. The descending aorta is tethered, in contrast, to the relatively mobile ascending aorta and aortic arch.[9] In classic blunt acceleration-deceleration injury, stretch, shear, torsion forces, and extrinsic vascular compression against neighboring structures as well as the water-hammer effect of high-pressure reflection of noncompressible blood in the face of acute aortic obstruction all may contribute to injury ranging from subintimal hemorrhage to total aortic disruption.[9]

The mechanism of blunt injury to intra-abdominal structures can be classified into compression forces and deceleration forces. Compression or concussive forces may result from direct blows or external compression against a fixed object; for example, a seat belt or the spinal column. The most common sequelae are tears or subcapsular hematomas to the solid viscera. These forces may also deform hollow organs, such as the small bowel, and transiently increase intraluminal pressure, resulting in rupture.

Deceleration forces cause stretching and linear shearing between relatively fixed and free objects. These longitudinal shearing forces tend to rupture supporting structures at the junction between free and fixed segments. Classic deceleration injuries include hepatic lacerations along the ligamentum teres and renal arterial intimal injuries. Additionally, as bowel loops travel from their mesenteric attachments, thrombosis and mesenteric tears to the splanchnic vessel may result.

Penetrating Trauma

The damage caused by penetrating trauma is directly related to the amount of kinetic energy that is supplied by the projectile or penetrating object. Lower-velocity injuries, such as stab wounds, usually lead to damage to the directly contacted structures and tissues. In contrast, higher-velocity ballistic injuries have an additional pressure wave component, which creates further tissue damage.[10] The full extent of injury, therefore, may not be initially apparent by recognition of entry and exit wounds. Of note, there is considerable literature supporting the delay of aggressive fluid resuscitation in hypotensive penetrating injury until operative intervention.[11]

What viscera are most often implicated in blunt abdominal trauma?

Splenic Injury

In cases of blunt abdominal trauma, the spleen is the most often affected organ, representing 40% of injuries to solid viscera. As with all cases of suspected abdominal trauma, initial management is guided by hemodynamic stability of the patient. ATLS protocol–driven care and timely clinical and/or imaging studies (ultrasound/FAST and/or helical computed tomographic [CT] scan) will guide patient triage to the OR, ICU, or less acute setting. Splenic injury, even rupture, may present along a spectrum from asymptomatic to diffuse abdominal tenderness, with or without hemodynamic instability. The decision to operate for splenic trauma depends largely on the hemodynamic stability of the patient. The grading of splenic injury ranges from I to V, depending on the presence and size of subcapsular hematoma, intraparenchymal laceration, laceration of segmental or hilar vessels, or complete avulsion.[12] The critical care issues in these patients are largely ongoing hemorrhage, if managed nonoperatively, so close hemodynamic monitoring with frequent laboratory assessment for bleeding is a must. Splenic artery aneurysms may also form after trauma and represent a potential source of brisk hemorrhage.

Hepatic Injury

Hepatic injury may occur in isolation or alongside other injuries. Nonoperative management is widely used in the hemodynamically stable patient, but is also increasingly being employed in more hemodynamically unstable patients as well.[13] The grading of hepatic injuries follows a similar pattern to that of the spleen, with grades I through VI ranging from small subcapsular hematoma to hepatic vascular avulsion. Renal, pancreatic, and small- and large-bowel injuries may also be seen.

What is the role of interventional radiology in the management of traumatic vascular injuries?

Endovascular homeostatic techniques involving embolization or stenting without the associated surgical stress intuitively confer benefit. The key question of what clinical scenarios of hemodynamic control offer better outcomes with minimally invasive management over open-surgery approaches remains controversial with a lack of robust supporting evidence at this time. There is some evidence pointing toward equal outcomes with interventional management of hepatic and splenic injuries.[13,14] Direct examination of pelvic and retroperitoneal injuries is difficult during laparotomy, and surgical exploration and control of hemorrhage in these anatomic areas are technically challenging.[15] Therefore, currently, although interventional radiologic management of pelvic bleeding in the hemodynamically unstable patient is gaining acceptance, the standard approach to other organ injuries remains surgery.[1,16]

On the first postoperative day, a right carotid bruit is noted. What is the concern and how should this be managed?

The concern here would be carotid artery dissection. Traumatic blunt vascular injuries to head and neck vessels occur in motor vehicle accidents because of rapid deceleration resulting in stretching of the internal carotid artery over the lateral masses of the cervical vertebrae or hyperflexion of the neck causing compression of the artery between the mandible and cervical spine. Vertebral dissections can occur as a result of excessive rotation, distraction, or flexion-extension injuries and are often associated with fractures extending into the transverse foramen or facet joint dislocations.

Presenting symptoms define the laterality of the cerebrovascular injury and isolate it to the respective extracranial arterial supply. Carotid injuries typically present with a contralateral sensory or motor deficit, and vertebral injuries present with ataxia, vertigo, emesis, and possible visual field deficits. Intra-arterial angiography was traditionally the mainstay of diagnostic imaging but has given way to other modalities such as ultrasound, CT angiography (CTA), and magnetic resonance imaging/magnetic resonance angiography (MRI/MRA) for both initial diagnosis and follow-up.[17,18] Pathopneumonic angiographic findings of dissection or aneurysm formation include a flame-shaped or tapered narrowing, "string sign." An MRI and MRA can demonstrate the luminal abnormalities seen with intra-arterial studies.

Multisection CTA provides high-resolution images of the arterial wall and vessel lumen and, in the setting of trauma, can also demonstrate the relationship of arterial injuries to bone structures of the cervical spine and skull base.

The natural history of blunt trauma causing vascular injuries in the neck is often initially occult, and even after this "silent period," devastating neurologic symptoms may be delayed for hours or even days. It has only recently become clear that these injuries are more common than previously appreciated and that disability secondary to cerebrovascular ischemia can be prevented by early intervention. Indeed, the overall incidence of blunt carotid and vertebral injury has been universally reported as less than 1% of all trauma admissions for blunt trauma, but this relatively small population of patients has a stroke rate ranging from 25% to 58% and mortality rates of 31% to 59%.[19,20] The index of suspicion for this type of injury should be high, and a low threshold for designated imaging may lead to earlier diagnosis. Aggressive screening protocols exist in trauma centers. Patients with cervical spine injury, diffuse axonal injury, basal skull fracture, Le Forte facial fracture, significant thoracic injury, or any neurologic deficit not explained by admission CT scanning should undergo additional imaging.

Intervention consists of anticoagulant and/or antiplatelet therapy, open repair or stenting, and hemodynamic management. A grading system exists with prognostic and therapeutic implications for blunt carotid injuries based on the angiographic appearance of the lesion. Grade I injuries are defined as irregularity of the vessel wall or dissection with less than 25% stenosis. Grade II injuries include those with intraluminal thrombus or a raised intimal flap, or dissections with intramural hematoma causing greater than 25% stenosis. Dissecting aneurysms are classified as grade III and complete occlusions as grade IV injuries. Grade V injuries are those associated with complete vessel transection and evidence of free contrast extravasation.

Severe head injuries are evenly distributed across the injury grades. However, the incidence of delayed stroke increased with injury grade from 3% with grade I injuries to 44% for grade IV, and therefore choice of intervention is often stratified according to grade.[21] Anticoagulant and/or antiplatelet medications (to which there are often contraindications in the severely injured trauma patient) represent the mainstay of medical treatment with excellent results in terms of stroke rate reduction. However, complications associated with anticoagulation range from 25% to 54% in the trauma population.[20] Most concerning is intracranial hemorrhage; however, more common are gastrointestinal bleeds, retroperitoneal hemorrhage, blunt solid organ injury with hemorrhage, or rebleeding from surgical wounds. In those patients with contraindications to anticoagulation or with evidence of hemodynamic insufficiency due to severe stenosis or occlusion, augmentation of cerebral blood flow is required on an urgent basis. Medical management with induced hypertension and hypervolemia can be employed. If symptoms persist despite maximal medical management, an intervention aimed at restoration of normal vessel diameter to improve cerebral perfusion should be considered.

Reconstruction with an in situ vein graft or extracranial to intracranial bypass may be technically feasible, although formal open repair has largely given way to the application of endovascular stents and covered stent grafts. Stent placement is associated with a risk of early or late thromboembolic complications or occlusion and requires periprocedural anticoagulation and continuation of single or combination antiplatelet therapy for several weeks subsequently.

Trauma and Surgical Intensive Care

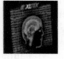
On postoperative day 3, the patient still has an external fixation device to the right tibia and develops swelling and tightness of the right lower extremity with pallor and diminished pulses.

What is the probable diagnosis and management?

These changes represent a probable acute compartment syndrome (ACS) of the extremity. The pathophysiology involves insult to compartment homeostasis, leading to increased tissue pressure, reduced capillary blood flow, local tissue hypoxia, and later necrosis. Older age confers a decreased risk presumptively due to weaker, less strong fascia. The vast majority of causes of traumatic ACS of the extremity are soft tissue injuries, ischemia, or fractures (open or closed), or a combination of these insults. Diagnosis is notoriously difficult, especially in the sedated, intubated patient, since the earliest clinical symptom is pain. Palpable tenseness, paresthesia, paresis, pallor, and pulselessness may also be associated with compartment syndrome. To confirm the clinical diagnosis, especially in difficult clinical situations, measurement of intracompartmental pressure may be useful. Normal resting intracompartmental pressure is 0 to 8 mm Hg. When intracompartmental pressure rises above capillary blood pressure, intracompartmental blood circulation ceases. The first clinical symptoms of ischemia appear at approximately an intracompartmental pressure of 20 to 30 mm Hg. Expert consensus opinion advocates for fasciotomy for absolute compartment pressures of 30 to 45 mm Hg.[22] Once the diagnosis of ACS has been established, urgent surgical decompression of the affected osseofascial compartments should be undertaken with the objective to relieve increased pressure. This can be done formally in the operating room or at the bedside.

A 72-year-old man with a known history of a 5.2-cm aneurysmal descending thoracic aorta presents to the ED with a 1-hour history of severe radiating back pain. His vital signs are stable. 3-D CTA demonstrates a contained rupture of his aortic aneurysm sac with a concomitant aortic dissection to the level of the renal arteries.

What is the mechanism of aneurysm and dissection formation?

Aneurysms can be categorized as true or false (pseudoaneurysm). True aneurysmal disease can occur anywhere within the vascular tree, but the vast majority develop within the arterial circulation. True aneurysms, resulting from a developing defect of the muscular layers of a contiguous arterial wall, can develop over time as a result of weakening of the wall caused by aging, smoking, hypertension, and atherosclerosis as well as occasionally infections, vasculitides, genetic conditions, and blunt trauma. The majority of true aneurysms are found in the aorta, of which 95% are infrarenal, and also in the cerebral circulation. Pseudoaneurysm, or false aneurysm, formation is a common complication of arterial injury. A pseudoaneurysm is a disruption of one or more layers of the arterial wall, resulting in leaking and external hematoma formation in communication with the arterial lumen. Approximately 0.6% of percutaneous femoral artery catheterization results in pseudoaneurysm formation.[23] When the wall stress from circulation exceeds the tensile strength of the vessel wall, rupture occurs. Wall stress is directly proportional to vessel diameter and blood pressure according to Laplace law, and therefore with increasing aneurysm size, risk of rupture or dissection increases. For example, the annual rupture rates for abdominal aortic aneurysms of less than 3 cm is 0.3%, whereas for abdominal aortic aneurysms greater than 7 cm the rupture rate is 31%.[24] The scenarios in which this would be seen include trauma patients with concomitant true aneurysm formation, where hemodynamic control would be the mainstay of treatment. Recognition of pseudoaneurysm formation after injury is paramount and should be followed with serial CTA or another imaging modality. Intervention should be considered on the basis of absolute size, increasing size, or worsening symptomatology.

The pathophysiology of arterial dissection involves a tear in the intimal vessel lining, with blood entering the media at this point of discontinuity. The force of systolic blood pressure will extend the intimal flap antegrade and/or retrograde and create a false lumen. With trauma, the inciting injury is often a wall hematoma rather than a weakness of collagen or elastin. Medical management would include pharmacotherapy to avoid extension of dissection by controlling the patient's heart rate and blood pressure as well as support of end-organ perfusion while awaiting definitive interventional or surgical management. The rate of acceleration of pulsatile flow ($\Delta P/\Delta t$) and the depth of intimal tear are the determinants of intimal flap extension; therefore, management must include rapid and strict heart rate and blood pressure control. The large inflammatory response accompanying dissection often leads to profound hypertension requiring multiple antihypertensive agents. Age, hypertension, connective tissue disorders, and trauma remain the leading risk factors for generation of arterial dissection.[25] Acute aortic dissection remains a morbid disease.

In contrast, chronic aortic dissections are complex lesions with a fairly predictable natural history depending on factors such as the baseline aortic diameter, the degree of false lumen thrombosis, the presence of a persistent communication, an underlying connective tissue disorder, and the control of hypertension. Medical management with antihypertensive therapy including β blockers is the treatment of choice for all stable chronic aortic dissections. Repair is indicated in the case of complications: aortic rupture, malperfusion syndromes, symptomatic dissections, asymptomatic dissections that become significantly aneurysmal or demonstrate a rapid growth rate. In this regard, serial imaging of the aorta is crucial to detect unstable lesions requiring surgery or an endovascular intervention.

What are the surgical options for this patient?

In general, the management of vascular injury can be categorized into surgical or medical. Surgery can be approached via an open or endovascular modality. The mainstays of medical management are supportive care, anticoagulation, and hemodynamic control.

Preoperatively, transesophageal echocardiography may be performed to assess the extent and type of injury and anti-impulse therapy with short-acting β blockade and potentially vasodilatory drugs should be started. Anti-impulse therapy has been shown to reduce in-hospital aortic rupture rates without adversely affecting the outcome of other injuries.

Open Repair

Conventional open repair of contained aortic rupture, elective aneurysm treatment, or traumatic aortic disruption with interposition grafting is the standard with which all other management strategies should be compared. Traditionally, simple aortic cross-clamping has been used, but more contemporary practice using extracorporeal lower body perfusion techniques lower the rate of paraplegia, which is as high as 30% with simple "clamp and sew" techniques with cross-clamp times longer than 30 minutes. Paradoxically, it is possible that young trauma victims have not developed significant vascular collateral flow and, therefore, are thought to be at higher risk of organ dysfunction distal to the aortic clamp site.

The spinal cord blood supply is through the anterior and posterior spinal arteries. The anterior two-thirds of the spinal cord is supplied by the anterior spinal artery arising from radicular and medullary branches of the posterior intercostal arteries off the aorta. The anterior spinal artery is well developed in the upper thorax and receives collateral flow from the left vertebral artery and the internal mammary artery through the intercostals, whereas in the lower thorax and abdomen, it is more dependent on collateral flow that it receives from the intercostals and lumbar arteries at these levels. The artery of Adamkiewicz comes off the aorta at approximately the level of the first lumbar vertebra (with much variation around T8 to L4) and is essential for the blood supply to the spinal cord in at least 25% of patients. Risk factors for postoperative paraplegia include increased cross-clamp time, the length of the aorta excluded, low distal perfusion pressure, systemic hypotension, the number of intercostal arteries ligated, increased body temperature, and increased cerebrospinal fluid pressure.

In addition to lower-body perfusion, several adjunctive measures can be used to reduce the risk of spinal cord ischemia during the management of thoracic aortic surgery, such as motor or somatosensory evoked potentials, lumbar cerebrospinal fluid drainage, and hypothermia. These modalities should certainly be considered in the perioperative care of these patients. Aside from the spinal cord, organ beds distal to the cross-clamp are also affected, most notably the mesentery, the kidneys, and the lower extremities. Monitoring of renal function, acid-base, liver enzymes, creatine kinase, arterial lactate, and serial examinations of the abdomen and lower extremities along with a low index of suspicion for abdominal compartment syndrome should be considered in the postoperative care plan.

Thoracic Endovascular Aortic Repair (TEVAR)

There are currently many reports of the efficacy of TEVAR for acute traumatic aortic disruption. Experience gleaned from the selective use of TEVAR in the repair of thoracic aortic aneurysms in high-risk patients has transformed the management of traumatic thoracic aortic injuries. Endovascular repair is the preferred management modality in many institutions. Although the long-term durability of these grafts in this younger subset of trauma patients is unknown, the accepted risk of chronic complications is offset by the benefits afforded by a less-invasive, less time-consuming technique where the added potential morbidity of an open repair is avoided.[26]

Complications occurring after TEVAR include endoleak, stent-graft collapse, stroke, embolization, bronchial obstruction, migration, paralysis, dissection, or rupture. Endoleaks are categorized as type I (leak around the proximal or distal end of the graft); type II (leak from an artery excluded by the graft that perfuses the vessel in a retrograde fashion between the wall of the aorta and the graft); type III (leak between modular components); and type IV (failure of graft integrity).

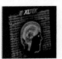 Three days after undergoing endovascular graft repair of the proximal descending aorta, the patient appears to be doing well. He is extubated, and his lumbar spinal drain has been removed. Over the course of the next 12 hours, he develops a metabolic acidosis as well as hypotension, requiring vasopressor therapy and volume resuscitation. The nurse informs you that the patient has had three episodes of melena.

What is the concern and how should this be investigated?

The main concern would be mesenteric ischemia from either a discrete thromboembolic event or a more prolonged and persistent low-flow state. Clinical examination, flow-based imaging, and serial laboratory studies focusing particularly on acid-base and lactate levels may show a trend. There should be a constant assessment of the need for bowel resection. Large-bore intravenous cannulas should be placed immediately in case of a massive upper or lower gastrointestinal bleed. Blood for transfusion should be made available in case of hemorrhagic shock. Invasive monitors should be considered and transfer to an ICU location should be arranged if the patient is in a poorly monitored location.

 A 23-year-old man is brought into the ED with two stab wounds to the anterior mediastinum. He was intubated in the field for obtundation. His vital signs are BP 50/10 mm Hg and HR 155 bpm. Oxygen saturation could not be obtained.

What is the appropriate management?

Securing the airway, fluid and vasopressor therapy, and rapid assessment and treatment of what must be assumed to be profound hemorrhagic hypovolemic shock from cardiac and/or great vessel trauma in the hope of survival are the goals of care.

Penetrating and Blunt Cardiac Trauma

The goals of penetrating cardiac trauma are immediate surgical intervention. Of those patients with penetrating stab wounds to the heart who reach the hospital, one-third have right ventricular injuries and one-quarter have left ventricular injuries. Coronary artery lacerations are also common.[27] Management involves fluid resuscitation and immediate transfer to the operating room or ED for thoracotomy. The majority of blunt cardiac trauma is seen with motor vehicle accidents. The compression and deceleration forces that are at play in blunt aortic injuries are similar to those resulting in cardiac trauma. An abrupt change in pressures within and surrounding the heart can cause disruption to the fairly static and fixed components of the heart; namely, the cardiac free wall, the septum, the coronary arteries, and the valvular apparatus. More often, and less morbidly, myocardial contusion to the anterior right ventricle may also occur.

Chest radiography, serum troponin levels, and electrocardiographic (ECG) monitoring can be used to screen trauma patients for cardiac contusion. If these tests are reassuring, they essentially rule out significant cardiac injury in young patients. If concern persists, echocardiography (either transthoracic or transesophageal) may be used to assess regional myocardial functionality. Cardiac injuries are graded according to the presence of structural injury and hemodynamic compromise. The management of such injuries spans a spectrum from conservative medical management to support the contractile state of the myocardium to percutaneous intervention to operative intervention.

Non–Aortic Great Vessel Injury

Blunt trauma to the great venous structures and the pulmonary arteries is rare, presumably because of their distensibility and low pressure, with the majority of injuries to these vessels being from penetrating injuries. Even with penetrating trauma the incidence of great vessel injury is in the order of 5%. Most commonly, exsanguination from pulmonary vessel hemorrhage into the thorax or pericardial tamponade is seen and requires appropriate management. As with other penetrating injuries, permissive hypotension has been shown to improve outcome until definitive surgical control has been achieved.

Penetrating (PAI) and Blunt Aortic Injury (BAI)

Penetrating aortic injury is unsurprisingly almost always fatal.

There is a spectrum of diseases related to BAI. Intervention must now be tempered in the context of other associated injuries. Minimal injuries have been successfully managed and may heal with appropriate medical management. Additionally, the increased use of and familiarity with endovascular aortic stenting techniques has simplified the repair of BAI and reduced the burden of organ dysfunction previously seen with open repair, at least in the relatively short term. Long-term data on the trauma population are sparse as to endovascular versus open techniques, but extrapolation from the elective aneurysm group may show an equalization of morbidity and mortality rates longitudinally.[28]

Broadly speaking, 75% of BAI victims die at the scene, with a further 5% presenting with instability, in whom the mortality rate is still 100%. The final 20% of patients with BAI, who often present later, have little or no hemodynamic perturbation. The mortality rate in this group is a more acceptable 25%.[27] It is in this group that timing and method of intervention warrant a balance of other injuries and there may be a role for delayed intervention, although optimal timing is still unclear.

! CRITICAL CONSIDERATIONS

- Vascular injuries often concomitantly exist in the setting of polytrauma. Immediate priority should be given to rapid assessment, diagnosis, and treatment of airway, breathing, and circulatory pathology.
- Damage control surgery with life and limb salvage and stabilization in the ICU setting has become the mainstay of traumatic vascular injury.

Trauma and Surgical Intensive Care

- Avoidance and aggressive correction of coagulopathy, acidosis, and hypothermia are imperative in the traumatic patient.
- Blunt and penetrating trauma through different mechanistic actions lead to a different clinical spectrum of injury.
- Abdominal injury following trauma affects most commonly the spleen, liver, bowel, and pancreas.
- Management of vascular injury may consist of formal open surgical repair, endovascular interventional radiologic options, or conservative management with appropriate surveillance, depending on anatomic site and severity
- Many imaging modalities may be used to assess injury including CT, angiography, and echocardiography.
- A low index of suspicion for end-organ manifestations of vascular compromise (mesenteric, ischemic, extremity compartment syndrome, neurologic deficit) should exist throughout the clinical course.
- Appropriate management of vascular traumatic injuries requires collaboration of surgical specialties (vascular, cardiac, trauma, general, orthopedic), radiology (diagnostic and interventional), and intensive care.

REFERENCES

1. American College of Surgeon. *ATLS, Advanced Trauma Life Support Program for Doctors.* Chicago, IL: ACS; 2008.
2. Duchesne JC, McSwain NE Jr, Cotton BA, et al. Damage control resuscitation: the new face of damage control. *J Trauma.* 2010;69:976-990.
3. Piper GL, Peitzman AB. Current management of hepatic trauma. *Surg Clin North Am.* 2010;90: 775-785.
4. Cirocchi R, Abraha I, Montedori A, et al. Damage control surgery for abdominal trauma. *Cochrane Database Syst Rev.* 2010;20:CD007438.
5. Sihler KC, Napolitano LM. Complications of massive transfusion. *Chest.* 2010;137:209-220.
6. Martini WZ. Coagulopathy by hypothermia and acidosis: mechanisms of thrombin generation and fibrinogen availability. *J Trauma.* 2009;67:202-208.
7. http://www.cdc.gov/injury/wisqars/leading_causes_death.html
8. Pfeifer R, Tarkin IS, Rocos B, Pape HC. Patterns of mortality and causes of death in polytrauma patients—Has anything changed? *Injury.* 2009;40:907-911.
9. Richens D, Field M, Neale M, et al. The mechanism of injury in blunt traumatic rupture of the aorta. *Eur J Cardiothorac Surg.* 2002;21:288-293.

10. Maiden N. Ballistics reviews: mechanisms of bullet wound trauma. *Forensic Sci Med Pathol.* 2009;5:204-209.
11. Bickell WH, Wall MJ Jr, Pepe PE, et al. Immediate versus delayed fluid resuscitation for hypotensive patients with penetrating torso injuries. *N Engl J Med* 1994;331:1105-1109.
12. Moore EE, Cogbill TH, Jurkovich GJ, et al. Organ injury scaling: spleen and liver. *J Trauma.* 1995;38:323-334.
13. Gaardner C, Naess PA, Eken T, et al. Liver injuries—Improved results with a formal protocol including angiography. *Injury.* 2007;38: 1075-1083.
14. Duchesne JC, Simmons JD, Schmeig RE Jr, et al. Proximal splenic artery angioembolization does not improve outcomes in treating blunt splenic injuries compared with splenectomy: a cohort analysis. *J Trauma.* 2008;65:1346-1353.
15. Frevert S, Dahl B, Lonn L. Update on the roles of angiography and embolisation in pelvic fracture. *Injury.* 2008;39:1290-1294.
16. Agolini SF, Shah K, Jaffe J, et al. Arterial embolization is a rapid and effective technique for controlling pelvic fracture hemorrhage. *J Trauma.* 1997;43:395-397.
17. Bok AP, Peter JC. Carotid and vertebral artery occlusion after blunt cervical injury: the role of

MR angiography in early diagnosis. *J Trauma.* 1996;40:968-972.

18. Fry WR, Dort JA, Smith RS, et al. Duplex scanning replaces arteriography and operative exploration in the diagnosis of potential cervical vascular injury. *Am J Surg.* 1994;168:693-695.

19. Berne JD, Norwood SH, McAuley CE, et al. The high morbidity of blunt cerebrovascular injury in an unscreened population: more evidence of the need for mandatory screening protocols. *J Am Coll Surg.* 2001;192:314-321.

20. Biffl WL, Moore EE, Ryu RK, et al. The unrecognized epidemic of blunt carotid arterial injuries: early diagnosis improves neurologic outcome. *Ann Surg.* 1998;228:462-470.

21. Biffl WL, Moore EE, Offner PJ, et al. Blunt carotid arterial injuries: implications of a new grading scale. *J Trauma.* 1999;47:845-853.

22. White TO, Howell GED, Will EM, et al. Elevated intramuscular compartment pressures do not influence outcome after tibial fracture. *J Trauma.* 2003;55:1133-1138.

23. Popovic B, Freysz L, Chometon F, et al. Femoral pseudoaneurysms and current cardiac catheterization: evaluation of risk factors and treatment. *Int J Cardiol.* 2010;141:75-80.

24. Choke E, Cockerill G, Wilson WRW. A review of biological factors implicated in abdominal aortic aneurysm rupture. *Eur J Vasc Endovasc Surg.* 2005;30:227-244.

25. Feldman M, Shah M, Elefteriades JA. Medical management of acute type A aortic dissection. *Ann Thorac Cardiovasc Surg.* 2009;15:286-293.

26. Gopaldas RR, Huh J, Dao TK, et al. Superior nationwide outcomes of endovascular versus open repair for isolated descending thoracic aortic aneurysm in 11,669 patients. *J Thorac Cardiovasc Surg.* 2010;140:1001-1010.

27. Cook CC, Gleason TG. Great vessel and cardiac trauma. *Surg Clin North Am.* 2009;89:797-820.

28. De Bruin JL, Baas AF, Buth J, et al. Long-term outcome of open or endovascular repair of abdominal aortic aneurysm. *N Engl J Med.* 2010;362:1881-1889.

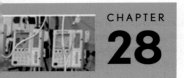

Abdominal Emergencies

28

Carlee Clark, MD

A 72-year-old man suffers from a recent left middle cerebral artery stroke. His lungs are mechanically ventilated. He develops progressive hypotension and tachycardia. His hemoglobin level has decreased from 10 mg/dL to 7.5 mg/dL over 24 hours. After several fluid boluses, the patient's blood pressure is 80/65 mm Hg. His heart rate is 120 bpm. The patient's nurse reports that the patient's stool is melenic.

What should be the first step in managing this patient?

The patient is suffering from a gastrointestinal bleed (GIB). Two large-bore intravenous catheters (16 gauge or larger) are necessary to initiate resuscitation with crystalloid and colloid fluids or blood products. When peripheral venous access cannot be obtained, a central venous line such as a Cordis catheter (Cordis Corp, Bridgewater, NJ) should be inserted. An arterial line should be inserted for beat-to-beat monitoring of systemic blood pressure. Four units of packed red blood cells (PRBCs) and 4 units of fresh-frozen plasma should be typed and crossed. Bedside assessment of end-organ perfusion and serial laboratory testing (basic metabolic profile, hemoglobin level, coagulation studies) guide transfusions and prevent delayed resuscitation and hypoperfusion. Vasoactive agents are administered during fluid resuscitation to maintain an adequate perfusion pressure.

This patient has a protected airway, but endotracheal intubation should be considered in patients with massive hemoptysis, shock, or obtundation. A nasogastric tube (NGT) should be placed to assess the site and rate of bleeding. If the abdomen is distended or if the patient complains of abdominal pain, a KUB (kidneys, ureters, and bladder) film should be performed and evaluated.

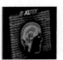

Two large-bore intravenous catheters, an arterial line, and an NGT are placed. The stomach is lavaged and 300 mL of bright red blood with coffee grounds appearance are observed. The patient's blood pressure has decreased to 70/55 mm Hg and his heart rate is 137 bpm. The gastrointestinal medicine service has been consulted.

What is the differential diagnosis for GI bleeding in this patient?

The differential diagnosis of GI bleeding in critically ill patients is broad (Table 28-1). Observation of bright red blood with coffee grounds appearance on NGT lavage suggests an upper gastrointestinal (UGI) source (originating proximal to the ligament of Treitz). UGI bleeding accounts for approximately 75% of GI bleeds and has a mortality rate of 20% to 30% in hospitalized patients.[1] Intensive care unit (ICU) patients whose lungs are mechanically ventilated

Table 28-1. Differential Diagnosis for Gastrointestinal Bleeding

Upper GI bleeding	Lower GI bleeding
Variceal bleeding	Intestinal obstruction
Esophageal varices	Intussusception
Gastric varices	Volvulus
	Incarcerated hernia
Mucosal bleeding	Painless bleeding
Peptic ulcer	Diverticular bleeding
Gastroduodenal erosions	Polyps
Stress-related mucosal damage	Vascular malformations
Mallory-Weiss tears	Inflammatory bowel disease
Esophagitis	Meckel diverticulum
Dieulafoy lesion	Nodular lymphoid hyperplasia
Vascular lesions	Bloody diarrhea
Arteriovenous malformations	Infectious colitis
	Ischemic colitis

for more than 48 hours have coagulopathy, a history of GI ulceration, or bleeding within the last 12 months or two of the following risk factors: sepsis, ICU admission longer than 7 days, occult bleeding of 6 days or longer, or daily use of 250 mg of hydrocortisone or an equivalent are at risk for stress-related mucosal damage.[2] A history of alcoholism, cirrhosis, or portal hypertension is often elicited in patients with variceal bleeding. Although melena is more common in patients with UGI bleeding, melena is also observed in patients with lower GI bleeding.

Should a proton pump inhibitor be prescribed?

Patients whose lungs are mechanically ventilated are at risk for mucosal damage and should be receiving medications to prevent stress gastritis. Prophylactic medications to prevent erosive gastritis include proton pump inhibitors, sucralfate, antacids, and histamine-2 receptor blockers. In patients who suffer from a GIB, a proton pump inhibitor infusion should be initiated. Pepsin is inactivated and cannot effectively lyse clots at pH levels greater than 6. Prescribing proton pump inhibitors with endoscopic hemostasis decreases the risk for rebleeding, the need for surgery, and mortality.[3,4] Eighty milligrams of omeprazole or pantoprazole are bolused intravenously to achieve rapid gastric acid suppression. An infusion is started at 8 mg per hour for 72 hours.[5]

Should the patient undergo an esophagogastroduodenoscopy (EGD)?

Seventy-five to 80% of UGI bleeding ceases with supportive care, but patients who are at high risk for rebleeding or death require endoscopic evaluation and treatment.[6-9] The Glasgow Blatchford Scale (GBS) score aids in predicting which patients are high risk. The GBS is an assessment tool developed to predict a patient's need for further medical or endoscopic treatment for UGI bleeding (Table 28-2). The GBS gives scores to multiple clinical and laboratory parameters, and 50% of patients with a score greater than 6 need endoscopic intervention.[10-12] Even without a recent BUN (blood urea nitrogen), the patient has a GBS score of 11 and should get an EGD for further evaluation and treatment. EGD identifies the location and type of bleeding in 90% of cases and decreases the mortality from hemorrhage.[13]

Trauma and Surgical Intensive Care

Table 28-2. Glasgow Blatchford Scale

Admission risk marker	Score component value
Blood Urea Nitrogen (BUN)	
≥ 6.5 < 8.0	2
≥ 8 < 10	3
≥ 10 < 25	4
≥ 25	6
Hemoglobin (g/L) for Men	
≥ 12 < 13	1
≥ 10 < 12	3
< 10	6
Hemoglobin (g/L) for Women	
≥ 10 < 12	1
< 10	6
Systolic Blood Pressure (mm Hg)	
100-109	1
90-99	2
< 90	3
Other Markers	
Pulse ≥ 100 bpm	1
Melena	1
Syncope	2
Hepatic disease	2
Cardiac disease	2

EGD also aids in the prognostication of patients with UGI bleeding. Multiple studies have taken into consideration clinical factors and findings on endoscopy to determine the risk of rebleeding and mortality (Table 28-3).[14-16] Risk of rebleeding and mortality increases with the number of indicators present.

A bleeding peptic ulcer is seen with EGD. The lesion is injected, sclerosed, and banded, yet the ulcer continues to bleed. The patient has received 6 units of PRBCs over 2 hours. A norepinephrine infusion is started for hypotension via a central line.

Table 28-3. Clinical and Endoscopic Prognostic Indicators for Upper Gastrointestinal Bleeding

Clinical indicators	Endoscopic indicators
Age > 60	Major stigmata
Severe comorbidities	Active bleeding
Onset of bleeding during hospitalization	Visible vessel
Emergency surgery	Adherent clot
Clinical shock	Ulcer location
Red blood emesis or nasogastric tube aspirate	Posterior duodenal bulb
Requiring > 5 units PRBCs	Higher lesser gastric curvature
	Ulcer size > 2 cm in diameter
	High-risk lesions
	Varices
	Aortoenteric fistula
	Malignancy

Which medical services should be consulted?

Experienced endoscopists achieve hemostasis in 90% of patients with UGI bleeding.[17-19] In patients who continue to bleed, arterial embolization by interventional radiologists or surgical intervention may be necessary. Surgery for acute GIB carries a mortality rate of 20% to 35%. Therefore, noninvasive intervention is often preferred prior to surgical intervention in unstable patients.[20,21]

Interventional radiology should be consulted for an angiogram and possible embolization in this patient. Transcatheter arteriograms are successful in localizing the bleeding vessel in 75% of cases.[22] Treatment with hemostatic therapy carries a long-term success rate of up to 65% with a low rate of complications.[23] There are few studies directly comparing efficacy, morbidity, and mortality of transcatheter interventions versus surgery, but transcatheter treatment for UGI bleeding does not increase mortality rate.[24,25]

 The interventional radiologist evaluates the patient and embolizes the left gastric artery without complication. The patient continues to require vasopressor therapy and returns to the neurologic ICU (NeuroICU). Twelve units of PRBCs have been administered over the past 24 hours.

How should the patient be managed in the ICU?

The proton pump inhibitor infusion should be continued for 72 hours to prevent upper GI rebleeding. Hematocrit levels should be evaluated every 4 hours for 24 hours. The patient's coagulation factors should be evaluated. The patient may develop a dilutional coagulopathy secondary to administration of PRBCs without the administration of plasma. A troponin level should be ordered to assess myocardial damage in the setting of his protracted anemia and hemodynamic instability. Urine output and serum creatinine are followed closely. Hypotension places this patient at risk for acute kidney injury (AKI) (Figure 28-1).

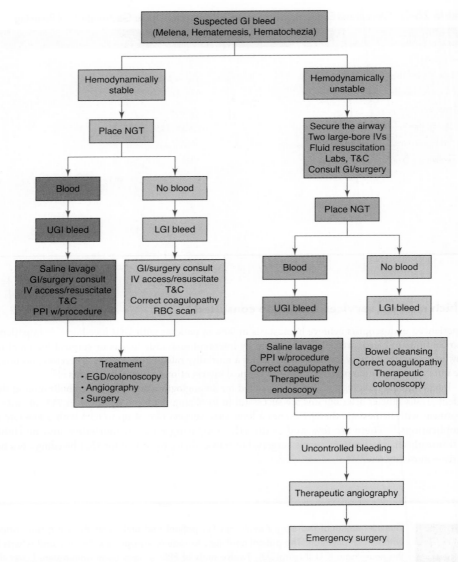

Figure 28-1. Algorithm for management of gastrointestinal (GI) bleeding. EGD, esophagoduodenoscopy; LGI, lower gastrointestinal; NGT, nasogastric tube; PPI, proton pump inhibitor; RBC, red blood cell; T&C, type and cross; UGI, upper gastrointestinal.

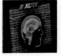

Abdominal compartment syndrome. A 65-year-old woman with a history of hypertension, pancreatitis, and smoking develops sepsis 5 days after a craniotomy for tumor resection. Her lungs are mechanically ventilated. Over the past 2 days, she has received 10 L of crystalloid fluid for hypotension. Her abdomen is distended; her urine output is decreasing; her peak airway pressures are increasing. Her bladder pressure is 15 mm Hg.

Table 28-4. World Society of the Abdominal Compartment Syndrome (WSACS) Definitions[29]

Intra-abdominal Pressure (IAP): Steady-state pressure within the abdominal cavity
Intra-abdominal Hypertension (IAH): A sustained IAP > 12 mm Hg (often causing occult ischemia) without obvious organ failure
Abdominal Compartment Syndrome (ACS): IAH > 20 mm Hg with at least one organ dysfunction or failure
Primary ACS: A condition associated with injury or disease in the abdominopelvic region; ie, tumors, bleeding, pancreatitis, ascites, obstruction, or ischemia
Secondary ACS: Conditions that do not originate in the abdominopelvic regions; ie, sepsis, burns, massive resuscitation

(From Malbrain ML, Cheatham M, Kirkpatrick A, et al. Results from the conference of experts on intraabdominal hypertension and abdominal compartment syndrome. I. Definitions. Intensive Care Med. 2006;32:1722-1732.)

What is the significance of a bladder pressure of 15 mm Hg?

A bladder pressure of 15 mm Hg suggests intra-abdominal hypertension (IAH) (Table 28-4). IAH is elevated intra-abdominal pressure (IAP). The normal IAP is 0 to 5 mm Hg, but it varies with body habitus and different disease states (Table 28-5). There are many risk factors for IAH (Table 28-6), and they include sepsis, large-volume resuscitation, abdominal masses, pancreatitis, and abdominal surgery. After aggressive volume resuscitation in patients with a capillary leak syndrome, abdominal and bowel wall edema occurs, increasing abdominal pressure. IAH increases patient morbidity and mortality rates.[26-29]

How is IAP measured?

There are several ways to measure IAP. Physical examination alone has not been shown to be sensitive in detecting IAH.[30,31] Direct measurement of IAP is possible, but requires placement of either a needle, catheter, or other pressure-monitoring device directly into the abdominal cavity. Direct measurement is complex and invasive. Measuring gastric or rectal pressures can make indirect estimations of IAP, but current standard of care is via bladder pressure measurement. Studies have shown bladder pressure measurements to be a cost-effective, safe, and accurate instrument for identifying IAH and guiding therapy.[32-36] Measurements are made by attaching a pressure-monitoring system to the injection port of a Foley catheter (Table 28-7). The Abdominal Compartment Syndrome World Congress currently recommends an intravesicular volume of 25 mL.[37] Previous recommendations suggested the use of 50 to 100 mL of normal saline, but studies have shown that larger injection volumes can lead to falsely elevated IAP.[38-40] Bladder pressures should be measured regularly in patients with or at risk for IAH to aid in diagnosis and management. The optimal frequency of bladder pressure monitoring has not been determined, but every 4 to 6 hours while critically ill should be sufficient.

Table 28-5. Intra-abdominal Pressures (mm Hg) Associated with Various Disease States

Normal adult	0-5
Typical intensive care unit patient	5-7
Postlaparotomy patient	10-15
Patient with septic shock	15-25
Patient with acute abdomen	25-45

Table 28-6. Risk Factors for Intra-abdominal Hypertension/Abdominal Compartment Syndrome

Acidosis (pH < 7.2)
Hypothermia (core temperature < 33°C)
Polytransfusion (> 10 U PRBCs/24 h)
Coagulopathy
Sepsis
Bacteremia
Intra-abdominal infection/abscess
Peritonitis
Liver dysfunction/cirrhosis with ascites
Mechanical ventilation
Positive end-expiratory pressure (PEEP) or auto-PEEP
Pneumonia
Abdominal surgery
Massive fluid resuscitation (> 5 L colloid or crystalloid/24 h)
Gastroparesis/gastric distention/ileus
Volvulus
Hemoperitoneum/pneumoperitoneum
Major burns
Major trauma
High body mass index (> 30)
Intra-abdominal or retroperitoneal tumors
Prone positioning
Massive incisional hernia repair
Acute pancreatitis
Distended abdomen
Damage control laparotomy
Laparoscopy with excessive inflation pressures
Peritoneal dialysis

(From Malbrain ML, Cheatham M, Kirkpatrick A, et al. Results from the conference of experts on intra-abdominal hypertension and abdominal compartment syndrome. I. Definitions. Intensive Care Med. 2006;32:1722-1732.)

Table 28-7. How to Measure Bladder Pressure

1. Measure at end expiration
2. Patient must be in the supine position
3. System needs to be zeroed at the iliac crest in the mid-axillary line
4. Inject 25 mL of normal saline (1 mL/kg for children up to 20 kg)
5. Measure after 30-60 s to allow for bladder relaxation
6. Measure only if the abdominal muscles are not actively contracting

What is the pathophysiology of IAH?

The pathophysiology of IAH is complex (Figure 28-2). An increase in IAP limits venous return and decreases left ventricular preload. Abdominal pressure increases systemic vascular resistance, resulting in increased afterload. Decreased preload and increased afterload result in decreased cardiac output. The cardiovascular system initially compensates with an elevation in the heart rate to maintain cardiac output. Abdominal pressure is transmitted to the thoracic cavity, which compresses the lungs and increases airway pressures. These physiologic changes can result in hypotension, which can lead to mesenteric ischemia and AKI and hypoxemia. Unfortunately, aggressive treatment often leads to worsening IAH and continued clinical deterioration (Figure 28-3).

Does an IAP of 15 mm Hg affect intracranial pressure (ICP) or cerebral perfusion pressure (CPP)?

An IAP of 15 mm Hg can affect ICP, CPP, and cerebral blood flow. An increased intrathoracic pressure elevates central venous pressures and decreases venous drainage from cerebral vessels. Cerebral venous congestion leads to elevated ICP, resulting in intracranial hypertension (ICP greater than 20 mm Hg). The pressure inside the cranium is directly proportional to the volume of its contents: blood, cerebrospinal fluid, and brain. Without adequate venous drainage, the volume inside the cranium increases. To compensate, cerebrospinal fluid shifts into the spinal column, but this is only a temporary solution. Eventually, the ICP will rise and stay elevated unless treated. Given her recent craniotomy and tumor removal, this patient needs to be evaluated for elevated ICP.

In nontraumatic brain injury patients, elevated IAP was associated with increased ICP and decreased CPP even at lower abdominal pressures.[41] A study of neurotrauma patients showed that ICP rose by artificially elevating IAP to an average of 15.5 mm Hg.[42] The concern for intracranial hypertension in this patient population comes from the relationship between ICP and CPP. CPP is the difference between mean arterial pressure (MAP) and ICP (CPP = MAP – ICP). An elevation in ICP without an increase in mean arterial pressure will result in decreased CPP, decreased oxygen delivery to the brain, progressive encephalopathy, and cell injury. Medical management for intracranial hypertension should be initiated in patients with IAH and elevated ICP. Intracranial hypertension secondary to brain injury or IAH may be refractory to medical therapy. Decompressive laparotomy has been shown to be useful in decreasing ICP in traumatic brain injury patients with refractory intracranial hypertension.[43,44]

Three hours later, the bladder pressure increases to 20 mm Hg. The patient remains hypotensive and oliguric with increased peak airway pressures. What is the significance of an increase in bladder pressure from 15 to 20 mm Hg?

Stratifying IAPs guides management to prevent end-organ damage and clinical deterioration.[37] An intra-abdominal pressure of 15 mm Hg is consistent with grade I IAH, and the recommended management is medical therapy (Table 28-8). An increase in IAP to 20 mm Hg indicates clinical deterioration. The patient now has grade II IAH. Suggested treatment is abdominal decompression if end-organ dysfunction is present. Hypotension, elevated airway pressures, and oliguria indicate end-organ dysfunction. The surgical service should be consulted to evaluate this patient.

If there is no surgeon available, how is IAH managed?

Until the surgical team is available to evaluate and possibly operate on the patient, medical management of IAH must be initiated (Figure 28-4). Medical management relies on nonoperative interventions to aid in reducing IAP. There are several medical treatment options to improve abdominal wall compliance, beginning with deepening sedation and analgesia. Most heavily sedated patients will relax their abdominal

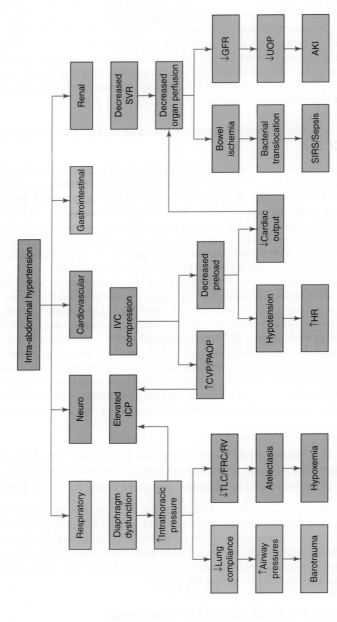

Figure 28-2. Pathophysiology of abdominal compartment syndrome. AKI, acute kidney injury; CVP, central venous pressure; FRC, functional residual capacity; GFR, glomerular filtration rate; HR, heart rate; ICP, intracranial pressure; IVC, inferior vena cava; PAOP, pulmonary artery occlusion pressure; RV, residual volume; SIRS, systemic inflammatory response syndrome; SVR, systemic vascular resistance; TLC, total lung capacity; UOP, urine output.

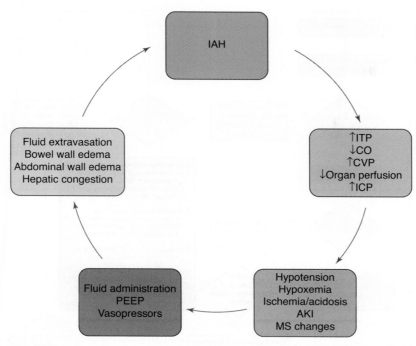

Figure 28-3. Illustration showing the cyclical nature of intra-abdominal hypertension (IAH)/abdominal compartment syndrome. AKI, acute kidney injury; CO, cardiac output; CVP, central venous pressure; ICP, intracranial pressure; ITP, intrathoracic pressure; MS, mental status; PEEP, positive end-expiratory pressure.

muscles, resulting in less ventilator dyssynchrony. If heavy sedation does not improve peak airway pressures or ventilation, neuromuscular blockade is considered. If abdominal muscle tension complicates IAH, paralysis will reduce the IAP.[45-47] The risks of prolonged neuromuscular blockade, namely, myopathy, are weighed against the benefits of IAP reduction. If there are no contraindications, an NGT, suppository, and enema can decompress the GI tract. Diuretics can decrease third spacing and abdominal wall edema but may compromise hemodynamics in a hypotensive patient. If the oliguria persists or anuria develops, initiation of continuous venovenous hemodialysis to aid in fluid removal or correction of acidemia may be necessary. Percutaneous abdominal decompression can decrease IAH or reverse abdominal compartment syndrome (ACS) when the patient has a fluid collection such as ascites, hematoma, or abscess.[48-52] Without current abdominal imaging, abdominal drainage carries an unacceptably high risk of accidental visceral

Table 28-8. Grading and Management of Intra-abdominal Hypertension

Grade	Bladder pressure (mm Hg)	Recommendation
I	12-15	Serial IAP monitoring and medical management to reduce IAP
II	16-20	Serial IAP monitoring and medical management to reduce IAP
III	21-25	Decompression if end-organ dysfunction present with monitoring of IAP post decompression
IV	> 22	Decompression if end-organ dysfunction present with monitoring of IAP post decompression

Abbreviation: IAP, intra-abdominal pressure.

Trauma and Surgical Intensive Care

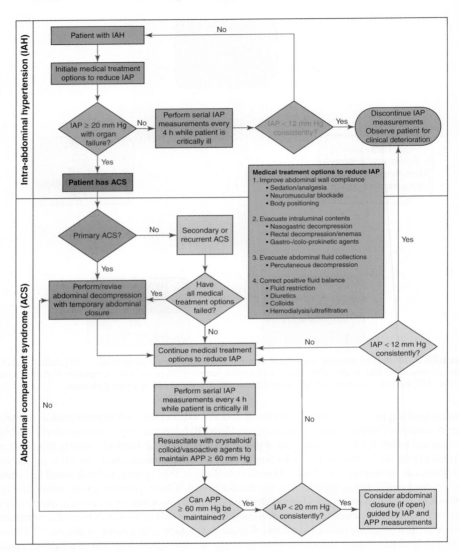

Figure 28-4. Intra-abdominal hypertension management algorithm. APP, abdominal perfusion pressure; IAP, intra-abdominal pressure. (*From Cheatham ML, Malbrain ML, Kirkpatrick A, et al. Results from the international conference of experts on intra-abdominal hypertension and abdominal compartment syndrome. II. Recommendations. Intensive Care Med. 2007;33:951-962.*)

perforation or bleeding; therefore, abdominal ultrasound or abdominal CT scanning may be of some benefit. It will help determine if the patient has primary or secondary ACS.

If the patient's IAP is 20 mm Hg, mean arterial pressure (MAP) is 65 mm Hg, and central venous pressure is 8 mm Hg, what are your hemodynamic goals to ensure organ perfusion?

Abdominal perfusion pressure (APP) should be calculated in patients with elevated bladder pressures. APP is calculated from the difference between the MAP and the IAP (APP = MAP − IAP).

Hemodynamic therapy targets an APP of 60 mm Hg. In patients with an IAP of 20 mm Hg, a MAP of 80 mm Hg will likely maintain adequate perfusion pressure to the abdominal organs, including the kidneys, liver, and intestines.[37,53-55] Maintaining adequate APP may improve survival, although no prospective randomized controlled trials have been completed. Strategies to maintain APP include fluid administration and vasopressor therapy. Maintaining adequate intravascular volume is an important concept in patients with IAH. Hypovolemia will further aggravate reductions in preload. The use of central venous pressure or pulmonary artery catheter measurements to guide therapy is controversial. The increase in intrathoracic pressure may falsely elevate both central venous and pulmonary pressures, making the use of these indices in fluid administration difficult.

 After placement of an NGT, 250 mL of bilious fluid is drained. Escalating doses of sedation and analgesics are given to the patient. The patient is hypotensive and oliguric. The IAP is 22 mm Hg. The abdominal CT scan shows peripancreatic inflammation and edema. The amylase level is 200 and the lipase level is 210.

What is the diagnosis?

The diagnoses of abdominal abscess, hematoma, perforated viscus, or obstruction of the intestines are unlikely because there is no evidence of a fluid collection, free air, or distention of the small bowel. Based on peripancreatic inflammation and edema, the radiologist confirms the diagnosis of pancreatitis. Several recent studies have suggested that patients with pancreatitis frequently develop IAH with worsening organ dysfunction.[56,57] ACS develops when fluid resuscitation for peripancreatic and retroperitoneal inflammation increases visceral edema; pancreatic fluid collections increase abdominal pressure, and paralytic ileus develops.[58] Patients with pancreatitis undergo surgery for debridement when there is infected necrosis or when an abscess or pseudocyst needs to be drained.

Should this patient be fed?

Historically, patients with pancreatitis have been placed on bowel rest, but this is quickly changing. Studies have shown that early enteral feeding may decrease the inflammatory response of pancreatitis.[59] Enteral feeding may also reduce/prevent the breakdown in gut mucosal defenses, which aid in preventing sepsis in pancreatitis patients.[60] The data suggest that enteral feeding decreases infection rates, need for surgical intervention, and shortens hospital stay. No effect on mortality has been proved. Pancreatic ileus is common and there are no current recommendations for jejunal versus gastric feedings. There are no specific recommendations to guide enteral feeding for moderate versus severe pancreatitis.[61] This patient has an acute abdominal process that requires the patient to remain supine and may require surgical therapy. Initiating enteral feeding at this time will increase the patient's risk for aspiration.

What is the disadvantage of elevating the head of the bed greater than 30 degrees?

Head of bed elevation greater than 30 degrees is standard of care for prevention of aspiration pneumonia in intubated and mechanically ventilated patients.[61,62] IAP, however, increases with increasing elevation of the head of the bed. Head of bed elevation of 20 degrees caused clinically significant increases in IAP by 2 mm Hg or more.[37] Bladder pressure measurements are made in the supine position. If head of bed is being elevated in between measurements, then the supine measurements of IAP will underestimate the "true" IAP. Prone positioning has also shown to increase IAP, and should not be used in a patient with IAH.[63-65] Further research is needed to truly understand the effects of body positioning on IAP. Until then, consider the potential risks of body positioning in patients with mild to moderate IAH.

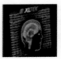

The patient becomes anuric, his oxygen saturation decreases to 92%, and his IAP increases to 25 mm Hg. He is sedated and paralyzed. His lactate level is 4 and his most recent arterial blood gas is 7.20/59/68/-6/94%. His BUN is 22 and his creatinine level is 3.4.

Should a surgeon be called to the bedside?

This patient has ACS. An elevation in lactate suggests abdominal organ hypoperfusion. Acidosis develops from azotemia, hyperlactatemia, and hypercarbia from a decrease in minute ventilation. This patient is developing multisystem organ failure. The patient's AKI has progressed to acute kidney failure. He may require dialysis to manage his fluid balance. Surgical decompression is the gold standard of treatment for ACS. At this point, a delay in surgical decompression increases the patient's mortality.[53]

The patient is taken to the operating room (OR), where a decompressive laparotomy is performed. The pancreas is not debrided. After laparotomy, the patient's hemodynamics improve, yet he remains anuric. Is the patient at risk for recurrent ACS?

After decompressive laparotomy, a temporary abdominal closure device is placed to protect the abdominal viscera and allow for continued expansion. All patients are at risk for recurrent ACS if the device is not large enough to accommodate the expanding viscera. Bladder pressures should continue to be monitored every 4 to 6 hours until the patient is clinically stable. Monitoring renal perfusion pressure and evaluating the patient for acute indications for renal replacement therapy are important.

Bowel obstruction. A 45-year-old woman is postoperative day 5 from a craniotomy for tumor resection. Her course has been complicated by respiratory failure. She develops abdominal distention and intermittent abdominal pain. The patient has had multiple abdominal surgeries for recurrent ventral hernias. She is fed via a nasoduodenal feeding tube. Her residual gastric volume has been increasing for the past 24 hours. Her abdominal examination is notable for tympany. The patient vomits 200 mL of bilious fluid. Her nurse reports that the patient had diarrhea yesterday but has not had flatus or a bowel movement for 24 hours.

What is in the differential diagnosis for increased residual volumes?

Increased residual volumes are observed with improper tube placement, feeding tube migration to the proximal stomach or esophagus, gastroparesis, and ileus. Ileus occurs after opioid administration, abdominal infection, and bowel edema. Bilious emesis and abdominal distention should arouse concern for something more serious than feeding tube displacement, ileus, or gastroparesis (Table 28-9). The history of diarrhea followed by absent flatus or bowel movements suggests a bowel obstruction. Intermittent pain and bilious emesis suggest an obstruction of the upper GI system rather than a colonic obstruction, but without imaging it remains unclear. Enteral feeds should be held when residual volumes are greater than 200 mL. Assessment of bowel motility and GI function is performed. Abdominal (upright and supine) films are ordered to evaluate distention of the stomach and intestines.

Table 28-9. Differential Diagnosis for Increased Residual Volumes

Large-bowel obstruction
Small-bowel obstruction
Visceral perforation
Constipation
Acute appendicitis
Cholangitis
Cholecystitis and biliary colic
Cholelithiasis
Diverticular disease
Gastroenteritis
Esophageal perforation, rupture, and tears

An 18-F nasogastric tube can be inserted to decompress the proximal GI tract via continuous low-wall suction. The patient is assessed for evidence of bowel ischemia.

The abdominal film (Figure 28-5) is obtained. Should this patient undergo emergency surgery?

The abdominal radiograph shows multiple loops of dilated small bowel, which suggests a small-bowel obstruction. Surgical management considers the clinical picture and classification of the small bowel (Table 28-10). Early treatment (< 36 hours) of a strangulated small-bowel obstruction improves survival.[66,67]

The terminology of partial versus complete obstruction is based on abdominal radiographic evidence, and 65% to 80% partial obstructions resolve without surgery.[68] It can be difficult to determine the degree of obstruction or the etiology from plain films and clinical evaluation (Table 28-11). The clinical feature of continuous abdominal pain is common in patients with strangulated bowel, but its presence is not definitive.

There are a number of radiographic studies and treatments that can aid in evaluating a patient with possible small-bowel obstruction (SBO). A small-bowel enteroclysis, which is a real-time radiographic examination with oral contrast, can be performed at the bedside. This should be performed without barium when there is concern of ischemia or perforation because barium can cause peritonitis if it enters the abdominal cavity.[69-71] Contrast-enhanced CT is becoming the study of choice for SBO evaluation. CT scan has a sensitivity and specificity of 82% to 100% for detecting cause of obstruction, location of a transition point, bowel wall edema, signs of ischemia, and extraluminal pathology.[71-73]

Postoperative adhesions and hernias cause 70% of SBO, and this patient has had multiple surgeries to repair ventral hernias (Figure 28-6). Postoperative adhesions develop in 95% of adult patients after abdominal surgery.[74] Common practice for nonstrangulated adhesive SBO involves the administration of Gastrografin. Gastrografin is a water-soluble, radiopaque, hypertonic liquid oral contrast that is used to diagnose and treat adhesive SBOs. It draws fluid into the lumen from the bowel wall, decreasing edema and promoting peristalsis. For patients with possible adhesive SBO, 100 mL of Gastrografin is given via NGT. The NGT is clamped for 2 hours. A repeat abdominal film is taken 4 to 12 hours later. If Gastrografin passed into the colon, then the SBO is partial. If Gastrografin is not in the colon after 6 hours, the obstruction is classified as complete.[75] Gastrografin passage into the colon is strongly

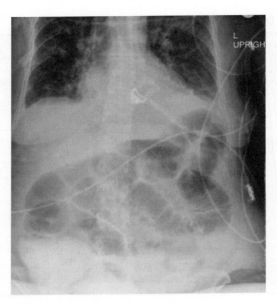

Figure 28-5. Radiograph of abdomen.

predictive of resolution of SBO. Administration of Gastrografin has been shown to decrease the duration of adhesive SBO and reduce mean hospital length of stay.[76-80]

Clinical and laboratory signs of strangulated bowel include increasing intensity and duration of abdominal pain, elevated arterial lactate levels, bloody stool, acidemia, and hemodynamic instability. Concern for strangulated bowel warrants immediate consultation of the surgical service.

 After placement of the NGT, the abdomen remains distended and the patient complains of pain. A hernia could not be localized through physical examination. Gastrografin is administered to the patient.

What are the complications of an SBO?

Complications such as dehydration, infection, ischemia, and perforation can follow SBO. Increased hydrostatic pressure inside the lumen compresses mucosal lymphatics and causes bowel wall lymphedema. Proteins and electrolytes extravasate across the capillary wall. Decreased venous return from intravascular volume depletion decreases cardiac output. End-organ failure may follow.

Table 28-10. Small-Bowel Obstruction Terminology

Partial	Small-bowel dilation with gas in the colon
Complete	Small-bowel dilation without gas in the colon
Simple	Obstruction with vascular supply spared
Strangulated	Obstruction with compromised vascular supply and ischemia

Table 28-11. Etiology of Small-Bowel Obstruction

Intraluminal	Foreign body
	Bezoar
	Gallstone
	Fecal impaction
Intramural	Adenoma
	Leiomyoma
	Intussusception
	Bowel wall thickening
	Hematoma
	Primary adenocarcinoma
	Metastatic disease
	Lymphoma
Extrinsic	Adhesions
	Hernia
	Adjacent mass or collection
	Volvulus

Native gut bacteria proliferate proximal to the obstruction. Bacteremia and abscess formation occur from bacterial translocation via the microcirculation to the abdominal cavity and mesenteric lymph nodes. Antibiotic therapy to cover gram-negative and anaerobic organisms is initiated in patients with SBO whose intestine may be compromised and who will be undergoing surgery. There are no data to support antibiotic prophylaxis in patients with an SBO who are managed conservatively.

After 6 hours, the abdominal radiograph shows Gastrografin in the colon. The patient continues to have abdominal pain with abdominal distention, but remains clinically stable. How should this patient be managed?

Radiographic evidence suggests this patient has a partial SBO. This can be treated successfully with conservative management in 73% to 90% of patients (Table 28-12).[68,81] Duration of conservative

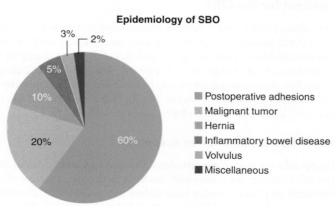

Epidemiology of SBO

3% — 2%
5%
10%
20%   60%

- Postoperative adhesions
- Malignant tumor
- Hernia
- Inflammatory bowel disease
- Volvulus
- Miscellaneous

Figure 28-6. Etiologies and epidemiology of small-bowel obstruction (SBO).

Table 28-12. Conservative Management of Small-Bowel Obstruction

Continuous gastric decompression with an 18-F nasogastric tube
Fluid resuscitation with Ringer lactate
Electrolyte replacement
Pain management
Frequent clinical reassessment for signs of bowel strangulation
Continuous urine output monitoring
Gastrografin administration

management varies, but may be continued for up to 5 days. If symptoms continue, further diagnostic studies or surgical intervention may be necessary (Figure 28-7).

The next morning the patient is febrile with a temperature of 38.5°C; the heart rate increases to 115 bpm; and the blood pressure decreases to 95/30 mm Hg. The patient's laboratory values are notable for an increase in white blood cell count to 17,000. What conditions explain the deterioration of the patient's clinical picture?

Leukocytosis, tachycardia, hypotension, and fever are consistent with a systemic inflammatory response. A diagnosis of strangulated small bowel, intestinal perforation, peritonitis, and abscess formation should be considered. Blood cultures should be sent and antibiotic therapy to cover gram-negative rods and anaerobic bacteria should be prescribed. Fluids should be administered to patients who are fluid responsive. Central venous access and direct blood pressure monitoring via an arterial line should be considered. Vasopressors should be titrated to target mean arterial blood pressures greater than 65 mm Hg. A bladder pressure should be measured because the patient is at risk for developing IAH. Further evaluation with a CT scan of the abdomen and pelvis should be performed.

After several fluid challenges, the patient's blood pressure increases to 107/64 mm Hg and the heart rate decreases to 96 bpm. A CT scan with oral and intravenous contrast shows acute appendicitis. The patient is scheduled for an emergent exploratory laparotomy and appendectomy. Why were the typical signs of appendicitis not present in this patient? What can you do to prepare the patient for the OR?

It is more difficult to obtain a history and to perform an abdominal examination in patients whose lungs are mechanically ventilated because they are often sedated and receiving analgesic medications. The patient is at risk for clinical deterioration during manipulation of the bowel during his OR course. The patient should be euvolemic. An arterial line should be placed. Two units of PRBCs should be typed and crossed because dissection of previous adhesions may be associated with intraoperative bleeding.

The patient has an uncomplicated OR course. The appendix was ruptured and the small bowel and proximal colon were distended. A bowel obstruction was not seen.

Why was a small-bowel obstruction suspected?

Perforation of the appendix can cause a paralytic ileus. The ileus appears as a partial SBO with administration of Gastrografin, but does not resolve with conservative therapy. A patient who has a ruptured appendix and peritonitis may have a similar presentation to a patient with strangulated bowel and ischemia. With a complicated abdominal history, partial SBO, and peritonitis, the patient should continue on antibiotics for 3 to 5 days.

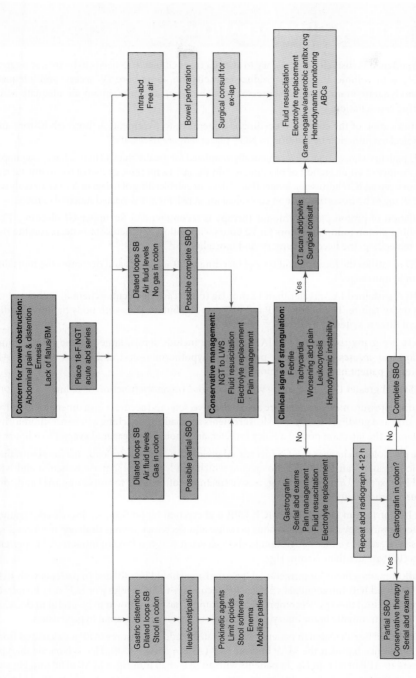

Figure 28-7. Algorithm for small-bowel obstruction (SBO) management: ABCs, airway, breathing, and circulation; abd, abdominal; antibx, antibiotics; BM, bowel movement; cvg, coverage; ex-lap, exploratory laparotomy; LWS, low wall suction; NGT, nasogastric tube; SB, small bowel.

> ## ! CRITICAL CONSIDERATIONS

- Hemodynamic instability secondary to anemia from GI bleeding needs to be treated aggressively with volume and blood product resuscitation, large-bore IV access, and adequate hemodynamic monitoring. Vasopressors may be necessary to maintain an adequate MAP during resuscitation.
- Identification of the source of bleeding is imperative to treatment. A thorough history and physical examination in addition to NGT placement are necessary.
- ICU patients whose lungs are mechanically ventilated for greater than 48 hours; have coagulopathy, history of GI ulceration or bleeding within the last 12 months; or two of the following risk factors: sepsis, ICU admission longer than 7 days, occult bleeding of 6 days or longer, or daily use of 250 mg of hydrocortisone or an equivalent are at risk for stress-related mucosal damage.
- Initiation of proton pump inhibitor therapy is recommended for upper GI bleeding. Prescribing proton pump inhibitors for 72 hours with endoscopic hemostasis decreases the risk for rebleeding, the need for surgery, and mortality.[3,4]
- EGD identifies the location and type of bleeding in 90% of cases and decreases the mortality from hemorrhage.[13]
- IAH: A sustained IAP greater than 12 mm Hg (often causing occult ischemia) without obvious organ failure. The normal IAP is 0 to 5 mm Hg, but it varies with body habitus and different disease states.
- There are many risk factors for IAH, and they include sepsis, large-volume resuscitation, abdominal masses, pancreatitis, peritonitis, hypothermia, and abdominal surgery. IAH increases patient morbidity and mortality.[26-28]
- ACS: IAH greater than 20 mm Hg with at least one organ dysfunction or failure.
- Bladder pressure measurements are a cost-effective, safe, and accurate instrument for identifying IAH and guiding therapy.[32-36] Measurements are made by attaching a pressure-monitoring system to the injection port of a Foley catheter, and should be measured every 4 to 6 hours.
- The physiologic changes in ACS (decreased preload, increased afterload, increased intrathoracic pressure) can result in hypotension, which can lead to mesenteric ischemia and AKI and hypoxemia. Unfortunately, aggressive treatment often leads to worsening IAH and continued clinical deterioration.
- An IAP of 15 mm Hg can affect ICP, CPP, and cerebral blood flow. An increased intrathoracic pressure elevates central venous pressure and decreases venous drainage from cerebral vessels. Cerebral venous congestion leads to elevated ICP, resulting in intracranial hypertension (ICP greater than 20 mm Hg).
- Medical management for intracranial hypertension should be initiated in patients with IAH and elevated ICP. Intracranial hypertension secondary to brain injury or IAH may be refractory to medical therapy. Decompressive laparotomy has been shown to be useful in decreasing ICP in traumatic brain injury patients with refractory intracranial hypertension.
- APP should be calculated in patients with elevated bladder pressures. APP is calculated from the difference between the MAP and the IAP (APP = MAP−IAP). Hemodynamic therapy targets an APP of 60 mm Hg. In patients with an IAP of 20 mm Hg, a MAP of 80 mm Hg will likely maintain adequate perfusion pressure to the abdominal organs, including the kidneys, liver, and intestines.[37,53-55]

- The terminology of partial versus complete obstruction is based on abdominal radiographic evidence, and 65% to 80% partial obstructions resolve without surgery. The clinical feature of continuous abdominal pain is common in patients with strangulated bowel, but its presence is not definitive.
- Contrast-enhanced CT is becoming the study of choice for SBO evaluation.
- Postoperative adhesions and hernias cause 70% of SBO.
- Common practice for nonstrangulated adhesive SBO involves the administration of Gastrografin. Gastrografin is a water-soluble, radiopaque, hypertonic liquid oral contrast that is used to diagnose and treat adhesive SBOs. It draws fluid into the lumen from the bowel wall, decreasing edema and promoting peristalsis.
- Complications such as dehydration, infection, ischemia, and perforation can follow obstruction of the small bowel.
- It is more difficult to obtain a history and to perform an abdominal examination in patients whose lungs are mechanically ventilated because they are often sedated and receiving analgesic medications.
- A patient who has a ruptured appendix and peritonitis may have a similar presentation to a patient with strangulated bowel and ischemia. With a complicated abdominal history, partial SBO and peritonitis, the patient should continue on antibiotics for 3 to 5 days.

REFERENCES

1. Pitcher JL. Therapeutic endoscopy and bleeding ulcers: Historical overview. *Gastrointes Endosc.* 1990;36:S2-S7.
2. Spirt MJ. Acid suppression in critically ill patients: What does the evidence support? *Pharmacotherapy.* 2003;23:S87-S93.
3. Bardou M, Toubouti Y, Benhaberou-Brun D, Rahme E, Barkun AN. Meta-analysis: proton-pump inhibition in high-risk patients with acute peptic ulcer bleeding. *Alimnet Pharmacol Ther.* 2005;21:677-686.
4. Khuroo MS, Farahat KL, Kagevi IE. Treatment with proton pump inhibitors in acute non-variceal upper gastrointestinal bleeding: a meta-analysis. *J Gastroenterol Hepatol.* 2005;20:11-25.
5. Baker DE. Peptic ulcer bleeding following therapeutic endoscopy: a new indication for intravenous esomeprazole. *Rev Gastroenterol Disord.* 2009;9:E111-E118.
6. Fallah M, Prakash C, Edmundowicz S. Acute gastrointestinal bleeding. *Med Clin North Am.* 2000;84:1183-1208.
7. Kandarpa K, Aruny J. Acute gastrointestinal bleeding. In: *Handbook of Interventional Radiologic Procedures.* 2nd ed. Baltimore, MD: Lippincott Williams & Wilkins; 1996:130-138.
8. Reuter S, Redman H, Cho K. Gastrointestinal bleeding. In: *Gastrointestinal Angiography.* 3rd ed. Philadelphia, PA: W. B. Saunders Co.; 1986.
9. Richter JM, Isselbacher KJ. Gastrointestinal bleeding. In: *Harrison's Principles of Internal Medicine.* 12th ed. New York, NY: McGraw-Hill; 1991:261-264.
10. Blatchford O, Murray WR, Blatchford M. A risk score to predict need for treatment for upper-gastrointestinal haemorrhage. *Lancet.* 2000;14;356:1318-1321.
11. Chen IC, Hung MS, Chiu TF, Chen JC, Hsiao CT. Risk scoring systems to predict need for clinical intervention for patients with nonvariceal upper gastrointestinal tract bleeding. *Am J Emerg Med.* 2007;25:774-779.
12. Stanlye AJ, Ashley D, Dalton HR, et al. Outpatient management of patients with low-risk upper-gastrointestinal haemorrhage: multicentre validation and prospective evaluation. *Lancet.* 2009;373:42-47.
13. Farrell JJ, Friedman LS: Gastrointestinal bleeding in older people. *Gastroenterol Clin North Am.* 2000;29:1-36.
14. Kollef MH, O'Brien JD, Zuckerman GR, Shannon W. BLEED: a classification tool to predict outcomes in patients with acute upper and lower gastrointestinal hemorrhage. *Crit Care Med.* 1997;25:1125-1132.

Trauma and Surgical Intensive Care

15. Rockall TA, Logan RFA, Devlin HB, Northfield TC. Risk assessment after acute upper gastrointestinal hemorrhage. *Gut.* 1996;38:316-321.

16. Corley DA, Stefan AM, Wolf M, et al. Early indicators of prognosis in upper gastrointestinal hemorrhage. *Am J Gastroenterol.* 1998;93:336-340.

17. Lau JY, Sung JJ, Lam YH, et al. Endoscopic retreatment compared with surgery in patients with recurrent bleeding after initial endoscopic control of bleeding ulcers. *N Engl J Med.* 1999;340: 751-756.

18. Chiu PWY, Lam CYW, Lee SW, et al. Effect of scheduled second therapeutic endoscopy on peptic ulcer rebleeding: a prospective randomized trial. *Gut.* 2003;52:1403-1407.

19. Wong SK, Yu LM, Lau JY, et al. Prediction of therapeutic failure after adrenaline injection plus heater probe treatment in patients with bleeding peptic ulcer. *Gut.* 2002;50:322-325.

20. Cochran TA. Bleeding peptic ulcer: surgical therapy. *Gastroeneterol Clin North Am.* 1993;22: 751-778.

21. Qvist P, Arnesen KE, Jacobsen CD, Rosseland AR. Endoscopic treatment and restrictive surgical policy in the management of peptic ulcer bleeding. Five year's experience in a central hospital. *Scand J Gastroenterol.* 1994;29:569-576.

22. Venclauskas L, Bratlie SO, Zachrisson K, et al. Is transcatheter arterial embolization a safer alternative than surgery when endoscopic therapy fails in bleeding duodenal ulcer? *Scand J Gastroeneterol.* 2010;45:1003-1004.

23. Millward SF. ACR Appropriateness criteria on treatment of acute non-variceal gastrointestinal tract bleeding. *J Am Coll Radiol.* 2008;5:550-554.

24. Larssen, L, Moger, T, Bjornbeth, B, Lygren I, Klow NI. Transcatheter arterial embolization in the management of bleeding duodenal ulcers: a 5.5-year retrospective of treatment and outcome. *Scand J Gastroeneterol.* 2008;43:217-222.

25. Irving JD, Northfield TC. Emergency arteriography in acute gastrointestinal bleeding. *Br J Med.* 1976;1:929-931.

26. Malbrain ML, Chiumello D, Pelosi P, et al. Prevalence of intra-abdominal hypertension in critically ill patients: a multicentre epidemiological study. *Intensive Care Med.* 2004;30:822-829.

27. Malbrain ML, Chiumello D, Pelosi P, et al. Incidence and prognosis of intra-abdominal hypertension in a mixed population of critically ill patients: a multiple-center epidemiological study. *Crit Care Med.* 2004;33:315-322.

28. Ivatury RR, Porter JM, Simon RJ, Islam S, John R, Stahl WM. Intra-abdominal hypertension after life-threatening penetrating abdominal trauma: prophylaxis, incidence, and clinical relevance to gastric mucosal pH and abdominal compartment syndrome. *J Trauma.* 1998;44:1016-1021.

29. Malbrain ML, Cheatham M, Kirkpatrick A, et al. Results from the conference of experts on intra-abdominal hypertension and abdominal compartment syndrome. I. Definitions. *Intensive Care Med.* 2006;32:1722-1732.

30. Kirkpatrick AW, Brenneman FD, McLean RF, Rapanos T, Boulanger BR. Is clinical examination an accurate indicator of raised IAP in critically injured patients? *Can J Surg.* 2000;43:207-211.

31. Sugrue M, Bauman A, Jones F, et al. Clinical examination is an inaccurate predictor of intraabdominal pressure. *World J Surg.* 2002;26:1428-1431.

32. Ivatury RR, Cheatham ML, Malbrain ML, Sugrue M, eds. *Abdominal Compartment Syndrome.* Georgetown, TX: Landes Biosciences; 2006.

33. Malbrain ML. Abdominal pressure in the critically ill: Measurement and clinical relevance. *Intensive Care Med.* 1999;25:1453-1458.

34. Malbrain ML. Abdominal pressure in the critically ill. *Curr Opin Crit Care.* 2000;6:17-29.

35. Malbrain ML, Jones F. Intra-abdominal pressure measurement techniques. In: Ivatury RR, Cheatham ML, Malbrain ML, Sugrue M, eds. *Abdominal Compartment Syndrome.* Georgetown, TX: Landes Biosciences; 2006:19-69.

36. Lui F, Sangosanya A, Kaplan LF. Abdominal compartment syndrome: clinical aspects and monitoring. *Crit Care Clin.* 2007;23:415-433.

37. Cheatham ML, Malbrain ML, Kirkpatrick A, et al. Results from the international conference of experts on intra-abdominal hypertension and abdominal compartment syndrome. II. Recommendations. *Intensive Care Med.* 2007;33:951-962.

38. De Waele J, Pletinckx P, Blot S, Hoste E. Saline volume in transvesical intra-abdominal pressure measurement: enough is enough. *Intensive Care Med.* 2006;32:455-459.

39. Fusco MA, Martin RS, Chang MC. Estimation of intra-abdominal pressure by bladder pressure measurement: validity and methodology. *J Trauma.* 2001;50:297-302.

40. Malbrain ML, Deeren DH. Effect of bladder volume on measured intravesical pressure: a prospective cohort study. *Crit Care.* 2006;10:R9.

41. Deeren DH, Dits H, Malbrain M. Correlation between intra-abdominal and intracranial pressure in nontraumatic brain injury. *Intensive Care Med.* 2005;31:1577-1581.

42. Citerio G, Vascotto E, et al. Induced abdominal compartment syndrome increases intracranial

pressure in neurotrauma patients. *Crit Care Med.* 2001;29:1466-1471.

43. Joseph DK, Dutton RP, Aarab B, Scalea TM. Decompressive laparotomy to treat intractable hypertension after traumatic brain injury. *J Trauma.* 2004;57:687-693; discussion 693-695.

44. Scalea TM, Bochicchio GV, Habashi N, et al. Increased intra-abdominal, intrathoracic, and intracranial pressure after severe brain injury: multiple compartment syndrome. *J Trauma.* 2007;62:647-656.

45. Parr MJ, Olvera CI. Medical management of abdominal compartment syndrome. In: Ivatury RR, Cheatham ML, Malbrain ML, Sugrue M, eds. *Abdominal Compartment Syndrome.* Georgetown, TX: Landes Biosciences; 2006:232-239.

46. De Waele J, Delaet I, Hoste E, Verholen E, Blot S. The effect of neuromuscular blockers on intraabdominal pressure. *Crit Care Med.* 2006;34:A70.

47. Mertens zur Borg IR, Verbrugge SJ, Kolkman KA. Anesthetic considerations in abdominal compartment syndrome. In: Ivatury RR, Cheatham ML, Malbrain ML, Sugrue M, eds. *Abdominal Compartment Syndrome.* Georgetown, TX: Landes Biosciences; 2006:254-265.

48. Corcos AC, Sherman HF. Percutaneous treatment of secondary abdominal compartment syndrome. *J Trauma.* 2001;51:1062-1064.

49. Reckard JM, Chung MH, Varma MK, Zagorski SM. Management of intraabdominal hypertension by percutaneous catheter drainage. *J Vasc Interv Radiol* 2005;16:1019-1021.

50. Gotlieb WH, Feldman B, Feldman-Moran O, et al. Intraperitoneal pressures and clinical parameters of total paracentesis for palliation of symptomatic ascites in ovarian cancer. *Gynecol Oncol.* 1998;71:381-385.

51. Sharpe RP, Pryor JP, Gandhi RR, Stafford PW, Nance ML. Abdominal compartment syndrome in the pediatric blunt trauma patient treated with paracentesis: report of two cases. *J Trauma.* 2002;53:380-382.

52. Parra MW, Al-Khayat H, Smith HG, Cheatham ML. Paracentesis for resuscitation-induced abdominal compartment syndrome: an alternative to decompressive laparotomy in the burn patient. *J Trauma.* 2006;60:1119-1121.

53. Cheatham ML, White MW, Sagraves SG, Johnson JL, Block EF. Abdominal perfusion pressure: a superior parameter in the assessment of intra-abdominal hypertension. *J Trauma.* 2000;49:621-626.

54. Malbrain ML. Abdominal perfusion pressure as a prognostic marker in intra-abdominal hypertension. In: Vincent JL, ed. *Yearbook of Intensive Care and Emergency Medicine.* New York, NY: Springer; 2000:792-814.

55. Cheatham ML, Malbrain ML. Abdominal perfusion pressure. In: Ivatury RR, Cheatham ML, Malbrain MLNG, Sugrue M, eds. *Abdominal Compartment Syndrome.* Georgetown, TX: Landes Biosciences; 2006:69-81.

56. Gecelter G, Fahoum B, Gardezi S, Schein M. Abdominal compartment syndrome in severe acute pancreatitis: an indication for a decompressing laparotomy. *Dig Surg.* 2002; 19:402-404; discussion 404-407.

57. Pupelis G, Austrums E, Snippe K, Berzins M. Clinical significance of increased intraabdominal pressure in severe acute pancreatitis. *Acta Chir Belg.* 2002;102:71-74.

58. De Waele JJ, Hoste E, Blot SI, Decruyenaere J, Colardyn F. Intra-abdominal hypertension in patients with severe acute pancreatitis. *Crit Care.* 2005;9:R452-R457.

59. Windsor AC, Kanwar S, Li AG, et al. Compared with parenteral nutrition, enteral feeding attenuates the acute phase response and improves disease severity in acute pancreatitis. *Gut.* 1998;42:431-435.

60. Lehocky P, Sarr MG. Early Enteral feeding in severe acute pancreatitis: can it prevent secondary pancreatic (super) infection? *Dig Surg.* 2000;17:571-577.

61. Mossner J, Teich N. Nutrition in acute pancreatitis. *Z Gastroenterol.* 2008;46:784-789.

62. Kollef MH. Ventilator-associated pneumonia: a multivariate analysis. *JAMA.* 1993;270:1965-1970.

63. Pelosi P, Tubiolo D, Mascheroni D, et al. Effects of the prone position on respiratory mechanics and gas exchange during acute lung injury. *Am J Respir Crit Care Med.* 1998; 157:387-393.

64. Hering R, Wrigge H, Vorwerk R, et al. The effects of prone positioning on intraabdominal pressure and cardiovascular and renal function in patients with acute lung injury. *Anesth Analg* 2001;92:1226-1231.

65. Hering R, Vorwerk R, Wrigge H, et al. Prone positioning, systemic hemodynamics, hepatic indocyanine green kinetics, and gastric intramucosal energy balance in patients with acute lung injury. *Intensive Care Med.* 2002;28:53-58.

66. Fevang BT, Fevang J, Stangeland L, Soreide O, Svanes K, Viste A. Complications and death after surgical treatment of small bowel obstruction: a 35-year institutional experience. *Ann Surg.* 2000;231:529-537.

67. Cox MR, Gunn IF, Eastman MC, Hunt RF, Heinz AW. The safety and duration of non-operative

treatment for adhesive small bowel obstruction. *Aust N Z J Surg.* 1993;63:367-671.

68. Seror D, Feigin E, Szold A, et al. How conservatively can postoperative small bowel obstruction be treated? *Am J Surg.* 1993;165:121-125; discussion 125-126.

69. Raptopoulos V, Schwartz RK, McNicholas MM, Movson J, Pearlman J, Joffe N. Multiplanar helical CT enterography in patients with Crohn's disease. *AJR Am J Roentgenol.* 1997;169:1545-1550.

70. Bodily KD, Fletcher JG, Solem CA, et al. Crohn disease: mural attenuation and thickness at contrast-enhanced CT enterography—correlation with endoscopic and histologic findings of inflammation. *Radiology.* 2006;238:505-516.

71. Diaz JJ Jr, Bokhari F, Mowery NT, et al. Guidelines for management of small bowel obstruction. *J Trauma.* 2008;64:1651-1664.

72. Cappell MS, Batke M. Mechanical obstruction of the small bowel and colon. *Med Clin North Am.* 2008;92:575-597.

73. Lappas JC, Reyes BL, Maglinte DD. Abdominal radiography findings in small bowel obstruction: relevance to triage for additional diagnostic imaging. *AJR Am J Roentgenol.* 2001;176:167-174.

74. Menzies D, Ellis H. Intestinal obstruction from adhesions: how big is the problem? *Ann R Coll Surg Engl.* 1990;72:60-63.

75. Schein M. Small bowel obstruction. In: Schein M, Rogers PN, eds. *Schein's Common Sense Emergency Abdominal Surgery.* New York, NY: Springer; 2005:179-190.

76. Abbas S, Bissett I, Parry BR. Oral water soluble contrast for the management of adhesive small bowel obstruction. *Cochrane Database Syst Rev.* 2006;2:1-25.

77. Biondo S, Pares D, Mora L, Marti Rague J, Kreisler E, Jaurrieta E. Randomized clinical study of Gastrografin administration in patients with adhesive small bowel obstruction. *Br J Surg.* 2003;90:542-546.

78. Tresallet C, Lebreton N, Royer B, Leyre P, Godiris-Petit G, Menegaux F. Improving the management of acute adhesive small bowel obstruction with CT-scan and water-soluble contrast medium: a prospective study. *Dis Colon Rectum.* 2009;52:1869-1876.

79. Burge J, Abbas S, Roadley G, et al. Randomized double blind controlled trial of the therapeutic effect of oral Gastrografin in adhesive small bowel obstruction. *A N Z J Surg.* 2005;75:672-674.

80. Farid, M, Fikry A, El Nakeeb A, et al. Clinical impacts of oral Gastrografin follow-through in adhesive small bowel obstruction (SBO). *J Surg Res.* 2010;162:170-176.

81. Roadley G, Cranshaw I, Young M, Hill AG. Role of Gastrografin In assigning patients to a non-operative course in adhesive small bowel obstruction. *A N Z J Surg.* 2004;74:830-832.

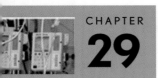

Genitourinary Emergencies

Francis Macchio, MD

Most patients with significant genitourinary injuries require prompt urologic consultation. The majority of these patients will have additional injuries within the chest, abdomen, or pelvis, which will also mandate immediate surgical evaluation. It is extremely rare for the genitourinary tract to be injured in isolation. Therefore, the initial management of genitourinary trauma should not be in isolation either. General trauma management, as explained in other chapters in this book, should be implemented upon arrival in order to identify and treat all life-threatening injuries.

In the intensive care unit (ICU), life-threatening injuries, such as traumatic shattered kidney or urosepsis from bladder rupture, are encountered much more frequently than an isolated injury to the external genitalia. Although situations such as a zipper injury or priapism might be considered a genitourinary emergency in the emergency department (ED), it would be extremely rare for someone to be admitted to an ICU solely under those circumstances. However, attention must be paid to the entire genitourinary system in the ICU. For example, it is more common in the ICU to have a patient with an injury to the external genitalia that accompanies a pelvic fracture. Timely recognition and appropriate treatment of all genitourinary emergencies are vital to minimizing associated morbidity, which may include renal insufficiency, sepsis, incontinence, decreased sexual function, impotence, and infertility. In addition, these less frequently encountered injuries are important because they will be relevant in some way, such as when not to place a Foley catheter in a trauma patient or when to complete a rape kit in a patient with pelvic injuries secondary to physical abuse.

Finally, it is always important to remember that even though the human body and medicine are broken down into systems, such as the genitourinary system, there is considerable overlap among them. Many topics pertaining to the genitourinary system are addressed elsewhere in this book, such as the management of renal failure and sepsis.

A 45-year-old man with a history of hypertension presents after being involved in an automobile accident. It is reported that he was not wearing a seat belt, but the air bag did deploy. Standard advanced trauma life support is initiated. He is drowsy from being intoxicated and intubated for airway protection. Initial vital signs include a heart rate of 102 bpm and blood pressure 115/75 mm Hg. On physical examination, no lacerations or abdominal distension can be appreciated. Significant bruising is noted along the left flank and back. A Foley catheter is passed without difficulty and initial urine collection shows no hematuria. Postintubation chest radiography shows fractures of the 11th and 12th ribs on the left as well as a mild pulmonary contusion also on the left. It is noted that despite aggressive crystalloid resuscitation, the patient's heart rate is now 112 bpm and blood pressure is 100/60 mm Hg, and a stat chest, abdomen, and pelvic computed tomographic (CT) scan with contrast is ordered. As the scan finishes, his heart rate is 125 bpm and blood pressure is 75/48 mm Hg. The CT scan result shows a grade IV kidney laceration on the left.

Describe the basic anatomy of the genitourinary system

The upper genitourinary tract consists of the kidneys and the ureters. Owing to the location of the liver, the right kidney extends lower than the left kidney. Substantial force is necessary to injure the kidneys, given their location and the fact that they are shielded by the lower ribs, back musculature, and perinephric fat. The ureters travel from the renal pelvis on the front of the psoas muscles and insert into the back of the bladder at the trigone.[1] Both the kidneys and ureters are located within the retroperitoneal space.

The lower genitourinary tract consists of the bladder, urethra, and the external genitalia. Since it is a hollow organ, the bladder is compact within the lower pelvis and is relatively protected when empty. However, when filled with urine, the bladder may expand up to the level of the umbilicus, where it is more at risk to injury. The male urethra runs through the prostate gland and is divided into anterior and posterior portions. The female urethra is shorter and more mobile than the male urethra. The male external genitalia are made up of the penis, testicles, scrotum, and the ejaculatory system. The female external genitalia are made up of the vagina, vulva, labia majora, labia minora, and the clitoris.[1]

What are the causes of renal injury?

The kidney is the most commonly injured organ of the genitourinary system. Renal injury occurs in approximately 1% to 5% of all traumas.[2] As explained above, significant force is required to harm the kidneys. Therefore, associated intra-abdominal injuries are also likely to occur. Ninety to 95% of renal injuries are the result of blunt trauma, such as motor vehicle accidents (MVAs), falls, direct blows, lower rib fractures, and bicycle accidents. Most severe are those that involve decelerating forces, which may cause avulsion of the renal pedicle or renal artery dissection.[1] The remainder of renal injuries is due to penetrating injuries, which tend to be more severe, have a higher number of associated organ injuries, and usually result in a higher nephrectomy rate.[3] It is important to note that preexisting renal disease makes renal injury more likely following trauma.[4] The Committee on Organ Injury Scaling of the American Association for the Surgery of Trauma (AAST) has developed a system for classifying the severity of renal injuries (Table 29-1).[5]

Table 29-1. American Association for the Surgery of Trauma Organ Injury Severity Scale for the Kidney

Scale	Type	Description
I	Contusion	Microscopic or gross hematuria, urologic studies normal
	Hematoma	Subcapsular, nonexpanding hematoma without parenchymal laceration
II	Hematoma	Nonexpanding perirenal hematoma confined to renal retroperitoneum
	Laceration	Laceration < 1 cm depth of renal cortex without urinary extravasation
III	Laceration	Laceration > 1 cm depth of renal cortex without collecting system rupture or urinary extravasation
IV	Laceration	Parenchymal laceration extending through renal cortex, medulla, and collecting system
	Vascular	Main renal artery or vein injury with contained hemorrhage
V	Laceration	Completely shattered kidney
	Vascular	Avulsion of renal hilum, devascularizing the kidney

(From Santucci RA, McAninch JW, Safir M, et al. Validation of the American Association for the Surgery of Trauma organ injury severity scale for the kidney. J Trauma. 2001;50:195-200.)

Describe the initial evaluation of renal injury

Injuries to organs that lie within the retroperitoneal space, such as the kidneys, may be difficult to identify since the area may be isolated from traditional physical examination, and these injuries may not present with signs and symptoms of classic peritonitis. Clinical signs of a potential renal injury are nonspecific and may include pain, bruising, abdominal or flank tenderness, posterior rib or spine fractures, hematuria, or other organ injury or shock. It is important to note that hematuria may not correlate with the degree of injury.[6] For example, injuries such as ureteropelvic junction disruption, renal pedicle damage, or segmental artery thrombosis may occur without hematuria.[7] On the other end of the spectrum, patients with preexisting renal disease had a higher degree of macroscopic hematuria, a lower rate of associated trauma to other abdominal organs, and their kidneys were more frequently injured by low-velocity impacts.[8]

In those patients who are hemodynamically stable, a CT scan with intravenous contrast is the modality of choice for the identification and staging of traumatic renal injury, both blunt and penetrating. It also gives a picture of the entire area around the kidney, in particular the retroperitoneum and other neighboring organs, and can identify any preexisting lesions.[9] For the most part, CT scan has replaced intravenous pyelography as the definitive study for suspected renal trauma not involving the ureters. Plain radiographs may identify injuries such as rib, spine, or pelvic fractures, which, as mentioned, may be associated with renal injury.

What are the indications for surgery?

Outside of a shattered kidney, a major renal vascular laceration, or a massive decelerating mechanism, genitourinary trauma is seldom life-threatening. As with all trauma situations, the initial screening of a trauma patient is to identify and manage any potential life-threatening injuries, as addressed in other chapters of this book. Injuries to the kidneys that result in shock, hemodynamic instability, or evidence of continued bleeding are indications for urgent surgical exploration.[10] Delaying surgery in these situations to obtain imaging studies in these patients may be deleterious. Special attention should be paid to penetrating renal injuries, particularly stabs and gunshot wounds. In these patients, if renal injury is clinically suspected or if hematuria is present, surgery should be strongly considered.[11] In renovascular injuries, nephrectomy is the treatment of choice unless there is a solitary kidney or the patient has sustained bilateral injuries.[12] The majority of patients with grade IV or grade V renal injury present with major associated injuries, with a resultant higher rate of renal exploration.[13] Interventional radiology arteriography with selective renal embolization for hemorrhage control is a reasonable alternative to surgery in selected hemodynamically stable patients.[14]

What are the postoperative concerns and complications?

Early complications consist of bleeding, infection, abscess, sepsis, urinary fistula, hypertension, urinary extravasation, and urinoma. After approximately 4 weeks, delayed complications include bleeding, hydronephrosis, renal calculi, pyelonephritis, hypertension, arteriovenous fistula, and pseudoaneurysms. If any of these complications are life-threatening, such as bleeding or sepsis, they should be handled immediately as explained elsewhere in the other chapters. Stable bleeding and pseudoaneurysms may be amenable to interventional radiology selective embolization.[15] Perinephric abscess may be drained percutaneously. Any of these complications may warrant reoperation. Acute renal failure may also occur, most commonly in those patients who experience hemodynamic instability.

Discuss the nonsurgical options of managing patients with renal injury

In hemodynamically stable patients, supportive care with bed rest and hydration is the preferred initial nonsurgical approach and is associated with a lower rate of nephrectomy, without any increase in

Table 29-2. American Association for the Surgery of Trauma Organ Injury Severity Scale for the Ureter

Grade	Description
I	Hematoma only
II	Laceration < 50% of circumference
III	Laceration > 50% of circumference
IV	Complete tear < 2 cm of devascularization
V	Complete tear > 2 cm of devascularization

(From Moore EE, Shackford SR, Pachter HL, et al. Organ injury scaling: Spleen, liver and kidney. J Trauma. 1989;29:1664-1666.)

morbidity.[16] In most cases, grade I and grade II renal injuries can be managed this way. Some studies advocate this treatment for grade III injuries as well.[17]

What are the causes of ureteral injury?

The ureters are small in size, mobile, and in a protected location, which makes injury rare. The majority (75%) of ureteral injuries are iatrogenic, with most occurring during urologic, general surgical, or gynecologic procedures. Blunt injury (18%) is the next most common mechanism; most commonly from a significant deceleration force with avulsion at the ureteropelvic junction resulting from a MVA or fall. The remainder of ureteral injuries are due to penetrating trauma (7%).[1] The AAST has also developed a system for classifying the severity of ureteral injuries (Table 29-2).[18]

Describe the initial evaluation of ureteral injury

Ureteral injury should be suspected in all penetrating abdominal injuries and in blunt injuries with a deceleration mechanism. Major intra-abdominal injuries are often associated with ureteral injury. It is important to note that as with renal injury, hematuria is not a consistent finding. Urinalysis is normal approximately 25% of the time.[19] Also, similar to renal injury, signs and symptoms of ureteral injury can be vague. Often, ureteral injury is not discovered until the late findings of fever, flank pain, and a palpable flank mass have set in.

Initial diagnosis of a ureteral injury may be difficult. When a CT scan is used to identify renal injury, it may also be used to identify ureteral injury. It is important to note that time must be allowed in order for the kidneys to excrete the intravenous contrast. When these delayed images are not diagnostic, intravenous pyelography may be used, although sensitivity ranges can vary greatly. Under surgical conditions, the ureters may be directly inspected. Retrograde pyelography may also be useful when the diagnosis is elusive.[19]

What is the management of ureteral injury?

Partial tears can be managed via ureteral stenting or via a nephrostomy tube for urinary diversion. Injuries above grade III are surgically repaired with debridement, stenting, and reconstruction. The specific type of reconstructive repair depends on the nature and site of the injury.[20]

What are the causes of bladder injury?

Urinary bladder injury may result from either blunt (67% to 86%) or penetrating (14% to 33%) injury.[21] Ruptures of the urinary bladder are most frequently seen in multitrauma patients with blunt injuries,

Table 29-3. American Association for the Surgery of Trauma Organ Injury Severity Scale for the Bladder

Grade		Description
I	Hematoma	Contusion, intramural hematoma
I	Laceration	Partial thickness
II	Laceration	Extraperitoneal bladder wall laceration < 2 cm
III	Laceration	Extraperitoneal (< 2 cm) or intraperitoneal (< 2 cm) bladder wall laceration
IV	Laceration	Intraperitoneal bladder wall laceration > 2 cm
V	Laceration	Intraperitoneal or extraperitoneal bladder wall laceration extending into the bladder neck or ureteral orifice

(From Moore EE, Shackford SR, Pachter HL, et al. Organ injury scaling: Spleen, liver and kidney. J Trauma. 1989;29:1664-1666.)

particularly following MVAs. The majority of patients with bladder rupture from blunt trauma are linked with pelvic fractures.[22] The propensity for bladder injury is related to the degree of distension at the time of impact.[23] When empty, the bladder is relatively protected unless the force of injury fractures the bony pelvis. When distended by urine, the bladder may extend up to the level of the umbilicus, where it is vulnerable to blunt trauma inflicted upon the lower abdomen. In an interesting combination, driving under the influence of alcohol predisposes to both accidents and a distended bladder.[24] The AAST has also developed a system for classifying the severity of bladder injuries (Table 29-3).[18]

Describe the initial evaluation of bladder injury

Signs and symptoms of bladder injury include lower abdominal pain, hematuria, inability to void, suprapubic bruising, and swelling of the scrotum, perineum, abdominal wall, or thighs. The combination of pelvic fracture and hematuria warrants immediate cystography in blunt trauma victims.[25] Retrograde cystography is considered the procedure of choice in evaluating bladder trauma.[26] The bladder must be distended sufficiently to ensure extravasation following rupture. Retrograde CT cystography may also be used, but has its limitations.[27] Intravenous pyelography, angiography, ultrasound, and standard CT scan are inadequate in assessing bladder injury following trauma.[28]

What is the management of bladder injury?

The primary goal in management of bladder injuries is to keep the bladder completely decompressed. Doing so facilitates healing by minimizing bladder wall tension. Urethral injury must be excluded prior to Foley catheter placement. Even in the presence of extensive extravasation, these patients can be managed safely by drainage only. Surgical involvement is needed for penetrating injuries, bladder entrapment by bone, or bladder neck injury.[29] Additional abdominal injuries should be considered when the diagnosis of bladder injury is made.

What are the causes of urethral injury?

Urethral injury is rare, comprising less than 1% of all genitourinary injuries. In males, anterior urethra injuries may be inflicted by direct blows, straddle injuries, instrumentation, or in conjunction with a penile fracture. Posterior urethral injuries usually occur in the setting of significant pelvic fractures, often caused by MVAs. The weakest point of the posterior urethra is the bulbomembranous junction, where the

Trauma and Surgical Intensive Care

Table 29-4. American Association for the Surgery of Trauma Organ Injury Severity Scale for the Urethra

Type	Description	Appearance
I	Contusion	Blood at the urethral meatus; normal urethrogram
II	Stretch injury	Elongation of the urethra without extravasation on urethrography
III	Partial disruption	Extravasation of contrast at injury site with contrast visualized in the bladder
IV	Complete disruption	Extravasation of contrast at injury site without visualization in the bladder; < 2 cm of urethral separation
V	Complete disruption	Complete transection with > 2 cm urethral separation, or extension into the prostate or vagina

(From Moore EE, Shackford SR, Pachter HL, et al. Organ injury scaling: Spleen, liver and kidney. J Trauma. 1989;29:1664-1666.)

majority of posterior disruptions occur. In females, urethral injuries are less common, given the anatomy. Overall, urethral disruption accompanies pelvic fracture in approximately 6% of cases in women and up to 25% in men. The risk of urethral injury is also influenced by the degree of pelvic fracture.[30] The AAST has also developed a system for classifying the severity of urethral injuries (Table 29-4).[18]

Describe the initial evaluation of urethral injury

Pain on urination or an inability to void point to a urethral injury. In the absence of blood at the meatus or hematoma, a urethral injury is unlikely and can be ruled out by bladder catheterization. However, if there is blood present at the meatus, the urethra must be imaged and no attempts at urethral catheterization should be made. In an unstable patient, a cautious attempt may be made, but should be aborted if any difficulty is encountered.[31] The catheter should remain in place if a urethral injury is suspected following its placement. Hematuria is nonspecific and may even be absent in cases of total transection.[32] An absent, high-riding, or boggy prostate may be associated with posterior urethral disruption. In this situation, the prostate shears away from the pelvis and migrates up, and blood fills the normal location of the prostate. Rectal and vaginal examinations must be included so as not to miss associated injuries or mechanisms. Retrograde urethrography is the test of choice for evaluating the urethra, in particular if a urethral injury is clinically suspected prior to Foley catheter insertion.

What is the management of urethral injury?

No treatment is required for type I urethral injury. Type II and type III injuries can be managed by suprapubic cystostomy or urethral catheterization. Endoscopic realignment or surgical exploration are considered for type IV and type V injuries and penetrating injuries.[1]

What are the causes of external genitalia injury?

An isolated injury to the external genitalia in the ICU is extremely rare. Most injuries of this type occur by blunt mechanisms such as direct blow, a fall from height, sporting accidents, straddle injury, MVAs, or by circulatory compromise inflicted by constricting objects. Penile fractures occur when the erect penis is bent abruptly and forcefully; typically through intercourse or assault. Blunt trauma to the scrotum can cause scrotal hematoma, testicular rupture, or traumatic dislocation.[33] Penetrating trauma to the external genitalia is frequently associated with complex injuries of other organs, such as pelvic fractures, which could potentially lead to an ICU admission.

Describe the initial evaluation of external genitalia injury

In females, with injury to the external genitalia, assault must be considered. Complete vaginal inspection and smears should be done.[34] As with urethral injury, hematuria indicates the need for retrograde urethrography. Local pain and swelling will be prominent.[35] In males, differing results surround the use of ultrasound in testicular trauma, and surgery is recommended if the diagnosis is unclear.[36]

What is the management of external genitalia injury?

Local hematoma and swelling of the external genitalia may be treated with ice packs and nonsteroidal analgesics such as ibuprofen 400 to 800 mg orally every 6 to 8 hours, not exceeding 3.2 g/24 hours. Surgical involvement is necessary for penile fracture, hematocele, testicular rupture, testicular dislocation, or penetrating injury to the external genitalia.

Why are these injuries important in the ICU?

Roughly one of every ten patients experiencing injuries serious enough to require admission to a trauma service also suffers injury to the genitourinary tract. The great majority of these injuries are from blunt trauma. Except in the rare instance of a shattered kidney or major renal vascular laceration with significant hemorrhage, genitourinary injuries seldom pose a threat to life. However, timely identification and management of genitourinary injuries minimize associated morbidity, which may range from incontinence and impotence to sepsis and renal failure. Of all genitourinary injuries, outside of those being life-threatening, the most debilitating has for decades been described as those affecting the posterior urethra, potentially leading to lifelong conditions with deleterious consequences compromising not only the ability to void and maintain urinary continence but also the ability to reproduce.[37]

Table 29-5 outlines the different diagnostic studies for each particular genitourinary organ injured.[1] As mentioned above, hemodynamic stability takes precedence. Obtaining these studies should not delay the emergency surgical care of life-threatening injuries if they are clinically suspected.

Table 29-5. Overview of Diagnostic Studies for Genitourinary Trauma

Injury	Main diagnostic study	Secondary studies
Kidney	CT scan with IV contrast	Intravenous pyelography
		Angiography
		Magnetic resonance imaging
Ureter	CT can with IV contrast and delayed images	Intravenous pyelography
		Retrograde pyelography
Bladder	Retrograde cystography	Computed tomographic cystography
Urethra	Retrograde urethrography	Magnetic resonance imaging
		Urethroscopy
		Suprapubic endoscopy
External genitalia	Direct inspection	Ultrasound
		Retrograde urethrography

(From Lynch TH, Martinez-Pineiro L, Plas E, et al. EUA guidelines on urological trauma. Eur Urol. 2005;47:1-15.)

A 72-year-old man has been in the neurologic ICU (NeuroICU, NICU) following an elective craniotomy for meningioma resection. His past medical history includes hypertension on metoprolol, non–insulin-dependent diabetes on metformin and glipizide, and benign prostatic hyperplasia status posttransurethral resection of the prostate 2 years ago. He was extubated without difficulty on postoperative day 1. Following extubation, his heart rate was 65 bpm, blood pressure 115/75 mm Hg, and central venous pressure 12 mm Hg. In addition to his home medications, he is on an intravenous hydromorphone patient-controlled analgesic (IVPCA) for pain control, which he has been using at least three times per hour. His Foley catheter was removed later that day with plans to discharge him to the neurosurgical floor the following day. On the morning of postoperative day 2, as you are signing the transfer orders, the nurse tells you that the patient has not urinated since the Foley catheter was removed 14 hours ago despite several attempts with the urinal. He also received midazolam 2 mg from the night staff early this morning for increasing agitation. His creatinine level is 1 mg/dL, which is exactly what it was preoperatively. At this time, his heart rate is 72 bpm, blood pressure is 130/90 mm Hg, and central venous pressure is 12 mm Hg.

What are the causes of acute urinary retention?

Acute urinary retention is the most common urologic emergency. It is frequently secondary to obstruction. In men older than 60 years old, the obstruction is often due to benign prostatic hyperplasia (BPH).[38] Table 29-6 lists the causes of acute urinary retention, which in some cases are intermingled.[39,40]

Which medications are associated with acute urinary retention?

Anticholinergic and sympathomimetic agents, which are widely used in the ICU, are two of the main groups of medications connected to acute urinary retention.[41] Opiates, also widely used in the ICU, can reduce detrusor contractility and bladder sensation.[42] Methylnaltrexone, a peripherally acting opioid-receptor antagonist used in the treatment of opioid-induced constipation, is currently being investigated as a treatment for opioid-induced urinary retention.[43] Table 29-6 lists the classes of medications linked to acute urinary retention.[40]

What is the evaluation of acute urinary retention?

As the name implies, acute urinary retention presents with the sudden failure to urinate, often accompanied with abdominal or suprapubic discomfort, and an overall feeling of distress.[44] There is little change in serum creatinine since this problem develops rapidly over a few hours. Important history to consider includes hematuria, dysuria, previous episodes, masses, surgery radiation, and medications. On physical examination, the bladder may be palpable or tender. A major difference between acute and chronic urinary retention is that chronic retention is often painless. A rectal examination for masses should be performed. In addition, a vaginal examination should be performed in females. If neurologic impairment is suspected, a neurologic examination should be completed to assess lower extremity function including reflexes, strength, and sensation. Further testing is established based on history and physical examination. For example, an ultrasound or CT scan may identify suspected masses or a complete blood count for screening a potential infection. Interestingly, prostate-specific antigen is of little value since it is often elevated in situations of acute urinary retention.[45]

What is the management of acute urinary retention?

The goal of therapy is immediate bladder decompression by transurethral catheterization and treatment of the underlying etiology. Urosepsis and renal failure are the most feared complications and

Table 29-6. Causes of Acute Urinary Retention

Benign prostatic hypertrophy
Trauma
Constipation
Prostate cancer
Postoperative
Urethral stricture
Neurologic disorder
Medications   Anticholinergics, Sympathomimetics, Opioids, Antidepressants, Antiarrhythmics, Antiparkinsonians, Hormones, Antipsychotics, Antihistamines, Muscle relaxants
Infection
Urolithiasis
Psychologic issues
Malignancy
Spinal cord compression
Phimosis
Pelvic mass
Malpositioned urinary catheter
Diabetic neuropathy
Cerebral vascular accident

(From Murray K, Massey A, Feneley RC. Acute urinary retention—A urodynamic assessment. Br J Urol. 1984;56:468-473; and Curtis LA, Dolan TS, Cespedes RD. Acute urinary retention and urinary incontinence. Emerg Med Clin North Am. 2001;19:591-619.)

are especially prevalent in the ICU setting. A 14- to 18-gauge catheter is typically used. A larger and stiffer catheter may be needed when dealing with benign prostatic hyperplasia, the most common cause of acute urinary retention. A smaller, more flexible catheter may be necessary when dealing with patients whose urethras have had prior instrumentation and may have developed scar tissue.[40] As with urethral trauma, this procedure should not be forced, and urologic expertise may be needed. Placement of a suprapubic catheter by a urologist may be required in cases of irregularities that prohibit passage of a transurethral catheter.[46] Suprapubic needle aspiration of the bladder may be necessary in emergency situations. Both urethral and suprapubic catheters have their own advantages and disadvantages as listed in Table 29-7.[46,47] Regardless of the method used, rapid and complete decompression of the obstructive bladder is safe and effective in most patients. Hematuria, hypotension, and post–obstructive diuresis may occur following the procedure, but are rarely clinically significant in otherwise healthy patients. However, they should be anticipated in hypovolemic and critically ill patients.[45] Prophylactic antibiotics are not indicated. Urologists vary in terms of how long

Table 29-7. Comparing Advantages of Urethral and Suprapubic Catheters in the Treatment of Acute Urinary Retention [46,47]

Urethral	Suprapubic
Easier placement	More comfortable
No risk of bowel perforation	Less urinary tract infections
More familiar management	Reduced sphincter dysfunction
	No risk of urethral stricture
	Patients still able to void

(From Ichsan J, Hunt DR. Suprapubic catheters: A comparison of suprapubic versus urethral catheters in the treatment of acute urinary retention. Aust N Z J Surg. 1987;57:33-36; and Horgan AF, Prasad B, Waldron DJ, et al. Acute urinary retention. Comparison of suprapubic and urethral catheterization. Br J Urol. 1992;70:149-151.)

to leave catheters in—from immediate removal up to 2 weeks.[48] α Blockers function to relieve the mechanical obstruction associated by benign prostatic hyperplasia by relaxation of the bladder neck smooth muscle. Men catheterized for acute urinary retention can void more successfully after catheter removal if treated with tamsulosin, and are less likely to need recatheterization.[49]

Further management, including medical and surgical treatment of recurrent episodes, is in the hands of urology and will likely be handled outside of the ICU. The majority of men who experience an episode of acute urinary retention will have repeat occurrences. The key to definitive treatment is to correct the underlying etiology. For men with moderate symptoms of benign prostatic hyperplasia, transurethral resection of the prostate is more effective than other treatments in reducing the rate of treatment failure and improving genitourinary symptoms.[50] Prostatectomy is rarely indicated in treating acute retention due to prostate issues, and patients are at an increased risk of developing postoperative complications. Waiting for at least a month following an episode of acute urinary retention is recommended.[51]

 A 21-year-old college athlete comes to the ED with intense scrotal pain of sudden onset. He states that it began abruptly while practicing with his team. He denies all medical problems. Initial vital signs include a heart rate of 96 bpm and blood pressure 135/85 mm Hg. On physical examination, his scrotum is swollen and extremely tender. It can be noted that the left testis is higher than the right testis.

What are the causes of acute scrotal pain?

Acute scrotal pain may be caused by testicular torsion, appendiceal torsion, epididymitis, inguinal hernia, direct trauma, mumps, and idiopathic edema. Of these, testicular torsion is the most serious. If the fixation of the lower pole of the testes is insufficient or absent, the testis may twist on the spermatic cord, which houses the testicular vessels. This movement, therefore, may produce ischemia from reduced arterial blood flow and venous outflow obstruction. The onset of pain is typically sudden, associated with nausea and vomiting, and frequently coupled with physical activity. Neonates and postpubescent males are most likely affected.[52]

What is the evaluation of acute scrotal pain?

Clinical diagnosis is extremely important since time is of the essence. Classically, the affected testis will be swollen, elevated, and often oriented transversely instead of longitudinally owing to the rotation and shortening of the spermatic cord. The cremasteric reflex will be absent on the affected side. Normally, the testis will rise upon touching of the ipsilateral upper thigh. With torsion, the spermatic cord is already shortened, owing to rotation, and unable to rise further. It is important to note that this reflex may be normal with both torsion of the appendix testis and with epididymitis.[53] Color Doppler ultrasonography will definitively diagnose testicular torsion, as well as rule out torsion of the appendix or epididymitis.[54]

What is the management of testicular torsion?

Immediate surgical exploration should be undertaken for testicular torsion. Irreversible damage is thought to occur after 12 hours. Longer periods may result in infarction and an increased need for orchiectomy.[55] Manual detorsion of the testicle is another option, particularly when surgery is not a readily available option. In most cases, the testis rotates medially and, therefore, is detorsed by rotating it laterally toward the thigh. This should lead to pain relief, the return of a longitudinal orientation, and the return of normal arterial flow by Doppler examination. However, surgery should still be undertaken in order to fixate the testis as well as rule out any residual torsion.[56]

! CRITICAL CONSIDERATIONS

- In the trauma setting, the genitourinary tract is hardly ever injured by itself. Associated abdominal and pelvic injuries are likely to occur, which take precedence and require immediate surgical evaluation.

- Following assessment and management of life-threatening injuries, timely recognition and appropriate treatment of genitourinary trauma are vital to minimizing associated genitourinary morbidity. Most patients with significant genitourinary injuries require urgent urologic consultation.

- Hematuria is an important marker for potential injury to the genitourinary system. However, the degree of hematuria does not correlate with the severity of injury and in some instances, may even be absent despite significant injury.

- Surgery is the treatment for all genitourinary trauma in which the patient is hemodynamically unstable, particularly when dealing with penetrating trauma. In hemodynamically stable patients, correct imaging is key to detailing further management.

- The kidney is the most commonly injured organ of the genitourinary system and patients with preexisting renal disease are more susceptible. Injury to the ureters is often iatrogenic. Bladder and urethral trauma are highly linked with pelvic fractures. When dealing with trauma to the external genitalia, the possibility of abuse must always be considered.

- Acute urinary retention is the most common urologic emergency. Urosepsis and renal failure are major complications. Patients with benign prostatic hyperplasia and prior urethral instrumentation are at highest risk. A large number of medications used in the ICU setting are known to cause acute urinary retention.

- Immediate bladder decompression by transurethral catheterization is the definitive treatment for acute urinary retention. Suprapubic access may be necessary where transurethral catheterization is complicated or dangerous. Hematuria, hypotension, and post–obstructive diuresis may follow decompression, which must be anticipated in patients who are hypovolemic or critically ill.

- Testicular torsion is the most serious cause of acute scrotal pain and swelling. It must be diagnosed, clinically or with ultrasonography, as soon as possible. Irreversible damage to the affected testis will occur after 12 hours. Surgery is the definitive treatment, although manual detorsion may temporarily correct the problem.

REFERENCES

1. Lynch TH, Martinez-Pineiro L, Plas E, et al. EUA guidelines on urological trauma. *Eur Urol.* 2005;47:1-15.
2. Baverstock R, Simons R, McLoughlin M. Severe blunt renal trauma: a 7-year retrospective review from a provincial trauma centre. *Can J Urol.* 2001;8:1372-1376.
3. Ersay A, Akgun Y. Experience with renal gunshot injuries in a rural setting. *Urology.* 1999;54:972-975.
4. Giannopolous A, Serafetinides E, Alamanis C, et al. Urogenital lesions diagnosed incidentally during evaluation for blunt renal injuries. *Prog Urol.* 1999;9:464-469.
5. Santucci RA, McAninch JW, Safir M, et al. Validation of the American Association for the Surgery of Trauma organ injury severity scale for the kidney. *J Trauma.* 2001;50:195-200.
6. Buchberger W, Penz T, Wicke E, et al. Diagnosis and staging of blunt kidney trauma. A comparison of urinalysis, i.v. urography, sonography and computed tomography. *Rofo Fortschr Geb Rontgenstr Neuen Bildgeb Verfahr.* 1993;158:507-512.
7. Eastham JA, Wilson TG, Ahlering TE. Radiographic evaluation of adult patients with blunt renal trauma. *J Urol.* 1992;148:266-269.
8. Schmidlin FR, Iselin CE, Naimi A, et al. The higher injury risk of abnormal kidneys in blunt renal trauma. *Scand J Urol Nephrol.* 1998;32:388-392.
9. Kawashima A, Sandler CM, Corriere Jr JN, et al. Imaging of renal trauma: a comprehensive review. *Radiographics.* 2001;21:557-574.
10. American College of Surgeons Committee on Trauma. *Advanced Trauma Life Support for Doctors.* 8th ed. Chicago, IL: American College of Surgeons; 2008:121.
11. Mee SL, McAninch JW, Robinson AL, et al. Radiographic assessment of renal trauma: a 10-year prospective study of patient selection. *J Urol.* 1989;141:1095-1098.
12. Tillou A, Romero J, Asensio JA, et al. Renal vascular injuries. *Surg Clin North Am.* 2001;81:1417-1430.
13. Santucci RA, McAninch JM. Grade IV renal injuries: evaluation, treatment, and outcome. *World J Surg.* 2001;25:1565-1572.
14. Hagiwara A, Sakaki S, Goto H, et al. The role of interventional radiology in the management of blunt renal injury: a practical protocol. *J Trauma.* 2001;51:526-531.
15. Heyns CF, Van Vollenhoven P. Selective surgical management of renal stab wounds. *Br J Urol.* 1992;69:351-357.
16. Schmidlin FR, Rohner S, Hadaya K, et al. The conservative treatment of major kidney injuries. *Ann Urol (Paris).* 1997;31:246.
17. el Khader K, Mhidia A, Ziade J, et al. Conservative treatment of stage III kidney injuries. *Acta Urol Belg.* 1998;66:25-28.
18. Moore EE, Shackford SR, Pachter HL, et al. Organ injury scaling: spleen, liver and kidney. *J Trauma.* 1989;29:1664-1666.
19. Elliott SP, McAninch JW. Ureteral injuries from external violence: the 25-year experience at San Francisco General Hospital. *J Urol.* 2003;170:1213-1216.
20. Morey AF, Bruce JE, McAninch JW. Efficacy of radiographic imaging in pediatric blunt trauma. *J Urol.* 1996;156:2014-2018.
21. Corriere JN Jr, Sandler CM. Management of the ruptured bladder: seven years of experience with 111 cases. *J Trauma.* 1986;26:830-833.
22. Castle WN, Richardson JR Jr, Walton BJ. Unsuspected intraperitoneal rupture of bladder presenting with abdominal free air. *Urology.* 1986;28:521-523.
23. Vaccaro JP, Brody JM. CT cystography in the evaluation of major bladder trauma. *Radiographics.* 2000;20:1373-1381.
24. Dreitlein DA, Suner S, Basler J. Genitourinary trauma. *Emerg Med Clin North Am.* 2001;19:569-590.
25. Morey AF, Iverson AJ, Swan A, et al. Bladder rupture after blunt trauma: guidelines for diagnostic imaging. *J Trauma.* 2001;51:683-686.
26. Sandler CM, Goldman SM, Kawashima A. Lower urinary tract trauma. *World J Urol.* 1998;16:69-75.
27. Hsieh GH, Chen RJ, Fang JF, et al. Diagnosis and management of bladder injury by trauma surgeons. *Am J Surg.* 2002;184:143-147.
28. Festini G, Gregorutti S, Reina G, et al. Isolated intraperitoneal bladder rupture in patients with

alcohol intoxication and minor abdominal trauma. *Ann Emerg Med.* 1991;20:1371-1372.

29. Morey AF, Hernandez J, McAninch JW. Reconstructive surgery for trauma of the lower urinary tract. *Urol Clin North Am.* 199;26:49-60.

30. Koratim MM. Pelvic fracture urethral injuries: the unresolved controversy. *J Urol.* 1999;161:1433-1441.

31. Dixon MD. Diagnosis and acute management of posterior urethral disruptions. In: McAninch JW, ed. *Traumatic and Reconstructive Urology.* Philadelphia, PA: Saunders: 1996;347-355.

32. Antoci JP, Schiff M Jr. Bladder and urethral injuries in patients with pelvic fractures. *J Urol* 1982;128:25-26.

33. Shefi S, Mor Y, Dotan ZA, et al. Traumatic testicular dislocation: a case report and review of published reports. *Urology.* 1999;54:744-745.

34. Okur H, Kucikaydin M, Kazez A, et al. Genitourinary tract injuries in girls. *Br J Urol.* 1996;78:446-449.

35. Haas CA, Brown SL, Spirnak JP. Penile fracture and testicular rupture. *World J Urol.* 1999;17:101-106.

36. Pavlica P, Barozzi L. Imaging of the acute scrotum. *Eur Radiol.* 2001;11:220-228.

37. Trafford HS. Traumatic rupture of the posterior urethra. *Br J Urol.* 1955;27:165-171.

38. Fong YK, Milani S, Djavan B. Natural history and clinical predictors of clinical progression in benign prostatic hyperplasia. *Curr Opin Urol* 2005;15:35-38.

39. Murray K, Massey A, Feneley RC. Acute urinary retention—A urodynamic assessment. *Br J Urol.* 1984;56:468-473.

40. Curtis LA, Dolan TS, Cespedes RD. Acute urinary retention and urinary incontinence. *Emerg Med Clin North Am.* 2001;19:591-619.

41. Verhamme KM, Sturkenboom MC, Stricker BH, et al. Drug-induced urinary retention: incidence, management and prevention. *Drug Safety.* 2008;31:373-388.

42. Raz S, Zeigler M, Caine M. Pharmacological receptors in the prostate. *Br J Urol.* 1973;45:663-667.

43. Rosow CE, Gomery P, Chen TY, et al. Reversal of opioid-induced bladder dysfunction by intravenous naloxone and methylnaltrexone. *Clin Pharmacol Ther.* 2007;82:48-53.

44. Thomas K, Chow K, Kirby RS. Acute urinary retention: a review of the aetiology and management. *Prostate Cancer Prostatic Dis.* 2004;7: 32-37.

45. Nyman MA, Schwenk NM, Silverstein MD. Management of urinary retention: rapid versus gradual decompression and risk of complications. *Mayo Clin Proc.* 1997;72:951-956.

46. Ichsan J, Hunt DR. Suprapubic catheters: a comparison of suprapubic versus urethral catheters in the treatment of acute urinary retention. *Aust N Z J Surg.* 1987;57:33-36.

47. Horgan AF, Prasad B, Waldron DJ, et al. Acute urinary retention. Comparison of suprapubic and urethral catheterization. *Br J Urol.* 1992;70:149-151.

48. Taube M, Gajraj H. Trial without catheter following acute retention of urine. *Br J Urol.* 1989;63:180-182.

49. Lucas MG, Stephenson TP, Nargund V. Tamsulosin in the treatment of urinary retention from benign prostatic hyperplasia. *Br J Urol Int.* 2005;95:354-357.

50. Wasson JH, Reda DJ, Bruskewitz RC, et al. A comparison of transurethral surgery with watchful waiting for moderate symptoms of benign prostatic hypertension. The Veteran Affairs Cooperative Study Group on Transurethral Resection of the Prostate. *N Engl J Med.* 1995;332:75-79.

51. Pickard R, Emberton M, Neal DE. The management of men with acute urinary retention. National Prostatectomy Steering Group. *Br J Urol.* 1998;81:712-720.

52. Cummings JM, Boullier JA, Sekhon D, et al. Adult testicular torsion. *J Urol.* 2002;167:2109-2110.

53. Edelsberg JS, Surh YS. The acute scrotum. *Emerg Med Clin North Am.* 1988;6:521-546.

54. al Mufti RA, Ogedegbe AK, Lafferty K. The use of Doppler ultrasound in the clinical management of acute testicular pain. *Br J Urol.* 1995;76:625-627.

55. Jarow JP, Sanzone JJ. Risk factors for male partner antisperm antibodies. *J Urol.* 1992;148:1805-1807.

56. Sessions AE, Rabinowitz R, Hulbert WC, et al. Testicular torsion: direction, degree, duration and disformation. *J Urol.* 2003;169:663-665.

Trauma and Surgical Intensive Care

CHAPTER 30

Critical Care Ultrasound

Oliver Panzer, MD

Fluid responsiveness. A 64-year-old man is admitted to the hospital with 2 days of worsening abdominal pain and intermittent fevers. He underwent a laparoscopic cholecystectomy. On postoperative day 1, the patient was hypotensive and oliguric. His blood pressure, heart rate, and urine output did not increase after administration of 3 L of lactated Ringer solution. His electrocardiogram showed a sinus rate of 120 bpm, his blood pressure was 89/45 mm Hg, and his central venous pressure was 12 mm Hg. Over the course of the morning, his mental status deteriorated, and his work of breathing increased. He was intubated and his lungs were mechanically ventilated. You are called by the resident physician in the postoperative anesthesia care unit and asked to guide further management.

How can an ultrasound examination assess volume responsiveness?

An intensivist assesses a patient's volume responsiveness to determine if a fluid bolus will increase a patient's stroke volume and cardiac output. Traditionally, static parameters of cardiac filling pressures, such as the central venous pressure (CVP) or the pulmonary artery occlusion pressure (PAOP), have been used as surrogates of a patient's volume status. Clinicians have also assessed volume status via echocardiographic parameters such as the left ventricular end-diastolic volume or estimated filling pressures. Most of these traditional parameters, however, poorly predict volume responsiveness because Frank-Starling forces, cardiopulmonary interactions, and changes in systolic, diastolic, intra-abdominal, and intrathoracic pressures influence the patient's response to volume loading.[1,2]

If a patient lies on the steep portion of the Frank-Starling curve, an increase in preload will increase the stroke volume (volume responsive). On the other hand, if the patient is on the flat portion of the Frank-Starling curve, an increase in preload will not increase stroke volume and indeed may reduce it (nonvolume responsive).

Volume assessment aided by dynamic parameters, in contrast to static measurements, recognizes the characteristic respirophasic changes that occur as a patient's intrathoracic pressure changes with positive-pressure ventilation (Figures 30-1 and 30-2). These changes are more dramatic in the hypovolemic patient and can be recognized via the arterial pressure waveform. During a positive-pressure breath with mechanical ventilation, right ventricular (RV) stroke volume drops for two main reasons. First, the RV has less preload owing to decreased venous return from an increased intrathoracic pressure. Second, there is a concomitant increase in afterload to the RV secondary to the pneumatic compression of the pulmonary capillaries. Simultaneously, during mechanical insufflation, the venous return to the left ventricle (LV) is increased as the pulmonary capillaries are compressed and blood is pushed to the left side of the heart. Therefore, LV stroke volume increases during mechanical inspiration. After two to three cardiac cycles (pulmonary transit time), the LV stroke volume falls as a consequence of the aforementioned reduction in RV stroke

528

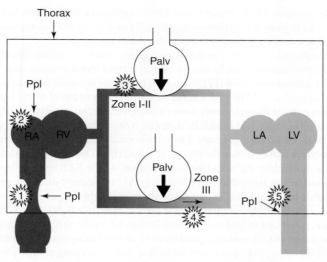

Figure 30-1. Cardiorespiratory interactions in hypovolemic patient during mechanical ventilation. RV preload decreases because the increased pleural pressures (1) compress the SVC and (2) compress the RA, whereas (3) the RV afterload is increased in the upper lung regions (West zones I and II). (4) In the dependent lung regions (West III), the pulmonary veins are squeezed and the blood pushed into LA. (5) Higher pleural pressures finally decrease LV afterload. LA, left atrium; LV, left ventricle; P_{alv}, alveolar pressure; P_{pl}, pleural pressure; RA, right atrium; RV, right ventricle; SVC, superior vena cava. *(From Michard F. Changes in arterial pressure during mechanical ventilation. Anesthesiology. 2005;103:419-428.)*

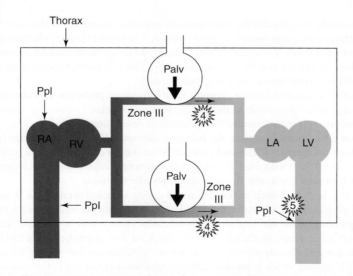

Figure 30-2. Cardiorespiratory interactions in hypervolemic patients during mechanical ventilation. The vena cava and RA are well filled and thus poorly compliant and compressible; therefore, changes in pleural pressure will have no effect. The pulmonary capillary bed is mainly consistent with West zone III areas; thus, the left preload will increase with insufflation (4) and LV afterload is decreased with increasing pleural pressures. LA, left atrium; LV, left ventricle; P_{alv}, alveolar pressure; P_{pl}, pleural pressure; RA, right atrium; RV, right ventricle. *(From Michard F. Changes in arterial pressure during mechanical ventilation. Anesthesiology. 2005;103:419-428.)*

Trauma and Surgical Intensive Care

volume and cardiac output. The converse is true for the expiratory phase of mechanical ventilation. As a patient becomes increasingly hypovolemic, this relationship becomes exaggerated and is manifested as arterial line waveform variation from inspiration to expiration.

Dynamic parameters such as the arterial pulse pressure variation, systolic blood pressure variation, and stroke volume variation can be assessed via an arterial blood pressure tracing.

Measuring the inferior vena cava (IVC) variation is another dynamic measurement that is noninvasive and easy to perform.[3,4] The IVC returns 80% of the venous blood to the right atrium (RA). It briefly passes through the thoracic cavity before joining the inferior aspect of the right atrium. The vena cava is a collapsible vessel, and as such its diameter is dependent on the internal distending pressure and the external compressing pressure. The intrathoracic vena cava's diameter is determined by the right atrial pressure (RAP) minus the pleural pressure (P_{pl}). During mechanical ventilation, the greater the P_{pl}, the more likely the vena cava is to collapse. As the RAP rises, collapse becomes less likely. This relationship can be evaluated by assessing IVC respiratory diameter and respirophasic variation. The higher the change in IVC diameter, the more likely the patient will respond to fluid loading with an increase in stroke volume (SV) and carbon monoxide (CO). Typical cutoff values that differentiate between responders and nonresponders depend on the method used: 12% (using max IVC diameter − minimal IVC diameter/mean diameter) or 18% (using max IVC diameter − min IVC diameter/min IVC diameter) IVC respiratory variability during mechanical ventilation.[3,4]

Respiratory variation of the superior vena cava (SVC) may also predict fluid responsiveness. In a study of 66 septic mechanically ventilated patients, SVC variability of greater than 36% predicted fluid-responsive hemodynamics with a 100% sensitivity and a 90% specificity.[5] However, this imaging is only readily obtainable with a transesophageal echocardiography (TEE) and therefore may have limited utility. IVC imaging has the advantage of being easily performed even by physicians untrained in echocardiography.[6]

How do I obtain the requisite ultrasound images? Where do I make the measurements?

The patient should be in a position that optimizes ultrasound windows. For evaluation of the IVC, the patient should be in a supine or semirecumbent position. The patient's legs may be bent to reduce tension on the abdominal wall. To produce a good ultrasound image there must be copious ultrasound gel between the skin surface and the ultrasound probe. This is important because air will limit the transmission of ultrasound waves, worsening image quality.

It is important to orient the probe properly. Each ultrasound probe has an index marker on one side, which at any time corresponds to the side of the screen marker (Figures 30-3 and 30-4) on the ultrasound machine. It is recommended that a consistent orientation be used.

Two probes are commonly used in the intensive care unit (ICU). A linear array probe (Figure 30-5A) has a high resolution, with limited penetration (at most 9 cm). The second probe is a phased array probe (Figure 30-5B) with a small footprint that generates high frame rates to analyze moving organs like the heart and is also able to penetrate deeply into the tissue.

Since the IVC is located deep in the abdominal cavity, a phased array probe is used. After the application of ultrasound gel, place the probe to the left of the patient's midline in the epigastric area along the longitudinal plane and angled slightly cranially. From top to bottom, the image obtained will show a short axis cut through the left liver lobe that has a homogeneous texture and is hypoechoic (gray color). Below and directly adjacent to the hepatic parenchyma you will see a longitudinal cut through the IVC lumen, which is anechoic (black). Identification of the IVC is enhanced by visualizing the hepatic veins draining from the liver parenchyma into the IVC just underneath the diaphragm. The IVC should continue cranially through the diaphragm into the right atrium. The diaphragm image is a crescent-shaped hyperechoic (very white) line that moves with respiration. This image of the diaphragm is a landmark that separates the intra-abdominal from intrathoracic cavities. If the IVC is not visualized, tilt the probe to the right or left side of the patient until the images come

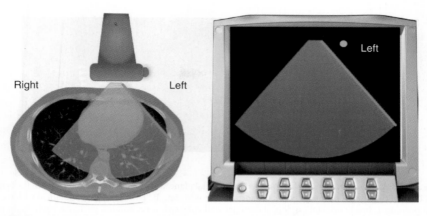

Figure 30-3. Index marker and screen marker correlation in the transverse plane. The left side of the patient corresponds to the right side of the screen.

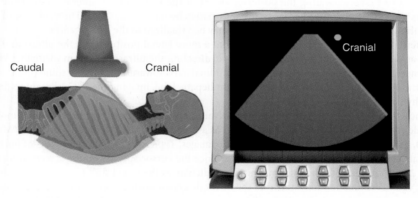

Figure 30-4. Index marker and screen marker correlation in the longitudinal plane. The cranial part of the patient corresponds to the right side of the screen.

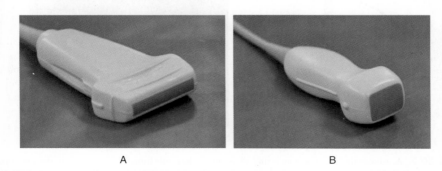

A   B

Figure 30-5. **A.** Linear array probe 5-10 MHz. **B.** Phased array probe 3-5 MHz.

Trauma and Surgical
Intensive Care

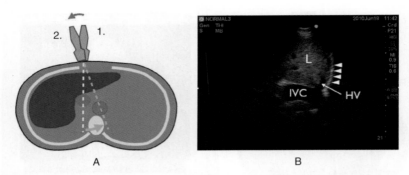

Figure 30-6. **A.** To scan the IVC in the longitudinal/sagittal plane, the probe is placed anteriorly in the epigastric space (1). By tilting the probe medially (2), the aorta comes into view. **B.** This is the image obtained with the probe held in position 1. Image orientation: top, abdominal wall/epigastric area; bottom, posterior/back. Right (screen marker), cranial; left, caudal. L, liver; IVC, inferior vena cava; HV, hepatic vein; arrows, diaphragm.

into view. The IVC should be differentiated from the abdominal aorta, which lies in close proximity. The aorta is usually deeper and to the patient's left side. Additionally, it has a clear hyperechoic layer of connective tissue separating the posterior aspect of the liver and the anterior wall of the aorta, whereas the IVC is directly adjacent to the liver parenchyma (Figure 30-6). The venous wall of the IVC is thinner than the aortic wall. Pulsations may be visualized in the IVC or aorta.

Alternatively, the IVC can be visualized from a more lateral position with the ultrasound probe placed at the patient's right anterior axillary line, directing the ultrasound beam medially (with the index marker pointing to the head in the longitudinal axis) toward the patient's spine (Figure 30-7). The ultrasound beam will pass through the right hepatic lobe, imaging the IVC adjacent to the liver parenchyma.

Once the IVC is identified, respirophasic variations are assessed via time-motion mode, or M-mode. This mode analyzes real-time images as a function of time, along only one line (M-mode cursor), making dynamic events appear on static images. Typically, the picture consists of horizontal black (anechoic) or white (hyperechoic) bands. Once the cursor appears on the screen, you place it within 2 to 3 cm distal to the diaphragm, perpendicular to the vessel wall (Figure 30-8). Also, the hepatic vein–IVC junction may not cross the M-mode cursor during respirations since it would lead to a false-positive test result. The IVC will be shown as a continuous anechoic band that varies in size depending on the degree of collapsibility during the respiratory cycle (Figure 30-9). Observing the ventilator or patient's chest is necessary to determine inspiration and expiration. After the widest and

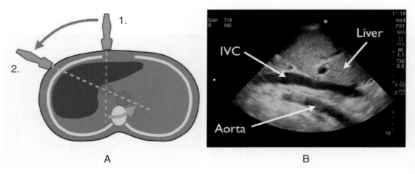

Figure 30-7. **A.** To scan the IVC in a more frontal plane, move the probe from the anterior (1) to the lateral position (2). In this plane, the inferior vena cava (IVC) and the aorta are lying next to each other. **B.** Image orientation: top, right lateral chest; bottom, patient midline. Right (screen marker), cranial; left, caudal.

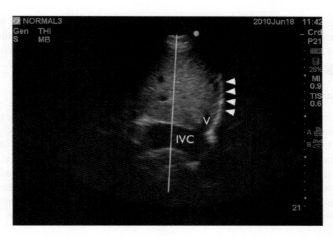

Figure 30-8. Measuring inferior vena cava (IVC) variability: the M-mode cursor is placed 2-3 cm distally from the diaphragm (*arrows*) and distally to the hepatic vein (V). With respiratory efforts the organs will move, and if the hepatic vein junction comes to lie underneath the cursor line, it will create a false widening of the IVC on the M-mode picture.

narrowest point of the IVC diameter is measured using the caliper function, the collapsibility index is calculated as described above.

What are the limitations of using the IVC variation?

Assessment of IVC variation is most reliable when patients are intubated and synchronous with mechanical ventilation. The sensitivity and specificities for predicting fluid responsiveness are not as strong in spontaneously ventilating patients.

Visualization of the IVC may be limited in obese patients. Air limits ultrasound penetration, so tissue emphysema, bowel loops, and recent laparotomy will all effect image quality. Well-aerated lung tissue may also extend into the costophrenic angles and come to lie between the ultrasound probe and

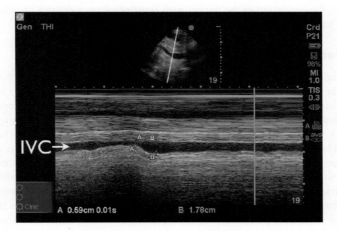

Figure 30-9. Calculation of the inferior vena cava (IVC) collapsibility index: *A* is during expiration and *B* is during inspiration during mechanical ventilation. In this example, the patient is fluid responsive with a collapsability index of 60% (maxIVCdiameter− minIVCdiameter/meanIVCdiameter, 1.78 cm − 0.59 cm/1.19 cm = > 60%).

the liver and will intermittently obscure the picture. Finally, respiratory variations in the IVC have only been studied in patients without increased intra-abdominal pressures. One could safely assume that if the patient has abdominal hypertension or even compartment syndrome, the compliance of the IVC is limited and subsequent analysis of variation in diameter may not be accurate.

What can I use if the patient is breathing spontaneously?

One technique that has repeatedly been shown to be useful is the passive leg raise test. This test is performed by elevating a patient's legs either manually or by tilting the bed cranially from a semirecumbent position and measuring a dynamic parameter before and after the test.[7] When using this method, the patient is challenged with increased preload with the advantage of total reversibility by putting the legs down. If there is a significant improvement in the measured dynamic parameter with leg elevation, the patient likely is volume responsive. Investigators have used the pulse-pressure variation, the aortic flow variation via esophageal Doppler,[8] or the velocity time integral (VTI) variation in the left ventricular outflow tract (LVOT) via the Apical 5 chamber view[9] to determine fluid responsiveness.

Chest ultrasonography. The patient develops acute respiratory distress. Chest radiography shows nonspecific opacifications and is relatively unchanged compared to the past several days.

Is there a role for performing a sonographic examination of the chest?

Yes, ever since Lichtenstein published his first paper on using chest ultrasonography to rule out a pneumothorax in 1995,[10] its popularity has been steadily rising as it has established itself as a possible alternative to computed tomography (CT). Chest ultrasonography can be quickly performed at the bedside, providing real-time results while avoiding time delays, ionizing radiation, and potentially risky patient transportation. It has been used to diagnose pulmonary edema, lung consolidations, large pleural effusions, and pneumothoraces. Furthermore, an easy-to-use algorithm for the systematic approach to the evaluation of the patient with acute respiratory distress or failure using ultrasound findings has-been published.[11]

How do I scan a patient's chest?

The patient should be in the supine or semirecumbent position. Two different probes may be used: the phased array probe or the longitudinal probe. The phased array probe has a small footprint, which makes imaging between the ribs straightforward. This probe can identify deeper structures in the chest, making it useful to determine the extent of a large pleural effusion or lung consolidation (Figure 30-10A). Some intensivists suggest that the linear array probe is sufficient. It better visualizes, with higher resolution, proximal structures such as the pleura, intercostal arteries, and the periphery of the lung (Figure 30-10B). It has great utility for procedural superficial needle placement.

It is advisable to start with the phased array probe since more structures can be visualized at once. First, the diaphragm should be identified to clearly determine the extent of the intrathoracic space. Second, the chest and lung should be scanned sequentially along longitudinal lines (from cranial to caudal) with the probe held perpendicularly to the chest wall. Each hemithorax should be divided into six scanning zones (Figure 30-11). The three large areas from the lateral edge of the sternum to the anterior axillary line, the anterior axillary line to the posterior axillary line, and from the posterior axillary line to the spine should be divided into superior and inferior regions. These regions make

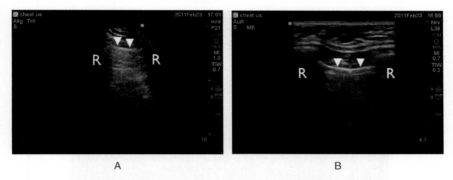

Figure 30-10. A. Picture obtained with phased array probe. R, ribs; *arrow*, pleural line. **B.** Picture obtained with linear array probe.

up the six scanning zones. The ultrasonographer examines the anterior chest wall to identify signs of a pneumothorax or pulmonary edema, then examines the lateral chest wall for pleural effusions and consolidations, which tend to develop in the dependent areas.[12] The posterior scan zone may be accessed by rolling the patient slightly and orienting the probe anteriorly. Other approaches have been described; however, all used the delineated chest wall sections for orientation.[13]

What is a normal lung pattern on ultrasound?

When scanning the lung or abdomen, the diaphragm should initially be identified in order to differentiate the thorax from the abdomen. Next, the ribs should be identified. They are superficial and produce a clean black acoustic shadow. A hyperechoic "sliding line" moving synchronously with respiration can be seen between the ribs about 0.5 cm deeper than the proximal rib surface (Figure 30-12). This line is called the pleural line, and the sliding movement is produced by the parietal and visceral pleurae sliding against each other during respiration. Using the time-motion mode (M-mode), the "seashore sign"[10] can be appreciated (Figure 30-13). Underneath the pleural line, motionless horizontal hyperechoic lines, called A-lines, appear repeatedly in fixed intervals and are generated by subpleural air (Figure 30-12). A-lines are a reverberation artifact created by the soft tissue–air interface at

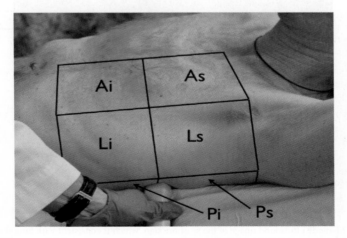

Figure 30-11. The scanning zones on the chest. The hemithorax is divided into three zones: anterior (A), lateral (L), and posterior (P). Each zone is divided into a superior (eg, As) and inferior segment (eg, Ai).

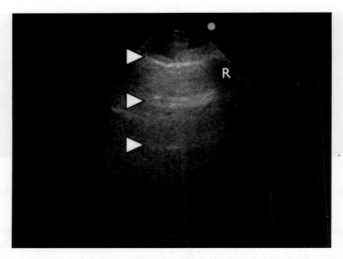

Figure 30-12. Normal lung pattern with A-lines (*arrows*); the first arrow represents the pleural line. R, rib.

the pleura and are normal. A normal chest ultrasound is defined by the presence of lung sliding and A-lines and referred to as an A-profile.[11]

Occasionally, vertically oriented B-lines will be seen. They tend to be seen in the dependent lung zones and are usually nonpathologic. B-lines (also know as "comet tails" or "lung rockets") are ultrasound artifacts caused by the reflection of ultrasound beams within thickened interlobular septa just under the pleura and are seen as hyperechoic vertical lines arising at the pleural line.[14] These lines span the entirety of the ultrasound image without fading, are well defined, efface A-lines, and move with the visceral pleura. They may be part of a normal lung picture if they occur occasionally, mostly representing, for example, a lung fissure. Their significance changes as they become more numerous; typically more than three in one window or when they appear in nondependent lung zones (Figure 30-14).

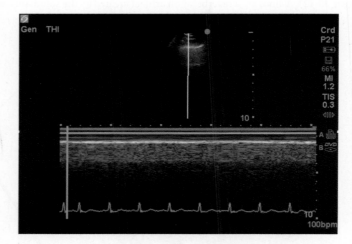

Figure 30-13. M-mode ultrasound image of the seashore sign, which is consistent with lung sliding. Above the pleura (bright white horizontal line) continuous bands indicate no movement of tissue over time (chest wall), whereas the granular pattern below the pleura is caused by constantly moving lung tissue with respirations.

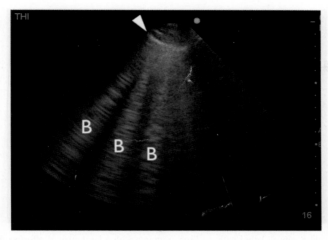

Figure 30-14. B-Lines. B-lines are hyperechoic and originate at the pleural line (*arrow*), efface A-lines, travel through the entire ultrasound image, and move with respiration. B, B-line.

What findings would raise your suspicion for a pathologic process?

Pleural effusions and alveolar consolidations are easily detected by chest ultrasonography (Figure 30-15). Interstitial pulmonary edema, pneumothoraces, and pulmonary emboli can also be imaged but require more expertise.

Pleural effusions are present in up to 60% of medical ICU patients and 40% are present upon admission.[15] Effusions appear as an anechoic layer of fluid separating the two pleural membranes. The fluid collection is typically dependent, resting upon the diaphragm. You can often differentiate between a transudative or exudative effusion. A transudate is totally anechoic and is clearly defined with sharp borders, whereas an exudate, parapneumonic effusion, or empyema is hypoechoic, with much less differentiation.

When lung becomes consolidated it generates an echotexture very similar to liver tissue. This pattern is called hepatization. Since the alveoli are filled with fluid and not air, A-lines will not be generated.[11] Most lung consolidations will have some degree of pleural effusion surrounding them. Often, small hyperechoic spots that are accentuated during inspiration can be appreciated. These spots are air bronchograms (Figure 30-16).[12]

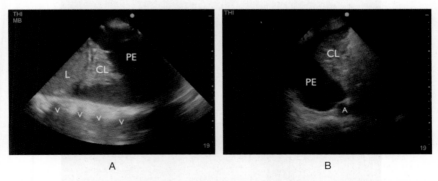

Figure 30-15. A. Simple pleural effusion (PE) with consolidated lung (CL) with the adjacent diaphragm and liver (L) taken in the frontal plane. **B.** Simple PE with consolidated lung taken in a transverse plane, like a slice of a CT scan. Since fluid conducts ultrasound waves well, the descending thoracic aorta (A) is also seen.

Trauma and Surgical Intensive Care

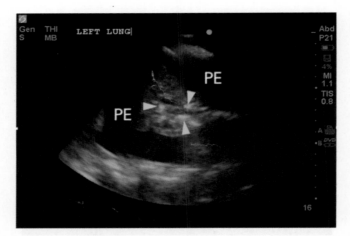

Figure 30-16. Alveolar consolidation with air bronchograms with a large pleural effusion. *Yellow arrows*: air bronchograms. PE, pleural effusion. Image orientation: top, left lateral chest wall; bottom, thoracic spine. Right side (screen marker), cranial; left side, diaphragm/caudal.

Once the lung is injured and the pathology extends to the periphery, the ultrasound image will have an increasing number of B-lines. When B-lines are separated by 7 mm, they correlate with thickened interlobular septa, and when 3 mm apart or almost confluent, they tend to represent alveolar flooding or ground-glass opacities (Figure 30-17).[16] Depending on the type and the extent of the pathologic process, the B-lines may be localized or disseminated.

The definitive diagnosis of a pneumothorax using ultrasound is not easy. The real value of chest ultrasonography in this instance is in its negative predictive value to rule out a pneumothorax.[10] The absence of lung sliding alone carries a low positive predictive value because many things such as acute respiratory distress syndrome (ARDS), atelectasis, pleural adhesions, phrenic palsy, or mainstem or esophageal intubation may cause this.

The only sign that confirms and quantifies a pneumothorax is a "lung point."[17] It is characterized by a normal lung pattern (A-profile: lung sliding in the presence of A-lines) alternating with the A'-profile

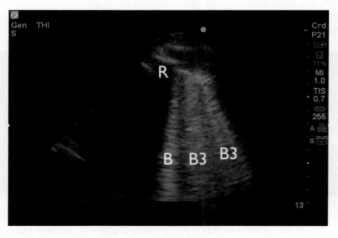

Figure 30-17. Alveolar consolidation: multiple B- and confluent B-lines (B3) are seen. R, rib; B, single B-line; B3, confluent B-lines consistent with ground-glass opacities on CT.

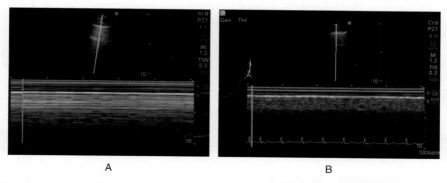

Figure 30-18. A. Sign of a possible pneumothorax: the stratosphere or bar code sign. Compared to the normal lung profile, the M-mode picture of a pneumothorax has only continuous bands throughout the picture, indicating lack of tissue movement (ie, lung sliding). **B.** For comparison, the seashore sign during lung sliding.

(absent lung sliding in the presence of A-lines) during the respiratory cycle within the same acoustic window. The M-mode facilitates the detection of the lung point. The image shows the regular seashore sign intermittently replaced by the "stratosphere sign"; that is, continuous straight lines throughout the entire M-mode picture (Figure 30-18). By marking the lung point in all intercostal spaces on the patient's chest wall, the extent of the partial pneumothorax may be assessed.

The presence or absence of pleural artifacts, lung sliding, and an alveolar consolidation or pleural effusion can be combined to create certain profiles that indicate different pathologic conditions. The *A-profile* is characterized by A-lines with lung sliding; the *A'-profile* is similar but without lung sliding. The *B-profile* is characterized by B-lines (more than three per view between two ribs) and lung sliding; the *B'-profile* is the same without lung sliding. The *A/B-profile* shows mostly A-lines on one side of the chest and mostly B-lines on the other half. The *C-profile* is consistent with anterior lung consolidation.[11]

In which clinical scenario may chest ultrasonography be of particular benefit?

Lung ultrasound may clarify equivocal chest radiographs that are limited by artifacts such as rotation and differences in penetration. In addition, chest ultrasonography may reduce the number of chest radiographs and CT scans performed and radiation exposure to critically ill patients.[18]

In the setting of acute dyspnea, an algorithm such as the bedside-lung-ultrasound-in-emergency (BLUE) protocol can guide diagnosis.[11] This three-step algorithm is quick and can be performed at the bedside.

First, the anterior chest is examined for lung sliding. The presence of lung sliding excludes a pneumothorax with a specificity of 100%. Second, anterior B-lines are assessed. The B-profile (see above) suggests pulmonary edema, and in the majority of cases, edema will be cardiogenic in origin (95% specificity). If an A/B-, C-, or B'-profile is noted, pneumonia is more likely. The sensitivity of a pneumonia diagnosis, however, only reaches 89% if all profiles are found together, which is unlikely. Thus, pneumonia is difficult to diagnose with ultrasound. If normal patterns are observed with chest ultrasonography, pulmonary thromboembolism should be ruled out. If there is no evidence of deep venous thrombosis with a normal profile, assessment for the presence of a posterior consolidation with or without some pleural effusion should be undertaken (posterolateral alveolar/pleural syndrome [PLAPS]). In cases in which PLAPS is present, pneumonia may be responsible for the acute respiratory distress. If PLAPS is absent, chronic obstructive pulmonary disease (COPD) or asthma should be considered (Figure 30-19).

Trauma and Surgical Intensive Care

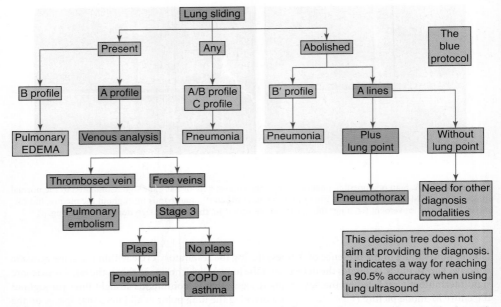

Figure 30-19. Decision tree using lung ultrasonography to guide diagnosis of acute severe dyspnea. First (stage 1), the anterior chest wall is examined and evaluated regarding the presence of lung sliding and B-lines. Second, the lateral chest wall is scanned (stage 2). *(From Lichtenstein DA, Mezière GA. Relevance of lung ultrasound in the diagnosis of acute respiratory failure: the BLUE protocol. Chest. 2008;134:117-125.)*

Lung ultrasonography can assess focal or disseminated disease in patients with ARDS/acute lung injury (ALI) and, therefore, help titrate positive end-expiratory pressure (PEEP) to avoid hyperinflation of the normal lung parenchyma.[19] The changes of lung aeration scores based on ultrasound findings correlate with changes found on chest CT scans after interventions like pleural drainage or antimicrobial therapy for ventilator-associated pneumonia.[20]

Diagnosis should integrate the patient's clinical picture with ultrasound findings. Generating a narrow differential diagnosis prior to ultrasonography scanning may prevent unnecessary treatment. For example, most healthy human beings will show signs of volume responsiveness but are in perfect homeostasis and will not need treatment or intervention. However, in the setting of an oliguric or hypotensive patient, these signs suggest a need for volume loading. In our patient, we found scattered B-lines in all segments of his chest. His transthoracic echocardiogram (TTE) showed a hyperdynamic heart with no signs of fluid responsiveness. A subsequent CT scan of his chest showed a picture consistent with early ARDS/ALI, possibly secondary to his intra-abdominal sepsis.

What are the limitations of chest ultrasonography?

Chest ultrasonography requires training and acquisition of specific skills to have a clinical impact. It has been shown that the learning curve is steep and quick (under 6 weeks) for proficiency in diagnosing simple pathologies like pleural effusions, alveolar consolidations, and alveolar interstitial syndrome.[21] Presumably, it may take longer to diagnose a pneumothorax.

Lung ultrasonography is limited by the fact that lesions or pathologies surrounded by normally aerated parenchyma will not be seen, since air is considered impermeable to ultrasound waves. Obese patients or those with thick chest walls, subcutaneous emphysema, and thoracic wound dressings may have suboptimal images.

! CRITICAL CONSIDERATIONS

- Respirophasic intrathoracic pressure alterations lead to variations in stroke volume, particularly in hypovolemic patients, and are the physiologic basis for predicting volume responsiveness.
- Using dynamic parameters like the IVC variation as a predictor for volume responsiveness only has been validated in mechanically ventilated patients mounting no spontaneous respiratory efforts.
- The IVC may be pictured in an anterior or lateral approach. The measurements of its diameter variation should be performed 2 to 3 cm distally to the diaphragm.
- When performing chest ultrasonography it is important to visualize the diaphragm first to differentiate the intra-abdominal from the intrathoracic cavity.
- The chest should be scanned along longitudinal planes through the different chest zones to allow for systematic description of findings.
- A normal lung pattern on chest ultrasonography is the presence of lung sliding and A-lines.
- Pleural effusions and lung consolidations are easily identified with chest ultrasonography. However, even interstitial pulmonary edema, pneumothoraces, and pulmonary emboli can be diagnosed but require more expertise.
- Ultrasound scores based on pathologic signs in the different chest zones have been shown to be helpful in adjusting ventilator settings in ARDS/ALI patients.
- In the acutely dyspneic patient, the BLUE protocol is a valuable bedside tool, helping to quickly differentiate between common etiologies and to guide clinical management.
- Findings on critical care ultrasonography should always be integrated into the specific clinical scenario to help clarify the diagnosis.

REFERENCES

1. Kumar A, Anel R, Bunnell E, et al. Pulmonary artery occlusion pressure and central venous pressure fail to predict ventricular filling volume, cardiac performance, or the response to volume infusion in normal subjects. *Crit Care Med.* 2004;32:691-699.
2. Marik PE, Baram M, Vahid B. Does central venous pressure predict fluid responsiveness? A systematic review of the literature and the tale of seven mares. *Chest.* 2008;134:172-178.
3. Feissel M, Michard F, Faller J-P, Teboul J-L. The respiratory variation in inferior vena cava diameter as a guide to fluid therapy. *Intensive Care Med.* 2004;30:1834-1837.
4. Barbier C, Loubieres Y, Schmit C, et al. Respiratory changes in inferior vena cava diameter are helpful in predicting fluid responsiveness in ventilated septic patients. *Intensive Care Med.* 2004;30:1-7.
5. Vieillard-Baron A, Chergui K, Rabiller A, et al. Superior vena caval collapsibility as a gauge of volume status in ventilated septic patients. *Intensive Care Med.* 2004;30:1734-1739.
6. Jardin F, Vieillard-Baron A. Ultrasonographic examination of the venae cavae. *Intensive Care Med.* 2006;32:203-206.
7. Monnet X, Teboul JL. Passive leg raising. *Intensive Care Med.* 2008;34:659-663.
8. Lafanechere A, Pene F, Goulenok C, et al. Changes in aortic blood flow induced by passive leg raising predict fluid responsiveness in critically ill patients. *Crit Care.* 2006;10:R132.
9. Soubrier S, Saulnier F, Hubert H, et al. Can dynamic indicators help the prediction of fluid responsiveness in spontaneously breathing critically ill patients? *Intensive Care Med.* 2007;33:1117-1124.
10. Lichtenstein DA, Menu Y. A Bedside ultrasound sign ruling out pneumothorax in the critically ill: Lung sliding. *Chest* 1995;108:1345-1348.
11. Lichtenstein DA, Mezière GA. Relevance of lung ultrasound in the diagnosis of acute respiratory failure: The BLUE protocol. *Chest.* 2008;134:117-125.

Trauma and Surgical Intensive Care

12. Lichtenstein DA, Lascols N, Meziere G, Gepner AS. Ultrasound diagnosis of alveolar consolidation in the critically ill. *Intensive Care Med.* 2004;30:276-281.

13. Bouhemad B, Zhang M, Lu Q, Rouby JJ. Clinical review—Bedside lung ultrasound in critical care practice. *Crit Care.* 2007;11:205.

14. Lichtenstein D, Mezière G, Biderman P, Gepner A. The comet-tail artifact: an ultrasound sign ruling out pneumothorax. *Intensive Care Med.* 1999;25:383-388.

15. Mattison LE, Coppage L, Alderman DF, Herlong JO, Sahn SA. Pleural effusions in the medical ICU: prevalence, causes, and clinical implications. *Chest.* 1997;111:1018-1023.

16. Lichtenstein DA, Mezière G, Lascols N, et al. Ultrasound diagnosis of occult pneumothorax. *Crit Care Med.* 2005;33:1231-1238.

17. Lichtenstein D, Meziere G, Biderman P, Gepner AXES. The "lung point": an ultrasound sign specific to pneumothorax. *Intensive Care Med.* 2000;26:1434-1440.

18. Peris A, Tutino L, Zagli G, et al. The use of point-of-care bedside lung ultrasound significantly reduces the number of radiographs and computed tomography scans in critically ill patients. *Anesth Anal.* 2010;111:687-692.

19. Bouhemad B, Brisson H, Le-Guen M, Arbelot C, Lu Q, Rouby JJ. Bedside ultrasound assessment of positive end-expiratory pressure–induced lung recruitment. *Am J Respir Crit Care Med.* 2011;183:341-347.

20. Arbelot C, Ferrari F, Bouhemad B, Rouby JJ. Lung ultrasound in acute respiratory distress syndrome and acute lung injury. *Curr Opin Crit Care.* 2008;14:70-74.

21. Lichtenstein D, Goldstein I, Mourgeon E, Cluzel P, Grenier P, Rouby JJ. Comparative diagnostic performances of auscultation, chest radiography, and lung ultrasonography in acute respiratory distress syndrome. *Anesthesiology.* 2004;100:9-15.

Cardiovascular Problems

Section Editor: Joseph E. Parrillo, MD, FCCP

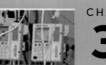

CHAPTER

31

Acute Coronary Syndrome

Joanne Mazzarelli, MD
Steven Werns, MD

A 67-year-old man with a history of hypertension, hyperlipidemia, and tobacco use was found by family members with left-sided paralysis, rightward eye deviation, and change in mental status and was brought to the emergency department (ED). Computed axial tomography (CAT) of the brain performed in the ED (Figure 31-1) showed a large acute nonhemorrhagic right hemispheric infarct within the vascular territory of the right middle cerebral artery. The infarct involved large portions of the frontal, temporal, and parietal lobes as well as underlying basal ganglia structures. The proximal right middle cerebral artery was hyperdense, consistent with thrombosis within the vessel. The patient was not administered thrombolytic therapy because of the unknown onset of symptoms. The local ED physicians decided to transfer the patient immediately to the nearest tertiary medical center. On arrival to the intensive care unit, the patient was awake and alert but with a left hemiparesis and left hemineglect. Upon admission he complained of dyspnea but no chest pain.

Heart rate (HR) was 77 bpm and regular, blood pressure (BP) 89/55 mm Hg, respiratory rate (RR) 15 breaths/min, temperature (T) 36.5°C (97.7°F), and arterial oxygen saturation (SaO$_2$) 98% on 6 L oxygen. Cardiovascular examination was notable for jugular venous distention with an estimated jugular venous pressure of 9 cm H$_2$O. The first and second heart sounds were noted to be normal and regular. There was a III/VI holosystolic murmur at the apex. The lungs were clear to auscultation bilaterally. Initial laboratory test results were notable for a blood urea nitrogen (BUN) of 65 mg/dL, creatinine of 1.5 mg/dL, white blood cell (WBC) count of 16,700/μL, hemoglobin (Hb) of 12.2 g/dL, and platelets of 413,000/μL. Cardiac biomarkers were elevated with a creatinine kinase of 821 U/L, a troponin T of 4.33 ng/mL, and a creatine kinase MB (CK-MB) of 12.0 ng/mL. An electrocardiogram (ECG) and chest x-ray were performed on admission (Figures 31-2 and 31-3).

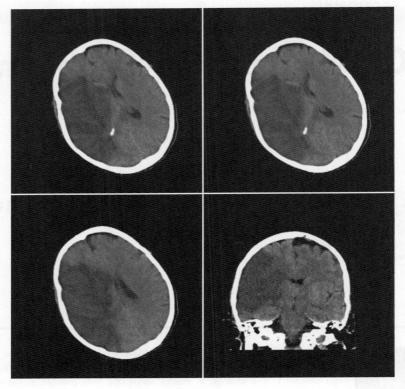

Figure 31-1. Computed axial tomography (CAT) scan of the brain.

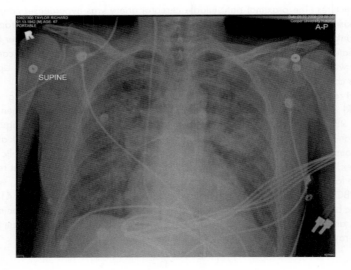

Figure 31-2. Chest x-ray.

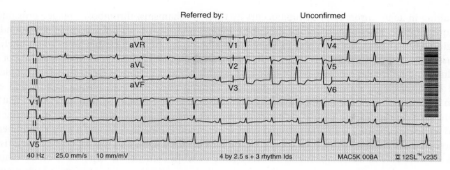

Figure 31-3. Twelve-lead electrocardiogram.

What should be the first step in managing this patient?

This patient presents with acute ischemic stroke and myocardial infarction. There is evidence of hemodynamic deterioration; therefore, a decision regarding management of acute coronary syndrome (ACS) must be made quickly. Management of acute ischemic stroke is discussed in Chapter 5.

How would you classify this patient's clinical presentation? How do you define acute coronary syndrome?

This patient presents with ECG and laboratory evidence of myocardial infarction. The initial ECG showed ST depressions anteriorly, which should alert the clinician to the possibility of posterior wall ST-segment elevation myocardial infarction. In this clinical scenario it would be appropriate to place "posterior" ECG leads, which can be accomplished by placing three electrodes—V_7, V_8, and V_9—in the left posterior axillary line at the fifth interspace, at the left midscapular line at the fifth interspace, and at the left paraspinal border at the fifth interspace, respectively. Significant ST elevation in leads V_7 through V_9 is defined as at least 0.5 mm in two or more of the leads, based on the increased distance between the posterior chest wall and the heart. Q waves wider than 0.04 second or deeper than one-quarter of the amplitude of the succeeding R wave are considered pathologic in leads V_7 through V_9.[1,2]

Acute coronary syndrome is a spectrum of clinical syndromes and includes unstable angina (UA), non–ST-segment-elevation myocardial infarction (NSTEMI), and ST-segment-elevation myocardial infarction (STEMI). Variant angina, also known as Prinzmetal angina, can manifest as ST-segment-elevation on the electrocardiogram and elevated serum troponin levels but is pathologically distinct from acute coronary syndrome. Although the pathogenesis and clinical presentation of UA and NSTEMI are similar, the presence of serum cardiac biomarkers, troponin I, or troponin T distinguishes NSTEMI from UA. In patients with NSTEMI, the degree of myocardial injury is severe enough to cause detectable serum levels of troponin I, troponin T, or CK-MB.

The Pathogenesis of ACS

It is well established that coronary atherosclerosis is by far the most common cause of acute myocardial ischemia, with thrombosis as the trigger for myocardial infarction. Less common causes of myocardial ischemia include coronary artery dissection, coronary arteritis, coronary artery vasospasm, emboli, and rarely myocardial bridging. Until recently, the majority of our understanding of the mechanisms of conversion from chronic to acute coronary artery disease had largely been limited to postmortem data. In 1912, Dr. James Herrick published an autopsy study that associated the clinical presentation of acute infarction with a thrombotic coronary occlusion.[3] Coronary artery occlusion resulting in acute coronary syndrome occurs by three mechanisms: thrombosis, plaque erosion, or plaque rupture. Plaque morphology described angiographically or via intravascular ultrasound or angioscopy has been instrumental in identifying atherosclerotic plaques that were more likely to cause acute coronary syndrome, the so-called vulnerable plaque. However, our understanding of the cellular and molecular mechanisms of how a vulnerable plaque develops is far from being complete.

Histopathologic and angioscopic studies have demonstrated that both plaque rupture and erosion leading to thrombosis are the most common causes of acute coronary syndrome. Plaques that are more likely to rupture are termed *vulnerable plaques* or *thin-cap fibroatheromas.* They are characterized as being eccentric, with a larger lipid core, fewer smooth muscle cells, and a greater number of macrophages.[4-6] Plaque with a lipid core often contains oxidized lipids and macrophage-derived tissue factor, which makes the plaque highly thrombogenic when its contents are exposed to blood. This in turn activates the clotting cascade, as well as platelet adhesion, activation, and aggregation.[7] It is thought that plaque rupture accounts for > 70% of fatal acute myocardial infarctions and/or sudden cardiac death. The smaller concentration of smooth muscle cells is thought to weaken the mechanical resistance of the plaque. Plaque rupture generally occurs where the plaque is thinnest and has the highest degree of inflammatory cells (ie, foam cells). In an eccentric plaque this typically occurs at the shoulder region, which is the junction between the plaque and the area of the vessel wall that is less diseased.[8]

Plaque erosion refers to a thin-cap fibroatheroma that literally develops a fissure or defect in the fibrous cap, thereby exposing the thrombogenic core to flowing blood.[9] Erosions occur over plaques that are rich in smooth muscle cells and proteoglycans. Luminal thrombi occur in denuded areas lacking surface endothelium. Unlike plaques prone to rupture, plaques prone to erosion typically lack a necrotic core of lipid but rather are composed of macrophages and lymphocytes. Lastly, calcified nodules are plaques with luminal thrombi showing calcified nodules protruding into the lumen through a disrupted thin fibrous cap. There is absence of endothelium at the site of the thrombus as well as lack of inflammatory cells (macrophages and T lymphocytes). There is little or no necrotic core and typically there is no obvious rupture of the lesion. However, there are superficial, dense, calcified nodules within the intima, which appear to be erupting through fibrous tissue into the lumen, possibly causing the thrombus.[10]

Numerous postmortem studies have identified ruptured plaque as the cause of thrombosis in acute myocardial infarction. Richardson et al studied 85 coronary thrombi postmortem and found a disrupted atheromatous plaque beneath 71 (84%) of the thrombi.[11] Studies comparing coronary angiograms before and after the onset of the acute coronary syndrome confirmed that the majority of culprit lesions demonstrate a luminal stenosis of < 70% on the initial angiogram. However, the lesions with a less severe degree of luminal stenosis (< 50%) on the initial angiogram were more likely to be the cause of acute coronary syndrome.[12-16] The composition and vulnerability of plaque rather than its volume or the consequent severity of stenosis produced have emerged as being the most important determinants of the development of the thrombus-mediated acute coronary syndromes.[8] In addition, both angiographic studies and intravascular ultrasound of plaque morphology in patients presenting with acute coronary syndrome have shown that multiple complex or ruptured plaques exist simultaneously. This implies a systemic process in the pathogenesis of plaque rupture.[17] The relationship between systemic markers of inflammation and the acute coronary syndromes is beyond the scope of this chapter.[18]

The clinical presentation and outcome depend on the location, severity, and duration of myocardial ischemia. Unstable angina and NSTEMI are typically caused by partial coronary artery obstruction by a thrombus, while STEMI is caused by complete coronary artery obstruction. The clinical presentation can, of course, be mediated by other factors such as vascular tone or the presence of collaterals.[19] It is noteworthy that many coronary arteries apparently occlude silently without causing myocardial infarction, probably because of a well-developed collateral circulation at the time of occlusion.[20] Morphological studies suggest that plaque progression beyond 40% to 50% cross-sectional luminal narrowing may occur secondary to repeated asymptomatic plaque ruptures, which may lead to healing with infiltration of smooth muscle cells.[7,18]

Are there triggers to plaque rupture that could explain this patient's simultaneous ischemic stroke and myocardial infarction?

Acute coronary syndrome is not likely to occur at random. The first study that looked at external triggers of ACS such as time of day, occupation of the patient, and physical effort was published by Masters in 1960. It was a retrospective review of 2600 patients. Although the study lacked formal statistical analysis, it concluded that there was no link between such external triggers and the onset of ACS.[21] In 2006, Strike et al performed a prospective observational study of 295 patients with electrocardiographic and biochemically verified ACS. Ten percent of patients reported physical exertion 1 hour before symptom onset, whereas 17.4% of patients reported anger in the 2 hours prior to symptom onset. Both types of triggers were more commonly associated with STEMI than with other forms of ACS.[22] The possible link between physical or emotional stress and acute coronary syndrome is not well understood. Physical exertion and mental stress may have similar effects on cardiovascular functioning in that both can trigger an increase in heart rate, blood pressure, coronary vasoconstriction, plasma catecholamine levels, and platelet activation.[23] During exercise or periods of stress, there is activation of the sympathetic nervous system with subsequent release of norepinephrine from myocardial sympathetic nerves in addition to circulating epinephrine and norepinephrine. Sympathetic stimulation leads to α_1-mediated vasoconstriction and β_2-mediated vasodilatation. The net physiologic response is dilation of the epicardial coronary arteries and microvessels.[24] Patients with impaired endothelial function and clinical risk factors for coronary artery disease exhibit an enhanced α-adrenergic vasoconstriction. When nitric oxide endothelium–dependent vasodilatation is impaired, vasoconstriction predominates, which in turn increases shear stress at the atherosclerotic plaque. A possible consequence is plaque rupture at the shoulder region.[25-27]

What are some examples of acute coronary syndrome with normal epicardial arteries?

What has been described above is the pathogenesis of acute coronary syndrome due to plaque disruption. However, coronary angiography may demonstrate normal coronary arteries in patients with chest pain, ECG abnormalities, and/or positive cardiac biomarkers. There are five major causes of ACS: thrombus, mechanical obstruction, dynamic obstruction, inflammation, and increased oxygen demand.[28] Takotsubo syndrome, also known as broken heart syndrome, is defined as transient reversible left ventricular (LV) apical ballooning of acute onset without coronary artery stenosis that clinically mimics acute coronary syndrome. It is associated with typical chest pain and ECG changes consistent with ischemia or infarction. Tsuchihashi et al performed a multicenter retrospective review of 88 patients (12 men and 76 women), aged 67 ± 13 years, who fulfilled the following criteria: (1) transient LV apical ballooning, (2) no significant angiographic stenosis, and (3) no known cardiomyopathies. Chest pain occurred in 67% of patients, and 56% of patients had a significant elevation in creatine kinase; of the 43 patients who had troponin T measured, 72% of them had a significant elevation. Electrocardiogram findings included ST elevation (90%), Q waves (27%), T-wave inversion (44%). Fifteen percent of patients developed cardiogenic shock. All patients had angiogram-confirmed nonobstructive epicardial coronary arteries (stenosis < 50%). During cardiac catheterization, only 10 patients were found to have coronary vasospasm. Based on chart review, the authors concluded that 20% of patients had a recent psychological stressor, 7% had an associated neurogenic condition, and 33% had a recent minor or major physiologic stress such as surgery.[29]

It has been proposed that stress-induced cardiomyopathy is a catecholamine-driven process. Wittstein et al performed a prospective study on 19 patients who presented with stress-induced cardiomyopathy. On hospital day 1 or 2, plasma levels of catecholamine among patients with stress cardiomyopathy were 2 to 3 times the values among patients with Killip class III myocardial infarction and 7 to 34 times the published normal values.[30]

Other causes of acute coronary syndrome with normal coronary arteries include coronary artery embolism (eg, in patients with atrial fibrillation or prosthetic heart valves)[31]; coronary artery spasm

Table 31-1. Nonatherosclerotic Causes of Acute Myocardial Infarction

1. Embolic
a. Infective endocarditis
b. Nonbacterial thrombotic endocarditis
c. Mural thrombi
d. Prosthetic valve
e. Debris from calcified valve after manipulation of the valve
f. Atrial fibrillation
2. Inflammatory
a. Viral infection
i. Coxsackie B
b. Syphilitic aortitis with narrowing of coronary ostia
c. Takayasu arteritis
d. Kawasaki disease
e. Giant cell arteritis
f. Therapeutic mediastinal radiation
3. Variant angina
4. Cocaine induced
5. Coronary artery dissection

(eg, in patients who abuse cocaine)[32]; and spontaneous coronary artery dissection (eg, in pregnant and postpartum women).[33] See Table 31-1.

Patients with coronary artery spasm (CAS), also known as variant or Prinzmetal angina, present with chest pain and concomitant ST-segment elevation. Prolonged vasospasm can result in frank myocardial infarction. It is commonly seen in young people who abuse cocaine. However, more recent reviews suggest that vagal withdrawal is most often the mechanism leading to spontaneous CAS. Other mechanisms responsible for CAS include increased sympathetic tone, abnormal nitric oxide synthase in dysfunctional endothelium, and enhanced phospholipase C enzyme activity inducing focal smooth muscle cell sensitivity.[34-36] Established therapies include calcium channel blockers, long-acting nitrates, and in rare intractable cases internal mammary artery grafting. CAS may be associated with life-threatening ventricular arrhythmias, which may be an indication for implantation of an automated defibrillator.[37]

This patient denied chest pain before or during his presentation. Is this typical in patients presenting with ACS? Does lack of chest pain in this patient's clinical presentation have clinical significance?

Acute coronary syndrome can present in varying ways. High-risk or probable high-risk chest pain is described as prolonged, lasting for more than 30 minutes, a pressure-like sensation, or chest heaviness with radiation to 1 or both shoulders or arms. It often occurs on exertion and is associated with nausea, vomiting, or diaphoresis.[38] However, a considerable proportion of patients who present with ACS do not have chest pain. The National Registry of Myocardial Infarction (NRMI) is a database to which 1674 US hospitals contribute data. Among patients with confirmed MI who were enrolled in the NRMI between 1994 and 1998, 33% (n = 142,445) had chest pain at the time of presentation to the hospital. Older patients, women, and diabetic patients were more likely to lack chest pain. Only 23% of patients without chest pain had ST elevation on the initial ECG.[39] Patients without chest pain but with myocardial infarction were less aggressively treated and had a 23.3% in-hospital mortality rate compared with 9.3% among patients with chest pain.[39] Other atypical symptoms such as dyspnea, nausea and vomiting, and syncope can be associated with ACS.

Describe the ECG changes seen on the patient's initial ECG. How does one differentiate an injury pattern from an infarct pattern on a 12-lead ECG? What are the ECG criteria for STEMI?

This patient has ST-segment depressions in V_1 through V_5. All patients with chest discomfort, anginal equivalent, or other symptoms consistent with ACS should have a 12-lead ECG within 10 minutes of arrival to the emergency department. An experienced physician should interpret the ECG immediately. Either serial ECGs at 5- to 10-minute intervals or continuous ST-segment monitoring should be performed in a patient with a nondiagnostic initial ECG if the patient remains symptomatic and there is high clinical suspicion for ACS. In patients with inferior STEMI, right-sided ECG leads should be obtained to screen for ST elevation suggestive of right ventricular infarction.[40] See Table 31-2.

Normally the ST segment on the ECG is at approximately the same baseline level as the PR segment or the TP segment. If coronary artery blood flow is sufficient to satisfy metabolic demands, then there is minimal alteration, if any, of the ST segment on the surface ECG. If there is partial obstruction of a coronary artery that prevents blood flow from increasing enough to meet the increased metabolic demand, the resulting ischemia is manifested by horizontal or downsloping ST-segment depression. This is typically called subendocardial ischemia. Often the ST segments return to normal once the metabolic demand has ceased. Hyperacute T waves might be the first manifestation of myocardial injury due to complete arterial occlusion. If the arterial occlusion persists without reperfusion, a myocardial infarction occurs and is represented as ST-segment deviation on the surface ECG.

This patient's electrocardiogram is consistent with posterior wall infarction. An ECG utilizing leads V_7, V_8, and V_9, which are placed on the posterior torso, would likely show ST-segment elevation. The standard 12-lead electrocardiogram is a relatively insensitive tool for detecting posterior infarction because these leads do not face the posterior wall of the left ventricle. Using leads V_7, V_8, and V_9, ECG criteria for ST elevation of the posterior wall is defined as an elevation of at least 0.5 mV in two or more of the leads. This lower voltage can be explained by the increased distance between the posterior chest wall and the heart.[2,41] Currently, the indications for thrombolytic therapy or percutaneous coronary intervention require identification of ST elevation on the standard 12-lead electrocardiogram. However, ST elevation may not be seen in up to 50% of patients with an MI because of occlusion of the left circumflex coronary artery.[4,42,43] Suspicion of left circumflex–related infarction should

Table 31-2. ECG Manifestations of Acute Myocardial Ischemia in the Absence of LVH or LBBB

ST elevation

New ST elevation at the J point in 2 contiguous leads[a] with the following cutoff points: ≥ 0.2 mV in men or ≥ 0.15 mV in women in leads V_2-V_3 and/or ≥ 0.1 mV in other leads

ST depression and T-wave changes

New horizontal or downsloping ST depression ≥ 0.05 mV in 2 contiguous leads[a] and/or T inversion ≥ 0.1 mV in 2 contiguous leads with prominent R wave or R/S ratio ≥ 1

Abbreviations: LBBB, left bundle branch block; LVH, left ventricular hypertrophy.

[a]Contiguous leads refer to lead groups such as anterior leads (V_1-V_6), inferior leads (II, III, and aVF), or lateral leads (I and aVL).

(Adapted from Thygesen K, Alpert JS, White HD, et al. Universal definition of myocardial infarction on behalf of the joint ESC/ACCF/AHA/WHF Task Force for the Redefinition of Myocardial Infarction. J Am Coll Cardiol. 2007;50:2173-2219.)

Cardiovascular Problems

occur if the standard 12-lead ECG shows an abnormal R wave in lead V_1, which may be defined as ≥ 0.04 seconds in duration and/or an R-to-S wave ratio of ≥ 1 in lead V_1 in the absence of preexcitation or right ventricular hypertrophy. In addition, the presence of anterior ischemia with ST-segment depression in leads V_1 and V_2 may suggest reciprocal electrical phenomena in the presence of a posterior infarction. Posterior wall infarction rarely occurs in isolation but rather is almost always associated with inferior or posterior lateral infarction. The term *posterior* to reflect the basal part of the LV wall that lies on the diaphragm is no longer recommended. It is preferable to refer to this territory as inferobasal.[44] In patients with ECG evidence of inferior wall MI, right-sided precordial leads should be recorded to detect ST-segment elevation in leads V_3R or V_4R, signs of right ventricular infarction.[45]

The location of the infarcted area can usually be determined by the standard 12-lead electrocardiogram and includes the left anterior descending artery (LAD), left circumflex artery (LCX), and right coronary artery (RCA). The LAD and its branches usually supply the anterior and anterolateral walls of the left ventricle and the anterior two-thirds of the septum. The LCX and its branches usually supply the posterolateral wall of the left ventricle. The RCA supplies the right ventricle, the inferior and true posterior walls of the left ventricle, and the posterior third of the septum. The usual ECG evolution of an STEMI is variable depending on the size of the MI, how quickly reperfusion is restored, and the location of the MI. See Table 31-3.

The first finding of ischemia on a 12-lead electrocardiogram can be hyperacute T waves, which appear as tall-amplitude primary T-wave abnormalities. These typically occur in the first 15 minutes of a transmural MI and therefore are rarely recorded. If transmural ischemia persists for more than a few minutes, the peaked T waves evolve into ST-segment elevation. The ST-segment elevation of myocardial infarction is usually upward convex. As acute infarction continues to evolve, the ST-segment elevation decreases and the T waves begin to invert. The T wave usually becomes progressively deeper as the ST-segment elevation subsides. Pathologic Q waves develop within the first few hours to days after an infarction. They are defined as having a duration ≥ 0.04 seconds or $> 25\%$ of the R-wave amplitude. However, ST-segment elevation that persists beyond 4 weeks is usually associated with the presence of a ventricular aneurysm.[46] See Table 31-3.

Table 31-3. Occluded Coronary Artery and Its Relationship to Anatomic Location and ECG Findings

Category	Anatomic location	ECG finding
Proximal LAD	Anteroseptal and anterior: proximal to first septal perforator	ST ⇑ V_1-V_6, I, aVL, and fascicular or bundle branch block
Mid-LAD	Anterior: distal to first septal perforator but likely proximal to large diagonal	V_1-V_6, aVL
Distal LAD	Anterolateral and apex: distal to first large diagonal branch	ST ⇑ V_1-V_4 or ST ⇑ I, aVL, V_5-V_6
Proximal RCA	Large inferior	ST ⇑ II, III, aVF
Left circumflex	Posterior	R/S ratio > 1 in V_1-V_2 with or without ST ⇓ in V_1-V_2
	Lateral	ST ⇑ V_5-V_6, I, aVL
	Right ventricular	ST ⇑ in V_1 or V_3R or V_4R
Distal RCA or LCX	Small inferior	ST ⇑ II, III, aVF only

Abbreviations: LAD, left anterior descending artery; LCX, left descending circumflex artery; RCA, right coronary artery. (Adapted from Topol EJ, Van De Werf F. Acute myocardial infarction: early diagnosis and management. In: Topol EJ, Califf RM, Prystowsky EN, et al, eds. Textbook of Cardiovascular Medicine. 3rd ed. Philadelphia, PA: Lippincott Williams & Wilkins; 2007:283-284; and Sgarbossa EB, Birnbaum Y, Parrillo JE. Electrocardiographic diagnosis of acute myocardial infarction: current concepts for the clinician. Am Heart J. 2001;141:507-517.)

Describe causes of ST elevation on a 12-lead ECG that are not associated with acute myocardial infarction

Typically the degree of ST elevation is determined by comparing it to the end of the PR segment. In certain populations, ST-segment elevation can be a normal finding or a normal variant. Early repolarization is an ECG finding that frequently occurs in young men and is described as an elevated takeoff of the ST segment at the junction between the QRS and ST segment (J point). It most commonly involves V_2 through V_5 but can be seen in II, III, and aVF. The ST segment is usually concave.[47,48]

Other causes of ST elevation not associated with acute myocardial infarction include left bundle branch block, left ventricular hypertrophy, acute pericarditis or myocarditis, Brugada syndrome, hyperkalemia, and arrhythmogenic right ventricular cardiomyopathy (Figure 31-4).

A 2-D echocardiogram was performed and revealed a severe abnormality of segmental wall motion and moderate to severe mitral regurgitation. Is echocardiography a useful tool in the diagnosis of acute coronary syndrome? What are the indications for echocardiography in ACS?

In the acute setting it is appropriate to consider 2-D echocardiography for the following indications: evaluation of acute chest pain with suspected myocardial ischemia in patients with nondiagnostic laboratory

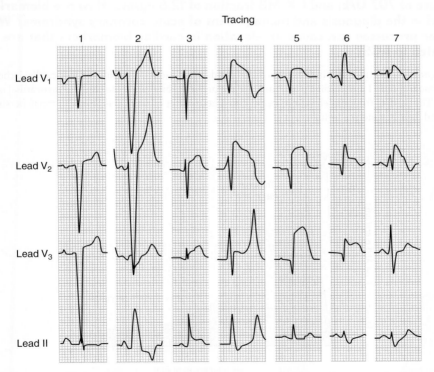

Figure 31-4. ST-segment elevation in various conditions. *Tracing 1*, left ventricular hypertrophy. *Tracing 2*, left bundle branch block. *Tracing 3*, acute pericarditis; note the PR depression in lead II. *Tracing 4*, hyperkalemia. *Tracing 5*, acute anteroseptal infarct. *Tracing 6*, acute anteroseptal infarction with right bundle branch block. *Tracing 7*, Brugada syndrome. *(Reprinted with permission from Wang K, Asinger RW, Marriot HJ. ST-segment elevation in conditions other than acute myocardial infarction. N Engl J Med. 2003;349:2128-2135.)*

markers and ECG and in whom a resting echocardiogram can be performed during pain; and evaluation of suspected complications of myocardial ischemia or infarction, including but not limited to acute mitral regurgitation, hypoxemia, abnormal chest x-ray, ventricular septal rupture, free wall rupture, cardiac tamponade, shock, right ventricular involvement, heart failure, or thrombus.[49] A 2-D echocardiogram alone should not be used to diagnose an acute coronary syndrome. However, there are several echocardiographic findings that may support the diagnosis of an acute coronary syndrome. In the setting of acute ongoing ischemia the echocardiogram may demonstrate hypokinesis of the affected wall, referred to as a segmental wall motion abnormality. Often the contralateral wall will appear hyperkinetic. However, if a segment is akinetic, dyskinetic, or severely hypokinetic, a single echocardiogram cannot differentiate ischemia with myocardial stunning from irreversible damage due to myocardial necrosis.

A transesophageal echo may be helpful in differentiating acute myocardial infarction from aortic dissection. Mitral regurgitation commonly occurs in the setting of acute myocardial infarction. Color Doppler echocardiography was performed within 48 hours of admission in a series of 417 consecutive patients with acute MI.[50] Mild mitral regurgitation was present in 29% of patients, moderate mitral regurgitation in 5%, and severe mitral regurgitation in 1%. Echocardiography performed in a cohort of 773 patients 30 days after an acute MI revealed that 50% of patients had mitral regurgitation.[51] Among 30-day survivors of an MI, during a mean follow-up period of 4.7 years, moderate to severe mitral regurgitation detected by echocardiography within 30 days of MI was associated with a 55% increase in the relative risk of death independent of age, gender, left ventricular ejection fraction, and Killip class.[51]

Initial labs on this patient revealed a troponin I of 11.6 ng/mL, creatinine kinase of 707 U/L, and CK-MB fraction of 12.6 ng/mL. How are biomarkers used in the diagnosis and management of acute coronary syndrome? What other processes can cause an elevation in cardiac biomarkers that are not related to ACS?

Myocardial infarction is defined as myocardial cell death as a result of prolonged myocardial ischemia. Cardiac troponin I and cardiac troponin T are the preferred biomarkers to confirm myocardial ischemia. The cardiac troponin elevations begin 2 to 4 hours after onset of symptoms and may persist for several days beyond the initial event (Figure 31-5).

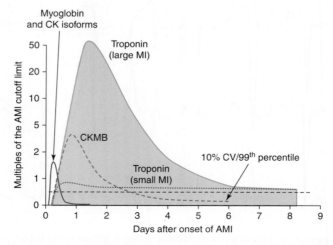

Figure 31-5. Timing of serum cardiac biomarkers in acute coronary syndrome (ACS). AMI, acute myocardial infarction; CK, creatine kinase; CV, coefficient of variation. (*Reprinted with permission from Jaffe AS, Babuin L, Apple FS. Biomarkers in acute cardiac disease: the present and the future. J Am Coll Cardiol. 2006;48(1):1-11.*)

Cardiac troponin offers little incremental value in classic STEMI. A more extensively studied group in which troponin is very common are high-risk patients with ACS (NSTEMI or UA). Cardiac troponin T and cardiac troponin I are sensitive[52,53] markers of cardiac injury, particularly when used with the recommended[54] diagnostic cutoff point of the 99th percentile of healthy controls.[55,56] An elevation in serum cardiac troponin in this group helps direct the use of antithrombotic and antiplatelet therapy (both will be discussed later).

Frequently, patients with end-stage renal disease will have chronically elevated levels of troponin, making it difficult to determine its utility in acute coronary syndrome. Keeping in mind that the most common cause of death among patients with end-stage renal disease is cardiovascular, these patients should be regarded as high risk. Therefore, despite the difficulty in determining chronic versus acute troponin levels, patients with end-stage renal disease will likely benefit from a more aggressive anti-thrombotic and interventional approach.[57,58] Creatine kinase, CK-MB fraction, and myoglobin have largely fallen out of favor as biomarkers to diagnose myocardial infarction.

An elevated cardiac troponin level in the absence of overt ischemic heart disease is a common finding in both acute and nonacute processes. When serum cardiac troponin is present but the clinical information does not suggest ACS, the clinician should look for other causes. See Table 31-4.

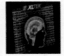

A 70-year-old woman is recovering in the neurology intensive care unit (ICU) after presenting with hypertensive emergency and thalamic hemorrhagic stroke 14 days earlier. She also has dyslipidemia, type 2 diabetes mellitus, and peripheral vascular disease and experienced a non–ST-segment-elevation inferior myocardial infarction 16 days ago for which she had a drug-eluting stent placed. While moving from the bed to the chair, she becomes diaphoretic and complains of chest pain. A 12-lead ECG is shown in Figure 31-6.

What does this ECG show and what are the initials steps in managing this patient?

It is not uncommon for patients who are critically ill in the ICU to have concomitant ACS. Continuous ECG monitoring is a key component to early detection and treatment of ACS in the critical care unit. This patient's ECG shows ST elevation in the inferior leads. Given that she recently had a drug-eluting stent placed for inferior wall MI, the clinician should immediately be concerned about subacute stent thrombosis. Since this patient presented with a hemorrhagic thalamic stroke, it is likely that antiplatelet agents such as aspirin and clopidogrel were appropriately held at admission. ST can occur acutely (within 24 hours), subacutely (within 30 days), late (within 1 year), or very late (beyond 1 year). According to the American College of Cardiology (ACC)/American Heart Association (AHA) 2007 Guidelines on Management of Patients with UA/NSTEMI, patients treated with bare-metal stents should remain on aspirin 162 to 325 mg/d and clopidogrel 75 mg/d for a minimum of 1 month and ideally for up to 1 year (class I recommendation).[59] For patients with UA/NSTEMI who are treated with a drug-eluting stent, aspirin 162 to 325 mg/d should be prescribed for at least 3 months after sirolimus-eluting stent implantation and for at least 6 months after paclitaxel-eluting stent implantation. Subsequently, aspirin should be continued indefinitely at a dose of 75 to 162 mg/d (class I recommendation). Clopidogrel 75 mg daily should be given for at least 12 months to all patients receiving drug-eluting stents after percutaneous coronary intervention (PCI) (class I recommendation).[58] This patient should be treated with aspirin, clopidogrel, and the appropriate anticoagulant when the neurologist deems it to be safe.

The frequency of stent thrombosis is greatest within 30 days after stent placement. The Dutch Stent Thrombosis Registry enrolled 1009 patients who received either a bare-metal or drug-eluting stent. Among 437 patients (2.1%) who presented with a definite stent thrombosis, 140 stent thromboses were acute, 180 were subacute, 58 were late, and 59 were very late. Along with several technical aspects of stent deployment, lack of aspirin, bifurcation lesions, ejection fraction < 30%, and younger age were associated

Cardiovascular Problems

Table 31-4. Non-ACS Causes of Elevated Troponin

Acute Disease	Chronic Disease
Cardiac or vascular	Infiltrative cardiac disease
1. Aortic dissection	1. Amyloidosis
2. Endocarditis	2. Sarcoidosis
3. Myocarditis	3. Hemochromatosis
4. Pericarditis	4. Scleroderma
5. Apical ballooning syndrome (takotsubo)	Hypertension
6. Acute decompensated heart failure	Hypothyroidism
7. Coronary vasospasm	Chronic renal insufficiency
8. Hypertrophic cardiomyopathy	
9. Tachyarrhythmia	
Neurologic	
1. Ischemic stroke	
2. Intracerebral hemorrhage	
3. Subarachnoid hemorrhage	
Respiratory	
1. Acute pulmonary embolism	
2. ARDS	
Infectious	
1. Sepsis	
Trauma	
1. Cardiac contusion	
2. Post-CABG	
3. Post-CPR	
4. Defibrillator discharge	
5. Burns	

Abbreviations: ARDS, acute respiratory distress syndrome; CABG, coronary artery bypass grafting; CPR, cardiopulmonary resuscitation. (Adapted from Kelley WE, Januzzi JL, Christenson RH. Increases of cardiac troponin in conditions other than acute coronary syndrome and heart failure. Clin Chem. 2009;55(12):2098-2112; and Jaffe AS, Babuin L, Apple FS. Biomarkers in acute cardiac disease: the present and the future. JACC. 2006;48(1):1-11.)

with stent thrombosis. The lack of clopidogrel therapy at the time of stent placement in the first 30 days after the index PCI was strongly associated with stent thrombosis (hazard ratio: 36.5; 95% confidence interval [CI]: 8.0-167.8).[60] In a substudy of the ACUITY trial published in 2009, the incidence of angiographically confirmed subacute stent thrombosis in 3405 moderate- and high-risk patients with acute coronary syndromes receiving stents (89.4% drug-eluting stents) was 1.4%.[61] Patients with acute and subacute stent thrombosis often present with STEMI. Immediate PCI is the treatment of choice if available. However, fibrinolytic therapy is also an option. Unfortunately, patients who have STEMI due to stent thrombosis have worse outcomes when compared with patients with STEMI due to de novo plaque rupture. One retrospective study showed that the successful reperfusion rate was lower in patients with stent thrombosis and the distal embolization rate was higher in patients with stent thrombosis when compared with patients with de novo plaque rupture.[62] In one real-world-experience study of

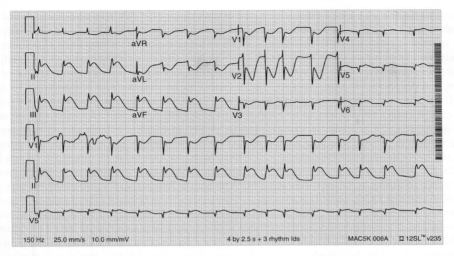

Figure 31-6. Twelve-lead electrocardiogram.

23,500 patients treated with drug-eluting stent, definite stent thrombosis developed in 301 (1.3%) and the mortality at 1-year follow-up was 16%.[63]

Which other medications are indicated in ACS, including UA/NSTEMI/STEMI and ACS due to stent thrombosis?

Oxygen

The body of literature regarding the use of supplemental oxygen in uncomplicated acute MI is small. In one small randomized controlled study in which 200 patients received either supplemental oxygen or compressed air, the mortality rate was higher in the oxygen group than in the control group (9/80 versus 3/77; PS = NS).[64] According to the ACC/AHA guidelines, the only class I indication for supplemental oxygen is if the patient's arterial saturation is < 90%. It is a class IIa indication to administer supplemental oxygen in the first 6 hours of an uncomplicated STEMI.[40]

Analgesics

Morphine sulfate (2-4 mg intravenously [IV] with increments of 2-8 mg IV repeated at 5- to 15-minute intervals) is the analgesic of choice for management of pain associated with ACS and is considered a class I indication according to the most recent ACC/AHA guidelines.[40] To date, there are no published randomized controlled trials that evaluate the use of morphine therapy in patients with acute MI. However, as a means of decreasing sympathetic tone during pain, morphine may be a useful agent in reducing the heart's metabolic demand. The CRUSADE Initiative, a nonrandomized, retrospective, observational registry, evaluated various therapies in over 17,000 patients presenting with non-STEMI. It showed that 29.8% of patients received morphine within 24 hours of presentation. Patients treated with any morphine had a higher adjusted risk of death (odds ratio [OR]: 1.48; 95% CI: 1.33-1.64) than patients not treated with morphine.[65]

Nitrates

Both intravenous and sublingual nitroglycerin are often used in the management of ACS.

According to the most recent ACC/AHA guidelines, there are two class I indications for the use of nitrates in an STEMI: (1) patients with ongoing ischemic discomfort should receive sublingual nitroglycerin, 0.4 mg every 5 minutes for a total of three doses, after which an assessment should be made about the need for intravenous nitroglycerin; and (2) intravenous nitroglycerin is indicated for relief of ongoing ischemic discomfort, control of hypertension, or management of pulmonary congestion.[40] Nitroglycerin has many beneficial physiologic effects, including vasodilation of peripheral arteries and veins and a reduction in pulmonary capillary wedge pressure, mean arterial pressure, and peripheral vascular resistance. The ultimate outcome is a decrease in myocardial oxygen demand. However, nitroglycerin should be used with caution in certain patients. Nitrates and other drugs that reduce preload should be avoided in patients with right ventricular infarction because adequate preload is necessary to maintain cardiac output. In addition, nitrates can produce severe hypotension in patients who have taken a phosphodiesterase inhibitor recently.[66] Generally, nitrates should not be administered to patients with systolic blood pressure below 90 mm Hg or 30 mm Hg below the baseline or if there is marked bradycardia or tachycardia.[67] Nitrates have not been shown to reduce mortality in patients with acute MI. The Fourth International Study of Infarct Survival (ISIS-4) enrolled 58,050 patients with suspected acute MI within 24 hours of presentation. Patients were randomized in a 2 × 2 × 2 fashion to an angiotensin-converting enzyme (ACE) inhibitor, magnesium, and 30 mg of oral mononitrate titrated to 60 mg daily or placebo for 28 days. Oral nitrates failed to produce a mortality benefit at 5 weeks or 1 year.[68] Similar findings were noted in the Gruppo Italiano per lo Studio della Sopravvivenza nell' infarto Miocardico-3 (GISSI-3) trial, which enrolled 19,394 patients with acute MI and randomized them to 6 weeks of nitrates, an ACE inhibitor, both, or neither. Nitrates were administered as IV glyceryl trinitrate for the first 24 hours, followed by transdermal or oral isosorbide mononitrate for 6 weeks. Nitroglycerin did not reduce the 6-week rates of death or clinical heart failure after MI.[69]

Aspirin

The efficacy of aspirin in patients with ACS is well established. Several different doses of aspirin have been shown to reduce mortality rate and vascular events in patients with ACS. The ISIS-2 trial demonstrated a 23% reduction in 5-week vascular mortality rate among patients with acute MI who were treated with aspirin 160 mg daily.[70] The absolute mortality reduction was 2.4 vascular deaths prevented per 100 patients treated. The Veterans Administration Cooperative Study demonstrated a 51% reduction in the principal end points of death and acute myocardial infarction at 12 weeks among patients with UA/NSTEMI who were randomized to 325 mg of aspirin daily.[71] A review of 4000 patients with unstable angina who were enrolled in randomized trials of aspirin versus placebo demonstrated a 5% absolute risk reduction in nonfatal stroke or MI or vascular death (9% versus 14%). This corresponds to 50 vascular events avoided per 1000 patients treated with aspirin for 6 months.[72] A recent trial randomized 25,087 patients with ACS (29.2% STEMI and 70.8% unstable angina or NSTEMI) to either low-dose aspirin (75-100 mg/d) or high-dose aspirin (100-325 mg/d). There was no significant difference between the two groups in either efficacy or bleeding. The current ACC/AHA practice guidelines recommend an initial aspirin dose of 162 to 325 mg followed by a maintenance dose of 75 to 162 mg daily.[40,59]

Would the use of β blockers be contraindicated in this patient?

Experimental data suggest that β blockers have several immediate beneficial physiologic effects during acute MI. The reduction in heart rate, systemic arterial pressure, and myocardial contractility may diminish myocardial oxygen demand in the first few hours of onset of acute MI. The benefit of β blocker therapy, either early or delayed, in ACS has been well described. A pooled analysis of 27 randomized trials indicated that early β blockade reduced mortality rate by 13% in the first week, with the greatest reduction in mortality rate occurring in the first 2 days.[73] The Thrombolysis in Myocardial Infarction (TIMI)-IIB study randomized 1434 patients who received tissue plasminogen activator (tPA) for acute STEMI to either immediate or deferred β blockade. Patients randomized to immediate therapy received three doses of 5 mg IV metoprolol, followed by 50 mg twice a day on day 1, then 100 mg twice a day. Patients randomized to deferred therapy received oral metoprolol 50 mg twice a day on day 6 followed by 100 mg twice a day thereafter. Overall, there was no difference in mortality rate between the immediate intravenous and deferred groups. However, there was a lower incidence of reinfarction (2.7% versus 5.1%; $P = .02$) and recurrent chest pain (18.8% versus 24.1%; $P < .02$) at 6 days in the immediate intravenous group.[74] A post-hoc analysis of the use of atenolol in the Global Utilization of Streptokinase and TPA for Occluded Arteries-1 (GUSTO-1) trial reported that adjusted 30-day mortality rate was significantly lower in atenolol-treated patients, but patients treated with intravenous and oral atenolol treatment versus oral treatment alone were more likely to die (OR: 1.3; 95% CI: 1.0-1.5; $P = .02$).[75]

The Clopidogrel and Metoprolol in Myocardial Infarction Trial-2 (COMMIT-CCS 2) of 45,852 patients with acute MI showed an increased risk of developing heart failure and cardiogenic shock in patients randomized to β-blocker therapy.[76] Patients were randomized to treatment with metoprolol (three intravenous injections of 5 mg each followed by 200 mg/d orally for up to 4 weeks) or placebo. Ninety-three percent of patients had STEMI and approximately 54% of patients received a fibrinolytic agent. There was no difference in the primary end point of death, reinfarction, or cardiac arrest by treatment group (9.4% for metoprolol versus 9.9% for placebo; $P = NS$). There was also no difference in the coprimary end point of all-cause mortality rate by hospital discharge (7.7% versus 7.8%; $P = NS$). Reinfarction was lower in the metoprolol group (2.0% versus 2.5%; $P = .001$). Death due to shock occurred more frequently in the metoprolol group (2.2%, n = 496, versus 1.7%, n = 384), while death due to arrhythmia occurred less frequently in the metoprolol group (1.7%, n = 388, versus 2.2%, n = 498). Cardiogenic shock was higher overall in the metoprolol group (5.0%, n = 1141, versus 3.9%, n = 885; $P < .0001$).[76]

Although acute oral β-blocker use in patients with STEMI undergoing fibrinolytic therapy or primary PCI is still a class I indication, the 2007 ACC/AHA Focused Update of the STEMI Guidelines downgraded it from the level of evidence A to the level of evidence B. Additionally, IV β blockers are no longer recommended in the absence of systemic hypertension.[77] The following relative contraindications should be considered before initiating β-blockers: heart rate < 60 bpm, systolic arterial pressure < 100 mm Hg, moderate or severe LV failure, signs of peripheral hypoperfusion, shock, PR interval > 0.24 second, second- or third-degree atrioventricular (AV) block, active asthma, and reactive airway disease.[77] β Blockers should not be administered to patients with cocaine-associated STEMI, because β blockade might exacerbate coronary artery vasospasm. β Blockers are contraindicated in patients with STEMI complicated by cardiogenic shock or severe left ventricular dysfunction.

In contrast to the use of early, aggressive β-blocker therapy, the long-term use of β blockers after occurrence of MI has favorable outcomes on mortality. The Carvedilol Post-infarct Survival Controlled Evaluation (CAPRICORN) trial was a randomized, placebo-controlled trial designed to test the long-term efficacy of carvedilol on morbidity and mortality in patients with LV dysfunction 3 to 21 days after MI who were already treated with ACE inhibitors. After an average follow-up period of 1.3 years, cardiovascular mortality was lower in the carvedilol arm (11% versus 14% for placebo; hazard ratio: 0.75; $P = .024$), as was all-cause mortality or nonfatal MI (14% versus 20%; hazard ratio: 0.71; $P = .002$).[78] This study supports the claim that β-blocker therapy after acute MI reduces mortality irrespective of reperfusion therapy or ACE inhibitor use.

Do calcium channel antagonists reduce mortality rate in patients with acute MI?

Calcium channel antagonists vary in the degree to which they produce vasodilation, decreased myocardial contractility, AV block, and sinus node slowing. Nifedipine and amlodipine have a greater effect on peripheral vasodilation, whereas verapamil and diltiazem have a greater effect on AV node and sinus node inhibition. Currently, there is no class I indication for the use of calcium channel antagonists in acute MI because there has been no proven mortality benefit demonstrated in individual clinical trials or pooled analyses.[79,80] There are two class III recommendations for the use of calcium channel antagonists in acute MI: (1) diltiazem and verapamil are contraindicated in patients with STEMI and associated systolic left ventricular dysfunction and congestive heart failure (CHF); and (2) nifedipine (immediate-release form) is contraindicated in the treatment of STEMI because of the reflex sympathetic activation, tachycardia, and hypotension associated with its use.[40]

This patient presented with ST elevation on her ECG. What options are available for reperfusion therapy for STEMI and when should it be performed? What are the contraindications to reperfusion therapy?

All patients with STEMI who present within 12 hours of symptom onset should be considered for reperfusion therapy with either fibrinolytics or PCI, with or without stent deployment. Early, complete, and sustained reperfusion after myocardial infarction is known to decrease 30-day mortality.

The preferred method for reperfusion in STEMI is PCI if it can be done in a timely manner. Early recognition and diagnosis of STEMI are key to achieving the desired door-to-needle (or medical contact–to-needle) time for initiation of fibrinolytic therapy of 30 minutes or door-to-balloon (or medical contact–to-balloon) time for PCI of < 90 minutes.[81] In patients receiving fibrinolysis, careful surveillance over the first 1 to 3 hours is critical to ensure that successful reperfusion occurs, as indicated by relief of symptoms and/or any hemodynamic or electrical instability, coupled with at least 50% resolution of the initial ST elevation. Achieving reperfusion in a timely manner correlates with improvement in ultimate infarct size, left ventricular function, and survival.[82-84] The ultimate goals are to restore adequate blood flow through the infarct-related artery to the infarct zone and to limit microvascular damage and reperfusion injury. The latter is accomplished with adjunctive and ancillary treatments, which will be discussed later.

What are the commonly used fibrinolytics?

Currently used fibrinolytic drugs are intravenously infused plasminogen activators that activate the blood fibrinolytic system. There are several well-known fibrinolytics with established efficacy for reducing short- and long-term mortality rate in patients with STEMI. The first large-scale trial to test thrombolytics was GISSI-1. In this trial, 11,712 patients were randomized to streptokinase or no treatment within 12 hours of presenting with acute MI. There was an 18% relative reduction in 21-day mortality rate for patients receiving streptokinase compared to placebo (10.7% versus 13%; $P = .0002$). The mortality benefit was greatest in the first hour. There was no difference in mortality when patients were treated beyond 6 hours.[85] Alteplase, recombinant tPA, is fibrin-specific. Fibrin-bound tPA has increased affinity for plasminogen, whereas unbound tPA in the systemic circulation does not extensively activate plasminogen.[86] GISSI-2 and ISIS-3 failed to demonstrate increased efficacy of alteplase over streptokinase.[87,88] The GUSTO-1 trial compared the effects of accelerated tPA with streptokinase on mortality in patients with acute MI. Forty-one thousand patients with acute MI who presented to more than 1000 hospitals within 6 hours of symptom onset were randomized to streptokinase plus either subcutaneous or intravenous heparin; accelerated alteplase with intravenous heparin; or a combination of streptokinase and alteplase.[89] There was a 14% reduction in mortality rate for accelerated tPA compared to the two streptokinase regimens ($P = .001$). The combined end point of death or disabling stroke was significantly lower in the accelerated tPA group (6.9%) than in the streptokinase groups (7.8%; $P = .006$).[89] The rate of stroke was 1.4%, which included intracerebral hemorrhage in 0.7%.[90]

A third agent, reteplase, is less fibrin-selective and has a longer half-life than alteplase. The GUSTO-3 trial enrolled 15,059 patients with acute MI and randomized them to either reteplase or alteplase. The average time from symptom onset to treatment with either drug was 2.7 hours. There was no significant difference between the two drugs in mortality rate, the incidence of stroke, or the combined end point of death or nonfatal, disabling stroke.[91] A follow-up study revealed that there was no difference in mortality rate at 1 year (11.2% versus 11.1%).[92]

Tenecteplase (TNK-tPA) is a genetically engineered fibrinolytic agent that has a longer plasma half-life and is 14 times more specific for fibrin. The ASSENT-2 trial directly compared tenecteplase with alteplase in 16,949 patients. At 30 days, there was no difference in mortality rate, the overall stroke rate, or the rate of intracerebral hemorrhage. The mortality rate at 1 year remained the same with the two agents (10.2%). The incidences of stroke were similar in the two treatment groups, with 1.78% occurring in the TNK-tPA group and 1.66% in the tPA group ($P = .55$).[93]

It is well established that patients who receive fibrinolytics within 1 hour of symptom onset, the so-called golden hour, derive the greatest mortality benefit.[94] All of the trials suggest that treatment beyond 12 hours confers no mortality benefit. Two large-scale randomized multicenter trials, LATE and Estuido Multicentrico Estrepoquinasa Republicass de Americas del Sur (EMARAS), evaluated the value of late thrombolysis, given 6 to 24 hours after the onset of symptoms.[95,96] In both studies, thrombolytics given at 12 to 24 hours showed no mortality benefit. The Fibrinolytic Therapy Trialist's Collaborative Group performed a meta-analysis of all randomized thrombolytic trials for suspected acute myocardial infarction enrolling 1000 or more patients. There was an 18% relative reduction in mortality rate to 35 days in the fibrinolytic-treated patients compared with controls (9.6% versus 11.5%; $P < .00001$) (Figure 31-7). Significant treatment benefit was seen up to 12 hours, but not in patients presenting more than 12 hours after symptom onset. Mortality rate reduction with thrombolytic therapy was demonstrated in all age groups except those aged 75 years or older. Fibrinolytic therapy was associated with a small but significant increase in strokes (1.2% versus 0.8%; $P < .00001$).[97] See Table 31-5.

Absolute and relative contraindications should be considered prior to initiating fibrinolytic therapy (Table 31-6). Intracranial hemorrhage is the major risk factor associated with fibrinolytic therapy. In GUSTO-1, the largest fibrinolytic study, there was a 1.8% risk of severe bleeding, defined as bleeding that caused hemodynamic compromise that required treatment. Also, 11.4% of patients suffered moderate bleeding, defined as bleeding that required blood transfusion but did not lead to hemodynamic compromise requiring intervention. The most common source of bleeding was related to procedures such as coronary angiography (17%), pulmonary artery catheter insertion (43%), and intra-aortic balloon pump placement (50%).[98] The NRMI-2 database accrued 71,073 patients who received reperfusion therapy for acute MI between 1994 and 1996. High-risk patients with ST-segment elevation were treated with thrombolytics (47.5%) or alternative forms of reperfusion therapy (9.3%) within 62 minutes and 226 minutes of hospital arrival, respectively. Intracranial hemorrhage was confirmed by computed tomography (CT) or magnetic resonance imaging in 625 patients (0.88%).[99] Several studies have proposed predictive models that assess the risk for intracranial hemorrhage (ICH) in patients receiving thrombolytic therapy. The following risk factors are associated with a

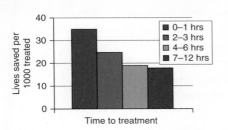
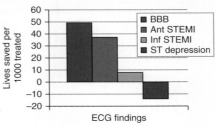

Figure 31-7. Impact of presenting electrocardiogram (ECG) and time to treatment on 35-day mortality in patients with ST-segment-elevation myocardial infarction (STEMI) receiving fibrinolytics. The impact of the presenting ECG and the time to treatment on the 35-day mortality of 58,600 patients enrolled in 9 randomized trials comparing various fibrinolytics, expressed as the number of lives saved per 1000 patients who received fibrinolytic therapy. Ant STEMI, anterior ST-segment-elevation myocardial infarction; BBB, bundle branch block; ECG, electrocardiogram; Inf STEMI, inferior ST-segment-elevation myocardial infarction. *(Adapted from Fibrinolytic Therapy Trialist's (FTT) Collaborative Group. Indications for fibrinolytic therapy in suspected acute myocardial infarction: collaborative overview of early mortality and major morbidity results from all randomized trials of more than 1000 patients. Lancet. 1994;343:311-322.)*

Table 31-5. Indications for Fibrinolytic Therapy in Acute Coronary Syndrome

Class I
1. In the absence of contraindications, fibrinolytic therapy should be administered to patients with STEMI with symptom onset within the prior 12 hours and ST elevation > 0.1 mV in at least two contiguous precordial leads or at least two adjacent limb leads or a presumably new LBBB.
Class IIa
1. In the absence of contraindications, it is reasonable to administer fibrinolytic therapy to patients with STEMI with symptom onset within the prior 12 hours and 12-lead ECG findings consistent with a true posterior MI.
2. In the absence of contraindications, it is reasonable to administer fibrinolytic therapy to patients with symptoms of STEMI beginning within the prior 12-24 hours who have continuing ischemic symptoms and ST elevation > 0.1 mV in at least two contiguous precordial leads or at least two adjacent limb leads.
Class III
1. Fibrinolytic therapy should not be administered to asymptomatic patients whose initial symptoms of STEMI began more than 24 hours earlier.
2. Fibrinolytic therapy should not be administered to patients whose 12-lead ECG shows only ST-segment depression except if a true posterior MI is suspected.

Abbreviations: ECG, electrocardiogram; LBBB, left bundle branch block; MI, myocardial infarction; STEMI, ST-segment-elevation myocardial infarction. (Adapted from Antman EM, Ange DT, Armstrong PW, et al. ACC/AHA guidelines for the management of patients with STEMI: a report of the American College of Cardiology/American Heart Association Task Force on Practice Guidelines [Committee to Revise the 1999 Guidelines for the Management of Patients with Acute Myocardial Infarction]. Circulation. 2004;110:e82-e292.)

Table 31-6. Absolute and Relative Contraindications to Fibrinolytics for STEMI

Absolute contraindications to fibrinolytics	Relative contraindications to fibrinolytics
1. Previous intracranial hemorrhage	1. Severe or uncontrolled hypertension (BP > 180/110 mm Hg)
2. Active bleeding	2. Previous ischemic stroke (> 3 mo)
3. Ischemic stroke within 3 mo	3. Recent internal bleeding (2-4 wk)
4. Suspected aortic dissection	4. Noncompressible vascular punctures
5. Trauma within 3 mo	5. Active menstruation
6. Intracranial neoplasm	6. Pregnancy
	7. Known intracranial pathology
	8. Prolonged CPR (> 10 min)
	9. Elevated INR (> 2)

Abbreviations: BP, blood pressure; CPR, cardiopulmonary resuscitation; INR, international normalized ratio; STEMI, ST-segment-elevation myocardial infarction. (Adapted from Topol EJ, Van De Werf FJ. Acute myocardial infarction: early diagnosis and management. In: Topol EJ, Califf RM, Prystowksy EN, et al, eds. Textbook of Cardiovascular Medicine. 3rd ed. Philadelphia, PA: Lippincott Williams & Wilkins; 2007:280-302.)

higher incidence of ICH: older age, female gender, systolic pressure > 160 mm Hg, diastolic pressure > 95 mm Hg, prior stroke, and excessive anticoagulation.[99-102]

When thrombolytic therapy for acute MI is administered, what other anticoagulants should be administered as ancillary therapy to reperfusion therapy?

Major limitations of fibrinolytic therapy are incomplete reperfusion or reocclusion of the infarct-related artery. Reperfusion of the infarct-related artery is determined angiographically and flow is categorized as 1 of 4 TIMI grades: grade 0 is complete occlusion, grade 1 is penetration of contrast material without distal perfusion, grade 2 is delayed perfusion of the entire artery, and grade 3 is normal flow. Initial reperfusion may be unsuccessful in as many as 20% of patients. Failure to achieve adequate reperfusion is associated with markedly increased mortality rate.[103-105] The original TIMI trial revealed that only 31% of occluded arteries were patent after administration of intravenous streptokinase.[103] In a substudy of GUSTO-1, 2431 patients underwent coronary angiography to assess patency of the infarct-related artery. Ninety minutes after initiation of accelerated tPA, 54% patients achieved adequate patency of the infarct-related artery as defined by TIMI grade 3 flow, compared to 31% of patients who received streptokinase plus unfractionated heparin (UFH).[103] Despite achieving TIMI grade 3 flow after fibrinolytic therapy, clinical outcomes and survival are related to the speed of epicardial flow and the state of myocardial perfusion. After rupture of a vulnerable plaque, the local milieu becomes rich in tissue factor, which subsequently activates the coagulation cascade and promotes platelet activation and aggregation. Ancillary anticoagulation therapy in patients with STEMI who do or do not receive reperfusion therapy acts to establish and maintain patency of the infarct-related artery. See Table 31-7.

Table 31-7. Recommendations for the Use of Anticoagulant Therapy in STEMI

Class I
For patients proceeding to primary PCI who have been treated with ASA and a thienopyridine, recommended supportive anticoagulant regimens include the following:
a. For prior treatment with UFH, additional boluses of UFH should be administered as needed to maintain therapeutic activated clotting time levels, taking into account whether GpIIb-IIIa receptor antagonists have been administered (level of evidence: C).
b. Enoxaparin for patients younger than 75 years of age, or patients at least 75 years of age. The initial intravenous bolus is eliminated and the subcutaneous dose is reduced. Renal dosing guidelines should be consulted. Maintenance dosing with enoxaparin should be continued for the duration of the index hospitalization, up to 8 days.
c. Fondaparinux. Renal dosing guidelines should be consulted. Maintenance dosing with fondaparinux should be continued for the duration of the index hospitalization, up to 8 days.
d. Bivalirudin is useful as a supportive measure for primary PCI with or without prior treatment with unfractionated heparin (level of evidence: B).
Class IIa
In STEMI patients undergoing PCI who are at high risk of bleeding, bivalirudin anticoagulation is reasonable (level of evidence: B).

Abbreviations: ASA, acetylsalicylic acid; GpIIb-IIIa, glycoprotein IIb/IIIa complex; PCI, percutaneous coronary intervention; STEMI, ST-segment-elevation myocardial infarction; UFH, unfractionated heparin. (Adapted from Kushner FG, Hand M, Smith SC et al. 2009 Focused updates: ACC/AHA guidelines for the management of patients with ST-elevation myocardial infarction [updating the 2004 guideline and 2007 focused update] and ACC/AHA/SCAI guidelines on percutaneous coronary intervention [updating the 2005 guideline and 2007 focused update]: a report of the American College of Cardiology Foundation/American Heart Association Task Force on Practice Guidelines. Circulation. 2009;120;2271-2306.)

Cardiovascular Problems

What is the role of glycoprotein IIb/IIIa antagonists in STEMI and when should they be initiated?

Much of the evidence supporting the use of glycoprotein IIb/IIIa antagonists in STEMI was generated before dual-antiplatelet therapy (aspirin plus a thienopyridine) was routinely administered to patients with STEMI. The results of recent clinical trials have raised questions regarding the utility of glycoprotein IIb/IIIa antagonists in addition to dual-antiplatelet therapy in patients with STEMI.[106-108] Based on these trials, the 2009 Joint STEMI/PCI Focused Update Recommendations assigned a class IIa recommendation to glycoprotein IIb/IIIa receptor antagonists (abciximab, tirofiban, eptifibatide) at the time of primary PCI (with or without stenting) in selected patients with STEMI. However, administration of a glycoprotein IIb/IIIa antagonist before patient arrival in the cardiac catheterization laboratory, referred to as upstream administration, received a class IIb recommendation.[81]

Use of antiplatelet therapy in patients with STEMI

Clopidogrel is an adenosine diphosphate receptor antagonist, a class of oral antiplatelet agents that block the $P2Y_{12}$ component of the adenosine diphosphate receptor and thus inhibit the activation and aggregation of platelets. A newer thienopyridine, prasugrel, was studied in the TRITON-TIMI 38 trial, which is discussed later in the text. Two randomized controlled trials, COMMIT-CCS 2 and CLARITY-TIMI 28, sought to determine the benefit of clopidogrel in combination with aspirin in patients with STEMI. CLARITY-TIMI 28, a trial sponsored by the manufacturer of clopidogrel, randomized 3491 patients who presented with STEMI within 12 hours of symptom onset to either clopidogrel (300 mg loading dose followed by 75 mg daily) or placebo. All patients received a fibrinolytic agent, aspirin, and when appropriate, heparin. Angiography was performed in 94% of patients a median of 84 hours after randomization. The primary end points consisted of patency of the infarct-related artery on angiography and death or recurrent MI before angiography. The incidence of this end point was significantly lower in the recipients of clopidogrel than in the recipients of the placebo (15% versus 22%). This difference was mostly a result of a difference in occlusion of the infarct-related artery (12% versus 18%). There was no difference in the rates of mortality or major bleeding between the two groups. COMMIT-CCS 2 randomized over 45,000 patients presenting with STEMI to either clopidogrel 75 mg daily plus 162 mg of aspirin or placebo plus aspirin 162 mg. Ninety-three percent of patients had ST-segment elevation or bundle branch block. Fifty-four percent of patients received fibrinolytics, and 3% underwent PCI. Compared to aspirin alone, dual-therapy recipients had significantly lower 30-day incidences of the primary composite end point of death, reinfarction, and stroke (9.2% versus 10.1%) and of death alone (7.5% versus 8.1%). A subgroup analysis revealed that the primary–end point benefit was restricted to recipients of fibrinolytic therapy. The incidence of major bleeding was about 0.6% in each group.[109] The 2009 Joint STEMI/PCI Focused Update Recommendations assigned a class I recommendation to administration of the loading dose of a thienopyridine in patients with STEMI for whom PCI is planned. Either of the following regimens was recommended: 300 to 600 mg of clopidogrel administered as early as possible before or at the time of primary or nonprimary PCI, or prasugrel 60 mg administered as early as possible before primary PCI. In patients with STEMI with a prior history of stroke and transient ischemic attack for whom primary PCI is planned, prasugrel is not recommended as part of a dual-antiplatelet therapy regimen (class III recommendation).[81] Clopidogrel 75 mg daily or prasugrel 10 mg daily for at least 12 months is a class I recommendation for patients with ACS who receive bare-metal or drug-eluting stents.[81]

What other options exist for patients presenting with STEMI who are not candidates for fibrinolytic therapy or PCI?

Fondaparinux is the preferred anticoagulant for patients with STEMI who do not receive reperfusion therapy. Otherwise, the recommendations included in the ACC/AHA guidelines apply to patients who do not receive reperfusion therapy; however, these patients have a higher risk for future adverse events.

Is this patient a candidate for PCI?

Fibrinolytic therapy is given to eligible patients if primary PCI cannot be performed in a timely fashion. Otherwise, PCI is the preferred method of reperfusion in patients with STEMI. Approximately 30% of patients presenting with STEMI have a contraindication to fibrinolytic therapy. Primary PCI has been compared with fibrinolytic therapy in more than 20 randomized trials. A meta-analysis of 23 randomized trials that directly compared percutaneous transluminal coronary angiography (PTCA) with fibrinolytic therapy in patients with STEMI concluded that primary PTCA was better than thrombolytic therapy at reducing overall short-term death (7% versus 9%; $P = .0002$), nonfatal reinfarction (3% versus 7%; $P < .0001$), stroke (1% versus 2%; $P = .0004$), and the combined end point of death, nonfatal reinfarction, and stroke (8% versus 14%; $P < .0001$).[110] However, the studies included in this meta-analysis were very heterogeneous in design and balloon angioplasty was the predominant method of PCI. High-risk patients, such as those with cardiogenic shock or anterior STEMI, seem to derive the greatest mortality benefit of PTCA versus fibrinolytic therapy.[111-114]

The DANAMI-2 trial randomized more than 1000 patients with STEMI and duration of symptoms < 12 hours (mean: 105 minutes) to either alteplase or PCI with stenting (93% of patients received stents). Patients who presented to non–PCI-capable facilities were transferred to a PCI-capable facility within 3 hours. The primary end point of mortality, reinfarction, or stroke at 30 days was significantly lower in the primary PCI group (8.0% versus 13.7%), prompting early termination of the study. This net benefit observed in the PCI group was largely driven by a strikingly lower rate of reinfarction in the PCI group (1.6% versus 6.3%; $P < .001$).[115]

The incidence of disabling stroke in the fibrinolytic and PCI groups was 2.0% versus 1.1% ($P = .15$), respectively. A subgroup analysis that risk-stratified patients according to TIMI risk score concluded that the mortality benefit of PCI was confined to high-risk patients (TIMI score ≥ 5).[116] A 3-year follow-up study demonstrated that the composite end point (death, clinical reinfarction, and disabling stroke) was reduced by PCI compared with fibrinolysis (19.6% versus 25.2%; $P = .006$).[117] Based on the current data, it is an ACC/AHA class I recommendation that patients with STEMI presenting to a hospital with PCI capability should be treated with primary PCI within 90 minutes of first medical contact. Patients with STEMI who present to a hospital without PCI capability and who cannot be transferred to a PCI center and undergo PCI within 90 minutes of first medical contact should be treated with fibrinolytic therapy within 30 minutes of hospital contact unless fibrinolytic therapy is contraindicated.[77]

PCI may be deferred in patients with an increased risk of bleeding from standard adjunctive anticoagulation and antiplatelet therapy that is administered during and after PCI. Is delayed PCI a reasonable option in patients who present with STEMI?

In the absence of reperfusion, angiographic studies of patients with STEMI suggest that occlusion of the infarct-related artery is present in 87% of patients at 4 hours, 65% at 12 to 24 hours, and 45% at 1 month after symptom onset.[118] Many patients with acute MI present to medical facilities more than 12 hours after the onset of symptoms. The late open artery hypothesis proposes that late opening of an occluded infarct-related artery may reduce adverse LV remodeling. However, despite modest improvement in LV function after late opening of an infarct-related artery, randomized clinical trials have not demonstrated a reduction in hard clinical outcomes such as death, recurrent MI, stroke, or New York Heart Association class IV heart failure among patients who underwent PCI 3 to 28 days after having an MI.[119-121] The 2007 ACC/AHA updated STEMI guidelines assigned a class IIa recommendation to performing PCI in a patent infarct-related artery more than 24 hours after STEMI. It is not recommended to perform PCI of a totally occluded infarct-related artery more than 24 hours after STEMI in asymptomatic patients with 1- or 2-vessel disease if they are hemodynamically and electrically stable and do not have evidence of severe ischemia.[77]

Patients who receive fibrinolytic therapy should be transferred immediately to the nearest PCI center. Reperfusion after administration of a fibrinolytic agent is assessed clinically and electrographically. Resolution of ST-segment elevation ≥ 50% and resolution of chest pain provide evidence of successful reperfusion after fibrinolytic therapy. However, fibrinolytic-treated patients with STEMI who meet high-risk criteria such as cardiogenic shock, hemodynamic or electrical instability, or persistent ischemic symptoms should be considered for rescue PCI (Figure 31-8). In contrast, facilitated PCI, defined as either a full dose of a fibrinolytic drug or a half-dose of a fibrinolytic drug plus a GpIIb-IIIa antagonist before planned PCI, is not recommended because it has been associated with increases in mortality rate, nonfatal reinfarction, urgent target lesion revascularization and stroke, and a trend toward a higher rate of major bleeding.[122-124]

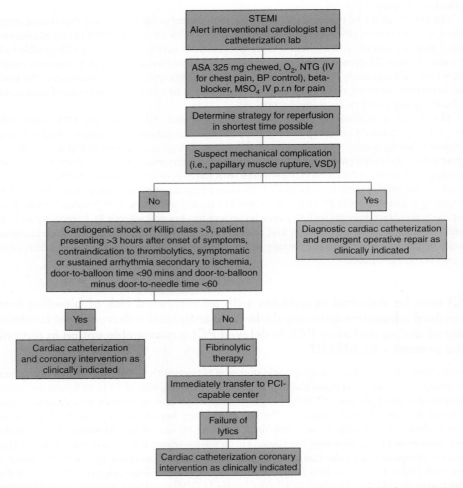

Figure 31-8. Algorithm for treatment of patients with ST-segment-elevation myocardial infarction (STEMI). ASA, acetylsalicylic acid; BP, blood pressure; IV, intravenously; MSO$_4$, morphine sulfate; NTG, nitroglycerin; PCI, percutaneous coronary intervention; VSD, vascular septal defect.

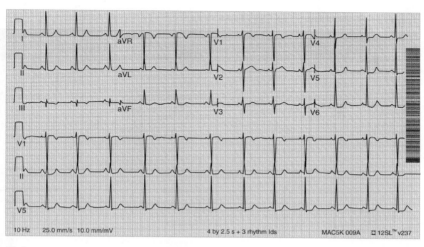

Figure 31-9. Twelve-lead electrocardiogram when patient was chest pain–free.

 A 54-year-old woman with type 2 diabetes mellitus, dyslipidemia, and temporal lobe epilepsy was admitted to the neurology ICU for status epilepticus, which was attributed to medication nonadherence. On day 2 of her admission and after being stabilized, she complained of chest pain. A 12-lead ECG was performed and cardiac biomarkers were drawn. Troponin I is 2.4 ng/mL (Figures 31-9 and 31-10).

What is this patient experiencing? What should be part of the immediate management of this patient?

This patient is having an NSTEMI as defined by her symptoms, ECG findings, and elevated troponin I level. Treatment algorithms are the same for NSTEMI and UA, with the former being defined

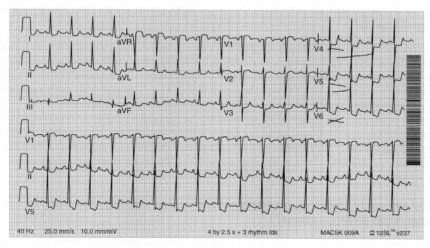

Figure 31-10. Twelve-lead electrocardiogram when patient had chest pain.

Table 31-8. TIMI Risk Score Calculation

TIMI risk score	All-cause mortality, new or recurrent MI, or severe recurrent ischemia requiring urgent revascularization through 14 days
0-1	4%-7%
2	8.3%
3	13.2%
4	19.9%
5	26.2%
6-7	40.9%

One point is given for each of the following variables: age 65 y or older; at least 3 risk factors for CAD; prior coronary stenosis of 50% or more; ST-segment deviation on ECG presentation; at least 2 anginal events in previous 24 h; use of aspirin in previous 7 d; and elevated serum cardiac biomarkers.

Abbreviations: CAD, coronary artery disease; ECG, electrocardiogram; MI, myocardial infarction; TIMI, thrombolysis in myocardial infarction.

as having an elevated serum troponin I or T level. A number of risk assessment tools have been developed to assist in assessing the risk of death and ischemic events in patients with UA/NSTEMI, thereby providing a basis for therapeutic decision making. The TIMI risk score incorporates 7 risk indicators into a predictive model for the composite end points, all-cause mortality, new or recurrent MI, or severe recurrent ischemia prompting urgent revascularization within 14 days. It has been validated in the TIMI 11B trial and two separate cohorts of patients who were enrolled in the Efficacy and Safety of Subcutaneous Enoxaparin in Unstable Angina and Non-Q-Wave Myocardial Infarction (ESSENCE) trial.[125,126] The TIMI risk calculator can be accessed at www.timi.org. Other risk models, the GRACE score and PURSUIT, have been designed and validated.[127-129] The GRACE score can be accessed at www.outcomes-umassmed.org/grace and can be used at the bedside to determine the probability of in-hospital death as well as death and/or MI at 6 months. A higher GRACE score may prompt the clinician to employ an early invasive strategy. See Table 31-8.

The patient's ECG is essentially normal when she is pain-free but shows marked ST-segment depression during chest pain. Does this have any clinical significance?

Yes. Dynamic ECG changes are highly suggestive of acute ischemia. Importantly, transient ST-segment changes (≥ 0.5 mV) that develop during a symptomatic episode at rest and that resolve when the patient becomes asymptomatic strongly suggest acute ischemia and a very high likelihood of underlying severe coronary artery disease (CAD).[59] A completely normal ECG in a patient with chest pain does not exclude the possibility of ACS. Both ST-segment depression and T-wave inversion may be signs of myocardial ischemia. The amount of ST-segment depression or elevation is measured relative to the TP segment (the end of the T wave to the beginning of the P wave). It has been proposed that isolated ST-segment depression ≥ 1 mm measured at 80 milliseconds of the J point in ≥ 6 leads is 96.5% specific for acute MI.[130] A comprehensive differential diagnosis of the causes of ST-segment depression and T-wave inversion is listed in Table 31-9.

Should an early invasive or early conservative strategy be adopted in the management of this patient?

The early conservative strategy refers to maximal medical therapy with anti-ischemic and antithrombotic agents, followed by an exercise test, usually with myocardial perfusion imaging, in patients

Table 31-9. Differential Diagnosis for ST- and T-Wave Changes on a 12-Lead ECG

ST-segment depression	T- wave inversions
1. Myocardial ischemia or infarction	1. Normal variant
a. Acute subendocardial ischemia	a. Juvenile T wave
b. Reciprocal change in STEMI	b. Early repolarization
2. Left or right ventricular hypertrophy	2. Myocardial ischemia/infarction
a. Strain pattern	3. Cerebrovascular accident
3. Left or right bundle branch block	4. Left or right ventricular dysfunction
4. Digitalis effect	a. Strain pattern
5. Hypokalemia	b. Apical hypertrophy
	5. Idiopathic global T-wave inversions
	6. Secondary to left or right bundle branch block

Abbreviations: ECG, electrocardiogram; STEMI, ST-segment-elevation myocardial infarction. *(Adapted from Goldberger AL. Myocardial ischemia and infarction. In: Goldberger AL. Clinical Electrocardiography: A Simplified Approach. 7th ed. Philadelphia, PA: Mosby Elsevier; 2006.)*

who do not have recurrent symptoms. Patients with inducible ischemia are scheduled for a cardiac catheterization if there are no contraindications. The early invasive strategy entails both maximal medical therapy and early cardiac catheterization and possible revascularization within 48 hours of presentation. Several randomized trials have directly compared the early invasive strategy with the early conservative strategy in patients with UA/NSTEMI and have demonstrated better short-term and long-term outcomes in patients randomized to the early invasive strategy. The Fragmin and Fast Revascularization during Instability in Coronary Artery Disease III (FRISC II),[131] TACTICS-TIMI 18,[132] and Randomized Intervention Trial of Unstable Angina III (RITA III)[133] trials each demonstrated that the composite end point of death, MI, and refractory angina was less frequent among patients who were randomized to the early invasive strategy, with the greatest benefit observed in high-risk patients. High-risk features include elevated serum troponin levels; the extent of ST-segment depression and the number of leads with ST-segment depression; age older than 65 years; recurrent angina or ischemia despite intensive anti-ischemic therapy; recurrent angina or ischemia with CHF or new or worsening mitral regurgitation; a high-risk noninvasive stress test; left ventricular ejection fraction < 40%; hemodynamic instability; sustained ventricular tachycardia; PCI within the past 6 months; and prior coronary artery bypass graft (CABG) surgery.[59]

The ICTUS trial enrolled 1200 patients with UA/NSTEMI who were initially treated with aspirin and enoxaparin before randomized assignment to one of two strategies: an early invasive strategy within 48 hours that included abciximab for PCI or a selective invasive strategy. Patients who were assigned the latter strategy were selected for coronary angiography only if they had refractory angina despite medical treatment, if they had hemodynamic or rhythm instability, or if predischarge exercise testing demonstrated clinically significant ischemia. The trial failed to show a reduction in the composite end points of death, nonfatal MI, and rehospitalization for angina at 1 year among patients who were assigned to the early invasive strategy. After 4 years of follow-up, the rates of death and MI among the two groups of patients remained similar.[134] It is not clear why the results of ICTUS differ so much from previous trials. The more recent Timing of Intervention in Acute Coronary Syndromes (TIMACS) study randomized 3031 patients with UA/NSTEMI to undergo cardiac catheterization either within 24 hours of symptom onset or more than 36 hours later.[135] The median time to angiography was 14 hours for the early-intervention group and 50 hours for the delayed-intervention group. There was no difference between the groups in the composite end point of death, myocardial infarction, and stroke at 6 months.[135] The most recent guidelines regarding an early invasive versus conservative

Table 31-10. UA/NSTEMI: Indications for an Early Invasive versus Conservative Strategy

Class I	Class IIb
1. An early invasive strategy (ie, diagnostic angiography with intent to perform revascularization) is indicated in UA/NSTEMI patients who have refractory angina or hemodynamic or electrical instability	1. In initially stabilized patients, an initially conservative/selectively invasive strategy may be considered as a treatment strategy for UA/NSTEMI patients who have an elevated risk for clinical events including those who are troponin positive.
2. An early invasive strategy is indicated in initially stabilized UA/NSTEMI patients who have an elevated risk for clinical events	2. An invasive strategy may be reasonable in patients with chronic renal insufficiency.

Abbreviations: NSTEMI, non–ST-segment-elevation myocardial infarction; UA, unstable angina. (Adapted from Anderson JL, Adams CD, Antam EM, et al. ACC/AHA 2007 guidelines for the management of patients with unstable angina/non-ST-elevation myocardial infarction: a report of the American College of Cardiology/American Heart Association Task Force on Practice Guidelines. J Am Coll Cardiol. 2007;50:e1-e157.)

strategy in patients with UA/NSTEMI are listed in Table 31-10. An early invasive strategy (ie, diagnostic angiography with intent to perform revascularization) is not recommended in patients with extensive comorbidities such that the risks of revascularization are likely to outweigh the benefits of revascularization, or in patients with acute chest pain and a low likelihood of ACS (class III recommendation) (Figure 31-11).[59]

This patient remained hemodynamically stable and free of chest pain after medical therapy was initiated. What are the evidence-based guidelines regarding the use of antiplatelet therapy in this circumstance?

Both aspirin and thienopyridines have been shown to improve outcome in patients with ACS. As soon as there is a suspicion of ACS, 162 to 325 mg of a nonenteric formulation of aspirin should be given orally or chewed unless there is a contraindication.

The thienopyridines (ticlopidine, clopidogrel, and prasugrel) and ticagrelor, a cyclopentyl triazolopyrimidine, block the $P2Y_{12}$ adenosine diphosphate receptor on platelets. Clopidogrel requires in vivo biotransformation to an active metabolite. The active metabolite irreversibly blocks the $P2Y_{12}$ component of adenosine diphosphate receptors on the platelet surface, which prevents activation of the GpIIb-IIIa receptor complex and reduces platelet aggregation for the remainder of the platelet's life span, which is approximately 7 to 10 days. Prasugrel is a prodrug that is metabolized to both active and inactive metabolites. Platelet aggregation returns to baseline within 5 to 9 days after prasugrel is discontinued.

The efficacy of clopidogrel was studied in the Clopidogrel in Unstable Angina to Prevent Recurrent Events (CURE) trial, which randomized 12,562 patients with UA/NSTEMI to either clopidogrel (300-mg oral loading dose, then 75 mg daily) or placebo for a mean of 9 months; all patients also received aspirin (dose range, 75-325 mg).[136] The primary end point was cardiovascular death, MI, or urgent target-vessel revascularization at 30 days after PCI. The incidence of the 30-day composite end point was significantly lower among patients who received clopidogrel (4.5%) than among patients who received placebo (6.4%). The PCI-CURE trial studied a subset of patients (n = 2658) who underwent PCI.[137] Overall, including events before and after PCI, there was a 31% reduction in cardiovascular death or MI (*P* < .002). There was no difference between the groups in major bleeding.[137] Therefore, in patients with UA/NSTEMI who undergo PCI, pretreatment with clopidogrel followed by up to 1 year of clopidogrel therapy is beneficial in reducing major cardiovascular events. However, PCI-CURE did not adequately address the question of dose or timing of clopidogrel in relationship to PCI. The CREDO trial randomized 2116 patients to a 300-mg loading dose of clopidogrel or placebo (3-24 hours before PCI). Both groups received 325 mg of aspirin. The clopidogrel group received 75 mg of clopidogrel daily for 1 year. Although there was no

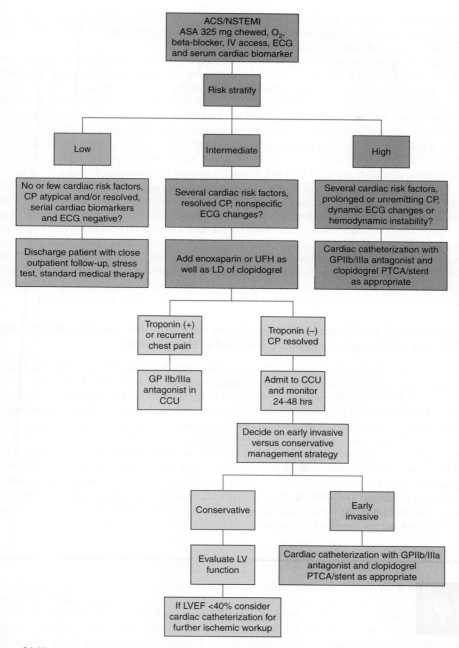

Figure 31-11. Treatment algorithm for patients with non–ST-segment-elevation myocardial infarction (NSTEMI)/unstable angina (UA). ACS, acute coronary syndrome; ASA, acetylsalicylic acid; CP, chest pain; CCU, cardiac care unit; ECG, electrocardiogram; GpIIb-IIIa, glycoprotein IIb/IIIa complex; IV, intravenous; LD, loading dose; LVEF, left ventricular ejection fraction; NSTEMI, non–ST-segment-elevation myocardial infarction; PTCA, percutaneous transluminal coronary angioplasty; UFH, unfractionated heparin. *(Adapted from Anderson JL, Adams CD, Antam EM, et al. ACC/AHA 2007 guidelines for the management of patients with unstable angina/non-ST-elevation myocardial infarction: a report of the American College of Cardiology/American Heart Association Task Force on Practice Guidelines. J Am Coll Cardiol. 2007;50:e1-e157.)*

Cardiovascular
Problems

difference between groups in the 28-day composite end point of death, MI, and urgent target-vessel revascularization, treatment with clopidogrel was associated with a 26.9% relative risk reduction in the 1-year composite end point of death, MI, and stroke.[138]

Prasugrel, a new thienopyridine, was compared with clopidogrel in a randomized, double-blind trial, TRITON-TIMI 38. It compared prasugrel (loading dose of 60 mg followed by maintenance dose of 10 mg) with clopidogrel (300-mg loading dose followed by 75-mg maintenance dose) in 13,608 patients with UA/NSTEMI (n = 10,074) or STEMI (n = 3534) who underwent PCI. All patients also received aspirin, and treatment with prasugrel or clopidogrel was continued for a median of 14.5 months. The primary end point, a composite of cardiovascular death, nonfatal MI, and nonfatal stroke, was less frequent among patients who received prasugrel (9.9% versus 12.1%; hazard ratio: 0.81; 95% CI: 0.73-0.90). The rate of major bleeding was higher in the prasugrel group (2.4% versus 1.8%; hazard ratio: 1.32; 95% CI: 1.03-1.68), as was the rate of life-threatening bleeding.[139]

Ticagrelor, which reversibly binds to the $P2Y_{12}$ platelet receptor and has not been approved for clinical use, exhibited greater efficacy than clopidogrel in the PLATO trial. Major bleeding events did not differ between the groups, although bleeding not related to coronary artery bypass grafting occurred more often with ticagrelor.[140] Both prasugrel and ticagrelor may have a quicker onset of action than clopidogrel and may prove to be very useful in patients who are clopidogrel-resistant. The current guidelines recommend a loading dose of 300 to 600 mg of clopidogrel in patients with UA/NSTEMI followed by 75 mg daily.[59] The duration of clopidogrel use may depend on whether or not the patient received a stent. Ideally, clopidogrel should be continued indefinitely if it is tolerated by the patient. However, adequate long-term data have not been sufficient to formulate a definite recommendation on the duration of therapy.

What kind of antithrombotic agents are available for use in patients with ACS, and which agent(s) should be used in this patient?

The efficacy of unfractionated heparin, low-molecular-weight heparins, fondaparinux, bivalirudin, and GpIIb-IIIa inhibitors has been extensively studied in patients with ACS. A discussion of the numerous trials is beyond the scope of this chapter. In the new era of clopidogrel use, the utility of GpIIb-IIIa inhibitors has been questioned. The current evidence base and expert opinion suggest that for patients with UA/NSTEMI in whom an initial invasive strategy is selected, *either* an intravenous GpIIb-IIIa inhibitor *or* clopidogrel should be added to acetylsalicylic acid (ASA) and anticoagulant therapy before diagnostic angiography for lower-risk, troponin-negative patients. In higher-risk and troponin-positive patients, both clopidogrel and a GpIIb-IIIa inhibitor should be started before angiography (class I recommendation).[59] For patients with UA/NSTEMI in whom an initial conservative strategy is selected, the addition of a GpIIb-IIIa inhibitor to anticoagulant and oral antiplatelet therapy may be reasonable for high-risk patients (class IIb recommendation).[59] Recommendations for antiplatelet and anticoagulant therapy are listed in Tables 31-11, 31-12, and 31-13.

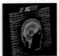 A 23-year-old man with a history of substance abuse is admitted to the neurology ICU with altered mental status and seizures. Before intubation he told the triage nurse he was having chest pain. Laboratory test results in the ED are remarkable for a urine drug screen positive for cocaine, acute renal failure, elevated CK and CK-MB, and a troponin I of 1.0. His ECG shows sinus tachycardia with ST depression of 0.5 mV in leads V_1 through V_4 with associated T-wave inversions.

Management of cocaine-induced ischemia

Cocaine-induced ischemic chest pain is often clinically indistinguishable from UA or NSTEMI. Cocaine-induced coronary artery vasoconstriction has been demonstrated in both in vivo[141-145] and

Table 31-11. Recommendations for Antiplatelet/Anticoagulant Therapy in Patients for Whom Diagnosis of UA/NSTEMI Is Likely or Definite

Antiplatelet Therapy Recommendations

Class I

1. Aspirin should be administered to patients with UA/NSTEMI as soon as possible after hospital presentation and continued indefinitely in patients not known to be intolerant of that medication.

2. Clopidogrel (loading dose followed by daily maintenance dose) should be administered to patients with UA/NSTEMI who are unable to take ASA because of hypersensitivity or major gastrointestinal intolerance.

3. For patients with UA/NSTEMI in whom an initial invasive strategy is selected, antiplatelet therapy in addition to aspirin should be initiated before diagnostic angiography (upstream) with either clopidogrel (loading dose followed by daily maintenance dose) or an intravenous GpIIb-IIIa inhibitor. Abciximab as the choice for upstream GpIIb-IIIa therapy is indicated only if there is no appreciable delay to angiography and PCI is likely to be performed; otherwise, IV eptifibatide or tirofiban is the preferred choice of GpIIb-IIIa inhibitor.

4. For patients with UA/NSTEMI in whom an initial conservative (ie, noninvasive) strategy is selected, clopidogrel (loading dose followed by daily maintenance dose) should be added to ASA and anticoagulant therapy as soon as possible after admission and administered for at least 1 mo and ideally up to 1 y.

Class IIa

1. For patients with UA/NSTEMI in whom an initial conservative strategy is selected and who have recurrent ischemic discomfort with clopidogrel, ASA, and anticoagulant therapy, it is reasonable to add a GpIIb-IIIa antagonist before diagnostic angiography.

2. For patients with UA/NSTEMI in whom an initial invasive strategy is selected, it is reasonable to initiate antiplatelet therapy with both clopidogrel (loading dose followed by daily maintenance dose) and an intravenous GpIIb-IIIa inhibitor. Abciximab as the choice for upstream GpIIb-IIIa therapy is indicated only if there is no appreciable delay to angiography and PCI is likely to be performed; otherwise, IV eptifibatide or tirofiban is the preferred choice of GpIIb-IIIa inhibitor.

Class III

1. Abciximab should not be administered to patients in whom PCI is not planned.

Abbreviations: ASA, acetylsalicylic acid; GpIIb-IIIa, glycoprotein IIb/IIIa complex; NSTEMI, non–ST-segment-elevation myocardial infarction; PCI, percutaneous coronary intervention; UA, unstable angina. (Adapted from Anderson JL, Adams CD, Antam EM, et al. ACC/AHA 2007 guidelines for the management of patients with unstable angina/non-ST-elevation myocardial infarction: a report of the American College of Cardiology/American Heart Association Task Force on Practice Guidelines. J Am Coll Cardiol. 2007;50:e1-e157.)

in vitro experiments.[146] In addition to its direct effect on vasomotor tone, cocaine promotes coronary thrombosis by increasing the response of platelets to arachidonic acid, thus increasing thromboxane A_2 production and platelet aggregation.[147] Chronic use of cocaine may promote accelerated atherosclerosis. Therefore, patients using cocaine who present with ischemic-like chest discomfort should be treated aggressively. If the initial ECG shows ST-segment elevation or depression, intravenous or sublingual nitroglycerin or an intravenous calcium channel blocker (such as diltiazem) should be administered immediately. If there is no improvement in the ECG, then fibrinolytic therapy or PCI should be considered after consultation with a cardiologist. If the initial ECG is nondiagnostic for ischemia, then nitroglycerin or a calcium channel blocker should be administered and the patient should be monitored for a minimum of 24 hours with serial ECGs and cardiac biomarkers as well as continuous ECG monitoring.[59] The use of β blockers in patients with cocaine-related chest discomfort remains controversial. Current recommendations support the use of calcium channel antagonists (diltiazem or verapamil) over β blockers in this setting.

Cardiovascular Problems

Table 31-12. Recommendations for Anticoagulation Therapy in Patients with UA/NSTEMI

Class I
1. For patients in whom an invasive strategy is selected, regimens with established efficacy at a level of evidence A includes enoxaparin and UFH, and those with established efficacy at a level of evidence B includes bivalirudin and fondaparinux.
2. For patients in whom a conservative strategy is selected, regimens using either enoxaparin or UFH or fondaparinux have established efficacy.
3. In patients in whom a conservative strategy is selected and who have an increased risk of bleeding, fondaparinux is preferable.
Class IIa
1. For patients with UA/NSTEMI in whom an initial conservative strategy is selected, enoxaparin or fondaparinux is preferable to UFH as anticoagulant therapy, unless CABG is planned within 24 hours.

Abbreviations: CABG, coronary artery bypass grafting; NSTEMI, non–ST-segment-elevation myocardial infarction; UA, unstable angina; UFH, unfractionated heparin. (Adapted from Anderson JL, Adams CD, Antam EM, et al. ACC/AHA 2007 guidelines for the management of patients with unstable angina/non-ST-elevation myocardial infarction: a report of the American College of Cardiology/American Heart Association Task Force on Practice Guidelines. J Am Coll Cardiol. 2007;50:e1-e157.)

Table 31-13. Doses for Antiplatelet/Anticoagulant Therapy in Patients with UA/NSTEMI

Drug	Initial medical treatment
Antiplatelet Drugs	
1. Aspirin	162-325 mg nonenteric formulation, orally or chewed
2. Clopidogrel	LD of 300-600 mg orally. MD of 75 mg orally per day
3. Ticlopidine	LD of 500 mg orally. MD of 250 mg orally twice daily
Anticoagulants	
1. Unfractionated heparin	LD of 60 U/kg (max 4000 U) as IV bolus. MD of IV infusion of 12 U/kg per hour (max 1000 U/h) to maintain aPTT at 1.5-2.0 times control (approximately 50-70 s)
2. Enoxaparin	LD of 30 mg IV bolus may be given. MD 1 mg/kg SC every 12 h. Extend dosing interval to 1 mg/kg every 24 h if estimated creatinine clearance < 30 mL/min
3. Fondaparinux	2.5 mg SC once daily. Avoid for creatinine clearance < 30 mL/min
4. Eptifibatide	LD of IV bolus of 180 μg/kg. MD of IV infusion of 2.0 μg/kg per minute; reduce infusion by 50% in patients with estimated creatinine clearance < 50 mL/min.
5. Tirofiban	LD of IV infusion of 0.4 μg/g per minute for 30 min. MD of IV infusion of 0.1 μg/kg per minute; reduce rate of infusion by 50% in patients with estimated creatinine clearance < 30 mL/ min
6. Bivalirudin	0.1 mg/kg bolus, 0.25 mg/kg per hour infusion

Abbreviations: aPTT, activated partial thromboplastin time; IV, intravenously; LD, loading dose; MD, maintenance dose; NSTEMI, non–ST-segment-elevation myocardial infarction; SC, subcutaneously; UA, unstable angina. (Adapted from Anderson JL, Adams CD, Antam EM, et al. ACC/AHA 2007 guidelines for the management of patients with unstable angina/non-ST-elevation myocardial infarction: a report of the American College of Cardiology/American Heart Association Task Force on Practice Guidelines. J Am Coll Cardiol. 2007;50:e1-e157.)

A 19-year-old man with a history of migraine headaches and recurrent syncope is admitted to the neurology ICU for monitoring after his third episode of syncope resulting in head trauma. On his third day of admission, the nurse pages you to say that he has ST-segment elevation on the monitor but does not complain of chest pain. A 12-lead ECG is performed and shows 2 mm of ST-segment elevation in the inferior leads, which quickly resolves after administration of sublingual nitroglycerin. The patient has no cardiac risk factors.

What is your next step?

This patient is experiencing variant or Prinzmetal angina. The exact mechanism for CAS in variant angina is unknown but may be due to increased vasomotor tone, vagal withdrawal, abnormal sympathetic activity, or endothelial dysfunction. Patients with either obstructive or nonobstructive coronary artery disease can have CAS.[148] Patients may have typical angina or be asymptomatic. Compared to patients with UA/NSTEMI, patients with variant angina are younger and have little or no cardiac risk factors. The attacks of angina usually resolve spontaneously without evidence of MI. However, a prolonged episode of vasospasm may result in complications such as MI, high-grade AV block, life-threatening ventricular tachycardia, or sudden death.[149,150]

The key to diagnosing variant angina due to CAS is recording transient ST-segment elevation that resolves when the chest pain resolves or after administration of nitroglycerin. Nitrates and calcium channel antagonists are the first line of therapy for CAS. Moderate to high doses of a calcium channel blocker should be prescribed (eg, verapamil 240-480 mg daily, diltiazem 180-360 mg daily, or nifedipine 60-120 mg daily). The addition of nitrates and/or a second calcium channel antagonist may be necessary if the CAS is severe and recurrent. Coronary angiography is recommended in patients with episodic chest pain accompanied by transient ST-segment elevation (class I recommendation).[59]

Overall, patients with variant angina due to CAS have an excellent prognosis with medical management. Occasionally, patients may need a permanent pacemaker to prevent transient AV block associated with ischemia during periods of prolonged coronary vasospasm. In this patient's case, the recurrent syncope should alert the clinician to ischemia-induced AV block or ventricular fibrillation during prolonged episodes of CAS, which may require a pacemaker or defibrillator.

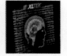

A 50-year-old woman was admitted to the neurology ICU after presenting with new-onset seizure activity. A CT scan of the brain showed a mass of unknown origin. She has no other medical problems. You enter the room to discuss your findings. She becomes hysterical. One hour later she complains of chest pain. An ECG is performed. Initial laboratory results are notable for a troponin level of 1.33 ng/mL (Figures 31-12 and 31-13).

What are your first steps in the management of this patient?

This patient's initial ECG shows diffuse T-wave inversions with a T-wave morphology that is suggestive of ischemia. Furthermore, the initial laboratory results are indicative of myocardial necrosis with a serum troponin level of 1.33 ng/mL. Despite having no identifiable cardiac risk factors, the patient's chest pain, ECG results, and increased troponin levels are consistent with NSTEMI. The fact that the T-wave inversions are diffuse rather than regional does not rule out ACS. Until further data can be collected, it is reasonable to treat this patient as if she is having an NSTEMI. Aspirin, clopidogrel, and anticoagulation should be initiated according to the UA/NSTEMI guidelines that were discussed earlier. Other medications such as β blockers should be started if appropriate. Given her lack of cardiac risk

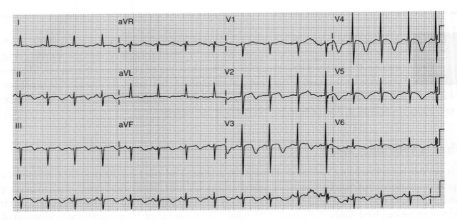

Figure 31-12. Initial 12-lead electrocardiogram.

factors and onset of chest pain after extreme emotional stress (ie, diagnosis of a brain mass), one should suspect a stress-induced cardiomyopathy, also known as apical ballooning syndrome, broken heart syndrome, or Takotsubo cardiomyopathy.

What is the differential diagnosis?

The differential diagnosis includes NSTEMI, coronary vasospasm, myocarditis, left ventricular hypertrophy, central nervous system disease, and pericarditis (stage III of ECG findings).

What diagnostic studies should be performed?

Coronary angiography should be performed to detect epicardial coronary artery occlusion. Left ventriculography will reveal akinesis of the left ventricular apex and/or the midportions of the left ventricle and a hypercontractile base. A 2-D echocardiogram would confirm these findings. Severe left ventricular dysfunction is common.

Generally, the diagnosis of stress-induced cardiomyopathy can be made if all four of the following criteria are met: (1) an ECG shows ST-segment elevation or T-wave inversions, or positive cardiac

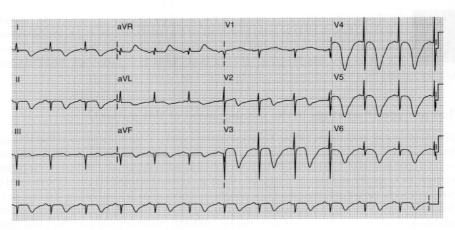

Figure 31-13. Twelve-lead elctrocardiogram several hours later.

biomarkers; (2) there is no angiographic evidence of coronary artery occlusion; (3) an echocardiogram shows *transient* hypokinesis, akinesis, or dyskinesis of the left ventricular wall from the midportion to the apex, with hypercontractility of the base; and (4) other diseases such as myocarditis have been excluded.[151,152]

What is the treatment, course of disease, and prognosis?

Stress-induced cardiomyopathy typically occurs in postmenopausal women, presents with chest pain and dyspnea, and is associated with emotional distress or critical illness. A systematic review performed in 2006 reported chest pain and dyspnea in 67.8% and 17.8% of the patients, respectively.[153] ECG changes included ST-segment elevation in 81.6% of the patients, T-wave abnormalities in 64.3%, and Q waves in 31.8%.[153] Cardiac biomarkers were usually mildly elevated, as reported in 86.2% of the patients.[153] The pathogenesis of stress-induced cardiomyopathy is unclear. Multivessel coronary vasospasm has been postulated but not proven. Other possible mechanisms include catecholamine excess.

Stress-induced cardiomyopathy is transient and initially requires supportive care. A proportion of patients can present with decompensated heart failure, cardiogenic shock, or lethal ventricular arrhythmias. In one study, the incidence of cardiogenic shock and ventricular fibrillation was reported to be 4.2% and 1.5%, respectively.[153]

Therapy for heart failure is indicated until recovery of LV function has been demonstrated by 2-D echocardiography. Recovery time varies but is usually 1 to 4 weeks. There is no official recommendation on the duration of therapy, but it should at least continue until LV systolic function has returned to normal on imaging studies. Prognosis is generally good despite the fact that many patients are critically ill at the onset of stress-induced cardiomyopathy. In-hospital mortality rates range between 0% and 8%.[151,154-156] Recurrence rates are unclear but were reported to be 3.5% in one study.[153]

A 68-year-old man has been in the neurology ICU for 5 days after suffering a hemorrhagic stroke. On hospital day 1, he was also noted to have an anterior wall STEMI that was treated conservatively without fibrinolytics or PCI. On day 5 of his admission, he became increasingly more tachypneic and hypotensive. A chest x-ray shows worsening pulmonary edema.

What is your differential diagnosis?

There are several mechanical complications that can occur after acute MI and that are often life threatening if not diagnosed and treated promptly. In addition to providing supportive care with vasopressor and/or vasoactive drugs, the first step in diagnosing this patient's worsening hemodynamic status is a 2-D echocardiogram. Two-dimensional echocardiography is crucial in diagnosing mechanical complications of acute MI, such as acute mitral regurgitation due to papillary muscle rupture, rupture of the interventricular septum, rupture of the left ventricular free wall, or cardiac tamponade.

An echocardiogram was performed in this patient and revealed papillary muscle rupture and severe mitral regurgitation (MR). What is the next step in this patient's management?

Ischemic MR frequently occurs in the setting of acute MI due to ischemic papillary muscle displacement, left ventricular dilatation of an aneurysm, or rupture of a papillary muscle or chordae.

Transient moderate MR can occur in up to 14% of patients with acute MI during periods of ischemia.[157] One study showed that mild MR (8.5% mortality rate) and moderate to severe MR (20.8% mortality rate) in the setting of acute MI were the strongest independent predictors of 1-year mortality.[158] The diagnosis of severe acute MR should be suspected in any patient after acute MI who develops hypotension and pulmonary edema. The absence of a loud systolic murmur does not exclude severe MR. Treatment of acute severe MR includes inotropic support, afterload reduction, an intra-aortic balloon pump, and emergency mitral valve surgery. Despite these treatments, mortality rate remains high.

Ventricular Septal Rupture

Prior to the use of reperfusion therapy, ventricular septal rupture occurred in approximately 2% of acute infarctions and probably accounted for 10% of cardiac ruptures.[159] However, the incidence of ventricular septal rupture was only 0.2% among patients who received fibrinolytic therapy in the GUSTO-1 trial. Sixty-seven percent of the patients with ventricular septal rupture in the GUSTO-1 trial developed cardiogenic shock. The mean time from onset of MI to ventricular septal rupture was approximately 1 day.[160] Septal rupture is seen with equal frequency in anterior and nonanterior infarctions. Clinical manifestations include chest pain, hypotension, dyspnea, and a harsh holosystolic murmur. The diagnosis is made by 2-D echocardiography with color Doppler imaging and/or insertion of a pulmonary artery balloon catheter to document a left-to-right shunt. Vasodilators, inotropic agents, and an intra-aortic balloon pump are used to initially stabilize the patient, but surgical repair portends the greatest survival benefit. In the GUSTO-1 trial surgical repair was performed at a median of 3.5 days after the onset of MI. Patients selected for surgery had better outcomes than patients treated medically (n = 35; 30-day mortality rate, 47% versus 94%).[160] However, it might be reasonable to delay surgery in patients who are hemodynamically stable without evidence of cardiogenic shock.

Left Ventricular Free Wall Rupture

Rupture of the left ventricular free wall may manifest in any of several ways: pericardial tamponade with acute hemodynamic collapse and immediate death, gradual onset of tamponade and hypotension, or subacute formation of a pseudoaneurysm with recurrent chest discomfort.[161] Risk factors for LV free wall myocardial rupture include anterior location of the infarction, a large transmural MI, absence of collateral blood flow, age older than 70 years, and female gender.[162,163] Rupture usually occurs between 5 days and 2 weeks after acute MI, and most often occurs in the anterior or lateral LV wall at the junction between normal and infarcted myocardium. The incidence of rupture among a series of 1378 patients was 3.3% among patients treated with fibrinolytic therapy and 1.8% among patients treated with PCI.[163] The goal of therapy is to stabilize the patient with fluids, inotropic support, vasopressors, pericardiocentesis, and an intra-aortic balloon pump until surgical repair is feasible.

 A 39-year-old male smoker was admitted to the neurology ICU with a subarachnoid hemorrhage. An admission ECG showed diffuse ST-segment depression, T-wave flattening, and QT prolongation.

What is your next step in the management of this patient?

ECG changes in the acute phase of subarachnoid hemorrhage (SAH), cerebral infarction, and intracerebral hemorrhage have been reported. Abnormal ECG findings include ST-segment elevation and depression, T-wave inversions and flattening, repolarization abnormalities, and QT prolongation. ECG changes that appear ischemic such as ST-segment depressions or T-wave inversions can occur in patients with and without underlying coronary artery disease. A systematic review of ECG changes in patients with acute stroke published in 2002 reviewed 29 observational, experimental, prospective, and retrospective studies. The studies were extremely heterogeneous. Patient populations were categorized as having "known heart disease" and "no known heart disease," terms that were loosely defined across studies. Details regarding ECG interpretation were vague. However, the incidence of ST-segment elevation in patients with SAH and no known heart disease was 31%; 35% had ST-segment depression, 19% had T-wave inversions, 27% had unspecified ST-segment or T-wave changes, and 4% had pathologic Q waves. There were very limited data regarding ECG changes in patients with ICH, cerebral infarction, or transient ischemic attack.[164] A descriptive study that confirmed SAH by CT scan found that 55% of patients had either T-wave inversions or T-wave flattening, despite no detectable cardiac abnormalities at autopsy.[165] When interpreting ECG changes in acute stroke patients, age, cardiac history, and ancillary data such as cardiac biomarkers are crucial in distinguishing a true ischemic event from neurogenic-mediated cardiac damage.

Is there a relationship between ECG abnormalities and early mortality in patients with ischemic stroke with no history or evidence of heart disease?

Very few studies have reported on this possible correlation. One small prospective study published in 2004 followed 162 patients (mean age: 62.4 ± 14 years) for 4 weeks after a first ischemic stroke was confirmed by CT.[166] A detailed medical history and clinical information were obtained from each patient. During the 4-week follow-up period, 44 of 162 patients died. Clinical characteristics and ECG changes were compared in survivors and nonsurvivors. Patients were excluded if they had any signs or symptoms of coronary artery disease; use of cardiac drugs; cerebral infarction due to cardiac embolism, SAH, or ICH; cerebral tumors; left ventricular hypertrophy; or left bundle branch block or right bundle branch block on ECG. ECGs were interpreted by a cardiologist who was blinded to the study. Sixty-five percent of all patients had ischemic-like ECG changes. Survivors had a significantly lower frequency of ischemic-like ECG changes when compared with nonsurvivors (60% versus 77%; $P = .044$). Thirty-three percent of survivors and 61% of nonsurvivors had ST-segment depression or ST-segment elevation ($P = .001$). By univariate analysis, predictors of early mortality were advanced age ($P = .01$), presence of ST-segment changes ($P = .001$), and abnormal U waves ($P = .03$). Multivariate analysis showed that age older than 65 years and presence of ST-segment changes were the only significant predictors for early mortality.[166] Although these data suggest that ischemic-like ECG changes are independent predictors of mortality, the results are difficult to interpret because no effort was made to diagnose asymptomatic coronary artery disease. Interestingly, 33% of patients had atrial fibrillation (AF), but the presence of AF had no predictive value for mortality. Previous studies have shown that AF and conduction defects are associated with threefold and fivefold increases in mortality in patients with cerebrovascular events.[167]

Christensen et al studied the admission ECGs of 1070 patients with cerebral infarction (n = 692), ICH (n = 155), or transient ischemic attack (n = 223) and followed them for 3 months. In multivariate analyses, 3-month mortality in patients with ischemic stroke was predicted by atrial fibrillation (OR: 2.0; 95% CI: 1.3-3.1), atrioventricular block (OR: 1.9; 95% CI: 1.2-3.9), ST-segment elevation (OR: 2.8; 95% CI: 1.3-6.3), ST-segment depression (OR: 2.5; 95% CI: 1.5-4.3), and inverted T waves (OR: 2.7; 95% CI: 1.6-4.6). These findings were independent of age or stroke severity.[168]

Cardiovascular Problems

! CRITICAL CONSIDERATIONS

- The ACSs—UA, NSTEMI, and STEMI—all share a common pathophysiology: erosion or rupture of an atherosclerotic plaque that precipitates either nonocclusive or occlusive coronary artery thrombosis.

- A 12-lead ECG should be performed and interpreted immediately in patients complaining of chest pain. If the initial ECG is nondiagnostic and STEMI is strongly suspected, continuous monitoring or serial ECGs at 5- to 10-minute intervals should be performed.

- Right-sided ECG should be performed in patients who have inferior MI to screen for right ventricular infarct.

- Indications for fibrinolytics in patients with STEMI include (1) symptom onset within the previous 12 hours and ST elevation > 0.1 mV in at least two contiguous precordial leads or at least two adjacent leads or with a presumably new left bundle branch block.

- Fibrinolytic therapy should be given within 30 minutes of presentation.

- Intracranial hemorrhage should be ruled out in any patient with a change in neurologic status during or after fibrinolytic therapy.

- Nitrates can be used for relief of ischemic chest pain, but they have no proven mortality benefit.

- Aspirin has a proven mortality benefit in patients with ACS and should be administered at a dose of 162 to 325 mg chewed.

- Clopidogrel in addition to aspirin has been shown to improve angiographic and clinical outcomes in patients with STEMI, NSTEMI, or UA. A loading dose of 300 or 600 mg should be administered to patients with STEMI, NSTEMI, or UA.

- A meta-analysis of 23 randomized trials concluded that the rates of short-term death, nonfatal reinfarction, stroke, and the combined end point of all three were lower for primary coronary intervention than for fibrinolytic therapy in patients with STEMI.

- Primary percutaneous coronary intervention is the preferred method of revascularization in patients with STEMI under the following circumstances: the diagnosis of STEMI is uncertain; fibrinolysis is contraindicated; the door-to-balloon time can be achieved in < 90 minutes and the difference between the door-to-balloon time and door-to-needle time is < 60 minutes; and the patient is in Killip class III or IV (pulmonary edema or cardiogenic shock).

- In patients with acute MI, early administration of β blockers reduces the rate of reinfarction and chronic administration improves survival. However, β blockers should not be administered to patients who are hypotensive or with other signs of shock.

- Diltiazem and verapamil are contraindicated in patients with STEMI and associated systolic left ventricular dysfunction and CHF.

- An early invasive strategy (coronary angiography with possible PTCA) is favored in patients with unstable angina or NSTEMI who have any of the following high-risk indicators: recurrent angina or ischemia despite intensive anti-ischemic therapy; elevated troponin levels; new or presumably new ST-segment depression; recurrent angina or ischemia with CHF or new or worsening mitral regurgitation; a high-risk noninvasive stress test; left ventricular ejection fraction < 40%; hemodynamic instability; sustained ventricular tachycardia; PCI within the past 6 months; and prior CABG surgery.

- Echocardiography is not useful in diagnosing ACS in patients with chest pain. However, it is essential in diagnosing mechanical complications of acute MI.
- Elevated serum cardiac biomarkers and ST-segment elevation and/or depression can occur in the absence of ACS.
- Postmyocardial complications include cardiogenic shock, CHF, left ventricular free wall rupture, ventricular septal rupture, ischemic mitral regurgitation, and papillary muscle rupture causing acute mitral regurgitation.
- ECG findings suggestive of ACS are often present in patients presenting with subarachnoid hemorrhage, cerebral infarction, and intracerebral hemorrhage even in the absence of underlying coronary artery disease.

REFERENCES

1. Matetzky S, Freimark D, Feinberg MS, et al. Acute myocardial infarction with isolated ST-segment elevation in posterior chest leads V_{7-9}. *J Am Coll Cardiol.* 1999;34:748-753.

2. Matetzky S, Freimark D, Chouraqui P, et al. The significance of ST-segment elevations in posterior chest leads (V_7–V_9) in patients with acute inferior myocardial infarction: application for thrombolytic therapy. *J Am Coll Cardiol.* 1998;31:506-511.

3. Herrick JB. Clinical features of sudden obstruction of the coronary arteries. *JAMA.* 1912;59:2015-2002.

4. Ward MR, Pasterkamp G, Yeung AC, et al. Arterial remodeling: mechanisms and clinical implications. *Circulation.* 2000;102:1186-1191.

5. Falk E. Stable versus unstable atherosclerosis: clinical aspects. *Am Heart J.* 1999;138:S421-S425.

6. Davies MJ. The pathophysiology of acute coronary syndromes. *Heart.* 2000;83:361-366.

7. Ni M, Chen WQ, Zhang Y. Animal models and potential mechanisms of plaque destabilisation and disruption. *Heart.* 2009;95(17):1393-1398.

8. Falk E, Shah PK, Fuster V. Coronary plaque disruption. *Circulation.* 1995;92(3):657-671.

9. Schaar JA, Muller JE, Falk E, et al. Terminology for high-risk and vulnerable coronary artery plaques. Report of a meeting on the vulnerable plaque, June 17 and 18, 2003, Santorini, Greece. *Eur Heart J.* 2004;25:1077-1082.

10. Virmani R, Burke AP, Farb A, et al. Pathology of the unstable plaque. *Prog Cardiovasc Dis.* 2002;44(5):349-356.

11. Richardson PD, Davies MJ, Born GVR. Influence of plaque configuration and stress distribution on fissuring of coronary atherosclerotic plaques. *Lancet.* 1989;2:941-944.

12. Ambrose JA, Winters SL, Arora RR, et al. Angiographic evolution of coronary artery morphology in unstable angina. *J Am Coll Cardiol.* 1986;7:472-478.

13. Ambrose JA, Tannenbaum, MA, Alexopoulos D, et al. Angiographic progression of coronary artery disease and the development of myocardial infarction. *J Am Coll Cardiol.* 1988;12:56-62.

14. Little WC, Constantinescu M, Applegate RJ, et al. Can coronary angiography predict the site of a subsequent myocardial infarction in patients with mild-to-moderate coronary artery disease? *Circulation.* 1988;78:1157-1166.

15. Giroud D, Li JM, Urban P, et al. Relation of the site of acute myocardial infarction to the most severe coronary arterial stenosis at prior angiography. *Am J Cardiol.* 1992;69:729-732.

16. Casscells W. Vulnerable atherosclerotic plaque: a multifocal disease. *Circulation.* 2003;107(16):2072-2075.

17. Goldstein JA, Demetriou D, Grines CL et al. Multiple complex coronary plaques in patients with acute myocardial infarction. *N Engl J Med.* 2000;343:915-922.

18. Mann J, Davies MJ. Mechanisms of progression in native coronary artery disease: role of healed plaque disruption. *Heart.* 1999;82:265-268.

19. Fuster V, Lewis A. Conner Memorial Lecture: mechanisms leading to myocardial infarction: insights from studies of vascular biology. *Circulation.* 1994;90:2126-2146.

20. Danchin N. Is myocardial revascularisation for tight coronary stenoses always necessary? *Lancet.* 1993;342:224-225.

21. Master AM. The role of effort and occupation (including physicians) in coronary occlusion. *JAMA.* 1960;174:942-948.

22. Strike PC, Perkins-Porras L, Whitehead DL, et al. Triggering of acute coronary syndromes by physical exertion and anger: clinical and sociodemographic characteristics. *Heart.* 2006;92:1035-1040.

23. Muller JE, Tofler GH, Stone PH. Circadian variation and triggers of onset of acute coronary cardiovascular disease. *Circulation.* 1989;79:733-743.

24. Heusch G, Baumgart D, Camici P, et al. α-Adrenergic coronary vasoconstriction and myocardial ischemia in humans. *Circulation.* 2000;101:689-693.

25. Nabel EG, Ganz P, Gordon JB, et al. Dilation of normal and constriction of atherosclerotic coronary arteries caused by the cold pressor test. *Circulation.* 1988;77:43-52.

26. Zeiher AM, Drexler H, Wollschläger H, et al. Endothelial dysfunction of the coronary microvasculature is associated with impaired coronary blood flow regulation in patients with early atherosclerosis. *Circulation.* 1991;84:1-10.

27. Zeiher AM, Krause T, Schächinger V, et al. Impaired endothelium-dependent vasodilation of coronary resistance vessels is associated with exercise-induced myocardial ischemia. *Circulation.* 1995;91:2345-2352.

28. Braunwald E. Unstable angina: an etiologic approach to management [editorial]. *Circulation.* 1998;98:2219-2222.

29. Tsuchihashi K, Ueshima K, Uchida T, et al. Transient left ventricular apical ballooning without coronary artery stenosis: a novel heart syndrome mimicking acute myocardial infarction. Angina pectoris-myocardial infarction investigations in Japan. *J Am Coll Cardiol.* 2001;38:11-18.

30. Wittstein IS, Thiamann DR, Lima JA, et al. Neurohumoral features of myocardial stunning due to sudden emotional stress. *N Engl J Med.* 2005;352:539-548.

31. Prizel KR, Hutchins GM, Bulkley BH. Coronary artery embolism and myocardial infarction. *Ann Intern Med.* 1978;88:155-161.

32. Minor RL Jr, Scott BD, Brown DD, et al. Cocaine induced myocardial infarction in patients with normal coronary arteries. *Ann Intern Med.* 1991;115:797-806.

33. Borczuk AC, van Hoeven KH, Factor SM. Review and hypothesis: the eosinophil and peripartum heart disease (myocarditis and coronary artery dissection)—coincidence or pathogenetic significance? *Cardiovasc Res.* 1997;33:527-532.

34. Cannon CP, Braunwald E. Unstable angina and non-ST elevation myocardial infarction. In: Libby P, Bonow RO, Mann DL, Zipes DP, eds. *Braunwald's Heart Disease.* 8th ed. Philadelphia, PA: Saunders Elsevier; 2008:1319-1351.

35. Egashira K, Katsuda Y, Mohri M, et al. Basal release of endothelium-derived nitric oxide at site of spasm in patients with variant angina. *J Am Coll Cardiol.* 1996;27:1444-1449.

36. Nakano T, Osanai T, Yomita H, et al. Enhanced activity of variant phospholipase C-1 protein (R257H) detected in patients with coronary artery spasm. *Circulation.* 2002;105:2024-2029.

37. Stern S, Bayes de Luna A. Coronary artery spasm: a 2009 update. *Circulation.* 2009;119(18):231-234.

38. Swap CJ, Nagurney JT. Value and limitations of chest pain history in the evaluation of patients with suspected acute coronary syndromes. *JAMA.* 2005;294:2623-2639.

39. Canto JG, Shlipak MG, Rogers WJ, et al. Prevalence, clinical characteristics, and mortality among patients with myocardial infarction presenting without chest pain. *JAMA.* 2000;283:3223-3322.

40. Antam EM, Anbe DT, Armstrong PW, et al. ACC/AHA guidelines for the management of patients with ST-elevation myocardial infarction: a report of the American College of Cardiology/American Heart Association Task Force on Practice Guidelines (Committee to Revise the 1999 Guidelines for the Management of Patients with Acute Myocardial Infarction). *Circulation.* 2004;110:e82-e292.

41. Elek R, Herman LM, Griffith GC. A study of unipolar left back leads and their application to posterior myocardial infarction. *Circulation.* 1953;7:656-668.

42. Berry C, Zalewski A, Kovach R, et al. Surface electrocardiogram in the detection of transmural myocardial ischemia during coronary artery occlusion. *Am J Cardiol.* 1989;63:21-26.

43. Huey BL, Beller GA, Kaiser DL, et al. A comprehensive analysis of myocardial infarction due to left circumflex artery occlusion: comparison with infarction due to right coronary artery and left anterior descending artery occlusion. *J Am Coll Cardiol.* 1988;12:1156-1166.

44. Bayés de Luna A, Wagner G, Birnbaum Y, et al. A new terminology for the left ventricular walls and for the location of myocardial infarcts that present Q wave based on the standard of cardiac magnetic resonance imaging. A statement for healthcare professionals from a committee appointed by the International Society for Holter and Noninvasive Electrocardiography. *Circulation.* 2006;114:1755-1760.

45. Lopez-Sendon J, Coma-Canella I, Alcasena S, Seoane J, Gamallo C. Electrocardiographic findings in acute right ventricular infarction: sensitivity and specificity of electrocardiographic alterations in right precordial leads V4R, V3R, V1, V2 and V3. *J Am Coll Cardiol.* 1985;6:1273-1279.

46. O'Keefe JH, Hammill SC, Freed MS, et al, eds. *The Complete Guide to ECGs: A Comprehensive Study Guide to Improve ECG Interpretation Skills.* 2nd ed. Royal Oak, MI: Physician's Press; 2002.

47. Goldberger AL. Basic ECG waves. In: Golderberg AL, ed. *Clinical Electrocardiography: A Simplified Approach.* 7th ed. Philadelphia, PA: Mosby.; 2006.

48. Wagner GS, Lim TH. Myocardial ischemia, injury, and infarction. In: Wagner GS, Gibert M, Haisty WK, Lim TH, Marriott HJL, Wang TY, eds. *Marriott's Practical Electrocardiography.* 8th ed. Baltimore, MD: Williams & Wilkins; 1994:145-149.

49. Douglas PS, Khandheria, B, Stainback RF, et al. ACCF/ASE/ACEP/ASNC/SCAI/SCCT/SCMR 2007 appropriateness criteria for transthoracic and transesophageal echocardiography: a report of the American College of Cardiology Foundation Quality Strategic Directions Committee Appropriateness Criteria Working Group, American Society of Echocardiography, American College of Emergency Physicians, American Society of Nuclear Cardiology, Society for Cardiovascular Angiography and Interventions, Society of Cardiovascular Computed Tomography, and the Society for Cardiovascular Magnetic Resonance endorsed by the American College of Chest Physicians and the Society of Critical Care Medicine. *J Am Coll Cardiol.* 2007;50:187-204.

50. Feinberg MS, Schwammenthal E, Shlizerman L, et al. Prognostic significance of mild mitral regurgitation by color Doppler echocardiography in acute myocardial infarction. *Am J Cardiol.* 2000;86:903-907.

51. Burst F, Enriquez-Saarano M, Nkomo VT, et al. Heart failure and death after myocardial infarction in the community: the emerging role of mitral regurgitation. *Circulation.* 2005;111:295-301.

52. Apple FS, Wu AHB, Jaffe AS. European Society of Cardiology and American College of Cardiology guidelines for redefinition of myocardial infarction: how to use existing assays clinically and for clinical trials. *Am Heart J.* 2002;144:981-986.

53. Babuin L, Jaffe AS. Troponin: the biomarker of choice for the detection of cardiac injury. *CMAJ.* 2005;173:1191-1202.

54. Thygesen K, Alpert JS, White HD, et al. Universal definition of myocardial infarction. *Circulation.* 2007;116:2634-2653.

55. Luepker RV, Apple FS, Christenson RH, et al. Case definitions for acute coronary heart disease in epidemiology and clinical research studies: a statement from the AHA Council on Epidemiology and Prevention; AHA Statistics Committee; World Heart Federation Council on Epidemiology and Prevention; the European Society of Cardiology Working Group on Epidemiology and Prevention; Centers for Disease Control and Prevention; and the National Heart, Lung, and Blood Institute. *Circulation.* 2003;108:2543-2549.

56. James S, Armstrong P, Califf R. Troponin T levels and risk of 30-day outcomes in patients with the acute coronary syndrome: prospective verification in the GUSTO-IV trial. *Am J Med.* 2003;115:178-184.

57. Januzzi JL Jr, Snapinn SM, DiBattiste PM, Jang IK, Theroux P. Benefits and safety of tirofiban among acute coronary syndrome patients with mild to moderate renal insufficiency: results from the Platelet Receptor Inhibition in Ischemic Syndrome Management in Patients Limited by Unstable Signs and Symptoms (PRISM-PLUS) trial. *Circulation.* 2002;105:2361-2366.

58. Januzzi JL, Cannon CP, DiBattiste PM, Murphy S, Weintraub W, Braunwald E. Effects of renal insufficiency on early invasive management in patients with acute coronary syndromes (the TACTICS-TIMI 18 trial). *Am J Cardiol.* 2002;90:1246-1249.

59. Anderson JL, Adams CD, Antam EM, et al. ACC/AHA 2007 guidelines for the management of patients with unstable angina/non-ST-elevation myocardial infarction: a report of the American College of Cardiology/American Heart Association Task Force on Practice Guidelines. *J Am Coll Cardiol.* 2007;50:e1-e157.

60. Van Werkum JW, Heestermans AA, Zomer AC, et al. Predictors of coronary stent thrombosis: the Dutch Stent Thrombosis Registry. *J Am Coll Cardiol.* 2009;53(16):1399-1409.

61. Aoki J, Lansky AJ, Mehran R, et al. Early stent thrombosis in patients with acute coronary syndromes treated with drug-eluting and bare metal stents: the Acute Catheterization and Urgent Intervention Triage Strategy trial. *Circulation.* 2009;119:687.

62. Chechi T, Vecchio S, Vittori G, et al. ST-segment elevation myocardial infarction due to early and late stent thrombosis a new group of high-risk patients. *J Am Coll Cardiol.* 2008;51(25):2396-2402.

63. de la Torre-Hernandez JM, Alfonso F, Hernandez F, et al. Drug-eluting stent thrombosis: results from the multicenter Spanish registry ESTROFA (Estudio ESpanol sobre TROmbosis de stents FArmacoactivos). *J Am Coll Cardiol.* 2008;51(10):986-990.

64. Rawles JM, Kenmure AC. Controlled trial of oxygen in uncomplicated myocardial infarction. *BMJ.* 1976;1:1121-1123.

65. Meine TJ, Roe MT, Chen AY, et al. Association of intravenous morphine use and outcomes in acute coronary syndromes: results from the CRUSADE

Quality Improvement Initiative. *Am Heart J.* 2005;149(6):1043-1049.

66. Cheitlin MD, Hutter AM Jr, Brindis RG, et al. ACC/AHA expert consensus document. Use of sildenafil (Viagra) in patients with cardiovascular disease. American College of Cardiology/ American Heart Association. *J Am Coll Cardiol.* 1999;33:273-282.

67. Come PC, Pitt B. Nitroglycerin-induced severe hypotension and bradycardia in patients with acute myocardial infarction. *Circulation.* 1976;54: 624-628.

68. ISIS-4 (Fourth International Study of Infarct Survival) Collaborative Group. ISIS-4: a randomised factorial trial assessing early oral captopril, oral mononitrate, and intravenous magnesium sulphate in 58,050 patients with suspected acute myocardial infarction. *Lancet.* 1995;345:669-685.

69. GISSI-3. Effects of lisinopril and transdermal glycerol trinitrate singly and together on 6-week mortality and ventricular function after AMI. Gruppo Italiano per lo Studio della Sopravvivenza nell' infarto Miocardico. *Lancet.* 1994;343:1115-1122.

70. ISIS 2 Collaborative Group. Randomised trial of intravenous streptokinase, oral aspirin, both, or neither among 17,187 cases of suspected acute myocardial infarction: ISIS-2. *Lancet* 1988;2:349-360.

71. Lewis HD Jr, Davis JW, Archibald DG, et al. Protective effects of aspirin against acute myocardial infarction and death in men with unstable angina. Results of a Veterans Administration Cooperative Study. *N Engl J Med.* 1983;309(7):396-403.

72. Antiplatelet Trialists' Collaboration. Collaborative overview of randomised trials of antiplatelet therapy: I. Prevention of death, myocardial infarction, and stroke by prolonged antiplatelet therapy in various categories of patients. *BMJ.* 1994;308:81-106.

73. Yusuf S, Wittes J, Friedman L. Overview of results of randomized clinical trials in heart disease. Treatment following myocardial infarction. *JAMA.* 1988;260:2088-2093.

74. Roberts R, Rogers WJ, Mueller HS, et al. Immediate versus deferred beta-blockade following thrombolytic therapy in patients with acute myocardial infarction. Results of the Thrombolysis in Myocardial Infarction (TIMI) II-B Study. *Circulation.* 1991;83:422-437.

75. Pfisterer M, Cox JL, Granger CB, et al. Atenolol use and clinical outcomes after thrombolysis for acute myocardial infarction: the GUSTO-I experience. Global Utilization of Streptokinase and TPA (alteplase) for Occluded Coronary Arteries. *J Am Coll Cardiol.* 1998;32:634-640.

76. Chen ZM, Pan HC, Chen YP, et al. COMMIT (ClOpidogrel and Metoprolol in Myocardial Infarction Trial) Collaborative Group. Early intravenous then oral metoprolol in 45,852 patients with acute myocardial infarction: randomised placebo-controlled trial. *Lancet.* 2005;366:1622-1632.

77. Antman EM, Hand M, Armstrong PW, et al. 2007 Focused update on the ACC/AHA 2004 guidelines for the management of patients with ST-elevation myocardial infarction. *J Am Coll Cardiol.* 2008;(51):210-247.

78. Dargie HJ. Effect of carvedilol on outcome after myocardial infarction in patients with left-ventricular dysfunction: the CAPRICORN randomised trial. *Lancet.* 2001;537:1385-1390.

79. Held P, Yusof S, Furberg C. Calcium channel blockers in acute myocardial infarction and unstable angina: an overview. *BMJ.* 1989;299:1187-1192.

80. Yusuf S, Wittes J, Friedman L. Overview of results of randomized clinical trials in heart disease. II. Unstable angina, heart failure, primary prevention with aspirin, and risk factor modification. *JAMA.* 1988;260:2259-2263.

81. Kushner FG, Hand M, Smith SC, et al. 2009 Focused updates: ACC/AHA guidelines for the management of patients with ST-elevation myocardial infarction (updating the 2004 guideline and 2007 focused update) and ACC/AHA/SCAI guidelines on percutaneous coronary intervention (updating the 2005 guideline and 2007 focused update): a report of the American College of Cardiology Foundation/American Heart Association Task Force on Practice Guidelines. *Circulation.* 2009;120:2271-2306.

82. Schroder R, Dissmann R, Bruggemann T, et al. Extent of early ST segment elevation resolution: a simple but strong predictor of outcome in patients with acute myocardial infarction. *J Am Coll Cardiol.* 1994;24:384-391.

83. Anderson DR, White HD, Ohman ME, et al. Predicting outcome after thrombolysis in acute myocardial infarction according to ST-segment resolution at 90 minutes: a substudy of the GUSTO III trial. *Am Heart J.* 2002;144:81-88.

84. Armstrong PW, Collen D, Antman E. Fibrinolysis for acute myocardial infarction: the future is here and now. *Circulation.* 2003;107:2533-2537.

85. Effectiveness of intravenous thrombolytic treatment in acute myocardial infarction. Gruppo Italiano per lo Studio della Sopravvivenza nell' infarto Miocardico (GISSI). *Lancet.* 1986;1:397-402.

86. Anderson HV, Willerson JT. Thrombolysis in acute myocardial infarction. *N Engl J Med.* 1993; 329:703.

87. GISSI-2: a factorial randomised trial of alteplase versus streptokinase and heparin versus no heparin among 12,490 patients with acute myocardial infarction. Gruppo Italiano per lo Studio della Sopravvivenza nell'Infarto Miocardico. *Lancet.* 1990;336(8707):65-71.

88. ISIS-3 (Third International Study of Infarct Survival) Collaborative Group. ISIS-3: a randomised comparison of streptokinase vs tissue plasminogen activator vs anistreplase and of aspirin plus heparin vs aspirin alone among 41,299 cases of suspected acute myocardial infarction. *Lancet.* 1992;339(8796):753-770.

89. The GUSTO Investigators. An international randomized trial comparing four thrombolytic strategies for acute myocardial infarction. *N Engl J Med.* 1993;329(10):673-682.

90. Gore JM, Granger CB, Simoons ML, et al. Stroke after thrombolysis. Mortality and functional outcomes in the GUSTO-I trial. Global Use of Strategies to Open Occluded Coronary Arteries. *Circulation.* 1995;92(10):2811-2818.

91. The Global Use of Strategies to Open Occluded Coronary Arteries (GUSTO III) Investigators. A comparison of reteplase with alteplase for acute myocardial infarction. *N Engl J Med.* 1997;337(16):1118-1123.

92. Topol EJ, Ohman EM, Armstrong PW, et al. Survival outcomes 1 year after reperfusion therapy with either alteplase or reteplase for acute myocardial infarction: results from the Global Utilization of Streptokinase and t-PA for Occluded Coronary Arteries (GUSTO) III Trial. *Circulation.* 2000;102(15):1761-1765.

93. ASSENT-2 Investigators. Single-bolus tenecteplase compared with front-loaded alteplase in acute myocardial infarction: the ASSENT-2 double-blind randomised trial. *Lancet.* 1999;354:716-722.

94. Boersma E, Maas AC, Deckers JW, et al. Early thrombolytic treatment in acute myocardial infarction: reappraisal of the golden hour. *Lancet.* 1996;348:771-775.

95. LATE Study Group. Late assessment of fibrinolytic efficacy (LATE) study with alteplase 6-24 hours after onset of acute myocardial infarction. *Lancet.* 1993;324:759-766.

96. Estuido Multicentrico Estrepoquinasa Republicass de Americas del Sur (EMERAS). Randomized trial of late thrombolytics in patients with suspected acute myocardial infarction. *Lancet.* 1993;342:767-772.

97. Fibrinolytic Therapy Trialist's (FTT) Collaborative Group. Indications for fibrinolytic therapy in suspected acute myocardial infarction: collaborative overview of early mortality and major morbidity results from all randomized trials of more than 1000 patients. *Lancet.* 1994;343:311-322.

98. Crenshaw BS, Granger CB, Birnbaum Y, et al. Risk factors, angiographic patterns, and outcomes in patients with ventricular septal defect complicating acute myocardial infarction. GUSTO-I (Global Utilization of Streptokinase and TPA for Occluded Coronary Arteries) Trial Investigators. *Circulation.* 2000;101(1):27-32.

99. Gurwitz JH, Gore JM, Goldberg RJ, et al. Risk for intracranial hemorrhage after tissue plasminogen activator treatment for acute myocardial infarction. Participants in the National Registry of Myocardial infarction 2. *Ann Intern Med.* 1998;129:597-604.

100. Brass LM, Lichtman JH, Wang Y, Gurwitz JH, Radford MJ, Krumholz HM. Intracranial hemorrhage associated with thrombolytic therapy for elderly patients with acute myocardial infarction: results from the Cooperative Cardiovascular Project. *Stroke* 2000;31:1802-1811.

101. Simoons ML, Maggioni AP, Knatterud G, et al. Individual risk assessment for intracranial hemorrhage during thrombolytic therapy. *Lancet.* 1993;342:1523-1528.

102. Sloan MA, Guigliano RP, Thompson SL. Prediction of intracranial hemorrhage in the InTIME-II trial. *J Am Coll Cardiol.* 2001;37:372-384.

103. The TIMI Study Group. The Thrombolysis in Myocardial Infarction (TIMI) trial: phase I findings. *N Engl J Med.* 1985;312:932-936.

104. The GUSTO Angiographic Investigators. The effects of tissue plasminogen activator, streptokinase, or both on coronary-artery patency, ventricular function, and survival after acute myocardial infarction. *N Engl J Med.* 1994;330:516.

105. Braunwald E. The open-artery theory is alive and well—again. *N Engl J Med.* 1993;329:1650-1652.

106. Mehilli J, Kastrati A, Schulz S, et al. Abciximab in patients with acute ST-segment-elevation myocardial infarction undergoing primary percutaneous coronary intervention after clopidogrel loading: a randomized double-blind trial. *Circulation.* 2009;119:1933-1940.

107. Van't Hof AW, Ten Berg J, Heestermans T, et al. Prehospital initiation of tirofiban in patients with ST-elevation myocardial infarction undergoing primary angioplasty (On-TIME 2): a multicentre, double-blind, randomised controlled trial. *Lancet.* 2008;372:537-546.

108. Stone GW, Witzenbichler B, Guagliumi G, et al. Bivalirudin during primary PCI in acute myocardial infarction. *N Engl J Med.* 2008;358:2218-2230.

109. (ClOpidogrel and Metoprolol in Myocardial Infarction Trial) Collaborative Group. Addition of clopidogrel to aspirin in 45,852 patients with acute myocardial infarction: randomised placebo-controlled trial. *Lancet.* 2005;366:1607-1621.

110. Keeley EC, Boura JA, Grines CL. Primary angioplasty versus intravenous thrombolytic therapy for acute myocardial infarction: a quantitative review of 23 randomised trials. *Lancet.* 2003;361:13-20.

111. Hochman JS, Sleeper LA, Webb JG, et al, for the Should We Emergently Revascularize Occluded Coronaries for Cardiogenic Shock (SHOCK) Investigators. Early revascularization in acute myocardial infarction complicated by cardiogenic shock. *N Engl J Med.* 1999;341:625-634.

112. Wu AH, Parsons L, Every NR, Bates ER, for the Second National Registry of Myocardial Infarction. Hospital outcomes in patients presenting with congestive heart failure complicating acute myocardial infarction: a report from the Second National Registry of Myocardial Infarction (NRMI-2). *J Am Coll Cardiol.* 2002;40:1389-1394.

113. Stone GW, Grines CL, Browne KF, et al. Influence of acute myocardial infarction location on in-hospital and late outcome after primary percutaneous transluminal coronary angioplasty versus tissue plasminogen activator therapy. *Am J Cardiol.* 1996;78:19-25.

114. Van't Hof AW, Henriques J, Ottervanger JP, et al. No mortality benefit of primary angioplasty over thrombolytic therapy in patients with nonanterior myocardial infarction at long-term follow-up: results of the Zwolle trial. *J Am Coll Cardiol.* 2003;41:369A.

115. Andersen HR, Nielsen TT, Rasmussen K, et al. A comparison of coronary angioplasty with fibrinolytic therapy in acute myocardial infarction. *N Engl J Med.* 2003;349(8):733-742.

116. Thune JJ, Hoefsten DE, Lindholm MG, et al. Simple risk stratification at admission to identify patients with reduced mortality from primary angioplasty. *Circulation.* 2005;112(13):2017-2021.

117. Busk M, Maeng M, Rasmussen K, et al. The Danish multicentre randomized study of fibrinolytic therapy vs primary angioplasty in acute myocardial infarction (the DANAMI-2 trial): outcome after 3 years follow-up. *Eur Heart J.* 2008;29(10):1259-1266.

118. Betriu A, Castaner A, Sanz GA, et al. Angiographic findings 1 month after myocardial infarction: a prospective study of 259 survivors. *Circulation.* 1982;65(6):1099-1105.

119. Schomig A, Mehilli J, Antoniucci D, et al. Mechanical reperfusion in patients with acute myocardial infarction presenting more than 12 hours from symptom onset: a randomized controlled trial. *JAMA.* 2005;293(23):2865-2872.

120. Hochman JS, Lamas GA, Buller CE, et al. Coronary intervention for persistent occlusion after myocardial infarction. *N Engl J Med.* 2006;355(23):2395-2407.

121. Steg PG, Thuaire C, Himbert D, et al. DECOPI (DEsobstruction COronaire en Post-Infarctus): a randomized multi-centre trial of occluded artery angioplasty after acute myocardial infarction. *Eur Heart J.* 2004;25(24):2187-2194.

122. Assessment of the Safety and Efficacy of a New Treatment Strategy with Percutaneous Coronary Intervention (ASSENT-4 PCI) Investigators. Primary versus tenecteplase-facilitated percutaneous coronary intervention in patients with ST-segment elevation acute myocardial infarction (ASSENT-4 PCI): randomised trial. *Lancet.* 2006;367:569-578.

123. Ellis SG, Tendera M, de Belder MA, et al. Facilitated PCI in patients with ST-elevation myocardial infarction. *N Engl J Med.* 2008;358(21):2205-2217.

124. Kastrati A, Mehilli J, Schlotterbeck K, et al. Early administration of reteplase plus abciximab vs abciximab alone in patients with acute myocardial infarction referred for percutaneous coronary intervention: a randomized controlled trial. *JAMA.* 2004;291(8):947-954.

125. Antman EM, Cohen M, Bernink PJ, et al. The TIMI risk score for unstable angina/non-ST elevation MI: a method for prognostication and therapeutic decision making. *JAMA.* 2000;284:835-842.

126. Cohen M, Demers C, Gurfinkel EP, et al. A comparison of low-molecular-weight heparin with unfractionated heparin for unstable coronary artery disease. Efficacy and Safety of Subcutaneous Enoxaparin in Non-Q-Wave Coronary Events Study Group. *N Engl J Med.* 1997;337:447-452.

127. Granger CB, Goldberg RJ, Dabbous O, et al. Predictors of hospital mortality in the global registry of acute coronary events. *Arch Intern Med.* 2003;163:2345-2353.

128. Eagle KA, Lim MJ, Dabbous OH, et al. A validated prediction model for all forms of acute coronary syndrome: estimating the risk of 6-month postdischarge death in an international registry. *JAMA.* 2004;291:2727-2733.

129. Boersma E, Pieper KS, Steyerberg EW, et al. Predictors of outcome in patients with acute coronary syndromes without persistent ST-segment elevation. Results from an international trial of 9461 patients. The PURSUIT Investigators. *Circulation.* 2000;101:2557-2567.

130. Menown IB, Mackenzie G, Adgey AA. Optimizing the initial 12-lead electrocardiographic diagnosis of acute myocardial infarction. *Eur Heart J.* 2000;21:275-283.

131. Invasive compared with non-invasive treatment in unstable coronary-artery disease: FRISC II prospective randomised multicentre study. FRagmin and Fast Revascularisation during InStability in Coronary artery disease Investigators. *Lancet.* 1999;354(9180):708-715.

132. Cannon CP, Weintraub WS, Demopoulos LA, et al. Comparison of early invasive and conservative strategies in patients with unstable coronary syndromes treated with the glycoprotein IIb/IIIa inhibitor tirofiban. *N Engl J Med.* 2001;344(25):1879-1887.

133. Fox KA, Poole-Wilson PA, Henderson RA, et al. Interventional versus conservative treatment for patients with unstable angina or non-ST-elevation myocardial infarction: the British Heart Foundation RITA 3 randomised trial. Randomized Intervention Trial of unstable Angina. *Lancet.* 2002;360(9335):743-751.

134. Hirsch A, Windhausen F, Tijssen JG, et al. Long-term outcome after an early invasive versus selective invasive treatment strategy in patients with non-ST-elevation acute coronary syndrome and elevated cardiac troponin T (the ICTUS trial): a follow-up study. *Lancet.* 2007;369(9564):827-835.

135. Mehta SR, Granger CB, Boden WE, et al, for the TIMACS Investigators. Early versus delayed invasive intervention in acute coronary syndromes. *N Engl J Med.* 2009;360:2165.

136. Yusuf S, Zhao F, Mehta SR, et al. Effects of clopidogrel in addition to aspirin in patients with acute coronary syndromes without ST-segment elevation. *N Eng J Med.* 2001;345(7):494-502.

137. Mehta SR, Yusuf S, Peters RJ, et al. Effects of pretreatment with clopidogrel and aspirin followed by long-term therapy in patients undergoing percutaneous coronary intervention: the PCI-CURE study. *Lancet.* 2001;358(9281):527-533.

138. Steinhubl SR, Berger PB, Mann JT 3rd, et al. Early and sustained dual oral antiplatelet therapy following percutaneous coronary intervention: a randomized controlled trial. *JAMA.* 2002;288:2411-2420.

139. Wiviott SD, Braunwald E, McCabe CH, et al. Prasugrel versus clopidogrel in patients with acute coronary syndromes. *N Engl J Med.* 2007;357(20):2001-2015.

140. Wallentin L, Becker RC, Budaj A, et al. Ticagrelor versus clopidogrel in patients with acute coronary syndromes. *N Engl J Med.* 2009;361:1045-1057.

141. Flores ED, Lange RA, Cigarroa RG, et al. Effect of cocaine on coronary artery dimensions in atherosclerotic coronary artery disease: enhanced vasoconstriction at sites of significant stenoses. *J Am Coll Cardiol.* 1990;16:74-79.

142. Lange RA, Cigarroa RG, Yancy CWJ, et al. Cocaine-induced coronary-artery vasoconstriction. *N Engl J Med.* 1989;321:1557-1562.

143. Zimmerman FH, Gustafson GM, Kemp HGJ. Recurrent myocardial infarction associated with cocaine abuse in a young man with normal coronary arteries: evidence for coronary artery spasm culminating in thrombosis. *J Am Coll Cardiol.* 1987;9:964-968.

144. Bedotto JB, Lee RW, Lancaster LD, et al. Cocaine and cardiovascular function in dogs: effects on heart and peripheral circulation. *J Am Coll Cardiol.* 1988;11:1337-1342.

145. Brogan WC, Lange RA, Kim AS, Moliterno DJ, Hillis LD. Alleviation of cocaine-induced coronary vasoconstriction by nitroglycerin. *J Am Coll Cardiol.* 1991;18:581-586.

146. Loper KA. Clinical toxicology of cocaine. *Med Toxicol Adverse Drug Exp.* 1989;4:174-185.

147. Togna G, Tempesta E, Togna AR, Dolci N, Cebo B, Caprino L. Platelet responsiveness and biosynthesis of thromboxane and prostacyclin in response to in vitro cocaine treatment. *Haemostasis.* 1985;15:100-107.

148. Stern S, Bayes de Luna A. Coronary artery spasm: a 2009 update. *Circulation.* 2009;119:2531-2534.

149. Fukai T, Koyanagi S, Takeshita A. Role of coronary vasospasm in the pathogenesis of myocardial infarction: study in patients with no significant coronary stenosis. *Am Heart J.* 1993;126:1305-1311.

150. MacAlpin RN. Cardiac arrest and sudden unexpected death in variant angina: complications of coronary spasm that can occur in the absence of severe organic coronary stenosis. *Am Heart J.* 1993;125:1011-1017.

151. Bybee KA, Kara T, Prasad A, et al. Systematic review: transient left ventricular apical ballooning: a syndrome that mimics ST-segment elevation myocardial infarction. *Ann Intern Med.* 2004;141(11):858-865.

152. Prasad A, Lerman A, Rihal CS. Apical ballooning syndrome (Tako-Tsubo or stress cardiomyopathy): a mimic of acute myocardial infarction. *Am Heart J.* 2008;155(3):408-417.

153. Gianni M, Dentali F, Grandi AM, et al. Apical ballooning syndrome or takotsubo cardiomyopathy: a systematic review. *Eur Heart J.* 2006;27:1523-1529.

154. Suchihashi K, Ueshima K, Uchida T, et al. Transient left ventricular apical ballooning without

coronary artery stenosis: a novel heart syndrome mimicking acute myocardial infarction. Angina Pectoris-Myocardial Infarction Investigations in Japan. *Am Coll Cardiol.* 2001;38(1):11-18.

155. Sharkey SW, Lesser JR, Zenovich AG. Acute and reversible cardiomyopathy provoked by stress in women from the United States. *Circulation.* 2005;111(4):472-479.

156. Akashi YJ, Goldstein DS, Barbaro G. Takotsubo cardiomyopathy: a new form of acute, reversible heart failure. *Circulation.* 2008;118:2754.

157. Lavie CJ, Gersh BJ. Mechanical and electrical complications of acute myocardial infarction. *Mayo Clin Proc.* 1990;65(5):709-730.

158. Pellizzon GG, Grines C, Cox DA, et al. Importance of mitral regurgitation in patients undergoing percutaneous coronary interventions for acute myocardial infarction: the Controlled Abciximab and Device Investigation to Lower Late Angioplasty Complications (CADILLAC) trial. *J Am Coll Cardiol.* 2004;43:1368-1374.

159. Reeder GS. Identification and treatment of complications of myocardial infarction. *Mayo Clin Proc.* 1995;70(9):880-884.

160. Crenshaw BS, Granger CB, Birnbaum Y, et al. Risk factors, angiographic patterns, and outcomes in patients with ventricular septal defect complicating acute myocardial infarction. GUSTO-I (Global Utilization of Streptokinase and TPA for Occluded Coronary Arteries) Trial Investigators. *Circulation.* 2000;101(1):27-32.

161. Raitt MH, Kraft CD, Gardner CJ, et al. Subacute ventricular free wall rupture complicating myocardial infarction. *Am Heart J.* 1993;126:946-955.

162. Becker RC, Hochman JS, Cannon CP, et al. Fatal cardiac rupture among patients treated with thrombolytic agents and adjunctive thrombin antagonists: observations from the Thrombolysis and Thrombin Inhibition in Myocardial Infarction 9 Study. *J Am Coll Cardiol.* 1999;33(2):479-487.

163. Moreno R, Lopez-Sendon J, Garcia E, et al. Primary angioplasty reduces the risk of left ventricular free wall rupture compared with thrombolysis in patients with acute myocardial infarction. *J Am Coll Cardiol.* 2002;39(4):598-603.

164. Khechinashvili G, Asplund K. Electrocardiographic changes in patients with acute stroke: a systematic review. *Cerebrovasc Dis.* 2002;14: 67-76.

165. Yamour BJ, Sridharan MR, Rice JF, et al. Electrocardiographic changes in cerebrovascular hemorrhage. *Am Heart J.* 1980;99(3):294-300.

166. Dogan A, Tunc M, Ozturk M. Electrocardiographic changes in patients with ischaemic stroke and their prognostic importance. *Int J Clin Pract.* 2004;58(5):436-440.

167. Dimant J, Grop D. Electrocardiographic changes and myocardial damage in patients with acute cerebrovascular accidents. *Stroke.* 1977;8:448-455.

168. Christensen H, Fogh Christensen A, Boysen G. Abnormalities on ECG and telemetry predict stroke outcome at 3 months. *J Neurol Sci.* 2005; 234:(1-2):99-103.

CHAPTER

32

Arrhythmias: Rhythm Disturbances in Critically Ill Patients

Tracy Walker, MD
Andrea M. Russo, MD

A variety of different rhythm disturbances may be seen in critically ill patients in an intensive care unit (ICU). These arrhythmias include supraventricular and ventricular tachyarrhythmias, which result from acute illness, electrolyte abnormalities, or drug use. Arrhythmias may also be preexisting and can be worsened by extrinsic factors or metabolic abnormalities in the acute setting. In addition, bradyarrhythmias may occur and may potentially be worsened by drugs or metabolic abnormalities. This chapter will review common types of bradyarrhythmias and tachyarrhythmias seen in the intensive care setting and offer diagnostic approaches and options for acute treatment.

 Bradyarrhythmias. A 78-year-old woman presents to the emergency room and is admitted to the ICU with complaints of dizziness and chest pain over the past week with mild right-side weakness noted on the morning of admission, which resolved prior to arrival at the hospital. Past medical history is remarkable for hypertension, hypothyroidism, paroxysmal atrial fibrillation, peptic ulcer disease, and coronary artery disease. Admission medications include Synthroid 25 µg daily, amiodarone 200 mg daily, metoprolol 50 mg twice daily, aspirin 81 mg daily, warfarin 5 mg daily, and isosorbide 60 mg daily. Vital signs on arrival include a heart rate of 40 bpm, blood pressure of 70/30 mm Hg, oral temperature of 37.1°C (98.7°F), pulse oximetry of 99% on room air, and respiratory rate of 16 breaths/min. The presenting rhythm is shown in Figure 32-1. Physical examination revealed an elderly diaphoretic woman in mild distress. Cardiac examination was remarkable for a non-displaced point of maximal impulse (PMI) with a bradycardic S_1 and S_2, which was physiologically split, with a II/VI systolic ejection murmur at the left upper sternal border. Lungs were clear to auscultation and percussion (A&P). Extremities were cool and clammy. Neurologic examination was remarkable for the absence of any weakness or other neurologic deficits.

What is the presenting rhythm?

The presenting rhythm is marked sinus bradycardia (Figure 32-1). Sinus bradycardia is defined as a heart rate less than 60 bpm. There is a P wave before every QRS complex with a constant PR interval. In this case, bradycardia may be related to medications, although underlying sinus node dysfunction cannot be excluded.

Cardiovascular Problems

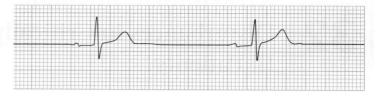

Figure 32-1. The presenting rhythm is sinus bradycardia in the 40s.

How are bradyarrhythmias classified?

Electrical activation of the heart originates in the sinoatrial (SA) node at a rate of 60 to 100 bpm. If the SA node fails to generate an impulse, a subsidiary pacemaker (the atrioventricular [AV] node) takes over but at a slower rate (typically < 60 bpm). Bradyarrhythmias are due to either failure of impulse formation in the SA node (sinus node dysfunction) or failure of impulse conduction out of the SA node through the AV node and His-Purkinje system. In the intensive care setting, the most common manifestation of sinus node dysfunction is sinus bradycardia, which may be associated with "brady-tachy syndrome." AV conduction abnormalities include first-degree AV block or delay, which represents slowing of conduction through the AV node and His-Purkinje system, as well as second- and third-degree AV block. The latter includes "dropped beats," described in more detail later.

What are potential causes of sinus bradycardia?

Sinus bradycardia can be a sign that the sinus node itself is dysfunctional. Sinus bradycardia can also be due to increased vagal tone, myocardial ischemia, an intracranial process (such as increased intracranial pressure, meningitis, or brain tumor), eye surgery, hypothermia, hypothyroidism, hypoxia, hyperkalemia, and some infectious diseases. Excessive vagal tone can occur with endotracheal suctioning, abdominal distention, vomiting, the Valsalva maneuver (straining), cervical or high thoracic spinal injuries, and pain. During sleep, heart rate can decrease to 35 to 40 bpm with pauses up to 2 seconds, which is not considered pathologic and does not necessarily require permanent pacing unless individuals also have symptomatic bradycardia while awake. Obstructive sleep apnea can also cause worsening bradycardia or promote pauses while individuals are asleep. Many drugs can also suppress the automaticity of the sinus node and slow the heart rate.

How would you treat this patient?

This patient is showing signs of hypoperfusion, and atropine can be used to increase the heart rate. If atropine fails to increase the heart rate, isoproterenol, transcutaneous pacing, or transvenous pacing can then be utilized. If transcutaneous pacing is needed in an urgent situation, sedation is required as this is a painful procedure. Permanent pacemaker implantation is recommended if symptomatic bradycardia persists without reversible causes. Symptoms may include lightheadedness, dizziness, presyncope, loss of consciousness, excessive fatigue, and hypotension. In this case, it is also feasible that hypotension may have led to transient cerebral hypoperfusion resulting in a transient neurologic deficit that resolved prior to arrival. Medications in this patient, including amiodarone and the β blocker, are likely contributing to bradycardia. Secondary causes of bradycardia, such as hypothyroidism, should also be excluded.

Permanent pacing may be indicated if bradycardia is the result of drug therapy considered necessary for the treatment of other disorders such as coronary artery disease or atrial arrhythmias. Indications for permanent pacing in the setting of sick sinus syndrome (SSS) are noted in Table 32-1.[1] In this case, antiarrhythmic therapy with amiodarone was necessary to treat atrial arrhythmias and β-blocker therapy was indicated for the treatment of atrial arrhythmias and coronary artery disease.

Table 32-1. Recommendations for Permanent Pacing in Sinus Node Dysfunction (SND)

CLASS I

1. Permanent pacemaker implantation is indicated for SND with documented symptomatic bradycardia, including frequent sinus pauses that produce symptoms *(level of evidence: C)*.

2. Permanent pacemaker implantation is indicated for symptomatic chronotropic incompetence *(level of evidence: C)*.

3. Permanent pacemaker implantation is indicated for symptomatic sinus bradycardia that results from required drug therapy for medical conditions *(level of evidence: C)*.

CLASS IIa

1. Permanent pacemaker implantation is reasonable for SND with heart rate < 40 bpm when a clear association between significant symptoms consistent with bradycardia and the actual presence of bradycardia has not been documented *(level of evidence: C)*.

2. Permanent pacemaker implantation is reasonable for syncope of unexplained origin when clinically significant abnormalities of sinus node function are discovered or provoked in electrophysiologic studies *(level of evidence: C)*.

CLASS IIb

1. Permanent pacemaker implantation may be considered in minimally symptomatic patients with chronic heart rate < 40 bpm while awake *(level of evidence: C)*.

CLASS III

1. Permanent pacemaker implantation is not indicated for SND in asymptomatic patients *(level of evidence: C)*.

2. Permanent pacemaker implantation is not indicated for SND in patients for whom the symptoms suggestive of bradycardia have been clearly documented to occur in the absence of bradycardia *(level of evidence: C)*.

3. Permanent pacemaker implantation is not indicated for SND with symptomatic bradycardia due to nonessential drug therapy *(level of evidence: C)*.

(Adapted from Epstein AC, DiMarco JP, Ellenbogen KA, et al. ACC/AHA/HRS 2008 guidelines for device-based therapy of cardiac rhythm abnormalities: a report of the American College of Cardiology/American Heart Association Task Force on Practice Guidelines [Writing Committee to Revise the ACC/AHA/NASPE 2002 Guideline Update for Implantation of Cardiac Pacemakers and Antiarrhythmia Devices]: developed in collaboration with the American Association for Thoracic Surgery and Society of Thoracic Surgeons. Circulation. 2008;117:e350-408.)

What is "brady-tachy syndrome"?

"Brady-tachy syndrome," also known as "sick sinus syndrome," is severe bradycardia associated with paroxysms of tachycardia, the latter of which most commonly include atrial fibrillation. After cessation of the tachycardia, there is typically a postconversion pause (Figure 32-2A). This pause may be prolonged, lasting several seconds, and may result in symptoms of lightheadedness, dizziness, fatigue, or loss of consciousness. Intermittent marked bradycardia or pauses may also occur during atrial fibrillation and can be symptomatic, requiring permanent pacing to allow continued treatment with AV nodal blocking drugs to control rapid rates during atrial fibrillation (Figure 32-2B).

How do you treat brady-tachy syndrome?

Patients with "brady-tachy syndrome" require that the tachycardia rate be controlled, and this is accomplished with AV nodal blocking drugs, which slow the ventricular response during atrial fibrillation. In addition, antiarrhythmic drugs to help maintain sinus rhythm may also be utilized, which will be discussed in a later section. However, medications utilized to control the rhythm may also worsen bradycardia and promote pauses. A permanent pacemaker is indicated in this situation to prevent worsening bradycardia. Indications for permanent pacing in the setting of SSS are noted in Table 32-1.[1]

Cardiovascular Problems

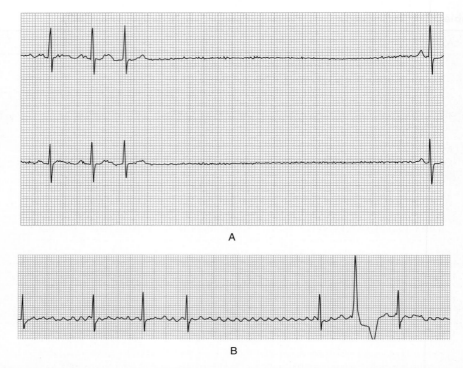

Figure 32-2. Sick sinus syndrome. **A.** Post-conversion pauses may occur, leading to symptoms including lightheadedness, presyncope, or loss of consciousness. A 4.3-second post-conversion pause is illustrated. **B.** Intermittent pauses during atrial fibrillation may also occur, and this may require permanent pacing to allow treatment of rapid rates during atrial fibrillation with atrioventricular nodal blocking therapy.

What are electrocardiographic manifestations of first-, second-, and third-degree AV block?

First-degree AV block is defined as a fixed prolongation of the PR interval to greater than 200 milliseconds. This represents prolonged conduction, without any dropped beats (Figure 32-3).

Second-degree AV block is classified as either Mobitz type I (Wenckebach) or Mobitz type II. In Mobitz type I AV block, the PR interval progressively prolongs prior to the occurrence of a P wave that does not conduct to the ventricles ("dropped beat") (Figure 32-4). The QRS complex is often narrow but may also be wide with preexisting underlying bundle branch block. The R-R intervals prior to the pause progressively shorten. The R-R interval after the pause is greater than the R-R interval prior to the pause. The pause is less than the preceding two R-R intervals.

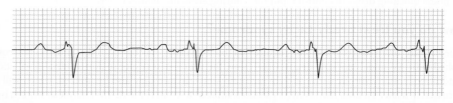

Figure 32-3. First-degree atrioventricular conduction delay is illustrated in this rhythm strip with a PR interval measuring 260 milliseconds.

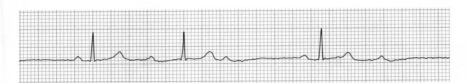

Figure 32-4. Mobitz type I second-degree atrioventricular block. This is manifest by gradual prolongation of the PR interval prior to the dropped beat. The PR interval after the dropped beat is shorter than the one prior to the dropped beat.

Mobitz type II AV block has a fixed PR interval with one P wave that does not conduct to the ventricles (Figure 32-5).[2] The R-R interval of the pause is equal to two of the preceding R-R intervals. The QRS complex is usually wide, although rarely it can be narrow.

In third-degree AV block, the atria and ventricles are dissociated and firing at their own rates. Typically, the atrial rate will be faster than the ventricular rate (Figure 32-6). If the block is above the His-Purkinje system, the QRS complex is typically narrow, with a rate of 40 to 60 bpm. If the block is below the His-Purkinje system, the QRS complex will be wide, with a rate less than 40 bpm. On occasion, the level of block may occur within the His-Purkinje system ("intra-His block") and the QRS complex may be narrow, but this is a rare finding.

What can cause AV block?

In Mobitz type I AV block, the site of block is usually within the AV node. In Mobitz type II block, the site of block is typically below the AV node, either within the His-Purkinje system or within the bundle branches. Type III heart block can occur within the AV node or below the AV node.

The SA node is supplied by the right coronary artery in 60% of patients and the left circumflex artery in 40%. The AV node is supplied by the right coronary artery in 90% of patients and the left

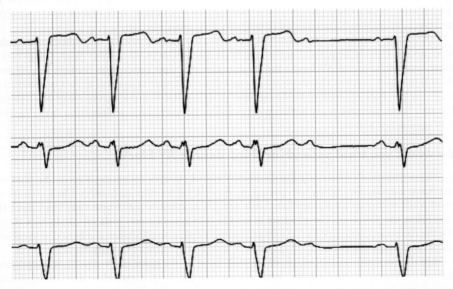

Figure 32-5. Mobitz type II second-degree atrioventricular block. There is a fixed PR interval prior to the dropped beat.

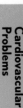

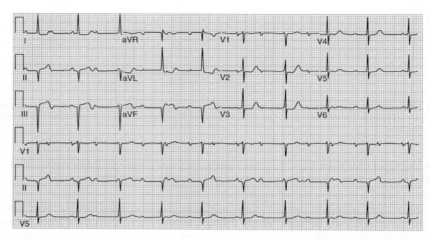

Figure 32-6. Complete heart block in the setting of an acute inferior wall myocardial infarction. There is dissociation of atrial and ventricular depolarizations. It should also be noted that the QRS complexes are narrow in this example, suggesting that the atrioventricular node may be the site of block. As this is often related to increased vagal tone in the setting of inferior injury, it is often reversible.

circumflex artery in 10%.[3] The His bundle is supplied by the SA nodal branch of the right coronary artery and septal perforators of the left anterior descending artery. The left anterior descending artery also supplies the bundle branches. Therefore, patients who present with an acute myocardial infarction (MI) can develop sinus brachycardia or first-, second-, or third-degree heart block. Patients with AV block related to an acute inferior wall MI often have complete heart block with a narrow QRS complex, and AV conduction commonly returns within days following the MI. Transient AV block may be related to ischemia or increased vagal tone in these patients. In contrast, patients who have heart block related to an acute anterior wall MI typically have occlusion of a very proximal portion of the left anterior descending artery with a wide QRS complex and bundle branch block, signifying more severe conduction disease related to extensive myocardial damage.

Both second- and third-degree heart block can occur in young healthy individuals as a result of increased vagal tone. Ischemia and underlying heart disease can produce heart block. Drugs may be another common cause of AV block, and medications that slow conduction through the AV node include β blockers, calcium channel blockers, and digoxin. Other drugs also impact on conduction through the His-Purkinje system, including class I and III antiarrhythmic agents. Heart block can also occur after aortic or mitral valve replacement owing to extensive surgical dissection in the region of the AV conduction system.

How would you treat second- or third-degree AV block?

For a hemodynamically unstable patient with heart block, temporary pacing is recommended with either transcutaneous or transvenous pacing. Atropine 1 mg intravenously every 3 to 5 minutes can be used while setting up for pacing. Care must be used, as atropine may worsen any heart block that occurs below the AV node. The presence of a wide QRS complex may indicate conduction disease below the AV node. Dopamine 5 to 20 μg/kg per minute continuous infusion can be added to enhance the heart rate. Isoproterenol infusion may also be utilized to enhance His-Purkinje conduction.

Once the patient is stabilized, an underlying cause of the heart block should be investigated, including assessment of medications. After discontinuing a drug, it should be kept in mind that it takes five half-lives for most of the drug to wash out and therefore determine if the drug caused the bradycardia. Ischemia should also be ruled out as a potential cause of the underlying conduction disturbance. Following an acute myocardial infarction, it may take hours to days for the conduction abnormality to resolve, particularly in the setting of an acute inferior wall MI. Indications for implantation of a permanent pacemaker in the setting of acquired AV block according to the American College of Cardiology (ACC)/American Heart Association (AHA)/Heart Rhythm Society (HRS) guidelines are outlined in Table 32-2, and indications for permanent pacing after the acute phase of MI are outlined in Table 32-3.[1]

Table 32-2. Recommendations for Acquired Atrioventricular Block in Adults

Class I

1. Permanent pacemaker implantation is indicated for third-degree and advanced second-degree AV block at any anatomic level associated with bradycardia with symptoms (including heart failure) or ventricular arrhythmias presumed to be due to AV block *(level of evidence: C)*.

2. Permanent pacemaker implantation is indicated for third-degree and advanced second-degree AV block at any anatomic level associated with arrhythmias and other medical conditions that require drug therapy that results in symptomatic bradycardia *(level of evidence: C)*.

3. Permanent pacemaker implantation is indicated for third-degree and advanced second-degree AV block at any anatomic level in awake, symptom-free patients in sinus rhythm, with documented periods of asystole ≥ 3.0 s or any escape rate < 40 bpm, or with an escape rhythm that is below the AV node *(level of evidence: C)*.

4. Permanent pacemaker implantation is indicated for third-degree and advanced second-degree AV block at any anatomic level in awake, symptom-free patients with AF and bradycardia with one or more pauses of at least 5 s or longer *(level of evidence: C)*.

5. Permanent pacemaker implantation is indicated for third-degree and advanced second-degree AV block at any anatomic level after catheter ablation of the AV junction *(level of evidence: C)*.

6. Permanent pacemaker implantation is indicated for third-degree and advanced second-degree AV block at any anatomic level associated with postoperative AV block that is not expected to resolve after cardiac surgery *(level of evidence: C)*.

7. Permanent pacemaker implantation is indicated for third-degree and advanced second-degree AV block at any anatomic level associated with neuromuscular diseases with AV block, such as myotonic muscular dystrophy, Kearns-Sayre syndrome, Erb dystrophy (limb-girdle muscular dystrophy), and peroneal muscular atrophy, with or without symptoms *(level of evidence: B)*.

8. Permanent pacemaker implantation is indicated for second-degree AV block with associated symptomatic bradycardia regardless of type or site of block *(level of evidence: B)*.

9. Permanent pacemaker implantation is indicated for asymptomatic persistent third-degree AV block at any anatomic site with average awake ventricular rates of 40 bpm or faster if cardiomegaly or LV dysfunction is present or if the site of block is below the AV node *(level of evidence: B)*.

10. Permanent pacemaker implantation is indicated for second- or third-degree AV block during exercise in the absence of myocardial ischemia *(level of evidence: C)*.

Class IIa

1. Permanent pacemaker implantation is reasonable for persistent third-degree AV block with an escape rate > 40 bpm in asymptomatic adult patients without cardiomegaly *(level of evidence: C)*.

2. Permanent pacemaker implantation is reasonable for asymptomatic second-degree AV block at intra- or infra-His levels found at electrophysiologic study *(level of evidence: B)*.

3. Permanent pacemaker implantation is reasonable for first- or second-degree AV block with symptoms similar to those of pacemaker syndrome or hemodynamic compromise *(level of evidence: B)*.

4. Permanent pacemaker implantation is reasonable for asymptomatic type II second-degree AV block with a narrow QRS. When type II second-degree AV block occurs with a wide QRS, including isolated right bundle branch block, pacing becomes a class I recommendation *(level of evidence: B)*.

(continued)

Table 32-2. Recommendations for Acquired Atrioventricular Block in Adults *(Continued)*

Class IIb

1. Permanent pacemaker implantation may be considered for neuromuscular diseases such as myotonic muscular dystrophy, Erb dystrophy (limb-girdle muscular dystrophy), and peroneal muscular atrophy with any degree of AV block (including first-degree AV block), with or without symptoms, because there may be unpredictable progression of AV conduction disease *(level of evidence: B)*.

2. Permanent pacemaker implantation may be considered for AV block in the setting of drug use and/or drug toxicity when the block is expected to recur even after the drug is withdrawn *(level of evidence: B)*.

Class III

1. Permanent pacemaker implantation is not indicated for asymptomatic first-degree AV block *(level of evidence: B)*.

2. Permanent pacemaker implantation is not indicated for asymptomatic type I second-degree AV block at the supra-His (AV node) level or that which is not known to be intra- or infra-Hisian *(level of evidence: C)*.

3. Permanent pacemaker implantation is not indicated for AV block that is expected to resolve and is unlikely to recur (eg, drug toxicity, Lyme disease, or transient increases in vagal tone or during hypoxia in sleep apnea syndrome in the absence of symptoms) *(level of evidence: B)*.

Abbreviations: ACC, American College of Cardiology; AF, atrial fibrillation; AHA, American Heart Association; AV, atrioventricular; HRS, Heart Rhythm Society; LV, left ventricular; NASPE, North American Society of Pacing and Electrophysiology. *(Adapted from Epstein AC, DiMarco JP, Ellenbogen KA, et al. ACC/AHA/HRS 2008 guidelines for device-based therapy of cardiac rhythm abnormalities: a report of the American College of Cardiology/American Heart Association Task Force on Practice Guidelines [Writing Committee to Revise the ACC/AHA/NASPE 2002 Guideline Update for Implantation of Cardiac Pacemakers and Antiarrhythmia Devices]: developed in collaboration with the American Association for Thoracic Surgery and Society of Thoracic Surgeons. Circulation. 2008;117:e350-e408.)*

Table 32-3. Recommendations for Permanent Pacing after the Acute Phase of MI

Class I

1. Permanent ventricular pacing is indicated for persistent second-degree AV block in the His-Purkinje system with alternating bundle branch block or third-degree AV block within or below the His-Purkinje system after ST-segment elevation MI *(level of evidence: B)*.

2. Permanent ventricular pacing is indicated for transient advanced second- or third-degree infranodal AV block and associated bundle branch block. If the site of block is uncertain, an electrophysiologic study may be necessary *(level of evidence: B)*.

3. Permanent ventricular pacing is indicated for persistent and symptomatic second- or third-degree AV block *(level of evidence: C)*.

Class IIb

1. Permanent ventricular pacing may be considered for persistent second- or third-degree AV block at the AV node level, even in the absence of symptoms *(level of evidence: B)*.

Class III

1. Permanent ventricular pacing is not indicated for transient AV block in the absence of intraventricular conduction defects *(level of evidence: B)*.

2. Permanent ventricular pacing is not indicated for transient AV block in the presence of isolated left anterior fascicular block *(level of evidence: B)*.

3. Permanent ventricular pacing is not indicated for new bundle branch block or fascicular block in the absence of AV block *(level of evidence: B)*.

4. Permanent ventricular pacing is not indicated for persistent asymptomatic first-degree AV block in the presence of bundle branch or fascicular block *(level of evidence: B)*.

Abbreviation: AV, atrioventricular. *(Adapted from Epstein AC, DiMarco JP, Ellenbogen KA, et al. ACC/AHA/HRS 2008 guidelines for device-based therapy of cardiac rhythm abnormalities: a report of the American College of Cardiology/American Heart Association Task Force on Practice Guidelines [Writing Committee to Revise the ACC/AHA/NASPE 2002 Guideline Update for Implantation of Cardiac Pacemakers and Antiarrhythmia Devices]: developed in collaboration with the American Association for Thoracic Surgery and Society of Thoracic Surgeons. Circulation. 2008;117:e350-e408.)*

Narrow Complex Tachycardias. Following acute treatment with atropine for marked sinus bradycardia, blood pressure increased to 110/70 mm Hg. However, a narrow complex tachycardia with a rate of 180 bpm was noted in the ICU (Figure 32-7).

What is the differential diagnosis for a regular narrow complex tachycardia?

The differential diagnosis for regular narrow complex tachycardias includes sinus tachycardia, atrial tachycardia, atrial flutter, AV nodal reentrant tachycardia, AV reciprocating tachycardia (AVRT), and junctional tachycardia.

How do you distinguish these tachycardias on ECG?

The presence or absence of P waves on the 12-lead ECG and the relationship of the P wave to the QRS complex are useful in the diagnosis and determination of the likely mechanism of the narrow complex tachycardia (Figure 32-8).

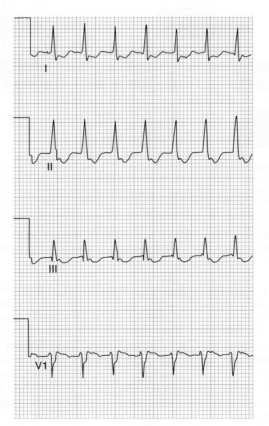

Figure 32-7. Rhythm strip of supraventricular tachycardia. There is the suggestion of a retrograde P wave just at the end of the QRS complex in leads II and III, and a "pseudo-R wave" in V_1, consistent with typical atrioventricular nodal reentry.

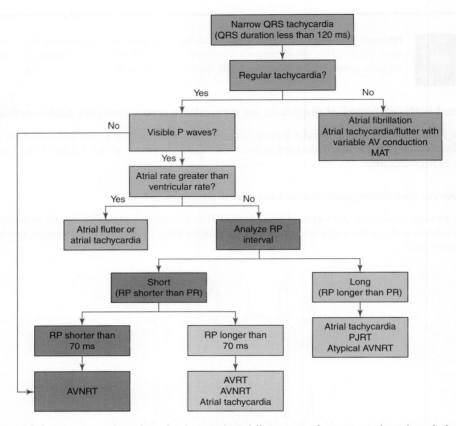

Figure 32-8. Narrow complex tachycardia: distinguishing different types of supraventricular tachycardia based on the presence or absence of P waves and the relationship of P waves to the QRS complex. AV, atrioventricular; AVNRT, AV nodal reentry; AVRT, AV reciprocating tachycardia/concealed bypass tract; MAT, multifocal atrial tachycardia; PJRT, paroxysmal junctional reentrant tachycardia. *(From Blomstrom-Lundqvist C, Scheinman M, Aliot E, et al. ACC/AHA/ESC guidelines for the management of patients with supraventricular arrhythmias—executive summary: a report of the American College of Cardiology/American Heart Association Task Force on Practice Guidelines and the European Society of Cardiology Committee for Practice Guidelines [Writing Committee to Develop Guidelines for the Management of Patients with Supraventricular Arrhythmias]. Circulation. 2003;108:1871-1909.)*

Sinus tachycardia is due to increased automaticity within the SA node. As a result, the onset and termination of this tachycardia will be gradual. The P wave precedes the QRS complex and usually has a "long RP" interval. However, if first-degree AV conduction delay is present, the P wave could be closer to the preceding QRS with a somewhat shorter RP interval compared to the PR interval (Figure 32-9). The rate of sinus tachycardia can range from 100 to 180 bpm, depending on the age of the patient, with a maximum rate estimated to be 220 minus the patient's age. The P waves have a morphology similar to sinus rhythm, although the P waves may become more peaked as the rhythm accelerates. Taller P waves often represent a focus higher in the SA node. In most instances, the PR interval shortens with an increase in heart rate due to increased catecholamines and enhanced conduction through the AV node.

Atrial flutter is a macro-reentrant atrial arrhythmia that rotates around the coronary sinus ostium in either a counterclockwise or clockwise fashion.[4] Flutter waves are best identified in leads II, III, aVF,

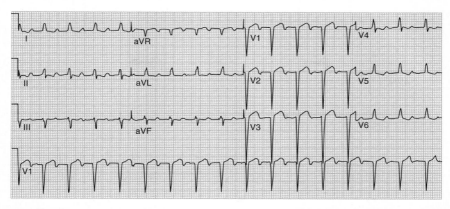

Figure 32-9. Sinus tachycardia. The rate is > 100 bpm, and there is one P wave before every QRS complex. The P-wave axis is positive in leads I, II, and aVF, or inferiorly directed, consistent with an origin from the sinus node within the right atrium. In this example, first-degree atrioventricular delay is also noted.

and V_1. The atrial rate can range from 250 to 350 bpm with a sawtooth contour. The flutter waves are positive in V_1 and negative in leads II, III, and aVF during counterclockwise flutter (Figure 32-10). In clockwise flutter, the flutter waves are negative in V_1 and positive in leads II, III, and aVF. The ventricular rate depends on the ability of the AV node to conduct to the ventricle. If the AV node is not diseased, conduction can occur on a 2:1 basis, resulting in a ventricular rate of approximately 150 bpm. In rare circumstances, 1:1 conduction during atrial flutter may occur. If the AV node is diseased, then conduction to the ventricles can be in a 4:1 ratio, with a ventricular rate of approximately 75 bpm, or even slower. AV nodal blocking drugs will also slow the ventricular rate during atrial flutter.

Atrioventricular nodal reentrant tachycardia (AVNRT) is a narrow complex tachycardia with a rate usually ranging from 150 to 250 bpm. The AV node has two pathways, a slowly conducting pathway with a short refractory period and a fast-conducting pathway with a long refractory period (Figure 32-11A). In sinus rhythm, the fast pathway is utilized. When a precisely timed premature atrial beat occurs, it can be blocked from conducting antegrade down the fast pathway owing to refractoriness within the fast pathway. This premature atrial beat then conducts slowly down the slow pathway.

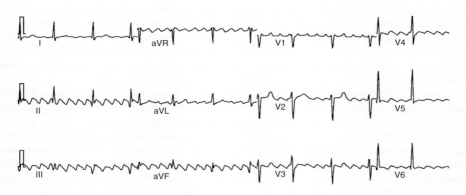

Figure 32-10. Typical atrial flutter. The "flutter waves" have a negative axis inferiorly and are positive in V_1, consistent with typical or counterclockwise atrial flutter.

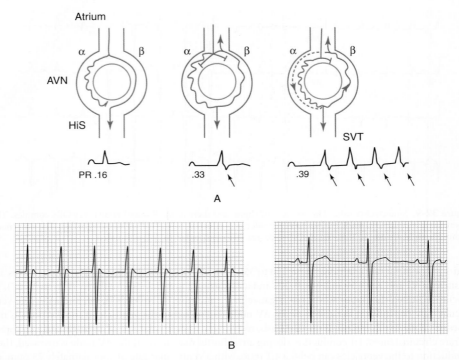

Figure 32-11. Atrioventricular nodal reentrant tachycardia (AVNRT). **A.** Schematic for typical AV nodal reentry. SVT, supraventricular tachycardia. *(From Josephson ME. Clinical Cardiac Electrophysiology: Techniques and Interpretations. 3rd ed. Philadelphia, PA: Lippincott Williams & Wilkins; 2002.)* **B.** A pseudo-RSr' is better seen in V$_1$ on the rhythm strip during AVNRT, which is not present in sinus rhythm.

By the time the impulse reaches the His-Purkinje system, the fast pathway has recovered excitability and the impulse not only travels antegrade through the His-Purkinje system to the ventricle but also conducts retrograde up the fast pathway to the atrium. This creates the slow–fast reentrant circuit otherwise known as "typical AVNRT." Because the atria and ventricles are activated simultaneously, the P wave is buried within the narrow QRS and therefore is not easily identified on ECG. A "pseudo-r" wave in lead V$_1$ and "pseudo-s" wave in the inferior leads represent the retrograde P wave (Figure 32-11B). If the onset of the arrhythmia is captured, the ECG will show a long PR interval or "jump" (as illustrated in the second schematic of panel A in Figure 32-11), representing the premature atrial beat traveling down the slow pathway.[5] The onset and termination of typical AVNRT are abrupt.

Atypical AVNRT occurs when antegrade conduction is down the fast pathway and retrograde conduction is up the slow pathway. Since ventricular activation occurs before atrial activation, the ECG demonstrates inverted P waves in the inferior leads and a long RP interval (Figure 32-12).

AV reciprocating tachycardia is a macro-reentrant tachycardia utilizing the normal His-Purkinje system in the antegrade direction and an accessory pathway in the retrograde direction. During sinus rhythm in patients with manifest Wolff-Parkinson-White (WPW) syndrome, simultaneous conduction down the accessory pathway and AV node produces a short PR interval and a delta wave (slurred upstroke of the QRS) on a 12-lead ECG (Figure 32-13). The initial slurred upstroke of the QRS complex is the delta wave, and this represents ventricular activation by the accessory pathway. However, in many cases, the accessory pathway does not conduct in the antegrade direction and can only function

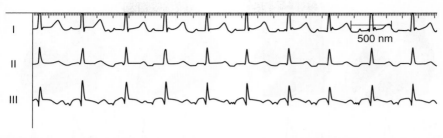

Figure 32-12. Atypical atrioventricular nodal reentrant tachycardia. A long RP tachycardia is demonstrated. P waves have a negative axis inferiorly, or superiorly directed, consistent with retrograde conduction up the slow pathway.

in a retrograde fashion. This is called a "concealed" accessory pathway and no delta wave is present in sinus rhythm. As the accessory pathway is still capable of conducting retrograde, supraventricular tachycardia (SVT) can still occur.

A premature atrial or ventricular beat can initiate AV reciprocating tachycardia, also referred to as "orthodromic tachycardia" (Figure 32-14). Orthodromic AV reciprocating tachycardia is the most common type of tachycardia using an accessory pathway. This is a narrow complex tachycardia that conducts antegrade down the AV node and retrograde activation up the accessory pathway, which produces a retrograde P wave within the ST segment. The delta wave is not seen in orthodromic AV tachycardia since the accessory pathway is being utilized in the retrograde direction. The ventricular rate typically ranges from 180 to 220 bpm.

In antidromic reciprocating tachycardia, there is antegrade conduction down the accessory pathway with retrograde conduction up the His-Purkinje system and AV node. This produces a wide QRS complex on the ECG.

Nonparoxysmal junctional tachycardia is thought to be due to enhanced automaticity in or near the bundle of His.[6] The ventricular rate ranges from 70 to 120 bpm. The tachycardia has a gradual

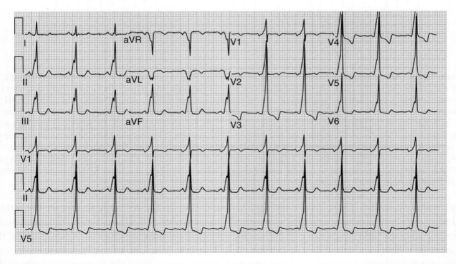

Figure 32-13. Wolff-Parkinson-White syndrome. There is a short PR interval with a slurred upstroke of the QRS complex, representing ventricular preexcitation. The delta wave is positive in V_1-V_6, with a negative delta wave in aVL, consistent with a left free wall accessory pathway.

Cardiovascular Problems

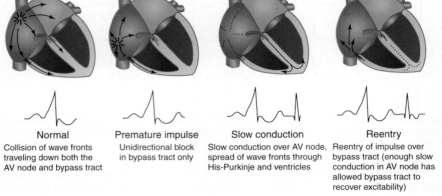

Normal
Collision of wave fronts
traveling down both the
AV node and bypass tract

Premature impulse
Unidirectional block
in bypass tract only

Slow conduction
Slow conduction over AV node,
spread of wave fronts through
His-Purkinje and ventricles

Reentry
Reentry of impulse over
bypass tract (enough slow
conduction in AV node has
allowed bypass tract to
recover excitability)

A

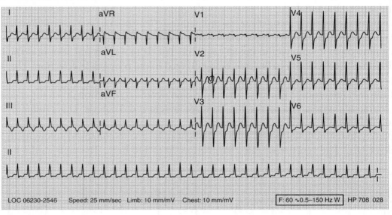

B

Figure 32-14. Atrioventricular reciprocating tachycardia (AVRT). **A.** A schematic of AV reciprocating tachycardia is shown where the AV node is used for antegrade conduction, and retrograde conduction occurs up the accessory pathway, resulting in a narrow QRS complex. The first panel illustrates pre-excitation with a ventricular depolarization produced by fusion over the accessory pathway and intrinsic conduction system, resulting in a delta wave. An atrial premature depolarization (APD) then blocks antegrade in the accessory pathway with conduction down the AV node, giving rise to a narrow QRS complex. The impulse then conducts retrograde up the accessory pathway in the last panel. *(From Josephson ME. Clinical Cardiac Electrophysiology: Techniques and Interpretations. 3rd ed. Philadelphia, PA: Lippincott Williams & Wilkins; 2002.)* **B.** Twelve-lead electrocardiogram of AVRT. Retrograde conduction occurs up the accessory pathway, resulting in a short RP tachycardia and retrograde P wave within the ST segment.

onset and termination. There can be retrograde conduction up the AV node to capture the atrium and ventricle simultaneously, resulting in inverted P waves in leads II, III, and aVF, which can occur before or after the QRS (Figure 32-15). When the retrograde P wave is before the QRS complex, the PR interval is short and less than 120 milliseconds. This may look similar to AV nodal reentry and often cannot be easily distinguished from this arrhythmia, especially if the onset of the tachycardia is not available.

Focal atrial tachycardia has an atrial rate ranging from 150 to 200 bpm (Figure 32-16). Focal atrial tachycardia arises from a single location in either the right or left atrium. The most common site of

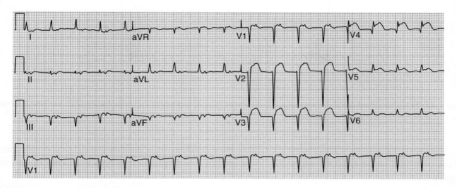

Figure 32-15. Junctional tachycardia. There is a retrograde P wave after the QRS complex, with a negative P-wave axis noted in the inferior leads. In this case, the junctional tachycardia occurred in the setting of anterior injury.

origin in the right atrium is from the crista terminalis.[7] The ostium of the pulmonary veins is the most common site in the left atrium.[8] Depending on the site of origin, the P-wave morphology may or may not be similar to the sinus P wave. If the origin is at the superior aspect of the crista terminalis, the P wave will be similar to the sinus P wave and therefore it might be difficult to distinguish this from sinus tachycardia. There is generally an abrupt onset and termination, with acceleration and deceleration occurring over 3 to 4 beats. Typically, focal atrial tachycardia has a long RP interval, but as the rhythm accelerates, this interval may shorten.

Multifocal atrial tachycardia may be seen in patients with diseased atria, who may also have acute or chronic lung disease. There are multiple areas within the atria that have abnormal or ectopic foci. The ECG will therefore have at least three morphologically different P waves. The PR interval varies because the foci that generate the P waves arise from different locations in the atria, at varying distances from the AV conduction system (Figure 32-17). The R-R interval can also vary with this rhythm, and it may often be confused with atrial fibrillation owing to its irregularity. Close observation will reveal distinct P waves of varying morphologies, distinguishing this from atrial fibrillation.

What are common causes or precipitants of narrow complex tachycardias?

Sinus tachycardia is a physiological response by the body to stress with a "flight-or-fight" response. Other causes include fever, volume depletion, shock, sepsis, hyperthyroidism, hypoxia, anemia, chronic pulmonary disease, and acidosis, to name a few.

Atrial flutter can occur in patients with congenital heart disease (septal defects), pulmonary disease, hyperthyroidism, or myocardial infarction or after atrial fibrillation ablation. It may also be seen after cardiac surgery or can be idiopathic in the absence of known structural heart disease.

Most patients with AVNRT and AVRT do not have any underlying structural heart disease. These arrhythmias are most often seen in otherwise young, healthy individuals. However, the first detection may occur in patients who are hospitalized unexpectedly for other medical problems.

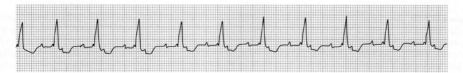

Figure 32-16. Atrial tachycardia. Atrial tachycardia with 2:1 atrioventricular conduction is noted on this rhythm strip.

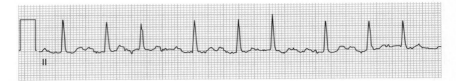

Figure 32-17. Multifocal atrial tachycardia. The P waves have at least three morphologies with varying PR intervals, often with very irregular R-R intervals.

Nonparoxysmal junctional tachycardia may be a marker for a serious underlying condition. It occurs during digoxin toxicity, acute MI, myocarditis, and hypokalemia and following open-heart surgery.

Focal atrial tachycardia can occur in structurally normal or abnormal hearts (ischemic or nonischemic cardiomyopathies) and can be seen in patients with obstructive lung disease. It can occur with electrolyte abnormalities and drug toxicity, such as with digoxin or theophylline. Multifocal atrial tachycardia is often seen in patients with either acute or chronic lung diseases such as pneumonia, pulmonary embolism, or chronic obstructive pulmonary disease. Medications (theophylline), electrolyte abnormalities (hypokalemia or hypomagnesemia), myocardial infarction, and sepsis can exacerbate multifocal atrial tachycardia.

What maneuvers/medications can be used to differentiate these rhythms?

Carotid sinus massage or adenosine can slow or block conduction through the AV node, which helps identify the arrhythmia mechanism for various supraventricular arrhythmias (Figure 32-18). During these maneuvers, a 12-lead ECG or rhythm strip should be recorded continuously. If the

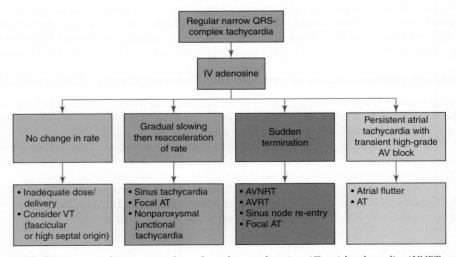

Figure 32-18. Response of narrow complex tachycardias to adenosine. AT, atrial tachycardia; AVNRT, atrioventricular nodal reentrant tachycardia; AVRT, atrioventricular reciprocating tachycardia; IV, intravenous; VT, ventricular tachycardia. (*From Blomstrom-Lundqvist C, Scheinman M, Aliot E, et al. ACC/AHA/ESC guidelines for the management of patients with supraventricular arrhythmias-executive summary: a report of the American College of Cardiology/American Heart Association Task Force on Practice Guidelines and the European Society of Cardiology Committee for Practice Guidelines [Writing Committee to Develop Guidelines for the Management of Patients with Supraventricular Arrhythmias]. Circulation. 2003;108:1871-1909.*)

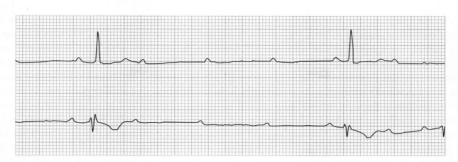

Figure 32-19. Atrioventricular (AV) block after adenosine administration. Adenosine 12 mg intravenously was administered in this patient during sinus rhythm to determine if there was any evidence for preexcitation following block in the AV node. Transient high-grade AV block was noted, which resolved spontaneously within seconds.

arrhythmia terminates abruptly with adenosine, it is most likely AVNRT, AVRT, or occasionally focal atrial tachycardia. If the ventricular rated during the arrhythmia slows but fails to terminate and multiple P waves are visualized for each QRS complex, then the arrhythmia represents atrial flutter or atrial tachycardia. The tachycardia will continue in the atrium, as the ventricles are not required as part of the reentrant circuit. Adenosine or other AV blocking agents will block in the AV node, allowing better identification of the underlying P-wave or flutter-wave morphology. It should also be noted that AV block will occur when adenosine is administered in sinus rhythm. Figure 32-19 demonstrates temporary high-grade AV block after adenosine administration.

How do you manage these rhythms?

Since sinus tachycardia is a physiologic response to stress, management would involve identifying and treating the underlying cause. β Blocker therapy is generally not used to treat sinus tachycardia except in special circumstances, such as acute myocardial infarction, thyrotoxicosis, and congestive heart failure.

For a hemodynamically unstable patient with atrial flutter, emergent synchronized cardioversion with low energy (25-100 joules) may be required to convert the rhythm to sinus. Intravenous ibutilide can also emergently convert atrial flutter to sinus rhythm. Ibutilide does carry a low risk of prolonging the QT interval and causing torsades de pointes. Therefore, ibutilide should only be used by trained personnel in an intensive care or other closely monitored settings. Anticoagulation status needs to be considered before attempted conversion, as detailed below.

Most patients with atrial flutter are hemodynamically stable. Rate control can be achieved with AV nodal blocking agents. Conversion to sinus rhythm can be achieved through overdrive pacing or external direct-current (DC) cardioversion, or pharmacologically with antiarrhythmic drugs, including class IA, IC, or III agents. It should be noted that class I and class III drugs can also slow the flutter rate in the atrium, making it more likely that 1:1 atrioventricular conduction might occur. Therefore, an AV nodal blocking drug (such as a β blocker or calcium channel blocker) should typically be used with these membrane-active antiarrhythmic agents. As with atrial fibrillation, atrial flutter has been associated with thrombus formation and increased risk of stroke.[9,10] Therefore, patients with atrial flutter should be anticoagulated in the same manner as those with atrial fibrillation. If the duration of the atrial flutter is unknown or greater than 48 hours, anticoagulation is required 3 weeks before and 4 weeks after cardioversion, including electrical or pharmacologic conversion.[11] If the arrhythmia duration is unknown or longer than 48 hours and more urgent conversion is needed, transesophageal echocardiography is indicated to first exclude left atrial thrombus.

Cardiovascular Problems

AVNRT relies on the AV node for continuation of the arrhythmia. For acute termination of the arrhythmia in an unstable patient, DC synchronized cardioversion with 150 to 200 joules may rarely be required. For a stable patient with AVNRT, blocking the AV node with vagal maneuvers (such as carotid massage or Valsalva) can terminate this arrhythmia. Adenosine works by prolonging AV nodal conduction. Adenosine 6 mg intravenous (IV) bolus followed by 12 mg IV, if the first dose is unsuccessful, usually terminates the arrhythmia. It should be noted that smaller doses may be utilized for termination of the arrhythmia if adenosine is administered centrally. The drug should be infused as close as possible to the skin (rather than through a port in an IV line far from the patient), as this drug has a very short half-life. Calcium channel blockers (such as verapamil or diltiazem) or β blockers are generally used if adenosine fails to terminate the arrhythmia. These calcium channel blockers and β blockers can also be used to prevent recurrences. For long-term treatment of AVNRT, catheter ablation is an option for "cure."

Wolff-Parkinson-White syndrome is defined as the WPW pattern on ECG in conjunction with a tachyarrhythmia (80% AVRT, 15%-30% atrial fibrillation, 5% atrial flutter). Vagal maneuvers and adenosine slow and block the conduction through the AV node and should be used as first-line therapy to terminate orthodromic AVRT, which has a narrow QRS complex. If the patient does not have congestive heart failure, intravenous verapamil can be used with a 5-mg bolus every 10 to 15 minutes for a total of 15 mg. Direct-current cardioversion can be employed if vagal maneuvers or adenosine fails to work, although this is very rarely needed.

Accessory pathways can rapidly conduct in an antegrade fashion to the ventricles during antidromic AVRT (which has a wide complex tachycardia). If antidromic AVRT is suspected, then AV nodal blocking agents including verapamil are contraindicated. Intravenous procainamide should be given with a loading dose of 10 mg/kg over 25 minutes followed by 1 to 4 mg/min continuous infusion. As procainamide can cause hypotension, close blood pressure monitoring is required during the infusion. The dose must be adjusted for renal dysfunction. If the patient is hemodynamically unstable, immediate cardioversion should be utilized.

Atrial fibrillation can also occur in the setting of WPW syndrome and may conduct very rapidly down the accessory pathway, which can degenerate into ventricular fibrillation. Atrial fibrillation in a patient with WPW syndrome should be treated with intravenous procainamide or ibutilide. If the patient is hemodynamically unstable, DC cardioversion is recommended.

With respect to long-term treatment, catheter ablation is curative therapy for patients with Wolff-Parkinson-White syndrome and supraventricular tachycardia. For those who decline catheter ablation, antiarrhythmic drugs can be used.

The management for nonparoxysmal junctional tachycardia should be aimed at treating the underlying condition. When digoxin is the offending agent, the drug should be withheld. In the setting of digoxin toxicity, ventricular arrhythmias or AV block may occur, and digoxin-specific antibody Fab fragments should be initiated. Hyperkalemia in digoxin toxicity has a 50% mortality rate when the levels are between 5.0 and 5.5 mEq/dL.[12] Therefore, a potassium level greater than 5.0 mEq/dL is an indication for digoxin-specific antibody Fab fragment therapy. Efforts should be made to correct hypokalemia or hypomagnesemia. An accelerated junctional tachycardia can occur during or after an acute myocardial infarction; therefore, ischemia should also be ruled out as a cause of the nonparoxysmal junctional tachycardia.

Focal atrial tachycardia may be difficult to treat medically. The mechanism of this arrhythmia may be a result of abnormal automaticity, triggered activity, or reentry.[13] Direct-current cardioversion is seldom successful. Adenosine can terminate some atrial tachycardias, depending on the arrhythmia mechanism.[14] β Blockers and calcium channel blockers can be used to control the ventricular rate and may terminate the arrhythmia. Class IC (flecainide) and class III (sotalol and amiodarone) agents may be effective in terminating this arrhythmia.[15] Coronary artery disease must be excluded prior to initiation of a class IC antiarrhythmic drug. Because of potential drug side effects and the high success rate of catheter ablation, ablation is often a good option for patients with incessant focal atrial tachycardia.[11]

Atrial fibrillation

What Are the Risks for Developing Atrial Fibrillation?

Atrial fibrillation is the most common arrhythmia seen in the intensive care unit setting, particularly in the elderly.[16,17] Risk factors for developing atrial fibrillation include hypertension, coronary artery disease, diabetes, valvular heart disease, and heart failure. Atrial fibrillation can also occur in patients with structurally normal hearts. Reversible causes of atrial fibrillation include hypoxia, cardiac ischemia, infection, hyperthyroidism, electrolyte disturbances, drugs (such as theophylline and digitalis), alcohol, sleep deprivation, obesity, and increased sympathetic tone. One must always consider an acute pulmonary embolism as the cause of atrial fibrillation, and this arrhythmia may rarely be the only sign. Atrial fibrillation is frequently seen in the postoperative period following cardiac and noncardiac surgery. In one study the incidence of postoperative atrial fibrillation following noncardiac surgery was 4.1%.[18] There is a 10% to 65% incidence of atrial fibrillation following open-heart surgery.[19]

How Is Atrial Fibrillation Classified?

According to the ACC/AHA/European Society of Cardiology (ESC) guidelines, atrial fibrillation is classified as paroxysmal, persistent, or permanent.[20] Paroxysmal atrial fibrillation is defined as recurrent atrial fibrillation (two or more episodes) that terminates spontaneously within 7 days. Persistent atrial fibrillation applies to recurrent atrial fibrillation with a duration of longer than 7 days that is not self-terminating. Persistent atrial fibrillation can terminate spontaneously after 7 days or can be cardioverted, either electrically or pharmacologically. Atrial fibrillation is considered "long-standing persistent" if it is present for longer than 1 year. It is considered "permanent" if cardioversion has failed or has not been attempted. The term "lone" atrial fibrillation has been used to apply to patients younger than 60 years old without evidence of structural heart disease.

How Would You Evaluate a Patient with Atrial Fibrillation?

Atrial fibrillation may be symptomatic or asymptomatic. The patient should be questioned regarding symptoms of palpitations, shortness of breath, lightheadedness, fatigue, or chest pain. History should also include the presence or absence of known heart disease, other contributing diseases, family history of atrial fibrillation, current medications, and social history (particularly alcohol intake). However, the patient may be intubated and unable to give any history.

It is important to determine the duration of the atrial fibrillation to help guide management, as this is related to the need for anticoagulation and safety of cardioversion. In addition to a 12-lead ECG, a transthoracic echocardiogram is indicated to evaluate for valvular abnormalities, left atrial size, left ventricular systolic function, and wall thickness, which will help guide medical therapy. For atrial fibrillation of unknown duration or lasting longer than 48 hours with plans for cardioversion, a transesophageal echocardiogram is recommended to exclude left atrial appendage thrombus. Transesophageal echocardiography may also occasionally aid in the diagnosis of a large pulmonary embolism. If the patient has an implantable pacemaker or defibrillator, interrogation of the device may help determine the duration of the atrial arrhythmia. A chest x-ray can also be performed to exclude an infectious process.

What Are the ECG Findings of Atrial Fibrillation?

The ECG will not show P waves, but rather "fibrillatory" waves. The ventricular rate typically ranges from 100 to 170 bpm with irregular R-R intervals in the absence of AV nodal blocking drugs. If there is normal conduction through the AV node, the QRS complex will be narrow. A wide QRS complex during atrial fibrillation represents either a preexisting bundle branch block, a rate-related aberrancy, or conduction through an accessory pathway. Comparison with an old ECG is always helpful.

How Do You Treat Atrial Fibrillation?

Indications for immediate cardioversion include hemodynamic compromise (hypotension), pulmonary edema, cardiac ischemia, or WPW syndrome with very rapid conduction down the accessory pathway. Direct-current cardioversion is painful and requires the patient to be heavily sedated with a short-acting anesthetic. The external defibrillator should be synchronized to the QRS complex to prevent induction of ventricular fibrillation during electrical conversion of atrial fibrillation. The starting energy for conversion of atrial fibrillation is 100 joules, with energies up to 360 joules if initial attempts are unsuccessful. Intravenous ibutilide can also result in conversion to sinus rhythm, but it must be administered cautiously in a monitored setting by trained personnel because of the risk of hypotension and torsades de pointes.

If the patient is hemodynamically stable, the determination of rate vs rhythm control should be made along with decisions regarding anticoagulation and timing of conversion. Anticoagulation status and the need for transesophageal echocardiography have been previously discussed in the atrial flutter section, and this also pertains to atrial fibrillation. Anticoagulation should be continued for at least 4 weeks after cardioversion. The timing and duration of anticoagulation are detailed in the ACC/AHA/ESC guidelines and summarized in Table 32-4.[20] Attempts at conversion to sinus rhythm are contraindicated if transesophageal echocardiography demonstrates the presence of left atrial thrombus. In this case, therapeutic anticoagulation should be continued for at least 4 weeks until the thrombus resolves. Repeat transesophageal echocardiography can be performed to document resolution of the thrombus prior to cardioversion. The risks and benefits of anticoagulation must always be taken into account when determining plans for rhythm vs rate control and whether or not cardioversion will be attempted. If a patient is not considered a candidate for even short-term anticoagulation, cardioversion should not be attempted.

If rate control is elected, a β blocker, calcium channel blocker (verapamil or diltiazem), or digoxin can be utilized. To obtain adequate rate control, more than one agent may be required. Standard drugs and dosing regimens are outlined in Table 32-5.

Digoxin is renally excreted and the dose should be adjusted based on the patient's creatinine clearance. Digoxin is less effective in states of increased sympathetic tone and therefore may not significantly slow the ventricular rate in a shock state. Calcium channel blockers have a negative inotropic effect and are therefore contraindicated in patients with decompensated congestive heart failure or severe left ventricular systolic dysfunction. β Blockers should be avoided in patients with asthma or severe chronic obstructive pulmonary disease.

Intravenous amiodarone can be used if pharmacologic cardioversion is desired. Pharmacologic cardioversion carries a similar risk of thromboembolism as electrical cardioversion. Therefore, a transesophageal echocardiogram should be performed to rule out intracardiac thrombus before initiating any antiarrhythmic drugs in the absence of an adequate duration of anticoagulation. The loading dose of amiodarone is a 150-mg bolus over 10 to 15 minutes followed by a continuous infusion of 1 mg/min for the first 6 hours, then 0.5 mg/min for the next 18 hours. Amiodarone may cause hypotension, requiring the dose to be decreased or the infusion to be discontinued. Amiodarone's potential side effects include hepatic, pulmonary, and thyroid toxicities. Baseline liver function and thyroid function tests should be performed. Pulmonary function tests would not be feasible in a critically ill patient, but a chest x-ray should be examined for any serious underlying pulmonary disease. Before beginning any antiarrhythmic medication, a cardiology or electrophysiology consultation should be considered.

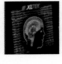

Ventricular Arrhythmias: Wide Complex Tachycardias. A 75-year-old man with a known history of coronary artery disease, remote anterior wall MI, status post–coronary artery bypass surgery (3 vessels) in 2002, and recent stenting to a saphenous vein graft presents to the emergency department with shortness of breath, chest pain, and syncope

Table 32-4. Recommendations for Antithrombotic Therapy to Prevent Ischemic Stroke and Systemic Embolism in Patients with AF Undergoing Cardioversion

Class I

1. For patients with AF of 48-h duration or longer, or when the duration of AF is unknown, anticoagulation (INR 2.0-3.0) is recommended for at least 3 wk prior to and 4 wk after cardioversion, regardless of the method (electrical or pharmacologic) used to restore sinus rhythm (*level of evidence: B*).

2. For patients with AF of > 48-h duration requiring immediate cardioversion because of hemodynamic instability, heparin should be administered concurrently (unless contraindicated) by an initial intravenous bolus injection followed by a continuous infusion in a dose adjusted to prolong the activated partial thromboplastin time to 1.5-2 times the reference control value. Thereafter, oral anticoagulation (INR 2.0-3.0) should be provided for at least 4 wk, as for patients undergoing elective cardioversion. Limited data support subcutaneous administration of low-molecular-weight heparin in this indication (*level of evidence: C*).

3. For patients with AF of < 48-h duration associated with hemodynamic instability (angina pectoris, myocardial infarction, shock, or pulmonary edema), cardioversion should be performed immediately without delay for prior initiation of anticoagulation (*level of evidence: C*).

Class IIa

1. During the 48 h after onset of AF, the need for anticoagulation before and after cardioversion may be based on the patient's risk of thromboembolism (*level of evidence: C*).

2. As an alternative to anticoagulation prior to cardioversion of AF, it is reasonable to perform transesophageal echocardiography (TEE) in search of thrombus in the left atrium (LA) or left atrial appendage (LAA) (*level of evidence: B*).

    2a. For patients with no identifiable thrombus, cardioversion is reasonable immediately after anticoagulation with unfractionated heparin (eg, initiated by intravenous bolus injection and an infusion continued at a dose adjusted to prolong the activated partial thromboplastin time to 1.5-2 times the control value until oral anticoagulation has been established with an oral vitamin K antagonist [eg, warfarin] as evidenced by an INR ≥ 2.0) (*level of evidence: B*). Thereafter, continuation of oral anticoagulation (INR 2.0-3.0) is reasonable for a total anticoagulation period of at least 4 wk, as for patients undergoing elective cardioversion (*level of evidence: B*). Limited data are available to support the subcutaneous administration of a low-molecular-weight heparin in this indication (*level of evidence: C*).

    2b. For patients in whom thrombus is identified by TEE, oral anticoagulation (INR 2.0-3.0) is reasonable for at least 3 wk prior to and 4 wk after restoration of sinus rhythm, and a longer period of anticoagulation may be appropriate even after apparently successful cardioversion, because the risk of thromboembolism often remains elevated in such cases (*level of evidence: C*).

3. For patients with atrial flutter undergoing cardioversion, anticoagulation can be beneficial according to the recommendations as for patients with AF (*level of evidence: C*).

Abbreviations: AF, atrial fibrillation; INR, international normalized ratio. (*Adapted from Fuster V, Ryden LE, Cannom DS, et al. ACC/AHA/ESC 2006 guidelines for the management of patients with atrial fibrillation. J Am Coll Cardiol. 2006;48:854-906.*)

while driving. He is admitted to the ICU. Vital signs on arrival included a blood pressure of 90/50 mm Hg and a heart rate of 160 bpm. Examination was remarkable for a laceration on his forehead, laterally displaced PMI with a tachycardic S_1 and S_2, clear lung fields, and normal neurologic examination. Head computed tomography scan was unremarkable. His ECG upon presentation is shown in Figure 32-20.

What is the differential diagnosis for a wide complex tachycardia?

Wide complex tachycardias can be either of ventricular or supraventricular origin. Supraventricular tachycardias can have a wide QRS complex if there is a preexisting bundle branch block, a rate-related bundle branch block, or an accessory pathway. Antiarrhythmic agents can also prolong the

Table 32-5. Intravenously and Orally Administered Pharmacologic Agents for Heart Rate Control in Patients with Atrial Fibrillation

Drug in the acute setting	Loading dose	Maintenance dose
Esmolol	500 μg/kg IV over 1 min	60-200 μg/kg/min IV
Metoprolol	2.5-5 mg IV bolus over 2 min; up to 3 doses	N/A
Propranolol	0.15 mg/kg IV	N/A
Diltiazem	0.25 mg/kg IV over 2 min	5-15 mg/h IV
Verapamil	0.075-0.15 mg/kg IV over 2 min	N/A
Digoxin	0.25 mg IV q2h, up to 1.5 mg	0.125-0.375 mg daily IV
Nonacute setting and chronic maintenance therapy		
Metoprolol		25-100 mg PO bid
Propranolol		80-240 mg PO daily in divided doses
Diltiazem		120-360 mg PO daily in divided doses
Verapamil		120-360 mg PO daily in divided doses

QRS duration, and sometimes greater widening of the QRS may be evident at faster heart rates, particularly if the patient is taking a class IC antiarrhythmic drug. Tachycardias of ventricular origin include monomorphic ventricular tachycardia, polymorphic ventricular tachycardia, and ventricular fibrillation.

How do you differentiate a tachycardia of ventricular origin from a supraventricular tachycardia with aberration?

Approximately 80% of wide complex tachycardias are ventricular tachycardias (VTs), with more than 95% of these patients having had a prior MI.[21,22] A potentially fatal mistake is the misdiagnosis of a

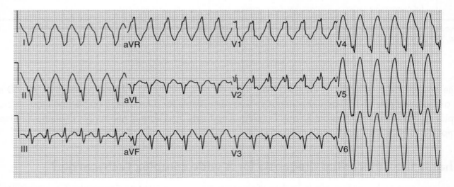

Figure 32-20. Twelve-lead electrocardiogram is consistent with monomorphic ventricular tachycardia (VT). This VT has a right bundle branch pattern in V_1 and QS in V_6, with a right superior axis, occurring in a patient with a prior anterior wall myocardial infarction.

monomorphic ventricular tachycardia as a supraventricular tachycardia and treating it with AV nodal blocking drugs, such as calcium channel blockers. This may result in hypotension and degeneration of VT to ventricular fibrillation in a patient with VT. Therefore, whenever a wide complex tachycardia is encountered, it should be presumed to be VT until proven otherwise.

The ECG characteristics can help to distinguish VT from supraventricular tachycardia with aberrancy. Features that favor VT but that are not always seen on the ECG are AV dissociation, marked change in axis, precordial concordance, and fusion or capture beats.[23] AV dissociation, capture and fusion beats, and precordial concordance are demonstrated in Figure 32-21. If the patient is hemodynamically stable, it is important to obtain a 12-lead ECG to aid in diagnosis. A comparison with an

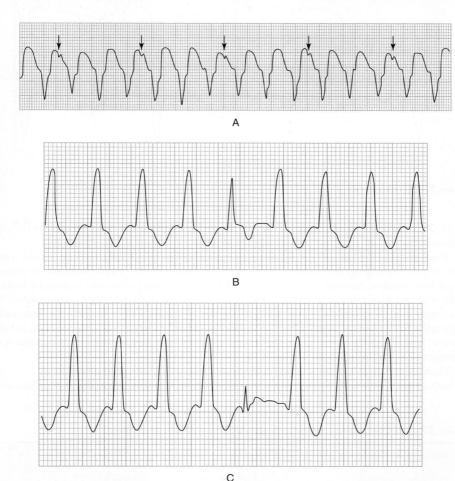

Figure 32-21. Criteria for distinguishing ventricular tachycardia (VT) from supraventricular tachycardia with aberration. **A.** This rhythm strip demonstrated atrioventricular dissociation. The arrows point to the P waves, which are dissociated from the QRS complexes. **B.** This rhythm strip demonstrates a fusion beat. This represents activation of the ventricle from a combination of the VT beat and a beat with intrinsic conduction. **C.** This rhythm strip demonstrates a capture beat, which represents a beat conducted to the ventricles from the intrinsic conduction system alone. It has a narrow QRS complex. **D.** Concordance. All QRS complexes (noted by the arrows) are positive across the precordium, consistent with a ventricular origin of the premature beats. In fact, this morphology suggests an epicardial origin of ventricular ectopy.

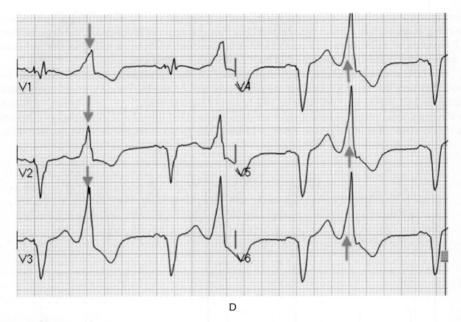

D

Figure 32-21. (*Continued.*)

old ECG should be attempted if one is available, although this may not always be feasible at the time of presentation.

Monomorphic VT can occur in the setting of myocardial scar, including a left ventricular aneurysm, or in the setting of a structurally normal heart. Monomorphic VT may be sustained or nonsustained. Nonsustained monomorphic VT is defined as three or more consecutive ventricular beats at a rate of greater than or equal to 100 bpm lasting less than 30 seconds. Sustained monomorphic VT lasts longer than 30 seconds or results in hemodynamic compromise prior to that time. Ventricular tachycardia arises from the ventricular myocardium and therefore has a wide QRS complex, but this is not a "typical" bundle branch block appearance compared to a supraventricular tachycardia with aberrancy or a preexisting bundle branch block.

There are certain ECG criteria to help distinguish VT from SVT with aberration[24] (Table 32-6). For VT with a right bundle branch morphology, the QRS duration is usually greater than 140 milliseconds

Table 32-6. ECG Criteria to Help Distinguish VT from SVT with Aberration

1. If RS complex absent from all precordial leads, then VT
2. If RS present, and the longest precordial RS interval > 100 ms in one or more precordial lead(s), then VT
3. If atrioventricular dissociation present, then VT
4. If morphologic criteria for VT present both in precordial leads V_1-V_2 and V_6, then VT. If morphologic criteria for VT not present, then the diagnosis of SVT with aberrant conduction is made by exclusion.

Abbreviations: ECG, electrocardiographic; SVT, supraventricular tachycardia; VT, ventricular tachycardia.(*Adapted from Brugada P, Brugada J, Mont L, Smeets J, Andries EW. A new approach to the differential diagnosis of a regular tachycardia with a wide QRS complex. Circulation. 1991;83:1649-1659.*)

with the R-to-S ratio less than 1 in V_6. VT with a left bundle branch morphology generally has a QRS duration of greater than 160 milliseconds, an R-wave duration in V_1 of less than 30 milliseconds, the onset of the R wave to the nadir of the S wave in lead V_1 greater than 60 milliseconds, or notching of the S wave in V_1 or V_2.[25] If the QRS complexes are either all-positive or all-negative (known as concordance) in the precordial leads (V_1-V_6), this would be more consistent with VT (Figure 32-21D). AV dissociation in VT exists because the atria and ventricles are firing at different rates without any relationship between the two (Figure 32-21A). Fusion beats represent simultaneous activation from a supraventricular and ventricular origin resulting in a QRS complex that has a combined morphology of the ventricular tachycardia and a normal sinus QRS complex (Figure 32-21B). Capture beats are sinus or supraventricular beats that conduct to the ventricle with a narrow QRS complex during ventricular tachycardia (Figure 32-21C).

An accelerated idioventricular rhythm can also frequently be seen in the ICU setting (Figure 32-22). This may be related to ischemia or reperfusion. The rate is typically less than 100 bpm and the rhythm has a wide complex. The ECG criteria used to distinguish this rhythm from SVT with aberrancy are identical to those criteria used for VT with a more rapid rate.

Polymorphic VT has wide QRS complexes that have varying morphologies and often phasic variation in axis around the baseline. The ventricular rate ranges from 150 to 250 bpm. Polymorphic VT can be associated with a normal or prolonged QT interval (Figure 32-23). When preceded by a long QT interval, this is referred to as "torsade de pointes," or *twisting of the points* (Figure 32-23A). Polymorphic VT associated with ischemia may be associated with a normal QT interval (Figure 32-23B).

Prolonged QT intervals can be acquired or congenital. Certain drugs and electrolyte abnormalities can prolong the QT interval and predispose to torsades de pointes. Table 32-7 outlines some major drug categories that can lead to QT prolongation and torsades de pointes. An extensive list of drugs that can cause prolongation of the QT interval is available on the website www.torsades.org. Polymorphic VT with a long QT interval can develop during periods of bradycardia or a pause that follows a premature beat. In patients with congenital long QT syndrome, the development of polymorphic VT or torsades de pointes may occur during periods of adrenergic stress, such as sudden awakening, exertion, or emotional stress in some patients. Central nervous system injury, including brain tumor, may also result in QT prolongation with diffuse T-wave inversion.

Supraventricular tachycardia can present with a wide QRS complex and can mimic VT. When the heart rate accelerates, conduction can be delayed in one of the bundle branches, leading to right or left bundle branch block. Sometimes P waves can be seen preceding the wide QRS complexes. The relationship between P waves and QRS complexes will not be helpful if the patient is in atrial

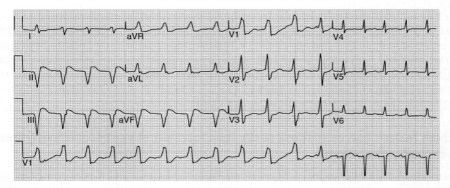

Figure 32-22. Accelerated idioventricular rhythm. The wide complex rhythm has a rate in the 90s and a right bundle branch morphology with right superior axis consistent with ventricular tachycardia. Prior to termination, a fusion beat (sixth beat from the right) is noted.

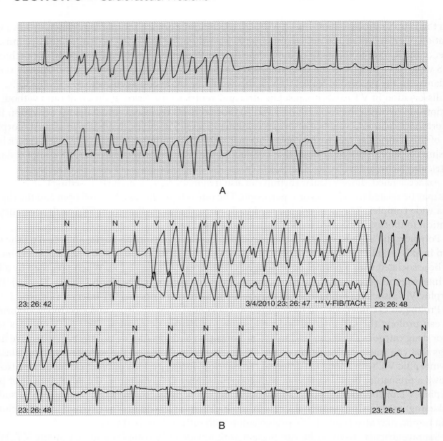

Figure 32-23. Polymorphic ventricular tachycardia (VT). **A.** This is an example of torsades de pointes with polymorphic VT (or twisting of the QRS complexes around the baseline) and a preceding long QT interval. This patient developed acute renal failure while on sotalol, which is an antiarrhythmic drug that can prolong the QT interval and that is renally excreted. **B.** This is polymorphic VT without a preceding long QT interval that developed in a patient with ongoing ischemia and recent inferior wall myocardial infarction.

fibrillation. If atrial fibrillation conducts aberrantly, the rhythm would be irregularly irregular. On occasion, patients with WPW syndrome can also have atrial fibrillation with rapid conduction down the accessory pathway, and this may also mimic VT. However, there is often marked beat-to-beat variation in the width and morphology of the QRS complexes in patients with preexcited atrial fibrillation (Figure 32-24). The latter rhythm may be extremely rapid and potentially life threatening, as the accessory pathway does not have the normal "slowing" properties of the AV node and very rapid rates can bombard the ventricle, degenerating into ventricular fibrillation.

Which factors can contribute to the development of ventricular arrhythmias in critically ill patients?

Electrolyte abnormalities including hypokalemia, hypomagnesemia, and hypocalcemia can, either alone or in combination, precipitate ventricular arrhythmias. Electrolytes should be aggressively repleted. A 12-lead ECG should be obtained and the QT interval measured. The patient's medication list should be checked for any QT-prolonging drugs. Ischemia, hypoxia, and acid-base disturbances

Table 32-7. Major Categories of Drugs That Can Cause QT Prolongation and Torsades de Pointes

Drugs that can prolong the QT interval and potentially induce torsades	
Antipsychotic drugs	Antidepressants
Thioridazine	Paroxetine
Butyrophenones, such as haloperidol	Sertraline
Phenothiazines	Venlafaxine
Quetiapine	Other
Risperidone	Cipsapride
Ziprasidone	Droperidol
Antiarrhythmic drugs	Pentamidine
Amiodarone (rarely)	Methadone
Sotalol	HIV protease inhibitors
Dofetilide	Phenytoin
Quinidine	Antibiotics
Procainamide	Erythromycin
Disopyramide	Levofloxacin
Flecainide	Moxifloxacin
Ibutilide	Sparfloxacin
Antihistamines	
Terfenadine	
Astemizole	
Fluoxetine	

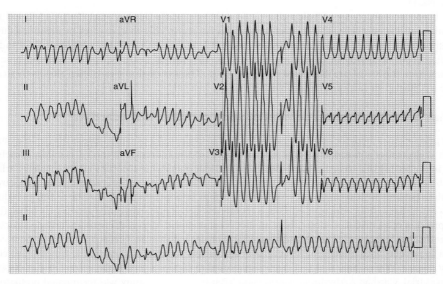

Figure 32-24. Atrial fibrillation with ventricular preexcitation. Very rapid conduction down the accessory pathway is noted, often with rates greater than 300 bpm.

should also be excluded. Some patients in the ICU setting may be receiving catecholamines for hemodynamic support. Endogenous or exogenous catecholamines are known to precipitate ventricular arrhythmias. When exogenous catecholamines are thought to be the culprit, the dose should be lowered or discontinued if feasible. Intravascular catheters should be checked for correct placement within the heart, as mechanical irritation between the catheter and the ventricular myocardium can induce ventricular ectopy, nonsustained VT, or sustained VT.

What is the clinical significance of ventricular tachycardia?

Nonsustained VT can occur in structurally abnormal hearts (ischemic heart disease, hypertrophic heart disease, valvular disease, dilated cardiomyopathy) or in structurally normal hearts. Nonsustained ventricular arrhythmias in the setting of an acute myocardial infarction may be related to ischemia or reperfusion, and this appears to have no long-term adverse prognostic significance. On the other hand, the presence of nonsustained VT occurring greater than 72 hours after an MI appears to portend a worse prognosis. Ventricular tachycardia occurring greater than 1 week after an MI on ambulatory monitoring has been associated with increased mortality rate and increased risk for sudden cardiac death.[26] The presence of nonsustained VT and reduced left ventricular systolic function are well-established independent predictors of mortality after an MI.[27]

Sustained ventricular arrhythmias may be seen in patients with ischemic heart disease and acute MI. Sustained monomorphic VT occurring greater than 48 hours after an MI is a strong independent predictor of 6-week mortality.[28] Sustained ventricular arrhythmias complicate 2% to 20% of acute MIs and are associated with increased in-hospital mortality rate.[29] However, it has been suggested that sustained VT/ventricular fibrillation (VF) in the peri-infarct period (24-48 hours) is not associated with any increased long-term mortality risk, although this is still somewhat controversial.[30,31] Both early (< 2 days) and late (> 2 days) occurrences of sustained VT and VF were associated with a higher risk of later mortality in the Global Utilization of Streptokinase and TPA for Occluded Arteries-1 (GUSTO-1) study ($P < .001$).[31] Among patients who survived hospitalization in this study, no significant difference was found in 30-day mortality rate between the VT/VF and no VT/VF groups, although after one year, the mortality rate was significantly higher in the VT alone and VT/VF groups ($P < .0001$).[31]

There are some types of "idiopathic" VT—right ventricular outflow tract (RVOT) VT, left ventricular outflow tract (LVOT) VT, or left ventricular fascicular VT—that may first be identified during monitoring in the ICU. These arrhythmias are considered benign in nature, with low risk of sudden cardiac death occurring in the setting of a structurally normal heart. Salvos of monomorphic VT arising from the RVOT are illustrated in Figure 32-25. These arrhythmias are often effectively treated with a β blocker or calcium channel blocker.

What is the acute management of wide complex tachycardias?

The primary treatment for nonsustained VT is first to evaluate for potential causes. Reversible causes, such as electrolyte abnormalities or ischemia, should first be addressed. If the VT is mildly symptomatic in the setting of a structurally normal heart without underlying coronary artery disease, a trial of a β blocker may be considered. β Blockers are also useful for primary prevention of sudden cardiac death in patients with asymptomatic ventricular ectopy or nonsustained VT in the setting of reduced left ventricular systolic function. Although membrane-active antiarrhythmic agents may be useful in suppression of ventricular ectopy, these are not recommended in the setting of underlying structural heart disease because of potential adverse effects or proarrhythmia. "Proarrhythmia" is more common in patients with underlying structural heart disease, reduced left ventricular function, or coronary disease. When antiarrhythmic agents were used to suppress ventricular ectopy in a multicenter clinical trial, Cardiac Arrhythmia Suppression Trial (CAST), the study was terminated prematurely because there was an increased mortality rate in the treated group.[32] In some situations, particularly

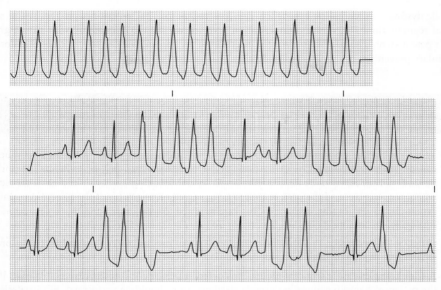

Figure 32-25. Rhythm strips demonstrating a wide complex tachycardia. Salvos of monomorphic ventricular tachycardia (VT) are noted with ventricular premature depolarizations having an identical morphology as the runs of VT. This occurred in a young woman with a structurally normal heart and repetitive monomorphic VT arising from the right ventricular outflow tract. This type of VT is benign and was responsive to β-blocker therapy.

in the absence of structural heart disease or with recurrent VT requiring frequent implantable cardioverter defibrillator shock therapy, catheter ablation should be considered if medications are not tolerated or are ineffective.[22]

In hemodynamically stable sustained monomorphic VT, a 12-lead ECG, history, and laboratory studies should be performed. The history should include questions regarding ischemic heart disease, prior MI, and drug therapy, particularly with antiarrhythmic drugs. Identification of reversible causes, such as ischemia or hypokalemia, should be evaluated and treated. Treatment options include synchronized DC cardioversion with sedation and/or IV antiarrhythmic drugs (amiodarone, procainamide, lidocaine). A bolus of amiodarone 150 mg over 10 minutes followed by a continuous infusion of 1.0 mg/min for 6 hours, then 0.5 mg/min may be administered. Intravenous amiodarone can cause hypotension, which requires a dose reduction or discontinuation of the drug. If VT is thought to be ischemic in nature, then IV lidocaine may be effective.[33] Lidocaine is dosed at a 1- to 1.5-mg/kg bolus over 2 to 3 minutes with a continuous infusion at 1 to 4 mg/min. Lidocaine can cause neurotoxicity, which is dose-dependent. Monitoring of daily lidocaine levels may be useful, particularly in the setting of hepatic disease or a low cardiac output state. Hemodynamically unstable monomorphic VT or pulseless VT should be treated promptly with DC cardioversion.

Sustained polymorphic VT is an unstable and hemodynamically poorly tolerated rhythm, and prompt DC cardioversion is required. Once cardioverted, the QT interval should be measured. If the QT interval is normal, acute ischemia should be suspected and urgent angiography may be considered. Administration of β blockers to reduce ischemia should also be considered. If the QT interval is prolonged, any QT-prolonging drugs should be discontinued and any electrolyte abnormalities corrected. If bradycardia or pause-dependent polymorphic VT is suspected, pacing or IV isoproterenol should be initiated. For patients with congenital long QT syndrome and torsades de pointes, β-blocker therapy should be initiated and an implantable defibrillator should be strongly considered for prevention of sudden cardiac death.

In the case presented in this section, the rhythm was effectively terminated following administration of IV amiodarone. Echocardiography following conversion revealed moderate left ventricular

Cardiovascular Problems

systolic dysfunction with a left ventricular ejection fraction of 42%, anterior hypokinesis, and mild mitral regurgitation. Diagnostic catheterization revealed no change in anatomy with patent grafts and a patent stent. The patient underwent insertion of an implantable cardioverter-defibrillator for secondary prevention of sudden cardiac death.

! CRITICAL CONSIDERATIONS

- When evaluating a patient with symptomatic bradycardia, a search for potential offending causes (such as AV nodal blocking drugs, electrolyte abnormalities, or ischemia) should be undertaken. Sinus node suppressant or AV nodal blocking agents should be withheld whenever possible, and the patient should be observed on telemetry. If the patient remains symptomatic with bradycardia, or if drugs are required to treat other conditions, permanent pacing may be required.

- Patients with recurrent SVT may be treated with either medical therapy or catheter ablation as first-line treatment, after the acute episode has been terminated.

- A wide complex tachycardia should be considered as possible VT until proven otherwise. If the patient is hemodynamically unstable, cardioversion should be performed. ECG criteria to help distinguish VT from SVT with aberration are useful in the hemodynamically stable patient presenting with a wide complex tachycardia.

- Polymorphic VT associated with a preceding long QT interval should be treated by cardioversion if it results in hemodynamic compromise prior to spontaneous conversion. A search for potential offending drugs or electrolyte abnormalities should be performed.

- In patients with sustained or nonsustained VT, a search for underlying heart disease should be performed. This should include a 2-D echocardiogram and evaluation to exclude ischemic heart disease in most patients.

REFERENCES

1. Epstein AC, DiMarco JP, Ellenbogen KA, et al. ACC/AHA/HRS 2008 guidelines for device-based therapy of cardiac rhythm abnormalities: a report of the American College of Cardiology/American Heart Association Task Force on Practice Guidelines (Writing Committee to Revise the ACC/AHA/NASPE 2002 Guideline Update for Implantation of Cardiac Pacemakers and Antiarrhythmia Devices): developed in collaboration with the American Association for Thoracic Surgery and Society of Thoracic Surgeons. *Circulation*. 2008;117:e350-e408.

2. O'Keefe J, Hammil S, Freed M, Pogwizd S. *The Complete Guide to ECG: A Comprehensive Study Guide to Improve ECG Interpretation Skills*. 2nd ed. Sudbury, MA: Physician's Press; 2002.

3. Pejković B, Krajnc I, Anderhuber F, Kosutić D. Anatomical aspects of the arterial blood supply to the sinoatrial and atrioventricular nodes of the human heart. *J Int Med Res*. 2008;36(4):691-698.

4. Saoudi N, Cosio F, Waldo A, et al. A classification of atrial flutter and regular atrial tachycardia according to electrophysiological mechanisms and anatomical bases: a statement from a Joint Expert Group from the Working Group of Arrhythmias of the European Society of Cardiology and the North American Society of Pacing and Electrophysiology. *Eur Heart J*. 2001;22(14):1162-1182.

5. Josephson ME. *Clinical Cardiac Electrophysiology: Techniques and Interpretations*. 3rd ed. Philadelphia, PA: Lippincott Williams & Wilkins; 2002.

6. Lee KL, Chun HM, Liem LB, et al. Effect of adenosine and verapamil in catecholamine-induced accelerated atrioventricular junctional rhythm: insights into the underlying mechanism. *Pacing Clin Electrophysiol*. 1999;99:1034-1040.

7. Kalman JM, Olgin JE, Karch MR, et al. "Cristal tachycardias": origin of right atrial tachycardias from the crista terminalis identified by intracardiac echocardiography. *J Am Coll Cardiol.* 1998;31:451-459.

8. Kistler PM, Sanders P, Fynn SP, et al. Electrophysiological and electrocardiographic characteristics of focal atrial tachycardia originating from the pulmonary veins: acute and long-term outcomes of radiofrequency ablation. *Circulation.* 2003;108:1968-1975.

9. Dunn MI. Thrombolism with atrial flutter. *Am J Cardiol.* 1998;82:580-583.

10. Seidl K, Hauer B, Schwick NG, et al. Risk of thromboembolic events in patients with atrial flutter. *Am J Cardiol.* 1998;82:580-583.

11. Blomstrom-Lundqvist C, Scheinman M, Aliot E, et al. ACC/AHA/ESC guidelines for the management of patients with supraventricular arrhythmias—executive summary: a report of the American College of Cardiology/American Heart Association Task Force on Practice Guidelines and the European Society of Cardiology Committee for Practice Guidelines (Writing Committee to Develop Guidelines for the Management of Patients with Supraventricular Arrhythmias). *Circulation.* 2003; 108:1871-1909.

12. Bismuth C, Gaultier M, Conso F, Efthymiou ML. Hyperkalemia in acute digitalis poisoning: prognostic significance and therapeutic implications. *Clin Toxicol.* 1973;6:153-162.

13. Wellens H, Brugada P. Mechanisms of supraventricular tachycardia. *Am J Cardiol.* 1988;62:10D-15D.

14. Chen SA, Chiang CE, Yang CJ, et al. Sustained atrial tachycardia in adult patients; electrophysiological characteristics, pharmacological response, possible mechanisms, and effects of radiofrequency ablation. *Circulation.* 1994;90:1262-1278.

15. Kuck KH, Kunze KP, Schluter M, et al. Encainide versus flecainide for chronic atrial and junctional ectopic tachycardia. *Am J Cardiol.* 1988;62: 37L-44L.

16. Trappe HJ, Brandts D, Weismueller P. Arrhythmias in intensive care patients. *Curr Opin Crit Care.* 2003;9:345-350.

17. Go AS, Hylek EM, Phillips KA, et al. Prevalence of diagnosed atrial fibrillation in adults: national implications for rhythm management and stroke prevention: the AnTicoagulation and Risk Factors in Atrial Fibrillation (ATRIA) Study. *JAMA.* 2001;285:2370-2375.

18. Polanczyk CA, Goldman L, Marcantonio ER, Oray EJ, Lee TH. Supraventricular arrhythmia in patients having noncardiac surgery: clinical correlates and effect on length of stay. *Ann Intern Med.* 1998;129(4):279-285.

19. Maisel WH, Rawn JD, Stevenson WG. Atrial fibrillation after cardiac surgery. *Ann Intern Med.* 2001;135(12):1061-1073.

20. Fuster V, Ryden LE, Cannom DS, et al. ACC/AHA/ESC 2006 guidelines for the management of patients with atrial fibrillation. *J Am Coll Cardiol.* 2006;48:854-906.

21. Gupta AK, Thakur RK. Wide QRS complex tachycardia. *Med Clin North Am.* 2001;85:245.

22. Zipes D, Camm AJ, Borggrefe M, et al. ACC/AHA/ESC 2006 guidelines for management of patients with ventricular arrhythmias and the prevention of sudden cardiac death-executive summary: a report of the American College of Cardiology/American Heart Association Task Force and the European Society of Cardiology Committee for the Practice Guidelines (Writing Committee to Develop Guidelines for Management of Patients with Ventricular Arrhythmias and the Prevention of Sudden Cardiac Death). *J Am Coll Cardiol.* 2006;48:1064-1108.

23. Edhouse J, Morris F. ABC of clinical electrocardiography: broad complex tachycardia—part I. *BMJ.* 2002;324:719-722.

24. Brugada P, Brugada J, Mont L, Smeets J, Andries EW. A new approach to the differential diagnosis of a regular tachycardia with a wide QRS complex. *Circulation.* 1991;83:1649-1659.

25. Kindlwall KE, Brown J, Josephson ME. Electrocardiographic criteria for ventricular tachycardia in wide complex left bundle branch block morphology tachycardias. *Am J Cardiol.* 1988;61:1279-1283.

26. Bigger JT Jr, Fleiss JL, Rolnitzky LM. Prevalence, characteristics and significance of ventricular tachycardia detected by 24 hour continuous electrocardiographic recordings in the late hospital phase of acute myocardial infarction. *Am J Cardiol.* 1986;58(13):1151-1160.

27. Mukharji J, Rude RE, Poole WK, et al. Risk factors for sudden death after acute myocardial infarction: two year follow-up. *Am J Cardiol.* 1984;54:31-36.

28. Volpi A, Cavalli A, Turato R, Barlera S, Santoro E, Negri E. Incidence and short-term prognosis of late sustained ventricular tachycardia after myocardial infarction: results of the Gruppo Italiano per lo Studio della Sopravvivenza nell'Infarto Miocardico (GISSI-3) data base. *Am Heart J.* 2001;142:87-92.

29. Piccini JP, Berger JS, Brown DL. Early sustained ventricular arrhythmias complicating acute myocardial infarction. *Am J Med.* 2008;121:797-804.

Cardiovascular Problems

30. Volpi A, Cavalli A, Franzosi MG, et al. One-year prognosis of primary ventricular fibrillation complicating acute myocardial infarction. The GISS (Gruppo Italiano per lo Studio della Streptochinasi nell'Infarto Miocardico) investigators. *Am J Cardiol.* 1989;63:1174-1178.

31. Newby KH, Thompson T, Stebbins A, Topol EJ, Califf RM. Sustained ventricular arrhythmias in patients receiving thrombolytic therapy: incidence and outcomes. The GUSTO Investigators. *Circulation.* 1998;98;2567-2573.

32. Echt DS, Liebson PR, Mitchell LB, et al. Mortality and morbidity in patients receiving encainide, flecainide, or placebo. The Cardiac Arrhythmia Suppression Trial. *N Engl J Med.* 1991;324:781-788.

33. Nasir N Jr, Taylor A, Doyle TK, et al. Evaluation of intravenous lidocaine for the termination of sustained monomorphic ventricular tachycardia in patients with coronary artery disease with or without healed myocardial infarction. *Am J Cardiol.* 1994;74:1183-1186.

CHAPTER

33

Congestive Heart Failure

Fredric Ginsberg, MD
Joseph E. Parrillo, MD

A 72-year-old woman is admitted to the intensive care unit (ICU) with a 9-hour history of left-sided weakness and tachypnea. She has had hypertension for over 15 years. There is no history of current chest pain or previous neurologic illness. Physical examination shows that she is awake and mildly lethargic. Pulse is regular at 80 bpm. Blood pressure is 210/110 mm Hg in both arms. Respiratory rate is 34 breaths/min. Temperature is 37°C. There is no pallor or jaundice. Jugular venous pressure is not elevated. Carotid pulses are brisk. Lungs show rales bilaterally. Cardiac examination shows normal heart tones without murmur. There is an S_3 gallop. Abdomen is soft without mass. There is no peripheral edema. Neurologic examination shows the patient to be lethargic. There is a left hemiparesis.

Laboratory shows normal complete blood cell count and chemistry profile. Serum B-natriuretic peptide (BNP) is elevated at 700 pg/mL. Serum troponin I is elevated at 0.10. Electrocardiogram (ECG) shows sinus rhythm with left ventricular hypertrophy and repolarization abnormality. Chest radiography shows cardiomegaly with signs of pulmonary edema. Emergency computed tomography scan of the head shows signs of acute right hemisphere ischemic infarction.

What are the initial steps in the therapy for this patient's cardiac and medical illness?

This patient has evidence of an acute cerebrovascular accident involving the right hemisphere. In addition, tachypnea, pulmonary rales, and S_3 gallop on examination are consistent with the diagnosis of heart failure, which is confirmed by abnormalities of the chest radiograph and serum BNP level. The immediate goals of therapy for heart failure are to improve dyspnea, optimize blood pressure, reduce lung congestion, and improve cardiac output. Medical treatments to reverse or prevent myocardial injury are instituted, and a search for reversible causes of heart failure needs to occur (see the box below). Drug therapy is initiated in order to improve hemodynamic status while preserving neurologic and renal function. Therapies should not increase the risk of myocardial ischemia and necrosis or promote the occurrence of arrhythmia. Careful serial assessment of patient status is mandatory to guide pharmacologic therapy following signs of heart failure on physical examination. Pulmonary rales, S_3 gallop, elevated jugular venous pressure, urine output, and pulse oximetry are important signs to follow.

Unlike chronic systolic heart failure, there is a paucity of controlled study data and few evidence-based guidelines for the treatment of acute heart failure. Strategies are based on small studies, experience, observation, and consensus of opinion. Initial therapies include supplemental oxygen and assessment of the need for ventilatory assistance with external positive airway pressure (continuous positive airway pressure or bilevel positive airway pressure) or endotracheal intubation with mechanical ventilation. External positive pressure

619

Cardiovascular Problems

Goals of Therapy during Hospitalization for Acute Heart Failure

Clinical

- Decreased dyspnea and orthopnea, improved exercise tolerance
- Improved pulmonary function and oxygenation
- Diuresis
- Decreased body fluid weight and edema
- Systolic blood pressure maintained > 80 mm Hg

Laboratory

- Normalized serum electrolyte levels
- Optimized renal function
- Decreased serum B-natriuretic peptide levels

Hemodynamics

- Pulmonary capillary wedge pressure < 16–18 mm Hg
- Central venous pressure < 8 mm Hg
- Normalized cardiac index

Improved prognosis

- Treatment of ischemia
- Evidence-based pharmacologic therapy initiated

ventilation improves oxygenation and pulmonary compliance and decreases work of breathing. This may prevent the need for endotracheal intubation. The latter may be required for patients with severe hypercapnia, acidosis, and respiratory muscle fatigue.[1]

Initial medical therapy includes intravenous morphine, which acts as a vasodilator, lowers blood pressure, and often reduces heart rate. Intravenous loop diuretics offer rapid and effective relief of dyspnea and tachypnea and often lead to rapid decongestion of the lungs. Although no randomized clinical trials exist, the use of loop diuretics is supported by a long history of clinical success. These agents increase renal excretion of salt and water. Furosemide is most often used, in a dose of 20 to 80 mg intravenously every 6 to 12 hours, titrated to adequate urine output. The onset of action of intravenous bolus furosemide is 30 minutes and peak effect occurs at 1 to 2 hours. The half-life of the medication is 6 hours, so twice-daily dosing is usually required after the patient has been stabilized.[2] Other loop diuretics that may be used are bumetanide and torsemide (Table 33-1). These drugs may be helpful in patients with suboptimal responses to furosemide.[3,4]

Table 33-1. Parenteral Loop Diuretics Used for the Treatment of Acute, Severe Heart Failure

	Initial IV dose	Maximum IV bolus dose
Bumetanide	1.0 mg	4-8 mg
Furosemide	40 mg	160-200 mg
Torsemide	10 mg	100-200 mg

Table 33-2. Continuous IV Infusion of Loop Diuretics

	Dose
Bumetanide	1 mg IV load, then 0.5-2 mg/h
Furosemide	40 mg IV load, then 10-40 mg/h
Torsemide	20 mg IV load, then 5-20 mg/h

Patients with chronic heart failure or associated chronic renal insufficiency may exhibit resistance to oral or intravenous bolus loop diuretics. This occurs as a result of delayed oral absorption and reduced amounts of drug delivered to the renal tubule, resulting in reduced responsiveness to the drug's diuretic effect. This resistance is associated with a poorer prognosis.[1] Constant delivery of diuretics with intravenous infusions over 8 hours has been shown to result in superior diuresis and natriuresis when compared to intravenous bolus administration with a low incidence of ototoxicity[5] (Table 33-2). Hypokalemia, alkalosis, and hypomagnesemia are frequent side effects of loop diuretics and can potentiate the occurrence of arrhythmias. Electrolyte levels must be carefully monitored during aggressive diuretic therapy. Diuretics may worsen renal function because of alterations in renal hemodynamics. Some degree of azotemia may need to be accepted to obtain adequate relief of dyspnea and edema. The dose of loop diuretics should be titrated to the response of the patient's symptoms, and should be reduced as symptoms improve.

Diuretics of other classes can be added to potentiate the effect of loop diuretics. Metolazone and thiazides act distally in the renal tubule. These have synergistic effects when used in combination with loop diuretics. Aldosterone blockers such as spironolactone or eplerenone can also be added[6] (Table 33-3).

This patient is also significantly hypertensive, which aggravates the heart failure syndrome by increasing left ventricular afterload. Patients with chronic hypertension and left ventricular hypertrophy also commonly have abnormalities of left ventricular diastolic function. Intravenous vasodilators are very useful in patients with hypertension and acute heart failure. Intravenous nitroglycerin is an effective systemic and coronary vasodilator. It is very useful in heart failure caused by acute coronary ischemia, as it improves coronary blood flow. Intravenous nitroglycerin is effective in lowering preload and pulmonary capillary wedge pressure, thereby reducing pulmonary congestion without increasing oxygen demand. It is also an arterial dilator at high doses, but is less effective at reducing afterload than nitroprusside. Dosage ranges between 5 and 200 μg/min. A major limitation of the use of intravenous nitroglycerin is the rapid development of tolerance to the drug's effect, often occurring after only 24 hours of therapy. Having a "nitrate-free" period during the daily dosage regimen may be required to limit the development of tolerance.

Intravenous sodium nitroprusside is a powerful venous and arterial dilator. It is very effective in treating hypertension-related heart failure complicated by pulmonary edema, as well as severe heart failure due to acute mitral regurgitation. This drug causes significant reduction of afterload and preload, leading to decreased right atrial pressure, decreased systemic vascular resistance and mean systemic blood pressure, decreased pulmonary capillary wedge pressure, and increased cardiac index in patients with heart failure and left ventricular dysfunction. Nitroprusside should be used in the ICU setting, preferably with invasive monitoring, including a pulmonary artery catheter and arterial line. Dosage range is 0.3 to 5.0 μg/kg per minute. Limitations of nitroprusside use include inducing a coronary "steal" syndrome in patients with active coronary ischemia.[2] In addition, toxic metabolites can accumulate with more prolonged administration. In patients with significant hepatic dysfunction, thiocyanate levels rise, and in patients with renal dysfunction, cyanide is generated.

Nesiritide (BNP) is another parenteral vasodilator that can be used in the treatment of acute heart failure. BNP is a hormone produced by ventricular and atrial myocytes in response to cardiac chamber

Table 33-3. Oral Diuretics Recommended for Use in Chronic Heart Failure

Drug	Initial daily dose	Maximum daily dose	Duration of action
Loop Diuretics			
Bumetanide	0.5-1.0 mg once or twice	10 mg	4-6 h
Furosemide	20-40 mg once or twice	600 mg	6-8 h
Torsemide	10-20 mg once	200 mg	12-16 h
Thiazide Diuretics			
Chlorothiazide	250-500 mg once or twice	1000 mg	6-12 h
Chlorthalidone	12.5-25 mg once	100 mg	24-72 h
Hydrochlorothiazide	25 mg once or twice	200 mg	6-12 h
Indapamide	2.5 mg once	5 mg	36 h
Metolazone	2.5 mg once	20 mg	12-24 h
Aldosterone Antagonists			
Spironolactone	12.5-25 mg once	50 mg[a]	2-3 d
Eplerenone	12.5-25 mg once	50 mg	16-24 h

[a]Higher doses may occasionally be used with close monitoring of serum creatinine and potassium.

dilatation and myofibril stretch. Human BNP is manufactured by recombinant DNA technology and is available as nesiritide, a formulation for intravenous use. Its hemodynamic effects are systemic venous and arterial dilation, coronary vasodilation, natriuresis, and diuresis. Its effects include rapid reduction in pulmonary capillary wedge pressure and mean right atrial pressure, exceeding the effects of intravenous nitroglycerin when compared directly.[7] It is not proarrhythmic and does not induce tolerance.[8] It can potentiate the effects of loop diuretics. Some patients do not respond to nesiritide. Significant hypotension may limit its use in some patients.[2] Because the hypotensive effects of nesiritide are less marked than nitroprusside, nesiritide can be used without invasive hemodynamic monitoring and can be initiated in emergency department settings. Nesiritide is initiated as an intravenous bolus dose of 2 μg/kg followed by infusion of 0.01 μg/kg per minute. Nesiritide was compared to dobutamine in patients with severe heart failure: nesiritide infusion was associated with less tachycardia and ventricular arrhythmia.[9] In another study, there was a trend toward improved survival with nesiritide,[10] and mortality and rehospitalization rates at 6 months were lower with nesiritide.[8] Nesiritide effectively relieves dyspnea and reduces left ventricular filling pressures and it may be safer than the inotropes milrinone and dobutamine (Table 33-4).

A review of multicenter randomized controlled trials of the use of nesiritide in patients with acute decompensated heart failure raised questions about the drug's safety. A meta-analysis of three randomized trials of nesiritide suggested a slight increase in mortality rate in patients given nesiritide versus a placebo control group.[11] There is a concern that this may be mediated through an adverse effect on renal function.[12] However, a retrospective review of patients receiving intravenous vasoactive medications for acute heart failure indicated that mortality rates, adjusted for clinical variables, were equivalent for patients receiving nitroglycerin and nesiritide. Patients who received intravenous nesiritide or intravenous nitroglycerin had a lower in-hospital mortality rate compared with patients who received dobutamine or milrinone.[13]

Table 33-4. A Comparison of Hemodynamic Effects of Parenteral Vasodilators and Inotropic Agents

	Nitroprusside	Nesiritide	Dobutamine	Milrinone
Mechanism of action	Balanced vasodilator	Vasodilator, natriuretic	β_1 stimulator	PDE inhibitor
Heart rate	–	–	slight ↑	slight ↑
Arrhythmia	–	–	+	+
Mean RA pressure	↓	↓	↓	↓↓
LVEDP	↓↓	↓↓	↓	↓↓
Mean arterial pressure	↓	↓	–	↓
SVR	↓↓	↓↓	↓	↓↓
Cardiac index	↑	↑	↑↑	↑↑
Inotropic effect	–	–	↑↑	↑
Hypotension	+	+	–	+
Direct Na^+ excretion	–	+	–	–
Other considerations	Increased cyanide and thiocyanate levels with prolonged infusion	Cannot follow serum BNP level during infusion	Difficult to use in patients on chronic β-blocker therapy	More vasodilator response at higher doses

Abbreviations: –, minimal or no effect; +, positive effect; ↑, mild increase; ↓, mild decrease; ↑↑, moderate increase; ↓↓, moderate decrease; BNP, B-natriuretic peptide; LVEDP, left ventricular end-diastolic pressure; PDE, phosphodiesterase; RA, right atrial; SVR, systemic vascular resistance.

A special panel, convened to review the safety of nesiritide, recommended that it be used only in patients admitted to the hospital with acute decompensated heart failure who were dyspneic at rest. This medication should not be used to replace diuretics, and there is no evidence that it enhances renal function.

Inotropic drugs are used for some patients with acute heart failure. Specific indications for these agents include persistent hypotension, low cardiac index, and signs of end-organ hypoperfusion, such as mental confusion; cold, clammy skin; or oliguria. Dobutamine and milrinone are commonly used inotropic drugs. The choice of agent depends on the specific clinical circumstances.[14,15] Dobutamine is a potent β_1 agonist with β_2- and α-agonist properties. Its major effect is to increase myocardial contractility. It also has venodilator properties. At doses of 2.5 to 15 μg/kg per minute, dobutamine will lower systemic vascular resistance and pulmonary capillary wedge pressure. Dobutamine causes a slight rise in heart rate and increases cardiac output. It increases myocardial oxygen demand. High doses are associated with vasoconstriction.

A limitation of dobutamine use is that in patients with heart failure, β receptors may be chronically down regulated, blunting its hemodynamic effects. In addition, dobutamine leads to increased myocardial oxygen demand and oxygen consumption, which is detrimental in patients with active coronary ischemia or following acute myocardial infarction. Increased ventricular arrhythmia has been associated with dobutamine use.[9] Also, tolerance to dobutamine effects has been demonstrated in patients with infusions lasting over 24 hours, theoretically due to induction of β-receptor down-regulation.[16]

Cardiovascular Problems

Milrinone is an inotropic agent that inhibits phosphodiesterase in the myocyte, which leads to increased intracellular cyclic adenosine monophosphate and calcium. It thus acts "downstream" from the β receptor. Hemodynamic effects include reduction of mean right atrial pressure and reduction in pulmonary and systemic vascular resistances. In heart failure, stroke volume and cardiac output are increased with a slight fall in mean systemic arterial pressure. Milrinone acts as a coronary vasodilator, and there is no net increase in myocardial oxygen consumption. Milrinone tends to lower arterial blood pressure, peripheral vascular resistance, and pulmonary capillary wedge pressure more than dobutamine. Milrinone's action is more prolonged. There is no tolerance or attenuation of its effect. Milrinone is started as a bolus dose, 50 to 75 μg/kg, with a maintenance infusion of 0.375 to 0.75 μg/kg per minute. Doses need to be reduced in patients with renal failure. Its use is limited in patients with hypotension (see Table 33-4).

Patients who do not respond to dobutamine may have a favorable response to milrinone. In the setting of acute heart failure, milrinone is used more often than dobutamine in view of its more potent vasodilator properties. In addition, its effects are not primarily mediated through β receptors, which is an important consideration in patients receiving concomitant β-blocker therapy. Milrinone and other inotropic agents are not indicated for routine use in patients with decompensated heart failure.[17]

In a study of class III/IV heart failure patients, a 14-day dobutamine infusion was associated with an *increased* risk of morbid events and higher short-term mortality rate. Another study compared 12-hour-per-day infusions of dobutamine and nitroprusside given over an average of 20 days, and nitroprusside showed better relief of symptoms and increased survival when compared with dobutamine.[18] No clinical studies have shown improved short-term or medium-term outcomes with inotropic therapy. The use of inotropic agents has been consistently associated with a *worse* prognosis for survival.[2] These negative outcomes with inotropic agents are felt to be related to their propensity to activate the sympathetic nervous system, increasing myocardial oxygen demand, exacerbating serious cardiac arrhythmias, increasing myocardial ischemia, and causing myonecrosis. Therefore, the use of inotropic agents should be restricted to short-term therapy (ie, < 72 hours) in patients with severe heart failure and problematic hypotension or critical end-organ hypoperfusion. Clinical examples where inotropic agents may be useful include cardiogenic shock due to acute myocardial infarction or right ventricular myocardial infarction, patients awaiting cardiac transplantation, or patients with end-stage heart failure. The decision to use inotropic agents in this circumstance is one that should be carefully individualized.

Vasopressors include dopamine and norepinephrine. Dopamine infusions at 1 to 5 μg/kg per minute lead to increased renal blood flow. At doses of 3 to 7 μg/kg per minute, dopamine causes increased myocardial contractility and heart rate through stimulation of β receptors. Vasoconstriction occurs at higher doses, 5 to 20 μg/kg per minute.[9] Dopamine is a less useful agent for treatment of heart failure because it causes tachycardia, coronary vasoconstriction, increased afterload, and increased oxygen consumption. Dobutamine generally will lead to a greater rise in cardiac output than dopamine in patients with heart failure. Dopamine can be used when significant hypotension is part of the hemodynamic picture in order to restore adequate arterial pressure for end-organ perfusion. Although dopamine at low doses is frequently added to inotropic therapy in an attempt to increase renal blood flow and augment diuresis, no controlled trials have demonstrated dopamine's usefulness in this setting. No significant benefit of "renal dose dopamine" has been shown in preventing acute renal failure in high-risk patients or in the treatment of established renal failure.[16]

Norepinephrine is a sympathomimetic agent with strong α-agonist and weak β-agonist effects. In patients with heart failure, norepinephrine's main effect is to raise blood pressure by increasing systemic vascular resistance with little effect on cardiac output. Dosage range is 0.2 to 1 μg/kg per minute. It will increase myocardial oxygen demand. Its use in the setting of heart failure is restricted to patients with the most severe hypotension, unresponsive to dopamine, or in patients with complicating illnesses such as sepsis.[16] Norepinephrine should be weaned off and discontinued as early as possible. (See Figure 33-1 for an algorithm for medical therapy of acute heart failure.)

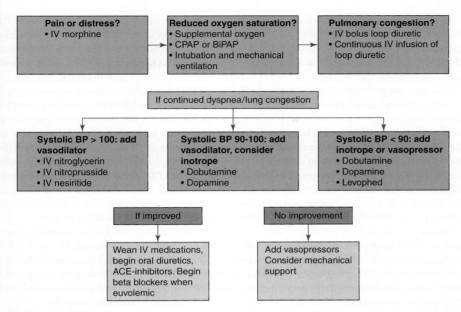

Figure 33-1. Management decisions in the therapy of acute heart failure. ACE, angiotensin-converting enzyme; BiPAP, bilevel positive airway pressure; BP, blood pressure; CPAP, continuous positive airway pressure; IV, intravenous. (*Adapted from Dickstein K, Cohen-Solal A, Filippatos G, et al. ESC Guidelines for the diagnosis and treatment of acute and chronic heart failure 2008. Eur Heart J. 2008;29:2388-2442.*)

Is a pulmonary artery catheter mandatory for effective management of this patient?

It is important to note that findings on physical examination may be insensitive indicators of hemodynamic status. Tailoring pharmacologic therapy to hemodynamic measurements obtained by placing a pulmonary artery catheter is often helpful and necessary to determine precise baseline measurements of cardiac output and other hemodynamic parameters, which then guides intensive intravenous drug therapy. In one study, clinical assessment of patients with severe heart failure was compared to measured pulmonary capillary wedge pressure and cardiac index. The severity of symptoms and findings on physical examination did not predict the hemodynamic status as defined by invasive monitoring.[19] Although pulmonary artery pressure monitoring has not been shown to improve prognosis in patients with heart failure, significant adverse effects have also not been demonstrated in these patients. When a pulmonary artery (PA) catheter is used in acute heart failure, hemodynamic targets of therapy include lowering pulmonary capillary wedge pressure to less than 18 mm Hg and lowering mean right atrial pressure to less than 8 mm Hg, with optimization of cardiac output.[20]

Aggressive therapy with parenteral vasodilators and diuretics, tailored to an early response in hemodynamic measurements obtained by bedside PA catheter monitoring, has been advocated as an effective method to obtain more rapid and sustained improvement in patients with acute severe heart failure.[3,4] When pulmonary capillary wedge pressure is reduced to less than 16 mm Hg and right atrial pressure reduced to less than 8 mm Hg, most patients will improve acutely. Additional hemodynamic goals include reducing systemic vascular resistance to less than 1200 dynes/s per cm^{-5}, improving cardiac index to greater than 2.6 L/min per m^2, and maintaining systolic blood pressure greater than 80 mm Hg. Pulmonary capillary wedge pressure can be lowered to a normal value of 10 to 12 mm Hg in many patients with significant left ventricular dysfunction, without untoward effects.[3,21]

Cardiovascular Problems

Improvement in hemodynamics can be obtained with aggressive intravenous vasodilator therapy. The choice of agents (intravenous nitroprusside, intravenous nitroglycerin, or nesiritide) depends on matching the specific hemodynamics and clinical picture of the patient's presentation with the predicted effects of each vasodilator.[7,22-24] After the initial derangement in hemodynamics has improved with therapy, a transition to oral therapy is then instituted to attempt to obtain sustained improvement in cardiac function.

Placement of a pulmonary artery catheter enables the clinician to accurately measure pulmonary capillary wedge pressure, cardiac output, and mixed venous oxygen saturation. Knowledge of these parameters helps to assess the effectiveness of therapy. Whether to *routinely* use PA catheters to assess and manage patients with acute heart failure has been long debated. The ESCAPE trial evaluated the routine use of PA catheterization in patients hospitalized with acute exacerbation of chronic heart failure and left ventricular systolic dysfunction.[25] There was no difference in the primary end point of days alive out of the hospital during 6 months after discharge in groups managed with or without a PA catheter. There were no subgroups identified where use of the PA catheter was beneficial. However, there was a trend noted in improving the initial diuresis, with less deterioration of renal function, in the PA catheter group.[20] The authors concluded that there was no indication for the *routine* use of PA catheters in the setting of acute heart failure.

Although not a routine procedure, the PA catheter is often an essential tool in the management of patients with acute severe heart failure. Indications for PA catheter use include the presence of cardiogenic shock, differentiating pulmonary from cardiac causes of dyspnea, defining hemodynamic parameters if one is unsure by clinical signs and symptoms, and determining management of patients who are not responding to initially prescribed therapies. Pulmonary catheter placement is also necessary as part of an evaluation when considering the implantation of a ventricular assist device.

In this patient, placement of a PA catheter is not indicated initially, as clinical assessment clearly indicates the presence of heart failure with pulmonary congestion. Shock and renal complications are not present.

 On the second hospital day, the patient's blood pressure is 130/75 mm Hg on intravenous nitroglycerin. Pulmonary edema has resolved and the patient has a good diuresis with intravenous bolus furosemide. She is now complaining of intermittent mild central chest discomfort. Left hemiparesis has significantly improved.

Serial ECGs show new, deep T-wave inversions in leads V_1 through V_6. Troponin level has trended down to the normal range. Resting echocardiogram shows moderate concentric left ventricular hypertrophy, a dilated left ventricle with global left ventricular (LV) hypokinesis, and a left ventricular ejection fraction reduced at 35%. There is no significant valve stenosis or regurgitation. Carotid ultrasound shows no significant stenosis of either internal carotid artery.

What are the next steps in evaluation and management?

The presence of chest pain, elevation of serum troponin, and new ECG changes suggest that acute myocardial ischemia is contributing to this patient's heart failure and LV dysfunction. It is important to determine the presence, extent, and severity of coronary artery disease in this setting.

Coronary artery disease can lead to acute heart failure via a number of different mechanisms. Acute ischemia leads to acute left ventricular diastolic dysfunction and elevation of left ventricular filling pressures. Acute ischemia can also cause "stunning," that is, reversible myocardial dysfunction due to severe and prolonged ischemia, which persists for some time after normal blood flow is restored. Acute myocardial infarction leads to necrosis of myocardial tissue and acute left ventricular systolic dysfunction due to loss of contractile tissue. The mechanical complications of myocardial infarction, papillary muscle rupture with acute, severe mitral valve regurgitation, and rupture of the

intraventricular septum will lead to acute severe heart failure and cardiogenic shock. Chronic ischemia can also cause myocardial contractile dysfunction without infarction, a process termed *hibernation*. Often, acute myocardial ischemia is superimposed on a ventricle impaired by chronic ischemia
and infarction, so that multiple mechanisms are usually operative in patients with chronic coronary
disease presenting with acute heart failure.[1,26]

Patients with acute heart failure due to myocardial infarction or acute myocardial ischemia have a
poor prognosis. In a large registry of 5573 consecutive patients with acute myocardial infarction, 42%
of patients had heart failure or left ventricular systolic dysfunction during hospitalization.[27] Patients
with heart failure tended to be older, were more commonly female, and were more likely to have
had previous myocardial infarction or coronary bypass surgery. Comorbidities were present more
commonly, including peripheral arterial disease, hypertension, diabetes mellitus, and previous stroke.
In-hospital mortality rate for these patients was 13%, versus 2.3% for patients with acute myocardial
infarction without heart failure or left ventricular dysfunction. Mortality rate was 13% to 21% for
patients with lung congestion and left ventricular ejection fraction less than 40%. Other complications also occurred more commonly in these patients, including atrial and ventricular arrhythmias,
reinfarction, and stroke (Figure 33-2).

In a European observational study, it was noted that 13% of patients hospitalized with acute coronary syndrome (ACS) without prior history of heart failure presented with heart failure on admission.[28] An additional 5.6% developed heart failure later during hospitalization. The incidence of acute
heart failure of 15.6% was identical in patients with ST-segment-elevation myocardial infarction
and non–ST-segment-elevation myocardial infarction. Prognosis for these patients was poor, with
in-hospital mortality rate of 12% for patients with heart failure on admission and 17.8% if heart failure developed during the hospitalization. This represents a three- to fourfold increased mortality
rate compared with patients with ACS without heart failure. These patients not only have a high in-
hospital mortality rate but also have a high morbidity and mortality rates after discharge, with an 8.5%
additional 6-month mortality rate and with 24% of patients being rehospitalized within 6 months.[26]

Several important points need to be stressed regarding acute heart failure due to acute ischemia.
Patients may develop acute heart failure even without significant left ventricular systolic dysfunction and
without acute necrosis. The majority of patients with ACS and heart failure will not have left ventricular
systolic dysfunction at discharge, and only a minority of these patients develop chronic heart failure.

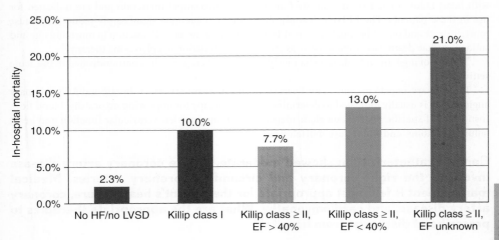

Figure 33-2. Hospital mortality rate related to the presence of heart failure in patients with acute myocardial
infarction. EF, left ventricular ejection fraction; HF, heart failure; LVSD, left ventricular systolic dysfunction; Killip
class I, no evidence of heart failure; Killip class II or higher, heart failure present.

In patients with acute heart failure due to acute myocardial infarction, rapid reperfusion is the cornerstone of therapy. Urgent coronary angiography is indicated to determine the most appropriate revascularization strategy.[26] This may be achieved with thrombolytic therapy, acute coronary angioplasty, or urgent coronary artery bypass surgery. In the GRACE study, revascularization therapies were associated with a lower mortality rate in patients with acute coronary syndrome and acute heart failure.[28]

Early aggressive pharmacologic therapies are also indicated. Acute treatment should include the use of intravenous diuretics and intravenous nitroglycerin (see above). β Blockers should be given early to patients with heart failure and ischemic chest pain, hypertension, or tachyarrhythmias. They should be used with caution in patients with severe heart failure and hypotension. Generally, β blockers should be continued in patients who were taking these drugs prior to hospitalization. Intra-aortic balloon counterpulsation should be used in patients with signs and symptoms of continued ischemia despite aggressive medical therapies.

In patients who develop heart failure or significant left ventricular systolic dysfunction (ejection fraction < 40%) after myocardial infarction, a number of pharmacologic therapies have been shown in large placebo-controlled randomized studies to improve mortality and reduce repeat hospitalization. β Blockers should be part of standard post–myocardial infarction therapy in these patients. For example, in the Carvedilol Post-infarct Survival Controlled Evaluation (CAPRICORN) study, a significant 23% relative risk reduction was achieved using the β blocker carvedilol.[29] The SAVE study was the first trial to show that the use of an angiotensin-converting enzyme (ACE) inhibitor (captopril) was beneficial in post–myocardial infarction patients with ejection fractions less than 40%.[30] There was a 5% absolute mortality rate reduction in 42 months of follow-up. Another trial showed that treatment with the ACE inhibitor ramipril, begun 3 to 10 days after myocardial infarction in patients with post–myocardial infarction heart failure, resulted in a significant mortality benefit at 15 months of follow-up.[31] Another trial showed that treatment with the ACE inhibitor trandolapril in patients after myocardial infarction with ejection fractions less than 35% resulted in a significantly improved survival at 2 to 4 years of follow-up.[32] Therefore, β blockers and ACE inhibitors should be started early and continued long-term. In the VALIANT study, a high dose of the angiotensin receptor blocker valsartan was as effective as an ACE inhibitor in improving survival and reducing cardiovascular morbidity rate.[33] Angiotensin receptor blockers are thus recommended in post–myocardial infarction patients with heart failure who are intolerant to ACE inhibitors.

Aldosterone blockers have also been shown to be effective in improving prognosis in patients with heart failure or left ventricular dysfunction after myocardial infarction and are indicated for use in these patients. The EPHESUS study showed that eplerenone significantly reduced all-cause mortality rate and repeat hospitalizations at 16 months of follow-up.[34] Reduction in mortality rate and sudden cardiac death was noted as early as 30 days after initiation of eplerenone therapy.[35]

The use of digoxin and calcium channel blocking agents is generally contraindicated in the acute setting.[36]

In summary, in patients with acute heart failure due to coronary artery disease and ACS, coronary angiography is usually indicated to determine the best therapy for improving myocardial blood flow. Institution of specific pharmacologic management will improve left ventricular function and heart failure symptoms, and will reduce mortality risk.

Cardiac catheterization showed moderate, diffuse coronary artery disease involving the right coronary and circumflex coronary arteries. Medical management is felt most appropriate for the patient's heart failure, coronary artery disease, and cardiomyopathy. What are the appropriate therapies to prescribe at discharge from hospital?

The medical treatment of chronic systolic heart failure is based on results of many large, randomized, placebo-controlled trials (see below). Long-term goals of treatment are to improve symptoms and functional capacity, to prevent rehospitalization, and to prolong survival. Medical therapies accomplish these

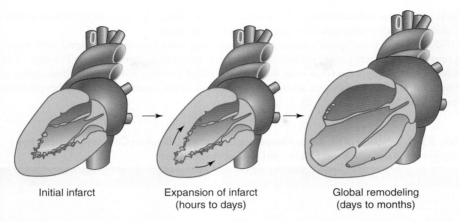

Initial infarct   Expansion of infarct   Global remodeling
                               (hours to days)   (days to months)

Figure 33-3. Pictorial representation of remodeling of the left ventricle in response to injury such as acute myocardial infarction. Over a period of days to months after transmural infarction, the left ventricle becomes dilated with decreased wall thickness and progressive impairment of systolic function.

by stabilizing or reversing the process of progressive LV dilatation and worsening systolic function, termed remodeling (Figure 33-3), as well as reducing the risk of sudden arrhythmic death. Therapies that accomplish "reverse remodeling" have been shown to improve long-term prognosis. These medications need to be initiated during hospitalization. Doses are then titrated up at subsequent outpatient evaluations.

Besides coronary artery disease, other common causes of LV systolic dysfunction and chronic heart failure include severe hypertension, chronic mitral or aortic valve regurgitation, and idiopathic dilated cardiomyopathy. Less common etiologies are familial cardiomyopathy, alcoholic cardiomyopathy, peripartum cardiomyopathy, myocarditis, diabetic cardiomyopathy, and cardiomyopathy seen in some patients with hyperthyroidism or severe obesity.[37-39] Regardless of the cause, chronic systolic heart failure is treated with a standard pharmacologic approach.

Pharmacologic treatment of heart failure involves combinations of multiple medications. Several drug classes have been shown to improve symptoms and functional capacity, decrease the need for repeat hospitalizations, and improve mortality rate (see below). Therapies are aimed at improving fluid balance as well as reversing the neurohormonal activation responsible for progressive decline in left ventricular function. Pharmacologic agents need to be started early in the course of the disease to prevent or attenuate the process of remodeling.

Diuretics are routinely used in patients with signs or symptoms of fluid retention.[6] Diuretics are continued once patients are euvolemic, to prevent reaccumulation of fluid. A flexible dosing schedule, based on daily weights, is very effective in maintaining a euvolemic state while reducing the frequency of diuretic side effects.

Angiotensin-converting enzyme inhibitors act to decrease the effects of the activation of the renin-angiotensin system by blocking the conversion of angiotensin I to angiotensin II, which has deleterious effects in heart failure. Many studies have shown benefits of ACE inhibitor therapy in post–myocardial infarction patients as well as patients with cardiomyopathy and heart failure. The SOLVD trial using enalapril in patients with class II/III heart failure and ejection fractions less than 35% showed a 10% relative risk reduction in mortality at 3.5 years.[40] Enalapril given to patients with asymptomatic left ventricular dysfunction (ejection fractions < 35%) resulted in a reduction in the development of clinical heart failure and a statistically significant reduction in heart failure hospitalizations at 3 years.[41] A meta-analysis performed of 32 trials, involving 7105 patients, using captopril, enalapril, ramipril, quinapril, or lisinopril found that ACE inhibitors reduce the risk of death and hospitalization due to heart failure.[42] These results indicate that the positive effects of ACE inhibitors are likely to be a class effect, and not specific to a particular agent.

Side effects of these agents include cough, worsening renal function in patients with underlying renal disease or renal artery stenosis, angioneurotic edema, and hyperkalemia. The dose of ACE inhibitors should be increased as renal function and blood pressure allow. Studies have shown that medium doses of ACE inhibitors, when compared to low doses, significantly reduce hospitalization rates for heart failure[43] (Table 33-5).

Table 33-5. Inhibitors of the Renin-Aldosterone System and β Blockers Commonly Used for the Treatment of Patients with Heart Failure with Low Ejection Fractions

Drug	Initial daily dose(s)	Maximum dose(s)
ACE inhibitors		
Captopril	6.25 mg 3 times	50 mg 3 times
Enalapril	2.5 mg twice	10-20 mg twice
Fosinopril	5-10 mg once	40 mg once
Lisinopril	2.5-5 mg once	20-40 mg once
Perindopril	2 mg once	8-16 mg once
Quinapril	5 mg twice	20 mg twice
Ramipril	1.25-2.5 mg once	10 mg once
Trandolapril	1 mg once	4 mg once
Angiotensin receptor blockers		
Candesartan	4-8 mg once	32 mg once
Losartan	25-50 mg once	50-100 mg once
Valsartan	20-40 mg twice	160 mg twice
Aldosterone antagonists		
Spironolactone	12.5-25 mg once	25 mg once or twice
Eplerenone	25 mg once	50 mg once
β Blockers		
Bisoprolol	1.25 mg once	10 mg once
Carvedilol	3.125 mg twice	25 mg twice (50 mg twice for patients > 85 kg)
Metoprolol succinate extended-release (metoprolol CR/XL)	12.5-25 mg once	200 mg once

Abbreviation: ACE, angiotensin-converting enzyme. *(From Nieminen MS, Bohm M, Cowie MR, et al. Executive summary of the guidelines on the diagnosis and treatment of acute heart failure. The Task Force on Acute Heart Failure of the European Society of Cardiology. Eur Heart J. 2005;26:384-416.)*

β-Blockers are very important medications to include in the treatment of patients with acute heart failure, especially if coronary artery disease and ischemia are present. Catecholamine levels are increased in heart failure, and higher levels correlate with worse disease severity. Catecholamines have direct negative effects on the myocardium, including induction of myocyte hypertrophy and apoptosis.[44] Clinically, these effects are evident as left ventricular dilation, increased ischemia, peripheral vasoconstriction, and cardiac arrhythmia.

β Blockers interfere with catecholamine-mediated activation of cardiac β receptors, thereby attenuating β-receptor–mediated increases in heart rate and oxygen consumption. Sympathetic nervous system–mediated effects on remodeling can be prevented or attenuated. In addition, the newer agent carvedilol also blocks α receptors, which mediate vasoconstriction and increase cardiac contractility.

Several large trials using β blockers in thousands of patients with chronic heart failure, or in post–myocardial infarction patients with ejection fractions less than 40%, have demonstrated significant and consistent reductions in the need for repeat rehospitalization for heart failure. Mortality rates are significantly improved. The BHAT study showed a relative 26% reduction in mortality at 2 years in post–myocardial infarction patients treated with propranolol.[45,46] The CIBIS II trial using bisoprolol showed a 34% relative risk reduction in hospitalizations and mortality at 16 months of therapy.[47] The MERIT-HF study showed a relative reduction of 33% in these end points at 12 months using long-acting metoprolol succinate.[48] Patients with more severe heart failure, class III/IV symptoms, with severely reduced ejection fractions less than 25% were studied in the COPERNICUS trial.[49] These patients began therapy with carvedilol in-hospital. At 10.4 months of follow-up, a 35% relative mortality reduction was seen, with improvement in mortality beginning as early as 3 weeks after initiation of therapy. In these trials, β-blockers were not discontinued more frequently than placebo for perceived side effects, and there was no increased risk of heart failure exacerbation due to β-blocker therapy when compared to placebo, even in the early phases of drug administration.[49,50] Several trials with carvedilol have shown an approximate 6% absolute increase in left ventricular ejection fraction after a minimum of 2 years of therapy.[51]

In patients with heart failure due to systolic dysfunction, β blockers should be instituted early once patients are deemed euvolemic, and titrated up to maximal recommended doses (eg, metoprolol succinate 200 mg daily or carvedilol 25 mg bid) or maximally tolerated doses. They are useful in patients with ischemic and nonischemic cardiomyopathy. β Blockers should be instituted in "compensated" patients as well, as these patients have a high likelihood of disease progression to symptomatic heart failure within 12 months. This therapy is indicated to be combined with ACE inhibitors in all patients with chronic systolic dysfunction (see Table 33-5).

Angiotensin receptor blockers (ARBs) work to counter the effects of angiotensin II at the tissue level by blocking angiotensin II receptors. Multiple studies have shown benefits of these medications in patients with heart failure. Large numbers of patients in controlled trials have been studied; these drugs have been as well studied as ACE inhibitors. Most often, ARBs were used as a substitute for ACE inhibitors. More recently, they have been evaluated as medications given in combination with ACE inhibitors and β blockers.

The use of candesartan in heart failure patients (mean ejection fraction of 27%) showed equivalent mortality rates and similar exercise tolerance and functional class to patients treated with enalapril at 3.5 years.[52] A study using losartan compared with captopril in patients with ejection fractions less than 40% showed no difference in mortality or heart failure admissions. Losartan was better tolerated because of the lower incidence of problematic cough.[53] When valsartan was used as a substitute for ACE inhibitor therapy, there was a relative 33% risk reduction in mortality when compared with placebo.[54] In the CHARM study, candesartan was prescribed for patients with ejection fractions less than 40%. A 17.5% relative risk reduction in cardiovascular death and congestive heart failure admissions was seen when this ARB was used as a substitute for ACE inhibitors.[55] When candesartan was added on to therapy with ACE inhibitors and β blockers, a 10% relative risk reduction was seen.[56]

In conclusion, ARBs are an appropriate choice for patients who cannot be maintained on ACE inhibitors because of side effects such as cough. Patients with angioneurotic edema during ACE inhibitor therapy can often be successfully treated with ARBs without developing this complication.[57,58] Adding ARB therapy onto ACE inhibitors and β blockers likely achieves a small additional benefit (see Table 33-5).

Aldosterone antagonists work to counteract the salt and water retention caused by aldosterone. In addition, this hormone is involved in the pathogenesis of progressive myocardial fibrosis, which occurs in heart failure. In the RALES trial, the aldosterone antagonist spironolactone was given to patients with severe, class III/IV heart failure with ejection fractions less than 35%. A 24% relative risk reduction in mortality was seen in treated patients over 2 years, with reduced cardiovascular death and reduced need for rehospitalization.[59] These medications are contraindicated in patients with renal insufficiency and creatinine levels over 2.5 mg/dL or in patients with baseline potassium levels greater than 5.0 mmol/L.

An analysis of a large Canadian health care database showed a substantial increase in the frequency of spironolactone use after the RALES study was published. This increased use was temporally associated with a two- to three fold increased rate of hospitalization for hyperkalemia.[60] These authors stressed the need for careful monitoring of serum electrolytes after aldosterone blockers are initiated. They should be reserved for patients with severe, symptomatic left ventricular systolic dysfunction. Spironolactone should be initiated at low doses, such as 12.5 mg daily or every other day, especially in elderly patients (see Table 33-5).

Hydralazine/isosorbide dinitrate (ISDN) combination therapy was associated with mortality improvement when compared to placebo in one study in the era prior to the advent of ACE inhibitors and β-blocker therapy for heart failure.[61] A retrospective analysis of this study suggested that African American patients may have benefited preferentially. More recently, the A-HeFT study enrolled over 1000 self-described black patients with class II to IV heart failure and ejection fractions less than 45%.[62] The use of the combination of hydralazine with ISDN, titrated to a dose of 75 mg hydralazine plus 40 mg ISDN given three times daily, was associated with a 40% relative risk reduction in mortality at 10 months and a 33% relative risk reduction in first hospitalization for heart failure. This therapy was used as add-on treatment to β blockers, ACE inhibitors, and spironolactone. A hydralazine/ISDN combination tablet is now commercially available and is approved for treatment of heart failure in black patients with heart failure and left ventricular systolic dysfunction.

Digoxin works by inhibiting the myocyte sodium/potassium pump, leading to increased intracellular calcium levels and increased inotropy. However, digoxin is a relatively weak inotropic agent. In addition, it has vagotonic effects. The use of digoxin in heart failure has been studied in large numbers of patients. A decreased need for rehospitalization for heart failure was seen with this therapy. However, there was no improvement in overall mortality.[63] Therefore, digoxin is indicated only for patients with symptomatic heart failure.[6] It is also useful in heart failure patients with atrial fibrillation, to help control the ventricular rate. Digoxin is not useful in the setting of acute heart failure, and it should be avoided in patients with hypokalemia, bradycardia, or heart block.

This patient's heart failure was treated with lisinopril 10 mg daily, carvedilol 3.125 mg bid, and spironolactone 25 mg daily. At discharge from the hospital, physical examination showed a blood pressure of 120/75 mm Hg, sinus rhythm at 65/min, clear lungs, and no cardiac murmur. She will see her outpatient physician regularly to monitor hypertension and to titrate the doses of lisinopril and carvedilol upward.

In what way could this patient's heart failure and cardiomyopathy be related to her acute neurologic event?

Acute and reversible myocardial dysfunction, termed *neurogenic stunned myocardium (NSM)*, can occur in patients with acute intracranial illness, independent of preexisting heart disease.[64] It has been most commonly reported in association with acute subarachnoid hemorrhage, but it can also occur with intracranial hemorrhage, acute ischemic stroke, and head trauma.[65]

In 1954, Burch et al first described ECG abnormalities in 17 patients with acute stroke, 14 of whom had central nervous system hemorrhage.[66] These changes included increased T-wave amplitude, deep T-wave inversions, prolonged QT interval, and prominent U waves. In 1960, Cropp and Manning reported similar ECG changes suggestive of acute myocardial infarction or ischemia in 15 of 29 cases of subarachnoid hemorrhage.[67] In addition to ECG abnormalities, echocardiography showed regional or global left ventricular wall motion abnormalities and confirmed the presence of NSM. Patients with wall motion abnormalities were shown to be more likely to have elevation of serum cardiac enzymes, severe neurologic deficit, and higher mortality rate.[68-70] In a group of patients with subarachnoid hemorrhage accompanied by ST-segment elevation in the precordial leads on ECG, without a history of heart disease, left ventriculography showed a dilated left ventricle with a large apical wall motion abnormality, which subsequently improved over several weeks.[71] Coronary angiography showed normal coronary arteries, confirming the neurogenic etiology of the cardiomyopathy.

Histopathology from autopsy specimens or endomyocardial biopsies in patients with NSM has shown myocytolysis and myofibrillar degeneration in the subendocardium.[68,71] This pattern is termed *contraction band necrosis,* reflecting myocyte death with hypercontracted sarcomeres.[72]

Subsequent reports describe ECG abnormalities mimicking acute myocardial infarction or ischemia in 50% to 90% of patients with subarachnoid hemorrhage.[65,69,73] Elevation of serum cardiac biomarkers is a highly sensitive and specific marker for this condition. Elevation of creatine kinase-MB (CK-MB) and troponin is seen in 20% to 50% of patients with subarachnoid hemorrhage and is more likely to occur in patients with more severe neurologic injury. Myocardial enzyme elevation is associated with overt left ventricular dysfunction.[68,69,74,75] In patients with ischemic stroke without known ischemic heart disease, elevation of troponin I was seen in 10% of patients. These patients tended to be older, had more severe strokes, and had more heart failure and renal disease. Elevation of troponin was associated with a threefold increased mortality risk.[76]

NSM occurs in 20% to 30% of patients with subarachnoid hemorrhage, usually early in the course of the illness.[65,72,77] It is more likely to occur in patients with more severe neurologic deficits. Left ventricular function is easily assessed at the bedside with echocardiography. Left ventricular wall motion abnormalities usually involve basal and midventricular segments, but can be global or even predominantly involve the left ventricular apex, similar to what is seen in stress-induced cardiomyopathy.[72] Right ventricular dysfunction may also be seen.[78] NSM is generally transient, resolving within weeks.

Because the ECG changes and wall motion abnormalities mimic ischemia due to coronary artery disease, coronary angiography may be necessary to exclude this diagnosis in older patients with preexisting risk factors for coronary artery disease. Life-threatening ventricular arrhythmias can occur in a small percentage of patients, especially if QT prolongation is present. The risk of cerebral vasospasm is also higher in patients with NSM.[68,79]

NSM is felt to be initiated by injury to the hypothalamus, causing a surge in adrenergic output from the brain. This, in turn, leads to an increase in local norepinephrine release in the myocardium. This results in myocyte calcium overload and contraction band myonecrosis.[65,71] Nuclear cardiac studies in patients with NSM and subarachnoid hemorrhage showed normal perfusion with abnormal sympathetic innervation. This supports the concept that cardiac adrenergic-mediated neuronal damage is responsible for the cardiomyopathy.[80]

Treatment of NSM is supportive. β-Adrenergic blocking drugs and α-blocking drugs (eg, phentolamine) may be of benefit.[74] In patients with severe NSM and cardiogenic shock, the use of intra-aortic balloon counterpulsation should be considered. Full hemodynamic and cardiac supportive measures are indicated as left ventricular function is likely to improve. Differentiation from acute myocardial infarction is important. NSM should be strongly suspected in patients with more severely depressed left ventricular ejection fractions (< 40%) with only modest elevation of troponin.[81] Definitive neurosurgical management of subarachnoid hemorrhage or intracranial hemorrhage should not be delayed in the presence of NSM.

Cardiovascular Problems

! CRITICAL CONSIDERATIONS

- The diagnosis of acute heart failure is made by history and physical examination findings, supported by laboratory testing (serum BNP level) and imaging with chest radiography and echocardiography.
- Placement of a pulmonary artery catheter may be necessary to define the hemodynamic status when the clinical picture is unclear, and to better assess the patient's response to management.
- Initial steps in the management of acute heart failure include adequate oxygen delivery, optimizing blood pressure and cardiac output, and evaluating for cardiac ischemia or acute myocardial infarction. Pharmacologic agents that may be used include intravenous loop diuretics, parenteral vasodilators, and inotropes.
- Transitioning the patient from intravenous to oral medications occurs after patients have been stabilized.
- The classes of oral medications indicated for the treatment of chronic heart failure include β blockers, angiotensin-converting enzyme inhibitors, angiotensin receptor blockers, aldosterone blockers, the combination of hydralazine and isosorbide dinitrate, and digoxin.
- In patients with documented acute left ventricular dysfunction, an evaluation for coronary artery disease is mandatory, and revascularization strategies are necessary when there is severe ischemia. This may involve coronary angioplasty or coronary artery bypass surgery.
- Acute cardiac injury mimicking myocardial infarction can occur in the setting of acute brain injury, typically with high-grade aneurysmal subarachnoid hemorrhage cases, which is called neurogenic stunned myocardium. This syndrome is reversible with judicious use of inotropic agents and supportive care usually within the first week of hemorrhage.

REFERENCES

1. Nieminen MS, Bohm M, Cowie MR, et al. Executive summary of the guidelines on the diagnosis and treatment of acute heart failure. The Task Force on Acute Heart Failure of the European Society of Cardiology. *Eur Heart J.* 2005;26:384-416.
2. Jain P, Massie B, Gattis W, et al. Current medical treatment for the exacerbation of chronic heart failure resulting in hospitalization. *Am Heart J.* 2003;145:S3-S17.
3. Steimle A, Stevenson L, Chelimsky-Fallick, C, et al. Sustained hemodynamic efficacy of therapy tailored to reduce filling pressures in survivors with advanced heart failure. *Circulation.* 1007;96:1165-1172.
4. Philbin EF, Rocco TA Jr, Lindenmuth NW, et al. Systolic versus diastolic heart failure in community practice: clinical features, outcomes, and the use of angiotensin-converting enzyme inhibitors. *Am J Med.* 2000;109:605-613.
5. Dormans T, Van-Meyel J, Gerlag P, et al. Diuretic efficacy of high dose furosemide in severe heart failure: bolus injection versus continuous infusion. *J Am Coll Cardiol.* 1996;28:376-382.
6. Hunt S, Abraham WT, Chin M, et al. ACC/AHA 2005 guideline update for the diagnosis and management of chronic heart failure in the adult-summary article. *Circulation.* 2005;112(12):1825-1852.
7. Publication Committee for the VMAC Investigators. Intravenous nesiritide versus nitroglycerin for treatment of decompensated congestive heart failure: a randomized controlled trial. *JAMA.* 2000;287:1531-1540.
8. Silver M, Horton D, Ghali J, et al. Effect of nesiritide versus dobutamine on short-term outcomes in the treatment of patients with acute decompensated heart failure. *J Am Coll Cardiol.* 2002;39:798-803.
9. Burger A, Horton D, LeGemtel T, et al. Effect of nesiritide (B-type natriuretic peptide) and dobutamine on ventricular arrhythmias in the treatment of patients with acutely decompensated congestive heart failure: the PRECEDENT study. *Am Heart J.* 2002;144:1102-1108.

10. Abraham W, Adams K, Fonarow G, et al. Comparison of in-hospital mortality in patients treated with nesiritide versus other parenteral vasoactive medications for acutely decompensated heart failure: an analysis from a large prospective registry database. *J Card Fail*. 2003;9:S81.

11. Sackner-Bernstein JD, Kowalski M, Fox M, Aaronson K. Short-term risk of death after treatment with nesiritide for decompensated heart failure. *JAMA*. 2005;293:1900-1905.

12. Sackner-Bernstein JD, Skopicki HA, Aarronson KD. Risk of worsening renal function with nesiritide in patients with acutely decompensated heart failure. *Circulation*. 2005;111:1487-1491.

13. Abraham WT, Adams KF, Fonarow GC, et al. In-hospital mortality in patients with acute decompensated heart failure requiring intravenous vasoactive medications. *J Am Coll Cardiol*. 2005;4(1):57-64.

14. Leier C, Binkley P. Parenteral inotropic support for advanced congestive heart failure. *Prog Cardiovasc Dis*. 1998;41:207-224.

15. Shah M, Hasselblad V, Stinnett S, et al. Hemodynamic profiles of advanced heart failure: association with clinical characteristics and long-term outcomes. *J Card Fail*. 2001;7:105-113.

16. Chattergee K, DeMarco T. Role of nonglycosidic inotropic agents. Indications, ethics, and limitations. *Med Clin North Am*. 2003;87(2):391.

17. Cuffe M, Califf R, Adams K, et al. Short-term intravenous milrinone for acute exacerbation of chronic heart failure: a randomized control trial. *JAMA*. 2002;287:1541-1547.

18. O'Connor C, Gattis W, Uretsky B, et al. Continuous intravenous dobutamine is associated with an increased risk of death in patients with advanced heart failure: insights from the Flolan International Randomized Survival Trial (FIRST). *Am Heart J*. 1999;138:78-86.

19. Stevenson L. Tailored therapy for hemodynamic goals for advanced heart failure. *Eur J Heart Fail*. 1999;1:251-257.

20. Stevenson LW. Are hemodynamic goals viable in tailoring heart failure therapy? *Circulation*. 2006;113:1020-1027.

21. Stevenson L, Tillisch J. Maintenance of cardiac output with normal filling pressures in patients with dilated heart failure. *Circulation*. 1986;74:1303-1308.

22. Colucci W, Wright R, Jaski B, et al. Milrinone and dobutamine in severe heart failure: differing hemodynamic effects and individual patient responsiveness. *Circulation*. 1986;73(III):175-183.

23. Jaski B, Fifer M, Wright R, et al. Positive inotropic and vasodilator actions of milrinone in patients with severe congestive heart failure. *J Clin Invest*. 1985;75:643-649.

24. Colucci W, Elkayam U, Horton D, et al. Intravenous nesiritide, a natriuretic in the treatment of decompensated congestive heart failure. *N Engl J Med*. 2002;343:246-253.

25. The ESCAPE Investigators and ESCAPE Study Coordinators. Evaluation study of congestive heart failure and pulmonary artery catheterization effectiveness. *JAMA*. 2005;294(13):1625-1633.

26. Velazquez EJ, Pfeffer MA. Acute heart failure complicating acute coronary syndromes. *Circulation*. 2004;109:440-442.

27. Velazquez EJ, Francis GS, Armstrong PW, et al. An international perspective on heart failure and left ventricular systolic dysfunction complicating myocardial infarction: the VALIANT registry. *Eur Heart J*. 2004;25:1911-1919.

28. Steg PG, Dabbous DH, Feldman LJ, et al. Determinants and prognostic impact of heart failure complicating acute coronary syndromes. *Circulation*. 2004;109:494-499.

29. The CAPRICORN Investigators. Effect of carvedilol on outcome after myocardial infarction in patients with left ventricular dysfunction: the CAPRICORN randomized trial. *Lancet*. 2001;357:1385-1390.

30. Pfeffer M, Braunwald E, Moye L, et al. Effect of captopril on mortality and morbidity in patients with left ventricular dysfunction after myocardial infarction. *N Engl J Med*. 1992;327:669-677.

31. The Acute Infarction Ramipril Efficacy (AIRE) Study Investigators. Effect of ramipril on mortality and morbidity of survivors of acute myocardial infarction with clinical evidence of heart failure. *Lancet*. 1003;342:821-828.

32. Kober L, Torp-Pedersen C, Carlsen JE, et al. A clinical trial of the angiotensin-converting-enzyme inhibitor trandolapril in patients with left ventricular dysfunction after myocardial infarction. *N Engl J Med*. 1995;333:1670-1676.

33. Pfeffer MA, McMurray JJV, Velazquez EJ. Valsartan, captopril, or both in myocardial infarction complicated by heart failure, left ventricular dysfunction, or both. *N Engl J Med*. 2003;349(20):1893-1903.

34. Pitt B, Remme W, Zannad F, et al. Eplerenone, a selective aldosterone blocker, in patients with left ventricular dysfunction after myocardial infarction. *N Engl J Med*. 2003;348:1309-1321.

35. Pitt B, White H, Nicolau J. Eplerenone reduces mortality 30 days after randomization following acute myocardial infarction in patients with left ventricular systolic dysfunction and heart failure. *J Am Coll Cardiol*. 2005;46(3):424-430.

36. Gheorghiade M, Zannad F, Sopko G. Acute heart failure syndromes. *Circulation*. 2005;112:3958-3968.

Cardiovascular Problems

37. Asbun J, Villarreal FJ. The pathogenesis of myocardial fibrosis in the setting of diabetic cardiomyopathy. *J Am Coll Cardiol.* 2006;47:693-700.

38. Fadel BM, Ellahham S, Ringel MD. Hyperthyroid heart disease. *Clin Cardiol.* 2000;23:402-408.

39. Alpert MA. Obesity cardiomyopathy: pathophysiology and evolution of the clinical syndrome. *Am J Med Sci.* 2001;321(4):225-236.

40. The SOLVD Investigators. Effect of enalapril on survival in patients with reduced left ventricular ejection fractions and congestive heart failure. *N Engl J Med.* 1991;325:293-302.

41. The SOLVD Investigators. Effect of enalapril on mortality and the development of heart failure in asymptomatic patients with reduced left ventricular ejection fractions. *N Engl J Med.* 1992;327:685-691.

42. Garg R, Yusuf S. Overview of randomized trials of angiotensin converting enzyme inhibitors on mortality and morbidity in patients with heart failure. *JAMA.* 1995;273:1450-1456.

43. Aronow WS. Epidemiology, pathophysiology, prognosis, and treatment of systolic and diastolic heart failure. *Cardiol Rev.* 2006;14:108-124.

44. Packer M. Current role of beta-adrenergic blockers in the management of chronic heart failure. *Am J Med.* 2001;110(7A):81S-84S.

45. BHAT Trial Research Group. A randomized trial of propranolol in patients with acute myocardial infarction. I. Mortality results. *JAMA.* 1982;747:1707-1714.

46. BHAT Trial Research Group. A randomized trial of propranolol in patients with acute myocardial infarction. II. Morbidity results. *JAMA.* 1983;250:2814-2819.

47. CIBIS II Investigators. The Cardiac Insufficiency Bisoprolol study II: a randomized trial. *Lancet.* 1999;353:9-13.

48. The MERIT-HF Study Group. Effects of controlled release metoprolol on total mortality, hospitalizations and well-being in patients with heart failure. *JAMA.* 2000;283:1295-1302.

49. Packer M, Coats A, Fowler M, et al. Effect of carvedilol on survival in severe chronic heart failure. *N Engl J Med.* 2001;344:1651-1658.

50. Krum H, Roecker E, Mohacsi P, et al. Effects on initiating carvedilol in patients with severe chronic heart failure. Results from the COPERNICUS Study. *JAMA.* 2003;289:712-718.

51. Bristow M, Gilbert E, Abraham W, et al. Carvedilol produces dose related improvements in left ventricular function and survival in subjects with chronic heart failure. *Circulation.* 1996;94:2807-2816.

52. The RESOLVD Pilot Study Investigators. Comparison of candesartan, enalapril, and their combination in congestive heart failure. *Circulation.* 1999;100:1056-1064.

53. Pitt B, Poole-Wilson P, Segal R, et al. Effect of losartan compared with captopril on mortality in patients with symptomatic heart failure: randomized trial—the Losartan Heart Failure Survival Study (ELITE II). *Lancet.* 2000;355:1582-1587.

54. Cohn J, Tognoni G. A randomized trial of the angiotensin receptor blocker valsartan in chronic heart failure. *N Engl J Med.* 2001;345:1667-1675.

55. Granger C, McMurray J, Yusuf S, et al. Effects of candesartan in patients with chronic heart failure and reduced left ventricular systolic function intolerant to angiotensin-converting enzyme inhibitors. The CHARM Alternative Trial. *Lancet.* 2003;362:772-776.

56. McMurray J, Ostergren J, Swedberg K, et al. Effects of candesartan in patients with chronic heart failure and reduced left ventricular systolic function taking angiotensin-converting enzyme inhibitors. The CHARM—added trial. *Lancet.* 2003;362:759-766.

57. Manohair P, Pina I. Therapeutic role of angiotensin II receptor blockers in the treatment of heart failure. *Mayo Clin Proc.* 2003;78:334-338.

58. Sharma D, Buyse M, Pitt B, et al. Meta-analysis of observed mortality data from all controlled double-blind multiple dose studies of losartan in heart failure. *Am J Cardiol.* 2000;85:187-192.

59. Pitt B, Zannad F, Remme W, et al. The effect of spironolactone on morbidity and mortality in patients with severe heart failure. *N Engl J Med.* 1999;341:709-717.

60. Juurlink DN, Mamdani NM, Lee DS, et al. Rates of hyperkalemia after publication of the randomized Aldactone study. *N Engl J Med.* 2004;351:543-551.

61. Cohn J, Archibald D, Ziesche S, et al. Effect of vasodilator therapy on mortality in chronic congestive heart failure. Results of a Veteran Administration Cooperative Study. *N Engl J Med.* 1986;314:1547-1552.

62. Taylor AL, Zieche S, Yancy C, et al. Combination of isosorbide dinitrate and hydralazine in blacks with heart failure. *N Engl J Med.* 2004;351:2049-2057.

63. The Digitalis Investigation Group. The effect of digoxin on mortality and morbidity in patients with heart failure. *N Engl J Med.* 1997;336:525-533.

64. Oppenheimer S. The heart of the matter. *Cerebrovasc Dis.* 2002;14(2):65-66.

65. Bybee KA, Prasad A. Stress-related cardiomyopathy syndromes. *Circulation.* 2008;118:397-409.

66. Burch GE, Meyers R, Abildskov JA. A new electrocardiographic pattern observed in cerebrovascular accidents. *Circulation.* 1954;9:719-723.

67. Cropp GJ, Manning GW. Electrocardiographic changes simulating myocardial ischemia and infarction associated with spontaneous intracranial hemorrhage. *Circulation.* 1960;22:25-38.

68. Mayer, S, Lin J, Homma, S, et al. Myocardial injury and left ventricular performance after subarachnoid hemorrhage. *Stroke.* 1999;30(4):780-786.

69. Nilesh P, Venkatesh B, Cross D, et al. Cardiac troponin I predicts myocardial dysfunction in aneurysmal subarachnoid hemorrhage. *J Am Coll Cardiol.* 2000;36:1328-1335.

70. Pollick C, Cujec B, Parker S, Tator C. Left ventricular wall motion abnormalities in subarachnoid hemorrhage: an echocardiographic study. *J Am Coll Cardiol.* 1988;12:600-605.

71. Kono T, Morita H, Kuroiwa T, et al. Left ventricular wall motion abnormalities in patients with subarachnoid hemorrhage: neurogenic stunned myocardium. *J Am Coll Cardiol.* 1994;24:636-640.

72. Lee V, Connolly HM, Fulgham JR, et al. Takotsubo cardiomyopathy in aneurysmal subarachnoid hemorrhage: an underappreciated ventricular dysfunction. *J Neurosurg.* 2006;105:264-270.

73. Di Pasquale G, Andreoli A, Lusa AM, et al. Cardiac complications of subarachnoid hemorrhage. *J Neurosurg Sci.* 1998;42(Suppl 1):33-36.

74. Macmillan CSA, Grant IS, Andrews PJD. Pulmonary and cardiac sequelae of subarachnoid hemorrhage: time for active management? *Intensive Care Med.* 2002;28:1012-1023.

75. Tung P, Kopelnik A, Banki N, et al. Predictors of neurocadiogenic injury after subarachnoid hemorrhage. *Stroke.* 2004;35:548-553.

76. Jensen J, Kristensen SR, Bak S, et al. Frequency and significance of troponin T elevation in acute ischemic stroke. *Am J Cardiol.* 2007;99:108-112.

77. Banki N, Kopelnik A, Tng P, et al. Prospective analysis of prevalence, distribution and rate of recovery of left ventricular systolic dysfunction in patients with subarachnoid hemorrhage. *J Neurosurg.* 2006;105:15-20.

78. Dujardin KS, McCully RB, Wijdicks EFM, et al. Myocardial dysfunction associated with brain death: clinical, echocardiographic and pathologic features. *J Heart Lung Transplant.* 2001;20:350-357.

79. Solenski NJ, Haley EC Jr, Kassel NF, et al. Medical complications of aneurismal subarachnoid hemorrhage: a report of the multicenter, cooperative aneurysm study. *Crit Care Med.* 1995;23:1007-1017.

80. Banki NM, Kopelnik, A, Dae MW, et al. Acute neurocardiogenic injury after subarachnoid hemorrhage. *Circulation.* 2005;112:3314-3319.

81. Schubert A. Cardiovascular therapy of neurosurgical patients. *Best Pract Res Clin Anaesthesiol.* 2007;21(4):483-496.

CHAPTER 34

Cardiogenic Shock and Intra-aortic Balloon Pump

Simon K. Topalian, MD
Joseph E. Parrillo, MD

A 69-year-old man who has hypertension and diabetes mellitus had a motor vehicle accident and suffered head trauma. He had a brief loss of consciousness. After evaluation in the emergency department, he was admitted to the neurology intensive care unit (ICU) for observation. The night of the admission, he developed severe substernal chest pain and quickly became diaphoretic. His blood pressure was 95/63 mm Hg, with a pulse rate of 60 bpm. He was in moderate distress and looked pale and clammy. The 12-lead electrocardiogram (ECG) showed acute inferolateral ST-segment-elevation myocardial infarction (STEMI) (Figure 34-1).

After consultation with the cardiologist, the patient was taken directly to the cardiac catheterization laboratory for emergent coronary angiography and angioplasty. This showed a total occlusion of a dominant proximal left circumflex (LCX) artery that was successfully opened with aspiration thrombectomy and stenting (Figure 34-2A, B). Left ventriculography showed a severe inferior and lateral wall hypokinesis with an ejection fraction of 30%.

The patient remained hypotensive despite being administered dopamine at 10 μg/kg per minute. Right heart catheterization revealed a pulmonary capillary wedge pressure of 28 mm Hg and a cardiac index of 1.8 L/min per m².

At this point, an intra-aortic balloon pump (IABP) was placed and the patient was transferred back to the ICU. His blood pressure remained stable. The dopamine was weaned off after several hours and the IABP was discontinued 24 hours later. His echocardiogram showed severe hypokinesis of the inferior and lateral wall.

This patient had acute myocardial infarction (AMI) complicated by cardiogenic shock (CS). How is CS defined?

CS is defined as persistent tissue hypoperfusion secondary to cardiac dysfunction in the presence of adequate left ventricular filling pressure. The clinical signs include hypotension, cold extremities, tachycardia, decreased urinary output, and altered mental status. Hemodynamically, there is hypotension, defined as a systolic blood pressure less than 90 mm Hg for more than 30 minutes, a low cardiac index (< 1.8 L/min per m² without support or < 2-2.2 L/min per m² with support), and finally an elevated filling pressure (pulmonary capillary occlusion pressure > 15 mm Hg, left ventricular end-diastolic pressure > 18 mm Hg, or right ventricular end-diastolic pressure > 10-15 mm Hg).[1-3]

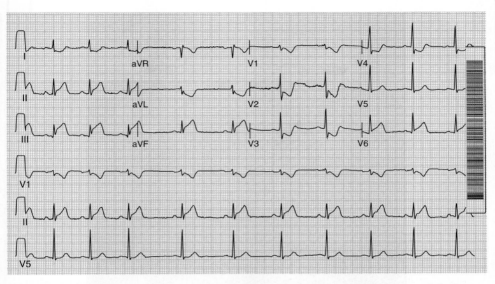

Figure 34-1. A 12-lead electrocardiogram showing acute inferolateral ST-segment-elevation myocardial infarction.

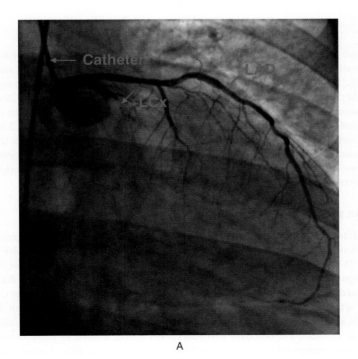

A

Figure 34-2. A. An occluded left circumflex (LCx) artery. **B.** LCx artery after revascularization. It was a large dominant vessel supplying a large area of myocardium. LAD, left anterior descending artery; OM, obtuse marginal branches.

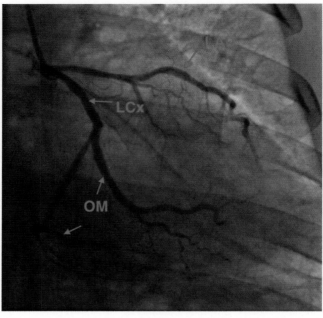

B

Figure 34-2. (*Continued.*)

CS, a major complication of AMI, remains the most common cause of mortality in hospitalized patients presenting with AMI. Its incidence has remained stable over the years and ranges between 7.1% and 8.6%.[4-6] It carries a very poor prognosis. The in-hospital mortality rate, although improved, is still high, varying between 47.9% and 60%.[6,7] Only one-third of patients manifest CS upon presentation. The majority develop CS hours later, on average 7 hours, raising the question of the golden hours to prevent it. Cardiogenic shock complicates 4.2% of patients with STEMI and 2.5% of patients with non–ST-segment-elevation myocardial infarction (NSTEMI).[8] In the latter, CS tends to occur later after presentation (76.3 hours in NSTEMI versus 9.6 hours in STEMI). The patients are usually elderly and have hypertension, dyslipidemia, diabetes mellitus, prior MI, azotemia, peripheral arterial disease, and extensive coronary artery disease.

What is the pathophysiology that leads to CS after AMI?

As mentioned before, CS is a serious complication of AMI. In the SHould we emergently revascularize Occluded Coronaries for cardiogenic shocK (SHOCK) Trial Registry, left ventricular pump failure accounted for 78.5% of CS cases complicating MI. Mechanical complications accounted for the remainder: acute mitral regurgitation, 6.9%; ventricular septal defect, 3.9%; isolated right ventricular defect, 2.8%; and tamponade and cardiac rupture, 1.4% (Figure 34-3).[7] Table 34-1 summarizes the causes of CS.

Typically after a massive AMI or with recurrent ischemia or infarction extension, left ventricular function is acutely depressed with decreased contractility, cardiac output, and blood pressure. A vicious cycle ensues. First, coronary perfusion is decreased, leading to more ischemia. Second, the compensatory mechanism involving the activation of the sympathetic and renin-angiotensin system leads to vasoconstriction, tachycardia, and fluid retention. This results in more stress on the heart, increased oxygen demand with worsening ischemia and cardiac output, and finally pulmonary edema. Figure 34-4 illustrates the paradigm of CS.[1,3]

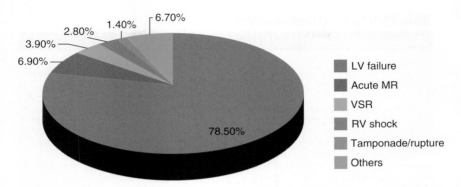

Figure 34-3. Major shock categories. LV, left ventricular; MR, mitral regurgitation; RV, right ventricular; VSR, ventricular septal rupture. *(Data from Hochman JS, Buller CE, Sleeper LA, et al. Cardiogenic shock complicating acute myocardial infarction—etiologies, management and outcome: a report from the SHOCK Trial Registry. SHould we emergently revascularize Occluded Coronaries for cardiogenic shocK? J Am Coll Cardiol. 2000; 36(3 Suppl A): 1063-1070.)*

At a cellular level, the metabolism is shifted from aerobic to anaerobic glycolysis with production of lactic acid. The intracellular calcium rises and the sodium competes to expel it. The end result is myonecrosis, mitochondrial swelling, and subsequent plasma membrane rupture.[9]

Findings of varying degrees of reduced ejection fraction, increased left ventricular size, and decreased systemic vascular resistance (SVR) in CS after an AMI raised the question of other mechanisms, mainly inflammatory, in CS development. In the SHOCK trial, one-fifth of the patients had clinical evidence of systemic inflammatory response syndrome[10] such as fever, leukocytosis, and low SVR. Inflammatory markers with myocardial depressant properties such as tumor necrosis factor α and interleukin 6 were elevated after MI and CS.[11] Nitric oxide (NO), produced by nitric oxide synthase (NOS), is an endogenous vasodilator. The inducible NOS[12] is expressed at pathologic levels in the myocytes and is associated with myocardial dysfunction.[13,14] The non–isoform-specific NOS inhibitor, N-monomethyl-L-arginine (L-NMMA), showed positive hemodynamic improvement as well as mortality benefit in a small study[15,16]; however, it failed to reproduce the same benefit in a larger trial.[17]

How should a patient who develops CS after an AMI be initially managed?

A high index of suspicion and early recognition of CS are the most important aspects in the initial care. Rapid assessment with history, physical examination, and chest radiography is key. Signs of tissue hypoperfusion and heart failure include low blood pressure, tachycardia, agitation, confusion, cyanosis, and cool and clammy skin. The 12-lead electrocardiogram (ECG) is the main modality used in diagnosing AMI, ischemia, and arrhythmias. Rapid echocardiographic assessment is very helpful to evaluate left and right ventricular function as well as the presence of mechanical complications such as acute mitral regurgitation, ventricular septal rupture, cardiac rupture, and tamponade.

Major differential diagnoses to consider in patients with CS include hemorrhage, sepsis, aortic dissection, and massive pulmonary embolism.

The definitive treatment of patients with CS secondary to AMI or ischemia remains rapid coronary revascularization. While waiting for this intervention, patients ought to be stabilized. Sedation, airway protection, and intubation with mechanical ventilation may be needed to correct hypoxemia and reduce the work of breathing.[1,18,19]

The goal of initial medical management of CS is to maintain adequate arterial pressure for tissue perfusion. Intravenous fluid challenges should be given with caution, especially in patients with pulmonary edema.

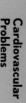

Cardiovascular Problems

Table 34-1. Causes of Cardiogenic Shock

Acute myocardial infarction
Pump failure
Large infarct
Smaller infarction with preexisting left ventricular dysfunction
Infarction extension
Severe recurrent ischemia
Mechanical complications
Acute mitral regurgitation
Ventricular septal defect
Free wall rupture
Pericardial tamponade
Right ventricular infarction
Other conditions
End-stage cardiomyopathy
Myocarditis
Myocardial contusion
Prolonged cardiopulmonary bypass
Septic shock with severe myocardial depression
Left ventricular outflow obstruction
Aortic stenosis
Hypertrophic cardiomyopathy
Obstruction to left ventricular filling
Mitral stenosis
Left atrial myxoma
Acute mitral regurgitation (chordal rupture)
Acute aortic regurgitation
Acute massive pulmonary embolism
Acute stress cardiomyopathy
Pheochromocytoma
Excess β blocker or calcium channel blocker

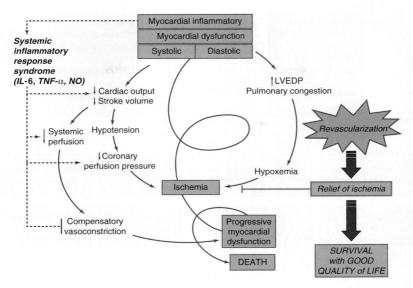

Figure 34-4. Cardiogenic shock (CS) pathogenesis. The classic paradigm, as illustrated by Hollenberg et al,[1] is shown in black and the inflammatory component by the dashed lines. IL-6, interleukin 6; LVEDP, left ventricular end-diastolic pressure; NO, nitric oxide; TNF-α, tumor necrosis factor α. *(Reproduced with permission from Reynolds HR, Hochman JS. Cardiogenic shock: current concepts and improving outcomes. Circulation. 2008;117(5):686-697.)*

Figure 34-5 outlines the American College of Cardiology/American Heart Association (ACC/ AHA) practice guidelines to treat low cardiac output shock. Dopamine, an inotrope and vasopressor, is the initial drug of choice to be used. Norepinephrine is a more potent vasoconstrictor and should be used for patients with more-severe hypotension. These medications increase the systemic vascular resistance and heart rate, hence increasing the myocardial oxygen demand, leading to worsening myocardial ischemia and arrhythmias. Dosages should be adjusted to the lowest dose.[1,18,20] Dobutamine has a more inotropic effect. It should be added, commonly in combination with vasopressors, to improve cardiac output.[18] Intravenous vasopressin can also be used.[21]

A subset of patients, termed as having *nonhypoperfusion cardiogenic shock* or *preshock*, manifest signs of tissue hypoperfusion with systolic blood pressure greater than 90 mm Hg. These patients have elevated pulmonary artery occlusion pressure, a low cardiac index, and high systemic vascular resistance. Their in-hospital mortality rate is 43%. They should be identified early, so appropriate and urgent diagnostic and therapeutic measures can be prescribed.[22]

Pulmonary artery (PA) catheterization can assist in precise measurement of filling pressure, volume status, and cardiac output. Hemodynamic evaluation helps guide fluid management and the use of inotropic agents and vasopressors. The use of PA catheterization is an ACC/AHA class I recommendation in hypotensive patients not responding to fluid administration or when mechanical complications of MI are suspected. It is a class IIa recommendation for patients in CS who have persistent signs of hypoperfusion and in patients receiving inotropic and vasopressor drugs.[20,23]

As alluded to, the final and definitive treatment of patients with CS complicating AMI is rapid coronary revascularization. What is the best way to achieve it?

The majority of patients presenting with AMI who develop CS do so several hours after infarction and hospital presentation.[4,6,7,24] The delayed onset results from reinfarction, recurrent ischemia, infarction extension, or decompensation of left ventricular function in a noninfarcted zone because of metabolic

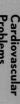

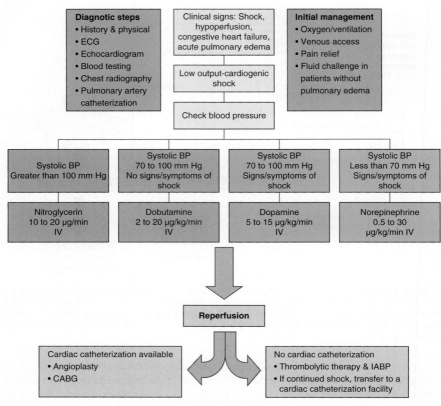

Figure 34-5. Emergency management of complicated ST-segment-elevation myocardial infarction. BP, blood pressure; CABG, coronary artery bypass grafting; ECG, electrocardiogram; IABP, intra-aortic balloon pump; IV, intravenous. *(Modified with permission from Antman EM, Anbe DT, Armstrong PW, et al. ACC/AHA guidelines for the management of patients with ST-elevation myocardial infarction—executive summary. A report of the American College of Cardiology/American Heart Association Task Force on Practice Guidelines [Writing Committee to revise the 1999 guidelines for the management of patients with acute myocardial infarction]. J Am Coll Cardiol. 2004;44(3): 671-719.)*

derangement. The above-mentioned strategies are used to stabilize patients. They should be undertaken at shock onset or even before to maintain adequate tissue perfusion. The ultimate and final therapy of CS secondary to myocardial infarction is rapid restoration of flow in the infarct-related artery.[25] Primary coronary intervention (PCI) has shown its superiority over fibrinolytic therapy to achieve flow.[26]

The landmark SHOCK trial randomized 302 patients with CS due to AMI and left ventricular failure either to emergency revascularization (ERV) with PCI or coronary artery bypass grafting (CABG) surgery or to initial medical stabilization (IMS) with drug therapy and IABP. The 30-day mortality rate trended in favor of the ERV group (47% versus 56%), but the difference was not statistically significant. However, late mortality rates were statistically in favor of ERV.[27,28] At 6 months, 1 year, and 6 years, an absolute survival difference of 13% was seen in the ERV group.[28,29] At 6 years, overall survival was 32.8% in the ERV group and 19.6% in the IMS group. In the hospital survivors, the 6-year survival rate was 62.4% in the ERV group and 44.4% in the IMS group. Patients who were transferred to hospitals with revascularization capabilities also had better outcome with ERV.[30] Quality-of-life measures were also better.[31] The positive benefit with early mechanical revascularization was translated in the ACC/AHA practice guidelines. Both PCI and CABG are class I recommendations for patients younger than 75 years old with STEMI or AMI with left bundle branch block who develop shock within 36 hours of onset.[20,32]

The relatively small number of elderly patients aged older than 75 years in the SHOCK trial may explain the worse outcome in this category of patients receiving ERV.[27-29] However, their outcome in the SHOCK Trial Registry was better than patients who were not revascularized.[33] While in the SHOCK trial CABG was performed in 36% and PCI in 64% of revascularizations, the real-world practice is different. Invasive procedures are still underutilized in patients with CS.[6,7]

Fibrinolytics are not as effective in restoring coronary perfusion in patients with STEMI and CS[1,18] because of decreased penetration of the coronary thrombus by fibrinolytics in hypotensive patients, a greater reocclusion rate, and a longer time to achieve patency.[1,18,19] Fibrinolytic therapy did not improve survival in patients with CS.[18] The addition of IABP to lytic therapy showed a lower mortality rate compared to lytics alone (49% vs 67%).[34,35] The patients at high risk of developing CS after fibrinolysis are elderly patients, those with Killip II/III heart failure, and those with lower blood pressure.[36] The use of thrombolytics for CS is a class I recommendation only in patients with STEMI not amenable to invasive therapy with PCI or CABG.[20] It is also recommended in patients who are admitted to hospitals without cardiac catheterization laboratories and when there will be unavoidable delays in transfer to tertiary care centers.

What are the hemodynamic effects of IABP?

IABP has been the most widely used left ventricular assist device for several decades. Its concept is based on the fact that coronary perfusion occurs during diastole. The initial experiments took place in the 1950s and 1960s.[37,38] In 1962, Moulopoulos et al designed a carbon dioxide (CO_2)-filled balloon that was placed in the descending aorta and that filled during diastole.[39] The theoretical benefits were increased coronary and systemic blood flow and a lower end-diastolic pressure. Subsequently, a helium-filled balloon replaced the CO_2-filled balloon. In 1968, the first positive human experience was reported in five patients with CS.[40] Over the years, further improvements in the design of the IABP took place. Wire-guided and prefolded IABPs were developed, allowing percutaneous insertion. Smaller balloons led to fewer vascular complications.

The IABP is inserted most commonly in the catheterization laboratory[41,42] using a percutaneous approach. The size of the balloon depends on the height of the patient. It is placed distal to the left subclavian artery proximally and above the origin of the renal arteries distally (Figure 34-6). The balloon is connected to a console that operates inflation and deflation. Balloon inflation and deflation are triggered by either the pressure waveform or electrocardiogram or pacer rhythm. Inflation occurs at the aortic valve closure and deflation at the end of diastole and aortic valve opening.

Figure 34-7 illustrates the systemic hemodynamic changes that the IABP creates during a cardiac cycle.[43] When the balloon inflates at the onset of diastole, the diastolic perfusion pressure is augmented substantially (diastolic augmentation). This will lead to increased coronary blood flow velocity.[44-46] When it deflates at the onset of systole, the afterload wall stress is reduced (assisted systole), leading to improved forward flow and stroke volume, especially in low cardiac output states.[44,47] The left ventricular end-diastolic pressure (EDP) and left ventricular filling pressure are decreased.[48] The net result is lowering myocardial oxygen demand with a smaller effect on myocardial oxygen supply. Hence, myocardial ischemia improves, as does left ventricular function.[49]

Several parameters can affect the hemodynamic changes seen with IABP, such as tachycardia, arrhythmias, intravascular volume status, aortic compliance, left ventricular function and reserve, the presence of coronary artery disease, and adjunctive pharmacotherapy.

For optimal benefit and reduction in afterload as well as maximal enhancement of diastolic perfusion pressure, timing of inflation and deflation is critical. Inflation should occur at the aortic valve

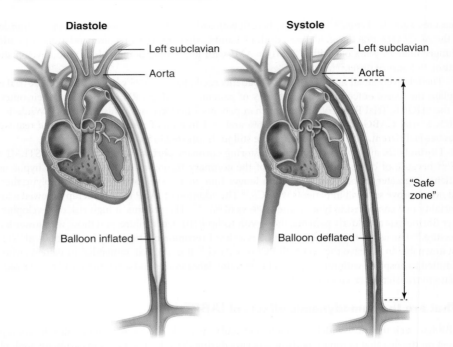

Figure 34-6. Location of intra-aortic balloon during inflation and deflation. Ideally the tip should be a few centimeters distal to the origin of the left subclavian artery and the proximal portion above the origin of the renal arteries, the "safe zone." *(Reproduced with permission from Turi ZG. Intra-aortic balloon counterpulsation. In: Parrillo JE, Dellinger RP, eds. Critical Care Medicine—Principles of Diagnosis and Management in the Adult. 3rd ed. Philadelphia, PA: Mosby Elsevier; 2008.)*

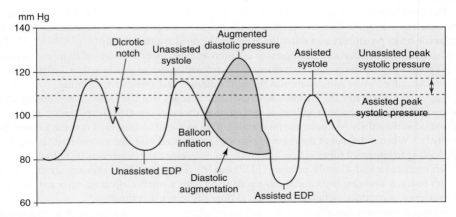

Figure 34-7. Hemodynamic response to intra-aortic balloon pump. The console is set to trigger at 1:2. Unassisted and assisted systole and diastole are seen. With balloon inflation, the diastolic pressure is augmented (area under curve in blue), the end-diastolic pressure (EDP) is decreased, and the systolic pressure (and thus afterload) is decreased. *(Reproduced with permission Turi ZG. Intra-aortic balloon counterpulsation. In: Parrillo JE, Dellinger RP, eds. Critical Care Medicine—Principles of Diagnosis and Management in the Adult. 3rd ed. Philadelphia, PA: Mosby Elsevier; 2008.)*

closure and deflation at the end of diastole and beginning of mechanical systole. The trigger of balloon operation can be achieved using the aortic pressure waveform or the electrocardiogram (including paced rhythm).

Figure 34-8 illustrates the different errors in the timing of either inflation or deflation. Early inflation (Figure 34-8A) leads to an increase in afterload. The left ventricular end-systolic pressure and the wall stress rise, leading to increased myocardial oxygen demand and decreased stroke volume. With late inflation (Figure 34-8B), stroke volume is reduced, as well as the augmented diastolic pressure. Early deflation (Figure 34-8C) results in suboptimal afterload reduction and suboptimal coronary perfusion. It can also lead to retrograde coronary flow with worsening ischemia. With late deflation (Figure 34-8D), the assisted peak systolic pressure is delayed and decreased. The afterload reduction is almost absent. Inflated or partially inflated balloon leads to resistance to the left ventricular ejection with increased myocardial oxygen consumption.

Anticoagulation, usually with heparin, is recommended when the IABP is in place, especially if patients are receiving less than 1:1 counterpulsation. There is a theoretical risk of clot formation on the balloon and on the arterial sheath.

Major complications related directly to IABP account for 2.6% to 2.8%,[42,50,51] while all IABP-related complications are around 7%. The relatively low complication rate is mainly a result of the development of a smaller catheter diameter, percutaneous insertion, and adjunctive medical therapy. The rate of IABP-related mortality is 0.05%, of severe bleeding requiring blood transfusion or surgical intervention is 0.8%, and of major limb ischemia is 0.9%.[50] Independent predictors of major complications related to IABP are female gender, presence of peripheral vascular disease, age (older than 75 years old), and small body surface (body surface area < 1.65 m²).

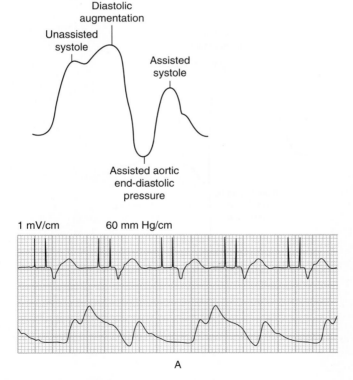

Figure 34-8. A. Early inflation. **B.** Late inflation. **C.** Early deflation. **D.** Late deflation.

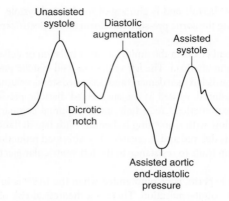

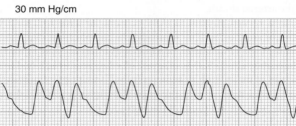

B

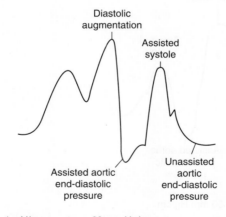

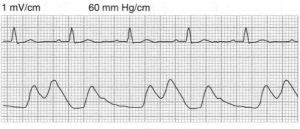

C

Figure 34-8. (*Continued.*)

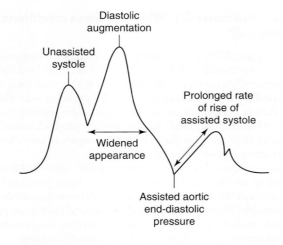

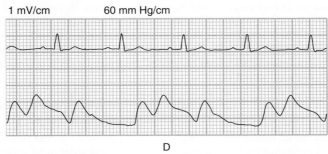

D

Figure 34-8. (*Continued.*)

What are the clinical indications and what is the role of IABP in patients with AMI complicated by CS?

The efficacy of IABP in AMI complicated by CS has not been evaluated in randomized clinical trials.

In the Benchmark Registry of IABP, CS was the indication for counterpulsation in 19% of patients. However, among patients with AMI, CS accounted for 27% of the indications, with a 39% mortality rate.[42,50,51] The other indications for IABP included hemodynamic instability, weaning off cardio-pulmonary bypass, refractory unstable angina, and preoperative use in high-risk patients. Balloon counterpulsation seemed to improve outcomes in patients with STEMI and CS who were treated with thrombolytic therapy but did not have any effect on revascularization outcome.[35,52-54] Current ACC/AHA practice guidelines list IABP as a class I recommendation for patients with low cardiac output states, hypotension, and CS not responding quickly to other measures.[20] IABP is also recommended for patients with AMI complicated by severe mitral regurgitation or ventricular septal rupture, before urgent cardiac surgery, and in patients with right ventricular infarction not responding to fluid challenge and inotropic therapy.

Contraindications to IABP are significant aortic regurgitation, abdominal aortic aneurysm, and aortic dissection. Relative contraindications include severe peripheral vascular disease, uncontrolled septicemia, and bleeding disorders.[18]

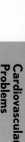

Complicated AMI can also cause CS. What are these conditions and how are these conditions managed?

- Right ventricular infarction (RVI). Ten percent to 15% of inferior wall myocardial infarctions are complicated by hemodynamically significant RVIs. RVI accounts for 2.8% of cases of CS in the SHOCK Trial Registry.[7] Acute right ventricular (RV) dysfunction leads to decreased preload and decreased cardiac output and causes CS. Also, RV dilatation shifts the intraventricular septum to the left, further compromising cardiac output and worsening CS.[55] CS caused by isolated RVI has a very high mortality rate,[56] although it is less than shock caused by left ventricular failure (53% versus 61%). Shock patients due to RVI are younger and have a lower prevalence of multivessel coronary artery disease and anterior MI.

  Diagnosis should be suspected in patients presenting with inferior AMI with hypotension, clear lung fields, and an elevated jugular venous pressure. Right precordial ECG shows ST-segment elevation, although this finding can be transient. Echocardiogram shows a dilated and hypokinetic right ventricle. Hemodynamic data show elevated right atrial pressure, exaggerated right atrial x descent, and right atrial/pulmonary artery occlusion pressure greater than 0.8. The right coronary artery is the culprit vessel in the majority of cases.

  Intravenous nitroglycerin should not be given. Initial therapy should be infusion of intravenous normal saline; however, large amounts of fluid can cause significant RV dilatation with subsequent impairment of left ventricular output. Inotropic agents, particularly dobutamine, and IABP may be required for patients who don't respond to fluid challenges.[20] Temporary transvenous pacing may be needed to correct conduction abnormalities, such as heart block, common with RVI.

  Most patients with RVI manifest spontaneous early hemodynamic improvement and later recovery of RV function.[57,58] Urgent revascularization with PCI is now the cornerstone of therapy. With successful reperfusion, RV function returns to normal within 3 to 5 days.[59]

- Acute severe mitral regurgitation (MR) accounts for 6.9% of CS after AMI.[7,60] Acute MR is more likely to complicate inferior and/or posterior AMI and is due to infarction and rupture of papillary muscle. It happens within the first 24 hours or between the third and fifth days after AMI. Patients develop acute pulmonary edema in the setting of inferior AMI. The MR murmur can be absent or faint because of the rapid equalization of pressure between the left ventricle and left atrium. Right heart catheterization reveals a large v wave in the pulmonary capillary wedge pressure.

  Diagnosis is made by echocardiography. Transesophageal echocardiogram may be needed to see the ruptured papillary muscle or torn chordae. Prompt diagnosis and aggressive support are vital. Inotropes and vasodilators should be tried. Intra-aortic balloon pump has a very beneficial role in this situation. It decreases afterload and increases forward flow into the aorta. It appears to lower aortic impedance with improvement of cardiac output and a slight decrease in regurgitant fraction.[61] Acute severe MR is associated with high in-hospital mortality rate, in the range of 55%.[60] Patients who underwent urgent mitral valve surgery had more IABP use. Their mortality was 40%.

- Ventricular septal rupture can complicate anterior or inferior wall MI. It accounts for 3.9% of CS after AMI[7] and occurs within the first 24 hours. Patients develop CS and pulmonary edema. A loud holosystolic murmur is the hallmark physical examination finding. Doppler echocardiography will confirm the diagnosis with evidence of left-to-right shunting at the ventricular level and shows RV volume overload. Urgent surgical intervention is a class I recommendation in the ACC/AHA guidelines. This complication is associated with a very high mortality rate.[62]

- Left ventricular wall rupture and cardiac tamponade are uncommon, but lethal, complications of AMI. They accounted for 1.4% of CS in the SHOCK Trial Registry, with a 62% mortality rate.[7,63] The true incidence is difficult to ascertain, as the majority of patients will die immediately after rupture from electromechanical dissociation. The incidence of free wall rupture has decreased in the era of thrombolytic and primary angioplasty. Diagnosis is made by echocardiography that shows the effusion and sometimes the rupture. Urgent surgery with repair of ventricular rupture (patch) has resulted in survival in some patients.

! CRITICAL CONSIDERATIONS

- Cardiogenic shock is still a common and lethal complication of AMI. Its incidence is 7.1% to 8.6%, with in-hospital mortality rates between 48% and 60%.

- Left ventricular pump failure is the most common cause of CS after AMI. Other causes of CS after AMI include RV infarction and mechanical complications. End-stage cardiomyopathy, myocarditis, advanced valvular heart disease, and stress cardiomyopathy can also be causes of CS.

- Early assessment and prompt action are keys in the management of CS after AMI. In patients presenting with AMI, persistent hypotension with signs of tissue hypoperfusion are indicators of CS. ECG, chest radiography, 2-D echocardiography, and sometimes PA catheterization are part of diagnostic procedures. Stabilization of patients includes oxygenation, adequate volume status, and arrhythmia control. Vasopressors such as dopamine, norepinephrine, or vasopressin and inotropic agents might be needed to preserve adequate tissue perfusion.

- Early rapid revascularization has the best outcome on mortality in all patients with CS after AMI. Effort should be made to direct these patients to a tertiary care center with catheterization laboratory facilities. Revascularization can be achieved by angioplasty or bypass surgery. Intra-aortic balloon pump, a left ventricular assist device, can provide hemodynamic support for these patients. The survival benefit, however, relies on early reperfusion.

- If a cardiac catheterization laboratory is not readily available, fibrinolytics should be administered in combination with placement of an IABP.

- The hemodynamic benefits of IABP are increasing the diastolic perfusion pressure and decreasing afterload and filling pressure, thus lowering myocardial oxygen demand and improving myocardial ischemia.

- For the optimal benefit of IABP, inflation should occur at the beginning of diastole and the dicrotic notch and deflation at the end of diastole and the beginning of mechanical systole.

- IABP is recommended in low output states and persistent hypotension despite medical therapy. Absolute contraindication include moderate to severe aortic regurgitation, abdominal aortic aneurysm, and aortic dissection. Major complications related to IABP account for less than 3%.

- IABP has a major role in CS secondary to mechanical complications of AMI and in RV infarction.

REFERENCES

1. Hollenberg SM, Kavinsky CJ, Parrillo JE. Cardiogenic shock. *Ann Intern Med.* 1999;131(1): 47-59.
2. Topalian S, Ginsberg F, Parrillo JE. Cardiogenic shock. *Crit Care Med.* 2008;36(1 Suppl):S66-S74.
3. Reynolds HR, Hochman JS. Cardiogenic shock: current concepts and improving outcomes. *Circulation.* 2008;117(5):686-697.
4. Holmes DR Jr, Bates ER, Kleiman NS, et al. Contemporary reperfusion therapy for cardiogenic shock: the GUSTO-I trial experience. The GUSTO-I Investigators. Global Utilization of Streptokinase

and Tissue Plasminogen Activator for Occluded Coronary Arteries. *J Am Coll Cardiol.* 1995;26(3): 668-674.

5. Goldberg RJ, Samad NA, Yarzebski J, Gurwitz J, Bigelow C, Gore JM. Temporal trends in cardiogenic shock complicating acute myocardial infarction. *N Engl J Med.* 1999;340(15):1162-1168.

6. Babaev A, Frederick PD, Pasta DJ, Every N, Sichrovsky T, Hochman JS. Trends in management and outcomes of patients with acute myocardial infarction complicated by cardiogenic shock. *JAMA.* 2005;294(4):448-454.

7. Hochman JS, Buller CE, Sleeper LA, et al. Cardiogenic shock complicating acute myocardial infarction—etiologies, management and outcome: a report from the SHOCK Trial Registry. SHould we emergently revascularize Occluded Coronaries for cardiogenic shocK? *J Am Coll Cardiol.* 2000;36(3 Suppl A):1063-1070.

8. Holmes DR Jr, Berger PB, Hochman JS, et al. Cardiogenic shock in patients with acute ischemic syndromes with and without ST-segment elevation. *Circulation.* 1999;100(20):2067-2073.

9. Kloner RA, Bolli R, Marban E, Reinlib L, Braunwald E. Medical and cellular implications of stunning, hibernation, and preconditioning: an NHLBI workshop. *Circulation.* 1998;97(18):1848-1867.

10. Kohsaka S, Menon V, Lowe AM, et al. Systemic inflammatory response syndrome after acute myocardial infarction complicated by cardiogenic shock. *Arch Intern Med.* 2005;165(14):1643-1650.

11. Zhang C, Xu X, Potter BJ, et al. TNF-alpha contributes to endothelial dysfunction in ischemia/reperfusion injury. *Arterioscler Thromb Vasc Biol.* 2006;26(3):475-480.

12. Herrero P, Magarinos M, Molina I, et al. Squeeze involvement in the specification of *Drosophila* leucokinergic neurons: different regulatory mechanisms endow the same neuropeptide selection. *Mech Dev.* 2007;124(6):427-440.

13. Hochman JS. Cardiogenic shock complicating acute myocardial infarction: expanding the paradigm. *Circulation.* 2003;107(24):2998-3002.

14. Feng Q, Lu X, Jones DL, Shen J, Arnold JM. Increased inducible nitric oxide synthase expression contributes to myocardial dysfunction and higher mortality after myocardial infarction in mice. *Circulation.* 2001;104(6):700-704.

15. Cotter G, Kaluski E, Blatt A, et al. L-NMMA (a nitric oxide synthase inhibitor) is effective in the treatment of cardiogenic shock. *Circulation.* 2000;101(12):1358-1361.

16. Cotter G, Kaluski E, Milo O, et al. LINCS: L-NAME (a NO synthase inhibitor) in the treatment of

refractory cardiogenic shock: a prospective randomized study. *Eur Heart J.* 2003;24(14):1287-1295.

17. Alexander JH, Reynolds HR, Stebbins AL, et al. Effect of tilarginine acetate in patients with acute myocardial infarction and cardiogenic shock: the TRIUMPH randomized controlled trial. *JAMA.* 2007;297(15):1657-1666.

18. Ellis TC, Lev E, Yazbek NF, Kleiman NS. Therapeutic strategies for cardiogenic shock, 2006. *Curr Treat Options Cardiovasc Med.* 2006;8(1):79-94.

19. Duvernoy CS, Bates ER. Management of cardiogenic shock attributable to acute myocardial infarction in the reperfusion era. *J Intensive Care Med.* 2005;20(4):188-198.

20. Antman EM, Anbe DT, Armstrong PW, et al. ACC/AHA guidelines for the management of patients with ST-elevation myocardial infarction—executive summary. A report of the American College of Cardiology/American Heart Association Task Force on Practice Guidelines (Writing Committee to revise the 1999 guidelines for the management of patients with acute myocardial infarction). *J Am Coll Cardiol.* 2004;44(3):671-719.

21. Mann HJ, Nolan PE Jr. Update on the management of cardiogenic shock. *Curr Opin Crit Care.* 2006;12(5):431-436.

22. Menon V, Slater JN, White HD, Sleeper LA, Cocke T, Hochman JS. Acute myocardial infarction complicated by systemic hypoperfusion without hypotension: report of the SHOCK trial registry. *Am J Med.* 2000;108(5):374-380.

23. Menon V, Hochman JS. Management of cardiogenic shock complicating acute myocardial infarction. *Heart.* 2002;88(5):531-537.

24. Webb JG, Sleeper LA, Buller CE, et al. Implications of the timing of onset of cardiogenic shock after acute myocardial infarction: a report from the SHOCK Trial Registry. SHould we emergently revascularize Occluded Coronaries for cardiogenic shocK? *J Am Coll Cardiol.* 2000;36(3 Suppl A):1084-1090.

25. Ross AM, The GUSTO Angiographic Investigators. The effects of tissue plasminogen activator, streptokinase, or both on coronary-artery patency, ventricular function, and survival after acute myocardial infarction. *N Engl J Med.* 1993;329(22): 1615-1622.

26. Keeley EC, Boura JA, Grines CL. Primary angioplasty versus intravenous thrombolytic therapy for acute myocardial infarction: a quantitative review of 23 randomised trials. *Lancet.* 2003;361(9351):13-20.

27. Hochman JS, Sleeper LA, Webb JG, et al. Early revascularization in acute myocardial infarction complicated by cardiogenic shock. SHOCK Investigators.

SHould We Emergently Revascularize Occluded Coronaries for Cardiogenic Shock. *N Engl J Med.* 1999;341(9):625-634.

28. Hochman JS, Sleeper LA, White HD, et al. One-year survival following early revascularization for cardiogenic shock. *JAMA.* 2001;285(2):190-192.

29. Hochman JS, Sleeper LA, Webb JG, et al. Early revascularization and long-term survival in cardiogenic shock complicating acute myocardial infarction. *JAMA.* 2006;295(21):2511-2515.

30. Jeger RV, Tseng CH, Hochman JS, Bates ER. Inter-hospital transfer for early revascularization in patients with ST-elevation myocardial infarction complicated by cardiogenic shock—a report from the SHould we revascularize Occluded Coronaries for cardiogenic shocK? (SHOCK) trial and registry. *Am Heart J.* 2006;152(4):686-692.

31. Ohman EM, Chang PP. Improving quality of life after cardiogenic shock: do more revascularization! *J Am Coll Cardiol.* 2005;46(2):274-276.

32. Eagle KA, Guyton RA, Davidoff R, et al. ACC/AHA 2004 guideline update for coronary artery bypass graft surgery: a report of the American College of Cardiology/American Heart Association Task Force on Practice Guidelines (Committee to Update the 1999 Guidelines for Coronary Artery Bypass Graft Surgery). *Circulation.* 2004;110(14):e340-e437.

33. Dzavik V, Sleeper LA, Cocke TP, et al. Early revascularization is associated with improved survival in elderly patients with acute myocardial infarction complicated by cardiogenic shock: a report from the SHOCK Trial Registry. *Eur Heart J.* 2003;24(9):828-837.

34. Trost JC, Hillis LD. Intra-aortic balloon counterpulsation. *Am J Cardiol.* 2006;97(9):1391-1398.

35. Sanborn TA, Sleeper LA, Bates ER, et al. Impact of thrombolysis, intra-aortic balloon pump counterpulsation, and their combination in cardiogenic shock complicating acute myocardial infarction: a report from the SHOCK Trial Registry. SHould we emergently revascularize Occluded Coronaries for cardiogenic shocK? *J Am Coll Cardiol.* 2000; 36(3 Suppl A):1123-1129.

36. Hasdai D, Califf RM, Thompson TD, et al. Predictors of cardiogenic shock after thrombolytic therapy for acute myocardial infarction. *J Am Coll Cardiol.* 2000;35(1):136-143.

37. Kantrowitz A. Experimental augmentation of coronary flow by retardation of the arterial pressure pulse. *Surgery.* 1953;34(4):678-687.

38. Clauss RH, Birtwell WC, Albertal G, et al. Assisted circulation: I. The arterial counterpulsator. *J Thorac Cardiovasc Surg.* 1961;41:447-458.

39. Moulopoulos SD, Topaz S, Kolff WJ. Diastolic balloon pumping (with carbon dioxide) in the aorta—a mechanical assistance to the failing circulation. *Am Heart J.* 1962;63:669-675.

40. Kantrowitz A, Tjonneland S, Freed PS, Phillips SJ, Butner AN, Sherman JL Jr. Initial clinical experience with intraaortic balloon pumping in cardiogenic shock. *JAMA.* 1968;203(2):113-118.

41. Torchiana DF, Hirsch G, Buckley MJ, et al. Intraaortic balloon pumping for cardiac support: trends in practice and outcome, 1968 to 1995. *J Thorac Cardiovasc Surg.* 1997;113(4):758-764; discussion 764-769.

42. Cohen M, Urban P, Christenson JT, et al. Intra-aortic balloon counterpulsation in US and non-US centres: results of the Benchmark Registry. *Eur Heart J.* 2003;24(19):1763-1770.

43. Turi ZG. Intra-aortic balloon counterpulsation. In: Parrillo JE, Dellinger RP, eds. *Critical Care Medicine—Principles of Diagnosis and Management in the Adult.* 3rd ed. Philadelphia, PA: Mosby Elsevier; 2008.

44. Kern MJ, Aguirre FV, Tatineni S, et al. Enhanced coronary blood flow velocity during intraaortic balloon counterpulsation in critically ill patients. *J Am Coll Cardiol.* 1993;21(2):359-368.

45. Takeuchi M, Nohtomi Y, Yoshitani H, Miyazaki C, Sakamoto K, Yoshikawa J. Enhanced coronary flow velocity during intra-aortic balloon pumping assessed by transthoracic Doppler echocardiography. *J Am Coll Cardiol.* 2004;43(3):368-376.

46. Zehetgruber M, Mundigler G, Christ G, et al. Relation of hemodynamic variables to augmentation of left anterior descending coronary flow by intraaortic balloon pulsation in coronary artery disease. *Am J Cardiol.* 1997;80(7):951-955.

47. Kveim M, Cappelen C Jr, Frooysaker T, Hall KV. Intra-aortic balloon pumping in the treatment of cardiogenic shock following open-heart surgery. *Scand J Thorac Cardiovasc Surg.* 1976;10(3):231-235.

48. Lee MS, Makkar RR. Percutaneous left ventricular support devices. *Cardiol Clin.* 2006;24(2):265-275, vii.

49. Weber KT, Janicki JS. Intraaortic balloon counterpulsation. A review of physiological principles, clinical results, and device safety. *Ann Thorac Surg.* 1974;17(6):602-636.

50. Ferguson JJ 3rd, Cohen M, Freedman RJ Jr, et al. The current practice of intra-aortic balloon counterpulsation: results from the Benchmark Registry. *J Am Coll Cardiol.* 2001;38(5):1456-1462.

51. Stone GW, Ohman EM, Miller MF, et al. Contemporary utilization and outcomes of intra-aortic balloon counterpulsation in acute myocardial infarction: the benchmark registry. *J Am Coll Cardiol.* 2003;41(11):1940-1945.

52. Sjauw KD, Engstrom AE, Vis MM, et al. A systematic review and meta-analysis of intra-aortic balloon pump therapy in ST-elevation myocardial infarction: should we change the guidelines? *Eur Heart J.* 2009;30(4):459-468.

53. Anderson RD, Ohman EM, Holmes DR Jr, et al. Use of intraaortic balloon counterpulsation in patients presenting with cardiogenic shock: observations from the GUSTO-I Study. Global Utilization of Streptokinase and TPA for Occluded Coronary Arteries. *J Am Coll Cardiol.* 1997;30(3): 708-715.

54. Barron HV, Every NR, Parsons LS, et al. The use of intra-aortic balloon counterpulsation in patients with cardiogenic shock complicating acute myocardial infarction: data from the National Registry of Myocardial Infarction 2. *Am Heart J.* 2001;141(6):933-939.

55. Goldstein JA. Pathophysiology and management of right heart ischemia. *J Am Coll Cardiol.* 2002;40(5):841-853.

56. Jacobs AK, Leopold JA, Bates E, et al. Cardiogenic shock caused by right ventricular infarction: a report from the SHOCK registry. *J Am Coll Cardiol.* 2003;41(8):1273-1279.

57. Laster SB, Shelton TJ, Barzilai B, Goldstein JA. Determinants of the recovery of right ventricular performance following experimental chronic right coronary artery occlusion. *Circulation.* 1993;88(2):696-708.

58. Dell'Italia LJ, Lembo NJ, Starling MR, et al. Hemodynamically important right ventricular infarction:

59. Bowers TR, O'Neill WW, Grines C, Pica MC, Safian RD, Goldstein JA. Effect of reperfusion on biventricular function and survival after right ventricular infarction. *N Engl J Med.* 1998;338(14):933-940.

60. Thompson CR, Buller CE, Sleeper LA, et al. Cardiogenic shock due to acute severe mitral regurgitation complicating acute myocardial infarction: a report from the SHOCK Trial Registry. SHould we use emergently revascularize Occluded Coronaries in cardiogenic shocK? *J Am Coll Cardiol.* 2000; 36(3 Suppl A):1104-1109.

61. Dekker AL, Reesink KD, van der Veen FH, et al. Intra-aortic balloon pumping in acute mitral regurgitation reduces aortic impedance and regurgitant fraction. *Shock.* 2003;19(4):334-338.

62. Menon V, Webb JG, Hillis LD, et al. Outcome and profile of ventricular septal rupture with cardiogenic shock after myocardial infarction: a report from the SHOCK Trial Registry. SHould we emergently revascularize Occluded Coronaries in cardiogenic shocK? *J Am Coll Cardiol.* 2000; 36(3 Suppl A):1110-1116.

63. Slater J, Brown RJ, Antonelli TA, et al. Cardiogenic shock due to cardiac free-wall rupture or tamponade after acute myocardial infarction: a report from the SHOCK Trial Registry. Should we emergently revascularize occluded coronaries for cardiogenic shock? *J Am Coll Cardiol.* 2000;36(3 Suppl A):1117-1122.

follow-up evaluation of right ventricular systolic function at rest and during exercise with radionuclide ventriculography and respiratory gas exchange. *Circulation.* 1987;75(5):996-1003.

Pulmonary Diseases

R. Phillip Dellinger, MD, FCCP

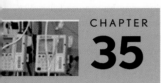

CHAPTER

35

The Neurocritical Care Airway

Laura McPhee, DO
David B. Seder, MD

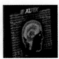
A 58-year-old hypertensive man is evaluated in the emergency department after being found on the floor in his home with left hemiparesis, a left frontotemporal scalp laceration, and somnolence. Because the patient does not remember the onset of symptoms and the mechanism of injury is uncertain, a rigid cervical collar is placed by emergency medical services in the field. Computed tomography (CT) of the head demonstrates a right thalamic intracerebral and intraventricular hemorrhage involving the right lateral and third ventricles. There is no skull fracture, cervical spine injury, or gross cervical misalignment. Initially, he is interactive and speaks clearly. The blood pressure is rapidly controlled, and preparations are made for transfer to the intensive care unit (ICU). But before transfer occurs he becomes progressively obtunded, with a symmetric increase in bilateral lower-extremity tone. He begins to struggle with respiration, making grunting sounds and activating accessory muscles on inspiration. It is not known when he last ate, and examination of the oropharynx reveals a blunted gag reflex and weak cough.

Does this patient need to be intubated?

Yes, for several reasons. He is in a period of acute neurologic decline, with an inadequate airway to provide for oxygenation and ventilation. He has dangerously dulled airway protective reflexes and could have a full stomach, putting him at risk for large-volume gastric aspiration. He will require an urgent invasive procedure (ventriculostomy placement), will be transported between units, and will undergo further imaging studies, requiring flat positioning on the bed. All of these factors suggest he should be intubated. Of interest is that a patient with the *same neurologic examination* can sometimes be safely *extubated* in the recovery period—safely monitored in an ICU, with no procedures or transfers planned, an empty stomach, and no clinical decline anticipated.

Neurocritical care patients include trauma victims with facial or cervical spinal injuries and patients in whom bleeding, seizures, or anatomic complications may cause progression from a state of relative stability to brain herniation and/or cardiopulmonary arrest in a matter of minutes. Furthermore, hypoxemia, hypoventilation, and hyperventilation are all powerful mediators of cerebral blood flow and tissue perfusion, so maintenance of a state of respiratory homeostasis is critical to preventing secondary brain injury.

Finally, aspiration before or during intubation can lead to fever, pneumonia, acute respiratory distress syndrome, and systemic inflammation, each associated with worse neurologic outcomes and increased mortality rate. These concerns, which suggest that intubation may be required for many acutely ill neurology patients, are balanced by the principles of preserving an accurate neurologic examination and avoiding the complications of intubation whenever possible.

Indications for endotracheal intubation in the neurocritically ill are often categorized according to three general criteria[1]:

1. Failure to maintain or protect the airway
2. Failure of oxygenation or ventilation
3. An anticipated course of clinical deterioration

These principles are discussed further below.

What constitutes failure to protect the airway?

Is it appropriate to intubate *every* patient with abnormal airway protection? No, although in the *acute phase* of a neurologic injury, endotracheal intubation is often indicated and may be lifesaving. Airway protection is a matter of some controversy, in part because of its complexity. A normal airway protective mechanism involves:

1. Coordinated oropharyngeal sensory and muscle activity to move oral secretions, liquids, or food in a posterior and inferior direction (away from the larynx) into the upper esophagus, and the rapid activation of esophageal peristalsis to clear the oropharynx
2. A tight lower esophageal sphincter and low gastric pH
3. Elevation and anterior displacement of the glottis during swallowing, with tight closure and approximation of vocal cords and folds
4. A robust sensory response to solids and liquids at the glottis and lower airways, as well as intact cough centers and efferent nervous pathways to the effector muscles
5. Adequate respiratory muscle strength and tidal volume to generate a strong cough
6. Healthy bronchial epithelium with intact villi that clear foreign substances from the smaller, distal airways
7. Maintaining the airway open during airflow—an active, not passive, process involving pharyngeal dilator muscles

Many patients have impaired execution of these multifold functions but, because of circumstances or redundancy in the system, do not require artificial airways. Nonetheless, patients with incomplete or failed airway protective mechanisms are at high risk of aspirating food, secretions, and gastric contents. A clinically unstable patient with severely impaired airway protection requires

Table 35-1. Semiquantitative Assessment of Need for Airway Care

Spontaneous cough	Gag	Sputum quantity
0: Vigorous	0: Vigorous	0: None
1: Moderate	1: Moderate	1: 1 pass
2: Weak	2: Weak	2: 2 passes
3: None	3: None	3: ≥ 3 passes

Sputum viscosity	Suctioning frequency (last 8 h)	Sputum character
0: Watery	0: > 3 h	0: Clear
1: Frothy	1: 2-3 h	1: Tan
2: Thick	2: 1-2 h	2: Yellow
3: Tenacious	3: < 1 h	3: Green

intubation, while a clinically stable patient with severely impaired airway protection can often be managed with careful feeding (often through a tube) and high-quality nursing, speech-language pathology, and respiratory care.

Routinely applied airway assessment measures include the Glasgow Coma Scale (GCS) score, strength of cough, quantity and character of oral and respiratory secretions, and an evaluation of oropharyngeal coordination and sensation. An airway protection score has been proposed (Table 35-1).[2,3] Assessment of the gag reflex is routine but does not correlate well with laryngeal closure and airway protection[4,5]; the gag reflex may be absent in up to 37% of healthy subjects.[6]

In the acute setting, a GCS score less than or equal to 8 has been described as both sensitive and specific for predicting the need for endotracheal intubation,[7] applied not only in trauma but also in patients with stroke, intoxication, and other etiologies of altered mental status.[1] Several studies have demonstrated that patients with GCS less than or equal to 8 commonly have airway obstruction, hypoxemia, and hypoventilation,[8] resulting from pooled secretions, anatomic compression, or foreign-body aspiration. While the GCS is routinely employed in the emergency department and by emergency medical services (EMS) as part of a triage process to assess patients for intubation, the GCS was not developed for this purpose and does not address *any* of the primary issues related to airway protection—cough, the ability to manage secretions in the upper airway, or the acuity or anticipated course of the primary neurologic process. In the ICU, a more sophisticated assessment of the airway is expected, should take into account all of the issues discussed above, and be balanced by the known repercussions of endotracheal intubation: confounding of the neurologic examination, an increased need for neuromonitoring and imaging, a need for vasopressors or fluids to counteract the vasodilatory properties of sedation and analgesia, and ventilator-associated pneumonia.

What constitutes a failure of oxygenation or ventilation?

It is sometimes simple to identify oxygenation or ventilatory failure, such as when a brainstem or spinal cord injury completely eliminates respiratory efforts, when a patient struggles unsuccessfully to breathe against an excessive workload, or when the oxyhemoglobin saturation cannot be maintained despite high inspired oxygen fraction (FIO_2). Other forms of respiratory failure are more subtle, however. Mild hypoventilation and hypercarbia that would be well tolerated in a patient with simple chronic obstructive pulmonary disease exacerbation may lead rapidly to an intracranial pressure (ICP) crisis in a patient with intracerebral hemorrhage or hydrocephalus. Similarly, modestly increased work of breathing that would ordinarily be well tolerated might compromise the ischemic penumbra of a stroke patient with heart failure. In these cases, critical care of the neurologically ill differs significantly from other patients. The neurointensivist must at all times recall that oxygen and carbon dioxide tensions in the cerebral vasculature are potent mediators of blood flow, ICP, and secondary neurologic injury.

Arterial blood gases should be measured in patients with a poor level of arousal, on mechanical ventilation, with significant or suspected respiratory compromise, or with elevated ICP. When cerebral blood flow is jeopardized, when there is elevated ICP or poor intracranial compliance, or when a procedure that jeopardizes ventilation, such as bronchoscopy or tracheostomy, is performed, we recommend continuous capnography and a dynamic assessment of the effects of arterial carbon dioxide and oxygen levels on brain perfusion and ischemia.

It is difficult to provide 100% oxygen to a patient without an endotracheal or tracheostomy tube in place. Oxygen supplementation depends on a variety of factors including the percent oxygen provided, flow rate through the tubing and mask of the device, minute ventilation of the patient, and admixture of room air through leaks in the system or in the upper airways. Commonly employed oxygen delivery devices and their estimated oxygen delivery are described in Table 35-2.

Acute hypoxemic respiratory failure is defined as failure to maintain a partial pressure of arterial oxygen (Pao_2) at 60 mm Hg despite the administration of maximal supplemental oxygen. While these low oxygen levels are usually well tolerated in patients with normal brains, there is reason to view this definition and standard of care with suspicion when brain injury or perfusion is a concern. In traumatic brain injury (TBI), hypoxia (defined as an oxygen saturation as measured by pulse oximetry [Spo_2] ≤ 90%), with a median duration of only 11.5 to 20 minutes, is an independent predictor of mortality.[9] Low brain tissue oxygen ($Pbto_2$) is associated with brain ischemia and poor neurologic outcome in TBI.[10,11] In healthy individuals, autoregulation of cerebral blood flow maintains oxygenation by shunting blood into ischemic regions to maintain a constant Pao_2, but in the injured brain, this mechanism is frequently absent.

Oxygen delivery within an ischemic region is already marginal, and tolerating borderline blood oxygen may increase cerebral infarction size or worsen hypoperfusion in a brain with ischemia due to ICP crisis. Furthermore, and against classical teaching regarding oxygen delivery, there is some evidence to suggest that brain tissue oxygen levels can be significantly increased by increasing the dissolved partial pressure of oxygen in blood, even when oxyhemoglobin is fully saturated.[12] The Brain Trauma Foundation (BTF) guidelines state "oxygenation should be monitored and hypoxia (Pao_2 < 60 mm Hg or O_2 saturation < 90%) avoided" (level III).[13] The American Stroke Association recommends maintaining oxygen saturation levels greater than or equal to 95% in acute ischemic stroke (level V).[14]

Table 35-2. Oxygen Delivery Devices and Actual Tracheal Oxygen Delivery

		"Intended" FIO_2	Actual FIO_2	
Oxygen Delivery System			Quiet Breathing	Hyperventilating
Nasal prongs	3 L/min		22.4%	22.7%
	10 L/min		46.4%	30.5%
	15 L/min		60.9%	36.2%
Face mask	10 L/min	0.60	53.4%	41%
	15 L/min	1.0	68.1%	50.2%
Venturi mask	4 L/min	0.28	24.2%	21.4%
	8 L/min	0.40	36.4%	29.4%

(Adapted with permission from Gibson RL, Comer PB, Beckham RW, McGraw CP. Actual tracheal oxygen concentrations with commonly used oxygen equipment. Anesthesiology 1976;44:71-77.).

Hypoventilation and hypercarbia in a patient with acute brain injury and elevated ICP constitute an emergency, and failure to provide adequate ventilation may result in vasodilation, increased cerebral blood volume, increased ICP, central downward brain herniation, and death. Conversely, iatrogenic hyperventilation can result in a dramatic increase in the volume of ischemic brain,[15] and even the auto-hyperventilation seen in many brain injuries has recently been associated with decreased $Pbto_2$.[16] Clinicians should attempt to maintain adequate but not excessive ventilation, and should be aware of the effects of changes in ventilation on brain perfusion and ICP in real time.

What are the major concerns during intubation?

The major concerns during intubation are the successful placement of the airway device; avoidance of large-volume aspiration; maintenance of hemodynamic, respiratory, and metabolic homeostasis; management of intracranial pressure; and protection of the cervical spine.

Preparation for intubation in the neurology ICU routinely includes:

1. Assessment of the airway and review of existing records describing the airway
2. Decompression of the stomach, if appropriate
3. Consideration of cervical spinal injury, and a plan to minimize spinal manipulation accordingly (see below)
4. Consideration of intracranial pressure, and a plan to minimize ICP and cerebral perfusion pressure (CPP) fluctuations during laryngoscopy, endotracheal tube (ETT) placement, and the administration of vasodilator medications
5. Spo_2, blood pressure, and ICP monitoring, and potentially capnography
6. Assembly of routine airway equipment, special equipment, and suction
7. Careful consideration of intubating medications to provide excellent sedation, analgesia, amnesia, and muscle relaxation without introducing hypotension, hypoxemia, or ICP crisis
8. Establishment of adequate intravenous access for medications, fluids, and vasopressors if necessary
9. Proper positioning of the patient
10. Determination, based on risk to the patient, of whether the intubation will be performed by a trainee or by the most experienced person present

How is ICP managed during intubation?

Patients with intracranial hypertension are at risk for both ICP crisis and critically low CPP during intubation. Clinicians should pay special attention to the adequacy of sedation and analgesia during laryngoscopy, to head-of-the-bed positioning, and to the maintenance of adequate blood pressure and oxygenation during intubation of these patients.

Direct laryngoscopy is a noxious stimulus that causes sympathetic stimulation, potentially triggering tachycardia, hypertension, bronchospasm, and increased ICP.[17] A crucial starting point to controlling ICP is to leave the head of the bed up 30 to 45 degrees during preparation for intubation, and lay the patient flat only during the procedure, then immediately return the bed to its elevated position. If necessary, the patient can be placed in reverse Trendelenburg positioning throughout the intubation. Medications that blunt the ICP rise associated with laryngoscopy are discussed in more detail below.

Hypotension, hypoxemia, and hypercarbia cause vasodilation and an increase in cerebral blood volume, leading to a rise in ICP. Preoxygenation is vital, as it washes out nitrogen in the lungs and prolongs the time to oxyhemoglobin desaturation. The patient's minute ventilation should be maintained throughout the procedure to avoid CO_2 retention—a matter of urgency in patients with central nervous system mass lesions.[18] Adequate intravenous access is critically important to managing hemodynamic changes during intubation, and we suggest routine infusion of isotonic crystalloid during the procedure. Vasopressors should be readily available in the event of hypotension to maintain adequate CPP.

What medications can be used in brain-injured patients during intubation?

Intubation can be performed under sedation assistance (absence of neuromuscular blockade) or rapid sequence (coadministration of neuromuscular blockade and sedatives) (Table 35-3). Rapid-sequence intubation is suggested when the stomach may be full to minimize the risk of distending the stomach with air, triggering vomiting and gastric aspiration.

Fentanyl has a rapid onset and short duration of action and reduces the hypertensive response to laryngoscopy.[19] Because it suppresses the sympathetic response to hypotension, caution must be used in shock states or hypovolemia. Fentanyl derivatives such as remifentanil, sufentanil, and alfentanil are increasingly utilized worldwide and may be more efficacious in blunting the tachycardic response.[17]

Lidocaine at a dose of 1.5 mg/kg intravenously blunts ICP rise during laryngoscopy by reducing tachycardia, airway hyperactivity, cerebral blood flow, cerebral vascular resistance, and cerebral metabolism.[20] It can, however, also decrease mean arterial pressure (MAP) and CPP.[21,22] The use of lidocaine to reduce ICP during intubation is controversial,[19,23] but has been shown to be effective in patients with cerebral neoplasms,[24] closed head injuries,[25] and known elevated ICPs.[26] Its side-effect profile includes hypotension, a decreased seizure threshold, and a low incidence of ventricular tachyarrhythmias.[27]

Pretreatment with low-dose nondepolarizing neuromuscular blocking agents prior to the administration of succinylcholine is often recommended in order to prevent fasciculation and ICP rise.[28-30] This practice may be effective, but it is not supported by published data.[17,31]

Etomidate is one of the most commonly used medications for facilitating endotracheal intubation,[32] with powerful sedative and muscle relaxant properties. It is a γ-aminobutyric acid (GABA) agonist without analgesic properties. Etomidate is popular because of its hemodynamically neutral effects and a tendency to reduce ICP and cerebral oxygen demand while purportedly preserving CPP.[32-34] Side effects include increases in airway resistance, myoclonus, nausea, and vomiting; reduction of the seizure threshold; and adrenal insufficiency. The clinical sequelae of this well-described adrenal insufficiency are unknown; there is growing concern about the use of etomidate in septic patients, in whom an increased mortality rate has been observed.[35,36]

Propofol is a GABA agonist that delivers sedation and anesthesia but not analgesia. It reduces airway resistance, has anticonvulsive and antiemetic effects, and suppresses sympathetic activity. This includes a reduction in cardiac inotropy, systemic vascular resistance, intracranial pressure (by decreasing cerebral blood flow), cerebral blood volume, and cerebral metabolism.[37] Propofol provides deeper anesthesia than etomidate and creates intubating conditions similar to succinylcholine when used with a nondepolarizing neuromuscular blocker or opiate.[17] However, propofol causes a reduction in systolic blood pressure by 15% to 33%.[38] Extreme caution should be exercised when using propofol as an induction agent in patients who require a higher cerebral perfusion pressure and those patients with known cardiomyopathy or low ejection fraction.

Thiopental causes sedation and amnesia through its GABA-agonist properties. It decreases cerebral blood flow, cerebral metabolism, cardiovascular contractility, systemic vascular resistance, and venous return to the heart. Major side effects include hypotension, allergic reactions (2%), laryngospasm, bronchospasm, hypersalivation, and immune suppression.

Ketamine is a "dissociative" anesthetic that provides sedation, amnesia, and analgesia. It is an appealing agent in critical illness because it does not cause vasodilation or hypotension. Ketamine binds to catecholamine receptors, causing an increase in heart rate, cardiac output, contractility, mean arterial pressure, and cerebral blood flow.[39] Prior studies have demonstrated that ketamine increases

Table 35-3. Commonly Used Medications for Induction

Drug	Dose	Onset of action	Duration of effect	Indications	Precautions
Fentanyl	1-2 μ/kg IV push over 1-2 min	Within 2-3 min	30-60 min	Preinduction, blunts ICP rise	Respiratory depression, hypotension, rare muscle wall rigidity
Lidocaine	1-1.5 mg/kg IV 2-3 min before intubation	45-90 s	10-20 min	Preinduction, blunts ICP rise	Avoid if allergic or high-grade heart block if no pacemaker
Etomidate	0.3 mg/kg IV push	30-60 s	3-5 min	Induction, sedation; good in hypotension. Decreases CBF, ICP; preserves CPP	Decreases seizure threshold, decreases cortisol synthesis; avoid in sepsis
Propofol	2 mg/kg very slow IV push	9-50 s	3-10 min	Induction, sedation, reduces ICP and airway resistance, anticonvulsive effects	Hypotension, myocardial depression
Ketamine	2 mg/kg IV push	1-2 min	5-15 min	Induction, analgesia, sedation, amnesia, bronchodilatory effects; good in hypotension	Catecholamine surge, possible increase in ICP, "reemergence" phenomenon if not pretreated with benzodiazepines
Thiopental	3 mg/kg IV push	30-60 s	5-30 min	Normotensive, normovolemic status epilepticus or increased ICP patients	Hypotension, bronchospasm
Succinylcholine	1.5-2 mg/kg IV push	30-60 s	5-15 min	Preferred paralytic unless contraindicated	Caution in hyperkalemia, myopathy, neuropathy/denervation; avoid if history of malignant hyperthermia
Rocuronium	0.6 mg/kg IV push	45-60 s	45-70 min	Paralysis when succinylcholine contraindicated	Caution in DMV and DI
Vecuronium	0.1 mg/kg IV push	Within 3 min	35 min	Least preferred paralytic for RSI	Caution in DMV and DI

Abbreviations: CBF, cerebral blood flow; CPP, cerebral perfusion pressure; DI, difficult intubation; DMV, difficult mask ventilation; ICP, intracranial pressure; IV, intravenously; RSI, rapid-sequence intubation.

ICP,[40-45] and some authors have recommended against its use in patients with intracranial hypertension. This recommendation is probably obsolete, however, as improvements in CPP have been clearly demonstrated despite elevated ICP when ketamine was used in conjunction with a GABA agonist.[46-49] Clinicians should be aware of the potential for dangerous agitation with ketamine when it is given with inadequate sedation, and that it has been poorly studied in the neurocritically ill.

Neuromuscular blocking agents cause profound skeletal muscle relaxation, creating ideal intubating conditions, and have hemodynamically neutral effects. They are always employed in conjunction with sedation. Succinylcholine is a depolarizing agent that activates the acetylcholine receptor, resulting in defasciculation and transient skeletal muscle paralysis. It has the shortest onset and duration of action (typically < 5 minutes) of all the neuromuscular blockers. Side effects include hyperkalemia, myalgias, and rarely malignant hyperthermia in genetically susceptible patients. Some studies suggest that succinylcholine increases intracranial pressure,[50] but this has been disputed.[31,51] The effect of succinylcholine on ICP is transient and of questionable significance[17,52] and should not preclude its use when needed.

Neurocritically ill patients may be at higher risk for succinylcholine-induced hyperkalemia.[53-55] Conditions leading to an upregulation of acetylcholine receptors cause greater potassium efflux from myocytes with nerve depolarization. This includes patients with disuse atrophy, such as stroke or TBI patients with a sudden onset of weakness or paralysis, occurring after as little as 24 to 72 hours of immobility, and patients with upper or lower motor neuron defects.[56] This risk may be averted by "precurization"—administration of a small dose of nondepolarizing neuromuscular blockers a few minutes before the succinylcholine—or by simply using a nondepolarizing agent instead.

How should I reduce the risk of aspiration during intubation?

Take care not to inflate the stomach during bag-mask ventilation (BMV). When appropriate, nasogastric decompression of the stomach should be performed prior to intubation, although a nasogastric tube may make mask ventilation more difficult. Downward cricoid pressure was described in 1961 as resulting in occlusion of the esophageal lumen posteriorly against the vertebral column[57] and is routinely applied during BMV and rapid-sequence intubation to help prevent the instillation of air into the stomach and regurgitation of gastric contents. Recent data suggest that the technique actually compresses the postcricoid hypopharynx, not the esophagus.[58] Although limited data confirm that the maneuver actually reduces the risk of aspiration,[59-64] cricoid pressure is typically well tolerated, may be helpful, and is unlikely to cause harm. It should not be applied when the cervical spine is unstable, and its use should be terminated if there is difficulty with mask ventilation, airway visualization, or active vomiting.

How do I predict a difficult airway?

Because both hypoxemia and hypercarbia often result in secondary brain injury, early recognition of a potentially difficult airway or difficult BMV is critically important. Difficult BMV is more dangerous than difficult intubation, since a patient who is difficult to intubate can typically be maintained indefinitely by BMV. When a difficult airway is identified, it is always appropriate to seek the most expert help available to perform the intubation or provide "backup" for the intubator. Important techniques for managing difficult airways include the use of special equipment designed to facilitate placement of the ETT, placement of temporizing airway devices, and surgical airways. Factors identified as predictive of difficult mask ventilation and difficult airway are listed in Tables 35-4 and 35-5.

What devices are available to facilitate intubation of a difficult airway?

Clinicians frequently performing endotracheal intubation should develop true expertise with a modest number of intubating techniques and airway adjunct devices. Commonly employed techniques

Table 35-4. Risk Factors for Difficult Mask Ventilation

- Age older than 55 y
- Male gender
- Body mass index > 26 kg/m^2
- Presence of beard
- Lack of teeth
- History of snoring
- Mallampati class IV airway

include bimanual laryngoscopy, videoscopic laryngoscopy, blind intubation using a light wand or intubating stylet, and fiberoptic intubation. Airway adjunct devices are multifold but include the gum elastic "bougie" or Eschmann stylet, light wands, articulating laryngoscope blades, intubating laryngeal mask airways, retrograde intubation kits, and an assortment of videoscopes. In particular, the GlideScope has been shown to increase the success rate of endotracheal intubation among untrained personnel when compared to direct laryngoscopy with a Macintosh blade (success rate 93% versus 51%; $P < .01$).[65] Airway adjuncts are summarized in Table 35-6.

"Temporizing" supraglottic devices can be inserted if the airway cannot be intubated or to oxygenate and ventilate while preparations are made for intubation. The most common device is the laryngeal mask airway (LMA), an inflatable latex mask placed blindly into the hypopharynx. While not considered a permanent or "definitive" airway as it does not protect against aspiration, the device requires minimal experience to competently employ and may be extremely helpful if a skilled intubator is not available, if the airway is difficult, or if a beard or facial anomaly makes BMV difficult.

A true emergency arises when a patient cannot be intubated or ventilated. In this situation, an immediate surgical airway may be necessary. A needle, wire-guided, or surgical cricothyrotomy should be performed. Tracheostomy is a more complex and time-consuming procedure and should be reserved for nonemergent situations (see Chapter 39).

What is the best way to stabilize the cervical spine during intubation?

Any patient with a confirmed or suspected unstable cervical spine needs to be immediately and carefully placed in a rigid cervical collar or other stabilization device. Manual in-line axial stabilization and gentle traction of the head and neck by an assistant are mandatory if the patient requires *any* manipulation of the head or neck. During airway management, cervical subluxation occurs during chin lift, jaw thrust, BMV, and tracheal intubation,[66,67] as well as maneuvers such as cricoid pressure and head turning. Mask ventilation was found in one study to cause more cervical spine displacement than any method used for tracheal intubation.[68]

Table 35-5. Risk Factors for Difficult Intubation

- Difficulty opening mouth (interincisor distance 3 cm or less)
- Thyromental distance < 3 ordinary fingerbreadths (6 cm or less)
- Short, thick neck
- Large incisors or "buckteeth"
- Neck fixed in flexion and limited neck mobility
- Mallampati class IV airway
- Obesity
- Extreme head/neck radiation changes, scarring, masses

Table 35-6. Airway Adjuncts

Gum elastic bougie	60-cm malleable rod placed through difficult-to-visualize vocal cords. Endotracheal tube (ETT) advanced over bougie
Lighted stylet or light wand	Placed blindly. ETT advanced over device when anterior neck displays a bright red light, indicating tracheal placement
Articulating laryngoscope blades	Bullard scope: rigid fiberoptic laryngoscope that facilitates oral or nasal intubations; McCoy scope: similar to Macintosh blade but has hinged tip operated by lever that elevates epiglottis
Intubating laryngeal mask airway (LMA)	Rigid and wider tube that allows for placement of modified ETT through mask
Retrograde intubation kit	Cricothyroid incision made and guidewire passed upward through vocal cords into mouth and ETT passed over wire/catheter
Video scope (eg, McGrath, Storz laryngoscope, GlideScope)	Camera at distal tip of laryngoscope displays vocal cords. ETT placed with video visualization
Flexible bronchoscope	Camera at distal tip of bronchoscope displays vocal cords. ETT advanced over scope through vocal cords

If direct laryngoscopy is employed, the cervical collar must be removed for intubation, as greater subluxation occurs with a collar in place than with in-line stabilization. Laryngeal visualization is also improved after the cervical collar is removed.[69,70] The collar should be carefully reapplied immediately following intubation.

In-line stabilization places the patient's head and neck into neutral position. Unfortunately, no accepted definition of this ideal position exists.[71] One study demonstrated that a mean of 4 cm of occiput elevation off the bed was required to assume a position as if someone was standing looking straight ahead.[72] A magnetic resonance imaging study determined that occiput elevation of at least 2 cm was required to maximize the spinal canal/spinal cord ratio at C5 and C6.[73] To perform in-line cervical stabilization, the patient is supine with the head and neck in neutral position. With the assistant at the head of the bed, each mastoid process is grabbed with the fingertips and the occiput is cradled in the palms. With the assistant at the side of the bed, stabilization can be provided by cradling the mastoids in the palms and grasping the occiput with the fingertips.[74]

Cricoid pressure causes cervical spine displacement in cadaver studies.[75] Without posterior support, cricoid pressure is associated with a mean neck displacement of 4.6 mm (range 0-8 mm).[76] Consequently, if cricoid pressure is necessary for intubation, it must be performed bimanually, with concomitant posterior support of the neck.[77] This modification should also be applied with the BURP (backward-upward-rightward pressure) maneuver. Many of the same rescue techniques used for a difficult airway are applied during a difficult intubation in a patient with cervical spine injury (see Figures 35-1 and 35-2).

Because the least amount of cervical spine motion detected fluoroscopically after a midcervical spine injury is with fiberoptic nasal intubation,[66] this approach may be preferable when severe cervical instability is suspected and when time and expertise are available to perform the intubation accordingly.

What airway concerns should be considered prior to extubation?

Traditional weaning parameters such as respiratory rate, tidal volume, rapid shallow breathing index, minute ventilation, negative inspiratory force, and the Pao_2-to-Fio_2 ratio do not predict successful

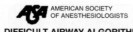

AMERICAN SOCIETY
OF ANESTHESIOLOGISTS

DIFFICULT AIRWAY ALGORITHM

1. Assess the likelihood and impact of basic management problems:
   A. Difficult ventilation
   B. Difficult intubation
   C. Difficulty with patient cooperation or consent
   D. Difficult tracheostomy

2. Actively pursue opportunities to deliver supplemental oxygen throughout the process of difficult airway management

3. Consider the relative merits and feasibility of basic management choices:

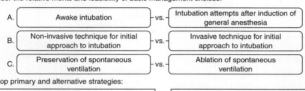

4. Develop primary and alternative strategies:

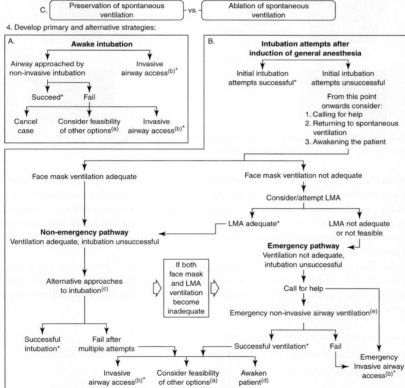

* **Confirm ventilation, tracheal intubation, or LMA placement with exhaled CO$_2$**

a. Other options include (but are not limited to): surgery utilizing face mask or LMA anesthesia, local anesthesia infiltration or regional nerve blockade. Pursuit of these options usually implies that mask ventilation will not be problematic. Therefore, these options may be of limited value if this step in the algorithm has been reached via the emergency pathway.

b. Invasive airway access includes surgical or percutaneous tracheostomy or cricothyrotomy.

c. Alternative non-invasive approaches to difficult intubation include (but are not limited to): use of different laryngoscope blades, LMA as an intubation conduit (with or without fiberoptic guidance), fiberoptic intubation, intubating stylet or tube changer, light wand, retrograde intubation, and blind oral or nasal intubation.

d. Consider re-preparation of the patient for awake intubation or canceling surgery.

e. Options for emergency non-invasive airway ventilation include (but are not limited to): rigid bronchoscope, esophageal-tracheal combitube ventilation, or transtracheal jet ventilation.

Figure 35-1. The American Society of Anesthesiologists' (ASA's) difficult airway algorithm. LMA, laryngeal mask airway.

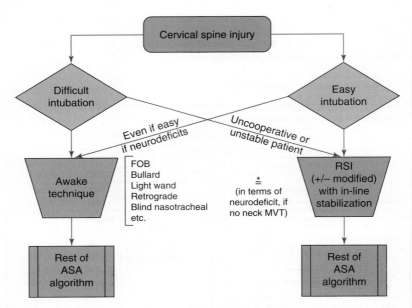

Figure 35-2. The American Society of Anesthesiologists' cervical spine injury algorithm. FOB, fiberoptic bronchoscope; MVT, movement; RSI, rapid-sequence intubation.

extubation in the neurocritically ill,[78,79] probably because the patients often do not have respiratory failure—most are better characterized as having airway failure. Clinicians anticipating extubation are repeatedly faced with the difficult task of predicting the ability of an intubated patient to protect his or her airway. Moreover, it is rare for these patients to rapidly normalize their airway protective reflexes—most will recover to some degree but remain at high risk for aspiration for a variable period of time following extubation.

There are a few reasonable approaches to this problem. The first, supported by a large, single-center observational trial in which patients that were extubated despite low GCS scores had significantly lower mortality rate,[2] is to attempt extubation once the patient meets traditional weaning criteria. These patients should be:

a. In the recovery phase of the acute illness

b. In an environment where good-quality nursing and respiratory care is performed

c. Without copious secretions

d. Able to mount a vigorous cough

The second is to perform early tracheostomy and percutaneous feeding tube placement. This approach removes the uncertainty of determining when the airway is safe and offers the advantages of allowing for minimization of sedation,[80] early disconnection from the ventilator, increased ability to perform physical and occupational therapy, and protection against large-volume aspiration. Early tracheostomy delivers multiple advantages for severely injured patients, but those who have a faster recovery than anticipated may undergo unnecessary procedures, accruing the risks of those procedures without any benefit. A third, commonly practiced approach is to perform tracheostomy only after a failed trial of extubation. In the absence of compelling evidence of superiority of one of these approaches, most clinicians practice a combination of them, based on patient- and institution-specific factors.

Postextubation laryngeal edema is a feared cause of reintubation, and a cuff-leak test prior to extubation may predict laryngeal edema and postextubation stridor.[81-86] Although overly aggressive administration of the cuff-leak test may lead to unnecessary delays in extubation, a meta-analysis of 14 randomized trials suggested lower rates of reintubation when corticosteroids were administered prior to extubation.[87] As such, it is reasonable to use the prophylactic administration of corticosteroids 12 hours prior to extubation in patients who fail a cuff-leak test or are suspected for other reasons of having laryngeal edema. While the presence of cuff leak (on patients who previously had cuff leak) may be a reassuring sign, absence of cuff leak is not an absolute contraindication for extubation.

What is the risk of aspiration following extubation?

Aspiration associated with brain injury is predicted by a "wet" voice after swallowing liquids, incomplete oral-labial closure, and a high National Institute of Health Stroke Scale score.[14] Up to 70% of stroke patients aspirate as evidenced by videofluoroscopic swallowing studies,[88,89] more than half of whom aspirate silently (subglottic penetration of a bolus without elicitation of a cough reflex).[90] This leads to a sevenfold risk of aspiration pneumonia in stroke patients who aspirate compared to those who do not, and a sixfold greater risk in those with silent aspiration compared to those who cough with aspiration.[90] Aspiration pneumonia due to dysphagia is a leading cause of death in patients with neurologic disorders.[91] It is therefore imperative to assess a patient's ability to swallow following extubation prior to any oral intake, and to tailor the patient's diet and feeding accordingly.

Conclusions

Airway management in patients with acute brain injury offers unique challenges, and a cautious, thoughtful clinical approach is necessary to minimize harm. Clinicians who approach the neurocritical care airway with respect, consistency, and meticulous preparedness will minimize secondary brain injury and provide their patients with the greatest chance of a good neurologic recovery.

! CRITICAL CONSIDERATIONS

- Neurologically unstable patients facing transfers, imaging, and procedures often require intubation, although airway protection and mechanical ventilation come at the cost of sedation and losing an accurate neurologic examination.
- Airway management in the neurocritically ill should focus first and foremost on avoiding excessively low or high blood pressure, arterial carbon dioxide levels, and arterial oxygen tension. Such abnormalities of homeostasis have profound effects in the injured brain and are an important cause of secondary injury.
- Direct laryngoscopy is a noxious stimulus that may increase intracranial pressure. Medications, especially sedation and analgesia, may be used to blunt the ICP rise. The bed should be placed flat for as brief a period as possible around intubation.
- Neurologic patients may be at greater risk of succinylcholine-induced hyperkalemia, especially those with prolonged immobility or paralysis.

- Manual in-line axial stabilization must be performed during all stages (including bag-mask ventilation) of intubating a patient with an unstable cervical spine. The cervical collar should be removed during intubation with continuous axial stabilization in place, and cricoid pressure must not be applied.
- Many patients can be successfully extubated despite a low GCS score, provided the cough reflex is strong and secretions are minimal.
- Prophylactic steroids may reduce the risk of laryngeal edema after extubation in patients with a failed cuff-leak test.

REFERENCES

1. Roppolo LP, Walters K. Airway management in neurological emergencies. *Neurocrit Care.* 2004;1(4):405-414.
2. Coplin WM, Pierson DJ, Cooley KD, Newell DW, Rubenfeld GD. Implications of extubation delay in brain-injured patients meeting standard weaning criteria. *Am J Respir Crit Care Med.* 2000;161(5):1530-1536.
3. Manno EM, Rabinstein AA, Wijdicks EF, et al. A prospective trial of elective extubation in brain injured patients meeting extubation criteria for ventilatory support: a feasibility study. *Crit Care.* 2008;12(6):R138.
4. Bleach NR. The gag reflex and aspiration: a retrospective analysis of 120 patients assessed by videofluoroscopy. *Clin Otolaryngol.* 1993;18(4):303-307.
5. Moulton C, Pennycook A, Makower R. Relation between Glasgow coma scale and the gag reflex. *BMJ.* 1991;303(6812):1240-1241.
6. Davies AE, Kidd D, Stone SP, MacMahon J. Pharyngeal sensation and gag reflex in healthy subjects. *Lancet.* 1995;345(8948):487-488.
7. Chan B, Gaudry P, Grattan-Smith TM, McNeil R. The use of Glasgow Coma Scale in poisoning. *J Emerg Med.* 1993;11(5):579-582.
8. Dunham CM, Barraco RD, Clark DE, et al. Guidelines for emergency tracheal intubation immediately after traumatic injury. *J Trauma.* 2003;55(1):162-179.
9. Jones PA, Andrews PJ, Midgley S, et al. Measuring the burden of secondary insults in head-injured patients during intensive care. *J Neurosurg Anesthesiol.* 1994;6(1):4-14.
10. Bardt TF, Unterberg AW, Hartl R, Kiening KL, Schneider GH, Lanksch WR. Monitoring of brain tissue Po$_2$ in traumatic brain injury: effect of cerebral hypoxia on outcome. *Acta Neurochir.* 1998;71:153-156.
11. Narotam PK, Morrison JF, Nathoo N. Brain tissue oxygen monitoring in traumatic brain injury and major trauma: outcome analysis of a brain tissue oxygen-directed therapy. *J Neurosurg.* 2009;111(4):672-682.
12. Rosenthal G, Hemphill JC 3rd, Sorani M, et al. Brain tissue oxygen tension is more indicative of oxygen diffusion than oxygen delivery and metabolism in patients with traumatic brain injury. *Crit Care Med.* 2008;36(6):1917-1924.
13. Brain Trauma Foundation; American Association of Neurological Surgeons; Congress of Neurological Surgeons; Joint Section on Neurotrauma and Critical Care, AANS/CNS, Bratton SL, Chestnut RM, Ghajar J, et al. Guidelines for the management of severe traumatic brain injury. I. Blood pressure and oxygenation. *J Neurotrauma.* 2007;24(1):S7-S13.
14. Adams HP Jr, Adams RJ, Brott T, et al. Guidelines for the early management of patients with ischemic stroke: a scientific statement from the Stroke Council of the American Stroke Association. *Stroke.* 2003;34(4):1056-1083.
15. Coles JP, Fryer TD, Coleman MR, et al. Hyperventilation following head injury: effect on ischemic burden and cerebral oxidative metabolism. *Crit Care Med.* 2007;35(2):568-578.
16. Carrera E, Schmidt JM, Fernandez L, et al. Spontaneous hyperventilation and brain tissue hypoxia in patients with severe brain injury. *J Neurol Neurosurg Psychiatry.* 2010;81:793-797.
17. Reynolds SF, Heffner J. Airway management of the critically ill patient: rapid-sequence intubation. *Chest.* 2005;127(4):1397-1412.
18. Seder DB, Mayer SA. Critical care management of subarachnoid hemorrhage and ischemic stroke. *Clin Chest Med.* 2009;30(1):103-122, viii-ix.
19. Feng CK, Chan KH, Liu KN, Or CH, Lee TY. A comparison of lidocaine, fentanyl, and esmolol for attenuation of cardiovascular response to laryn-

goscopy and tracheal intubation. *Acta Anaesthesiol Sinica.* 1996;34(2):61-67.

20. Salhi B, Stettner E. In defense of the use of lidocaine in rapid sequence intubation. *Ann Emerg Med.* 2007;49(1):84-86.

21. Asfar SN, Abdulla WY. The effect of various administration routes of lidocaine on hemodynamics and ECG rhythm during endotracheal intubation. *Acta Anaesthesiol Belg.* 1990;41(1):17-24.

22. Vaillancourt C, Kapur AK. Opposition to the use of lidocaine in rapid sequence intubation. *Ann Emerg Med.* 2007;49(1):86-87.

23. Robinson N, Clancy M. In patients with head injury undergoing rapid sequence intubation, does pretreatment with intravenous lignocaine/lidocaine lead to an improved neurological outcome? A review of the literature. *Emerg Med J.* 2001;18(6):453-457.

24. Bedford RF, Persing JA, Pobereskin L, Butler A. Lidocaine or thiopental for rapid control of intracranial hypertension? *Anesth Analg.* 1980;59(6):435-437.

25. Donegan MF, Bedford RF. Intravenously administered lidocaine prevents intracranial hypertension during endotracheal suctioning. *Anesthesiology.* 1980;52(6):516-518.

26. Grover VK, Reddy GM, Kak VK, Singh S. Intracranial pressure changes with different doses of lignocaine under general anaesthesia. *Neurol India.* 1999;47(2):118-121.

27. Hine LK, Laird N, Hewitt P, Chalmers TC. Meta-analytic evidence against prophylactic use of lidocaine in acute myocardial infarction. *Arch Intern Med.* 1989;149(12):2694-2698.

28. Martin R, Carrier J, Pirlet M, Claprood Y, Tetrault JP. Rocuronium is the best non-depolarizing relaxant to prevent succinylcholine fasciculations and myalgia. *Can J Anaesth.* 1998;45(6):521-525.

29. Schreiber JU, Lysakowski C, Fuchs-Buder T, Tramer MR. Prevention of succinylcholine-induced fasciculation and myalgia: a meta-analysis of randomized trials. *Anesthesiology.* 2005;103(4):877-884.

30. Motamed C, Choquette R, Donati F. Rocuronium prevents succinylcholine-induced fasciculations. *Can J Anaesth.* 1997;44(12):1262-1268.

31. Clancy M, Halford S, Walls R, Murphy M. In patients with head injuries who undergo rapid sequence intubation using succinylcholine, does pretreatment with a competitive neuromuscular blocking agent improve outcome? A literature review. *Emerg Med J.* 2001;18(5):373-375.

32. Bergen JM, Smith DC. A review of etomidate for rapid sequence intubation in the emergency department. *J Emerg Med.* 1997;15(2):221-230.

33. Giese JL, Stanley TH. Etomidate: a new intravenous anesthetic induction agent. *Pharmacotherapy.* 1983;3(5):251-258.

34. Moss E, Powell D, Gibson RM, McDowall DG. Effect of etomidate on intracranial pressure and cerebral perfusion pressure. *Br J Anaesth.* 1979;51(4):347-352.

35. Cuthbertson BH, Sprung CL, Annane D, et al. The effects of etomidate on adrenal responsiveness and mortality in patients with septic shock. *Intensive Care Med.* 2009;35(11):1868-1876.

36. Jabre P, Combes X, Lapostolle F, et al. Etomidate versus ketamine for rapid sequence intubation in acutely ill patients: a multicentre randomised controlled trial. *Lancet.* 25 2009;374(9686):293-300.

37. Aitkenhead AR, Pepperman ML, Willatts SM, et al. Comparison of propofol and midazolam for sedation in critically ill patients. *Lancet.* 1989;2(8665):704-709.

38. Hug CC Jr, McLeskey CH, Nahrwold ML, et al. Hemodynamic effects of propofol: data from over 25,000 patients. *Anesth Analg.* 1993;77(4 Suppl):S21-S29.

39. Reich DL, Silvay G. Ketamine: an update on the first twenty-five years of clinical experience. *Can J Anaesth.* 1989;36(2):186-197.

40. Wyte SR, Shapiro HM, Turner P, Harris AB. Ketamine-induced intracranial hypertension. *Anesthesiology.* 1972;36(2):174-176.

41. Gardner AE, Dannemiller FJ, Dean D. Intracranial cerebrospinal fluid pressure in man during ketamine anesthesia. *Anesth Analg.* 1972;51(5):741-745.

42. Langsjo JW, Maksimow A, Salmi E, et al. S-ketamine anesthesia increases cerebral blood flow in excess of the metabolic needs in humans. *Anesthesiology.* 2005;103(2):258-268.

43. Schwedler M, Miletich DJ, Albrecht RF. Cerebral blood flow and metabolism following ketamine administration. *Can Anaesthetist Soc J.* 1982;29(3):222-226.

44. Takeshita H, Okuda Y, Sari A. The effects of ketamine on cerebral circulation and metabolism in man. *Anesthesiology.* 1972;36(1):69-75.

45. Werner C, Kochs E, Rau M, Blanc I, Am Esch JS. Dose-dependent blood flow velocity changes in the Basal cerebral arteries following low-dose ketamine. *J Neurosurg Anesthesiol.* 1990;2(2):86-91.

46. Albanese J, Arnaud S, Rey M, Thomachot L, Alliez B, Martin C. Ketamine decreases intracranial pressure and electroencephalographic activity in traumatic brain injury patients during propofol sedation. *Anesthesiology.* 1997;87(6):1328-1334.

47. Bourgoin A, Albanese J, Wereszczynski N, Charbit M, Vialet R, Martin C. Safety of sedation with

ketamine in severe head injury patients: comparison with sufentanil. *Crit Care Med.* 2003;31(3):711-717.

48. Sakai K, Cho S, Fukusaki M, Shibata O, Sumikawa K. The effects of propofol with and without ketamine on human cerebral blood flow velocity and CO$_2$ response. *Anesth Analg.* 2000;90(2): 377-382.

49. Strebel S, Kaufmann M, Maitre L, Schaefer HG. Effects of ketamine on cerebral blood flow velocity in humans. Influence of pretreatment with midazolam or esmolol. *Anaesthesia.* 1995;50(3):223-228.

50. Lanier WL, Milde JH, Michenfelder JD. Cerebral stimulation following succinylcholine in dogs. *Anesthesiology.* 1986;64(5):551-559.

51. Kovarik WD, Mayberg TS, Lam AM, Mathisen TL, Winn HR. Succinylcholine does not change intracranial pressure, cerebral blood flow velocity, or the electroencephalogram in patients with neurologic injury. *Anesth Analg.* 1994;78(3):469-473.

52. Mace SE. Challenges and advances in intubation: rapid sequence intubation. *Emerg Med Clin North Am.* 2008;26(4):1043-1068, x.

53. Khan TZ, Khan RM. Changes in serum potassium following succinylcholine in patients with infections. *Anesth Analg.* 1983;62(3):327-331.

54. Schaner PJ, Brown RL, Kirksey TD, Gunther RC, Ritchey CR, Gronert GA. Succinylcholine-induced hyperkalemia in burned patients. 1. *Anesth Analg.* 1969;48(5):764-770.

55. Dronen SC, Merigian KS, Hedges JR, Hoekstra JW, Borron SW. A comparison of blind nasotracheal and succinylcholine-assisted intubation in the poisoned patient. *Ann Emerg Med.* 1987;16(6):650-652.

56. Martyn JA, Richtsfeld M. Succinylcholine-induced hyperkalemia in acquired pathologic states: etiologic factors and molecular mechanisms. *Anesthesiology.* 2006;104(1):158-169.

57. Sellick BA. Cricoid pressure to control regurgitation of stomach contents during induction of anaesthesia. *Lancet.* 1961;2(7199):404-406.

58. Rice MJ, Mancuso AA, Gibbs C, Morey TE, Gravenstein N, Deitte LA. Cricoid pressure results in compression of the postcricoid hypopharynx: the esophageal position is irrelevant. *Anesth Analg.* 2009;109(5):1546-1552.

59. Ellis DY, Harris T, Zideman D. Cricoid pressure in emergency department rapid sequence tracheal intubations: a risk-benefit analysis. *Ann Emerg Med.* 2007;50(6):653-665.

60. Neilipovitz DT, Crosby ET. No evidence for decreased incidence of aspiration after rapid sequence induction. *Can J Anaesth.* 2007;54(9): 748-764.

61. Brimacombe JR, Berry AM. Cricoid pressure. *Can J Anaesth.* 1997;44(4):414-425.

62. Lerman J. On cricoid pressure: "may the force be with you." *Anesth Analg.* 2009;109(5):1363-1366.

63. Ovassapian A, Salem MR. Sellick's maneuver: to do or not do. *Anesth Analg.* 2009;109(5):1360-1362.

64. Kluger MT, Short TG. Aspiration during anaesthesia: a review of 133 cases from the Australian Anaesthetic Incident Monitoring Study (AIMS). *Anaesthesia.* 1999;54(1):19-26.

65. Nouruzi-Sedeh P, Schumann M, Groeben H. Laryngoscopy via Macintosh blade versus GlideScope: success rate and time for endotracheal intubation in untrained medical personnel. *Anesthesiology.* 2009;110(1):32-37.

66. Brimacombe J, Keller C, Kunzel KH, Gaber O, Boehler M, Puhringer F. Cervical spine motion during airway management: a cinefluoroscopic study of the posteriorly destabilized third cervical vertebrae in human cadavers. *Anesth Analg.* 2000;91(5):1274-1278.

67. Donaldson WF 3rd, Heil BV, Donaldson VP, Silvaggio VJ. The effect of airway maneuvers on the unstable C1-C2 segment. A cadaver study. *Spine.* 1997;22(11):1215-1218.

68. Hauswald M, Sklar DP, Tandberg D, Garcia JF. Cervical spine movement during airway management: cinefluoroscopic appraisal in human cadavers. *Am J Emerg Med.* 1991;9(6):535-538.

69. Gerling MC, Davis DP, Hamilton RS, et al. Effect of surgical cricothyrotomy on the unstable cervical spine in a cadaver model of intubation. *J Emerg Med.* 2001;20(1):1-5.

70. Majernick TG, Bieniek R, Houston JB, Hughes HG. Cervical spine movement during orotracheal intubation. *Ann Emerg Med.* 1986;15(4):417-420.

71. McGill J. Airway management in trauma: an update. *Emerg Med Clin North Am.* 2007;25(3): 603-622, vii.

72. Schriger DL, Larmon B, LeGassick T, Blinman T. Spinal immobilization on a flat backboard: does it result in neutral position of the cervical spine? *Ann Emerg Med.* 1991;20(8):878-881.

73. De Lorenzo RA, Olson JE, Boska M, et al. Optimal positioning for cervical immobilization. *Ann Emerg Med.* 1996;28(3):301-308.

74. Crosby ET. Airway management in adults after cervical spine trauma. *Anesthesiology.* 2006;104(6): 1293-1318.

75. Donaldson WF 3rd, Towers JD, Doctor A, Brand A, Donaldson VP. A methodology to evaluate motion of the unstable spine during intubation techniques. *Spine.* 1993;18(14):2020-2023.

76. Gabbott DA. The effect of single-handed cricoid pressure on neck movement after applying manual in-line stabilisation. *Anaesthesia.* 1997;52(6): 586-588.

77. Yentis SM. The effects of single-handed and bimanual cricoid pressure on the view at laryngoscopy. *Anaesthesia.* 1997;52(4):332-335.

78. Ko R, Ramos L, Chalela JA. Conventional weaning parameters do not predict extubation failure in neurocritical care patients. *Neurocrit Care.* 2009;10(3):269-273.

79. Navalesi P, Frigerio P, Moretti MP, et al. Rate of reintubation in mechanically ventilated neurosurgical and neurologic patients: evaluation of a systematic approach to weaning and extubation. *Crit Care Med.* 2008;36(11):2986-2992.

80. Nieszkowska A, Combes A, Luyt CE, et al. Impact of tracheotomy on sedative administration, sedation level, and comfort of mechanically ventilated intensive care unit patients. *Crit Care Med.* 2005;33(11):2527-2533.

81. Jaber S, Chanques G, Matecki S, et al. Post-extubation stridor in intensive care unit patients. Risk factors evaluation and importance of the cuff-leak test. *Intensive Care Med.* 2003;29(1):69-74.

82. Ochoa ME, Marin Mdel C, Frutos-Vivar F, et al. Cuff-leak test for the diagnosis of upper airway obstruction in adults: a systematic review and meta-analysis. *Intensive Care Med.* 2009;35(7):1171-1179.

83. Chung YH, Chao TY, Chiu CT, Lin MC. The cuff-leak test is a simple tool to verify severe laryngeal edema in patients undergoing long-term mechanical ventilation. *Crit Care Med.* 2006;34(2):409-414.

84. De Bast Y, De Backer D, Moraine JJ, Lemaire M, Vandenborght C, Vincent JL. The cuff leak test to predict failure of tracheal extubation for laryngeal edema. *Intensive Care Med.* 2002; 28(9):1267-1272.

85. Kriner EJ, Shafazand S, Colice GL. The endotracheal tube cuff-leak test as a predictor for postextubation stridor. *Respir Care.* 2005;50(12): 1632-1638.

86. Miller RL, Cole RP. Association between reduced cuff leak volume and postextubation stridor. *Chest.* 1996;110(4):1035-1040.

87. McCaffrey J, Farrell C, Whiting P, Dan A, Bagshaw SM, Delaney AP. Corticosteroids to prevent extubation failure: a systematic review and meta-analysis. *Intensive Care Med.* 2009;35(6): 977-986.

88. Horner J, Massey EW. Silent aspiration following stroke. *Neurology.* 1988;38(2):317-319.

89. Linden P, Siebens AA. Dysphagia: predicting laryngeal penetration. *Arch Phys Med Rehabil.* 1983;64(6):281-284.

90. Daniels SK, Brailey K, Priestly DH, Herrington LR, Weisberg LA, Foundas AL. Aspiration in patients with acute stroke. *Arch Phys Med Rehabil.* 1998;79(1):14-19.

91. Marik PE. Aspiration pneumonitis and aspiration pneumonia. *N Engl J Med.* 2001;344(9): 665-671.

Mechanical Ventilation

36

Brian M. Fuller, MD

A 45-year-old man with no significant past medical history presents to the intensive care unit (ICU) status post motor vehicle collision. Upon presentation to the emergency department (ED), he was endotracheally intubated for airway protection, with a Glasgow Coma Scale (GCS) score of 7 (eye 1, verbal 2, motor 4). Intubation was accomplished without any incidence of hypotension or hypoxia; however, the patient was actively vomiting at presentation and vomitus was noted at his vocal cords during direct laryngoscopy. His trauma workup included computed tomography (CT) scans of the head, cervical spine, chest, abdomen, and pelvis, as well as a chest radiograph. Bifrontal contusions and suspected diffuse axonal injury (DAI) were demonstrated on CT. No other injuries were discovered. He presents to your ICU early in the night with the following settings on the mechanical ventilator: assist-control/volume-targeted mode (AC/VC), tidal volume of 650 mL, positive end-expiratory pressure (PEEP) of 5 cm H_2O, respiratory rate of 14, and a fraction of inspired oxygen (FIO_2) of 0.50. On these settings, you note that his peak inspiratory pressure is 29 cm H_2O and his inspiratory plateau pressure is 25 cm H_2O. The patient's vital signs are as follows: heart rate 115 bpm, blood pressure 120/80 mm Hg, respiratory rate 14 breaths/min, oxygen saturation 92%, and temperature 37.5°C (99.5°F). Also, as you review the graphics package on the ventilator, you note smooth waveforms, with no evidence of intrinsic PEEP or dyssynchrony. As you receive the report from the emergency medicine physician, you note the concerns for aspiration and you review his chest radiograph and chest CT, which both suggest aspiration to the bilateral lower lobes. You are happy with his current status, but you wonder how his head injury and potential lung injury will progress. As you settle in for an interesting call night, you notice that his inspiratory plateau pressure is now 35 cm H_2O and his FIO_2 is 0.80.

General overview of mechanical ventilation

Regardless of the indication for endotracheal intubation and initiation of mechanical ventilation, a mechanical ventilator, in and of itself, does not *treat* much. However, it does have great potential for harm. Effective mechanical ventilation should prioritize limitation of ventilator-induced lung injury (VILI) almost as much as oxygenation and maintenance of normal carbon dioxide levels should take less priority in the majority of patients.[1] Keen knowledge of basic and advanced principles will allow the clinician to use the mechanical ventilator for its maximum therapeutic potential and minimize iatrogenic injury while the process that led to respiratory failure is allowed to heal. It cannot be stressed enough that knowledge of cardiopulmonary physiology, heart-lung interactions, and the effects of mechanical ventilator settings on cerebral oxygenation and blood flow will allow the clinician flexibility when titrating support to an *individual* patient at the bedside. While the clinician should be intimately familiar with guidelines and large clinical trials, they are only as good as the response a particular patient has to a chosen therapy.

Table 36-1. Indications for Mechanical Ventilation

Physiologic reason	Clinical assessment	Normal value	Abnormal value suggesting need for mechanical ventilation
Hypoxemia	A-a gradient PaO_2/FIO_2 ratio SaO_2	25-65 350-400 98%	> 350 < 300 < 90%
Hypercarbia/inadequate alveolar ventilation	$Paco_2$	35-45 mm Hg	Acute increase from patient's baseline, pH < 7.15, mental status decline
Oxygen delivery/oxygen consumption imbalance	Elevated lactate Decreased mixed venous oxygen saturation	2.2 mg/dL 70%	> 4 mg/dL despite adequate resuscitation < 70% despite adequate acute resuscitation
Increased work of breathing	Minute ventilation Dead space fraction	5-10 L/min 0.15-0.30	> 15-20 L/min –
Inspiratory muscle weakness	NIP VC	80-100 cm H_2O 60-75 mL/kg	< 20-30 < 15-20
Acute decompensated heart failure	Jugular venous distention Pulmonary edema Decreased EF		Clinical judgment combined with the above factors

Abbreviations: A-a gradient, alveolar-arterial gradient; EF, ejection fraction; NIP, negative inspiratory pressure; VC, vital capacity.

What are the usual indications for mechanical ventilation?

Mechanical ventilation is instituted for a number of reasons (Table 36-1).[2] Most commonly, these indications are a combination of a failure to adequately oxygenate, ventilate, or meet the metabolic demands of a physiologically stressed patient. Type I respiratory failure is hypoxemic respiratory failure, defined as a partial pressure of oxygen in arterial blood (PaO_2) of less than 60 mm Hg. Type II respiratory failure is hypercarbic respiratory failure, defined as a partial pressure of carbon dioxide in arterial blood ($Paco_2$) greater than 50 mm Hg.[3] Mechanical ventilation may also be instituted to maintain normal blood pH, to decrease work of breathing, to assist left ventricular function in the setting of acute decompensated heart failure, or for airway protection in the setting of toxic overdose, traumatic brain injury, or any other significant acute central nervous system illnesses.

What are the main phases of the breath generated by a mechanical ventilator?

The breath generated by a mechanical ventilator can be separated into *four phases*[2,4] (Table 36-2):

> **Triggering:** Triggering represents the change from expiration to inspiration and occurs either because of a drop in circuit pressure or flow (when patient triggered) or because of elapsed time. *Sensitivity* refers to a preset threshold of pressure or flow. When this is reached, a mechanical breath is delivered. This can be manipulated by the clinician, and is usually set at −1 to −2 cm H_2O. In the setting of pressure triggering, airway pressure is reduced (by patient effort) in the proximal circuit, the expiratory valve closes, and the patient receives a breath. In the setting of flow triggering, the patient's inspiratory effort induces a disruption of the constant

Table 36-2. Breath Characteristics of the Five Basic Mechanical Ventilation Breaths

	Trigger	Target/Limit	Cycle
Volume control (VC)	Time	Flow/volume	Volume
Volume assist (VA)	Patient effort	Flow/volume	Volume
Pressure control (PC)	Time	Pressure	Time
Pressure assist (PA)	Patient effort	Pressure	Time
Pressure support (PS)	Patient effort	Pressure	Flow

flow in the ventilator inspiratory circuit. This change in flow signals the expiratory valve to close and the ventilator to deliver the next breath.

Inspiration: Pressurized gas is channeled from the ventilator to the patient after the exhalation valve closes. This phase can be controlled (or targeted, see below) based on volume or pressure. For example, AC/VC is volume control/targeted and AC/PC is pressure control/targeted. Choice of control variable is largely the discretion of the clinician, as either can be manipulated to achieve set goals. It should be noted, though, that in volume-targeted ventilation, excessive airway pressures can arise secondary to worsening pulmonary mechanics. In this situation, the pressure alarm will cause a pressure limit to cycle to expiration. In pressure-targeted ventilation, minute ventilation is not guaranteed. It is a function of the compliance and resistance of the respiratory system. The clinician, therefore, should monitor these physiologic changes closely to avoid untoward changes in either airway pressure or $Paco_2$ levels.

The pattern of inspiratory flow can be *square, decelerating,* or *sinusoidal* (Figure 36-1). Square inspiratory flow pattern results in a rapid rise to a preset level (set by the clinician) followed by constant flow until cycling occurs. Decelerating flow results in a rapid rise to a maximum level followed by a gradual decrease until cycling. This is secondary to the decrease in pressure difference (Δ pressure) between the ventilator and patient as inspiration progresses during pressure-targeted ventilation. All pressure-targeted breaths are of the decelerating flow pattern. Sinusoidal flow pattern most closely represents normal physiologic breathing. It results in flow that gradually increases, then decreases during inspiration. The choice of inspiratory flow pattern should be based on patient characteristics, and a few common clinical scenarios should be familiar to the clinician. Square flow over time results in a shorter inspiratory time (I time) and, therefore, longer expiratory time (E time). For this reason it can be preferred in patients with obstructive physiology (chronic obstructive pulmonary disease [COPD] or asthma).[5,6] It may also be tolerated better in patients with demand for high minute ventilation, such as those with severe metabolic acidosis or elevated intracranial pressure (ICP). In this situation, there is potential for dyssynchrony to occur during the progression of the inspiratory phase if decelerating flow is chosen. The tradeoff is higher peak airway pressures with a square wave form. Decelerating flow results in a longer I time and a better distribution of flow. With pulmonary pathophysiology involving heterogenous distribution of injury (acute lung injury as the prototype example), decelerating flow is likely the best choice. The length of inspiration depends on several factors. In pressure-targeted modes of ventilation, the clinician directly controls the I time and I-to-E ratio. In volume-targeted ventilation, the I time is a function of set tidal volume (V_T) and flow rate (V_T/inspiratory flow rate).

Cycling: This is the transition from inspiration to expiration. It can occur because of a decrease in flow, elapsed time, or delivered volume. *Flow-cycled breaths* are pressure-support (PS) breaths. When a predetermined decrement in flow occurs, inspiration is terminated and the patient cycles to expiration. This is typically set at 25% of initial flow, but can be manipulated

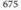

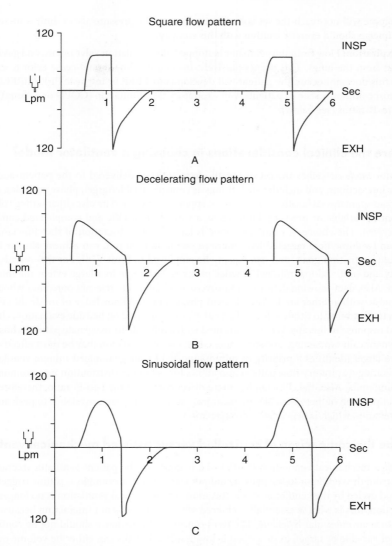

Figure 36-1. Inspiratory flow patterns. **A.** Square flow pattern. **B.** Decelerating flow pattern. **C.** Sinusoidal flow pattern.

based on different clinical conditions. For example, if a large leak occurs (bronchopleural fistula or ventilator circuit leak), it may be wise to set the cycle at a higher percentage of initial flow to terminate inspiration at the appropriate time. It should be noted that for safety reasons, PS can be cycled because of excessive pressures or elapsed time. In *time-cycled breaths*, inspiration is terminated after a preset interval, regardless of whether preset pressure has been achieved. Pressure-targeted ventilation is time cycled. In *volume-cycled breaths*, the clinician has selected the targeted tidal volume. Volume is delivered until that volume is reached. Airway pressure is directly dependent on the tidal volume and the mechanical characteristics of the patient's respiratory system. For safety reasons, volume-cycled breaths will be pressure cycled if airway pressures exceed the pressure alarm limit. In this situation, the delivered tidal volume will not reach the set volume target unless the pressure alarm limit is increased (the clinician should exercise caution with this strategy).

Expiration: Flow from the ventilator is stopped, the exhalation valve opens, and gas is allowed out from the lungs. This occurs passively. Inspiratory flow should cease prior to expiration. If this does not occur, the patient will develop auto-PEEP or intrinsic PEEP (iPEEP). This is most commonly seen in patients with expiratory flow limitation (COPD or asthma) or higher I-to-E ratios (see below).

What are the clinical considerations in choosing a ventilator mode?

A ventilator *mode* describes the set of breath characteristics delivered to the patient and patient-ventilator interactions, and includes such things as control variable/target, phase variables, and mandatory versus spontaneous breaths.[2,7] Two general approaches exist and involve either setting volume/flow as the control variable or pressure. From there, a variety of specific and complicated combinations can be derived. The choice of ventilator mode is largely at the discretion of the clinician. Pressure targeted and volume/flow targeted have more in common than not, can achieve similar frequency and minute ventilation goals, and can equally be employed to limit VILI. For this reason, clinician familiarity and unit and institutional practice patterns determine to a large extent the mode that is employed. Also, data showing definitive improvement in clinically relevant outcomes when comparing one mode with another are lacking. Patient physiology and knowledge of mode differences will allow greater flexibility to titrate safe mechanical ventilation based on bedside evaluation, clinical scenario, and response to therapy. When confronted with a difficult-to-oxygenate patient whose compliance is dynamically worsening, pressure-targeted modes of ventilation may be most effective. Setting a pressure target identifies a priority of minimizing VILI over guaranteed minute ventilation, and the decelerating inspiratory flow pattern also allows for better gas distribution into nonhomogenous injured lung units. Also, the clinician has more direct control of the I-to-E ratio, therefore allowing easier manipulation of these variables to maximize mean airway pressure relative to peak and plateau airway pressures, which is beneficial for oxygenation.

Describe the comparison of controlled versus assisted mechanical ventilation.

In *controlled* mechanical ventilation (CMV), the majority of the patient-ventilator interaction that occurs is from the ventilator to the patient, and not vice versa. For example, it is time triggered and is limited and cycled by the ventilator. While this mode of mechanical ventilation is no longer an available selection, this is what is essentially achieved when a patient is not interacting because of heavy sedation or neuromuscular blockade. The term *control* in this instance should not be confused with the control variable or target, as described below. *Assisted* breaths can either be volume or pressure targeted (AC/PC or AC/VC, for example). With these types of breaths, the clinician sets the target (tidal volume or pressure) and a respiratory rate. The patient can then trigger the ventilator and receive the set target each time, more frequently than the set rate on the ventilator. In this instance, the ventilator is doing work, specifically on the patient, and therefore *assisting* the breath after the patient triggers/initiates it. Assisted breaths also encompass intermittent mandatory ventilation, where the ventilator delivers a set number of breaths but the patient can also trigger spontaneous breaths, as well as pressure support ventilation, where the patient triggers all the breaths and the delivered volume is determined by the set pressure, patient effort, and mechanical characteristics of the respiratory system.

Controlled breaths versus spontaneously triggered breaths are undoubtedly different with respect to respiratory muscle function and viability, gas exchange properties, lung expansion, and hemodynamics.[8] A fully controlled breath must fully expand the lungs and chest wall without inspiratory muscle assistance. Spontaneous breathing also serves to maintain venous return by lowering pleural pressure and therefore right atrial pressure.[9] Diaphragmatic movement is more pronounced ventrally in the supine patient with spontaneous breathing. This favors atelectasis in dorsal lung units and a ventral distribution of ventilation, resulting in increased dead space ventrally and shunt dorsally.[10] In patients with vigorous respiratory muscle activity, a switch to fully controlled ventilation may be beneficial. In this setting, oxygen consumption (Vo_2) can decrease substantially, and by removing expiratory muscle contraction, end-expiratory lung volume can be preserved, which improves oxygenation.[8] The preservation of spontaneous breathing is of more benefit than harm in the great majority of patients. However, in the setting of very high demand, such as severe, early acute respiratory distress syndrome (ARDS), there may be a role for fully controlled breaths, but this should be titrated to the individual patient.[11-13]

Describe the basic airway pressures and respiratory system mechanics.

For a breath to occur, whether it be spontaneous or by positive pressure, a pressure gradient must exist from the airway opening to the alveoli.[2,4,7,14] The volumes delivered and pressures generated largely depend on the mechanical properties of the respiratory system: the lungs and chest wall, as well as the abdomen. Each of these components has mechanical properties that determine the overall behavior of the respiratory system. While the respiratory system can be quite complex, the main *variables* of interest are really only pressure, flow, and volume. Specifically, the ventilator must generate a *pressure* to cause *flow* and therefore increase lung *volume*.[14] The pressure required to do this reflects a combination of the pressures to inflate the lung and chest wall. This can be illustrated by the equation of motion[14,15]:

$$\text{Muscle pressure} + \text{ventilator pressure} = (\text{elastance} \times \text{volume}) + (\text{resistance} \times \text{flow})$$

The equation of motion illustrates several basic principles. A ventilator can only directly control one of the three variables at a time (pressure, volume, or flow). Despite its complexity, a ventilator is simply a machine controlling one of these three variables (*control* variables).[2,4,7] They are also referred to commonly as the "target" and are the variables that the ventilator holds constant despite changing respiratory system mechanics. For example, in pressure-control ventilation, pressure is the control variable or target and is held constant, while flow and tidal volume will vary based on the patient's respiratory mechanics. Control in this instance should not be confused with a controlled versus assisted breath, as above.

Compliance describes the ability or tendency of the respiratory system to expand in response to a delivered pressure and volume.[14,16] Simplistically, this is Δ volume/Δ pressure, and the compliance of the respiratory system (C_{RS}) is $\Delta V/\Delta P_{alveolar}$. Elastance is the inverse of compliance, or the ratio of pressure change to volume change, and describes the tendency to recoil. Resistance describes the impedance to airflow through the respiratory system, or the ratio of pressure change to flow change.

A pressure-volume (PV) curve (Figure 36-2) demonstrates key features of respiratory system mechanics.[17,18] The lower (LIP) and upper inflection points (UIP) reveal areas of reduced compliance secondary to low and high volumes, respectively (compliance is volume-dependent). As de-recruited alveoli are opened up, the lower inflection point transitions into the steeper (most compliant) portion of the PV curve. This is theoretically the physiologically most sound and safe portion to ventilate the patient, though where this lies in an individual patient can be difficult to elucidate. At higher tidal volumes, the upper inflection point represents a transition to overdistention, risk for barotrauma, and reduced compliance. This graphically represents a foundation for the concept of PEEP setting and VILI (discussed below).[19] The PV curve also demonstrates hysteresis: greater compliance during expiration versus inspiration. This reflects the fact that recruited alveoli are more compliant than recruiting or unrecruited alveoli and provides the foundation for the concept of recruitment maneuvers in

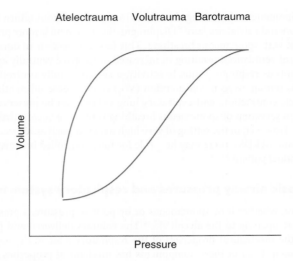

Figure 36-2. Pressure-volume curve.

PEEP setting, as well as advanced modes of mechanical ventilation, such as airway pressure release ventilation (APRV) and high-frequency oscillatory ventilation (HFOV). The normal lung and chest wall are remarkably compliant (200 mL/cm H_2O) and the normal compliance of the respiratory system is around 100 mL/cm H_2O (lung compliance and chest wall compliance added in series).[14] The severely injured lung may have compliance as low as 20 mL/cm H_2O or even lower. Unfortunately, C_{RS} that is displayed by the mechanical ventilator has to be interpreted with caution. This number represents a weighted average of many million alveolar units, and in pathophysiologic states exhibiting heterogenous injury distribution (acute lung injury), compliance, volume distribution, and potential for VILI vary greatly.[20,21] Resistance to airflow is determined by artificial and natural airways, as well as the rate and pattern of flow. Similar to compliance, resistance varies with volume, but also flow, and differs between inspiration and expiration.

The three most common airway pressures displayed for monitoring on a mechanical ventilator are peak airway pressure (P_{peak}), inspiratory plateau pressure (P_{PL}), and mean airway pressure (P_{mean})[15] (Figure 36-3). P_{peak} reflects C_{RS} as well as resistance. Elevated P_{peak} can lead to barotrauma,

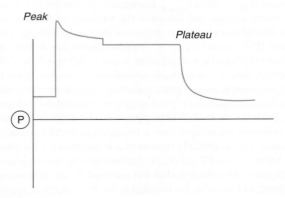

Figure 36-3. Peak and plateau pressures.

increased pulmonary vascular resistance, and right heart dysfunction, as well as decreased venous return.[22] Under no-flow conditions (inspiratory hold maneuver on the ventilator), resistance is eliminated, and this pressure reflects P_{PL}. The distending force of the lung is the transalveolar pressure, or alveolar pressure minus pleural pressure.[14,23] In the setting of elevated pleural pressure, such as elevated intra-abdominal pressure or reduced chest wall compliance, transalveolar pressure may be quite low; therefore, P_{PL} in the "safe" range may lead to significant underventilation.[23] Currently, without the ability to directly measure pleural pressure, the P_{PL} is the best reflection of transalveolar pressure and the distending pressure of an alveolus, and is an important reflection of potential for VILI. Of note, pleural pressure can be measured indirectly, via an esophageal balloon, and this pressure can be used in the calculation of transalveolar pressure.[24] P_{mean} is the average airway pressure over the respiratory cycle. Elevating the mean airway pressure should be viewed as a strategy to improve recruitment and oxygenation, with the goal being elevation to a greater extent relative to P_{peak} and P_{PL}.[25] If a patient has an elevated P_{peak} relative to P_{PL}, the problem lies in increased resistance, such as bronchoconstriction or endotracheal tube blockage or kink. If both P_{peak} and P_{PL} are elevated, then a compliance problem exists, such as worsening lung injury, pneumothorax, or elevated intra-abdominal pressures.

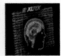 Because of a declining GCS score, your recently admitted patient has a repeat head CT scan, which reveals expansion of the hemorrhagic contusions in the bifrontal lobes, as well as worsening edema and intraventricular hemorrhage. The patient now has an external ventricular drain (EVD), ICP monitor, and brain tissue oxygen monitor placed. You have yet to manipulate his ventilator settings, and the high pressure alarm repeatedly is heard. A repeat chest radiograph now shows progression of his aspiration to diffuse, bilateral alveolar infiltrates consistent with ARDS. His airway pressures are now in the mid-40s and his oxygen saturation is 90% on an FIO_2 of 1.0. The arterial blood gas (ABG) shows the following: 7.27/50/58. Your fears are confirmed and you realize that your patient is now becoming one of the most challenging cases seen in the ICU: the difficult to oxygenate and ventilate patient with severe traumatic brain injury (TBI). You think quickly not only how to manipulate the ventilator to oxygenate and ventilate this patient but also how to do so *safely*, with a strategy to limit VILI and ICP while promoting brain oxygenation and cerebral blood flow.

What are the important mechanical ventilation strategies for this type of patient?

Knowledge of the general concepts of mechanical ventilation is of little use without knowledge of the patient at the bedside and defining the goals of therapy for that *individual* patient. With all critically ill patients, goals can be defined as oxygenation, limitation of VILI (perhaps just underneath oxygenation in order of importance), and ventilation. However, in the neurologically injured patient, we must add *limitation of secondary brain injury*.[26] This includes hypoxia, hypotension, prolonged periods of hypercapnia or hypocapnia, and elevated ICP. Manipulation of the mechanical ventilator can directly affect all of these.

Mechanical ventilation is common in the management of the neurologically injured patient.[27-29] Unfortunately, the direct generalization of many high-quality clinical trials is difficult in this patient population, as TBI is often an exclusion to trial enrollment.[30] To add to the complexity, protective ventilation strategies and the management of TBI have often been viewed as having competing and discordant therapeutic targets, such as permissive hypercapnia and PEEP setting to ameliorate VILI.[27] To this end, the ventilator must be adjusted to (1) improve brain oxygenation and (2) improve cerebral blood flow. At a very minimum, it must be adjusted to not *harm* cerebral oxygenation and blood flow. They are intimately linked, and inevitable overlap exists, but they will be discussed separately to provide a balanced approach with seemingly competing and potentially conflicting therapeutic strategies in the neurologically injured patient requiring evolving mechanical ventilation requirements.

Table 36-3. Mechanisms of Hypoxemia

Mechanism	Therapeutic strategy for reversal
Alveolar hypoventilation	Endotracheal intubation
Decreased FIO_2	Supplemental oxygen. Try to maintain $FIO_2 \leq 0.60$
Diffusion abnormality/increased DLCO	Reversal of pathologic process
V/Q mismatch	Alveolar recruitment, PEEP setting, reversal of hypoxic pulmonary vasoconstriction, inhaled nitric oxide, limit intrinsic PEEP
Shunt	Alveolar recruitment, PEEP setting, prone positioning, closure of patent foramen ovale
Decreased oxygenation of systemic venous blood (SvO_2)	Decrease oxygen consumption, hemodynamic support, increase cardiac output

Abbreviations: DLCO, diffusion capacity of the lung for carbon monoxide; FIO_2, fraction of inspired oxygen; PEEP, positive end-expiratory pressure; V/Q, ventilation/perfusion.

How can systemic and cerebral oxygenation be optimized?

Oxygenation should be the primary goal in any mechanically ventilated patient, especially the neurologically injured. Under normal conditions, alveolar ventilation is nearly equal to cardiac output, producing an overall ventilation-to-perfusion ($\dot{V}/\dot{Q}$) ratio close to unity.[31] While the exact causes of hypoxemia are innumerable, only a few physiologic mechanisms explain arterial hypoxemia (Table 36-3).[3] In the critically ill, mismatch between alveolar ventilation and perfusion and right-to-left shunt are by far the most common mechanisms. Diffusion is rarely the cause of hypoxia, unless severely impaired.

Oxygenation can be assessed several ways.[32] A noninvasive pulse oximeter allows assessment of arterial oxygen saturation (SaO_2). Arterial blood gas analysis gives us the PaO_2. Perhaps greater indicators for an oxygenation problem, calculation of the alveolar-arterial oxygenation (A-a) gradient, PaO_2-to-FIO_2 ratio, or oxygenation index (OI) gives the clinician greater insight into the extent of oxygenation failure.

Setting Oxygenation Goals

Normal SaO_2 and PaO_2 are greater than 95% and greater than 80 mm Hg, respectively. In the critically ill patient, these goals can sometimes be unattainable. Setting oxygenation goals in the critically ill can be largely empiric, but patient factors and available data should be considered. The majority of high-quality ARDS trials have allowed for an SaO_2 of 88% and a PaO_2 of 55 mm Hg.[30,33-36] It should be noted that at these levels, the patient is most certainly on the steep portion of the oxyhemoglobin dissociation curve and is in danger of a quick decline in arterial oxygenation with any decline in cardiopulmonary physiology, circuit disruption, or daily patient care activities. Hypoxemia not only will decrease cerebral oxygen delivery but also will result in cerebral vasodilation, therefore raising ICP. The Brain Trauma Foundation recommends keeping arterial oxygenation above a PaO_2 of 60 mm Hg. Other guidelines, including the UK transfer guidelines for brain injury, recommend even higher oxygenation targets (97.5 mm Hg).[37,38] Given the well-known association of hypoxemia with worse outcome[26,39-42] as well as the consideration of guideline recommendations, the neurologically injured patient should have these goals raised. Hypoxia should be avoided at all costs, and the ARDS Network (ARDSNet) targets are likely too low in this patient population. A target of a PaO_2 of 60%

and an Sao_2 of 92% at a minimum is likely reasonable, and these goals should be revisited based on individual patient physiology.

How can the mechanical ventilator be manipulated to improve oxygenation?

Fraction of Inspired Oxygen

Increasing the Fio_2 is perhaps the simplest and quickest way to improve arterial oxygenation and should be done immediately in the setting of life-threatening hypoxia. Unfortunately, simply increasing Fio_2 may be the least physiologic way to improve oxygenation from a pulmonary mechanics standpoint, and prolonged administration of high levels of oxygen has consequences.

Lung tissue is exposed to the highest concentrations of oxygen in the body. In animal and human studies, high fractions of inspired oxygen can cause lung injury, ranging from mild subjective symptoms to diffuse alveolar damage histologically indistinguishable from ARDS.[43,44] Exposure to elevated Fio_2 can reduce lung volumes secondary to absorptive atelectasis, increase intrapulmonary right-to-left shunt, and directly injure pulmonary parenchyma. The onset and rate of development are likely directly related to level of oxygen administration as well as duration.

Hypoxia is known to cause secondary brain injury, and the delivery of Fio_2 1.0 has been shown to increase brain tissue oxygenation.[45] Typically, the partial pressure of brain oxygen tension ($Pbto_2$) measured by a brain tissue oxygen probe improves almost immediately when Fio_2 is increased.[45] The administration of high levels of oxygen should be cautioned against, however. Despite some studies demonstrating reduced lactate levels and reduced lactate-to-pyruvate ratios, other studies have not reproduced these findings, and no good clinical studies demonstrate benefit of normobaric hyperoxia.[46-49] In addition, systemic hyperoxia has not been shown to improve cerebral metabolic rate or functional outcome.[50] Given these negative findings, as well as the well-known toxicity of hyperoxia, administration of prolonged levels of increased Fio_2 should be discouraged in favor of better ventilator management to maximize recruitment, PEEP effects, and the compliant portion of the PV curve. When Fio_2 exceeds 0.60, the clinician should manipulate the ventilator settings to improve oxygenation.

Positive End-Expiratory Pressure

Positive end-expiratory pressure (PEEP) maintains airway pressure above atmospheric pressure throughout the respiratory cycle by pressurization of the ventilator circuit. A full review of the topic is beyond the scope of this chapter, as the published literature on PEEP is extensive. However, the clinician should be aware of the pathophysiology pertinent to PEEP setting, advantages and side effects, approaches to PEEP setting, and the use of PEEP in the neurologically injured patient.

In patients with hypoxia due to atelectasis, alveolar edema, and/or volume loss (which causes most type I respiratory failure), PEEP serves to restore functional residual capacity (FRC), reduce intrapulmonary shunt, shift ventilation to a more compliant portion of the PV curve, and prevent end-expiratory volume loss (derecruitment).[51] PEEP recruits previously nonaerated lung tissue and homogenizes regional distribution of tidal ventilation. The net effect on gas exchange reflects the balance between recruitment and overdistention. In the setting of obstructive physiology or expiratory flow limitation, PEEP serves less to improve oxygenation and more to improve patient-ventilator synchrony and triggering (discussed below).[5,6,52]

PEEP is not without side effects. Given the heterogenous distribution of lung injury in acute lung injury (ALI)/ARDS, PEEP can overdistend more compliant lung units, contributing to VILI.[53] If PEEP leads to overdistention, it can augment dead space, increase pulmonary vascular resistance, and cause right heart dysfunction. It can also decrease venous return and, in the setting of volume depletion, decrease cardiac output.

The optimal way to set PEEP is widely debated and controversial, as is the optimal level of PEEP to use.[34-36,54-58] The literature reveals that PEEP has been set to maximal compliance, a level just exceeding the lower inflection point on a PV curve, the lowest PEEP to achieve adequate oxygenation, or a PEEP-F_{IO_2} combination table.[34,56,59,60] There is no widely accepted method to enhance clinical outcome. Before implementing any PEEP-setting strategy, an assessment of the risks and benefits and, most important, the potential to recruit alveolar units should be ascertained. Patients with primary pulmonary disorders, such as pneumonia or pulmonary contusions, usually have lung units with much less recruitability compared to patients with an extrapulmonary etiology of hypoxia, such as sepsis.[61] Villar et al set PEEP at 2 cm H_2O above the lower inflection point and demonstrated a mortality decrease from 53.3% to 32%.[56] Using higher PEEP, Ranieri demonstrated attenuation in cytokine response, suggesting decreased inflammatory signaling with higher PEEP.[58] These studies were done with simultaneous decreases in tidal volumes, however. The ALVEOLI trial was done to determine the isolated benefit of higher levels of PEEP in patients with ARDS. Despite improvement in oxygenation, the higher PEEP group showed no improvement in clinically relevant outcomes.[34] In two recently published trials, high PEEP was set based on a "lung open ventilation" protocol along with recruitment maneuvers and adjusted as high as possible to not exceed a P_{PL} of 28 to 30 cm H_2O. Both of these trials demonstrated improved oxygenation, but no mortality benefit.[35,36] Another physiologically attractive alternative is PEEP setting under the guidance of an esophageal balloon. The balloon is placed similarly to a nasogastric tube and is used to estimate pleural pressure in order to calculate transpulmonary pressure. Recent data show an improvement in oxygenation and compliance, but again no improvement in clinically relevant outcomes.[24] Data have shown wide variability with respect to lung recruitment and PEEP effect on lung recruitment. As such, individualizing PEEP setting is likely the most prudent approach.

PEEP can be set with or without recruitment maneuvers, with the aim being to open collapsed alveoli that may need higher, sustained inflation pressures to open. Clinical characteristics, such as etiology of ALI, can help assess potential for recruitment, but likely the easiest way to assess potential for alveolar recruitment is with a recruitment maneuver. After recruitment, alveoli are more compliant and easier to keep open. Recruitment maneuvers have been applied as sustained inflation pressures (30-40 seconds at 35-50 cm H_2O), as pressure-controlled breaths at increased PEEP levels, or as intermittent sighs.[35,55,59,62-65] They are generally very effective at improving oxygenation; however, they should be followed by an incremental increase in PEEP, or the effects will only be transient. In general, recruitment maneuvers are safe and tolerated well, but should likely be limited to patients early in the course of lung injury (more recruitability) with bilateral lung disease and no evidence of hypovolemia.

PEEP can adversely affect ICP and cerebral perfusion pressure (CPP), and PEEP setting in patients with neurologic injury has been a controversial topic.[26,27] By increasing intrathoracic pressure, and therefore juxtacardiac pressure, right atrial pressure can increase. This can impede venous outflow from the brain and lead to elevated ICP. Also, if PEEP decreases cardiac output, this can lead to hypotension and reduced cerebral blood flow. These effects are usually less significant in patients with reduced lung compliance. Also, if PEEP leads to overdistention, as opposed to alveolar recruitment, an increase in dead space can lead to elevated $Paco_2$ levels. Elevated ICP and reduced CPP have historically been viewed as (relative) contraindications to the use of increasing levels of PEEP. This has led to the observation of a lower threshold to simply increase the F_{IO_2} to combat hypoxia in this patient population. Fortunately, the literature demonstrates that PEEP is well tolerated in patients with TBI.[26,27,66,67] Early studies show that PEEP causes only modest, clinically insignificant changes in ICP.[68-71] In fact, PEEP set lower than ICP typically does not result in an increase in ICP, and if PEEP achieves alveolar recruitment, it can reduce ICP. Even in the setting of normal lung compliance (and therefore greater transmission of pressure to the intravascular space), PEEP has been shown to not significantly increase ICP. Furthermore, if PEEP results in alveolar recruitment, brain oxygenation may improve as a result.[72] Therefore, traumatic brain injury and elevated ICP should not be considered contraindications to PEEP setting in patients who need alveolar

Assess potential for recruitment (etiology of lung injury, CT morphology, response to recruitment maneuver)

Assess risk for potential adverse events (volume status, LV function, ICP and CPP and ability to control it)

If recruitable with acceptable risk-factor profile: PEEP set with or without a recruitment maneuver, and set PEEP based on either best compliance or guided by an esophageal balloon, as this approach makes the most physiologic sense

Keep P_{PL} at least < 30 cm H_2O or transpulmonary pressure < 25 H_2O

All changes in PEEP should be followed by a reassessment of overall hemodynamic status, right atrial pressure, pulmonary pressures, cardiac output (if monitored), ICP, and CPP

Figure 36-4. PEEP setting. CPP, cerebral perfusion pressure; CT, computed tomography; ICP, intracranial pressure; LV, left ventricular; PEEP, positive end-expiratory pressure; P_{PL}, inspiratory plateau pressure.

recruitment. The data and physiology dictate that the benefits likely outweigh the risks in the majority of patients.

In summary, PEEP serves to improve alveolar recruitment, decrease shunt, and improve oxygenation, as well as improve triggering in the setting of expiratory flow limitation. It has predictable physiologic effects, but the net hemodynamic effect of PEEP is some combination of volume status, ventricular function, and alveolar recruitment versus overdistention. There are several approaches to PEEP setting, but there is no convincing evidence that one method is superior to another. In the setting of TBI and/or elevated ICP, most data show that PEEP is well tolerated, and therefore should be attempted when necessary. PEEP setting and improving respiratory system mechanics should be favored over increasing FIO_2, as this approach has a higher risk versus benefit profile and is less physiologically sound management. When confronted with a neurologically injured patient with either hypoxemia or unacceptable levels of inspired oxygen, the approach given in Figure 36-4 can be used.

Partial Pressure of Brain Tissue Oxygen Tension

Cerebral monitoring has historically focused on ICP and CPP. However, with the knowledge that cerebral ischemia is associated with worse clinical outcomes, $Pbto_2$ monitoring allows the clinician continuous monitoring of cerebral oxygenation.[73] Despite an ongoing clinical debate regarding $Pbto_2$ monitoring, data suggest worse outcomes associated with low $Pbto_2$ levels.[74] Systemic oxygenation, pulmonary function, and cerebral oxygenation are strongly linked, given the basic physiology of oxygen transport from the lungs to the brain.[75] ALI is also an independent risk factor for cerebral hypoxia in the setting of TBI.[76] Given these facts, the care of patients with severe TBI should consider brain-lung interactions and that maneuvers that safely increase systemic oxygenation will likely increase $Pbto_2$ as well.

If monitored, $Pbto_2$ values of less than 15 mm Hg should be a concern. The first step in addressing persistently low $Pbto_2$ values should be the assessment of the invasive monitoring probe, as it may reside in dead tissue. Similarly, catheter fidelity must be maintained and assessed. While the absolute cutoff point of acceptable $Pbto_2$ is debatable, persistently low values have again been shown to be associated with worse outcomes.[74] Different threshold values likely exist for different patients and conditions, and other clinical questions remain (such as what defines "acceptable" brain oxygenation). Mechanical ventilator strategies to increase $Pbto_2$ parallel strategies to increase Pao_2: manipulation of FIO_2, PEEP setting, manipulation of the I-to-E ratio to increase mean airway pressure, advanced mechanical ventilation modes, and rescue therapies such as inhaled nitric oxide.

 Upon insertion and calibration of the EVD, ICP monitor, and brain tissue oxygen monitor, the patient's ICP is 35 mm Hg, CPP 55 mm Hg, and $PbtO_2$ 13 mm Hg. You institute standard medical therapy for elevated ICP with good results. To address the hypoxia and elevated airway pressures, you PEEP set (without using a recruitment maneuver). Also, citing the data from large ARDSNet trials that showed that low tidal volume ventilation was associated with $PaCO_2$ levels in the 40s, you figured you could decrease his tidal volume safely. You set tidal volume to 6 mL/kg based on ideal body weight (IBW). After some time, his ICP is 20 mm Hg, CPP is 60 mm Hg, $PbtO_2$ is 19 mm Hg, and ABG is 7.29/48/80. Despite raising his PEEP to 15 cm H_2O, his P_{PL} is actually better now at 30 cm H_2O (you must have improved compliance by recruiting collapsed alveoli) and his FIO_2 is 0.60. Just as you begin to feel comfortable, you wonder if his lung injury will continue to worsen. As you walk through the unit, you see his P_{PL} is now 42 H_2O and his mean arterial pressure is falling, and you notice a large v wave on his central venous pressure (CVP) tracing, which reads 19 mm Hg. His ICP is creeping close to 30 mm Hg, and his $PbtO_2$ is 13 mm Hg. You are concerned his lung injury and airway pressures are harming forward blood flow.

What is the relationship between mechanical ventilation and blood flow?

Skilled management of a mechanical ventilator can influence both venous return and forward blood flow. Unfortunately, when learning mechanical ventilation, most clinicians do not think in terms of blood flow. However, positive pressure ventilation causes predictable physiologic changes, and cardiopulmonary function is intimately linked.[9,77] Cerebral autoregulation maintains cerebral blood flow constant over a mean arterial pressure ranging from around 50 to 150 mm Hg under *normal* conditions.[78,79] In the setting of traumatic brain injury, this autoregulation may be impaired. Cerebral blood flow can be altered by a change in the *venous outflow* or *arterial inflow* as well as changes in mean arterial pressure (and therefore CPP), among other factors (such as blood viscosity, arteriolar resistance, and microcirculatory function). Ventilator management can affect all of these parameters and the effect of ventilator settings on cerebral blood flow is underappreciated. Cerebral blood flow must be maintained in the neurologically injured patient, and with the knowledge of the detrimental effects of hypotension in patients with TBI, every change in the mechanical ventilator must be made with the knowledge of how the change may affect forward flow.[39-41] A full review of heart-lung interactions is beyond the scope of this chapter, but the clinician must be aware of some key points.

Venous Blood Compartment

Venous return and right ventricular function

The venous system is a low-pressure reservoir that contains about three-fourths of our total blood volume.[9,80] There is a primacy of preload in determining myocardial performance, and the determinants of venous return have been documented for over 50 years.[81] The mean systemic pressure is the upstream pressure in the venous reservoirs governing venous return, and the right atrial pressure is the backpressure for venous return. The venous drainage of the brain is a system without valves and communicates directly with the right atrium.[78,79] Therefore, venous return and cardiac function are in direct communication with the intracranial compartment. Positive pressure ventilation, by increasing right atrial pressure, can decrease venous return and cardiac output.

The right ventricle's (RV's) main function is to accept venous return and eject the optimum amount of blood into a (usually) highly compliant pulmonary vascular system.[77,80,82,83] This maintains a low right atrial pressure, thereby maximizing venous return and overall myocardial performance.

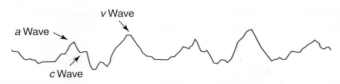

Figure 36-5. Large *v* wave on central venous pressure waveform tracing.

If airway pressure or lung volumes are elevated, pulmonary vascular resistance will increase, inducing RV dysfunction, the most severe manifestation of this being acute cor pulmonale (ACP).[84] ALI is a syndrome of the alveolar epithelium and capillary endothelium. As such, it is strongly associated with RV function.[85] RV dysfunction and/or ACP has been shown to be present in up to 35% of patients with ARDS and independently associated with increased mortality rate.[22,86,87] This incidence increases as P_{PL} increases. Given these findings, RV dysfunction should be suspected in *any* patient with ALI and ventilator settings should be adapted to unload the right ventricle, especially in the setting of elevated airway pressures.[88] Also, while not useful to predict preload responsiveness, the value of CVP and waveform morphology (large *v* wave, signifying tricuspid regurgitation) should both be followed closely, as should echocardiography[88] (Figure 36-5).

Similar to RV function, the left ventricle (LV) is affected by positive pressure ventilation. If mechanical ventilation induces decreased venous return, this will decrease LV preload several cardiac cycles later.[9,77] By decreasing LV transmural pressure, positive pressure ventilation decreases LV afterload and can therefore improve contractility. This is responsible for the positive effect of positive pressure ventilation in acute decompensated heart failure.

Putting it all together

Respiratory function alters cardiovascular function and cardiovascular function alters respiratory function.[9,77] In turn, they both can alter cerebral blood flow. The right and left ventricles are dependent in series (the left ventricle cannot pump what the right ventricle does not give it) and in parallel (they share a common septum and pericardial space). This is all affected by the mechanical ventilator. A positive pressure breath increases lung volume and increases intrathoracic pressure, which increases juxtacardiac pressure and therefore right atrial pressure. This can decrease venous return and therefore LV preload several cardiac cycles later. Improper use of excessive tidal volumes can elevate airway pressure, increase West lung zone I and zone II conditions, and therefore increase RV afterload.[85] PEEP, if it serves to recruit alveoli, can lower pulmonary vascular resistance and improve RV function. If it overdistends alveoli, it can increase dead space, increase pulmonary vascular resistance, and induce RV dysfunction.[85] These deleterious changes can impede venous outflow from the injured brain and further increase ICP.

To minimize the potential deleterious effects of mechanical ventilation on ICP and cerebral blood flow (CBF), secondary to venous return and RV dysfunction, the clinician should employ a low tidal volume ventilation strategy with tidal volumes set at 6 to 8 mL/kg IBW. This will limit the effect of excessive volumes on airway pressures and pulmonary vascular resistance. If this strategy results in permissive hypercapnia, it must be balanced with the effects of hypercapnia on ICP and RV function.[85] PEEP should be set as previously described. Suspect RV dysfunction in all patients with ALI and follow them with echocardiography. Follow the P_{PL} closely, and realize that a significant proportion of patients with an "acceptable" P_{PL} of less than 30 cm H_2O may still have RV dysfunction,[22] and continue to have high clinical suspicion of this. To avoid risk of RV dysfunction and/or ACP, if echocardiography is not routinely followed, P_{PL} should be kept at less than 27 cm H_2O. Realize that an elevated central venous pressure is only present in diseased states, as the primary function of the RV is to keep right atrial pressure low.[9,77] Follow CVP closely when RV dysfunction is suspected. If the patient has RV dysfunction, measures should be taken immediately for treatment, which will likely include some combination of inotropes/inodilators, pressors to maintain mean arterial pressure and CPP, inhaled afterload reducers, and judicious volume management.

Arterial Blood Compartment

The arterial blood flow responsible for cerebral blood volume, and therefore a component of ICP, is also governed by several factors, including blood pressure, viscosity, cerebral metabolic rate, and carbon dioxide and oxygen levels.[79] Skilled management of a mechanical ventilator can limit the potential for a decrease in mean arterial pressure and CPP, as discussed above. The majority of the following discussion will focus on CO_2 and O_2, however.

Carbon dioxide and cerebral blood flow

The $Paco_2$ represents a balance between CO_2 production ($\dot{V}co_2$) and CO_2 elimination ($Paco_2 = \dot{V}co_2/\dot{V}_E - V_D$, where $\dot{V}_E$ is minute ventilation and V_D is dead space.[89] In the setting of critical illness, elevated $Paco_2$ is usually secondary to decreased minute ventilation or increased dead space. While ALI is often viewed as an oxygenation problem, it is dead space that has been shown to directly correlate with mortality in this situation.[31,90] Permissive hypercapnia refers to a deliberate tolerance of elevated $Paco_2$ levels to limit lung stretch and VILI and is commonly used in a variety of patient populations, such as acute severe asthma and ARDS.[91] Increased $Paco_2$ has a variety of physiologic effects and data show that it is well tolerated, even at sometimes extreme levels.[89,91]

Cerebral blood flow is linearly related to $Paco_2$. For every mm Hg change in Pco_2, a 3% change in CBF can occur.[79] In the setting of TBI, cerebral blood flow is altered, and this is not a static phenomenon. Hypocapnia rapidly induces an increase in cerebrovascular resistance and a decrease in CBF (and a subsequent decrease in ICP). If hypocapnia is prolonged, vascular constriction can contribute to cerebral ischemia, promoting secondary brain injury.[92] For these reasons, prolonged hypocapnia cannot be recommended, and therefore hyperventilation is recommended only for life-threatening intracranial hypertension while other therapies are instituted.

Hypercapnia has the exact opposite effect. For patients with increased ICP, hypercapnia may be the cornerstone of the discordant and sometimes competing goals of safe mechanical ventilation, aimed at limiting tidal volumes and airway pressures.[26,27] These concerns are real, as increasing $Paco_2$ can certainly increase ICP. Examination of the high-quality protective ventilation clinical trials in ARDS reveals the $Paco_2$ levels from day 0 to day 7 to be in the normal to high 40s mm Hg range.[30] Also, high tidal volume ventilation in the setting of TBI has been shown to be associated with the development of ARDS, which not only has been shown to be associated with brain hypoxia but also increases morbidity and mortality rates in this patient population.[76,93] Given these findings, it is likely that the majority of patients with ALI and elevated ICP can safely be managed with a low tidal volume strategy. The balance between permissive hypercapnia and ICP will likely be a fine line and should be managed on a case-by-case basis. Knowing the physiology governing $Paco_2$ levels, $\dot{V}co_2$ can be decreased with proper sedation, fever and seizure control, and appropriate nutrition goals. Dead space in the ventilator circuit can easily be removed and is a simple solution, albeit with varying results. While alveolar recruitment and PEEP are often viewed as a strategy to ameliorate shunt and hypoxia, effective recruitment also decreases dead space, allowing more effective ventilation and less minute ventilation requirements. In the setting of ALI, manageable ICP, and adequate CPP, a $Paco_2$ high threshold of 55 mm Hg is a reasonable target, as this level will likely facilitate protective lung ventilation and can be acutely corrected should elevated ICP become an issue. In the setting of difficult-to-control ICP, normocapnia or slight hypocapnia should be maintained. If this is accomplished with a nonprotective lung ventilation strategy, the patient should be managed with the lowest tidal volumes and airway pressures as possible, and every attempt should be made for the safest ventilatory strategy as soon as possible. All patients with an ICP monitor and dynamically changing respiratory system mechanics and/

or ventilator settings should also be managed with an end-tidal CO_2 detector as well. Similarly, a direct, invasive CBF monitoring probe is available and can give readily available data on the effects of changing $Paco_2$ on CBF.

The echocardiogram shows clear evidence of RV dysfunction, which you attribute to his markedly elevated airway pressures. Given this, and his need for hemodynamic support, you choose to support his RV with afterload reduction with inhaled nitric oxide at 8 parts per million and inotropy with dobutamine at 5 µg/kg per minute, and to maintain pressure, norepinephrine at 8 µg/min. As day breaks and rounds are set to begin, your patient's ventilator settings are AC/PC, respiratory rate 20, I-to-E ratio 1:1, FIO_2 0.60, PEEP 10 cm H_2O, and drive pressure +25. His tidal volumes are around 6 mL/kg based on IBW. His central venous pressure is now 8 mm Hg, his prominent v wave is gone, and repeat echocardiograph after your interventions shows improved function of the right ventricle. Because of his 1:1 I-to-E ratio (which you did to help increase mean airway pressure to help with oxygenation), you look at his flow/time waveform and are pleased to see no evidence of breath stacking/auto-PEEP, and his end-tidal CO_2 monitor has continually revealed normocapnia. On these settings, his ABG is 7.30/45/90 and his ICP is 19 mm Hg, CPP 62 mm Hg, and $PbtO_2$ 18 mm Hg. You are pleased, given the patient's overnight course, but wonder about the effects his high tidal volumes and airway pressures had on organ dysfunction and brain-oriented outcomes.

What are the implications of ventilator-induced lung injury?

The majority of patients with ALI do not die of hypoxia, but rather multiple organ dysfunction syndrome (MODS).[94-97] While mechanical ventilation can be a life saving intervention, it has great potential for harm, and the clinician's focus should extend beyond normalization of gas exchange to providing safe and physiologically sound mechanical ventilation. Perhaps nowhere is this demonstrated more significantly than with the concept of VILI. Despite a uniform appearance on chest radiography, the distribution of ventilator defects and the distribution of injury is very heterogenous in ALI.[53,98] As such, applied airway pressures have a heterogenous distribution, leaving more compliant lung units overdistended and others collapsed and nonrecruited. CT scans have provided valuable insight into the pathoanatomy of ALI, showing alveolar units with normal gas tissue density (ventrally), alveolar units totally collapsed and potentially nonrecruitable (dorsally), and others in between, which likely remain recruitable and prone to repetitive opening and closing.[53,98] Respiratory system compliance is related to the amount of normally aerated lung tissue that remains, the so-called baby lung.[20] This heterogeneity leads to a maldistribution of ventilation, with some alveoli overdistended, others collapsed throughout the respiratory cycle, and others cyclically opening and closing. VILI is a spectrum, including barotrauma, atelectrauma, and volutrauma (stretch injury).[99] All of these can lead to biotrauma, or the decompartmentalization of the inflammatory response secondary to increased alveolar epithelial–capillary endothelial permeability. This results in the release of biologic inflammatory mediators and the spread of injury to distant organs, causing MODS and increased mortality. In an individual patient, it is likely some combination of these factors contributing to VILI.

Barotrauma represents extra-alveolar air from pneumothoraces, pneumomediastinum, subcutaneous emphysema, pneumoperitoneum, and pulmonary interstitial emphysema. While some controversy exists as to the exact pathophysiology of its development, it is likely a combination of excessive airway pressures and tidal volumes, coupled with at-risk patients, namely, those with expiratory flow limitation (asthma, COPD) and/or severe ALI. Atelectrauma refers to the repeated cyclic opening and closing of alveoli. Theoretically, this closure would occur at end expiration at low lung volumes, as the volumes drop below FRC and the LIP on a PV curve. Reopening occurs with each inspiratory cycle and this repetition is injurious to alveoli, causing shear injury. Overinflation of alveoli with high pressures and/or volumes (likely more significant) has been established to cause injury indistinguishable from ALI. Alveolar epithelial injury, capillary endothelial injury, and diffuse pulmonary edema can occur. Barotrauma, atelectrauma, and volutrauma likely all lead to some extent to biotrauma.

What is the evidence for excessive volume versus pressure?

So is it excessive pressure or volume, and what is the evidence?[100] Lung protective ventilation has been shown to improve outcome, but the exact mechanism of lung protective ventilation is not known.[30] Excessive stretch is known to cause lung injury, whether it is due to pressure or volume, and the addition of PEEP has been shown to ameliorate lung injury, likely by preventing atelectrauma.[101] By banding the chest and abdominal wall in rats (and therefore controlling pressure), Dreyfuss et al showed that it is perhaps higher tidal volumes that are most important, as the higher tidal volume group developed ALI regardless of airway pressures.[102] This evidence, coupled with clinical trials of low tidal volume ventilation, points to the importance of tidal volume as perhaps the greatest contributor to VILI. The effects of flow rate and respiratory rate on VILI has been described, but with less convincing evidence.[103-105] Numerous studies lend support to the concept of biotrauma, showing increased cytokines in bronchoalveolar lavage and serum in ALI. Data show increased levels of these markers with higher tidal volumes and airway pressures and without PEEP, and a decrease with the use of protective lung ventilation.[106-109]

Human studies support the concept of VILI and the importance of a protective ventilation strategy with low tidal volumes and the use of PEEP. Low tidal volume ventilation is the only intervention shown to consistently improve outcome in ALI, and support for protective lung ventilation to decrease VILI from several well-conducted clinical trials exists.[30,57,58] This includes data showing a decrease in inflammatory mediators in patients ventilated with a protective lung strategy. In the absence of a patient-specific factor to suggest otherwise, a protective ventilation strategy, consisting of low tidal volume ventilation, PEEP setting, and limitation of P_{PL}, should be attempted at all times. Emerging data suggest that these strategies should be employed not just in patients with ALI, but in all patients receiving mechanical ventilation, especially those with known risk factors for development of ALI.[110]

Can the brain be viewed as a target for VILI?

The brain and peripheral nervous system are affected by critical illness. Encephalopathy and critical illness polyneuropathy are well described in the literature. VILI leading to MODS is also well described; however, this organ dysfunction has historically focused on organs other than the brain, namely, the kidneys, lungs, and heart. This is despite the neurologic complications of mechanical ventilation existing in the literature for years and the extracranial complications of acute brain injury being well known.[29] Mounting data suggest that this focus should also include the brain, and clinicians should view the brain as an end organ in MODS.[111] Patients with brain injury have a known predisposition both to requiring mechanical ventilation and to progressing to ALI, and are therefore innately at risk for additional brain dysfunction secondary to mechanical ventilation and VILI. The brain as an end organ for VILI should be considered, and brain-lung interactions should be viewed as crucial. While it would be difficult to ascribe the effects of VILI as being more important than the sequelae of the neurologic injury itself, the effects of ventilator settings on brain function should be considered. Also, patients with acute neurologic injury frequently present with preexisting comorbidities. Given these facts, a paradigm shift should occur as no patient should be considered to have "isolated head injury."

Neurologic dysfunction in mechanically ventilated patients is a spectrum that includes delirium, dementia, cognitive decline, and loss of IQ, as well as mood and memory disorders.[112,113] These types of brain injuries can occur with alarming frequency and are likely underappreciated in the critical care population as a whole. Multiple studies show persistent cognitive deficits that exist years after liberation from mechanical ventilation. Similar findings exist with respect to quality of life, IQ loss, and mood and memory deficits.[114-118] Patients with ALI have brain atrophy and ventricular enlargement, suggesting neuronal cell damage of some etiology.[112]

The pathophysiology of this neurologic dysfunction is multifactorial. This includes the initial injury, hypoxia, hypotension, loss of central nervous system connectivity, persistent inflammation from nonprotective ventilation strategies, and metabolic abnormalities, such as hyper- and hypoglycemia.[111] Sedation regimen, specifically benzodiazepines, likely plays a factor as well.[113,119]

There is no specific treatment for VILI, but the clinician should focus on prevention, have a heightened awareness of the at-risk patient, and provide sound evidence-based and physiologic-centered care. Although specific recommendations on how to set the mechanical ventilator in brain-injured patients are lacking, care must taken to protect all organs with respect to VILI. Patients with ALI should have low tidal volume ventilation at 6 to 8 mL/kg of IBW. PEEP should be set as previously recommended, and P_{PL} should be limited to at least less than 30 cm H_2O. Given the heterogenous distribution of lung injury, there is likely no safe P_{PL}, and at any given value, there are likely some alveolar lung units that remain collapsed, while others are overdistended. P_{PL} should be kept as low as possible in patients with ALI. If monitored with an esophageal balloon, transalveolar pressure should be limited to at least less than 25 cm H_2O. Brain-injured patients may also benefit from continuous brain tissue oxygen monitoring, and optimization of brain oxygenation should be considered a potential aim for therapy. When appropriate and safe, all patients should be awakened daily, have daily spontaneous breathing trials, have target-based sedation to allow appropriate limitation of sedative infusions, have limited benzodiazepine exposure, and be monitored for delirium.[113] These interventions as a whole should result in decreased mortality, a decrease in all mechanisms of VILI, increased ventilator-free days, fewer ICU days, less sedation use, and less delirium.

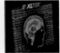 Your patient has stabilized for the moment, but as your attending enters the unit for rounds, the neighboring patient's high pressure alarm continues to sound. This patient has severe COPD and you remember that his previous pulmonary function tests (3 months prior to the rupture of his anterior communicating artery aneurysm) showed a severe obstructive ventilatory defect. You glance at the ventilator waveforms, shown in Figure 36-6. Your attending asks: "What are some of the considerations to approaching mechanical ventilation in patients with obstructive airway disease and expiratory flow limitation?"

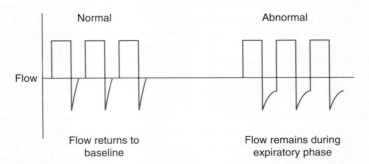

Figure 36-6. Intrinsic positive end-expiratory pressure (PEEP) in a patient with expiratory flow limitation.

Patients with obstructive lung disease and expiratory flow limitation (most commonly asthma and COPD) present unique challenges with respect to mechanical ventilation. Regardless of the specific disease that caused the pathology, the increase in airway resistance, loss of normal lung elastance, and airway narrowing lead to alveolar regions that have difficulty emptying and returning to resting end-expiratory lung volume, as well as increased inspiratory muscle workload.[5,6,52] Because of inadequate expiratory time, these patients are prone to air trapping and iPEEP, increased respiratory pump workload, and a variety of gas exchange abnormalities.

In the setting mentioned above, iPEEP can occur, as alveolar units with prolonged time constants are not allowed to empty to resting end-expiratory lung volume. This can have several cardiopulmonary consequences. By raising intrathoracic pressure and therefore right atrial pressure, venous return may be impaired. Of note, the effects of iPEEP and extrinsic PEEP (set on the ventilator) are similar from a hemodynamic, alveolar recruitment, and alveolar overdistention standpoint, as long as they produce similar changes in end-expiratory lung volume.[120,121] Because of compression of alveolar capillaries and increases in West zone I and zone II conditions, the high lung volumes may result in increased pulmonary vascular resistance and RV failure.[122] Overinflation also puts inspiratory muscles at a mechanical disadvantage, substantially increasing work of breathing and contributing to patient-ventilator dyssynchrony and inability to effectively trigger. In contrast to parenchymal pathology, the ventilation/perfusion mismatch is one largely of increased dead space, as opposed to shunt. This is secondary to capillary loss, as well as overinflation, which leads predominantly to hypoventilation and type II respiratory failure.[5,6,52] Hypoxemia may also occur due to ventilation and blood flow redistribution, but is not usually the etiology of the respiratory failure in the setting of expiratory flow limitation. If it does occur, it can contribute to increased pulmonary vascular resistance and RV failure as well.

These changes are in contrast to the patient with alveolar filling and consolidation, parenchymal pathology, and reduced compliance. The primary etiology of respiratory failure is type I, with hypoxia driven by shunt physiology. As outlined above, this patient population should benefit from alveolar recruitment with PEEP setting and judicious tidal volume management.

The goals of managing patients with expiratory flow limitation and obstructive physiology are largely the same as for patients with parenchymal lung injury and include oxygenation, protection against VILI, ventilation, preservation of respiratory muscle function, and prevention of secondary neurologic injury. Because of the physiology outlined above, the clinician should also add the following goal: allow for adequate expiratory time to limit the effects of iPEEP.

Unlike ALI, there are no large randomized controlled trials to guide the clinician in how to best employ mechanical ventilation in this setting. Instead, basic knowledge of mechanical ventilation and physiologic rationale help guide therapy and patient response. When mechanically ventilating this population, a reasonable approach to ventilator settings can have similarities to ALI. Tidal volume should be 6 to 8 mL/kg IBW and P_{PL} limited to at least less than 30 cm H_2O. Expiratory time should be long enough to limit iPEEP. The most effective way is to decrease respiratory rate. Expiratory time can also be extended by decreasing tidal volume and increasing flow rate (in volume-targeted ventilation), but the clinician should be aware that this is less effective and an increased flow rate results in increased airway pressure. Intrinsic PEEP should be monitored closely. This can be done by monitoring the flow/time waveform to assess for no flow before inspiration begins. If expiratory flow remains when inspiration begins, iPEEP is present. Also, an expiratory hold maneuver can stop flow in the ventilator circuit, allowing detection of iPEEP. The clinician should also make note of the purpose of extrinsic PEEP in this patient population. Unlike parenchymal lung injury, in which PEEP is delivered to maximize alveolar recruitment and eliminate shunt, PEEP in the setting of expiratory flow limitation is usually not needed for hypoxia/shunt. For a breath to occur, a pressure gradient must be overcome from the ventilator to the patient. This gradient is increased in the setting of iPEEP. The purpose of extrinsic PEEP is to therefore overcome this inspiratory threshold load imposed by iPEEP, assist in triggering, and ameliorate dyssynchrony. Intrinsic PEEP should be measured and the clinician should set extrinsic PEEP to some value less than this (perhaps as high as 80% of iPEEP).[120,121]

This will facilitate triggering while not adversely raising alveolar pressures. If set higher, extrinsic PEEP can raise alveolar pressure and produce overdistention. The net effect of tidal volume, respiratory rate, and iPEEP limitation can result in hypercapnia, which is generally very well tolerated in this patient population. However, despite a decrease in minute ventilation, if this strategy allows for decreased dead space, then ventilation may actually improve. In the neurologically injured patient, if ICP is a concern, permissive hypercapnia may not be tolerated. As in all instances, the balance will be a very fine one and the benefit of limiting iPEEP and tolerating higher $Paco_2$ levels must be weighed against secondary brain injury and elevated ICP. With these concerns, volume-targeted ventilation may be best in this patient population, given the strict control of minute ventilation it allows.

You dropped your COPD patient's respiratory rate and tidal volume and watched his airway pressure and iPEEP decrease nicely. Rounds begin with the patient who has the severe TBI that gave you trouble all night long. Before you get a word out, your attending sees how sick the patient is, notices your ventilator settings, and questions if you considered other, more complex modes of mechanical ventilation.

Describe other modes of mechanical ventilation.

The majority of patients, regardless of the etiology of their respiratory failure, can be managed with conventional modes of mechanical ventilation, such as volume- or pressure-targeted assist control. However, in certain clinical situations, other modes of mechanical ventilation can be used. The clinician should recognize that clinical outcome data for these modes of mechanical ventilation are not as robust. However, the physiologic rationale does make sense in certain clinical situations.

Airway Pressure Release Ventilation

Airway pressure release ventilation (APRV) has been described in the literature since 1987.[123] It is a time-triggered, pressure-targeted, time-cycled mode of mechanical ventilation that exactly resembles AC/PC with very extended I-to-E ratios if the patient is not spontaneously breathing.[10,25] It has been described as continuous positive airway pressure (CPAP) with an intermittent, time-cycled release phase to a set lower pressure. Whereas conventional modes of mechanical ventilation elevate airway pressure up from a set baseline to accomplish tidal ventilation, APRV employs very extended I-to-E ratios to maintain mean airway pressure and brief deflations to accomplish ventilation. The expiratory valve in APRV also facilitates spontaneous breathing throughout the ventilatory cycle, facilitating ventilation. Pressure high (P_{HIGH}) is the baseline airway pressure that occupies most of the ventilatory cycle. Pressure low (P_{LOW}) is the release pressure and is set at 0 cm H_2O. Time high (T_{HIGH}) is the length of time for which P_{HIGH} is maintained, and time low (T_{LOW}) is the length of time for which P_{LOW} is maintained.

While outcome data for APRV are lacking compared to conventional ventilation using protective lung strategies, the reported advantages of APRV include sustained alveolar recruitment with improved oxygenation, higher mean airway pressures accomplished with lower P_{peak} and P_{PL}, spontaneous breathing throughout the ventilatory cycle, and decreased use of sedation and neuromuscular blockade.[25] The maintenance of spontaneous breathing may improve $\dot{V}/\dot{Q}$ matching by preferential ventilation of dependent lung regions, and the higher mean airway pressure, relative to P_{peak} and P_{PL}, may limit VILI.

Alveolar recruitment is a pan-inspiratory phenomenon, and alveoli that are recruited are more compliant than recruiting or nonrecruited alveoli. With prolonged elevated pressures, APRV likely recruits alveoli that require a longer inflation with higher threshold opening pressures.[10,25] Sustained inflation maintains recruitment, decreases shunt and dead space, and uses the more compliant expiratory limb of the PV curve. Ventilation is determined by the stored kinetic energy at the high pressure, the intermittent release phase, and is augmented by spontaneous breathing. While minute ventilation is decreased with this mode of ventilation, ventilation is also improved by a decrease in dead space.

Clinical data are limited but have shown improved oxygenation, less shunt and dead space, and a decreased need for sedation and neuromuscular blockade.[25,124-127] Data on clinically relevant outcomes, such as mortality, mechanical ventilation days, and ICU days, are very limited and conflicting, with no high-quality trials specifically looking at the neurologically injured patient. This mode remains physiologically attractive for its effects on oxygenation and potential to limit VILI; however, no specific recommendations can be made given the lack of good outcome data.

High-Frequency Oscillatory Ventilation

Fundamentally, high-frequency oscillatory ventilation (HFOV) is very different from conventional bulk flow ventilation and uses respiratory frequencies much higher and tidal volumes much lower than conventional modes. It is similar to APRV in that it aims to elevate mean airway pressure to maximize recruitment and oxygenation while limiting P_{peak}.[128] Given the fact that tidal volume is often less than anatomic dead space, HFOV relies on gas transport mechanisms much different than those with bulk flow ventilation. These include some convective gas transport, but also molecular diffusion, pendelluft, coaxial flow, and Taylor dispersion.[129]

When initiating HFOV, the mean airway pressure should be set 2 to 5 cm H_2O higher than that on conventional ventilation. Prior to this, the patient's endotracheal tube should be verified to be patent, as heavy secretions or kinks in the endotracheal tube will significantly harm ventilation. The bias flow delivers fresh gas into the ventilator circuit at 40 to 60 L/min and helps maintain mean airway pressure.[129] HFOV relies on a piston-type mechanism to apply pressure, and this amplitude (Δ pressure), as well as frequency (hertz), helps determine ventilation. The Δ pressure is set to observe vibration down to the patient's thighs, and initial frequency is set at 5 hertz.

Similar to APRV, clinical outcome data on HFOV are limited. It is also physiologically attractive with respect to limitation of VILI and improvement in oxygenation, and promising data do exist with respect to oxygenation and perhaps improved outcome with the application of HFOV. This effect seems most beneficial when applied early in the course of ALI.[128,130,131] Limited data suggest that HFOV is safe in patients with elevated ICP and is well tolerated in this subgroup of patients.[28,132,133] In patients with mean airway pressures greater than 24 cm H_2O in whom protective lung ventilation strategies are failing with respect to oxygen requirements and airway pressures, HFOV should be considered. The clinician should note that these patients will require heavy sedation and/or neuromuscular blockade.

Pressure-Regulated Volume Control

Pressure-regulated volume control (PRVC) is a dual-control mode of ventilation that is very similar to AC/PC. It is a pressure-targeted breath, time cycled, with square pressure waveform and decelerating variable flow. Tidal volume is set on the ventilator, and a "test breath" is delivered. The ventilator then calculates the C_{RS} and adjusts the needed pressure delivered to achieve the set tidal volume. In this regard, tidal volume is used as a feedback control, which changes the pressure limit (usually breath to breath) as respiratory mechanics change. It maintains the advantage of guaranteed minute ventilation while limiting pressure and using a decelerating flow pattern.[7]

Proportional Assist Ventilation and Neurally Adjusted Ventilatory Assistance

Proportional assist ventilation (PAV) is an alternative mode of partial support, where the ventilator delivers pressure in proportion to the patient's effort.[134] The theory behind PAV is based on the equation of motion. Through a sophisticated software algorithm, the ventilator is able to know the flow, volume, airway resistance, and lung compliance, and therefore is able to calculate patient work of breathing. The ventilator responds to the *mechanical output* of the patient and will amplify patient effort with a preset proportional amount of pressure. The clinician sets the percent effort for the ventilator to provide support based on patient effort and desire.

Whereas PAV responds to a mechanical output, neurally adjusted ventilatory assistance (NAVA) responds to the *neural input* from the electrical activity of the diaphragm (Edi), and the patient retains all control of ventilator pattern. Pressure is delivered in proportion to the electrical activity of the diaphragm. This requires the placement of an esophageal electrode (similar to nasogastric tube placement). The ventilator is triggered based on Edi, therefore improving synchrony, as the time delay from patient effort to breath is very brief. In addition, the amount of ventilator assistance varies based on Edi. As such, to achieve greater assistance, the patient must increase Edi. Clinical data on NAVA are limited but have shown improved synchrony, preserved ventilatory pattern over a wide range of PEEP, and successful offload of respiratory muscles.[135-138]

Like many clinical situations involving choice of mechanical ventilator mode, the decision to use PAV or NAVA should be tailored to the individual patient. Patients with a high amount of dyssynchronous breaths and iPEEP secondary to obstructive physiology may benefit from a switch to these modes. These modes do not, however, ameliorate iPEEP, and extrinsic PEEP should be delivered appropriately. In patients recently intubated (< 48 hours), severely hypoxemic, or hemodynamically unstable, these modes should be avoided. Both modes require an intact ventilator drive, and ongoing assessments of pulmonary mechanics are a necessity. If sudden changes in respiratory system mechanics occur, the percent assist must be adjusted. Finally, as neither mode is controlling any factors in the equation of motion, neither mode can change the ventilator pattern (only assist level is being changed), and the clinician must give up a significant amount of control when using PAV and NAVA.

 Your attending concedes that clinical data seem to be stronger for your current strategy than for the above, more complex modes of mechanical ventilation. You finish rounds happy that the patient seems to have stabilized for the moment and go home wondering how to condense all of the clinical scenarios and complex physiology that just occurred.

! CRITICAL CONSIDERATIONS

- Institution of mechanical ventilation is done for many reasons, but for the most part, a mechanical ventilator does not treat disease. It should be managed safely while the inciting process is allowed to heal.
- A mechanical breath is separated into triggering, inspiration, cycling, and expiration.
- A ventilator mode describes the set of breath characteristics delivered to the patient and patient-ventilator interactions, and includes such things as control variable/target, phase variables, and mandatory versus spontaneous breaths.
- While respiratory system mechanics can be complex, the variables of interest are really only broken down into pressure, flow, and volume. Understanding the equation of motion will shed light on what a ventilator is controlling or targeting for a given breath.
- Pressure-volume curves demonstrate several key features, including the concepts of over-distention and derecruitment, compliance, and PEEP setting.
- While the individual diseases or syndromes causing hypoxemia are vast, they can be grouped into only a few true mechanisms.

- Oxygenation goals should be based on individual patient physiology. ARDSNet tolerance of Pao_2 of 55 mm Hg is likely too low for patients with ICP concerns, given the association of hypoxemia with secondary brain injury.
- PEEP serves to elevate the baseline pressure in the circuit and allows for recruitment of collapsed alveoli to minimize shunt and restore FRC. Optimal PEEP-setting strategy is controversial and should be done based on potential for recruitment balanced against risk of the potential for untoward PEEP effects. Most data point to the fact that PEEP is well tolerated in patients with elevated ICP.
- If brain tissue oxygenation is monitored, a level less than 15 mm Hg should cause concern.
- When setting mechanical ventilation, heart-lung interactions and forward blood flow should always be considered. This is true especially for RV function in the setting of ALI, as the incidence of RV dysfunction in these patients is high and associated with increased mortality.
- Hypocapnia and hyperventilation should only be reserved for emergent ICP elevations.
- In the setting of ALI, patients with manageable ICP elevations will likely tolerate mild permissive hypercapnia. This strategy should be weighed against the difficulty with which ICP can be controlled.
- There is no such thing as an isolated head injury. Brain-lung interactions should be considered in all patients with neurologic injury receiving mechanical ventilation, and the brain should be considered an end organ affected by VILI.
- Patients with expiratory flow limitation and iPEEP need prolonged expiratory time to relieve dynamic hyperinflation. The most efficient way to accomplish this is with a respiratory rate decrease.
- While most patients can be managed with conventional modes of mechanical ventilation, alternative modes such as APRV and HFOV can be considered for the difficult-to-oxygenate patient. PAV and NAVA can be considered as physiologically attractive modes to prevent respiratory muscle atrophy and promote synchrony.

Acknowledgements

I would like to thank Dr. William A. Knight IV from the University of Cincinnati for his thoughtful and very helpful review of this chapter, and Dr. Nicholas Mohr from the University of Iowa for aid with table and figure preparation.

REFERENCES

1. Marini JJ, Gattinoni L. Ventilatory management of acute respiratory distress syndrome: a consensus of two. *Crit Care Med.* 2004;32(1):250-255.
2. Cinel I, Smith J, Dellinger RP. General principles of mechanical ventilation. In: Parrillo JE, Dellinger RP, eds. *Critical Care Medicine: Principles of Diagnosis and Management in the Adult.* 3rd ed. Philadelphia, PA: Mosby Elsevier; 2008:153-176.
3. Gurka DP, Balk RA. Acute respiratory failure. In: Parrillo JE, Dellinger RP, eds. *Critical Care Medicine: Principles of Diagnosis and Management in the Adult.* 3rd ed. Philadelphia, PA: Mosby Elsevier; 2008:771-794.
4. Chatburn RL, Branson RD. Classification of mechanical ventilators. In: MacIntyre NR, Branson RD, eds. *Mechanical Ventilation.* 2nd ed. St. Louis, MO: Saunders Elsevier; 2009:1-45.

5. Marini J. Ventilatory management of obstructive airway disease. In: Parrillo JE, Dellinger RP, eds. *Critical Care Medicine: Principles of Diagnosis and Management in the Adult.* 3rd ed. Philadelphia, PA: Mosby Elsevier; 2008: 177-190.

6. MacIntyre NR. Management of obstructive airway disease. In: MacIntyre NR, Branson RD, eds. *Mechanical Ventilation.* 2nd ed. St. Louis, MO: Saunders Elsevier; 2009:297-305.

7. Branson RD. Modes of ventilator operation. In: MacIntyre NR, Branson RD, eds. *Mechanical Ventilation.* 2nd ed. St. Louis, MO: Saunders Elsevier; 2009:49-85.

8. Marini JJ. Spontaneously regulated vs. controlled ventilation of acute lung injury/acute respiratory distress syndrome. *Curr Opin Crit Care.* 2011;17(1):24-29.

9. Pinsky MR. Effect of mechanical ventilation on heart-lung interactions. In: Torbin MJ. *Principles & Practice of Mechanical Ventilation.* 2nd ed. New York: McGraw-Hill; 2006:729-757.

10. Habashi N, Andrews P. Ventilator strategies for posttraumatic acute respiratory distress syndrome: airway pressure release ventilation and the role of spontaneous breathing in critically ill patients. *Curr Opin Crit Care.* 2004;10(6):549.

11. Forel JM, Roch A, Marin V, et al. Neuromuscular blocking agents decrease inflammatory response in patients presenting with acute respiratory distress syndrome. *Crit Care Med.* 2006;34(11):2749-2757.

12. Papazian L, Forel JM, Gacouin A, et al. Neuromuscular blockers in early acute respiratory distress syndrome. *N Engl J Med.* 2010;363(12): 1107-1116.

13. Slutsky AS. Neuromuscular blocking agents in ARDS. *N Engl J Med.* 2010;363(12):1176-1180.

14. MacIntyre NR. Respiratory system mechanics. In: MacIntyre NR, Branson RD, eds. *Mechanical Ventilation.* 2nd ed. St. Louis, MO: Saunders Elsevier; 2009:159-170.

15. Lucangelo U, Bernabe F, Blanch L. Lung mechanics at the bedside: make it simple. *Curr Opin Crit Care.* 2007;13(1):64.

16. Kallet R, Katz J. Respiratory system mechanics in acute respiratory distress syndrome. *Respir Care Clin.* 2003;9(3):297-319.

17. Kallet R. Pressure-volume curves in the management of acute respiratory distress syndrome. *Respir Care Clin.* 2003;9(3):321-341.

18. Albaiceta GM, Blanch L, Lucangelo U. Static pressure-volume curves of the respiratory system: were they just a passing fad? *Curr Opin Crit Care.* 2008;14:80-86.

19. Hickling KG. The pressure-volume curve is greatly modified by recruitment. A mathematical model of ARDS lungs. *Am J Respir Crit Care Med.* 1998;158(1):194.

20. Gattinoni L, Pesenti A. The concept of "baby lung." *Intensive Care Med.* 2005;31(6):776-784.

21. Victorino JA, Borges JB, Okamoto VN, et al. Imbalances in regional lung ventilation: a validation study on electrical impedance tomography. *Am J Respir Crit Care Med.* 2004;169(7):791-800.

22. Jardin F, Vieillard-Baron A. Is there a safe plateau pressure in ARDS? The right heart only knows. *Intensive Care Med.* 2007;33(3):444-447.

23. Pelosi P, Luecke T, Rocco PR. Chest wall mechanics and abdominal pressure during general anaesthesia in normal and obese individuals and in acute lung injury. *Curr Opin Crit Care.* 2011;17(1):72-79.

24. Talmor D, Sarge T, Malhotra A, et al. Mechanical ventilation guided by esophageal pressure in acute lung injury. *N Engl J Med.* 2008;359(20):2095.

25. Habashi NM. Other approaches to open-lung ventilation: airway pressure release ventilation. *Crit Care Med.* 2005;33(Suppl.):S228-S240.

26. Young N, Rhodes JK, Mascia L, Andrews PJ. Ventilatory strategies for patients with acute brain injury. *Curr Opin Crit Care.* 2010;16(1):45-52.

27. Lowe GJ, Ferguson ND. Lung-protective ventilation in neurosurgical patients. *Curr Opin Crit Care.* 2006;12(1):3.

28. Nyquist P, Stevens RD, Mirski MA. Neurologic injury and mechanical ventilation. *Neurocrit Care.* 2008;9(3):400-408.

29. Mascia L, Sakr Y, Pasero D, Payen D, Reinhart K, Vincent JL. Extracranial complications in patients with acute brain injury: a post-hoc analysis of the SOAP study. *Intensive Care Med.* 2008;34(4): 720-727.

30. De Campos T. Ventilation with lower tidal volumes as compared with traditional tidal volumes for acute lung injury and the acute respiratory distress syndrome. The Acute Respiratory Distress Syndrome Network. *N Engl J Med.* 2000;342:1301-1308.

31. Gattinoni L, Carlesso E, Cressoni M. Assessing gas exchange in acute lung injury/acute respiratory distress syndrome: diagnostic techniques and prognostic relevance. *Curr Opin Crit Care.* 2011;17(1):18-23.

32. Jubran A, Tobin MJ. Noninvasive respiratory monitoring. In: Parrillo JE, Dellinger RP, eds. *Critical Care Medicine: Principles of Diagnosis and Management in the Adult.* 3rd ed. Philadelphia, PA: Mosby Elsevier; 2008:219-232.

33. Network T. Comparison of two fluid-management strategies in acute lung injury. *N Engl J Med* 2006;354:2564-2575.

34. Brower R, Lanken P, MacIntyre N, et al. Higher versus lower positive end-expiratory pressures in patients with the acute respiratory distress syndrome. *N Engl J Med*. 2004;351(4):327.

35. Meade MO, Cook DJ, Guyatt GH, et al. Ventilation strategy using low tidal volumes, recruitment maneuvers, and high positive end-expiratory pressure for acute lung injury and acute respiratory distress syndrome: a randomized controlled trial. *JAMA*. 2008;299(6):637.

36. Mercat A, Richard JCM, Vielle B, et al. Positive end-expiratory pressure setting in adults with acute lung injury and acute respiratory distress syndrome: a randomized controlled trial. *JAMA*. 2008;299(6):646.

37. Helmy A, Vizcaychipi M, Gupta A. Traumatic brain injury: intensive care management. *Br J Anaesth*. 2007;99(1):32-42.

38. Ireland TAoAoGBa. *Recommendations for the safe transfer of patients with brain injury*. http://www.aagbiorg/publications/guidelines/docs/braininjurypdf. 2006. Accessed January 5, 2011.

39. Wald SL, Shackford SR. The effect of secondary insults on mortality and long-term disability after severe head injury in a rural region without a trauma system. *J Trauma*. 1993;34(3):377.

40. McHugh GS, Engel DC, Butcher I, et al. Prognostic value of secondary insults in traumatic brain injury: results from the IMPACT study. *J Neurotrauma*. 2007;24(2):287-293.

41. Jones P, Andrews P, Midgley S, et al. Measuring the burden of secondary insults in head-injured patients during intensive care. *J Neurosurg Anesthesiol*. 1994;6(1):4.

42. Gentleman D, Jennett B. Hazards of inter-hospital transfer of comatose head-injured patients. *Lancet*. 1981;318(8251):853-855.

43. Demchenko IT, Welty-Wolf KE, Allen BW, Piantadosi CA. Similar but not the same: normobaric and hyperbaric pulmonary oxygen toxicity, the role of nitric oxide. *Am J Physiol Lung Cell Mol Physiol*. 2007;293(1):L229.

44. Altemeier WA, Sinclair SE. Hyperoxia in the intensive care unit: why more is not always better. *Curr Opin Crit Care*. 2007;13(1):73.

45. Diringer MN. Hyperoxia–good or bad for the injured brain? *Curr Opin Crit Care*. 2008;14(2):167.

46. Magnoni S, Ghisoni L, Locatelli M, et al. Lack of improvement in cerebral metabolism after hyperoxia in severe head injury: a microdialysis study. *J Neurosurg*. 2003;98(5):952-958.

47. Reinert M, Schaller B, Widmer HR, Seiler R, Bullock R. Influence of oxygen therapy on glucose-lactate metabolism after diffuse brain injury. *J Neurosurg*. 2004;101(2):323-329.

48. Reinert M, Barth A, Rothen H, Schaller B, Takala J, Seiler R. Effects of cerebral perfusion pressure and increased fraction of inspired oxygen on brain tissue oxygen, lactate and glucose in patients with severe head injury. *Acta Neurochir*. 2003;145(5):341-350.

49. Tolias CM, Reinert M, Seiler R, Gilman C, Scharf A, Bullock MR. Normobaric hyperoxia-induced improvement in cerebral metabolism and reduction in intracranial pressure in patients with severe head injury: a prospective historical cohort-matched study. *J Neurosurg*. 2004;101(3):435-444.

50. Diringer MN, Aiyagari V, Zazulia AR, Videen TO, Powers WJ. Effect of hyperoxia on cerebral metabolic rate for oxygen measured using positron emission tomography in patients with acute severe head injury. *J Neurosurg Pediatr*. 2007;106(4):526-529.

51. Cressoni M, Caironi P, Polli F, et al. Anatomical and functional intrapulmonary shunt in acute respiratory distress syndrome. *Crit Care Med*. 2008;36(3):669-675.

52. Dominguez-Cherit G, Posadas-Calleja JG, Borunda D. Chronic obstructive pulmonary disease. In: Parrillo JE, Dellinger RP, eds. *Critical Care Medicine: Principles of Diagnosis and Management in the Adult*. 3rd ed. Philadelphia, PA: Mosby Elsevier; 2008:811-826.

53. Rouby JJ, Puybasset L, Nieszkowska A, Lu Q. Acute respiratory distress syndrome: lessons from computed tomography of the whole lung. *Crit Care Med*. 2003;31(4 Suppl):S285-S295.

54. Gainnier M, Michelet P, Thirion X, Arnal JM, Sainty JM, Papazian L. Prone position and positive end-expiratory pressure in acute respiratory distress syndrome. *Crit Care Med*. 2003;31(12):2719-2726.

55. Girard TD, Bernard GR. Mechanical ventilation in ARDS: a state-of-the-art review. *Chest*. 2007;131(3):921-929.

56. Villar J, Kacmarek RM, Perez-Mendez L, Aguirre-Jaime A. A high positive end-expiratory pressure, low tidal volume ventilatory strategy improves outcome in persistent acute respiratory distress syndrome: a randomized, controlled trial. *Crit Care Med*. 2006;34(5):1311-1318.

57. Amato MBP, Barbas CSV, Medeiros DM, et al. Effect of a protective-ventilation strategy on mortality in the acute respiratory distress syndrome. *N Engl J Med*. 1998;338(6):347.

58. Ranieri VM. Effect of mechanical ventilation on inflammatory mediators in patients with acute respiratory distress syndrome: a randomized controlled trial. *JAMA*. 1999;282(1):54-61.

59. Halter JM, Steinberg JM, Schiller HJ, et al. Positive end-expiratory pressure after a recruitment maneuver prevents both alveolar collapse and recruitment/derecruitment. *Am J Respir Crit Care Med*. 2003;167(12):1620-1626.

60. Mols G, Priebe HJ, Guttmann J. Alveolar recruitment in acute lung injury. *Br J Anaesth*. 2006; 96(2):156-166.

61. Gattinoni L, Pelosi P, Suter PM, Pedoto A, Vercesi P, Lissoni A. Acute respiratory distress syndrome caused by pulmonary and extrapulmonary disease. Different syndromes? *Am J Respir Crit Care Med*. 1998;158(1):3.

62. Foti G, Cereda M, Sparacino M, De Marchi L, Villa F, Pesenti A. Effects of periodic lung recruitment maneuvers on gas exchange and respiratory mechanics in mechanically ventilated acute respiratory distress syndrome (ARDS) patients. *Intensive Care Med*. 2000;26(5):501-507.

63. Richard JC, Maggiore SM, Jonson B, Mancebo J, Lemaire F, Brochard L. Influence of tidal volume on alveolar recruitment. Respective role of PEEP and a recruitment maneuver. *Am J Respir Crit Care Med*. 2001;163(7):1609.

64. Nemer SN, Caldeira JB, Azeredo LM, et al. Alveolar recruitment maneuver in patients with subarachnoid hemorrhage and acute respiratory distress syndrome: a comparison of 2 approaches. *J Crit Care* 2010;26(1):22-27.

65. Pelosi P, Cadringher P, Bottino N, et al. Sigh in acute respiratory distress syndrome. *Am J Respir Crit Care Med*. 1999;159(3):872.

66. Zhang XY, Wang QX, Fan HR. Impact of positive end-expiratory pressure on cerebral injury patients with hypoxemia. *Am J Emerg Med*. 2010;29(7):699-703.

67. Huynh T, Messer M, Sing RF, Miles W, Jacobs DG, Thomason MH. Positive end-expiratory pressure alters intracranial and cerebral perfusion pressure in severe traumatic brain injury. *J Trauma*. 2002;53(3):488-492; discussion 492-493.

68. Frost E. Effects of positive end-expiratory pressure on intracranial pressure and compliance in brain-injured patients. *Survey Anesthesiol*. 1978; 22(5):440.

69. Burchiel KJ, Steege TD, Wyler AR. Intracranial pressure changes in brain-injured patients requiring positive end-expiratory pressure ventilation. *Neurosurgery*. 1981;8(4):443.

70. Cooper KR, Boswell PA, Choi SC. Safe use of PEEP in patients with severe head injury. *J Neurosurg*. 1985;63(4):552-555.

71. McGuire G, Crossley D, Richards J, Wong D. Effects of varying levels of positive end-expiratory pressure on intracranial pressure and cerebral perfusion pressure. *Crit Care Med*. 1997;25(6):1059.

72. Mascia L, Grasso S, Fiore T, Bruno F, Berardino M, Ducati A. Cerebro-pulmonary interactions during the application of low levels of positive end-expiratory pressure. *Intensive Care Med*. 2005;31(3):373-379.

73. Haitsma IK. Advanced monitoring in the intensive care unit: brain tissue oxygen tension. *Curr Opin Crit Care*. 2002;8:115-120.

74. Maloney-Wilensky E, Gracias V, Itkin A, et al. Brain tissue oxygen and outcome after severe traumatic brain injury: a systematic review. *Crit Care Med*. 2009;37(6):2057.

75. Rosenthal G, Hemphill JC, Sorani M, et al. The role of lung function in brain tissue oxygenation following traumatic brain injury. *J Neurosurg*. 2008;108(1):59-65.

76. Oddo M, Nduom E, Frangos S, et al. Acute lung injury is an independent risk factor for brain hypoxia after severe traumatic brain injury. *Neurosurgery*. 2010;67(2):338-344.

77. Pinsky MR. Heart-lung interactions. *Curr Opin Crit Care*. 2007;13(5):528.

78. Turtz AR. Intracranial monitoring. In: Parrillo JE, Dellinger RP, eds. *Critical Care Medicine: Principles of Diagnosis and Management in the Adult*. 3rd ed. Philadelphia, PA: Mosby Elsevier; 2008:281-288.

79. Turtz AR, Goldman HW. Head injury. In: Parrillo JE, Dellinger RP, eds. *Critical Care Medicine: Principles of Diagnosis and Management in the Adult*. 3rd ed. Philadelphia, PA: Mosby Elsevier; 2008:1385-1422.

80. Magder S. Hemodynamic monitoring in the mechanically ventilated patient. *Curr Opin Crit Care*. 2011;17(1):36-42.

81. Guyton AC, Lindsey AW, Abernathy B, Richardson T. Venous return at various right atrial pressures and the normal venous return curve. *Am J Physiol* 1957;189(3):609.

82. Calzia E, Ivanyi Z, Radermacher P. Determinants of blood flow and organ perfusion. *Funct Hemodynamic Monitor*. 2005:19-32.

83. Mebazaa A, Karpati P, Renaud E, Algotsson L. Acute right ventricular failure–from pathophysiology to new treatments. *Intensive Care Med*. 2004;30(2):185-196.

84. Jardin F, Vieillard-Baron A. Acute cor pulmonale. *Curr Opin Crit Care.* 2009;15(1):67-70.

85. Bouferrache K, Vieillard-Baron A. Acute respiratory distress syndrome, mechanical ventilation, and right ventricular function. *Curr Opin Crit Care.* 2011;17(1):30-35.

86. Vieillard-Baron A. Is right ventricular function the one that matters in ARDS patients? Definitely yes. *Intensive Care Med.* 2009;35(1):4-6.

87. Osman D, Monnet X, Castelain V, et al. Incidence and prognostic value of right ventricular failure in acute respiratory distress syndrome. *Intensive Care Med.* 2009;35(1):69-76.

88. Vieillard-Baron A. Assessment of right ventricular function. *Curr Opin Crit Care.* 2009;15(3): 254-260.

89. Curley G, Laffey JG, Kavanagh BP. Bench-to-bedside review: carbon dioxide. *Crit Care.* 2010;14:220.

90. Nuckton TJ, Alonso JA, Kallet RH, et al. Pulmonary dead-space fraction as a risk factor for death in the acute respiratory distress syndrome. *N Engl J Med.* 2002;346:1281-1286.

91. Laffey JG, Kavanagh BP. Carbon dioxide and the critically ill—too little of a good thing? *Lancet.* 1999;354(9186):1283-1286.

92. Curley G, Kavanagh BP, Laffey JG. Hypocapnia and the injured brain: more harm than benefit. *Crit Care Med.* 2010;38(5):1348-1359.

93. Mascia L, Zavala E, Bosma K, et al. High tidal volume is associated with the development of acute lung injury after severe brain injury: an international observational study. *Crit Care Med.* 2007;35(8):1815-1820.

94. Del Sorbo L, Slutsky AS. Acute respiratory distress syndrome and multiple organ failure. *Curr Opin Crit Care.* 2011;17(1):1-6.

95. Montgomery AB, Stager MA, Carrico CJ, Hudson LD: Causes of mortality in patients with the adult respiratory distress syndrome. *Am Rev Respir Dis.* 1985;132:485-489.

96. Stapleton RD, Wang BM, Hudson LD, Rubenfeld GD, Caldwell ES, Steinberg KP. Causes and timing of death in patients with ARDS. *Chest.* 2005;128(2):525.

97. Suchyta MR, Orme JF, Morris AH. The changing face of organ failure in ARDS. *Chest.* 2003;124(5):1871.

98. Pelosi P, Crotti S, Brazzi L, Gattinoni L. Computed tomography in adult respiratory distress syndrome: what has it taught us? *Eur Respir J.* 1996;9(5):1055-1062.

99. Stapleton RD, Steinberg, Kenneth P. Ventilator-induced lung injury. In: MacIntyre NR, Branson RD, eds. *Mechanical Ventilation.* 2nd ed. St. Louis, MO: Saunders Elsevier; 2009.

100. Dreyfuss D, Saumon G. Ventilator-induced lung injury. Lessons from experimental studies. *Am J Respir Crit Care Med.* 1998;157(1):294.

101. Webb H. Experimental pulmonary edema due to intermittent positive pressure ventilation with high inflation pressures. Protection by positive end-expiratory pressure. *Am Rev Respir Dis.* 1974;110(5):556-565.

102. Dreyfuss D, Soler P, Basset G, Saumon G. High inflation pressure pulmonary edema. Respective effects of high airway pressure, high tidal volume, and positive end-expiratory pressure. *American Rev Respir Dis.* 1988;137(5):1159.

103. Simonson DA, Adams AB, Wright LA, Dries DJ, Hotchkiss JR, Marini JJ. Effects of ventilatory pattern on experimental lung injury caused by high airway pressure. *Crit Care Med.* 2004;32(3):781.

104. Rich PB, Douillet CD, Hurd H, Boucher RC. Effect of ventilatory rate on airway cytokine levels and lung injury. *J Surg Res.* 2003;113(1): 139-145.

105. Hotchkiss J Jr, Blanch L, Murias G, et al. Effects of decreased respiratory frequency on ventilator-induced lung injury. *Am J Respir Crit Care Med.* 2000;161(2):463.

106. Chiumello D, Pristine G, Slutsky AS. Mechanical ventilation affects local and systemic cytokines in an animal model of acute respiratory distress syndrome. *Am J Respir Crit Care Med.* 1999; 160(1):109.

107. Haitsma JJ, Uhlig S, Göggel R, Verbrugge SJ, Lachmann U, Lachmann B. Ventilator-induced lung injury leads to loss of alveolar and systemic compartmentalization of tumor necrosis factor-α. *Intensive Care Med.* 2000;26(10):1515-1522.

108. Herrera MT, Toledo C, Valladares F, et al. Positive end-expiratory pressure modulates local and systemic inflammatory responses in a sepsis-induced lung injury model. *Intensive Care Med.* 2003;29(8):1345-1353.

109. Imai Y, Parodo J, Kajikawa O, et al. Injurious mechanical ventilation and end-organ epithelial cell apoptosis and organ dysfunction in an experimental model of acute respiratory distress syndrome. *JAMA.* 2003;289(16):2104.

110. Determann RM, Royakkers A, Wolthuis EK, et al. Ventilation with lower tidal volumes as compared with conventional tidal volumes for patients without acute lung injury: a preventive randomized controlled trial. *Crit Care.* 2010;14(1):R1.

111. Gonzalvo R, Marti-Sistac O, Blanch L, Lopez-Aguilar J. Bench-to-bedside review: brain-lung

interaction in the critically ill–a pending issue revisited. *Crit Care.* 2007;11(3):216.

112. Hopkins RO, Gale SD, Weaver LK. Brain atrophy and cognitive impairment in survivors of acute respiratory distress syndrome. *Brain Inj.* 2006;20(3):263-271.

113. Morandi A, Brummel NE, Ely EW. Sedation, delirium and mechanical ventilation: the "ABCDE" approach. *Curr Opin Crit Care.* 2011;17(1):43-49.

114. Herridge MS, Cheung AM, Tansey CM, et al. One-year outcomes in survivors of the acute respiratory distress syndrome. *N Engl J Med.* 2003; 348(8):683.

115. Davidson TA, Caldwell ES, Curtis JR, Hudson LD, Steinberg KP. Reduced quality of life in survivors of acute respiratory distress syndrome compared with critically ill control patients. *JAMA.* 1999;281(4):354.

116. Schelling G, Stoll C, Haller M, et al. Health-related quality of life and posttraumatic stress disorder in survivors of the acute respiratory distress syndrome. *Crit Care Med.* 1998;26(4):651.

117. Rothenhäusler HB, Ehrentraut S, Stoll C, Schelling G, Kapfhammer HP. The relationship between cognitive performance and employment and health status in long-term survivors of the acute respiratory distress syndrome: results of an exploratory study. *Gen Hosp Psychiatry.* 2001;23(2):90-96.

118. Schelling G, Stoll C, Vogelmeier C, et al. Pulmonary function and health-related quality of life in a sample of long-term survivors of the acute respiratory distress syndrome. *Intensive Care Med.* 2000;26(9):1304-1311.

119. Pandharipande P, Shintani A, Peterson J, et al. Lorazepam is an independent risk factor for transitioning to delirium in intensive care unit patients. *Anesthesiology.* 2006;104(1):21.

120. Brochard L. Intrinsic (or auto-) positive end-expiratory pressure during spontaneous or assisted ventilation. *Appl Physiol Intensive Care Med.* 2009:7-9.

121. Brochard L. Intrinsic (or auto-) PEEP during controlled mechanical ventilation. *Appl Physiol Intensive Care Med.* 2006:3-5.

122. Simmons DH, Linde LM, Miller JH, O'Reilly RJ. Relation between lung volume and pulmonary vascular resistance. *Circ Res.* 1961;9(2):465.

123. Stock MC, Downs JB, Frolicher DA. Airway pressure release ventilation. *Crit Care Med.* 1987; 15(5):462.

124. Putensen C, Zech S, Wrigge H, et al. Long-term effects of spontaneous breathing during ventilatory support in patients with acute lung injury. *Am J Respir Crit Care Med.* 2001;164(1):43.

125. Putensen C, Mutz NJ, Putensen-Himmer G, Zinserling J. Spontaneous breathing during ventilatory support improves ventilation-perfusion distributions in patients with acute respiratory distress syndrome. *Am J Respir Crit Care Med.* 1999;159(4):1241.

126. Sydow M, Burchardi H, Ephraim E, Zielmann S, Crozier TA. Long-term effects of two different ventilatory modes on oxygenation in acute lung injury. Comparison of airway pressure release ventilation and volume-controlled inverse ratio ventilation. *Am J Respir Crit Care Med.* 1994;149(6):1550.

127. Rathgeber J, Schorn B, Falk V, Kazmaier S, Spiegel T, Burchardi H. The influence of controlled mandatory ventilation (CMV), intermittent mandatory ventilation (IMV) and biphasic intermittent positive airway pressure (BIPAP) on duration of intubation and consumption of analgesics and sedatives. A prospective analysis in 596 patients following adult cardiac surgery. *Eur J Anaesthesiol.* 1997;14(6):576-582.

128. Chan KPW, Stewart TE. Clinical use of high-frequency oscillatory ventilation in adult patients with acute respiratory distress syndrome. *Crit Care Med.* 2005;33(Suppl):S170-S174.

129. Gentile MA, MacIntyre, Neil R. High-frequency ventilation. In: MacIntyre NR, Branson RD, eds. *Mechanical Ventilation.* 2nd ed. St. Louis, MO: Saunders Elsevier; 2009.

130. Chan KPW, Stewart TE, Mehta S. High-frequency oscillatory ventilation for adult patients with ARDS. *Chest.* 2007;131(6):1907.

131. Derdak S. High-frequency oscillatory ventilation for acute respiratory distress syndrome in adults: a randomized, controlled trial. *Am J Respir Crit Care Med.* 2002;166(6):801-808.

132. David M, Karmrodt J, Weiler N, Scholz A, Markstaller K, Eberle B. High-frequency oscillatory ventilation in adults with traumatic brain injury and acute respiratory distress syndrome. *Acta Anaesthesiol Scand.* 2005;49(2):209-214.

133. Bennett SS, Graffagnino C, Borel CO, James ML. Use of high frequency oscillatory ventilation (HFOV) in neurocritical care patients. *Neurocrit Care.* 2007;7(3):221-226.

134. Grasso S, Puntillo F, Mascia L, et al. Compensation for increase in respiratory workload during mechanical ventilation. Pressure-support versus proportional-assist ventilation. *Am J Respir Crit Care Med.* 2000;161(3):819.

135. Colombo D, Cammarota G, Bergamaschi V, De Lucia M, Corte FD, Navalesi P. Physiologic response to varying levels of pressure support and neurally adjusted ventilatory assist in patients

with acute respiratory failure. *Intensive Care Med.* 2008;34(11):2010-2018.

136. Piquilloud L, Vignaux L, Bialais E, et al. Neurally adjusted ventilatory assist improves patient–ventilator interaction. *Intensive Care Med.* 2011; 37(2):263-271.

137. Brander L, Leong-Poi H, Beck J, et al. Titration and implementation of neurally adjusted

ventilatory assist in critically ill patients. *Chest.* 2009;135(3):695.

138. Passath C, Takala J, Tuchscherer D, Jakob SM, Sinderby C, Brander L. Physiologic response to changing positive end-expiratory pressure during neurally adjusted ventilatory assist in sedated, critically ill adults. *Chest.* 2010; 138(3):578-587.

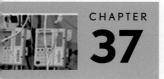

CHAPTER
37

Acute Respiratory Distress Syndrome

Maher Dahdel, MD
R. Phillip Dellinger, MD

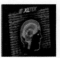

A 63-year-old man with no past medical history presented with a 3-day history of productive cough, hemoptysis, fever, and shortness of breath. In the emergency department (ED) the patient was mildly hypotensive and in severe respiratory distress, which required immediate intubation and initiation of mechanical ventilation. His laboratory workup revealed leukocytosis, mild renal insufficiency, and elevated serum lactate. His chest radiograph revealed dense consolidation in the right lower lung field with bilateral patchy infiltrates. The patient continued to be profoundly hypoxemic despite incremental increases in the mechanical ventilation support.

This is unfortunately a common clinical scenario for severe community-acquired pneumonia with associated sepsis and acute respiratory distress syndrome. In this chapter we will:

- Review the definitions, etiologies, and clinical aspects of acute respiratory distress syndrome (ARDS).
- Describe ventilator-induced lung injury and how it can be minimized.
- Review the role of steroid therapy and fluid management in ARDS.
- Review rescue strategies that may be considered in selected patients with ARDS.
- Describe outcome of ARDS survivors.
- Review neurogenic pulmonary edema.
- Review the effect of positive ventilation on cerebral perfusion.

How is the syndrome defined?

ARDS is an acute process of noncardiogenic pulmonary edema due to lung inflammation leading to hypoxemia. The American-European Consensus Conference (AECC)[1] defines ARDS as (1) acute onset (< 7 days); (2) partial pressure of oxygen in arterial blood (Pao_2)/fraction of inspired oxygen (Fio_2) less than or equal to 200 mm Hg (regardless of positive end-expiratory pressure [PEEP] level); (3) diffuse bilateral infiltrates on frontal chest radiograph, consistent with pulmonary edema; and (4) pulmonary capillary arterial occlusion pressure (PAOP) less than or equal to 18 mm Hg if measured, or in the absence of capability to measure PAOP, no clinical evidence of left atrial hypertension.

Acute lung injury (ALI) carries the same definition except a lesser degree of hypoxemia ($Pao_2/Fio_2 \leq 300$ mm Hg for ALI). The definitions of ARDS and ALI do not require mechanical ventilation and exclude chronic lung diseases.

Table 37-1. Common Causes of ALI/ARDS

Primary causes
Pulmonary infections
Aspiration injury
Trauma
Inhalation injury
Secondary causes
Severe sepsis
Shock
Acute pancreatitis
Transfusion-related lung injury
Anaphylaxis
Medications (opioids, tocolytics, chemotherapy)

Abbreviations: ALI, acute lung injury; ARDS, acute respiratory distress syndrome.

Etiologies of ARDS are divided into primary (initial insult comes from alveolar side of lung interstitium) and secondary or extrapulmonary (insult comes from blood side of lung interstitium) (Table 37-1).[2] The diagnosis of ARDS does not require a pulmonary artery (PA) catheter. Echocardiography, however, is often relied on in diagnosing systolic or diastolic dysfunction as the cause of pulmonary edema and in ruling out ALI/ARDS. Patients presenting with cardiogenic edema may have normal PAOP by the time a pulmonary artery catheter is placed (therapy had already been initiated).

Acute lung injury is quite common in the United States, perhaps affecting more than 200,000 people per year, with an associated mortality rate of 30% to 35% and a burden of subsequent morbidity and disability on survivors.[3]

What is the pathophysiology of the syndrome?

The clinical presentation follows an inflammatory response involving neutrophils, macrophages/monocytes, and lymphocytes undergoing adhesion, chemotaxis, and activation, as well as noncellular events, such as complement activation, coagulopathy, and kinin elaboration. Cytokines, lipid mediators, oxidants, proteases, nitric oxide, growth factors, neuropeptides, and protein synthesis may be involved in lung injury.

Clinical Manifestations

Gas exchange derangements

Following endothelium or epithelium injury, plasma moves into the lung interstitium and alveolar space, creating shunt and reducing lung compliance. The hallmark of ARDS is shunting, where inspired gas never reaches flooded alveoli and a substantial fraction of mixed venous blood, at low oxyhemoglobin saturation, traverses the pulmonary circulation without being exposed to oxygen, causing arterial hypoxemia that does not respond to increasing the F_{IO_2}. Dead space ventilation (decreased perfusion relative to ventilation) is also raised in ARDS. In addition to the adverse consequences on gas exchange, diseases characterized by interstitial and alveolar fluid accumulation reduce the compliance of the respiratory system, imposing a mechanical load on the patient with a resulting increase in the work of breathing.

Radiographic findings

The plain chest radiograph is useful in distinguishing ARDS from focal lung processes such as pneumonia or atelectasis. It is less helpful in separating ARDS from hydrostatic (high pulmonary capillary pressure) edema (usually, but not always, caused by heart disease).

Imaging patients with ARDS with chest computed tomography (CT) scans, although not frequently done clinically, often reveals the lungs to be composed of three compartments: one is relatively normal; another one has mild consolidation or atelectasis; and the third, in the more dependent area, has dense consolidation. The striking nonhomogeneity of lung flooding and consolidation on chest CT scans in patients with ARDS have important implications; the relatively normal part of the lung should be considered small ("baby" lung) rather than stiff in terms of the alveolar population receiving machine-delivered tidal volumes.[4] This has implications for mechanical ventilation as discussed below since the remaining aerated alveoli are subject to overdistention when excessive tidal volumes are used.

What would you do with this case? What would be an appropriate treatment approach?

The cornerstone of current management of ARDS consists of supportive therapy, including lung protective ventilation, and cardiovascular manipulation as needed. Supportive management of ARDS should be joined by aggressive diagnosis and treatment of the predisposing condition since the underlying problem (eg, sepsis) typically requires specific therapy.

Mechanical Ventilation

The majority of patients with ARDS will require intubation and mechanical ventilation to decrease the work of breathing and to apply PEEP. Some causes of ARDS, such as tocolytic-associated pulmonary edema, postictal pulmonary edema, and pulmonary edema associated with air emboli, tend to have a benign course and may respond simply to supportive therapy. Also, some patients will have rather mild ALI and may be successfully ventilated noninvasively (alert patients with near-drowning).[5,6]

Mechanical ventilation has been demonstrated to be injurious to the lung by both (1) overdistention of alveoli and (2) repeated recruitment (opening of closed lung during inspiration) and decruitment (closure of that same lung at end expiration), which amplifies lung injury.[7,8]

Lung Overdistention

Volutrauma is defined as overdistention of alveoli (rather than pressure, per se) and causes histopathologic, radiologic, and clinical findings of acute lung injury. It is determined by the transpulmonary pressure in the alveoli of concern. Computed tomographic studies show that in most patients, the ARDS lung is remarkably inhomogeneous, with some normally compliant and likely fragile alveoli (nondependent) and others that are flooded or collapsed (dependent). The loss of functional alveoli necessitates that, if the tidal volume is not reduced, alveoli that are open will be overdistended. Indeed, the apparently "stiff" lung of ARDS is better understood as gross overdistention of a few relatively normal alveoli rather than as caused by generalized parenchymal "stiffness." The mechanisms by which alveolar overstretching produces damage remain controversial, but inflammatory cytokines are found in lavage fluid and systemic blood following ventilation with excessive tidal volumes.[9]

The lung pressure-volume relationship in ARDS has a sigmoidal shape, with a lower inflection point (LIP) and an upper inflection zone (UIZ), and exhibits hysteresis (better compliance on the descending limb than the ascending limb) when the inflation and deflation limbs are compared (Figure 37-1). The UIZ signals progressively falling compliance, indicating that many alveoli have reached their normal limits of expansion and overdistention has become the predominant influence on compliance. It has been proposed that when the inflation curve reaches the UIZ, that lung is at risk.

The ARDS Network (ARDSNet) tested the relevance of overdistention in a clinical study using a simple method: limiting tidal volume to 6 mL/kg ideal body weight (IBW).[10] This important study entered 861 patients with both ALI and ARDS and randomized them to 6 versus 12 mL/kg IBW. The primary outcome measure, hospital mortality, markedly favored the lower tidal volume approach

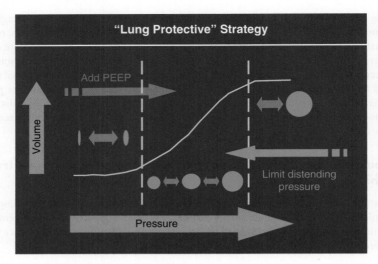

Figure 37-1. Lung protective strategy. Depicted are the two areas of concern during the mechanical ventilation of acute respiratory distress syndrome (ARDS), both amenable to lung protective strategy. On the lower portion of the pressure-volume curve is the lower inflection point where minimum positive end-expiratory pressure (PEEP) is needed to prevent clinically significant alveolar collapse. On the upper portion of the pressure-volume curve is the upper inflection zone where overdistention and volutrauma may occur. In between is the more compliant area of the pressure-volume curve where tidal excursion is desired. *(Courtesy of ARDSNet.)*

(39.8% versus 31.0%). A consequence of limiting the tidal volume in this manner is that the partial pressure of carbon dioxide in arterial blood ($Paco_2$) may rise above 40 mm Hg. Tolerating this respiratory acidosis is called permissive hypercapnia and is preferable to alveolar overdistention. Other ARDSNet ventilator strategies include reducing the tidal volume further, if needed, to keep the plateau pressure (P_{plat}) less than 30 cm H_2O; protocolized PEEP and FIO_2 settings to maintain the arterial saturation between 88% and 95%; and rate increases to as high as 35 breaths/min.

The ARDSNet protocol including low tidal volume ventilation has become the benchmark against which alternative approaches are compared.[10] The existing data support a dose-response relationship in which the lower the tidal volume, the lower the mortality rate.[11] However, very low tidal volumes are poorly tolerated in most patients and require significant sedation, which is problematic.

Recruitment/Derecruitment and the Lower Inflection Point

The LIP of the pressure-volume curve (see Figure 37-1) is the point where lower applied pressures will result in significant lung collapse. Many studies suggest that an appropriate level of PEEP (minimal PEEP) applied at the LIP can protect the injured ARDS lung by preventing repeated deflation-inflation across the LIP and the associated shear force injury. Locating the LIP requires constructing a compliance curve by measuring compliance at various PEEP settings following recruitment maneuvers.[7] The ARDS Network has tested a higher PEEP approach (superimposed on low tidal volume ventilation) and found no meaningful benefit or harm in this approach. It remains possible, however, that increasing PEEP only in the presence of improving compliance would be an appropriate, yet unconfirmed strategy.

Permissive Hypercapnia

Historically, physicians first attempted to ventilate patients with ARDS to a normal $Paco_2$. In patients with severe acute lung injury, however, this arbitrary goal has a mechanical cost because of inappropriately sized tidal volume and amplification of lung injury, as described above. Over the past decade, there has been increasing evidence that points to the safety and efficacy of allowing the $Paco_2$ to rise well above 40 mm Hg.[12] When patients with severe ARDS are ventilated with a lung protective strategy, $Paco_2$ may rise to 50 to 70 mm Hg (occasionally higher) and the pH falls accordingly. Despite the adverse effects of respiratory acidosis in the nonmechanically ventilated patient, very high levels of $Paco_2$ seem remarkably well tolerated by adequately sedated patients. One may allow the $Paco_2$ to rise gradually (5-10 mm Hg/h) in order to allow time for some cellular compensation. In patients without contraindications, sodium bicarbonate may be infused to raise the blood pH. Sodium bicarbonate delivers a substantial CO_2 load to a patient already marginally able to excrete what is produced endogenously and further risks volume overload and potassium depletion. Bicarbonate should be considered when ventilator strategy results in very low pH (ie, < 7.20).

Contraindications to permissive hypercapnia are the presence of increased intracranial pressure or active cardiac ischemia; also, the inspired gas must be oxygen enriched to prevent hypoxemia, and patients would be expected to require more sedation. Over time, in patients with good renal function, the kidney will retain bicarbonate in response to the respiratory acidosis as an endogenous compensation mechanism, making permissive hypercapnia easier to maintain.

Approach to Mechanical Ventilation

The principles that guide our ventilatory management of ARDS are (1) avoid alveolar overdistention targeting an initial tidal volume of 6 mL/kg IBW, tolerating hypercapnia if necessary[10]; (2) obtain and maintain an FIO_2 of less than or equal to 0.6 as soon as feasible; and (3) apply PEEP to avoid deflation/reinflation injury. Either volume- or time-cycled assist-control ventilation (ACV) is used. Since with pressure-control ventilation changes in lung elastance or airway resistance over time cause tidal volume to vary, it is typically deployed in a pressure-regulated volume-control (PRVC) or volume-guaranteed mode. In these circumstances the ventilator software adjusts pressure up or down in an attempt to keep tidal volume constant. PRVC ventilation in the distressed ARDS patient may require significant sedation, which, if necessary, in addition to aiding patient-ventilator synchrony, reduces the oxygen consumption and CO_2 production.

One of the management goals is to reduce the FIO_2 over the first 24 to 48 hours to less than 0.6 to avoid the potential for oxygen toxicity, and this can usually be accomplished by recruitment and increasing PEEP, using pulse oximetry as a guide. Positive end-expiratory pressure exploits the hysteresis of the inflation and deflation limbs of each breath to recruit alveoli on inspiration (by expanding collapsed units and translocating fluid from flooded units to the interstitial space) and then preventing derecruitment at end expiration. Recruitment maneuvers such as applying 40 cm H_2O continuous positive airway pressure for 40 seconds may increase lung opening, which can be held open by increased PEEP settings. The result is increased respiratory system compliance as a result of increased functional residual capacity and improved gas exchange because of oxygenation of perfused recruited air space.[13,14] Positive end-expiratory pressure may be initially set at 12 to 15 cm H_2O in a single step and then lowered over time as tolerated, or set lower after initial recruitment maneuvers and sequentially increased if recruitment-induced improvement in oxygenation is not maintained. Both methods require re-recruitment and return to previous PEEP setting if desaturation occurs. PEEP raises pleural pressure, which will produce an increase in juxtacardiac pressure; this raises right atrial pressure (downstream pressure for filling of the heart) and decreases the transmural filling pressure of the left ventricle, and hypotension may result. This, however, is uncommon, perhaps because the pleural pressure increment is slight because of a decrease in lung compliance due to ARDS. Significant hypotension can be treated by reducing the PEEP temporarily and by infusing fluids or vasoactive drugs to restore cardiac output. Just as shunt lesions are poorly responsive to increased FIO_2, so are they to reduced FIO_2, and it is usually possible to achieve the target of 0.6 early in the management of ARDS. If initial PEEP was set at 15 cm H_2O following recruitment and adequate oxygenation was achieved, PEEP can be decreased in steps of 2 cm H_2O, allowing at least 15 minutes between steps and seeking the least PEEP that maintains the recruitment-induced oxygenation improvement. An alternative to sustained higher inflation pressure over time for recruitment is incremental increases in PEEP with fixed tidal volume. This is a one-step maneuver that simultaneously increases end-expiratory lung volume (recruiting closed lung), with the increase in PEEP keeping some portion of the newly recruited lung from collapsing at end expiration. Reducing PEEP significantly, even for short periods of time, is often associated with alveolar derecruitment and rapid arterial hemoglobin desaturation. Thus, airway disconnections should be kept to a minimum, and when required or occurring, they should be followed by re-recruitment if recruitment had been used as part of the PEEP-setting strategy. When severely hypoxemic patients fail to respond to PEEP, one should suspect a focal lung process, such as lobar pneumonia or atelectasis. In some patients, PEEP must be raised higher than 15 cm H_2O (rarely much higher in order to get the F_{IO_2} below 0.6).

Once the PEEP is adjusted and the F_{IO_2} is lowered to 0.6, the tidal volume and rate should be reevaluated. A 0.3-second end-inspiratory pause should be used to determine P_{plat}. If P_{plat} exceeds 30 cm H_2O, the tidal volume (initially set at 6 cm H_2O IBW) should be reduced progressively, in decrements of 0.5 mL/kg IBW, until this target value of less than or equal to 30 cm H_2O is achieved. The initial respiratory rate of 20 breaths/min may need to be raised to reduce the work of breathing and help with CO_2 elimination, but the expiratory flow waveform should be inspected for the presence of end-expiratory flow (signaling auto-PEEP), which should be avoided. Respiratory rate should typically not exceed 35 to 40 breaths/min.

What are available salvage therapies for ARDS?

Prone Positioning

Multiple studies have shown that a substantial fraction of patients with ARDS exhibit improved oxygenation with prone positioning, because of a redistribution of lung perfusion and a change in regional diaphragm motion.[15] Prone positioning improves oxygenation by (1) shifting atelectatic lung from dependent higher blood flow to nondependent lesser blood flow areas, (2) facilitating secretion drainage from atelectatic lung, (3) relieving cardiac compression of lung, (4) optimizing the lung-tethering effect on functional residual capacity, and (5) facilitating the dorsal chest protective effect against gravity influence. There are, however, practical challenges. Special attention is necessary to prevent pressure necrosis of the nose, face, and ears and to ensure maintenance and patency of the endotracheal tube. Pressure on the eye could lead to retinal ischemia, especially in hypotensive patients. Some patients experience cardiac arrhythmias or hemodynamic instability on being turned. One controlled trial failed to show a survival benefit to prone ventilation, but a subset of more severely hypoxic patients may have benefited.[16] A subsequent study suggested benefit of prone positioning when initiated early in more severe ARDS and sustained for longer periods of time each day.[17,18] We recommend initial prone positioning for 14 to 16 hours before return to the supine position in patients with the most severe form of ARDS (F_{IO_2} of 0.8 or greater or $P_{plat} > 30$ cm H_2O despite low tidal volume strategy).

High-Frequency Ventilation

High-frequency ventilation is the application of mechanical ventilation with a respiratory rate of greater than 100 breaths/min with a small tidal volume. This type of ventilation may improve oxygenation in patients with refractory hypoxemia.[19] However, there is not sufficient evidence to conclude that high-frequency oscillatory ventilation reduces mortality or long-term morbidity rates in patients with ALI or ARDS.

Extracorporeal Gas Exchange

The use of venovenous extracorporeal membrane oxygenation (ECMO) has been an attractive strategy for the management of patients with acute lung injury. The Conventional Ventilatory Support versus Extracorporeal Membrane Oxygenation for Severe Adult Respiratory Failure (CESAR) trial has shown evidence of survival improvement in patients with severe but potentially reversible acute lung injury.[20] This strategy carries multiple technical difficulties; however, it is still a heroic salvage therapy for patients with isolated severe respiratory failure of reversible cause, in whom all other supportive measures have failed.

Inhaled Selective Pulmonary Vasodilator

Inhaled selective pulmonary vasodilators such as nitric oxide or prostacyclin have several potential salutary effects in ARDS.[21] They selectively vasodilate pulmonary capillaries and arterioles that subserve ventilated alveoli, diverting blood flow to these alveoli (and away from areas of shunt). The beneficial effects on oxygenation of inhaled nitric oxide (INO) initially take place at inspired concentrations of 1 to 10 ppm, but roughly one-third of patients will not respond at all. There are ample studies showing beneficial physiologic effects of inhaled nitric oxide, but two large, controlled studies failed to show a clinical outcome benefit.[22,23] Potential adverse effects of INO include methemoglobinemia and increased levels of nitrogen dioxide, neither of which is common unless high doses of INO (80 ppm) are used. It is not clear whether there is any role for inhaled nitric oxide or inhaled prostacyclin, but it is reasonable to try it in patients whose hypoxemia remains refractory to mechanical ventilation optimization and with contraindications or failure of prone positioning.

Steroids

As the pathophysiology of acute lung injury seems to be unregulated inflammatory response of the lung, corticosteroid therapy has been studied as a possible effective treatment of ARDS. However, several trials of high-dose steroids for a short period at the onset of ARDS failed to demonstrate benefit.

A subset of patients with ARDS will develop disordered healing with subsequent lung fibrosis. This so-called unresolving fibroproliferative phase will manifest as persistent infiltrates on chest radiography without evidence of infection, increasing airway pressures, a further fall in lung compliance, less responsiveness to PEEP, and rising minute ventilation requirements.[24]

Subsequent studies have shown that corticosteroids can ameliorate pulmonary inflammation at this phase. The current data on steroid use in patients with severe ARDS, although encouraging, need further validation in larger randomized trials before this therapy should be considered for general use in clinical practice. Decisions for steroid use in the circumstance of unresolving ARDS need to be individualized, and steroids should not routinely be used in this circumstance as no survival advantage was demonstrated in the ARDSNet trial.[25]

If methylprednisolone is administered for unresolving ARDS, it should be avoided after day 13 from the onset of ARDS, the dose should be modest (0.5 mg/kg every 6 hours) and tapered slowly, active infection should be ruled out, and the use of neuromuscular blocking agents concomitantly should be avoided.

Neuromuscular Blocking Agents

The administration of neuromuscular blocking agents in patients with ARDS improves oxygenation primarily when there is persistent patient-ventilator dyssynchrony.[26] When these agents are used, the lowest effective dose is recommended, and the duration should be as brief as possible. Intermittent dosing is preferred. If continuous infusion is used, a twitch monitor (ulnar or temporal) should be applied, and a minimum of "two out of four" responses after a train-of-four electrical stimulus maintained. The titration of neuromuscular blocking agents should be toward unassisted breathing. If this can be accomplished with "four out of four," that is ideal. Concomitant administration of corticosteroids should be avoided because of the increased risk of myopathy.

Hemodynamic and Circulatory Management of ARDS

If pulmonary edema is diminished in acute lung injury, ventilator, PEEP, and oxygen therapy can be reduced. Several studies initially reported data showing a correlation between survival and net diuresis or reduction in PAOP, and a prospective trial showed that reducing extravascular lung water decreased ventilator and intensive care unit (ICU) days in patients with ARDS.[27] However, diuresis and fluid restriction could compromise perfusion, potentially contributing to organ dysfunction, so the target should be to seek the lowest intravascular volume compatible with an adequate cardiac output. A large clinical trial supported that a fluid-conservative versus a fluid-liberal approach improved outcome.[28] Use of central venous pressure monitoring to achieve this goal was as equally effective as a pulmonary artery catheter.[29] In the absence of hypotension or tissue hypoperfusion (oliguria), central venous pressure should be maintained at less than 5 mm Hg.

The patient may have intracranial hypertension with abnormally elevated ICP. What is the relationship between high PEEP and ICP?

Increased intrathoracic pressure due to applied PEEP could theoretically decrease cerebral venous outflow, which could lead to increased intracranial pressure. Whether this actually occurs is uncertain. Observational studies with patients who had acute stroke or acute subarachnoid hemorrhage found that incremental elevation of applied PEEP was associated with diminished cerebral perfusion pressure due to decreased mean arterial pressure.[30,31] Another study that investigated 21 comatose patients with severe head injury or subarachnoid hemorrhage receiving ICP monitoring found that in patients with poor pulmonary compliance (as in ARDS), PEEP has no significant effect on cerebral and systemic hemodynamics, probably because the PEEP-induced increase in intrathoracic pressure is poorly transmitted to the pleural (juxtacardiac) space.[32]

Given the uncertainty that exists, it is prudent to monitor both the mean arterial blood pressure and the intracranial pressure (if available) whenever applied PEEP is used in a patient with an intracranial abnormality. Reduction of applied PEEP should be considered if the mean arterial blood pressure decreases or intracranial pressure increases.

Pathophysiology and Manifestation of Neurogenic Pulmonary Edema

Neurogenic pulmonary edema (NPE) needs special attention in the neurology ICU setting as a hybrid form of ARDS, although its pathophysiology and prognosis are significantly different. This entity characteristically presents within minutes to hours of a severe central nervous system insult and usually resolves within several days. It is believed to be caused by a severe acute generalized systemic rise in vascular resistance, producing a sudden surge in pulmonary capillary pressure, resulting in pulmonary capillary endothelial injury. By the time of diagnosis, the initial insult has typically abated but endothelial injury persists.

Neurogenic pulmonary edema presents with the same clinical and radiologic findings of acute pulmonary edema without the evidence of left ventricular dysfunction. This picture may be confused with aspiration pneumonitis because they both commonly occur in settings of altered consciousness. A clinical diagnosis is based largely on the occurrence of pulmonary edema in the appropriate setting and in the absence of another obvious cause. NPE usually occurs in association with elevated ICP, but elevated ICP is not a necessary condition.

The major causes of NPE are cerebral hemorrhage, epileptic seizure, and head injury. Less commonly it may occur in nonhemorrhagic stroke, brain tumors, Guillain-Barré syndrome, vertebral artery ligation, and hydrocephalus.[33]

Although NPE has been recognized for more than a century, its pathophysiologic mechanisms remain incompletely understood. Various theories have centered on potential roles for the hypothalamus and medulla,[34] elevated intracranial pressure, and activation of the sympathoadrenal system.

α-Adrenergic blockers such as phentolamine can prevent the development of NPE, suggesting an important role for sympathetic activation. Pulmonary venoconstriction can occur with intracranial hypertension or sympathetic stimulation and can elevate capillary hydrostatic pressure and produce pulmonary edema without affecting left atrial, systemic, or pulmonary capillary wedge pressures.

The outcome of patients with NPE is usually determined by the course of the neurologic insult that produced NPE, and specific treatment should focus on the underlying disorder. NPE is generally managed in a supportive and conservative fashion because many episodes of NPE are well tolerated and the majority of cases resolve within 48 to 72 hours. Positive pressure mechanical ventilation is commonly required, and the pulmonary edema is PEEP responsive; however, special attention should be given to the hypercapnia because it carries the risk of cerebral vasodilatation and exacerbation of elevated intracranial pressure. Maintenance of low cardiac filling pressures may decrease edema genesis, but care must be taken to avoid compromise of cardiac output and cerebral perfusion; pulmonary artery catheterization may be helpful in guiding therapy. NPE is generally considered a contraindication to lung harvesting for transplantation.

Prognosis and Outcome of ARDS

Negative cognitive, emotional, and quality-of-life outcomes have been reported in survivors of ARDS.[35,36] They found that these outcomes occurred in over 70% of patients at hospital discharge and over 40% at 1 and 2 years after discharge. The etiology of these impairments is likely multifactorial and includes hypoxemia, hypotension, sedative use, delirium, and inflammatory mediators.

! CRITICAL CONSIDERATIONS

- ARDS is defined by the following features: acute onset, bilateral infiltrates, no evidence of elevated left atrial pressure, and Pao_2/Fio_2 less than or equal to 200 mm Hg.
- Cardiogenic pulmonary edema and other causes of acute hypoxemic respiratory failure with bilateral infiltrates must be excluded before the diagnosis of ARDS is made.
- The hallmark of the syndrome is the accumulation of exudative fluid in both the interstitium and alveoli because of a lung injury, which causes gas exchange abnormalities and a decrease in lung compliance.
- The management incorporates the treatment of the underlying cause, support of gas exchange, and prevention of complications such as deep venous thrombosis and ventilator-associated pneumonia.
- The cornerstone in the mechanical ventilation of ARDS is the use of low tidal volume ventilation (< 6 mL/kg predicted body weight) to prevent overdistention injury.
- The recruitment of collapsed alveoli and maintaining an open state by applying adequate PEEP will avoid the deflation/reinflation injury and improve lung mechanics and oxygenation.
- Refractory hypoxemia can be managed by multiple strategies including the use of an inhaled selective pulmonary vasodilator, prone positioning, neuromuscular blocking agents, and ECMO.
- Neurogenic pulmonary edema needs special attention in the neurology ICU setting as a hybrid form of ARDS.

Acknowledgment

We wish to acknowledge Dr. Gregory A. Schmidt (University of Iowa) and the Society of Critical Care Medicine. Dr. Schmidt co-authored with RPD the syllabus chapter on Acute Respiratory Distress Syndrome published in the *Adult Multiprofessional Critical Care Review,* eds, JE Szalados and CG Rehm, Society of Critical Care Medicine, August 2007. Revision and update of some portions of that chapter were used in the preparation of the current manuscript.

REFERENCES

1. Bernard GR, Artigas A, Brigham KL, et al. The American-European Consensus Conference of ARDS: definitions, mechanisms, relevant outcomes, and clinical trial coordination. *Am J Respir Crit Care Med.* 1994;149:818-824.

2. Gattinoni L, Pelosi P, Suter PM, et al. Acute respiratory distress syndrome caused by pulmonary and extrapulmonary disease. *Am J Respir Crit Care Med.* 1999;159:3-11.

3. Rubenfeld GD, Caldwell E, Peabody E, et al. Incidence and outcomes of acute lung injury. *N Engl J Med.* 2005;353:1685-1693.

4. Gattinoni L, Pesenti A. The concept of "baby lung." *Intensive Care Med.* 2005;31:776-784.

5. Antonelli M, Conti G, Moro ML, et al. Predictors of failure of noninvasive positive pressure ventilation in patients with acute hypoxemic respiratory failure: a multi-center study. *Intensive Care Med.* 2001;27:1718-1728.

6. Patrick W, Webster K, Ludwig L, et al. Noninvasive positive-pressure ventilation in acute respiratory distress without prior chronic respiratory failure. *Am J Respir Crit Care Med.* 1996;153:1005-1011.

7. Amato MRP, Barbas CSV, Medeiros DM, et al. Beneficial effects of the "open lung approach" with low distending pressures in acute respiratory distress syndrome. *Am J Respir Crit Care Med.* 1995;152:1835-1846.

8. Benito S, LeMaire F. Pulmonary pressure-volume relationship in acute respiratory distress syndrome in adults: role of positive end-expiratory pressure. *Crit Care.* 1990;5:27.

9. Chiumello D, Pristine G, Slutsky A. Mechanical ventilation affects local and systemic cytokines in an animal model of acute respiratory distress syndrome. *Am J Respir Crit Care Med.* 1999;160:109-116.

10. Acute Respiratory Distress Syndrome Network. Ventilation with lower tidal volumes as compared with traditional tidal volumes for acute lung injury and the acute respiratory distress syndrome. *N Engl J Med.* 2000;342:1301-1308.

11. Kallet RH, Jasmer RM, Pittet JF, et al. Clinical implementation of the ARDS Network protocol is associated with reduced hospital mortality compared with historical controls. *Crit Care Med.* 2005;33:925-929.

12. Chonghaile MN, Higgins B, Laffey JG. Permissive hypercapnia: role in protective lung ventilatory strategies. *Curr Opin Crit Care.* 2005;11:56-62.

13. Fan E, Wilcox ME, Brower RG, et al. Recruitment maneuvers for acute lung injury. *Am J Respir Crit Care Med.* 2008;178:1156-1163.

14. Gattinoni L, Caironi P, Cressoni M, et al. Lung recruitment in patients with the acute respiratory distress syndrome. *N Engl J Med.* 2006;354:1775-1786.

15. Abroug F, Ouanes-Besbes L, Elatrous, et al. The effect of prone positioning in acute respiratory distress syndrome or acute lung injury: a meta-analysis. Areas of uncertainty and recommendations for research. *Intensive Care Med.* 2008;34:1002-1011.

16. Gattinoni L, Tognoni G, Pesenti A, et al. Effect of prone positioning on the survival of patients with acute respiratory failure. *N Engl J Med.* 2001;345:568-573.

17. Mancebo J, Fernandez R, Blanch L, et al. A multicenter trial of prolonged prone ventilation in severe acute respiratory distress syndrome. *Am J Respir Crit Care Med.* 2006;173:1233-1239.

18. Ward NS. Effects of prone position ventilation in ARDS. *Crit Care Clin.* 2002;18:35-44.

19. Derdak S, Mehta S, Stewart TE, et al. High-frequency oscillatory ventilation for acute respiratory distress syndrome in adults: a randomized, controlled trial. *Am J Respir Crit Care Med.* 2002;166:801-808.

20. Peek GJ, Mugford M, Tiruvoipati R, et al. Efficacy and economic assessment of conventional ventilatory support versus extracorporeal membrane oxygenation for severe adult respiratory failure (CESAR). *Lancet.* 2009;374(9698):1351-1363.

21. Walmrath D, Schneider T, Schermuly R, et al. Direct comparison of inhaled nitric oxide and aerosolized prostacyclin in acute respiratory distress syndrome. *Am J Respir Crit Care Med.* 1996;153(3):991-996.

22. Michael JR, Barton RG, Saffle JR, et al. Inhaled nitric oxide versus conventional therapy: effect on oxygenation in ARDS. *Am J Respir Crit Care Med.* 2000;157:1372-1380.

23. Rossiant R, Gerlach H, Schmidt-Ruhnke H, et al. Efficacy of inhaled nitric oxide in patients with severe ARDS. *Chest.* 1995;107:1107-1115.

24. Meduri GU, Chinn AJ, Leeper KV, et al. Corticosteroid rescue treatment of progressive fibroproliferation in late ARDS. Patterns of response and predictors of outcome. *Chest.* 1994;105:1516-1527.

25. Dellinger RP. Steroid therapy of septic shock: the decision is in the eye of the beholder. *Crit Care Med.* 2008;36:1987-1989.

26. Forel JM, Roch A, Papazian L. Paralytics in critical care: not always the bad guy. *Curr Opin Crit Care.* 2009;15(1):59-66.

27. Mitchell JP, Schuller D, Calandrino FS, et al. Improved outcome based on fluid management in critically ill patients requiring pulmonary artery catheterization. *Am J Respir Crit Care Med.* 1992;145:990-998.

28. The National Heart, Lung and Blood Institute Acute Respiratory Distress Syndrome (ARDS) Clinical Trials Network. Comparison of two fluid-management strategies in acute lung injury. *N Engl J Med.* 2006;354:2564-2575.

29. The National Heart, Lung and Blood Institute Acute Respiratory Distress Syndrome (ARDS) Clinical Trials Network. Pulmonary-artery versus central venous catheter to guide treatment of acute lung injury. *N Engl J Med.* 2006;354:2213-2224.

30. Georgiadis D, Schwarz S, Baumgartner RW, et al. Influence of positive end-expiratory pressure on intracranial pressure and cerebral perfusion pressure in patients with acute stroke. *Stroke.* 2001;32(9):2088-2092.

31. Muench E, Bauhuf C, Roth H, et al, Effects of positive end-expiratory pressure on regional cerebral blood flow, intracranial pressure, and brain tissue oxygenation. *Crit Care Med.* 2005;33(10):2367-2372.

32. Caricato A, Conti G, Della Corte F, et al. Effects of PEEP on the intracranial system of patients with head injury and subarachnoid hemorrhage: the role of respiratory system compliance. *J Trauma.* 2005;58(3):571-576.

33. Simon RP. Neurogenic pulmonary edema. *Neurol Clin.* 1993;11(2):309-323.

34. Baumann A, Audibert G, McDonnell J, Mertes PM. Neurogenic pulmonary edema. *Acta Anaesthesiol Scand.* 2007;51(4):447-455.

35. Hopkins RO, Weaver LK, Collingridge D. Two-year cognitive, emotional, and quality-of-life outcomes in acute respiratory distress syndrome. *Am J Respir Crit Care Med.* 2004;171:340-347.

36. Bernard GR. Acute respiratory distress syndrome. *Am J Respir Crit Care Med.* 2005;172:798-806.

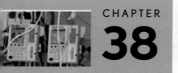

Deep Venous Thrombosis and Pulmonary Embolism

Ramya Lotano, MD
Hiren Shingala, MD

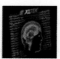

A 68-year-old man with a history of hypertension, type 2 diabetes mellitus, and coronary artery disease presents to the emergency department at 6:45 PM with sudden onset of right-sided weakness and difficulty swallowing and speaking. The patient's wife reports that the symptoms started at 6 PM. He was last noticed to be asymptomatic at 5 PM. He was brought to the emergency department by family members.

On arrival to the emergency department, his vital signs were as follows: blood pressure 180/100 mm Hg, heart rate 120 bpm, and respiratory rate 6 to 8 breaths/min. He had flaccid right upper and lower extremities. An emergent computed tomography (CT) scan of the head did not show an acute intracranial hemorrhage. Tissue plasminogen activator (tPA) was given per protocol and he was admitted to the intensive care unit (ICU).

What is the risk of venous thromboembolism in this patient?

Venous thromboembolism (VTE) is a common preventable complication in hospitalized patients. It includes a spectrum of disease, such as deep venous thrombosis (DVT) and pulmonary embolism (PE). General risk factors for DVT were first described by Virchow in the 19th century.[1] These include stasis, vascular wall abnormalities, and a hypercoagulable state; dynamic interaction between these factors leads to thrombosis (Figure 38-1).

The incidence of VTE is thought to be in excess of 600,000 cases per year in the United States.[2] The incidence of VTE is even higher in critically ill patients. In a prospective ultrasound study, DVT was detected in 33% of patients admitted to a medical ICU.[3] VTE carries a significant risk of morbidity and mortality. Most studies have shown that 15% to 20% of patients with PE have cardiovascular or respiratory compromise manifested by shock, syncope, respiratory distress, or hypoxemia.[4,5]

Most of the acute neurologic disorders often put patients in periods of prolonged immobilization, thus placing them at the highest risk for VTE. This is particularly true for patients with acute ischemic stroke and spinal cord injury. Studies that used I[125] fibrinogen as a screening method in patients with acute hemiplegic stroke have shown that the incidence of DVT is approximately 50% in the first 2 weeks in the absence of heparin prophylaxis.[6] The majority of these deep vein thromboses are asymptomatic and affect a paralyzed leg. The peak incidence of DVT is between day 2 and day 7.[7] The incidence of PE in patients with ischemic stroke has been estimated to be between 0.8% and 13%.[8,9] Mortality rate of untreated PE in unselected hospital patients is up to 30%.[10] One study has suggested that

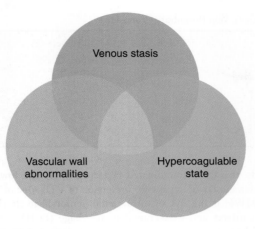

Figure 38-1. Virchow triad.

mortality rate of PE is even higher in patients with acute stroke.[11] The incidence of VTE in other neurocritical care conditions is listed in Table 38-1.

Options for prophylaxis against venous thromboembolism are being considered in the above patient. What is the best method to prevent VTE in this patient?

There are variety of methods available for prophylaxis against VTE. These methods are listed in Table 38-2.

Evidence for the use of physical methods to prevent DVT in patients with acute stroke is limited. A Cochrane review identified only two randomized controlled trials in this area.[16] It failed to show any conclusive benefits of physical methods (both graduated compression stockings [GCSs] and sequential compression devices [SCDs]) for DVT prophylaxis after acute stroke. As literature is scant, optimal timing and duration of the therapy remain unclear. Based on the evidence, we suggest that neither GCSs nor SCDs should be used as the only therapeutic strategy for prevention of VTE in patients with acute stroke.

Table 38-1. Incidence of Venous Thromboembolism (VTE) in Various Neurologic Critical Care Conditions

Clinical condition	Incidence of VTE
Acute ischemic CVA	0.8%-50%[6-9]
Subarachnoid hemorrhage	6.7%-18%[12,13]
Intracerebral hemorrhage	2.9%[12]
Traumatic brain injury	3.8%[12]
Spinal cord injury	9%-90%[14,15]

Abbreviation: CVA, cerebrovascular accident.

Table 38-2. Methods for Deep Vein Thrombosis Prophylaxis

Physical methods	Graduated compression stockings (GCSs)
	Sequential compression devices (SCDs)
Pharmacologic methods	Unfractionated heparin (UFH)
	Low-molecular-weight heparin (LMWH)
	Heparinoid
	Factor X inhibitors

Pharmacologic methods, mainly unfractionated heparin (UFH) and low-molecular-weight heparin (LMWH), remain the mainstay of therapy for prevention of VTE. One of the major concerns with the use of UFH or LMWH is the risk of intracranial hemorrhage (ICH), including hemorrhagic transformation of infarct and extracranial hemorrhage (ECH). Several studies have assessed UFH, LMWH, and heparinoids in VTE prophylaxis in patients with stroke. A systematic review by Kamphuisen and Agnelli[17] assessing the efficacy and risks of UFH and LMWH included 16 trials with 23,043 patients. They found that, compared to control, the use of high-dose UFH (> 15,000 units/d) was associated with a reduction in PE, but was associated with an increased risk of ICH and ECH. Use of low-dose UFH (≤ 15,000 units/d) was associated with a reduction in the risk of DVT, but not PE, without an increase in ICH or ECH. High-dose LMWH was associated with a reduction in both DVT and PE, but at the expense of an increased risk of ICH and ECH. Low-dose LMWH was associated with a reduction in both DVT and PE without an increase in the risk of ICH or ECH (Table 38-3). For low-dose LMWH, the number needed to treat for DVT was 7 and for PE was 38.

Several studies have compared UFH and LMWH for VTE prophylaxis in stroke patients.[18-20] A systematic review by Sandercock et al[21] comparing LMWH and UFH included 9 trials and 3137 patients. They suggested that compared to UFH, the use of LMWH or heparinoids is associated with a lower incidence of DVT. There was no significant difference in PE, ICH, hemorrhagic transformation of infarct, and death from all causes. However, the numbers of these events were very small. A meta-analysis by Shorr et al[22] suggested that the use of LMWH was associated with a reduction in proximal VTE and PE when compared to UFH. The risk of ICH, overall bleeding rate, and mortality rate were similar in both the UFH and the LMWH groups.

Table 38-3. Relative Risks of DVT, PE, ICH, and ECH Associated with Prophylaxis of UFH and LMWH to No Prophylaxis After Acute Ischemic Stroke

	DVT		PE		ICH		ECH	
	OR	95% CI	OR	95% CI	OR	95% CI	OR	95% CI
Low-dose UFH	0.17	0.11-0.26	0.83	0.53-1.31	1.67	0.97-2.87	1.58	0.89-2.81
High-dose UFH	No studies		0.49	0.29-0.83	3.86	2.41-6.19	4.74	2.88-7.78
Low-dose LMWH	0.34	0.19-2.59	0.36	0.15-0.87	1.39	0.53-3.57	1.44	0.13-16
High-dose LMWH	0.07	0.02-0.29	0.44	0.18-1.11	2.01	1.02-3.96	1.78	0.99-3.17

Abbreviations: CI, confidence interval; DVT, deep vein thrombosis; ECH, extracranial hemorrhage; ICH, intracranial hemorrhage; LMWH, low-molecular-weight heparin; OR, odds ratio; PE, pulmonary embolism; UFH, unfractionated heparin. (From Kamphuisen PW, Agnelli G. What is the optimal pharmacological prophylaxis for the prevention of deep-vein thrombosis and pulmonary embolism in patients with acute ischemic stroke? Thromb Res. 2007;119(3):265-274.)

In recent years, many newer options have become available for prevention of VTE in general medicine patients.[23] But to date, they have not been tested in specific neurologic conditions, including stroke.

Based on the available data, we recommend the use of LMWH as a primary method of DVT prophylaxis in patients with stroke unless contraindicated.

 The patient was placed on subcutaneous heparin for DVT prophylaxis. He had partial recovery of neurologic function within 24 to 48 hours. He was transferred to a neurologic floor on day 2. On day 4, he was transferred to a rehabilitation facility. On day 14, he developed acute shortness of breath associated with hypoxemia. You suspect pulmonary embolism.

What should you do next?

If acute PE is suspected, a careful assessment of the patient is necessary, including a history, a physical examination, a risk factor assessment, and laboratory/imaging studies (Table 38-4). Clinical features that may suggest DVT are leg pain, warmth, swelling, or redness.[24] Clinical features suggestive of acute PE are acute onset of dyspnea, pleuritic chest pain, tachycardia, and hypoxemia. Massive acute PE should be considered if the patient has acute-onset hypotension, severe hypoxemia, or cardiac

Table 38-4. Initial Investigations in a Patient with Suspected Acute Pulmonary Embolism

	Investigations	Comments
Clinical data	History and physical exam	• Helps in determining pretest probability of pulmonary emoblism
Labs	ABG	• Hypoxemia in massive pulmonary embolism • Not sensitive or specific
	Cardiac biomarkers—troponin and BNP	• Mainly used for risk stratification in massive/submassive pulmonary embolism • Not sensitive or specific
	D-dimer	• Used mainly in emergency room to rule out pulmonary embolism in low-risk situation • High negative predictive value in low-risk patients
Imaging	Chest x-ray	• Normal in most of the cases
	CT angiography	• Has become gold standard • Highly sensitive and specific
	Duplex ultrasound	• Might be normal in 30% patients with pulmonary embolism
	V/Q scan	• Highly sensitive • Normal chest x-ray is a prerequisite
	Pulmonary angiography	• The gold standard
Other	Echocardiogram	• Used for risk stratification based on right-heart strain

Abbreviations: ABG, arterial blood gas; BNP, B-natriuretic peptide; CT, computed tomography; V̇/Q̇, ventilation/perfusion.

arrest. The presence of clinical features of both DVT and PE is highly suggestive of the diagnosis, but is not specific.[24] Thus, further studies need to be done to make a final diagnosis.

Additional studies should be considered whenever acute PE is suspected. Electrocardiography (ECG) may reveal unexplained tachycardia, which is common in PE, but is nonspecific. An $S_1Q_3T_3$ pattern, right bundle branch block, or right-axis deviation on ECG might suggest massive PE, but these findings are nonspecific.[25] Arterial blood-gas analysis might show hypoxemia and/or respiratory alkalosis, although arterial Po_2 levels might be normal in patients with a PE.

D-Dimer assay can also be helpful to diagnose venous thrombosis and PE, but it is nonspecific. It can also be positive in cancer, trauma, infection, or other inflammatory states.[26] It is used mainly in the emergency department to rule out PE in low-risk patients.[26] The diagnostic value of the D-dimer assay in neurocritical care is not well established.

Other biomarkers may also provide valuable information in terms of severity of PE. Levels of cardiac troponins are often increased in massive PE and can be used for risk stratification, but they are not sensitive or specific and should not be used as the sole diagnostic tool.[27] Elevated levels of B-natriuretic peptide (BNP) may be seen in massive PE in response to ventricular stretching,[28] but these, too, are not sensitive or specific enough to be used as a diagnostic tool.

Chest radiography is routinely obtained in patients with acute shortness of breath and is typically normal in patients with PE.

Lately, multidetector CT angiography (MDCTA) of the chest has become the initial test of choice for diagnosis of acute PE (Figure 38-2). Sensitivity of helical CT angiography in the diagnosis of PE has been reported to be from 57% to 100%, and its specificity has been reported from 78% to 100%.[29,30] A recent study using MDCTA performed in outpatients with suspected PE has reported its sensitivity as 83% and specificity as 96%.[31] Sensitivity and specificity of MDCTA also depend on pretest clinical probability and location of the embolus. Patients with a high clinical suspicion of PE and negative MDCTA will require further testing to rule out PE. Advantages of MDCTA over ventilation/perfusion V̇/Q̇ scanning or conventional angiography include ease of performance, speed, and characterization of the right ventricle and pulmonary parenchyma. Given its advantages and high sensitivity and specificity, MDCTA has become the gold standard to diagnose or rule out PE. MDCTA does require administration of intravenous contrast, which can lead to nephrotoxicity in patients with elevated creatinine and needs to be kept in mind. There are no randomized controlled trials conducted in specific neurologic conditions to evaluate the efficacy of MDCTA in the diagnosis of

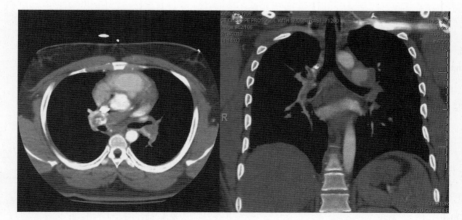

Figure 38-2. Multidetector computed tomography angiography showing pulmonary embolism in main pulmonary artery.

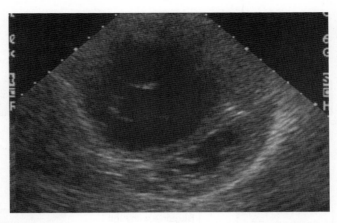

Figure 38-3. Short-axis view of an echocardiogram showing right ventricular dilatation in a patient with pulmonary embolism.

PE. But we do believe that findings from studies done in other patient populations can be extrapolated to neurologic patients.

Ventilation/perfusion scanning ($\dot{V}/\dot{Q}$ scan) had a major role in the diagnosis of PE a few years ago, but it has been largely replaced by MDCTA in recent years. It has good sensitivity and specificity. A normal $\dot{V}/\dot{Q}$ scan essentially rules out PE.[32] But there are some logistical issues with $\dot{V}/\dot{Q}$ scanning: patients are required to have a normal chest radiograph, and most of the patients in the ICU have an abnormal chest radiograph, thus limiting the value of the $\dot{V}/\dot{Q}$ scan as a diagnostic tool for PE in critical care setting.

Duplex ultrasonography of the lower extremity is often done, as most of the pulmonary emboli originate from lower extremities. It is positive in 10% to 20% of patients without any clinical features of DVT, and in 50% of patients with clinical features of DVT.[33] Thus, a negative duplex ultrasonography of lower extremities with high clinical suspicion does not rule out PE.[33]

Pulmonary angiography is the gold standard for diagnosis of PE, but it is an invasive procedure. Because the sensitivity and specificity of MDCTA have been similar to those of pulmonary angiography, MDCTA has largely replaced pulmonary angiography as a diagnostic tool for PE.

Echocardiography is a useful tool for risk stratification of massive and submassive PE. Some recent studies have suggested that right ventricular strain on echocardiography in normotensive patients puts these patients at higher risk of death. Signs of right ventricular strain on echocardiography include right ventricle dilation and right ventricle hypokinesis (Figure 38-3). Administration of thrombolytics has been suggested in this subgroup of patients but is debatable.[34,35] Echocardiography requires some training and can be done by intensivists.

Figure 38-4 shows general approach to a patient with suspected PE with CT angiography as the initial test.

The diagnosis of acute pulmonary embolism was confirmed by MDCTA. What do you do next in this patient's management?

Anticoagulation is the main therapy for a patient with acute PE. This must be considered on a case-by-case basis, taking into account the risk of intracranial bleed.

Points to consider prior to initiating treatment include:

- Whether anticoagulation should be initiated
- Which anticoagulant and what dose should be used based on clinical evidence supporting its use

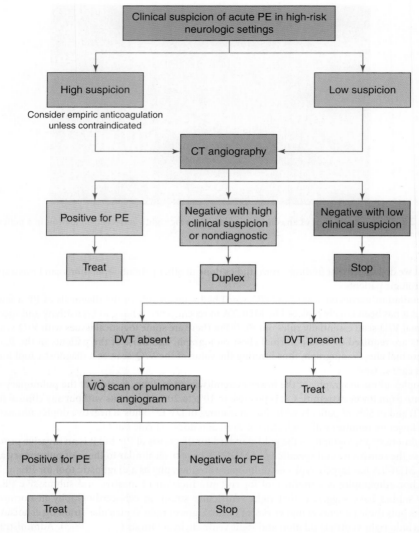

Figure 38-4. General approach to a patient with suspected pulmonary embolism (PE) with computed tomography (CT) angiography as the initial test. DVT, deep vein thrombosis; V̇/Q̇, ventilation/perfusion.

- Common complications
- Duration of therapy

Other aspects of treatment to consider include placement of an inferior vena cava filter, use of thrombolytics, and performance of an embolectomy. The efficacy of anticoagulant therapy depends on achieving a therapeutic level within the first 24 hours of therapy.[36-38]

Available therapeutic options include the following:[39]

- Subcutaneous (SC) LMWH
- Intravenous (IV) UFH

- SC UFH
- SC fondaparinux

Special Considerations in Anticoagulation in the Neurologic Critical Care Patient Population

Patients with acute or prior intracerebral hemorrhage

The availability of data or expert consensus regarding optimal treatment for VTE is poor in this patient population. In a review, the estimated risk of fatal PE in the acute ICH population with untreated DVT or nonfatal PE was about 25%.[40] This risk is too high to deny treatment for VTE to patients with good neurologic prognosis.

The risk of worsening ICH with or without anticoagulation is unknown. The estimated risk of recurrent ICH with anticoagulation is estimated to be 3% to 5%.[41] In the absence of anticoagulation the rate of ICH is 0.4% to 3%.[42]

Based on the above data and given the known efficacy of heparin and LMWH in the nonstroke patient population, patients with proximal DVT and nonfatal PE should be considered for treatment with heparin and LMWH. Subsequent treatment with a reduced dose of oral anticoagulation warfarin after 1 week with a target international normalized ratio (INR) of 2.0 (range of 2-2.5) for 3 months is recommended.[43,44] Aggressive management of blood pressure is critical to reduce the risk of subsequent bleeding.

In patients with recent ICH with nonmassive PE who have adequate cardiopulmonary reserve and negative ultrasonography for proximal DVT, the 3-month risk of recurrent PE is very low. In this population anticoagulation may be withheld.[45]

Patients with an unruptured intracranial aneurysm

Unruptured intracranial aneurysms are detected in approximately 3% of adults who undergo intracranial arterial imaging. Subarachnoid hemorrhage from a ruptured aneurysm is associated with 40% increase in short-term mortality and 50% increase in permanent neurologic injury. Rates of rupture vary according to size and location (posterior communicating artery); risk factors include age older than 60 years, female gender, and tobacco smoking.[46]

There are no randomized clinical trials reporting data supporting higher rupture rates with the use of anticoagulation. The available clinical trials in patients with ICH so infrequently include patients with subarachnoid hemorrhage; therefore, it is difficult to exclude higher rates of hemorrhage with anticoagulation. Therefore, the decision must be individualized according to the best clinical judgment of benefits versus risks.

Patients with brain tumors

Because of a hypercoagulable state, patients with brain tumors have a substantially high risk of developing VTE. There is concern, however, that antithrombotic agents can precipitate hemorrhage into the tumor site. The risk factors for developing VTE include age older than 60 years, large tumor size, neurosurgery within 2 months, leg paresis, and treatment with chemotherapy.[47,48]

Recommendations

1. Anticoagulation should be used in all patients except those who have a high rate of ICH, such as patients with metastatic renal cell carcinoma, melanoma, and choriocarcinoma. Given the high rate of recurrent VTE, patients with malignant glioma should be anticoagulated long-term.

2. For patients with brain tumors who have a high risk of hemorrhage as above, place an inferior vena cava filter if there is residual metastatic disease.

Inferior Vena Cava Filters

Inferior vena cava (IVC) filters are placed percutaneously via the jugular or femoral approach under fluoroscopy or ultrasound guidance. The filter is typically placed in the infrarenal position. In patients who demonstrate renal vein thrombosis, an IVC clot above the renal vein will require the filter to be placed in the suprarenal position.

Filter placement protects the pulmonary vascular bed but does nothing to decrease the predisposition to thromboembolism or lessen thrombosis. Small thrombi can pass through patent filters or through collaterals around obstructed vessels. Two types of filters are currently available: retrievable and nonretrievable filters.

The only validated indications for IVC filter placement are:

- An absolute contraindication to anticoagulation
- Failure of anticoagulation therapy (ie, recurrent thromboembolism despite therapeutic levels of anticoagulation)
- Venous thromboembolism in a patient with a high risk of bleeding

Complications of IVC filter placement include:

- Filter erosion through the IVC wall
- Filter embolization/migration[49]
- IVC obstruction by a subsequent clot[50]
- Local complications such as hematoma related to time of insertion
- Insertion site thrombosis
- Venous insufficiency

Prophylactic IVC filter placement may increase the relative risk of deep venous thrombosis after acute spinal cord injury.[51]

! CRITICAL CONSIDERATIONS

- Anticoagulation should be used in all patients except those who have a high rate of ICH, such as those with metastatic renal cell carcinoma, melanoma, and choriocarcinoma. Given the high rate of recurrent VTE, patients with malignant glioma should be anticoagulated long-term.
- For patients with brain tumors who have a high risk of hemorrhage, place an inferior vena cava filter if there is residual metastatic disease.
- Based on current available evidence, IVC filters are indicated in only a small proportion of patients who have venous thromboembolism.
- In situations where anticoagulation is contraindicated, the use of a retrievable filter is recommended. Anticoagulation should be initiated after filter placement as soon as it is safe to do so and the filter should then be removed shortly thereafter.[52]

REFERENCES

1. Virchow R. Thrombosis and emboli. In: Virchow R, ed. *Gesammelte Abhandlungen zur Wissenschaftlichen Medicin.* Frankfurt, Meidinger: Sohn & Co.;1856:1846-1856. Reprint edition: Virchow R 1998 (AC Matzdorff, WR Bell, transl. Canton, MA: Science History Publications).

2. Prevention of venous thrombosis and pulmonary embolism. NIH Consensus Development. *JAMA.* 1986;256(6):744-749.

3. Corrigan PW, Hirschbeck JN, Wolfe M. Memory and vigilance training to improve social perception in schizophrenia. *Schizophr Res.* 1995;17(3):257-265.

4. De Takats G. The urokinase pulmonary embolism trial. *Am J Surg.* 1973;126(3):311-313.

5. Value of the ventilation/perfusion scan in acute pulmonary embolism. Results of the prospective investigation of pulmonary embolism diagnosis (PIOPED). The PIOPED Investigators. *JAMA.* 1990;263(20):2753-2759.

6. Kelly J, Rudd A, Lewis R, Hunt BJ. Venous thromboembolism after acute stroke. *Stroke.* 2001;32(1):262-267.

7. Brandstater ME, Roth EJ, Siebens HC. Venous thromboembolism in stroke: literature review and implications for clinical practice. *Arch Phys Med Rehabil.* 1992;73(5-S):S379-S391.

8. The International Stroke Trial (IST): a randomised trial of aspirin, subcutaneous heparin, both, or neither among 19,435 patients with acute ischaemic stroke. International Stroke Trial Collaborative Group. *Lancet.* 1997;349(9065):1569-1581.

9. Davenport RJ, Dennis MS, Wellwood I, Warlow CP. Complications after acute stroke. *Stroke.* 1996;27(3):415-420.

10. Dalen JE, Alpert JS. Natural history of pulmonary embolism. *Prog Cardiovasc Dis.* 1975;17(4):259-270.

11. Wijdicks EF, Scott JP. Pulmonary embolism associated with acute stroke. *Mayo Clin Proc.* 1997;72(4):297-300.

12. Kim KS, Brophy GM. Symptomatic venous thromboembolism: incidence and risk factors in patients with spontaneous or traumatic intracranial hemorrhage. *Neurocrit Care.* 2009;11(1):28-33.

13. Ray WZ, Strom RG, Blackburn SL, Ashley WW, Sicard GA, Rich KM. Incidence of deep venous thrombosis after subarachnoid hemorrhage. *J Neurosurg.* 2009;110(5):1010-1014.

14. Attia J, Ray JG, Cook DJ, Douketis J, Ginsberg JS, Geerts WH. Deep vein thrombosis and its prevention in critically ill adults. *Arch Intern Med.* 2001;161(10):1268-1279.

15. Aito S, Pieri A, D'Andrea M, Marcelli F, Cominelli E. Primary prevention of deep venous thrombosis and pulmonary embolism in acute spinal cord injured patients. *Spinal Cord.* 2002;40(6):300-303.

16. Mazzone C, Chiodo GF, Sandercock P, Miccio M, Salvi R. Physical methods for preventing deep vein thrombosis in stroke. *Cochrane Database Syst Rev.* 2004(4):CD001922.

17. Kamphuisen PW, Agnelli G. What is the optimal pharmacological prophylaxis for the prevention of deep-vein thrombosis and pulmonary embolism in patients with acute ischemic stroke? *Thromb Res.* 2007;119(3):265-274.

18. Hillbom M, Erila T, Sotaniemi K, Tatlisumak T, Sarna S, Kaste M. Enoxaparin vs heparin for prevention of deep-vein thrombosis in acute ischaemic stroke: a randomized, double-blind study. *Acta Neurol Scand.* 2002;106(2):84-92.

19. Diener HC, Ringelstein EB, von Kummer R, et al. Prophylaxis of thrombotic and embolic events in acute ischemic stroke with the low-molecular-weight heparin Certoparin: results of the PROTECT Trial. *Stroke.* 2006;37(1):139-144.

20. Sherman DG, Albers GW, Bladin C, et al. The efficacy and safety of enoxaparin versus unfractionated heparin for the prevention of venous thromboembolism after acute ischaemic stroke (PREVAIL Study): an open-label randomised comparison. *Lancet.* 2007;369(9570):1347-1355.

21. Sandercock PA, Counsell C, Tseng MC. Low-molecular-weight heparins or heparinoids versus standard unfractionated heparin for acute ischaemic stroke. *Cochrane Database Syst Rev.* 2008(3):CD000119.

22. Shorr AF, Jackson WL, Sherner JH, Moores LK. Differences between low-molecular-weight and unfractionated heparin for venous thromboembolism prevention following ischemic stroke: a meta-analysis. *Chest.* 2008;133(1):149-155.

23. Garcia D, Libby E, Crowther MA. The new oral anticoagulants. *Blood.* 2010;115(1):15-20.

24. Tapson VF. Acute pulmonary embolism. *N Engl J Med.* 2008;358(10):1037-1052.

25. Stein PD, Terrin ML, Hales CA, et al. Clinical, laboratory, roentgenographic, and electrocardiographic findings in patients with acute pulmonary embolism and no pre-existing cardiac or pulmonary disease. *Chest.* 1991;100(3):598-603.

26. Stein PD, Hull RD, Patel KC, et al. D-Dimer for the exclusion of acute venous thrombosis and pulmonary embolism: a systematic review. *Ann Intern Med.* 2004;140(8):589-602.

27. Pruszczyk P, Bochowicz A, Torbicki A, et al. Cardiac troponin T monitoring identifies high-risk

group of normotensive patients with acute pulmonary embolism. *Chest.* 2003;123(6):1947-1952.

28. Melanson SE, Laposata M, Camargo CA Jr, et al. Combination of D-dimer and amino-terminal pro-B-type natriuretic peptide testing for the evaluation of dyspneic patients with and without acute pulmonary embolism. *Arch Pathol Lab Med.* 2006;130(9):1326-1329.

29. Rathbun SW, Raskob GE, Whitsett TL. Sensitivity and specificity of helical computed tomography in the diagnosis of pulmonary embolism: a systematic review. *Ann Intern Med.* 2000;132(3):227-232.

30. Hiorns MP, Mayo JR. Spiral computed tomography for acute pulmonary embolism. *Can Assoc Radiol J.* 2002;53(5):258-268.

31. Stein PD, Fowler SE, Goodman LR, et al. Multidetector computed tomography for acute pulmonary embolism. *N Engl J Med.* 2006;354(22):2317-2327.

32. Fedullo PF, Tapson VF. Clinical practice. The evaluation of suspected pulmonary embolism. *N Engl J Med.* 2003;349(13):1247-1256.

33. Kearon C, Ginsberg JS, Hirsh J. The role of venous ultrasonography in the diagnosis of suspected deep venous thrombosis and pulmonary embolism. *Ann Intern Med.* 1998;129(12):1044-1049.

34. Todd JL, Tapson VF. Thrombolytic therapy for acute pulmonary embolism: a critical appraisal. *Chest.* 2009;135(5):1321-1329.

35. Zamanian RT, Gould MK. Effectiveness and cost effectiveness of thrombolysis in patients with acute pulmonary embolism. *Curr Opin Pulm Med.* 2008;14(5):422-426.

36. Hull RD, Raskob GE, Pineo GF, et al. Subcutaneous low-molecular-weight heparin compared with continuous intravenous heparin in the treatment of proximal-vein thrombosis. *N Engl J Med.* 1992;326(15):975-982.

37. Raschke RA, Reilly BM, Guidry JR, Fontana JR, Srinivas S. The weight-based heparin dosing nomogram compared with a "standard care" nomogram. A randomized controlled trial. *Ann Intern Med.* 1993;119(9):874-881.

38. Raschke RA, Gollihare B, Peirce JC. The effectiveness of implementing the weight-based heparin nomogram as a practice guideline. *Arch Intern Med.* 1996;156(15):1645-1649.

39. Kearon C, Kahn SR, Agnelli G, Goldhaber S, Raskob GE, Comerota AJ. Antithrombotic therapy for venous thromboembolic disease: American College of Chest Physicians evidence-based clinical practice guidelines (8th edition). *Chest.* 2008;133(6 Suppl):S454-S545.

40. Kelly J, Hunt BJ, Lewis RR, Rudd A. Anticoagulation or inferior vena cava filter placement for patients with primary intracerebral hemorrhage developing venous thromboembolism? *Stroke.* 2003;34(12):2999-3005.

41. Eckman MH, Rosand J, Knudsen KA, Singer DE, Greenberg SM. Can patients be anticoagulated after intracerebral hemorrhage? A decision analysis. *Stroke.* 2003;34(7):1710-1716.

42. Bailey RD, Hart RG, Benavente O, Pearce LA. Recurrent brain hemorrhage is more frequent than ischemic stroke after intracranial hemorrhage. *Neurology.* 2001;56(6):773-777.

43. Kearon C, Ginsberg JS, Anderson DR, et al. Comparison of 1 month with 3 months of anticoagulation for a first episode of venous thromboembolism associated with a transient risk factor. *J Thromb Haemost.* 2004;2(5):743-749.

44. Kearon C, Gent M, Hirsh J, et al. A comparison of three months of anticoagulation with extended anticoagulation for a first episode of idiopathic venous thromboembolism. *N Engl J Med.* 1999;340(12):901-907.

45. Stein PD, Hull RD, Raskob GE. Withholding treatment in patients with acute pulmonary embolism who have a high risk of bleeding and negative serial noninvasive leg tests. *Am J Med.* 2000;109(4):301-306.

46. Wermer MJ, van der Schaaf IC, Algra A, Rinkel GJ. Risk of rupture of unruptured intracranial aneurysms in relation to patient and aneurysm characteristics: an updated meta-analysis. *Stroke.* 2007;38(4):1404-1410.

47. Marras LC, Geerts WH, Perry JR. The risk of venous thromboembolism is increased throughout the course of malignant glioma: an evidence-based review. *Cancer.* 2000;89(3):640-646.

48. Semrad TJ, O'Donnell R, Wun T, et al. Epidemiology of venous thromboembolism in 9489 patients with malignant glioma. *J Neurosurg.* 2007;106(4):601-608.

49. Owens CA, Bui JT, Knuttinen MG, et al. Intracardiac migration of inferior vena cava filters: review of published data. *Chest.* 2009;136(3):877-887.

50. Ahmad I, Yeddula K, Wicky S, Kalva SP. Clinical sequelae of thrombus in an inferior vena cava filter. *Cardiovasc Intervent Radiol.* 2010;33(2):285-289.

51. Gorman PH, Qadri SF, Rao-Patel A. Prophylactic inferior vena cava (IVC) filter placement may increase the relative risk of deep venous thrombosis after acute spinal cord injury. *J Trauma.* 2009;66(3):707-712.

52. Ingber S, Geerts WH. Vena caval filters: current knowledge, uncertainties and practical approaches. *Curr Opin Hematol.* 2009;16(5):402-406.

CHAPTER

39

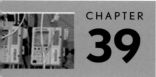

Percutaneous Tracheostomy

David B. Seder, MD
Jason A. Yahwak, MD

A 30-year-old man is admitted after an unhelmeted bicycling accident in which he suffered a skull fracture, traumatic subarachnoid and subdural hemorrhages, bifrontal contusions, and diffuse axonal injury. He was intubated without medications in the field, and on presentation, the Glasgow Coma Scale (GCS) score is 4. Computed tomography (CT) scan of the neck does not reveal bony injury to the cervical spine. A fiberoptic intracranial pressure (ICP) device is placed, and ICP, cerebral perfusion pressure (CPP), and brain tissue oxygen tension (PbtO$_2$) are monitored. On hospital day 5, the GCS score is 5, ICP is 18 mm Hg, CPP is 70 mm Hg, and PbtO$_2$ in the right frontal lobe near a contusion is 24 mm Hg. His cardiopulmonary status is stable. A rigid cervical collar is in place, and he is maintained on the controlled mechanical ventilation (CMV) mode at a set rate of 14 × 550 mL (actual respiratory rate [RR] is 21 beaths/min), fraction of inspired oxygen (FIO$_2$) of 0.35, and positive end-expiratory pressure (PEEP) of 5.

Is tracheostomy indicated?

This patient is certain to have a prolonged course of mechanical ventilation as a result of neurologic failure, and he should undergo tracheostomy. Although prolonged endotracheal intubation with a modern high-volume low-pressure cuffed tube is safe, infrequently resulting in subglottic stenosis or vocal cord injury,[1] tracheostomy offers several advantages in patients with severe brain injury. These include facilitation of weaning from mechanical ventilation,[2,3] prolonged access to the lower airways for secretions management, improved comfort,[4,5] and earlier mobilization for physical and occupational therapy. Tracheostomy often makes possible discontinuation of sedating medications,[5] facilitating the neurologic examination, and may allow brain-injured patients with good cardiopulmonary function to be completely disconnected from mechanical ventilation, preventing the common complications of atelectasis and respiratory muscle atrophy. Disadvantages include perioperative and long-term complications of the procedure and introduction of a potential reservoir of bacterial colonization into the airway. General indications for tracheostomy in the neurocritically ill are presented in Table 39-1.

What is the optimal timing of tracheostomy?

Optimal timing of tracheostomy in all patient groups is controversial. One randomized single-center trial in the medical intensive care unit (ICU) suggested lower mortality and other benefits when tracheostomy was performed by day 3 as opposed to day 14,[6] but this finding was not replicated in two subsequent multicenter randomized trials.[7,8] A meta-analysis suggested benefits to early tracheostomy in patients expected to receive mechanical ventilation for prolonged periods,[9] and multiple retrospective studies

Table 39-1. Indications for Tracheostomy in the Neurocritically Ill

Prolonged mechanical ventilation (cardiopulmonary etiology)
Inadequate airway protective reflexes
Weak cough and failure to expectorate respiratory secretions
Bulbar dysfunction
Prolonged coma
Upper airway obstruction or injury

suggest benefit when tracheostomy is performed before day 7, compared to delayed tracheostomy.[10-15] A recent multicenter randomized controlled trial showed a nonsignificant trend toward less ventilator-associated pneumonia in critically ill patients randomized to early tracheostomy vs prolonged mechanical intubation, while the secondary outcome measures of ventilator-free days, ICU-free days, and survival to ICU discharge favored early tracheostomy.[16] Recent trauma guidelines suggest early tracheostomy for patients with severe traumatic brain injury.[17] Considerations in the timing of tracheostomy are summarized in Table 39-2.

What are some important anatomic considerations of tracheostomy?

Open surgical tracheostomy and, to some degree, modified percutaneous tracheostomy offer direct visualization and palpation of the anatomic structures of the anterior neck, while a pure percutaneous technique relies on careful planning and palpation, familiarity with neck anatomy, and sometimes ultrasound and/or bronchoscopic guidance for optimal results. All three techniques are supported by a vast collective experience, and the experience of the surgeon or proceduralist[18,19] is a more important factor in preventing complications than the technique used or subspecialty of the physician.[20-22]

Tracheostomy is typically performed between the second and third tracheal rings, well above the innominate artery and below the thyroid isthmus. Major vessels traverse the anterior neck, including the innominate artery, inferior thyroid vein, and carotid artery, and significant anatomic variance in these structures is present within the population. Accidental puncture of large arteries and veins can be averted by routine ultrasonographic imaging prior to the procedure,[23,24] especially in obese patients. The surgical field should always be carefully palpated prior to incision and cannulation, but anatomically variant veins will be detected in only the thinnest patients without dissection or ultrasonographic imaging.

Table 39-2. Advantages and Disadvantages to Early Tracheostomy after Acute Brain Injury

Advantages	Disadvantages
Protection against large-volume aspiration	Small number of patients will have a tracheostomy unnecessarily
Discontinuation of sedation	Surgical complications
Allows vocal cords and folds to close	Does not protect against microaspiration
Early disconnection from mechanical ventilation	Procedure may transiently cause elevated intracranial pressure
Early mobilization	Stigma of the procedure

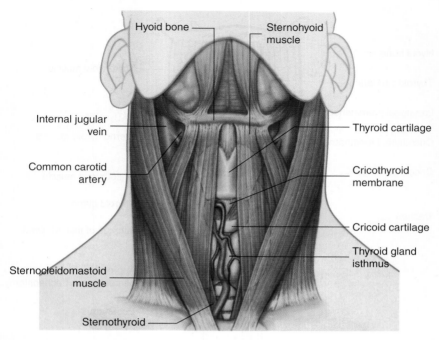

Figure 39-1. Normal neck anatomy. *(From Heffner JE, Sahn SA. The technique of tracheostomy and cricothyroidotomy. J Crit Illness. 1987;2(1):79-87.)*[26]

Normal neck anatomy is shown in Figures 39-1 and 39-2. The rigid cricoid cartilage is located just inferior to the vocal cords. At the base of this structure, typically superficial and easily palpated, is the cricothyroid membrane—the preferred location for an emergent surgical airway in nonintubated patients owing to its proximity to the skin. Tracheostomy is performed lower, owing to the potential for laryngeal injury with cricothyroidotomy and the tendency for a higher tracheostomy to interfere with laryngeal function. The anterior tracheal wall is cartilaginous and formed by 18 to 22 rings, while the posterior trachea is membranous, thin, and separates the trachea from the esophagus. When tracheomalacia is present, the trachea is collapsible, and anterior and posterior tracheal walls appose under downward pressure, so that bronchoscopic guidance or an open surgical technique should be employed to prevent esophageal injury or paratracheal placement and to facilitate the procedure.[25]

Tracheostomy tube selection

Clinicians should carefully consider the type and size of tracheostomy tube to be placed. In obese patients, a tube with inadequate depth is at risk of becoming dislodged, resulting in loss of the airway, or may become posteriorly angulated in the neck, resulting in partial airway occlusion against the tracheal wall and increasing the risk of suction trauma and subsequent tracheal stenosis. Conversely, thin patients whose tracheostomy tubes are overlong may suffer erosion of the stoma owing to angulation and pressure causing soft tissue injury, increasing the risk of tracheoinnominate fistula. In all cases, a midline insertion and appropriate angle within the airway are least likely to result in tracheal complications. Different commonly employed tubes have dramatically different inner and outer diameters, angulations, depths, and lengths. Tracheostomy tubes with fenestration (for speech), with variable ventilator interfaces, with and without cuffs, with adjustable lengths, with armor, and

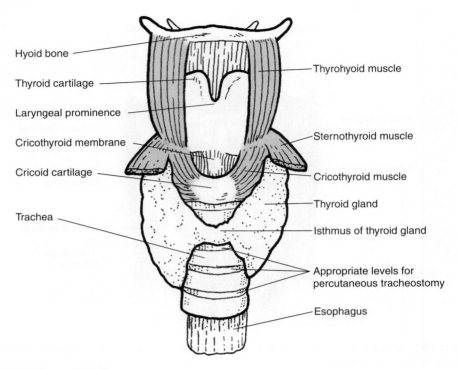

Figure 39-2. Normal neck anatomy.

with foam or air cuffs are all available from manufacturers, and familiarity with a variety of these products is advised.[27]

Who should perform tracheostomy?

Percutaneous and modified percutaneous tracheostomy techniques are routinely performed by surgeons, and increasingly by anesthesiologists and intensivists of various backgrounds.[19-21] The procedure is considered an advanced airway technique, building on expertise in endotracheal intubation, bronchoscopy, and other guidewire-based percutaneous techniques. Multiple percutaneous tracheostomy techniques and commercially produced kits are available, and both the American College of Chest Physicians[28] and European Respiratory Society[29] have published guidelines for training and certification of competency, typically requiring a minimum number of procedures and a period of supervised apprenticeship. Tracheostomy should be performed by an experienced operator,[18,19] with a system in place to provide protocolized tracheostomy care and long-term follow-up. Table 39-3 delineates elements of a successful percutaneous tracheostomy program.

How should percutaneous or modified percutaneous tracheostomy be performed?

Percutaneous or modified percutaneous tracheostomy performed at the bedside offers convenience and cost savings when compared to surgical techniques, with a similar safety profile.[21,30,31] In the brain-injured population, special attention should be paid to intracranial pressure, cervical spine

Table 39-3. An Institutional Approach to Safe Tracheostomy Management

Safety concern	Strategies for minimizing harm
Selection of appropriate candidates	Institutional guidelines clearly stratifying procedural risk, consideration of open tracheostomy or prolonged intubation when more appropriate
Attention to coagulopathy, appropriate tube selection, and special circumstances	Reversal of coagulopathy whenever possible, availability and familiarity with a wide variety of tracheostomy tubes, special measures for cervical spine protection and management of intracranial pressure
Safe procedural technique and conditions	Institutional standards for competency and credentialing, procedures closely supervised or performed by credentialed clinicians, proper equipment, and procedural conditions
Safe tracheostomy care	Institutional protocols and guidelines for tracheostomy management by nurses and respiratory therapists
Appropriate follow-up	Standardized outpatient follow-up for tracheal stenosis, vocal cord function, and skin problems related to tracheostomy

injury, and strict preservation of metabolic and hemodynamic homeostasis during the procedure. These issues are described in greater detail below.

Procedural Technique

The neck is examined and anatomic features noted. Is the trachea easily palpated? Note the thyroid and cricoid cartilage and the cricothyroid ligament. Are the cartilaginous rings easily palpated and rigid? Is the innominate artery palpable in or above the sternal notch, or are there thyroid anomalies that warrant further evaluation? Can the neck be moderately extended to bring the trachea closer to the skin surface? If obesity, deformity or anatomic irregularity, prior tracheostomy, or other concerns exist, then ultrasonographic or CT evaluation may be necessary prior to the procedure.[23,24] Surgical marking pens are often used to define procedural anatomy prior to incising the skin.

The neck is prepared in sterile fashion, and the skin and subdermal tissues overlying the second/third cartilaginous interspace is infused with a lidocaine-epinephrine mixture. After analgesia and sedation, a transverse incision is performed. In the pure percutaneous technique, the trachea is then cannulated without blunt dissection and a guidewire is inserted. In the modified technique, blunt dissection down to the trachea is performed and the trachea is cannulated under direct visualization prior to guidewire insertion. Not all proceduralists use bronchoscopic guidance to visualize the tracheal puncture,[21,32,33] but such visualization adds a measure of safety, especially when a pure percutaneous technique is used, in that tracheal placement is confirmed at the time of puncture, midline insertion is confirmed, and injury to the posterior tracheal wall or esophagus is avoided with certainty.

Confirmation of tracheostomy placement is critical, since most of the rare fatalities associated with the procedure occur either because of paratracheal placement or when the tube is dislodged from the airway and cannot be rapidly replaced. Tracheal insertion may be verified by direct visualization, capnography, ventilator pressure-volume waveforms, breath sounds and chest rise, or gas exchange—typically, multimodal verification is suggested. The tube is then sutured into place.

What are the complications of tracheostomy?

Percutaneous tracheostomy has a mortality rate below 1%.[34-36] Reported complications vary widely: a 2006 report described 1000 sequential percutaneous tracheostomy procedures using a single technique, including more than 50% in patients regarded as "high risk" owing to either hypoxemia, cervical spine injury, or coagulopathy, with an overall 1.5% incidence of significant periprocedural complications.[34] At the other extreme, a 2005 series reported 22.2% overall complications (though 90% of these were considered minor) in 474 patients using a mixed series of procedural techniques.[37] This wide variability in complications, which persists in review of other published case series, suggests that procedural safety may depend on the systematic application of a single safe technique (Table 39-4).

The most serious early complication of percutaneous tracheostomy is paratracheal insertion—potentially fatal if unrecognized, but easily avoided by systematic and multimodal assessment of tube position; by using longer tracheotomy tubes in obese patients, which seat securely in the trachea; by securing tubes appropriately; and by cautious perioperative manipulation and assessment. Great care should be taken to avoid early displacement of the tracheostomy tube, and protocols should be in place to manage tube malposition. If malposition occurs and the airway is lost, oral reintubation should be immediately performed to reestablish a definitive airway.

Pneumothorax and pneumomediastinum are uncommon. In older series, damage to the posterior tracheal wall was noted in up to 12% of procedures,[36,38] but this complication can be easily avoided by employing bronchoscopic guidance. Minor bleeding from the stoma is common, but because of the tamponading effect of the tracheostomy tube, it is self-limited, and when it continues, it can often be controlled by packing gauze circumferentially around the tube and then tightly into the stoma on the outside of the tube. Removal of the tracheostomy tube to evaluate bleeding should almost always be avoided unless arterial repair is clearly necessary or the airway has been lost. With the

Table 39-4. Complications of Tracheostomy and Their Management

Complication	Evaluation	Management	Frequency
Loss of the airway	Bronchoscopy or surgical	Immediate oral reintubation	Infrequent
Pneumothorax	Physical exam, CXR	Tube thoracostomy	Rare
Minor bleeding	Bronchoscopic verification that bleeding is external	Pack stoma circumferentially, reverse coagulopathy	Frequent
Stomal infection	Culture drainage	Antibiotics	Rare
Major bleeding	Bronchoscopy	Surgical exploration	Rare
TIF	Sternotomy	Overinflate cuff, apply direct manual pressure to artery	< 0.3%
Tracheal stenosis	Bronchoscopy	Laser, surgery, stent	Unknown; clinically significant stenosis is infrequent
Elevated ICP	ICP monitoring	Increase minute ventilation: remove bronchoscope, increase RR	Infrequent
Stomal ulceration	May need to remove tube to evaluate stoma fully	Stabilize tube, measures to prevent traction, protective dressings, consider prescription for cellulitis	Infrequent

Abbreviations: CXR, chest x-ray; ICP, intracranial pressure; RR, respiratory rate; TIF, tracheoinnominate artery fistula.

dilational technique, bleeding into the airway *after* completion of the procedure is unusual, though minor bleeding into the airway *during* the procedure is not uncommon. More significant hemorrhage can occur if blood vessels are damaged during insertion. This bleeding rarely requires surgical or endovascular repair. Patients undergoing open surgical tracheostomy are more likely to experience significant bleeding and wound infections.[36,39]

Life-threatening bleeding may occur in the setting of tracheoinnominate fistula (TIF). TIF is historically reported to occur in 0.3% of tracheostomies—typically within a month of the procedure.[36,38] In most patients, the innominate artery crosses the trachea anteriorly at approximately the ninth tracheal ring,[25] but anatomic variation is not uncommon, and the artery may ride in or above the sternal notch. Low-placed tracheostomy tubes or pressure necrosis, more commonly occurring at the tip of the tube than at the insertion site, can lead to erosion into the innominate artery. TIF can result from erosion, excessive traction on the tube, chronic overinflation of the tracheostomy cuff, excessive angulation of the tube, or stomal infection. If TIF occurs, the first responder should attempt superinflation of the cuff and anterior traction on the tube, to compress the innominate artery against the posterior sternum. It is also possible to insert a finger into the stoma and provide anterior compression of the innominate artery against the back of the sternum, though the airway must be maintained. Urgent sternotomy and surgical ligation of the artery or endovascular repair is then required to control bleeding.[40,41]

Tracheal stenosis may develop at the level of tracheostomy insertion, at the cuff, or at the tip of the tube.[36,38] The condition is usually a result of pressure necrosis of the tracheal wall from a tight-fitting tube, high-pressure cuff, off-midline insertion, or mechanical irritation due to frequent levering of the tube by poorly supported ventilator tubing or head movements. Pressure necrosis of the trachea leads to formation of a fibrous scar and transmural airway narrowing. Symptoms usually manifest 2 to 6 weeks after decannulation, but have been reported up to 6 months after tracheostomy removal. Patients may present with difficulty clearing secretions, exertional dyspnea, persistent cough, or stridor. Flattening of the inspiratory limb on the flow-volume loop suggests at least 80% narrowing of the tracheal lumen. Tracheal stenosis may be suggested by CT images, but should be confirmed by bronchoscopic visualization. Treatment involves laser excision, surgery, or tracheal stent placement.[38]

What special circumstances should be considered?

There are at least five factors to consider when determining risk for periprocedural complications of percutaneous tracheostomy. These circumstances are outlined below.

Coagulopathy

Although small series have suggested the safety of percutaneous tracheostomy in the settings of coagulopathy and thrombocytopenia, standard practice is the complete reversal of coagulopathy to an international normalized ratio (INR) of less than 1.5, a normal partial thromboplastin time (PTT), and platelets greater than 100,000 whenever possible. Under high-risk circumstances, it is occasionally necessary to consider tracheostomy in coagulopathic patients, such as those with mechanical heart valves, recent deep vein thrombosis/pulmonary embolism, or advanced liver disease. Although these procedures are often well tolerated, the actual risk of serious bleeding is unknown, and the decision to proceed with tracheostomy is based on careful accounting of the anticipated benefits of the procedure.[42-45]

Intracranial Hypertension

Several case series suggest that the percutaneous tracheostomy procedure causes a significant increase in ICP.[46,47] These increases may be due to pain, fear, or hypoventilation—all of which must be studiously avoided by proceduralists. Hypoventilation during tracheostomy of a patient with elevated ICP or poor intracranial compliance at baseline may result in catastrophic intracranial hypertension, so end-tidal CO_2 and ICP monitoring are therefore indicated when ICP is known or suspected to be elevated, when intracranial compliance is poor, or when brain imaging suggests mass effect. Under these circumstances, it is advisable to delay tracheostomy. If tracheostomy is performed, bronchoscopy time must be minimized,[48] patients may require modest hyperventilation prior to the procedure, the airway must never be compromised, and care must be taken to ensure that sedation and analgesia do not lead to hypotension. Deep sedation and excellent pain control are essential, so it is advisable to have vasopressors on hand at the onset of the procedure.

Cervical Spine Injury

Although case series suggest procedural success,[35,49,50] the safety of percutaneous tracheostomy in patients with an unstable or a suspected unstable cervical spine remains unknown, and the procedure should be undertaken with caution and trepidation. In-line cervical stabilization and posterior support are critical, and even modest downward pressure from the dilations must be absolutely avoided. Under these conditions, the modified percutaneous or open surgical techniques are preferred in order to minimize downward force. A newer percutaneous device (Ciaglia Blue Dolphin, Cook Medical, Bloomington, IN), based on balloon dilatation, may offer the advantage of substituting a radial vector of force for the usual tangential vectors, but safety data are not yet available in this population or with the device under these circumstances. Bronchoscopy is a crucial airway management measure in this population since neck manipulation must be minimized, and in the event of accidental loss of the airway, the bronchoscope facilitates safe reintubation.

Obesity

Percutaneous tracheostomy is frequently performed in obese and morbidly obese patients, but it is likely that their periprocedural complications are higher. One study evaluated 474 patients who underwent percutaneous tracheostomy, of whom 73 were obese (defined as body mass index [BMI] > 27.5), and found a higher complications rate among obese than nonobese patients (43.8% vs 18.2%; $P < .001$).[35] This finding was echoed in a series of 500 single-center tracheostomies performed in Canada, where patients with a BMI greater than or equal to 30 had a higher rate of complications (15% vs 8%; $P < .05$).[51] Conversely, one institution reported on 143 percutaneous tracheostomy experiences in morbidly obese patients (defined as having a BMI > 35), finding only 1.1% to have overall complications, including bleeding, and 5.6% to have conversion to an open procedure.[52]

When planning tracheostomy in obese patients, it is reasonable to consider preprocedure ultrasound evaluation of the neck to visualize vascular structures, thyroid tissue, and anatomic variants. Proceduralists should rigorously consider the shape and length of the tracheostomy tube, which can become anteriorly displaced or downward angulated if insufficiently long or deep.[27]

Severe Respiratory Failure

Although patients with high levels of FIO_2 and PEEP are sometimes considered "high risk," two publications suggest these patients can safely undergo percutaneous tracheostomy. The first evaluated 88 patients ventilated with high PEEP (> 7.5 mm Hg), finding no short- (1-hour) or long-term (24-hour) disturbances in oxygenation and no absolute or statistical difference in procedural complications when they were compared with 115 similar patients undergoing tracheostomy with low PEEP.[53] The second large series demonstrated an extremely low rate of procedural complications among 1000 patients, despite the inclusion of 150 patients with an FIO_2 greater than 0.5 and 110 patients with a PEEP greater than 10 mm Hg.[37] These authors suggest that tracheostomy be delayed when the FIO_2 is greater than 80% or the PEEP is greater than 15 cm H_2O.

Programmatic approach to tracheostomy

Tracheostomy offers many advantages to prolonged endotracheal intubation in the critically ill neuroscience patient, but its benefit depends on safety. Tracheostomy safety is improved by standardized care under institutional protocols and pathways and the standardized involvement of nurses and respiratory care practitioners. A tracheostomy program serves to decrease low-frequency, high-risk events and depends on appropriate patient selection, standardized procedural techniques by experienced practitioners, appropriate tube selection and management, and protocolized long-term management.[35,54-56] In the modern era of quality initiatives and the safety culture, such a program is considered a standard element of patient care.

! CRITICAL CONSIDERATIONS

- Tracheostomy is frequently indicated in patients with neurologic disease.
- Early tracheostomy (within 1 week of neurologic injury) may be appropriate when long-term mechanical ventilation or failure of airway protection is anticipated by experienced clinicians.
- Percutaneous tracheostomy is a viable alternative to open, surgical tracheostomy and is cost-effective, safe, and convenient to perform at the bedside.
- Percutaneous tracheostomy is routinely performed by intensivists, surgeons, and anesthesiologists who have advanced airway skills. Standards for training and the development of competency are published and widely available.
- Safe percutaneous tracheostomy depends on knowledge of anatomic and physiologic factors, on the experience of the proceduralist, and on a regimented system for performing the procedure.
- Bronchoscopy and ultrasound techniques may increase the safety of tracheostomy.
- Important complications of percutaneous tracheostomy include minor or catastrophic bleeding, loss of the airway, and tracheal injury, which may lead to stenosis.
- Special circumstances during tracheostomy include coagulopathy, obesity, and severe respiratory failure.
- Special circumstances frequently present in the neurocritically ill include known or suspected cervical spine injury and poor intracranial compliance or elevated intracranial pressure. These circumstances deserve special attention and preparation, but are not necessarily absolute contraindications to the procedure.
- Safe tracheostomy depends on a multidisciplinary programmatic approach, which involves protocolized nursing and respiratory therapy care. A systematic approach to tracheostomy and tracheostomy management is considered the standard of care.

REFERENCES

1. Dunham CM, LaMonica C. Prolonged tracheal intubation in the trauma patient. *J Trauma.* 1984;24:120-124.

2. Boynton JH, Hawkins K, Eastridge BJ, O'Keefe GE. Tracheostomy timing and the duration of weaning in patients with acute respiratory failure. *Crit Care.* 2004;8:R261-R267.

3. Pierson DJ. Tracheostomy and weaning. *Respir Care.* 2005;50:526-533.

4. Heffner JE. The role of tracheotomy in weaning. *Chest.* 2001;120;S477-S481.

5. Nieszkowska A, Combes A, Luyt CE, et al. Impact of tracheotomy on sedative administration, sedation level, and comfort of mechanically ventilated intensive care unit patients. *Crit Care Med.* 2005;33(11):2527-2533.

6. Rumbak MJ, Newton M, Truncale T, et al. A prospective randomized study comparing early percutaneous dilational tracheostomy to prolonged translaryngeal intubation (delayed tracheotomy) in critically ill medical patients. *Crit Care Med.* 2004;32(8):1689-1694.

7. Blot F, Similowski T, Trouillet JL, et al. Early tracheotomy versus prolonged endotracheal intubation in unselected severely ill ICU patients. *Intensive Care Med.* 2008;34(10):1779-1787.

8. Down J, Williamson W. Early vs late tracheostomy in critical care. *Br J Hosp Med (Lond).* 2009;70(9):510-513.

9. Griffiths J, Barber V, Morgan L, et al. Systematic review and meta-analysis of studies of the timing of tracheostomy in adult patients undergoing artificial ventilation. *BMJ.* 2005;330:1243.

10. Bouderka MA, Fakhir B, Bouaagad F, et al. Early tracheostomy versus prolonged endotracheal intubation in severe head injury. *J Trauma.* 2004;57:251-254.

11. Rodriguez JL, Steinberg SM, Luchetti FA, et al. Early tracheostomy for primary airway management in the surgical critical care setting. *Surgery.* 1990;108:655-659.

12. Lesnik I, Rappaport W, Fulginiti J, Witzke D. The role of early tracheostomy in blunt multiple organ trauma. *Am Surg.* 1992;58(6):346-349.

13. Koh WY, Lew TW, Chin NM, Wong MF. Tracheostomy in a neuro-intensive care setting: indications and timing. *Anaesth Intensive Care.* 1997;25(4):365-368.

14. Kane TD, Rodriguez JL, Luchette FA. Early versus late tracheostomy in the trauma patient. *Respir Care Clin North Am.* 1997;3(1):1-20.

15. Rodriguez JL, Steinberg SM, Luchetti FA, et al. Early tracheostomy for primary airway management in the surgical critical care setting. *Surgery.* 1990;108(4):655-659.

16. Terragni PP, Antonelli M, Fumagalli R, et al. Early vs late tracheotomy for prevention of pneumonia in mechanically ventilated adult ICU patients: a randomized controlled trial. *JAMA.* 2010;303(15):1483-1489.

17. Holevar M, Dunham JC, Brautigan R, et al. Practice management guidelines for timing of tracheostomy: the EAST Practice Management Guidelines Work Group. *J Trauma.* 2009;67(4):870-874.

18. Massick DD, Powell DM, Price PD, et al. Quantification of the learning curve for percutaneous dilatational tracheotomy. *Laryngoscope.* 2000;110(2 Pt 1):222-228.

19. Díaz-Regañón G, Miñambres E, Ruiz A, González-Herrera S, Holanda-Peña M, López-Espadas F. Safety and complications of percutaneous tracheostomy in a cohort of 800 mixed ICU patients. *Anaesthesia.* 2008;63(11):1198-1203.

20. Klein M, Agassi R, Shapira AR, Kaplan DM, Koiffman L, Weksler N. Can intensive care physicians safely perform percutaneous dilational tracheostomy? An analysis of 207 cases. *Isr Med Assoc J.* 2007;9(10):717-719.

21. Seder DB, Lee K, Rahman C, et al. Safety and feasibility of percutaneous tracheostomy performed by neurointensivists. *Neurocrit Care.* 2009;10(3):264-268.

22. Seybt MW, Blanchard AR, Gourin CG, Terris DJ. 100 consecutive collaborative percutaneous tracheostomies. *Otolaryngol Head Neck Surg.* 2007;136(6):934-937.

23. Flint AC, Midde R, Rao VA, Lasman TE, Ho PT. Bedside ultrasound screening for pretracheal vascular structures may minimize the risks of percutaneous dilatational tracheostomy. *Neurocrit Care.* 2009;11(3):372-376.

24. Sustić A. Role of ultrasound in the airway management of critically ill patients. *Crit Care Med.* 2007;35(5 Suppl):S173-S177.

25. Epstein S. Anatomy and physiology of tracheostomy. *Respir Care.* 2005;50(4):476-482.

26. Heffner JE, Sahn SA. The technique of tracheostomy and cricothyroidotomy. *J Crit Illness.* 1987;2(1):79-87.

27. Hess DR. Tracheostomy tubes and related appliances. *Respir Care.* 2005;50(4):497-510.

28. Ernst A, Silvestri GA, Johnstone D; American College of Chest Physicians. Interventional pulmonary procedures: guidelines from the American College of Chest Physicians. *Chest.* 2003;123(5):1693-1717.

29. Bolliger CT, Mathur PN, Beamis JF, et al. ERS/ATS statement on interventional pulmonology. European Respiratory Society/American Thoracic Society. *Eur Respir J.* 2002;19(2):356-373.

30. Cobean R, Beals M, Moss C, Bredenberg CE. Percutaneous dilatational tracheostomy. A safe, cost-effective bedside procedure. *Arch Surg.* 1996;131:265-271.

31. Higgins KM, Punthakee X. Meta-analysis comparison of open versus percutaneous tracheostomy. *Laryngoscope.* 2007;117(3):447-454.

32. Paran H, Butnaru G, Hass I, Afanasyv A, Gutman M. Evaluation of a modified percutaneous tracheostomy technique without bronchoscopic guidance. *Chest.* 2004;126(3):868-871.

33. Mallick A, Venkatanath D, Elliot SC, Hollins T, Nanda Kumar CG. A prospective randomised controlled trial of capnography vs. bronchoscopy for Blue Rhino percutaneous tracheostomy. *Anaesthesia.* 2003;58(9):864-868.

34. Silvester W, Goldsmith D, Uchino S, et al. Percutaneous versus surgical tracheostomy: a randomized controlled study with long-term follow-up. *Crit Care Med.* 2006;34(8):2145-2152.

35. Kornblith LZ, Burlew CC, Moore EE, et al. One thousand bedside percutaneous tracheostomies in the surgical intensive care unit: time to change the gold standard. *J Am Coll Surg.* 2011;212(2):163-170

36. Freeman BD, Isabella K, Lin N, Buchman T. A meta-analysis of prospective trials comparing percutaneous and surgical tracheostomy in critically ill patients. *Chest.* 2000;118:1412-1418.

37. Byhahn C, Lischke V, Meininger D, Halbig S, Westphal K. Peri-operative complications during percutaneous tracheostomy in obese patients. *Anaesthesia.* 2005;60(1):12-15.

38. Epstein, SK. Late complications of tracheostomy. *Respir Care.* 2005;50(4):542-549.

39. Antonelli M, Michetti V, Di Palma A, et al. Percutaneous translaryngeal versus surgical tracheostomy: a randomized trial with 1-yr double-blind follow-up. *Crit Care Med.* 2005;33(5):1015-1020.

40. Ridley RW, Zwischenberger JB. Tracheoinnominate fistula: surgical management of an iatrogenic disaster. *J Laryngol Otol.* 2006;120(8):676-680.

41. Allan JS, Wright CD. Tracheoinnominate fistula: diagnosis and management. *Chest Surg Clin N Am.* 2003;13(2):331-341.

42. Auzinger G, O'Callaghan GP, Bernal W, Sizer E, Wendon JA. Percutaneous tracheostomy in patients with severe liver disease and a high incidence of refractory coagulopathy: a prospective trial. *Crit Care.* 2007;11(5):R110.

43. Pandian V, Vaswani RS, Mirski MA, Haut E, Gupta S, Bhatti NI. Safety of percutaneous dilational tracheostomy in coagulopathic patients. *Ear Nose Throat J.* 2010;89(8):387-395.

44. Beiderlinden M, Eikermann M, Lehmann N, Adamzik M, Peters J. Risk factors associated with bleeding during and after percutaneous dilational tracheostomy. *Anaesthesia.* 2007;62(4):342-346.

45. Kluge S, Meyer A, Kühnelt P, Baumann HJ, Kreymann G. Percutaneous tracheostomy is safe in patients with severe thrombocytopenia. *Chest.* 2004;126(2):547-551.

46. Stocchetti N, Parma A, Songa V, Colombo A, Lamperti M, Tognini L. Early translaryngeal tracheostomy in patients with severe brain damage. *Intensive Care Med.* 2000;26(8):1101-1107.

47. Imperiale C, Magni G, Favaro R, Rosa G. Intracranial pressure monitoring during percutaneous tracheostomy "percutwist" in critically ill neurosurgery patients. *Anesth Analg.* 2009;108(2):588-592.

48. Reilly PM, Sing RF, Giberson FA, et al. Hypercarbia during tracheostomy: a comparison of percutaneous endoscopic, percutaneous Doppler, and standard surgical tracheostomy. *Intensive Care Med.* 1997;23(8):859-864.

49. Mayberry JC, Wu IC, Goldman RK, Chesnut RM. Cervical spine clearance and neck extension during percutaneous tracheostomy in trauma patients. *Crit Care Med.* 2000;28(10):3436-3440.

50. Ben Nun A, Orlovsky M, Best LA. Percutaneous tracheostomy in patients with cervical spine fractures—feasible and safe. *Interact Cardiovasc Thorac Surg.* 2006;5(4):427-429.

51. Kost KM. Endoscopic percutaneous dilatational tracheotomy: a prospective evaluation of 500 consecutive cases. *Laryngoscope.* 2005;115(10):1-30.

52. Heyrosa MG, Melniczek DM, Rovito P, Nicholas GG. Percutaneous tracheostomy: a safe procedure in the morbidly obese. *J Am Coll Surg.* 2006;202(4):618-622.

53. Beiderlinden M, Groeben H, Peters J. Safety of percutaneous dilational tracheostomy in patients ventilated with high positive end-expiratory pressure (PEEP). *Intensive Care Med.* 2003;29(6):944-948.

54. McGrath BA, Thomas AN. Patient safety incidents associated with tracheostomies occurring in hospital wards: a review of reports to the UK National Patient Safety Agency. *Postgrad Med J.* 2010;86(1019):522-525.

55. Garrubba M, Turner T, Grieveson C. Multidisciplinary care for tracheostomy patients: a systematic review. *Crit Care.* 2009;13(6):R177.

56. Blankenship DR, Kulbersh BD, Gourin CG, Blanchard AR, Terris DJ. High-risk tracheostomy: exploring the limits of the percutaneous tracheostomy. *Laryngoscope.* 2005;115(6):987-989.

Bronchoscopy in the ICU

Yousef Shweihat, MD
Wissam Abouzgheib, MD
Melvin R. Pratter, MD
Thaddeus Bartter, MD

A 27-year-old patient presents to the emergency department after a motor vehicle accident. He was taken out of a crumpled car. Emergency medical services reported that he was conscious when they arrived. On arrival, he has pain and swelling in the jaw area. During examination his mental status deteriorates, the swelling increases, and breathing becomes labored.

Should this patient be intubated? If so, how?

This patient should be intubated for several reasons. First, there is an alteration of mental status. Second, there is an injury of unknown severity, which may include the upper airway. Third, evaluation of the patient may involve both nonsurgical and surgical approaches, both of which would require relative immobility; airway control increases the safety of pharmacologic sedation. Fourth, agitation could lead to significant changes in intracranial pressure in this individual with an undefined intracranial status. Intubation ensures a secure airway. Failure to establish a secure airway can be the cause of significant morbidity related to airway injuries, hypoxemia and hypoxic brain injuries,[1] severe hypotension, and frank aspiration.[2] It can also result in death if associated with difficulty in ventilating the patient "noninvasively."[3]

Bronchoscopic intubation is the method of choice in a case such as this. When being secured, the airway in a critically ill patient should always be considered to be a "difficult airway,"[4] and bronchoscopy can facilitate intubation. In the scenario depicted above, there is a potential upper airway obstruction and there is a potential spinal injury; bronchoscopic intubation is strongly indicated. The capacity for bronchoscopic intubation cannot be an afterthought. Every institution should have in place an established protocol for management of the difficult airway, including access to equipment and expertise.[4]

The safety benefit from bronchoscopic intubation lies in the flexibility of the scope. Whereas with routine intubation a direct visual line to the vocal cords must be established, the bronchoscope can maintain visualization while following the arc to the posterior pharynx. The bronchoscope can be conformed to the body rather than conforming the body to a visual need, and when the bronchoscope is used the jaw thrust and manipulation of the head and neck are not required.

What is the method of bronchoscopic intubation?

Bronchoscopic intubation utilizes the scope as an introducer. Prior to bronchoscopy, an endotracheal tube (ETT) is preloaded onto the hilt of the bronchoscope. The bronchoscope is lubricated and passed through the vocal cords to the midtrachea. The preloaded endotracheal tube can then be passed over it. If resistance is met at the level of the larynx, rotating the ETT 30 to 90 degrees can change the position of the tube and facilitate its advancement through the vocal cords.

Endotracheal intubation via bronchoscopy offers another major benefit: visual confirmation both of placement within the trachea and of position. All other methods of confirmation (auscultation, observation for chest movement, and even CO_2 monitoring) have a margin of error, and none of them can confirm optimal positioning (2-3 cm above the main carina). Positioning the ETT using the fiberoptic scope confirms position and obviates the need for chest radiography.

The fiberoptic bronchoscope is an invaluable tool for positioning dual-lumen endotracheal tubes. These are used when single-lung ventilation is desired, when two different ventilation strategies are used for each lung, or for protection of one lung from a disease process in the other lung. The technique is basically an extension of the above-mentioned technique for intubation. The scope should be passed to the desired main bronchus instead of the midtrachea and the ETT advanced over it.

What is the preferable route for bronchoscopic intubation?

There are two routes of intubation, orotracheal and nasotracheal.[5] Each has a rationale. The nasotracheal route is generally easier, as the nasal passageways spill into the posterior pharynx directly above the vocal cords. The disadvantages of nasotracheal intubation are (1) there is a high incidence of sinusitis with nasotracheal intubation[6,7] (an accepted principle although still controversial in microbiologically based studies[8,9]) and (2) the nasal passageways often require a tube smaller than could be inserted via the oropharynx. Nasal intubation would be contraindicated in the presence of a nasal tumor or nasal trauma. In contrast to nasotracheal intubation, orotracheal intubation is the preferred route but is more difficult because of the loss of the nasal passages as a guide to the posterior pharynx. Orotracheal intubation can be rendered even more difficult by tongue swelling or oral trauma. Note also that during orotracheal intubation the nonparalyzed patient can bite and damage a bronchoscope if a bite block is not in place.

Does bronchoscopy play a role in endotracheal tube management apart from the initial intubation?

Apart from its utility in initial intubation and confirmation of placement, bronchoscopy can be used for endotracheal tube replacement, particularly if one is changing routes—nasal to oral or oral to nasal. In these cases, the bronchoscope with a preloaded endotracheal tube is passed through the alternate passageway and through the vocal cords. The balloon on the existing endotracheal tube is dropped, and the end of the bronchoscope is passed into the middle or distal trachea. The old endotracheal tube is then removed, and the new one is passed over the scope into the trachea.

In addition, one should not forget that once an endotracheal tube has been placed, the endotracheal tube becomes part of the patient's airway. When an airway problem occurs, problems pertaining to the endotracheal tube need to be considered. Perhaps the most common would be a marked increase in peak airway pressure. Three possible causes of this are partial obstruction of the lumen of the endotracheal tube with secretions, compression of the endotracheal tube from kinking or (if the tube is oral) from biting by the patient, and migration of the cuff to the distal end of the tube causing obstruction.

Six days after admission, intubation, and craniofacial surgery including drainage of a subarachnoid hemorrhage, the patient has developed new fever, worsening hypoxia, and increased secretions. On chest roentgenogram there is increased density at the right base with obliteration of right diaphragmatic shadow.

What is the definition of ventilator-associated pneumonia, and how should it be evaluated?

Ventilator-associated pneumonia (VAP), as defined by the American Thoracic Society (ATS) and Infectious Diseases Society of America (IDSA), is pneumonia that develops after 48 to 72 hours of intubation.[10] There is a significant difference in microbiologic etiology of early-onset (within 4 days of hospital admission) versus late-onset (after 4 days) hospital-acquired pneumonias[11]; the latter are mostly caused by resistant pathogens. VAP occurs in 10% to 20% of ventilated patients. In their most recent guidelines,[10] the ATS and IDSA consider VAP to be a subset of what is known as health care–associated pneumonia (HCAP), which encompasses hospital-acquired pneumonias, VAP, and pneumonias in patients who reside in long-term care facilities or have other risk factors for multidrug-resistant organisms. VAP shares epidemiologic and microbiologic characteristics in common with the other forms of HCAP, which makes it logical to group the three entities under one umbrella.

It has been recognized for years that VAP poses a diagnostic dilemma; there is no clinical presentation that is diagnostic of pneumonia in the critically ill. There are many causes of fever, both infectious and noninfectious. None of the other criteria mentioned above—increased phlegm, worsening of gas exchange, or pulmonary infiltrates—is sensitive or specific for VAP. These findings are therefore used only to raise the possibility of VAP, and the clinician is left with two options: (1) initiate and complete a course of broad-spectrum antibiotics or (2) begin with broad-spectrum coverage, try to get diagnostic bacteriologic material, and then narrow the spectrum of coverage to cover specifically identified organisms.

What are the available methods to obtain samples for cultures?

Bacteriologic diagnosis is preferable to clinical diagnosis.[10] It has long been recognized that a culture of organisms from the upper respiratory tract is not diagnostic of parenchymal lung pathogens, and there is now extensive literature on the methods and utility of obtaining cultures of organisms from the lower respiratory tract.[10,11] The two main techniques of culture of the lower respiratory tract are bronchoscopic bronchoalveolar lavage (BAL) and the use of a protected specimen brush (PSB). While both will be discussed below, the technique that has emerged as dominant is BAL.

What is the technique for BAL?

BAL is done in an attempt to bypass the upper respiratory tract (which is essentially always colonized by potential pathogens) and to sample organisms from the lower respiratory tract where they may play an active pathogenic role. The principles are simple. First, one must bypass the upper respiratory tract doing as little suctioning/contamination of the lumen of the bronchoscope as possible. Second, one must instill enough fluid to reach and sample alveoli. When a bronchoscope is wedged and alveoli are flushed with sterile saline, it is estimated that one can sample 1/100 of the alveoli in the lungs. There is evidence that the optimal volume for this is 120 mL.[12] Third, the collected sample must be analyzed using quantitative cultures. Using a specific cutoff of colonies per cubic millimeter limits the false positives of the technique, preventing low numbers of contaminating upper airway organisms from being considered clinically significant. There is a difference of opinion about some of the details of how BAL is done, but a reasonable and literature-backed protocol is listed in Table 40-1.[13]

What is the technique for PSB?

The PSB technique is a bronchoscopic technique in which a special catheter is used to obtain lower airway cultures. An inner catheter containing a sterile brush is housed in a larger outer catheter whose tip is capped with a pledget of soft material similar to bone wax. After the bronchoscope

Table 40-1. Technique for Bronchoalveolar Lavage

1.	Pass a clean bronchoscope into the airways using as little suctioning as possible.
2.	Avoid the use of lidocaine or flush the lumen if you did use it; lidocaine is bacteriostatic/-cidal and could cause false-negative results.[13]
3.	Wedge the bronchoscope into a subsegment of lung that represents the area of greatest abnormality on radiography. If the disease is diffuse, guide the scope to the segment with the most apparent purulence. If this cannot be identified, advance the scope to the right middle lobe or the lingula.
4.	Instill 120 mL of fluid into the airways. (If the wedge is tight, this should not cause cough.)
5.	Apply suction. This can be done with a sputum trap in line with the bronchoscopy suction or with a syringe connected to the suction port.
6.	If there is no yield, instill more fluid. Yields of 10 mL or greater should be adequate for culture.
7.	Make sure that the material is processed by the laboratory within an hour unless the sample is refrigerated.
8.	Colony counts of 10^4 or greater are considered to represent parenchymal infection and so are treated. Antibiotics are changed to cover the detected organisms or stopped if none are present in significant amounts.

is passed into the area of greatest radiologic abnormality, the PSB catheter is inserted through the suction channel of the bronchoscope. Deployment is telescopic. The outer catheter is passed into distal airways. Then the inner catheter is passed through the larger one, pushing the pledget out of place. Finally, the brush is passed beyond the end of the inner cannula and agitated to collect a specimen. All is then withdrawn in reverse order. The outer catheter is wiped to minimize upper airway contaminants, then the inner cannula is extended and wiped, and then the brush is extended and cut off with sterile scissors into a few milliliters of sterile saline in a sterile cup for quantitative culture.

How are samples handled?

Samples obtained by PSB or BAL should be handled in a sterile fashion and delivered to the laboratory as soon as possible. Most laboratories have their guidelines for delivering and processing samples. If a delay of more than 1 hour is expected in delivering the samples for processing, the samples need to be refrigerated. In case viral culture is needed, 3 to 5 mL of the BAL sample should be mixed with a viral transport medium and the solution refrigerated until inoculation.

Why is one technique better than the other?

Both techniques have similar accuracy, but there are several reasons for the emergence of BAL as the dominant method for culture of lower respiratory tract specimens. First, BAL is simpler and less expensive. Second, it samples a larger number of alveoli. (If one does use PSB, the criteria for significant colony counts drop by a factor of 10.) Third, BAL can be used to diagnose other possible causes of pulmonary infiltrates such as hemorrhage. Fourth, the PSB technique has a greater risk of pneumothorax than does BAL.

Finally, it should be noted that all of the above discussion has to do only with the culture of bacteria suspected to be responsible for infection. These steps do not apply to other infections such as tuberculosis and viral pneumonia or to noninfectious processes. For these other etiologies whose diagnosis does not depend on quantitative culture, one does not need to be so assiduous.

How does antibiotic treatment affect the results?

The results of BAL with quantitative culture can change antibiotic therapy. This knowledge should not change initial therapy; when the clinical suspicion for VAP is high or a patient is in apparent septic shock, broad-spectrum antibiotic therapy should be instituted as soon as possible. Waiting for confirmatory stains or cultures or withholding treatment for a few hours until a procedure is performed can lead to adverse outcomes.[11] Ideally, BAL should be performed as soon as the order for broad-spectrum coverage is placed. Too long a delay invalidates the results of BAL; somewhere between 24 and 48 hours after therapy is instituted, the number of recovered organisms is reduced by 50%.[14-16] BAL after treatment can lead to negative cultures or to colony counts below the threshold considered significant. Adjusting the threshold of a positive quantitative culture (eg, using 10 to the power 2 instead of the power 4 for BAL cultures), depending on the duration of antibiotic therapy and the pretest probability based on clinical suspicion, is warranted.[15] There is an exception to this rule; if a patient develops findings suspect for VAP while already on antibiotic therapy for a previous infection, the results of a BAL or PSB are not affected, and microbiology maintains the same threshold.[14] If BAL is not going to be available within a reasonable time after suspicion of VAP, then a tracheal aspirate could be obtained; to assume that it accurately represented distal airway flora would be fallacious, but to include antimicrobial coverage for every recovered tracheal organism would be reasonable.

 You arrive in the neurology intensive care unit (ICU) one morning and find that your resident is bronchoscoping all of the intubated patients in the ICU. He says that he needs the practice and that he is helping with airway toiletry.

Are you upset? Should you be? Do your resident's actions bear potential harm? What is the physiologic impact of bronchoscopy?

You should be upset. Although minor by surgical standards, bronchoscopy is an invasive procedure, and all invasive procedures bear risks that should be balanced by potential benefits. Bronchoscopy in the neurology ICU contains risks, some of which are quite evident and others that are less obvious. The physiologic changes associated with bronchoscopy have the potential to cause harm. Below is a summary of cardiovascular, respiratory, and central nervous system sequelae of bronchoscopy.

Systemic Cardiovascular Effects

When a tube of any sort is passed through the vocal cords, there is a reflexive physiologic response; intubation of any type is far from a neutral event. In one study, there was evidence of an adrenergic surge; there was a mean 40% increase in heart rate, a 30% increase in mean arterial pressure (MAP), and an 86% increase in pulmonary capillary wedge pressure.[17] The reflex is independent of route of cannulation (nares versus mouth) and is not ablated by paralysis or general anesthesia.[18,19] There is a blunting of the cardiovascular response to intubation when lidocaine is used for topical anesthesia.[20]

Respiratory Effects

Bronchoscopy changes work of breathing, pressures, and volumes within the lung. Transnasal cannulation of the trachea of a nonintubated patient leads to a decrease in inspiratory and expiratory flow, a decrease in vital capacity, and an increase in functional residual capacity.[21] These changes were similar when comparing the introduction of a bronchoscope or an ETT into the trachea and tend to resolve after removal of the scope or endotracheal tube.

Bronchoscopy through an ETT in a sedated and spontaneously breathing (ie, nonventilated) patient leads to a significant further decrease in flows and vital capacity and a marked increase in the work of breathing.[21,22]

Bronchoscopy of a patient on a ventilator can cause barotrauma. The bronchoscope within the lumen of the ETT causes an airway obstruction. The ventilator (particularly if set on a volume mode) can increase pressure to deliver flow, but expiratory flow remains a passive result of elastic recoil pressure. There can thus be a dramatic dichotomy between how much air is delivered and how much is exhaled, placing the patient at risk for marked hyperinflation and very high levels of positive end-expiratory pressure (PEEP). This imbalance becomes more marked as the outer diameter of the bronchoscope approaches the luminal diameter of the ETT, as elegantly outlined by Lindholm et al.[22] The authors documented that when a patient on a ventilator is being scoped through an ETT, levels of PEEP commonly reach 18 cm H_2O and can be as high as 35 cm H_2O.[22] Further complicating the physiology of bronchoscopy through an ETT is suction through the bronchoscope, which can have an opposite physiologic effect; suction can decrease the amount of lung inflation and, if sustained, even decrease functional residual capacity, tidal volume, and minute ventilation.

In clinical practice, the danger of barotrauma during bronchoscopy increases as the ETT size decreases. If one is using a standard bronchoscope, bronchoscopy through a 7.0 ETT (the ETT sizing refers to the inner diameter of the tube) is dangerous, and bronchoscopy through a 7.5 ETT is difficult. For an 8.0 ETT, there is less resistance and therefore less risk. The use of a smaller scope such as a pediatric scope will decrease airway obstruction and is fine for visual examination of the lower airways, but as scope diameter decreases, the capacity to suction through the scope decreases. Another variable that can be changed is the ventilator mode. With a volume mode, the ventilator increases pressure as needed to deliver a set volume. In contrast, with a pressure mode, the volume delivered decreases as physiology changes. Thus, with a pressure mode, increasing airflow obstruction decreases both the delivered and the exhaled tidal volumes and there is a lesser dichotomy between the two than would occur with a volume mode. (This ameliorates but does *not* correct the physiologic issues.) Based on the physiologic principles noted above, a suggested protocol for bronchoscopy through an endotracheal tube is documented in Table 40-2.

Central Nervous System Changes

Bronchoscopy in patients with intracranial pathology raises concerns regarding its safety in this population. It is known that suctioning through an endotracheal tube in adults with head trauma results in increased intracranial pressure (ICP) and a parallel increase in MAP with maintained to elevated cerebral perfusion pressure (CPP).[23] Respiratory therapy maneuvers and PEEP are known to increase ICP.[24] The effects specifically of bronchoscopy on ICP were demonstrated in studies of patients with severe head trauma done by Kerwin et al[25] and by Peerless et al.[26] In both studies, there were concomitant increases in both ICP and MAP such that CPP was maintained to slightly increased. The increase in ICP in both studies was generally more than 50% of baseline and was as great as 115% of baseline.

Table 40-2. Bronchoscopy of the Ventilated Patient: Minimizing Barotrauma

- If you have a choice, use the smallest scope that will achieve your goals.
- If the ETT is size 7.5 or smaller and a therapeutic bronchoscopy is indicated, consider changing the ETT to a larger size.
- Change the ventilator to a pressure mode.
- Decrease the respiratory rate to allow more time for exhalation.
- Use suction intermittently.
- Withdraw the scope at intervals.
- Watch for hypotension; if it occurs, it may be the hemodynamic sequela of markedly elevated PEEP.

Abbreviations: ETT, endotracheal tube; PEEP, positive end-expiratory pressure.

Most patients had recovery of their ICP to baseline within 15 minutes after the procedure ended. There were no reported side effects or complications from the procedure. In a retrospective study of patients with computed tomographic evidence of increased ICP secondary to metastatic lung cancer (ie, edema around tumor with or without midline shift), it was noted that a diagnostic fiberoptic bronchoscopy did not cause discernable morbidity or mortality within 1 week of the procedure.[27] Of note, there was no difference in the rate of complications between patients who received corticosteroids to decrease the ICP and those who did not.

What can be done to minimize fluctuations in intracranial pressure during bronchoscopy?

Although the literature to date has not documented increased morbidity/mortality rates related to increased intracranial pressures during bronchoscopy, it is difficult to believe that these changes will always be benign in patients with brain matter at risk. Most of the published studies are small and do not include patients with extreme baseline increases in ICP for whom the risk of a further increase may be greater. There are two main mechanisms for elevations in ICP during bronchoscopy: (1) the reflex response to tracheal stimulation and (2) dramatic increases in PEEP that can occur during the procedure.

Several studies have been done to evaluate whether medications or specific maneuvers can attenuate the reflex ICP response to tracheal stimulation. Topical lidocaine instilled through an ETT prior to suctioning has been shown to decrease by 50% the increase in ICP associated with suctioning.[28] Opiate administration prior to ETT suctioning results in significantly less increase in ICP when compared to no medication.[29] The addition of a paralytic agent had a significant additive value in attenuating the reflex in the same population.[29] In one study, hyperventilation prior to suctioning was shown to ablate the suction-related increase in ICP with little effect on CPP.[30] In another study, hyperventilation during bronchoscopy had almost the same effect.[31] (Note that because of obstruction of the ETT by the bronchoscope, as discussed above, hyperventilation during bronchoscopy is often not possible.)

As noted above, bronchoscopy of the ventilated patient can be associated with dramatic increases in PEEP, and this can lead to an elevated ICP. In contrast to the reflex elevation in vascular pressures, there is no reason to suspect that a PEEP-induced increase in ICP would be associated with an increase in MAP and relatively stable CPP. In fact, the opposite is more likely; it is known that high levels of PEEP can decrease cardiac output and blood pressure, factors that would tend to decrease CPP. The best way to avoid this PEEP-induced increase in ICP is to avoid bronchoscopy; the procedure should be performed only when clearly indicated. When bronchoscopy is indicated, the maneuvers noted in Table 40-2 might mitigate increases in PEEP. Other maneuvers specifically to decrease impact upon ICP include bronchoscopy with the patient in the sitting position and maneuvers to decrease or prevent cough. The sitting position will limit the transmission of PEEP and intrathoracic pressure to the head.[24] Cough can be attenuated with the use of opiates, which have a direct dampening effect on the cough reflex, or with lidocaine, which decreases airway sensitivity. Cough can be ablated by the use of paralysis prior to bronchoscopy.

Physiologic effects and complications are different. What are the known complications of bronchoscopy?

Like any other invasive procedure, bronchoscopy has its complications and risks that should be weighed against the benefits before a decision to use it. This is so despite the fact that it is generally considered a safe procedure with a low rate of complications.

These complications can be divided into the following:

1. Complications related to medications
   a. In the awake and nonintubated patient, the use of moderate sedation is the standard of care during bronchoscopy. Different medications can be used depending on local expertise, the

availability of certain drugs in the institution, and support of anesthesia. A commonly used combination includes midazolam and an opiate. Topical lidocaine is regularly used to decrease the cough reflex. The bronchoscopist should be aware of the side effects and duration of action of these sedative drugs and be knowledgeable about reversal agents. The most common complication of presedation is a decrease in ventilation causing hypoxia and hypercapnia. There are two possible mechanisms for sedation-related hypoventilation. One is depression of central respiratory drive.[32] The second (in nonintubated patients) is sedation-induced relaxation of the upper airway with oropharyngeal wall collapse. This obstruction can be relieved by the use of nasopharyngeal airway.[33] In the intubated patient, there is no risk of upper airway collapse, and respiration can be supported. This allows the bronchoscopist to use larger doses of sedatives and even, if appropriate, to use paralytics.

2. Complications related to the procedure

   a. Pneumothorax is the most common complication of bronchoscopy.[34] It can occur with or without biopsy, although the rate of pneumothorax is higher when parenchymal biopsies are obtained. Pneumothorax can be a life-threatening event, especially in the mechanically ventilated patient. The rule, rarely broken, is that a pneumothorax in a patient on positive pressure ventilation requires a chest tube.

   b. Bleeding is the next most common complication and is directly related to the platelet function and coagulation status when a mucosal or parenchymal biopsy is performed. It is not a frequent complication during BAL or removal of secretions even when thrombocytopenia exists,[35] but in the coagulopathic or thrombocytopenic patient, caution should be applied to minimize trauma to the airways.

   c. Bronchospasm and airway obstruction can occur in reaction to airway irritation by the bronchoscope.

3. Complications related to physiologic changes in the lung and distant organs

   a. Hypoxemia: Hypoxemia is very common (up to 50%)[36] during bronchoscopy and occurs to varying degrees. Multiple factors contribute to the severity. The level of sedation, the severity of a preexisting lung disease,[37] the length of procedure with the use of more suctioning,[38] and the volume of fluid/BAL instilled in the airway[39,40] can all affect the severity of hypoxemia. Hypoxemia can persist for 1 to 2 hours and sometimes longer after removal of the scope. The danger of hypoxemia lies in its potential to further limit oxygen delivery to organs at risk.

   b. Cardiac ischemia: The increases in blood pressure and heart rate observed during bronchoscopy increase the workload of the heart. This potential increase in demand results in increased oxygen consumption. There may be a concomitant decrease in blood oxygen as described directly above. If a patient has significant coronary artery disease with limited flow, bronchoscopy can precipitate an ischemic event. The rate of such ischemic events (depressed ST segments) can be as high as 17% in older patients,[41] but death from ischemic events is very rare.[34,41-43] The ischemic changes usually resolve within 30 minutes, with no sequelae in most patients.[41]

   c. Arrhythmias: In one study, a disturbance of cardiac rhythm occurred in 70% of patients.[44] Multiple abnormalities can be noted, and some of them can be life-threatening. They can range from simple first-degree block to ventricular asystole or ventricular fibrillation. It seems that the development of arrhythmias is related to the development of hypoxemia.[44,45] A history of cardiac disease or chronic lung disease did not seem to increase the risk of cardiac arrhythmias.[44]

Table 40-3. Contraindications to Bronchoscopy

- Severe hypoxemia ($PaO_2 < 60$) on maximal support
- Hemodynamic instability (uncontrolled hypertension or severe hypotension on pressors)
- Recent myocardial infarction
- Active cardiac ischemia
- Active cardiac arrhythmias
- Severely elevated or uncontrolled intracranial pressure

    d. Intracranial pressure: As discussed above, ICP is known to rise, but the literature implies that bronchoscopy is safe in the short term in patients with mild to moderate increases in ICP. One must remember that the studies that documented such safety included small numbers of patients with mean ICP moderately elevated.[25,26] It is always wise to consider increased ICP as a complication and to make every effort to minimize the rise in ICP as discussed above.

What are the contraindications?

Whether bronchoscopy is contraindicated in a certain patient remains a clinical decision and depends on the indication for bronchoscopy and the anticipated degree of risk. Bronchoscopy should only be performed if the results are likely to alter the clinical approach to the patient. No single rule applies without exception; a contraindication to bronchoscopy such as severe hypoxemia in a patient with collapsed lung due to mucus plugging may actually be an urgent indication. Common sense rules; for example, active cardiac ischemia or arrhythmia is a clear contraindication to diagnostic BAL for VAP. Table 40-3 lists some of the more common relative contraindications.

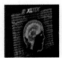

The same patient, after successful treatment of VAP with no residual fever and no leukocytosis, develops left lower lobe opacity. There is no worsening of oxygenation.

What is the role of bronchoscopy in diagnosis and management of atelectasis?

Atelectasis is common in the intubated critically ill ventilated patient and is a common indication for fiberoptic bronchoscopy.[46] It is known that the collapsed/atelectatic lung can serve as a focus for infection. The collapsed segment or lobe can also worsen hypoxemia not only by its lack of participation in gas exchange but also through shunting of blood from the right to the left circulation. In the nonhypoxic patient, whether treatment of atelectasis has any meaningful effect on significant clinical outcomes (ie, mortality, morbidity, length of intubation) is not really known. In the hypoxic patient, recruitment of atelectatic lung might lead to a significant improvement in oxygenation. Many studies have documented the effectiveness of fiberoptic bronchoscopy in reexpanding the atelectatic lung, with rates of success ranging from 19% in one study[47] to around 80% in others.[48-50]

    A landmark study by Marini et al looked at whether bronchoscopy plus aggressive chest physiotherapy (CPT) was preferable to aggressive CPT alone.[51] The answer was no, with bronchoscopy the inferior approach. Several findings were evident. There was no difference in volume recovery between the bronchoscopy-CPT and the CPT-only groups after the first intervention and still no difference at 48 hours. Bronchoscopy was complicated by more frequent desaturations that required medical intervention. Patients with air bronchograms showed a significantly lower volume recovery. There was no significant difference in oxygenation improvement between the two groups. In another study, a lack of secretions in the major airways (ie, patent airways that can correlate with the presence of air bronchograms on chest radiography) was noted to decrease the likelihood of reexpansion from 81% to 22%.[49] The conclusions to be drawn are clear: (1) atelectasis should be treated at least initially with CPT unless there is a clear contraindication to CPT, (2) there is no indication for bronchoscopy for a radiologic finding in the absence of a gas exchange defect, and (3) one must accept the potential for a deterioration postbronchoscopy if bronchoscopy is undertaken.

Despite the caveats noted above, bronchoscopy is at times indicated and is a rational approach to physiologically important atelectasis. Areas of atelectatic lung have a very low compliance and a very high opening pressure. When the ventilator is used to apply pressure using PEEP or recruitment maneuvers, that pressure is likely to cause overdistention of compliant nonatelectic alveoli before it can overcome the opening pressure of the atelectatic segments.[46] Some investigators have advocated the use of targeted inflation of the atelectatic lobe or segment, in which a bronchoscope is used to apply an opening pressure directly to an atelectatic segment of the lung. Described approaches to targeted insufflation include the use of a Swan-Ganz catheter through a flexible bronchoscope, a dedicated bronchoscope with a balloon cuff, and a balloon-cuffed rigid bronchoscope.[52-56] The simplest approach is to wedge a bronchoscope into the atelectatic segment and then use the suction channel of the wedged flexible bronchoscope as the delivery port for the insufflation of positive pressure.[54,57,58] The advantages of this approach include simplicity and the ready availability of equipment. The delivered pressure can be measured. Delivery of at least 30 cm H_2O (but not higher than 50 cm H_2O) to each segment is necessary for a duration of 20 to 60 seconds. Success of reexpansion ranges from 70% to 100% depending on the study population.

Targeted bronchoscopic insufflation for the management of atelectasis has not been compared with bronchoscopy alone, but in most of the above-mentioned studies it has been used when other conservative therapies could not be used or had failed. In the study by Haenel et al, a well-designed and aggressive respiratory physiotherapy protocol had been tried prior to bronchoscopy with insufflation.[57] When the insufflation data are combined with the conclusion from the Marini et al study that bronchoscopy is not superior to aggressive CPT,[51] one could argue that bronchoscopic insufflation should be attempted when CPT has failed or for patients who cannot tolerate CPT (eg, patients with trauma to the chest, hemothorax, or spinal cord).

Of note, bronchoscopy is more successful for therapy of lobar or segmental atelectasis than for subsegmental disease.[59] Unifocal subsegmental disease is also less likely to cause significant hypoxemia.

See Figure 40-1 for a suggested algorithm for treatment of atelectasis.

After the patient has been intubated for 12 days with slow improvement of mental status, a spontaneous breathing trial was performed per the ICU protocol and the patient passed the trial. The respiratory therapist performed a cuff-leak test and there was no apparent leak, raising the question of upper airway edema/obstruction.

What is the role of bronchoscopy in assessing the upper airway before/at the time of extubation? Is there a role for bronchoscopy for the diagnosis and management of post-extubation stridor?

A few hours of intubation are enough to induce ischemic injury to the laryngeal mucosa, with resultant edema.[60] This edema can be the cause of significant narrowing of the laryngeal lumen that is not apparent until extubation occurs. Symptoms usually develop when the airway lumen is narrowed to less than 50% of its original diameter.[61] The patient usually develops stridor, which may

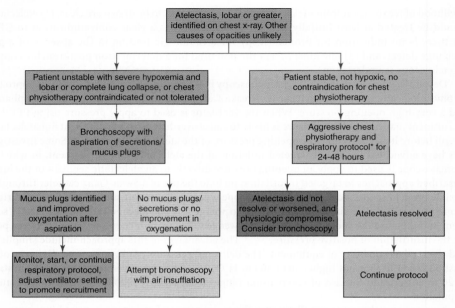

Figure 40-1. Evaluation and management of atelectasis. *Respiratory protocol can include but is not limited to the use of cough induction (eg, hypertonic saline nebulizers), suctioning, mucolytics, bronchodilators, hyperinflation therapy, increased positive end-expiratory pressure (PEEP) or noninvasive positive pressure ventilation (NIPPV) in non-intubated patients, kinetic beds, chest physiotherapy, and positional drainage.

be accompanied by the use of accessory muscles and respiratory distress. The rate of postextubation stridor (PES) varies in different populations but ranges from 3.5% up to 30% in one study.[62,63] PES and/or postextubation laryngeal edema have been identified as the cause of reintubation in 1% to 4% of extubated patients. For the subset of extubated patients who develop stridor, the rate of reintubation ranges from 18% to 69%.[64] The cuff-leak test has been described as a simple maneuver to predict upper airway obstruction.[65] The cuff of the endotracheal tube is deflated while the patient is on positive pressure ventilation. The lack of an air leak or the presence of only a minimal leak implies upper airway obstruction. Measured as a percentage of tidal volume, a leak that is less than 10% to 24% of the tidal volume implies obstruction.[63,66] Measured as an absolute volume, obstruction is suspected at a leak of less than 110 to 130 mL.[67,68] A positive test (low percentage or low volume of leaked air) has a low specificity; only 30% to 69% of patients develop postextubation stridor.[63,67] A negative test, on the other hand, has a high negative predictive value (no obstruction present) with a specificity approximating 99%.[67]

Many studies have examined the effect of corticosteroids on decreasing laryngeal edema and thus lowering the rate of reintubation. It seems that corticosteroids can decrease the rate of laryngeal edema and decrease the need for reintubation if used 7 hours (or longer) prior to a planned extubation in a patient with a positive cuff-leak test.[63] Differing doses, every 4 to 6 hours for 12 to 24 hours, have also been employed effectively.[69,70] Whereas only a portion of patients with postextubation stridor require reintubation, to treat all patients who fail the leak test with steroids will result in a lot of unnecessary treatment. Another logical approach that has not been studied prospectively is to extubate all patients who fail the leak test with a bronchoscope; the bronchoscope is passed through the ETT, and the vocal cords and upper airway are examined as the ETT is withdrawn. If significant edema exists and stridor develops, the tube can be advanced again and the patient can then be treated with steroids for 12 to 24 hours before a repeat trial of extubation over the bronchoscope. If no stridor and no major edema exist, extubation can be completed and the patient monitored for subsequent stridor or distress. The bronchoscopic approach requires a trained bronchoscopist with knowledge of normal laryngeal structures. As mentioned, this approach will probably limit the unnecessary use of steroids and at the same time decrease the rate of failed extubation with its increased morbidity and mortality rates.[71]

The patient had laryngeal edema. He was given steroids, and the spontaneous breathing trial was repeated. He failed. Tracheostomy is indicated for failure to wean.

What is the role of bronchoscopy in guiding interventional procedures in the ICU? What is the role of bronchoscopy in guiding percutaneous tracheostomy?

The bronchoscope is an invaluable tool for interventional procedures in the airway. These might include control of hemoptysis, debulking of obstructive tumors, and stenting of the airways. These procedures can be lifesaving if the airway pathology is the cause of respiratory failure. These instances are infrequent in a dedicated neurologic ICU. In contrast, tracheostomy is a relatively common airway intervention in a neurologic ICU. Tracheostomy can be accomplished by an open surgical approach or with a bedside approach, percutaneous dilational tracheostomy (PDT) (Table 40-4). PDT has emerged as the preferable and standard approach in most institutions; it has a better overall safety profile and is more cost-effective.[72-74] We think that the use of bronchoscopy for PDT is important. The greatest risk of PDT is perforation of the posterior tracheal wall.[75] This can be prevented with the use of bronchoscopy to guide insertion; when the bronchoscope is used, intraluminal position can be confirmed visually, eliminating this complication. No double-blinded trial has confirmed this, although the logic is unavoidable and several authors recommend bronchoscopy-guided PDT.[72,75-78] PDT has three important operators, a bronchoscopist, a therapist to hold the endotracheal tube, and the inserting physician.[72,75,79] The neck is prepared and draped. The patient is heavily sedated or briefly paralyzed. A bronchoscope is then passed through the ETT to the tip of the ETT. The ETT balloon is dropped, the ETT is loosened, and the ETT is slowly pulled back by the therapist until it is in a subglottic position and the early cartilaginous tracheal rings can be seen. A thin needle with lidocaine is used to numb the tissues and to locate a pathway that perforates the trachea between the second and third or third and fourth tracheal rings. This procedure is then repeated with a larger needle, through which a wire can be passed. Once the wire is in place, a shallow incision of about 1 cm is made in the dermis. After two dilations, a tracheostomy tube is passed over a trocar. Position is confirmed once more with the bronchoscope, the ventilator circuitry is moved to the tracheostomy tube, the ETT is removed, and the tracheostomy tube is sutured into place. There is a risk of hypoventilation during this procedure.[76] (See above regarding bronchoscopy through the ETT.) This can be mitigated by the use of a pediatric scope, which allows adequate ventilation around the ETT.

Are there any other uses for bronchoscopy in the ICU?

There are several other diagnostic and therapeutic indications for bronchoscopy. One is to evaluate the patient who fails weaning trials despite normalizing gas exchange and other clinical parameters.

Table 40-4. Suggested Technique for Percutaneous Dilational Tracheostomy

1.	Deeply sedate the patient. Short-term paralysis is optional.
2.	Prepare the neck, examine the anatomic location, clean, and drape.
3.	RT drops the ETT balloon and loosens the tube, and secures position by hand.
4.	Bronchoscopist advances the scope to the tip of the ETT.
5.	Bronchoscopist and RT retract the scope and ETT in synchrony until the first tracheal ring is visible. (For a thin patient, transillumination will help to identify correct ETT/scope positioning.)
6.	Using lidocaine and a 25-gauge needle, numb the skin and soft tissue of the anticipated suture site and then penetrate the trachea between the second and third or third and fourth rings. Identify and confirm this placement bronchoscopically, and inject lidocaine into the trachea. Retract the needle.
7.	Pass the larger needle for wire introduction using the trajectory identified with the 25-gauge needle. Confirm bronchoscopically.
8.	Pass the wire into the trachea and withdraw the needle over the wire.
9.	Make a small 1-cm incision in the dermis, not deeper than a few millimeters.
10.	Dilate twice over the wire using provided gradual dilators. Remove dilator after each dilation.
11.	Load the tracheostomy tube over a trocar and pass the unit over the wire. Some resistance is expected. Watch the tracheostomy tube enter the trachea with the bronchoscope.
12.	Withdraw the trocar and wire with one hand, keeping the other on the tracheostomy tube to secure it in place.
13.	Remove the bronchoscope from the ETT and briefly look through the tracheostomy tube to again confirm intraluminal position.
14.	Attach the ventilator to the tracheostomy tube after inserting the inner cannula and inflate the cuff.
15.	Take out the ETT.
16.	Secure the tracheostomy in place by both suturing it to the skin and applying a trach collar.

Abbreviations : ETT, endotracheal tube; RT, respiratory therapist.

These patients need to be evaluated for tracheal obstruction; two possibilities for this are granulation tissue and tracheomalacia.[80] Bronchoscopy is the diagnostic modality of choice. Another useful application of bronchoscopy that is not infrequently dealt with in cases of trauma is foreign body aspiration. Although rigid bronchoscopy is the tool with the most historical use for this indication, fiberoptic bronchoscopy is a useful initial tool, especially with the advent of multiple tools that can be applied through the working channel of a therapeutic fiberoptic bronchoscope. Finally, and not frequently encountered in the surgical or neurologic ICU, is the need for parenchymal lung tissue for diagnosis of chronic infectious or interstitial lung diseases. Fiberoptic bronchoscopy can provide some diagnostic tissue through performance of transbronchial biopsies. It is advised that this procedure be performed by the most experienced bronchoscopist available, especially if the patient is mechanically ventilated, since the rate of pneumothorax in mechanically ventilated patients can be up to 23%.[81]

REFERENCES

1. Lavery GG, McCloskey BV. The difficult airway in adult critical care. *Crit Care Med.* 2008;36(7):2163-2173.

2. Griesdale DE, Bosma TL, Kurth T, Isac G, Chittock DR. Complications of endotracheal intubation in the critically ill. *Intensive Care Med.* 2008;34(10):1835-1842.

3. Caplan RA, Posner KL, Ward RJ, Cheney FW. Adverse respiratory events in anesthesia: a closed claims analysis. *Anesthesiology.* 1990;72(5):828-833.

4. Matioc AA, Arndt G, Jofee A. The critical airway: the difficult airway in the adult critical care. *Crit Care Med.* 2009;37(3):1175-1176.

5. Dellinger RP. Fiberoptic bronchoscopy in adult airway management. *Crit Care Med.* 1990;18(8):882-887.

6. Salord F, Gaussorgues P, Marti-Flich J, et al. Nosocomial maxillary sinusitis during mechanical ventilation: a prospective comparison of orotracheal versus the nasotracheal route for intubation. *Intensive Care Med.* 1990;16(6):390-393.

7. Bach A, Boehrer H, Schmidt H, Geiss HK. Nosocomial sinusitis in ventilated patients. Nasotracheal versus orotracheal intubation. *Anaesthesia.* 1992;47(4):335-339.

8. Holzapfel L, Chevret S, Madinier G, et al. Influence of long-term oro- or nasotracheal intubation on nosocomial maxillary sinusitis and pneumonia: results of a prospective, randomized, clinical trial. *Crit Care Med.* 1993;21(8):1132-1138.

9. Rouby JJ, Laurent P, Gosnach M, et al. Risk factors and clinical relevance of nosocomial maxillary sinusitis in the critically ill. *Am J Respir Crit Care Med.* 1994;150(3):776-783.

10. American Thoracic Society; Infectious Diseases Society of America. Guidelines for the management of adults with hospital-acquired, ventilator-associated, and healthcare-associated pneumonia. *Am J Respir Crit Care Med.* 2005;171(4):388-416.

11. Torres A, Ewig S, Lode H, Carlet J. Defining, treating and preventing hospital acquired pneumonia: European perspective. *Intensive Care Med.* 2009;35(1):9-29.

12. Kelly CA, Kotre CJ, Ward C, Hendrick DJ, Walters EH. Anatomical distribution of bronchoalveolar lavage fluid as assessed by digital subtraction radiography. *Thorax.* 1987;42(8):624-628.

13. Chandan SS, Faoagali J, Wainwright CE. Sensitivity of respiratory bacteria to lignocaine. *Pathology.* 2005;37(4):305-307.

14. Souweine B, Veber B, Bedos JP, et al. Diagnostic accuracy of protected specimen brush and bronchoalveolar lavage in nosocomial pneumonia: impact of previous antimicrobial treatments. *Crit Care Med.* 1998;26(2):236-244.

15. Baker AM, Bowton DL, Haponik EF. Decision making in nosocomial pneumonia. An analytic approach to the interpretation of quantitative bronchoscopic cultures. *Chest.* 1995;107(1):85-95.

16. Prats E, Dorca J, Pujol M, et al. Effects of antibiotics on protected specimen brush sampling in ventilator-associated pneumonia. *Eur Respir J.* 2002;19(5):944-951.

17. Lundgren R, Haggmark S, Reiz S. Hemodynamic effects of flexible fiberoptic bronchoscopy performed under topical anesthesia. *Chest.* 1982;82(3):295-299.

18. Kaplan JD, Schuster DP. Physiologic consequences of tracheal intubation. *Clin Chest Med.* 1991;12(3):425-432.

19. Staender S, Marsch SC, Schumacher P, Schaefer HG. Haemodynamic response to fiberoptic versus laryngoscopic nasotracheal intubation under total intravenous anaesthesia. *Eur J Anaesthesiol.* 1994;11(3):175-179.

20. Stoelting RK. Circulatory changes during direct laryngoscopy and tracheal intubation: influence of duration of laryngoscopy with or without prior lidocaine. *Anesthesiology.* 1977;47(4):381-384.

21. Matsushima Y, Jones RL, King EG, Moysa G, Alton JD. Alterations in pulmonary mechanics and gas exchange during routine fiberoptic bronchoscopy. *Chest.* 1984;86(2):184-188.

22. Lindholm CE, Ollman B, Snyder JV, Millen EG, Grenvik A. Cardiorespiratory effects of flexible fiberoptic bronchoscopy in critically ill patients. *Chest.* 1978;74(4):362-368.

23. Rudy EB, Turner BS, Baun M, Stone KS, Brucia J. Endotracheal suctioning in adults with head injury. *Heart Lung.* 1991;20(6):667-674.

24. Lodrini S, Montolivo M, Pluchino F, Borroni V. Positive end-expiratory pressure in supine and sitting positions: its effects on intrathoracic and intracranial pressures. *Neurosurgery.* 1989;24(6):873-877.

25. Kerwin AJ, Croce MA, Timmons SD, Maxwell RA, Malhotra AK, Fabian TC. Effects of fiberoptic bronchoscopy on intracranial pressure in patients with brain injury: a prospective clinical study. *J Trauma.* 2000;48(5):878-882; discussion 882-883.

26. Peerless JR, Snow N, Likavec MJ, Pinchak AC, Malangoni MA. The effect of fiberoptic bronchoscopy on cerebral hemodynamics in patients with severe head injury. *Chest.* 1995;108(4):962-965.

27. Bajwa MK, Henein S, Kamholz SL. Fiberoptic bronchoscopy in the presence of space-occupying intracranial lesions. *Chest.* 1993;104(1):101-103.

28. Bilotta F, Branca G, Lam A, Cuzzone V, Doronzio A, Rosa G. Endotracheal lidocaine in preventing endotracheal suctioning-induced changes in cerebral hemodynamics in patients with severe head trauma. *Neurocrit Care.* 2008;8(2):241-246.

29. Kerr ME, Sereika SM, Orndoff P, et al. Effect of neuromuscular blockers and opiates on the cerebrovascular response to endotracheal suctioning in adults with severe head injuries. *Am J Crit Care.* 1998;7(3):205-217.

30. Kerr ME, Rudy EB, Weber BB, et al. Effect of short-duration hyperventilation during endotracheal suctioning on intracranial pressure in severe head-injured adults. *Nurs Res.* 1997;46(4):195-201.

31. Previgliano IJ, Ripoll PI, Chiappero G, et al. Optimizing cerebral perfusion pressure during fiberoptic bronchoscopy in severe head injury: effect of hyperventilation. *Acta Neurochir Suppl.* 2002; 81:103-105.

32. Kristensen MS, Milman N, Jarnvig IL. Pulse oximetry at fibre-optic bronchoscopy in local anaesthesia: indication for postbronchoscopy oxygen supplementation? *Respir Med.* 1998;92(3):432-437.

33. Chhajed PN, Aboyoun C, Malouf MA, et al. Management of acute hypoxemia during flexible bronchoscopy with insertion of a nasopharyngeal tube in lung transplant recipients. *Chest.* 2002;121(4):1350-1354.

34. Pue CA, Pacht ER. Complications of fiberoptic bronchoscopy at a university hospital. *Chest.* 1995;107(2):430-432.

35. Weiss SM, Hert RC, Gianola FJ, Clark JG, Crawford SW. Complications of fiberoptic bronchoscopy in thrombocytopenic patients. *Chest.* 1993;104(4):1025-1028.

36. Webb AR, Doherty JF, Chester MR, et al. Sedation for fibreoptic bronchoscopy: comparison of alfentanil with papaveretum and diazepam. *Respir Med.* 1989;83(3):213-217.

37. Shinagawa N, Yamazaki K, Kinoshita I, Ogura S, Nishimura M. Susceptibility to oxygen desaturation during bronchoscopy in elderly patients with pulmonary fibrosis. *Respiration.* 2006;73(1):90-94.

38. Petersen GM, Pierson DJ, Hunter PM. Arterial oxygen saturation during nasotracheal suctioning. *Chest.* 1979;76(3):283-287.

39. Pirozynski M, Sliwinski P, Radwan L, Zielinski J. Bronchoalveolar lavage: comparison of three commonly used procedures. *Respiration.* 1991;58(2): 72-76.

40. Pirozynski M, Sliwinski P, Zielinski J. Effect of different volumes of BAL fluid on arterial oxygen saturation. *Eur Respir J.* 1988;1(10):943-947.

41. Matot I, Kramer MR, Glantz L, Drenger B, Cotev S. Myocardial ischemia in sedated patients undergoing fiberoptic bronchoscopy. *Chest.* 1997;112(6): 1454-1458.

42. Suratt PM, Smiddy JF, Gruber B. Deaths and complications associated with fiberoptic bronchoscopy. *Chest.* 1976;69(6):747-751.

43. Dreisin RB, Albert RK, Talley PA, Kryger MH, Scoggin CH, Zwillich CW. Flexible fiberoptic bronchoscopy in the teaching hospital. Yield and complications. *Chest.* 1978;74(2):144-149.

44. Shrader DL, Lakshminarayan S. The effect of fiberoptic bronchoscopy on cardiac rhythm. *Chest.* 1978;73(6):821-824.

45. Katz AS, Michelson EL, Stawicki J, Holford FD. Cardiac arrhythmias. Frequency during fiberoptic bronchoscopy and correlation with hypoxemia. *Arch Intern Med.* 1981;141(5):603-606.

46. Kreider ME, Lipson DA. Bronchoscopy for atelectasis in the ICU: a case report and review of the literature. *Chest.* 2003;124(1):344-350.

47. Olopade CO, Prakash UB. Bronchoscopy in the critical-care unit. *Mayo Clin Proc.* 1989;64(10): 1255-1263.

48. Weinstein HJ, Bone RC, Ruth WE. Pulmonary lavage in patients treated with mechanical ventilation. *Chest.* 1977;72(5):583-587.

49. Lindholm CE, Ollman B, Snyder J, Millen E, Grenvik A. Flexible fiberoptic bronchoscopy in critical care medicine. Diagnosis, therapy and complications. *Crit Care Med.* 1974;2(5):250-261.

50. Stevens RP, Lillington GA, Parsons GH. Fiberoptic bronchoscopy in the intensive care unit. *Heart Lung.* 1981;10(6):1037-1045.

51. Marini JJ, Pierson DJ, Hudson LD. Acute lobar atelectasis: a prospective comparison of fiberoptic bronchoscopy and respiratory therapy. *Am Rev Respir Dis.* 1979;119(6):971-978.

52. Lee TS, Wright BD. Selective insufflation of collapsed lung with fiberoptic bronchoscope and Swan-Ganz catheter. *Intensive Care Med.* 1981;7(5): 241-243.

53. Millen JE, Vandree J, Glauser FL. Fiberoptic bronchoscopic balloon occlusion and reexpansion of refractory unilateral atelectasis. *Crit Care Med.* 1978;6(1):50-55.

54. Tsao TC, Tsai YH, Lan RS, Shieh WB, Lee CH. Treatment for collapsed lung in critically ill patients. Selective intrabronchial air insufflation using the fiberoptic bronchoscope. *Chest.* 1990;97(2):435-438.

55. Harada K, Mutsuda T, Saoyama N, Taniki T, Kimura H. Re-expansion of refractory atelectasis using a bronchofiberscope with a balloon cuff. *Chest.* 1983;84(6):725-728.

56. Susini G, Sisillo E, Bortone F, Salvi L, Moruzzi P. Postoperative atelectasis reexpansion by selective

insufflation through a balloon-tipped catheter. *Chest.* 1992;102(6):1693-1696.

57. Haenel JB, Moore FA, Moore EE, Read RA. Efficacy of selective intrabronchial air insufflation in acute lobar collapse. *Am J Surg.* 1992;164(5):501-505.

58. van Heerden PV, Jacob W, Cameron PD, Webb S. Bronchoscopic insufflation of room air for the treatment of lobar atelectasis in mechanically ventilated patients. *Anaesth Intensive Care.* 1995;23(2):175-177.

59. Snow N, Lucas AE. Bronchoscopy in the critically ill surgical patient. *Am Surg.* 1984;50(8):441-445.

60. Donnelly WH. Histopathology of endotracheal intubation. An autopsy study of 99 cases. *Arch Pathol.* 1969;88(5):511-520.

61. Mackle T, Meaney J, Timon C. Tracheoesophageal compression associated with substernal goitre. Correlation of symptoms with cross-sectional imaging findings. *J Laryngol Otol.* 2007;121(4):358-361.

62. Maury E, Guglielminotti J, Alzieu M, Qureshi T, Guidet B, Offenstadt G. How to identify patients with no risk for postextubation stridor? *J Crit Care.* 2004;19(1):23-28.

63. Cheng KC, Hou CC, Huang HC, Lin SC, Zhang H. Intravenous injection of methylprednisolone reduces the incidence of postextubation stridor in intensive care unit patients. *Crit Care Med.* 2006;34(5):1345-1350.

64. Wittekamp BH, van Mook WN, Tjan DH, Zwaveling JH, Bergmans DC. Clinical review: post-extubation laryngeal edema and extubation failure in critically ill adult patients. *Crit Care.* 2009;13(6):233.

65. Kemper KJ, Benson MS, Bishop MJ. Predictors of postextubation stridor in pediatric trauma patients. *Crit Care Med.* 1991;19(3):352-355.

66. Sandhu RS, Pasquale MD, Miller K, Wasser TE. Measurement of endotracheal tube cuff leak to predict postextubation stridor and need for reintubation. *J Am Coll Surg.* 2000;190(6):682-687.

67. Miller RL, Cole RP. Association between reduced cuff leak volume and postextubation stridor. *Chest.* 1996;110(4):1035-1040.

68. Jaber S, Chanques G, Matecki S, et al. Post-extubation stridor in intensive care unit patients. Risk factors evaluation and importance of the cuff-leak test. *Intensive Care Med.* 2003;29(1):69-74.

69. Francois B, Bellissant E, Gissot V, et al. 12-h pretreatment with methylprednisolone versus placebo for prevention of postextubation laryngeal oedema: a randomised double-blind trial. *Lancet.* 2007;369(9567):1083-1089.

70. Lee CH, Peng MJ, Wu CL. Dexamethasone to prevent postextubation airway obstruction in adults: a prospective, randomized, double-blind, placebo-controlled study. *Crit Care.* 2007;11(4):R72.

71. Epstein SK, Ciubotaru RL. Independent effects of etiology of failure and time to reintubation on outcome for patients failing extubation. *Am J Respir Crit Care Med.* 1998;158(2):489-493.

72. Melloni G, Muttini S, Gallioli G, et al. Surgical tracheostomy versus percutaneous dilatational tracheostomy. A prospective-randomized study with long-term follow-up. *J Cardiovasc Surg (Torino).* 2002;43(1):113-121.

73. Freeman BD, Isabella K, Lin N, Buchman TG. A meta-analysis of prospective trials comparing percutaneous and surgical tracheostomy in critically ill patients. *Chest.* 2000;118(5):1412-1418.

74. Freeman BD, Isabella K, Cobb JP, et al. A prospective, randomized study comparing percutaneous with surgical tracheostomy in critically ill patients. *Crit Care Med.* 2001;29(5):926-930.

75. Barba CA, Angood PB, Kauder DR, et al. Bronchoscopic guidance makes percutaneous tracheostomy a safe, cost-effective, and easy-to-teach procedure. *Surgery.* 1995;118(5):879-883.

76. Grundling M, Pavlovic D, Kuhn SO, Feyerherd F. Is the method of modified percutaneous tracheostomy without bronchoscopic guidance really simple and safe? *Chest.* 2005;128(5):3774-3775.

77. Marx WH, Ciaglia P, Graniero KD. Some important details in the technique of percutaneous dilatational tracheostomy via the modified Seldinger technique. *Chest.* 1996;110(3):762-766.

78. Shennib H, Baslaim G. Bronchoscopy in the intensive care unit. *Chest Surg Clin N Am.* 1996;6(2):349-361.

79. Polderman KH, Spijkstra JJ, de Bree R, et al. Percutaneous tracheostomy in the intensive care unit: which safety precautions? *Crit Care Med.* 2001;29(1):221-223.

80. Rumbak MJ, Walsh FW, Anderson WM, Rolfe MW, Solomon DA. Significant tracheal obstruction causing failure to wean in patients requiring prolonged mechanical ventilation: a forgotten complication of long-term mechanical ventilation. *Chest.* 1999;115(4):1092-1095.

81. Bulpa PA, Dive AM, Mertens L, et al. Combined bronchoalveolar lavage and transbronchial lung biopsy: safety and yield in ventilated patients. *Eur Respir J.* 2003;21(3):489-494.

Renal and Electrolyte Disorders

Section editor: Lawrence S. Weisberg, MD

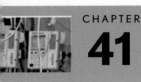

41

Acute Renal Failure

Jean-Sebastien Rachoin, MD
Lawrence S. Weisberg, MD

A 72-year-old man, recently treated for resistant *Escherichia coli* urosepsis, is sent to the emergency department from his nursing home because of new left-sided hemiparesis. He has a past history of chronic kidney disease (CKD), hypertension, and osteoarthritis. Medications include lisinopril 20 mg daily and naproxen 400 mg twice a day. On physical examination, he has a low-grade fever of 38°C (100.4°F), his initial blood pressure is 130/66 mm Hg, and his heart rate is 88 bpm. He is breathing at 28 breaths/min, and his hemoglobin oxygen saturation by pulse oximetry is 89% on supplemental oxygen by nasal cannula. He has a flaccid left hemiparesis and is stuporous.

He undergoes a computed tomogram (CT) of the head, which shows no hemorrhage. He has a CT angiogram of the chest, which shows no evidence of pulmonary embolism. His temperature rises quickly to 38.9°C (102°F), the blood pressure falls to 78/50 mm Hg, and the heart rate rises to 120 bpm. His initial white blood cell count is 29.9 with 44% bands, and a urine analysis shows pyuria and bacteriuria. Treatment is initiated with vancomycin, gentamicin, and cefepime. Intravenous normal saline is given by rapid infusion, according to the sepsis protocol. The patient is intubated and placed on mechanical ventilation. The serum creatinine, 1.6 mg/dL on arrival, increases to 2.0 mg/dL by the following day, and the blood urea nitrogen (BUN) has risen from 22 mg/dL to 36 mg/dL. Urine output has been about 20 mL/h for the past 8 hours.

The patient's daughter, a registered nurse, is in the room when you make rounds. She is aware of his history of chronic kidney disease, and wants to know if he is in "kidney failure." What do you tell her?

Although acute renal failure (ARF) is conceptually simple to characterize as "an abrupt decrease in renal function," a commonly accepted definition of ARF emerged only very recently.

An international group of experts convened in 2002 to develop a consensus definition of ARF in order to advance research in the field. They devised a staging classification for ARF—using changes in serum creatinine concentration and hourly urine output—and gave it the acronym RIFLE (Risk, Injury, Failure, Loss, and End-Stage) (Table 41-1).[1] Many investigators have since validated that classification scheme in various clinical settings, and a recent meta-analysis showed a graded impact on mortality by RIFLE stage.[2]

The RIFLE criteria represented real progress in the field of ARF research. Nonetheless, shortcomings of RIFLE were soon recognized: there was frequent discordance between the stage assignment by the serum creatinine and the urine output criteria.[3] In addition, smaller changes in serum creatinine (≥ 0.3 mg/dL)[4] over a short time (48 hours)[5] were shown to be associated with important clinical outcomes.

With the goal of refining the ARF definition, a second international group met in 2004. Their consensus produced the Acute Kidney Injury Network (AKIN) criteria.[6] They recommended that the term *acute kidney injury (AKI)* replace ARF, to reflect the fact that *failure* is at the extreme end

Table 41-1. Comparison of RIFLE and AKIN Criteria

Definitions				
	RIFLE[a] Stage		**AKIN[b] Stage**	
Risk	GFR ↓ 25% from baseline	1		SCr ≥ 0.3 mg/dL, or
	SCr ↑ 1.5-2 times baseline			SCr ↑ 1.5-2 times baseline
	UOP < 0.5 mL/kg per h for > 6 h			UOP < 0.5 mL/kg per h for > 6 h
Injury	GFR ↓ 50% from baseline	2		SCr ↑ 2-3 times
	SCr ↑ 2 times baseline			UOP < 0.5 mL/kg per h for > 12 h
	UOP < 0.5 mL/kg per h for > 12 h			
Failure	GFR ↓ 75%	3		SCr ↑ 3 times
	SCr ↑ 3 times baseline			SCr > 4 mg/dL or acute ↑ 0.5 mg/dL
	SCr > 4 mg/dL or acute ↑ 0.5 mg/dL			UOP < 0.3 mL/kg per h for ≥ 24 h
				Acute RRT
	UOP < 0.3 mL/kg per h for ≥ 24 h			
Loss[c]	Dialysis dependence > 4 wk			
ESRD[c]	Dialysis dependence > 3 mo			

Abbreviations: ESRD, end-stage renal disease; GFR, glomerular filtration rate; RRT, renal replacement therapy (see text); SCr, serum creatinine concentration; UOP, urine output.

[a] Change over 7 d compared to baseline.

[b] Change over 48 h.

[c] Outcome stages.

(From Bellomo R, Ronco C, Kellum JA, Mehta RL, Palevsky P. Acute renal failure—definition, outcome measures, animal models, fluid therapy and information technology needs: the Second International Consensus Conference of the Acute Dialysis Quality Initiative (ADQI) Group. Crit Care. 2004;8(4):R204-R212; and Mehta RL, Kellum JA, Shah SV, et al. Acute Kidney Injury Network: report of an initiative to improve outcomes in acute kidney injury. Crit Care. 2007;11(2):R31.)

of a broad spectrum of injury to the kidney.[6] They defined stages of AKI based on smaller changes in serum creatinine concentration (0.3 mg/dL) over shorter time period (48 hours). Table 41-1 compares the RIFLE and AKIN criteria.

The AKIN and RIFLE criteria agreed substantially in the classification of a large number of critically ill patients, and similarly correlated with mortality.[7] (Whether mortality is the proper outcome by which to validate a definition of AKI is open to question.[8])

It is important to recognize that these definitions of ARF or AKI were devised to facilitate research. From a practical standpoint, clinicians will diagnose AKI by a rise in the serum creatinine concentration and BUN over hours to days. Using this practical criterion, or either of the consensus definitions, our patient has AKI.

The daughter wants to know how common it is to develop acute kidney injury in this setting, and whether her father was at particular risk.

AKI is common in critically ill patients, and its frequency increases with severity of illness.[7] Overall, its occurrence varies from 5% in all hospitalized patients,[9] to 10% to 20% in patients after cardiac surgery,[10] to 20% in patients with sepsis, and up to 50% in patients with positive blood cultures.[11] AKI was diagnosed in 23% of patients with acute subarachnoid hemorrhage[12] and in 14% to 27% of patients after acute stroke.[13,14]

Risk factors for AKI in patients with strokes include age, underlying CKD, heart disease, stroke type (hemorrhagic more than ischemic), and severity.[13,14] In patients with subarachnoid hemorrhage, poor Hunt and Hess score on admission and higher admission serum creatinine concentration were associated with AKI (Table 41-2).[12]

The daughter wants to know whether the AKI itself will affect her father's prognosis.

AKI is associated with worse outcomes in critically ill patients as it aggravates morbidity and both short- and long-term mortality. In addition to the direct effects of kidney dysfunction (eg, volume overload, electrolyte and acid-base derangements, uremia), it also affects other organs at a distance both in space and time.

Table 41-2. AKI in Specific Settings Encountered in Neurology ICU

Clinical setting	Incidence	Risk factor	Impact
Stroke	14%-27%	• CKD • Age • Stroke type/severity	• ↑ 30-day and long-term mortality
Subarachnoid hemorrhage	23%	• Poor H&H scale (IV-V) • Higher admission SCr	• ↑ Mortality and cardiovascular outcomes
Rhabdomyolysis induced by seizures	Rare	• Prolonged seizure • Status epilepticus • CK > 15,000 • Volume depletion	• No long-term impact • Might require short-term RRT
CT angiography	3%-3.5%	• Worsening CKD	• No RRT
Mannitol	0%-11%	• CKD • Higher mannitol dose	• Unclear

Abbreviations: AKI, acute kidney injury; CK, creatine kinase; CKD, chronic kidney disease; CT, computed tomography; H&H, Hunt and Hess; ICU, intensive care unit; RRT, renal replacement therapy.

Animal data show that AKI induces or worsens acute lung injury by increasing pulmonary vascular permeability and neutrophil infiltration[15] via cytokine production.[16-18] Moreover, it leads to cardiac dysfunction by stimulating inflammation,[19] fibrosis,[20] and apoptosis.[15] The neurologic system may be affected by AKI, with reported increases in cerebral vascular permeability, inflammation, and functional impairment.[20] In addition, uremic toxins also have deleterious effects on the bone marrow and on liver function.[21] Thus, it is not surprising that AKI is reported to have an independent association with mortality.[11,22-24]

Until recently, it was generally thought that if patients survived their episode of AKI, their renal function was likely to recover to its baseline. It is now increasingly apparent that AKI predisposes to the development of CKD[22,25] and end-stage (dialysis-dependent) renal disease (ESRD),[25-27] the latter being more common in patients with underlying CKD and in older patients.

In a prospective study of patients admitted with acute subarachnoid hemorrhage, AKI was significantly associated with increased mortality rate.[12] In patients with acute stroke, AKI worsened both short-term[14] and long-term mortality.[13]

What is the likely cause of the patient's AKI?

The etiology of AKI can be divided into prerenal, postrenal, and renal causes (Table 41-3).

Prerenal failure is AKI due to altered renal hemodynamics, such that if normal renal perfusion were restored, the AKI would resolve immediately. Prerenal states often are evident by

Table 41-3. Causes of Acute Kidney Injury

- Prerenal
  - Absolute volume depletion
  - Decreased effective circulating volume
    - Congestive heart failure
    - Cirrhosis
  - "Renal autoregulatory failure"
- Postrenal
  - Ureteral obstruction
    - Stones
    - Tumor
    - Fibrosis
  - Bladder outlet obstruction
- Intrinsic renal disease
  - Acute tubular necrosis (ATN)
    - Toxic
    - Ischemic
    - Mixed
  - Acute glomerulonephritis (AGN)
  - Acute interstitial nephritis (AIN)
  - Acute renal vasculitis
  - Acute intratubular obstruction
    - Tumor lysis syndrome
    - Drug induced

history (eg, history of negative fluid balance or hemorrhage) or physical examination. It is important to recognize, however, that physical assessment of volume status may be quite unreliable,[28] and perhaps all the more so in critically ill patients, where the usual indices (vital signs, edema) may be misleading. In oliguric patients (urine output < 0.5 mL/kg per hour), the fractional excretion of sodium (FE_{Na}) may improve diagnostic accuracy: an FE_{Na} less than 1% is evidence of avid sodium reabsorption by functional renal tubules and is consistent with a prerenal state.[29,30] FE_{Na}, expressed as a percentage, is calculated from a "spot" urine and simultaneous plasma sample as follows:

$$FE_{Na} = \frac{U_{Na}}{P_{Na}} \div \frac{U_{Cr}}{P_{Cr}} \times 100$$

where U_{Na} is the urine sodium concentration, P_{Na} is the plasma sodium concentration (mEq/L), U_{Cr} is the urine creatinine concentration, and P_{Cr} is the plasma or serum creatinine concentration (mg/dL). Note that the FE_{Na} may be high in a volume-depleted patient who is undergoing diuresis[29] and may be low with some causes of intrinsic renal failure, most notably radiocontrast[31] and pigmenturia.[32]

Prerenal failure due to "renal autoregulatory failure" is a common phenomenon. The kidney depends on a variety of humoral mediators of vascular tone—among which are components of the renin-angiotensin system and vasodilatory prostaglandins—to autoregulate its blood flow over a wide range of mean arterial pressure and to autoregulate its glomerular filtration rate (GFR) over a wide range of renal blood flow. This complex autoregulation serves to maintain GFR in states of hemodynamic compromise.[33] Medications that interrupt renal autoregulation (eg, angiotensin-converting enzyme [ACE] inhibitors, angiotensin receptor blockers, and prostaglandin synthesis inhibitors) lead to prerenal AKI in the setting of modest volume depletion or hypotension that would otherwise be well tolerated.[34] Our patient was taking both an ACE inhibitor and a cyclooxygenase (COX) inhibitor and so is at risk for prerenal failure.

Postrenal failure is due to obstruction of the urinary tract distal to the renal collecting ducts. Common causes are listed in Table 41-3. In elderly men, the most common cause is bladder outlet obstruction from prostate enlargement. Stroke may amplify the tendency for bladder outlet obstruction. After stroke, bladder dysfunction is common, and bladder-emptying disorders may be more common after ischemic than hemorrhagic stroke.[35] Other factors that may predispose to bladder outlet obstruction include underlying autonomic neuropathy (eg, from diabetes mellitus) and medications with anticholinergic activity. Renal ultrasound has over 95% sensitivity for detecting urinary tract obstruction, manifested by dilation of the urinary collecting system (hydronephrosis with or without hydroureter).[36]

The classification of intrinsic or renal parenchymal causes of AKI follows a histologic nosology (see Table 41-3). Diagnosis is guided by urinalysis with microscopic examination of the sediment (Table 41-4).[37]

Among the types of intrinsic renal failure, acute tubular necrosis (ATN) is by far the most common in the intensive care unit (ICU).[38,39] ATN may be caused by a nephrotoxic or ischemic insult, or a combination of the two.[39,40] Common nephrotoxins include radiocontrast dye, aminoglycoside antibiotics, amphotericin, and endogenous pigments such as myoglobin and free hemoglobin. Ischemic insults include shock, sepsis, and major vascular surgery that may compromise renal perfusion. The likelihood of having ATN is proportional to the number of granular casts on urine microscopy; the positive predictive value of finding any casts approaches 100%.[37]

Of particular relevance to the neurology ICU (but not a factor in the current case) is the role of mannitol in the development of AKI. Mannitol infusion for treatment of increased intracranial pressure (ICP) is recognized to be associated with AKI,[41,42] especially with the use of very high doses.[42,43] High-dose mannitol seems to have a vasoconstrictive effect and also induces "osmotic nephrosis" in renal proximal tubule cells.[44] AKI also has been reported to result from hypertonic saline infusion for treatment of increased ICP.[45]

Table 41-4. Urinalysis in Intrinsic Renal Disease

Lesion	Urine Dipstick	Urine Sediment
ATN	Sp. gr. 1.010-1.020 1+ protein reaction	Many granular casts "Dirty" or "dusty" background
AGN	Sp. gr. 1.020-1.030 1-3+ protein reaction > 2+ heme reaction	RBCs > WBCs Dysmorphic RBCs RBC casts
AIN	Sp. gr. 1.010-1.020 1+ protein reaction	WBCs > RBCs WBC casts Eosinophiluria
Vasculitis	Sp. gr. variable 1-2+ protein reaction Variable heme reaction	Bland sediment or RBCs
Intratubular obstruction	Sp. gr. variable Variable heme reaction	Crystalluria

Abbreviations: AGN, acute glomerulonephritis; AIN, acute interstitial nephritis; ATN, acute tubular necrosis; RBCs, red blood cells; Sp. gr., specific gravity; WBCs, white blood cells.

Acute glomerulonephritis (AGN) and acute renal vasculitis are rare causes of AKI in critically ill patients.[11,46] AGN or renal vasculitis in a patient with a critical brain disorder should trigger a search for a systemic disease that might explain both phenomena, such as systemic lupus erythematosus and cryoglobulinemia. The suggested serologic evaluation of a patient suspected of having AGN or vasculitis is presented in Table 41-5.

Acute interstitial nephritis (AIN) is most commonly seen as an allergic reaction to a medication. The list of medications associated with AIN is long[47]; frequent culprits include β-lactam and sulfonamide antibiotics, loop-acting and thiazide diuretics, allopurinol, and nonsteroidal anti-inflammatory drugs.[47,48] Other causes of AIN include infections of various types and systemic conditions, such as lupus erythematosus, Sjögren syndrome, and sarcoidosis.[48] Classic associations with AIN include fever, generalized rash, and peripheral eosinophilia. Each of these is present in fewer than 50% of patients with drug-induced AIN, however, and the triad occurs in fewer than 5% of cases.[47] Thus, AIN should be suspected in any patient with otherwise unexplained AKI and an active urine sediment.

Table 41-5. Serologic Evaluation of Suspected Vasculitis or AGN

- C_3, C_4 complement components
- ANA, anti-dsDNA
- Anti-GBM antibody
- ANCA antibodies (MPO, PR3)
- Hepatitis serologies
- Cryoglobulins

Abbreviations: AGN, acute glomerulonephritis; ANA, antinuclear antibody; ANCA, antineutrophil cytoplasmic antibodies; dsDNA, double-stranded DNA; GBM, glomerular basement membrane.

This patient received two nephrotoxins, gentamicin and iodinated radiocontrast. What is the likelihood that either of these contributed to his AKI? Could the AKI have been prevented?

Aminoglycosides such as gentamicin can induce ATN in up to 20% of cases. Among the frequently used agents, amikacin may be less nephrotoxic than gentamicin or tobramycin.

The drugs accumulate in the renal proximal tubule cells and cause cellular necrosis.[49] Risk factors for nephrotoxicity are advanced age, liver failure, renal failure, peak concentration, and volume depletion.[49,50]

With aminoglycoside nephrotoxicity, the serum creatinine concentration starts to rise a week to 10 days after beginning treatment. The AKI often is accompanied by hypokalemia, hypomagnesemia, and a non-anion-gap metabolic acidosis.

Prevention of aminoglycoside-induced AKI is best achieved by minimizing drug exposure, single daily dosing (in patients with normal baseline renal function), frequent pharmacokinetic monitoring, and daily serum creatinine concentration.[49]

The time course of AKI in this case is incompatible with aminoglycoside nephrotoxicity.

Radiocontrast-induced nephropathy (RCIN) is the third most common cause of AKI in hospitalized patients.[51] Its exact incidence is reported to be quite variable, and it depends on the stringency of the definition of AKI and the number and severity of risk factors prevalent in the population under consideration.[52] Risk factors for RCIN are shown in Table 41-6.[52-57] The incidence of RCIN in patients with mild CKD is less than 5%,[58,59] and as high as 50% in patients with advanced CKD with diabetes mellitus.[60] All other factors being equal, it appears to be less common with intravenous than intra-arterial radiocontrast administration.[61,62] One retrospective study, using a liberal definition of AKI, found a 3% incidence of radiocontrast-induced injury in unselected patients with acute stroke undergoing CT angiography; none of the patients in that study required renal replacement therapy (RRT).[63]

After injection of iodinated contrast, the glomerular filtration rate falls immediately, but the consequent accumulation of creatinine in the blood may be slow enough that a change in serum creatinine concentration is not detectable for 24 or 48 hours. The serum creatinine concentration usually reaches a plateau within a few days to a week, followed by resolution in 2 to 4 weeks. About 10% of patients require RRT to manage the consequences of AKI[64]; however, permanent dialysis dependence solely as a consequence of RCIN is rare.

Table 41-6. Risk Factors for RCIN

- Patient factors
  - CKD
  - Diabetes mellitus
  - Volume depletion
  - CHF
  - Shock
  - Intra-arterial balloon-pump
  - Age > 75 y
  - Low hematocrit
- Procedure-related factors
  - High-osmolality radiocontrast
  - High-contrast volume
  - Intra-arterial administration

Abbreviations: CHF, congestive heart failure; CKD, chronic kidney disease; RCIN, radiocontrast-induced nephropathy.

Renal and Electrolyte Disorders

Table 41-7. Preventive Measures for Minimizing the Risk of RCIN

We recommend the following:

- Avoid high-osmolality contrast agents
- Minimize volume of contrast injected
- Optimize the patient's volume status:
  Volume expansion with 0.9% NaCl (1 mL/kg) starting up to 12 h before and continuing up to 12 h after (adjusted for volume status; see text)
- Stop intravenous diuretics before the procedure
- Stop COX inhibitors

We do not discourage the use of:

- N-acetylcysteine 600-1200 mg orally every 12 h starting the day before, for a total of 4 doses

Abbreviations: COX, cyclo-oxygenase; RCIN, radiocontrast-induced nephropathy.

Because RCIN results from a discrete, premeditated event, it has been considered the paradigm for prevention (Table 41-7). Notwithstanding decades of research into its prevention, however, few interventions have shown convincing benefit.[55,65] The only surefire way to prevent RCIN is to avoid contrast administration. Short of that, only two interventions have proven unequivocally effective: intravenous fluids and manipulation of the radiocontrast agents.

Intravenous administration of sodium chloride reduces the risk of RCIN. Normal (0.9%) saline seems to be more effective than half-normal (0.45%) saline, when administered at 1 mL/kg/h starting before the contrast injection and continuing for 24 hours.[66] There has been debate as to whether sodium bicarbonate is more effective than normal saline for the prevention of RCIN. Studies to date have yielded conflicting results,[67,68] so there is no basis for recommending sodium bicarbonate. Decompensated congestive heart failure probably is just as great a risk for RCIN as volume depletion. Thus, intravenous saline must be used cautiously in patients with impaired heart or renal function, and should be avoided in patients who are already fluid overloaded. The use of intravenous furosemide before contrast administration has been shown to be deleterious,[69] and this has led to the recommendation that even oral diuretics be held before contrast procedures.

The risk of RCIN appears to be related to the chemistry of the radiocontrast agent, its route of administration, and its dose. Radiocontrast agents vary according to their osmolality. Conventional high-osmolality agents have an osmolality of about 1200 mOsm/kg, and so-called low-osmolality agents about 600 mOsm/kg. The newest, iso-osmolar agents have an osmolality of about 300 mOsm/kg. There is little doubt that high-osmolality agents are more nephrotoxic than low-osmolality agents.[70,71] The additional benefits of iso-osmolar agents in this regard are unclear.[72,73] Recent studies have shown that intra-arterial rather than intravenous administration of contrast is associated with a greater risk of ARF.[61,62] Finally, the risk of RCIN in high-risk patients seems to be proportional to the volume of contrast administered.[53]

Other interventions intended to prevent RCIN have failed to show a consistent benefit. N-acetylcysteine (NAC, Mucomyst) showed great promise early on,[74] but subsequent studies have been equivocal.[75-78] Because oral NAC appears to have little if any toxicity, its use in this setting cannot be strongly discouraged. Other interventions shown to be of no benefit for prophylaxis of RCIN include natriuretic peptides,[79] dopaminergic agents,[55] and cessation of ACE inhibitors or angiotensin receptor blockers.[80] A single-center study on the use of prophylactic hemofiltration showed a reduction in 1-year mortality,[81] an outcome of dubious relationship to the intervention, and one that does not justify routine use of this invasive modality. Because COX inhibitors predispose animals to RCIN,[82] it is prudent to withhold them in patients about to receive a radiocontrast infusion.

In the present case, radiocontrast administration is very likely to have contributed to the development of nephrotoxic ATN. The additional probable cause is sepsis leading to ischemic ATN. This sort of multifactorial AKI is quite typical of critically ill patients.

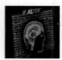

In support of the diagnosis of ATN, the urinalysis shows a specific gravity of 1.010 and more than 5 granular casts per high-power field. The patient's urine volume fell steadily, and over the next few days he became anuric.

What is the general medical treatment of AKI?

Table 41-8 shows the general approach to medical management of the patient with AKI.

Hemodynamic optimization will, by definition, reverse prerenal AKI[83] and may reduce the likelihood of progression from prerenal failure to ATN.[84] Regardless of the impact on renal function, however, critically ill patients in shock need adequate intravascular volume resuscitation in order to restore organ perfusion and cardiac output. The amounts and duration of fluid therapy are still controversial: fluid administration is clearly beneficial early in the course of the disease,[85] but overaggressive volume resuscitation has been associated with worse outcomes.[86] Furthermore, only half of the patients with circulatory failure respond to fluid,[87] and the determination of fluid responsiveness can be challenging.[88]

Hence, the need for fluid administration has to be carefully evaluated in order to not place patients at risk of pulmonary edema or abdominal compartment syndrome.[89] There does not seem to be any superiority of colloid over crystalloid fluid administration[90]; in fact, use of the colloid plasma expander hydroxyethyl starch has been associated with increased risk of AKI.[91]

Loop diuretics have been used to augment urine output and potentially treat AKI. Although they can facilitate fluid management, they do not shorten the course of AKI, reduce the need for dialysis, or improve hospital mortality rate.[92]

Low-dose dopamine has achieved mythic status for its purported effect to selectively improve renal perfusion, and thus to cure renal failure. So sturdy is this myth that low-dose dopamine has even been given the eponym "renal dose dopamine." A body of literature has accumulated over many years, however, showing conclusively that dopamine is of no benefit whatsoever in AKI, and may be associated with gut necrosis and digital gangrene.[93,94] Indeed, low-dose dopamine seems to worsen renal hemodynamics in patients with ARF.[95] We strongly discourage the use of low-dose dopamine in AKI.

In cases of probable or possible AIN, the culprit medication should be stopped immediately. Glucocorticoid therapy appears to be beneficial in about half of patients if initiated within the first

Table 41-8. Medical Management of the Patient with AKI

- Optimize systemic hemodynamics
- Stop medications that caused or perpetuate AKI
- Adjust dosage of medications for renal dysfunction
- Monitor/adjust electrolytes
- Monitor/adjust acid-base status
- Ensure adequate nutrition
- Monitor for indications for renal replacement therapy

Abbreviation: AKI, acute kidney injury.

2 weeks of diagnosis,[96] and is indicated in cases where the diagnosis is highly likely or confirmed by renal biopsy.

Dosage of all medications should be reviewed for the impact of the decreased renal function on their elimination. In that regard, it is important to recognize that formulas for estimating glomerular filtration rate (eg, the MDRD formula[97]) and creatinine clearance (eg, the Cockroft and Gault formula[98]) cannot be used with a serum creatinine concentration that is rising or falling on a daily basis. These formulas apply only in steady-state conditions; they will overestimate renal function with a rising serum creatinine concentration, resulting in overdosage.

Because of the central role of the kidney in maintaining homeostasis of "the internal environment," disorders of sodium, potassium, calcium, phosphorus, and acid-base balance are common in patients with AKI. Serum chemistries should be monitored at least daily; more frequent monitoring would depend on the severity of the renal dysfunction and comorbidities.

Adequate nutrition should be ensured, with a daily caloric intake of 25 to 35 kcal/kg, with 0.8 g/kg of protein for patients not yet on RRT.[99]

The patient's systemic hemodynamics improve, but the urine output falls progressively, the BUN and serum creatinine concentration continue to rise, and by the fifth hospital day he is started on intermittent hemodialysis (see Chapter 42). The serum chemistries improve.

On the 10th hospital day, the temperature rises to 39.1°C (102.3°F) and the systolic blood pressure falls to 88 mm Hg. Antibiotic coverage is broadened, intravenous fluids are administered, and eventually, vasopressors are required to maintain a mean arterial pressure of 70 mm Hg. His oxygenation deteriorates, and on the 12th hospital day, the patient dies.

! CRITICAL CONSIDERATIONS

- AKI is currently defined by a rise in BUN and serum creatinine concentration over hours to days. Consensus criteria, for research purposes, specify a rise in serum creatinine concentration of 0.3 mg/dL over 48 hours.
- AKI is common in critically ill patients, and risk factors include underlying CKD and severity of illness.
- Renal dysfunction affects multiple organs and can result in distant injuries. It impacts both short- and long-term prognosis and is associated with increased mortality rate and a higher likelihood for future chronic kidney disease and ESRD.
- The differential diagnosis of AKI includes prerenal, postrenal, and renal causes. The diagnostic approach depends on a careful history and physical examination and simple laboratory tests. The FE_{Na} is useful in discriminating oliguric prerenal failure from ATN, but its use has limitations.
- Radiocontrast nephropathy develops immediately after exposure to the agent in susceptible patients. Risk factors include underlying CKD, diabetes mellitus, and volume depletion, among others. It can be best prevented by avoiding radiocontrast administration. If that is not possible, it is important to ensure the patient's fluid status is optimized and that the lowest dose of low-osmolality dye is used.
- Aminoglycoside nephrotoxicity typically develops a week to 10 days into the course of treatment. Risk factors for aminoglycoside-induced nephropathy include advanced age, liver

failure, renal failure, peak concentration, and volume depletion. Pharmacokinetics should be carefully monitored.

- Medical treatment of AKI includes optimizing systemic hemodynamics, eliminating culprit medications, adjusting medication dosages for renal dysfunction, and monitoring for the metabolic complications of AKI. Adequate nutrition needs to be ensured. Diuretics may aid in fluid management but will not shorten the course of AKI. Low-dose dopamine has no place in the treatment or prevention of ARF.

- Formulas that estimate GFR or creatinine clearance based on the serum creatinine concentration do not apply to patients with AKI, either developing or resolving. Their use in that setting will lead to either overdosing or underdosing of renally eliminated medications.

REFERENCES

1. Bellomo R, Ronco C, Kellum JA, Mehta RL, Palevsky P. Acute renal failure—definition, outcome measures, animal models, fluid therapy and information technology needs: the Second International Consensus Conference of the Acute Dialysis Quality Initiative (ADQI) Group. *Crit Care.* 2004;8(4):R204-R212.

2. Ricci Z, Cruz D, Ronco C. The RIFLE criteria and mortality in acute kidney injury: a systematic review. *Kidney Int.* 2008;73(5):538-546.

3. Cruz DN, Bolgan I, Perazella MA, Bonello M, de Cal M, Corradi V. North East Italian Prospective Hospital Renal Outcome Survey on Acute Kidney Injury (NEiPHROS-AKI): targeting the problem with the RIFLE Criteria. *Clin J Am Soc Nephrol.* 2007;2(3):418-425.

4. Chertow GM, Burdick E, Honour M, Bonventre JV, Bates DW. Acute kidney injury, mortality, length of stay, and costs in hospitalized patients. *J Am Soc Nephrol.* 2005;16(11):3365-3370.

5. Lassnigg A, Schmidlin D, Mouhieddine M, Bachmann LM, Druml W, Bauer P. Minimal changes of serum creatinine predict prognosis in patients after cardiothoracic surgery: a prospective cohort study. *J Am Soc Nephrol.* 2004;15(6):1597-1605.

6. Mehta RL, Kellum JA, Shah SV, Molitoris BA, Ronco C, Warnock DG. Acute Kidney Injury Network: report of an initiative to improve outcomes in acute kidney injury. *Crit Care.* 2007;11(2):R31.

7. Bagshaw SM, George C, Bellomo R. A comparison of the RIFLE and AKIN criteria for acute kidney injury in critically ill patients. *Nephrol Dial Transplant.* 2008;23(5):1569-1574.

8. Weisberg LS, Rachoin JS. Redefine acute renal failure? Not yet, thanks. *Crit Care Med.* 2008;36(4):1370-1372.

9. Xue JL, Daniels F, Star RA, Kimmel PL, Eggers PW, Molitoris BA. Incidence and mortality of acute renal failure in Medicare beneficiaries, 1992 to 2001. *J Am Soc Nephrol.* 2006;17(4):1135-1142.

10. Kuitunen A, Vento A, Suojaranta-Ylinen R, Pettila V. Acute renal failure after cardiac surgery: evaluation of the RIFLE classification. *Ann Thorac Surg.* 2006;81(2):542-546.

11. Uchino S, Kellum JA, Bellomo R, Doig GS, Morimatsu H, Morgera S. Acute renal failure in critically ill patients: a multinational, multicenter study. *JAMA.* 2005;294(7):813-818.

12. Zacharia BE, Ducruet AF, Hickman ZL, Grobelny BT, Fernandez L, Schmidt JM. Renal dysfunction as an independent predictor of outcome after aneurysmal subarachnoid hemorrhage: a single-center cohort study. *Stroke.* 2009;40(7):2375-2381.

13. Tsagalis G, Akrivos T, Alevizaki M, Manios E, Theodorakis M, Laggouranis A. Long-term prognosis of acute kidney injury after first acute stroke. *Clin J Am Soc Nephrol.* 2009;4(3):616-622.

14. Covic A, Schiller A, Mardare NG, Petrica L, Petrica M, Mihaescu A. The impact of acute kidney injury on short-term survival in an Eastern European population with stroke. *Nephrol Dial Transplant.* 2008;23(7):2228-2234.

15. Kelly KJ. Distant effects of experimental renal ischemia/reperfusion injury. *J Am Soc Nephrol.* 2003;14(6):1549-1558.

16. Hoke TS, Douglas IS, Klein CL, He Z, Fang W, Thurman JM. Acute renal failure after bilateral nephrectomy is associated with cytokine-mediated pulmonary injury. *J Am Soc Nephrol.* 2007;18(1):155-164.

17. Klein CL, Hoke TS, Fang WF, Altmann CJ, Douglas IS, Faubel S. Interleukin-6 mediates lung injury following ischemic acute kidney injury or bilateral nephrectomy. *Kidney Int.* 2008;74(7):901-909.

18. Grigoryev DN, Liu M, Hassoun HT, Cheadle C, Barnes KC, Rabb H. The local and systemic inflammatory transcriptome after acute kidney injury. *J Am Soc Nephrol.* 2008;19(3):547-558.

19. Tokuyama H, Kelly DJ, Zhang Y, Gow RM, Gilbert RE. Macrophage infiltration and cellular proliferation in the non-ischemic kidney and heart following prolonged unilateral renal ischemia. *Nephron Physiol.* 2007;106(3):p54-p62.

20. Liu M, Liang Y, Chigurupati S, Lathia JD, Pletnikov M, Sun Z. Acute kidney injury leads to inflammation and functional changes in the brain. *J Am Soc Nephrol.* 2008;19(7):1360-1370.

21. Scheel PJ, Liu M, Rabb H. Uremic lung: new insights into a forgotten condition. *Kidney Int.* 2008;74(7):849-851.

22. Coca SG, Yusuf B, Shlipak MG, Garg AX, Parikh CR. Long-term risk of mortality and other adverse outcomes after acute kidney injury: a systematic review and meta-analysis. *Am J Kidney Dis.* 2009;53(6):961-973.

23. Liano F, Junco E, Pascual J, Madero R, Verde E. The spectrum of acute renal failure in the intensive care unit compared with that seen in other settings. The Madrid Acute Renal Failure Study Group. *Kidney Int Suppl.* 1998;66:S16-S24.

24. Metnitz PG, Krenn CG, Steltzer H, Lang T, Ploder J, Lenz K. Effect of acute renal failure requiring renal replacement therapy on outcome in critically ill patients. *Crit Care Med.* 2002;30(9):2051-2058.

25. Ishani A, Xue JL, Himmelfarb J, Eggers PW, Kimmel PL, Molitoris BA. Acute kidney injury increases risk of ESRD among elderly. *J Am Soc Nephrol.* 2009;20(1):223-228.

26. Hsu CY, Chertow GM, McCulloch CE, Fan D, Ordonez JD, Go AS. Nonrecovery of kidney function and death after acute on chronic renal failure. *Clin J Am Soc Nephrol.* 2009;4(5):891-898.

27. Schmitt R, Coca S, Kanbay M, Tinetti ME, Cantley LG, Parikh CR. Recovery of kidney function after acute kidney injury in the elderly: a systematic review and meta-analysis. *Am J Kidney Dis.* 2008;52(2):262-271.

28. Chung HM, Kluge R, Schrier RW, Anderson RJ. Clinical assessment of extracellular fluid volume in hyponatremia. *Am J Med.* 1987;83(5):905-908.

29. Steiner RW. Interpreting the fractional excretion of sodium. *Am J Med.* 1984;77(4):699-702.

30. Miller TR, Anderson RJ, Linas SL, Henrich WL, Berns AS, Gabow PA. Urinary diagnostic indices in acute renal failure: a prospective study. *Ann Intern Med.* 1978;89(1):47-50.

31. Fang LS, Sirota RA, Ebert TH, Lichtenstein NS. Low fractional excretion of sodium with contrast media-induced acute renal failure. *Arch Intern Med.* 1980;140(4):531-533.

32. Corwin HL, Schreiber MJ, Fang LS. Low fractional excretion of sodium. Occurrence with hemoglobinuric- and myoglobinuric-induced acute renal failure. *Arch Intern Med.* 1984;144(5):981-982.

33. Cupples WA, Braam B. Assessment of renal autoregulation. *Am J Physiol Renal Physiol.* 2007;292(4):F1105-F1123.

34. Abuelo JG. Normotensive ischemic acute renal failure. *N Engl J Med.* 2007;357(8):797-805.

35. Ersoz M, Tunc H, Akyuz M, Ozel S. Bladder storage and emptying disorder frequencies in hemorrhagic and ischemic stroke patients with bladder dysfunction. *Cerebrovasc Dis.* 2005;20(5):395-399.

36. Mostbeck GH, Zontsich T, Turetschek K. Ultrasound of the kidney: obstruction and medical diseases. *Eur Radiol.* 2001;11(10):1878-1889.

37. Perazella MA, Coca SG, Kanbay M, Brewster UC, Parikh CR. Diagnostic value of urine microscopy for differential diagnosis of acute kidney injury in hospitalized patients. *Clin J Am Soc Nephrol.* 2008;3(6):1615-1619.

38. Bonventre JV, Weinberg JM. Recent advances in the pathophysiology of ischemic acute renal failure. *J Am Soc Nephrol.* 2003;14(8):2199-2210.

39. Mehta RL, Pascual MT, Soroko S, Savage BR, Himmelfarb J, Ikizler TA. Spectrum of acute renal failure in the intensive care unit: the PICARD experience. *Kidney Int.* 2004;66(4):1613-1621.

40. Weisberg LS, Allgren RL, Genter FC, Kurnik BR. Cause of acute tubular necrosis affects its prognosis. The Auriculin Anaritide Acute Renal Failure Study Group. *Arch Intern Med.* 1997;157(16):1833-1838.

41. Gondim Fde A, Aiyagari V, Shackleford A, Diringer MN. Osmolality not predictive of mannitol-induced acute renal insufficiency. *J Neurosurg.* 2005;103(3):444-447.

42. Dziedzic T, Szczudlik A, Klimkowicz A, Rog TM, Slowik A. Is mannitol safe for patients with intracerebral hemorrhages? Renal considerations. *Clin Neurol Neurosurg.* 2003;105(2):87-89.

43. Perez-Perez AJ, Pazos B, Sobrado J, Gonzalez L, Gandara A. Acute renal failure following massive mannitol infusion. *Am J Nephrol.* 2002;22(5-6):573-575.

44. Dickenmann M, Oettl T, Mihatsch MJ. Osmotic nephrosis: acute kidney injury with accumulation of proximal tubular lysosomes due to administration of exogenous solutes. *Am J Kidney Dis.* 2008;51(3):491-503.

45. Forsyth LL, Liu-DeRyke X, Parker D Jr, Rhoney DH. Role of hypertonic saline for the management of intracranial hypertension after stroke and traumatic brain injury. *Pharmacotherapy.* 2008;28(4):469-484.

46. Silvester W, Bellomo R, Cole L. Epidemiology, management, and outcome of severe acute renal failure of critical illness in Australia. *Crit Care Med.* 2001;29(10):1910-1915.

47. Rossert J. Drug-induced acute interstitial nephritis. *Kidney Int.* 2001;60(2):804-817.

48. Michel DM, Kelly CJ. Acute interstitial nephritis. *J Am Soc Nephrol.* 1998;9(3):506-515.

49. Rougier F, Claude D, Maurin M, Maire P. Aminoglycoside nephrotoxicity. *Curr Drug Targets Infect Disord.* 2004;4(2):153-162.

50. Kasiakou SK, Sermaides GJ, Michalopoulos A, Soteriades ES, Falagas ME. Continuous versus intermittent intravenous administration of antibiotics: a meta-analysis of randomised controlled trials. *Lancet Infect Dis.* 2005;5(9):581-589.

51. Nash K, Hafeez A, Hou S. Hospital-acquired renal insufficiency. *Am J Kidney Dis.* 2002;39(5):930-936.

52. Murphy SW, Barrett BJ, Parfrey PS. Contrast nephropathy. *J Am Soc Nephrol.* 2000;11(1):177-182.

53. Goldfarb S, McCullough PA, McDermott J, Gay SB. Contrast-induced acute kidney injury: specialty-specific protocols for interventional radiology, diagnostic computed tomography radiology, and interventional cardiology. *Mayo Clin Proc.* 2009;84(2):170-179.

54. Solomon R, Deray G. How to prevent contrast-induced nephropathy and manage risk patients: practical recommendations. *Kidney Int Suppl.* 2006;(100):S51-S53.

55. Pannu N, Wiebe N, Tonelli M. Prophylaxis strategies for contrast-induced nephropathy. *JAMA.* 2006;295(23):2765-2779.

56. Barrett BJ, Parfrey PS. Clinical practice. Preventing nephropathy induced by contrast medium. *N Engl J Med.* 2006;354(4):379-386.

57. Parfrey P. The clinical epidemiology of contrast-induced nephropathy. *Cardiovasc Intervent Radiol.* 2005;28(Suppl 2):S3-S11.

58. Parfrey PS, Griffiths SM, Barrett BJ, Paul MD, Genge M, Withers J. Contrast material-induced renal failure in patients with diabetes mellitus, renal insufficiency, or both. A prospective controlled study. *N Engl J Med.* 1989;320(3):143-149.

59. Kelly AM, Dwamena B, Cronin P, Bernstein SJ, Carlos RC. Meta-analysis: effectiveness of drugs for preventing contrast-induced nephropathy. *Ann Intern Med.* 2008;148(4):284-294.

60. Manske CL, Sprafka JM, Strony JT, Wang Y. Contrast nephropathy in azotemic diabetic patients undergoing coronary angiography. *Am J Med.* 1990;89(5):615-620.

61. Weisbord SD, Mor MK, Resnick AL, Hartwig KC, Sonel AF, Fine MJ. Prevention, incidence, and outcomes of contrast-induced acute kidney injury. *Arch Intern Med.* 2008;168(12):1325-1332.

62. Weisbord SD, Mor MK, Resnick AL, Hartwig KC, Palevsky PM, Fine MJ. Incidence and outcomes of contrast-induced AKI following computed tomography. *Clin J Am Soc Nephrol.* 2008;3(5):1274-1281.

63. Krol AL, Dzialowski I, Roy J, Puetz V, Subramaniam S, Coutts SB. Incidence of radiocontrast nephropathy in patients undergoing acute stroke computed tomography angiography. *Stroke.* 2007;38(8):2364-2366.

64. Rihal CS, Textor SC, Grill DE, Berger PB, Ting HH, Best PJ. Incidence and prognostic importance of acute renal failure after percutaneous coronary intervention. *Circulation.* 2002;105(19):2259-2264.

65. Barrett BJ, Parfrey PS. Prevention of nephrotoxicity induced by radiocontrast agents. *N Engl J Med.* 1994;331(21):1449-1450.

66. Mueller C, Buerkle G, Buettner HJ, Petersen J, Perruchoud AP, Eriksson U. Prevention of contrast media-associated nephropathy: randomized comparison of 2 hydration regimens in 1620 patients undergoing coronary angioplasty. *Arch Intern Med.* 2002;162(3):329-336.

67. Maioli M, Toso A, Leoncini M, Gallopin M, Tedeschi D, Micheletti C. Sodium bicarbonate versus saline for the prevention of contrast-induced nephropathy in patients with renal dysfunction undergoing coronary angiography or intervention. *J Am Coll Cardiol.* 2008;52(8):599-604.

68. Merten GJ, Burgess WP, Gray LV, Holleman JH, Roush TS, Kowalchuk GJ. Prevention of contrast-induced nephropathy with sodium bicarbonate: a randomized controlled trial. *JAMA.* 2004;291(19):2328-2334.

69. Solomon R, Werner C, Mann D, D'Elia J, Silva P. Effects of saline, mannitol, and furosemide to prevent acute decreases in renal function induced by radiocontrast agents. *N Engl J Med.* 1994;331(21):1416-1420.

70. Barrett BJ, Carlisle EJ. Meta-analysis of the relative nephrotoxicity of high- and low-osmolality iodinated contrast media. *Radiology.* 1993;188(1):171-178.

71. Rudnick MR, Goldfarb S, Wexler L, Ludbrook PA, Murphy MJ, Halpern EF. Nephrotoxicity of ionic and nonionic contrast media in 1196 patients: a

randomized trial. The Iohexol Cooperative Study. *Kidney Int.* 1995;47(1):254-261.

72. Rudnick MR, Davidson C, Laskey W, Stafford JL, Sherwin PF. Nephrotoxicity of iodixanol versus ioversol in patients with chronic kidney disease: the Visipaque Angiography/Interventions with Laboratory Outcomes in Renal Insufficiency (VALOR) Trial. *Am Heart J.* 2008;156(4):776-782.

73. Heinrich MC, Haberle L, Muller V, Bautz W, Uder M. Nephrotoxicity of iso-osmolar iodixanol compared with nonionic low-osmolar contrast media: meta-analysis of randomized controlled trials. *Radiology.* 2009;250(1):68-86.

74. Tepel M, van der Giet M, Schwarzfeld C, Laufer U, Liermann D, Zidek W. Prevention of radiographic-contrast-agent-induced reductions in renal function by acetylcysteine. *N Engl J Med.* 2000;343(3):180-184.

75. Bagshaw SM, McAlister FA, Manns BJ, Ghali WA. Acetylcysteine in the prevention of contrast-induced nephropathy: a case study of the pitfalls in the evolution of evidence. *Arch Intern Med.* 2006;166(2):161-166.

76. Birck R, Krzossok S, Markowetz F, Schnulle P, van der Woude FJ, Braun C. Acetylcysteine for prevention of contrast nephropathy: meta-analysis. *Lancet.* 2003;362(9384):598-603.

77. Kay J, Chow WH, Chan TM, Lo SK, Kwok OH, Yip A. Acetylcysteine for prevention of acute deterioration of renal function following elective coronary angiography and intervention: a randomized controlled trial. *JAMA.* 2003;289(5):553-558.

78. Marenzi G, Assanelli E, Marana I, Lauri G, Campodonico J, Grazi M. N-acetylcysteine and contrast-induced nephropathy in primary angioplasty. *N Engl J Med.* 2006;354(26):2773-2782.

79. Kurnik BR, Allgren RL, Genter FC, Solomon RJ, Bates ER, Weisberg LS. Prospective study of atrial natriuretic peptide for the prevention of radiocontrast-induced nephropathy. *Am J Kidney Dis.* 1998;31(4):674-680.

80. Rosenstock JL, Bruno R, Kim JK, Lubarsky L, Schaller R, Panagopoulos G. The effect of withdrawal of ACE inhibitors or angiotensin receptor blockers prior to coronary angiography on the incidence of contrast-induced nephropathy. *Int Urol Nephrol.* 2008;40(3):749-755.

81. Marenzi G, Marana I, Lauri G, Assanelli E, Grazi M, Campodonico J. The prevention of radiocontrast-agent-induced nephropathy by hemofiltration. *N Engl J Med.* 2003;349(14):1333-1340.

82. Heyman SN, Brezis M, Epstein FH, Spokes K, Silva P, Rosen S. Early renal medullary hypoxic injury from radiocontrast and indomethacin. *Kidney Int.* 1991;40(4):632-642.

83. Himmelfarb J, Joannidis M, Molitoris B, Schietz M, Okusa MD, Warnock D. Evaluation and initial management of acute kidney injury. *Clin J Am Soc Nephrol.* 2008;3(4):962-967.

84. Schrier RW, Wang W, Poole B, Mitra A. Acute renal failure: definitions, diagnosis, pathogenesis, and therapy. *J Clin Invest.* 2004;114(1):5-14.

85. Rivers E, Nguyen B, Havstad S, Ressler J, Muzzin A, Knoblich B. Early goal-directed therapy in the treatment of severe sepsis and septic shock. *N Engl J Med.* 2001;345(19):1368-1377.

86. Wiedemann HP, Wheeler AP, Bernard GR, Thompson BT, Hayden D, deBoisblanc B. Comparison of two fluid-management strategies in acute lung injury. *N Engl J Med.* 2006;354(24):2564-2575.

87. Michard F, Teboul JL. Predicting fluid responsiveness in ICU patients: a critical analysis of the evidence. *Chest.* 2002;121(6):2000-2008.

88. Marik PE. Techniques for assessment of intravascular volume in critically ill patients. *J Intensive Care Med.* 2009;24(5):329-337.

89. Shear W, Rosner MH. Acute kidney dysfunction secondary to the abdominal compartment syndrome. *J Nephrol.* 2006;19(5):556-565.

90. Finfer S, Bellomo R, Boyce N, French J, Myburgh J, Norton R. A comparison of albumin and saline for fluid resuscitation in the intensive care unit. *N Engl J Med.* 2004;350(22):2247-2256.

91. Wiedermann CJ. Systematic review of randomized clinical trials on the use of hydroxyethyl starch for fluid management in sepsis. *BMC Emerg Med.* 2008;8:1.

92. Ho KM, Sheridan DJ. Meta-analysis of frusemide to prevent or treat acute renal failure. *BMJ.* 2006;333(7565):420.

93. Kellum JA, Decker JM. Use of dopamine in acute renal failure: a meta-analysis. *Crit Care Med.* 2001;29(8):1526-1531.

94. Bellomo R, Chapman M, Finfer S, Hickling K, Myburgh J. Low-dose dopamine in patients with early renal dysfunction: a placebo-controlled randomized trial. Australian and New Zealand Intensive Care Society (ANZICS) Clinical Trials Group. *Lancet.* 2000;356(9248):2139-2143.

95. Lauschke A, Teichgraber UK, Frei U, Eckardt KU. 'Low-dose' dopamine worsens renal perfusion in patients with acute renal failure. *Kidney Int.* 2006;69(9):1669-1674.

96. Gonzalez E, Gutierrez E, Galeano C, Chevia C, de Sequera P, Bernis C. Early steroid treatment improves the recovery of renal function in patients with drug-induced acute interstitial nephritis. *Kidney Int.* 2008;73(8):940-946.

97. Levey AS, Bosch JP, Lewis JB, Greene T, Rogers N, Roth D. A more accurate method to estimate glomerular filtration rate from serum creatinine: a new prediction equation. Modification of Diet in Renal Disease Study Group. *Ann Intern Med.* 1999;130(6):461-470.

98. Cockcroft DW, Gault MH. Prediction of creatinine clearance from serum creatinine. *Nephron.* 1976;16(1):31-41.

99. Chan LN. Nutritional support in acute renal failure. *Curr Opin Clin Nutr Metab Care.* 2004;7(2):207-212.

CHAPTER

42 Renal Replacement Therapies

Andrew Davenport, MD

A 26-year-old woman was admitted following a horse-riding accident. She had fractured her femur and suffered an intracranial hemorrhage. Postoperatively she required ventilation and then developed a respiratory tract infection, and on the third day of admission, her urine output had fallen to 0.5 mL/kg per hour, and her serum creatinine had risen from 0.5 mg/dL on admission to 1.24 mg/dL. At this stage her intracranial pressure (ICP), measured with an intraventricular catheter, remained elevated at 35 mm Hg, with a mean arterial blood pressure of 90 mm Hg. In view of the increase in creatinine and fall in urine output, a fluid challenge was given to try to prevent progression of acute kidney injury (AKI), to exclude a volume-responsive reversible cause of AKI (see Chapter 41). However, by the following day her urine output had fallen to 0.3 mL/kg per hour and her serum creatinine increased to 2.0 mg/dL.

Timing of initiating renal replacement therapy

As kidney function declines, the products of cellular metabolism accumulate, leading to retention of both the nitrogenous products of metabolism, typically assessed by the measurement of urea and creatinine but also potassium accumulation, and the development of a metabolic acidosis. Other potential toxins also accumulate,[1] leading to the term *azotemia* rather than *uremia*. This patient has AKI, and as such the time course of the illness is short, and only a limited amount of toxins will have accumulated. However, patients with AKI may have to be started on renal replacement therapy (RRT) because of hyperkalemia refractory to standard medical therapy or increasing pulmonary edema compromising oxygenation, and brain hypoxia (Table 42-1).

Historic data suggest that "early" initiation of RRT in AKI is associated with improved survival,[2-6] but the evidence base is not sufficiently robust to allow a specific recommendation and the decision to initiate RRT should remain a clinical one. Whereas the decision to initiate RRT is straightforward in those patients with refractory hyperkalemia, severe metabolic acidosis and volume overload, and/or overt azotemic symptoms, in the absence of these overt manifestations, there is debate as to the optimal time to initiate renal support (see Table 42-1). Early introduction of RRT as soon as a patient enters AKIN (Acute Kidney Injury Network) stage 3 (see Chapter 41) may be of benefit, so that the patient is not exposed to the potential deleterious effects of metabolic abnormalities and/or volume overload. However, early initiation of RRT will result in some patients suffering the adverse consequences of treatment, such as venous thrombosis and bacteremia secondary to vascular access catheters, hemorrhage from anticoagulants, and other treatment-related complications, in particular hypotension, which may exacerbate cerebral ischemic injury.

Table 42-1. Indications Generally Used to Start Renal Replacement Therapy in Standard Clinical Practice in Patients with Acute Kidney Injury (AKI)

Biochemical indications	
	Refractory hyperkalemia > 6.5 mEq/L
	Serum urea > 80 mg/dL
	Refractory metabolic acidosis pH ≤ 7.1
	Refractory electrolyte abnormalities: hyponatremia or hypernatremia and hypercalcemia
	Tumor lysis syndrome with hyperuricemia and hyperphosphatemia
	Urea cycle defects, and organic acidurias resulting in hyperammonemia, methylmalonic acidemia
Clinical indications	
	Urine output < 0.3 mL/kg for 24 h or absolute anuria for 12 h
	AKI with multiple organ failure
	Refractory volume overload
	End-organ damage: pericarditis, encephalopathy, neuropathy, myopathy, uremic bleeding
	To create intravascular space for plasma and other blood product infusions and nutrition
	Severe poisoning or drug overdose
	Severe hypothermia or hyperthermia

Initial reports, some dating back 50 years, suggested a clinical benefit of early initiation of RRT.[2-7] These and other studies formed the basis for standard clinical practice that dialytic support should be instituted when the serum urea reached 80 mg/dL.[2-7] However, not all studies have shown a survival advantage with early initiation.[8]

Although the current consensus from retrospective and observational studies suggests that "early" initiation of RRT in AKI may be associated with improved patient survival, this has not been proven.[8] In patients with acute traumatic brain injury (TBI), RRT not only adds complexity to patient management but also may cause additional complications in terms of changes in ICP and mean arterial blood pressure.[9] Thus, in cases of AKI developing in patients with TBI, early initiation of RRT should only be undertaken in cases of refractory hyperkalemia or pulmonary edema; as in the majority of cases, AKI is secondary to a prerenal insult, which may be volume responsive and recover, thus avoiding the necessity of RRT. However, additional toxic insults, such as aminoglycoside antibiotics and nonsteroidal anti-inflammatory drugs (NSAIDs), should either be avoided or minimized, and every effort should be made to reduce the risk of radiocontrast-induced AKI,[10] including minimizing the number of radiocontrast studies.[11]

If kidney function continues to deteriorate, then azotemic toxins accumulate over days, and these will be retained, leading to increased intracellular osmolality. If plasma osmolality is rapidly decreased during dialysis, then the osmolality gradient between plasma and the brain may lead to a movement of water into the brain, and so potentially increase brain edema.

Although there are no randomized clinical trials, it is probably advisable to initiate RRT before the serum urea nitrogen exceeds 40 to 50 mg/dL in cases of AKI, to limit the amount of cerebral edema caused by the fall in serum urea during RRT.[12]

When should renal replacement therapy be instituted in patients previously established on dialysis?

Patients with chronic kidney disease established on regular dialysis are susceptible to brain injury. These patients are at increased risk of subdural hemorrhage due to the prescription of coumarin anti-coagulants, intracerebral hemorrhage secondary to hypertension, and cerebral abscesses secondary to central venous dialysis access catheter-associated infections. These patients have chronically high levels of urea and other azotemic toxins, and as such, delaying dialysis treatments will lead to even higher chemistries, and thereby increase the risk of RRT-induced cerebral edema. So for this group of patients, RRT should be considered once the patient has been stabilized.[13]

Choice of Renal Replacement Therapy

The key strategy of any RRT is to remove small water-soluble solutes. Urea clearance from the plasma water is faster during hemodialysis treatments than urea movement from cells into the plasma water. As such, this sets up a urea gradient. In addition, water transport across cell membranes through aquaporin channels is some 20 times faster than the corresponding transcellular passage of urea through urea transporters.[14] This can result in an osmotic gradient developing between the plasma and the brain (Figure 42-1). Renal replacement therapy, particularly intermittent hemodialysis (HD), can lead to cerebral edema not only in acute experimental animal models of HD[15] but also in the out-patient setting of dialyzing healthy patients with end-stage kidney failure.[16] This swelling of the brain associated with HD is termed the *dialysis disequilibrium syndrome*.

Although RRT is primarily designed to remove small water-soluble toxins that accumulate in kidney failure, it is also used to correct the metabolic acidosis associated with kidney failure, and therefore

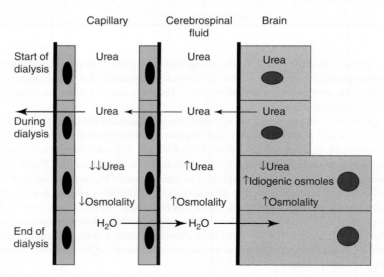

Figure 42-1. Schematic cartoon of the changes in urea concentration in different compartments during dialysis, leading to a concentration gradient with water passing into the brain.

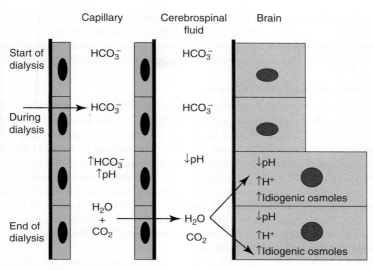

Figure 42-2. Schematic cartoon of the changes in bicarbonate concentration in different compartments during dialysis, leading to a concentration gradient with water passing into the brain.

dialysates either contain bicarbonate or lactate in supraphysiologic concentrations. The rapid correction or increase in plasma bicarbonate, rather than correcting intracellular acidosis, may paradoxically worsen intracellular acidosis,[17] as bicarbonate being charged does not readily cross lipid-rich cell membranes, unlike carbon dioxide (Figure 42-2). Intracellular acidosis increases cell swelling and will exacerbate any underlying cerebral edema. These changes in plasma bicarbonate compared to cerebrospinal fluid bicarbonate typically lead to changes in the respiratory center in the medulla, with alteration in breathing patterns in healthy outpatient dialysis subjects.[18] Thus, too rapid a correction of plasma bicarbonate in nonventilated brain-injured patients may potentially adversely affect cerebral oxygenation.

In addition, the connection of a patient to an extracorporeal circuit can lead to hypotension, which can potentially compromise cerebral perfusion. The passage of blood across the dialyzer, particularly those with a very negative surface charge (zeta potential), can lead to the generation of potent vasodilators, bradykinin, nitric oxide, and the anaphylotoxins C3a and C5a,[19] and it is now recognized that both cardiac and cerebral perfusion can fall within the first few minutes of initiating standard outpatient hemodialysis.[20,21] This effect on cardiac perfusion may be exacerbated in cases of subarachnoid hemorrhage or severe cerebral edema, owing to the associated neurogenic cardiac stunning. Bradykinin and complement activation by the extracorporeal circuit can be reduced by rinsing the circuit with isotonic bicarbonate rather than saline, and some centers advocate priming the dialyzer with albumin to coat the membrane to reduce membrane reactions. However, priming the circuit with blood, particularly aged blood, may exacerbate any reactions owing to the acidic nature of stored blood.[22] Similarly, angiotensin-converting enzyme inhibitors prevent bradykinin degradation, and as such should be avoided.

Several different modes of RRT are potentially available.

Peritoneal dialysis

Peritoneal dialysis (PD) is a form of continuous renal replacement therapy (CRRT), and as such the fall in serum urea and osmolality during treatment are slower than that compared to intermittent HD,[23] but even so the dialysis disequilibrium syndrome has still been reported during PD.[24] Peritoneal dialysate fluids are hyponatremic relative to blood, with a sodium concentration of 132 mEq/L, but are hypertonic owing to a high glucose content, varying from 13.6 to 38.6 g/dL, and so may cause patients to become hyponatremic. Large intraperitoneal volume exchanges of hypertonic glucose solutions can adversely impact cerebral perfusion and cerebral perfusion pressure by reducing right atrial filling and cardiac output.[25] To minimize these potential changes, peritoneal dialysis prescriptions should use the lowest glucose concentrations possible and avoid major swings in intraperitoneal volumes. This can best be achieved by using peritoneal dialysis cycler machines with a tidal exchange.

Intermittent hemodialysis/hybrid therapies

Brain edema occurs during routine outpatient thrice-weekly HD.[16] Thus, intermittent HD increases brain swelling in the patient with acute neurologic injury.[26] ICP increases not only because of changes in osmotic gradients and a rapid increase in arterial pH but also because of abrupt falls in mean arterial pressure, and thus cerebral perfusion pressure.[27] Intermittent RRT should therefore only be considered as a treatment option in cardiovascularly stable patients without changes of increased ICP or a midline shift on cerebral imaging (see Figure 42-1). Small solute removal is more efficient by diffusion down a concentration gradient rather than convection, where there is removal of plasma water and the solutes contained within it. Thus, urea removal is faster with hemodialysis than hemofiltration (Figure 42-3). Hence, hemofiltration or hemodiafiltration are preferable treatments, and the rate of urea and other small solute clearances can be further slowed by infusing the replacement fluids prefilter/-dialyzer rather than postfilter/-dialyzer (Figure 42-4).

If intermittent hemodialysis is the only renal replacement modality available, then the prescription should be modified to minimize cardiovascular instability, using a high sodium and calcium dialysate concentration, cooling the dialysate to 35°C, and minimizing changes in effective blood volume.[28] In addition, the rate of change in serum osmolality should be minimized by utilizing slower blood pump and dialysate flows, with smaller surface area dialyzer membranes, and lower dialysate bicarbonate concentrations,[29] thus moving from a standard intermittent hemodialysis prescription to one of slow extended dialysis, or a hybrid therapy. Whereas the standard practice for outpatient hemodialysis is thrice weekly, patients with acute brain injury should be treated daily, to minimize

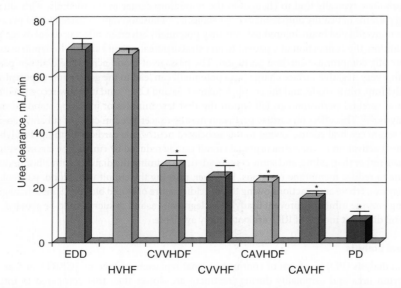

Figure 42-3. Urea clearance after 1 hour of treatment with slow extended hemodialysis (EDD), high-volume hemofiltration (HVHF) approximately 5 L/h, pumped continuous venovenous hemofiltration (CVVHF) and continuous venovenous hemodiafiltration (CVVHDF) approximately 2 L/h, continuous arteriovenous hemofiltration (CAVHF) and continuous arteriovenous hemodiafiltration (CAVHDF), and peritoneal dialysis (PD). Values expressed as mean (SEM). * P < .05 versus intermittent hemodialysis (IHD).

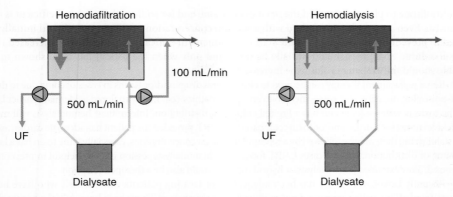

Figure 42-4. Differences between intermittent hemodialysis and hemodiafiltration. Ultrafiltration (UF) is much higher with hemodiafiltration, and to compensate for losses, dialysate is infused into the patient, and there is greater fluid movement within the dialyzer.

the peaks and troughs in blood urea, thus reducing the time-averaged urea concentration. Hypotension during intermittent hemodialysis is typically due to a high ultrafiltration rate leading to plasma volume depletion by being faster than compensatory refilling from extracellular fluid.

There are no randomized prospective trials that have investigated the optimum predialysis urea to minimize changes in ICP during dialysis; however, clinical practice suggests that a predialysis blood urea nitrogen less than 30 to 35 mg/dL reduces the risk of ICP increasing during treatment.[29]

Continuous dialysis/hemofiltration therapies

In patients with increased ICP, continuous forms of arteriovenous hemofiltration and/or dialysis have been shown to cause fewer changes in ICP and central perfusion pressure (CPP) than intermittent therapies[30,31] because of a combination of slower changes in plasma osmolality and greater cardiovascular stability (see Figure 42-2).[12] However, with the introduction of pumped venous hemofiltration, dialysis and hemodiafiltration, and in particular high-volume exchange, greater changes in osmolality have become possible (Figure 42-5). Thus, when performing CRRT in critically ill patients with AKI, hemofiltration is preferable to dialysis, as this leads to a slower rate of change in serum urea and other small solutes and also greater cardiovascular stability owing to additional cooling, particularly with predilutional fluid replacement[32] (see Figure 42-4). Sodium balance during hemofiltration tends to be positive, as the amount of sodium in the ultrafiltrate is typically less than that in the plasma. The ratio

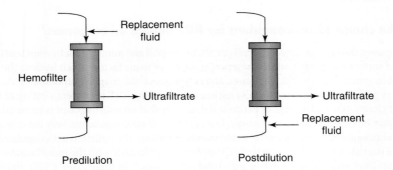

Figure 42-5. Predilutional fluid replacement and postdilutional fluid replacement.

of ultrafiltrate to plasma is termed the *sieving coefficient*, and for sodium the sieving coefficient is less than 1.0. Even so, a replacement fluid with a sodium concentration > 140 mmol/L should initially be used to prevent hyponatremia.[33] At the start of treatment, in critically ill patients with increased ICP, small volume exchanges should initially be used, and only when the patient has been shown to be stable should the exchange volume be increased.

Renal replacement therapy can be used to clear several drugs and/or toxins in cases of coma due to drug self-poisoning, toxicity, and some metabolic encephalopathies (eg, methylmalonic acidemia), particularly if the toxin is water-soluble and has a limited volume of distribution. Intermittent hemodialysis will more quickly remove such drugs and/or toxins compared to CRRT, provided the patient has adequate cardiovascular stability, but then may be followed by a rebound in plasma concentrations, especially if the toxin has a large volume of distribution. In such cases CRRT following a hemodialysis session may be helpful in preventing rebound. Slow extended hemodialysis or hybrid therapy would also be a therapeutic option.

Recently isovolemic CRRT has been advocated for treating patients without AKI who have been resuscitated after cardiac arrest and not regained consciousness.[34] There have been initial encouraging reports of increased survival for those patients treated for 8 hours with high-volume hemofiltration.[35]

Is the choice of dialysate or replacement fluid important?

In addition to inducing osmotic changes, the rapid diffusion during hemodialysis of supraphysiologic bicarbonate concentrations rapidly corrects plasma pH. Bicarbonate is charged, and cannot readily cross the blood-brain barrier (BBB). However, bicarbonate forms H_2CO_3 by reacting with hydrogen ions, which can dissociate into water and carbon dioxide, and carbon dioxide can readily cross the BBB. These fluxes of HCO_3^-, H_2CO_3, and carbon dioxide lead to changes in pH according to the Henderson-Hasselbalch equation, resulting in what is termed a *paradoxical* intracellular acidosis.[36] This then leads to a compensatory production of so-called intracellular osmoles and water movement into the brain, along a concentration gradient (see Figure 42-2).[18] Although lactate- or acetate-based dialysates and substitution fluids result in a slower increase in plasma bicarbonate, these fluids lead to an increase in lactate and/or acetate, with greater risk of hypotension and inotrope requirement. As such lower bicarbonate concentrations, 30-32 mEq/L, are recommended rather than standard bicarbonate of 35-40 mEq/L.

Intradialytic hypotension, which is relatively common during intermittent hemodialysis,[37] causes a reduction in CPP, with a consequent increase in ICP, owing to compensatory cerebral vasodilatation.[11] Cardiovascular stability during hemodialysis is greater when higher dialysate sodium concentrations are used, up to a maximum of 10 mmol/L greater than plasma sodium.[38] In addition, dialysate calcium concentrations of 2.7 to 3.0 mEq/L lead to fewer episodes of intradialytic hypotension than dialysate calcium concentrations of 2.5 mEq/L or less.

Cooling the dialysate improves cardiovascular stability during hemodialysis. Increased cooling can be achieved with predilutional fluid removal and during CRRT by not warming dialysates and/or replacement fluids.

Does the choice of anticoagulant for RRT impact on outcomes?

As blood passes through an extracorporeal circuit, neutrophil and monocyte activation leads to release of blebs of surface membrane, which are a potent source of tissue factor, which leads to the initiation of thrombin generation, platelet activation, and activation of the coagulation cascades. As such, the majority of patients require some form of anticoagulant during RRT to prevent clotting of the extracorporeal circuit. (One advantage of peritoneal dialysis is that no anticoagulant is required.) Anticoagulants may be either regional or systemic. During regional anticoagulation, only the extracorporeal circuit is anticoagulated, whereas with systemic anticoagulants, the patient is anticoagulated.

There is a risk of hemorrhage around ICP monitors, particularly with the more invasive intraventricular catheters and to a lesser extent with subdural devices.[39] In these cases, CRRT should preferably be anticoagulant free or a regional anticoagulant used.[12]

Anticoagulant-Free Extracorporeal Circuits

Clotting in the extracorporeal circuit often starts in areas of blood-air contact. Thus, for anticoagulant-free circuits, careful preparation of the circuit is required with complete flushing of all air, in particular from the dialyzer, and ensuring that all joints are airtight. Predilutional fluid replacement during hemofiltration and/or hemodiafiltration reduces the hemoconcentration along the dialyzer and dilutes both platelets and clotting factors, thus reducing the risk of circuit clotting compared to postdilutional fluid replacement (see Figure 42-4). The same effect of predilutional fluid replacement can be achieved during intermittent hemodialysis by the administration of regular isotonic saline boluses.

Unfractionated heparin is a highly negatively charged molecule and as such can adsorb to the dialyzer surface. Thus, several centers rinse the dialysis circuit with around 20,000 IU heparin in 1 L of isotonic saline for 60 minutes and then flush out the heparinized solution and dialyze patients without any additional anticoagulant. Hospal (Hospal AN69ST, Lyon, France) has altered the surface of a dialyzer in a deliberate attempt to increase heparin adsorption to allow priming with heparin but then dialysis without additional heparin.[40]

Regional Anticoagulants

Citrate, nafamostat, and prostacyclin all have very short half-lives and can be used as regional anticoagulants. The risk of bleeding is markedly reduced, as these agents provide anticoagulation for the extracorporeal circuit but do not systemically anticoagulate the patient. Nafamostat maleate, a serine protease inhibitor, is extensively used in Japan. Typically a loading dose of 20 to 40 mg is followed by an infusion of 20 to 40 mg/h, titrated to achieve an activated partial thromboplastin time ratio of around 1.5 to 2.0 times normal. Prostacyclin is a potent pulmonary vasodilator and is mainly limited to European practice. There is no simple monitoring test, and most patients are empirically started on an infusion of 2.5 to 5 ng/kg per minute. As it is such a potent vasodilator, hypovolemia should be corrected before starting treatment, and some centers increase vasopressor support as prostacyclin is started. In some cases prostacyclin has been reported to reduce CPP and increase ICP.[41]

Citrate is gaining popularity, particularly as an anticoagulant for CRRT, especially now that commercially available dialysates and replacement solutions have been developed specifically for citrate CRRT. Although citrate may occasionally accumulate—typically in cases of acute severe liver damage, cardiogenic shock, and extensive rhabdomyolysis—it is both a potent and an effective extracorporeal anticoagulant. The amount of citrate administered is adjusted according to the blood flow rate, and then as citrate chelates calcium, with loss of the calcium-citrate complex into the dialysate/ultrafiltrate effluent, calcium is then reinfused to maintain a normal systemic ionized calcium concentration.[42]

Systemic Anticoagulants

Systemic anticoagulants include heparins and the direct thrombin inhibitors. Traditionally, unfractionated heparin has been the standard anticoagulant for extracorporeal therapies. The main risk with systemic anticoagulants is one of hemorrhage, which is greatest in the first 24 hours following surgery and then falls over the subsequent 48 hours, but thereafter there remains an increased risk of bleeding compared to no anticoagulant or regional anticoagulants.[43] To reduce the risk of bleeding with unfractionated heparin (UFH), lower doses are now used, although the data suggesting that lower doses reduce the risk of bleeding are limited. During CRRT many centers use a loading dose of 500 IU followed by 500 IU/h, aiming for a systemic activated thromboplastin time ratio of 1.5 to 2.0 times normal.[44] More recently low-molecular-weight heparins (LMWHs) have been introduced. These have longer half-lives and a single bolus can be used for intermittent treatments (enoxaparin 0.5 mg/kg or tinzaparin 1500 to 4500 IU depending on duration of session). LMWHs require specialized anti-Xa activity monitoring, particularly for CRRT, when infusions are required.[45]

UFH is negatively charged and, particularly when contaminated with chondroitin sulfate, can increase bradykinin and C3a and C5a production as it passes through the dialyzer, risking hypotension.[46] In addition, patients may have allergic reactions to heparins, particularly if they have a porcine allergy. Occasionally patients may develop an autoimmune thrombocytopenia, termed *heparin-induced thrombocytopenia* (HIT), in which case patients are at increased risk of thrombosis. Management includes both withdrawal of all heparins and administration of an alternative systemic anticoagulant.

Direct thrombin inhibitors include lepirudin and argatroban and are typically used for cases of HIT. Lepirudin is an irreversible antagonist of thrombin, which has a very prolonged half-life in kidney failure, and as such is associated with a marked increased risk of bleeding. The plasma concentration of hirudin does not correlate linearly with the activated partial thromboplastin time, and thus monitoring of either plasma hirudin or the ecarin clotting time is recommended. Argatroban is a reversible thrombin antagonist and, as such, requires a bolus of 250 µg, followed by an infusion of around 2 µg/kg per minute titrated to achieve an activated partial thromboplastin ratio around 2.0.[47]

How should surges of increases in ICP be treated during renal replacement therapy?

When sustained surges in ICP occur during RRT, standard neurosurgical conservative management should first be instituted, checking that arterial oxygenation is adequate (Pao_2 of > 82.5 and $Paco_2$ of 49.5 to 55 mm Hg)[48] and the neck is not compressed.[49] Boluses of propofol and/or thiopentone can be administered if the CPP is high, whereas if the CPP is normal or low, then hypertonic saline and/or mannitol should be given. Deliberate ultrafiltration will also reduce CPP but may then result in a rebound in ICP.[27]

Individual centers differ in the concentrations of hypertonic saline they use (ranging from 3% to 10%),[50] and these can be infused during CRRT and other renal replacement therapies,[51] aiming for a serum sodium of 145 mmol/L, up to a maximum of 155 mmol/L, depending on the ICP response. If mannitol is infused during CRRT, then 100 mL of a 20% mannitol solution is effective when infused quickly over 10 to 15 minutes.[12]

! CRITICAL CONSIDERATIONS

- RRT adds complexity and risks to management of the neurocritical patient. Thus, initiation of RRT for AKI should be delayed unless the patient has hyperkalemia or develops pulmonary edema, whereas for patients already established on dialysis, RRT should be commenced once the patient is stabilized.

- Brain swelling during RRT tends to occur from rapid reduction in plasma osmolality owing to removal of urea and other small solutes. Thus, continuous forms of dialysis or slow hybrid forms of hemodialysis are advantageous compared to standard intermittent hemodialysis.

- Hypotension is a major risk with extracorporeal therapies. Hypotension due to the dialyzer interaction can be modified by avoiding angiotensin-converting enzyme inhibitors, priming the circuit with isotonic bicarbonate, and avoiding heparins. Hypotension due to a rapid ultrafiltration rate can be minimized by extending treatment session duration and giving more frequent treatments. The risk of intradialytic hypotension can also be reduced by high sodium and cooled dialysate.

- The risk of bleeding is greatest within the first 72 hours of trauma or postoperatively. Preferably, extracorporeal circuits should be anticoagulant free or a regional anticoagulant used, rather than systemic heparinization, in order to reduce the risk of bleeding.

REFERENCES

1. Vanholder R, Baurmeister U, Brunet P, Cohen G, Glorieux G, Jankowski J; European Uremic Toxin Work Group. A bench to bedside view of uremic toxins. *J Am Soc Nephrol.* 2008;19:863-870.

2. Teschan PE, Baxter CR, O'Brien TF, Freyhof JN, Hall WH. Prophylactic hemodialysis in the treatment of acute renal failure. *Ann Intern Med.* 1960;53:992-1016.

3. Parsons FM, Hobson SM, Blagg CR, McCracken CB. Optimum time for dialysis in acute reversible renal failure. Description and value of an improved dialyser with large surface area. *Lancet.* 1961;1:129-134.

4. Kleinknecht D, Jungers P, Chanard J, Barbanel C, Ganeval D. Uremic and non-uremic complications in acute renal failure: evaluation of early and frequent dialysis on prognosis. *Kidney Int.* 1972;1:190-196.

5. Conger JD. A controlled evaluation of prophylactic dialysis in post-traumatic acute renal failure. *J Trauma.* 1975;15:1056-1063.

6. Gillum DM, Dixon BS, Kelleher SP, et al. The role of intensive dialysis in acute renal failure. *Clin Nephrol.* 1986;25:249-255.

7. Gettings LG, Reynolds HN, Scalea T. Outcome in post-traumatic acute renal failure when continuous renal replacement therapy is applied early vs. late. *Intensive Care Med.* 1999;25:805-813.

8. Bouman CS, Oudemans-Van Straaten HM, Tijssen JG, et al. Effects of early high-volume continuous venovenous hemofiltration on survival and recovery of renal function in intensive care patients with acute renal failure: a prospective, randomized trial. *Crit Care Med.* 2002;30:2205-2211.

9. Davenport A, Will EJ, Davison AM, et al. Changes in intracranial pressure during hemofiltration in oliguric patients with grade IV hepatic encephalopathy. *Nephron.* 1989;53:142-146.

10. Brown JR, Block CA, Malenka DJ, O'Connor GT, Schoolwerth AC, Thompson CA. Sodium bicarbonate plus N-acetylcysteine prophylaxis: a meta-analysis. *JACC Cardiovasc Interv.* 2009;2:1116-1124.

11. Merten GJ, Burgess WP, Gray LV, et al. Prevention of contrast-induced nephropathy with sodium bicarbonate: a randomized controlled trial. *JAMA.* 2004;291:2328-2334.

12. Davenport A. Renal replacement therapy for the patient with acute traumatic brain injury and severe acute kidney injury. *Contrib Nephrol.* 2007;156:333-339.

13. Davenport A. Practical guidance for dialyzing a hemodialysis patient following acute brain injury. *Hemodial Int.* 2008;12:307-312.

14. Trinh-Trang-Tan MM, Cartron JP, Bankir L. Molecular basis for the dialysis disequilibrium syndrome: altered aquaporin and urea transporter expression in the brain. *Nephrol Dial Transplant.* 2005;20:1984-1988.

15. Arieff AI, Massry SG, Barrientos A, Kleeman CR. Brain water and electrolyte metabolism in uraemia: effects of slow and rapid hemodialysis. *Kidney Int.* 1973;4:177-187.

16. Winney RJ, Kean DM, Best JJ, Smith MA. Changes in brain water with hemodialysis. *Lancet.* 1986;8515:1107-1108.

17. Arieff AI, Guisado R, Massry SG, Lazarowitz VC. Central nervous system pH in uremia and the effects of hemodialysis. *J Clin Invest.* 1976;58:306-311.

18. Jones JG, Bembridge JL, Sapsford DJ, Turney JH. Continuous measurements of oxygen saturation during hemodialysis. *Nephrol Dial Transplant.* 1992;7:110-116.

19. Stoves J, Goode NP, Visvanathan R, et al. The bradykinin response and early hypotension at the introduction of continuous renal replacement therapy in the intensive care unit. *Artif Organs.* 2001;25:1009-1013.

20. Dasselaar JJ, Slart RH, Knip M, et al. Hemodialysis is associated with a pronounced fall in myocardial perfusion *Nephrol Dial Transplant.* 2009;24:604-610.

21. Provhovnik I, Post J, Uribarri J, Lee H, Sandu O, Langhoff E. Cerebrovascular effects of hemodialysis in chronic kidney disease. *J Cereb Blood Flow Metab.* 2007;27:1861-1869.

22. Coppo R, Amore A, Cirina P, et al. Bradykinin and nitric oxide generation by dialysis membranes can be blunted by alkaline rinsing solutions. *Kidney Int.* 2000;58:881-888.

23. Davenport A. Peritoneal dialysis for acute kidney injury. *Perit Dial Int.* 2008;28:423-424.

24. Pai MF, Hsu SP, Peng YS, Hung KY, Tsai TJ. Hemorrhagic stroke in chronic dialysis patients. *Renal Failure.* 2004;26:165-170.

25. Selby NM, Fonseca S, Hulme L, Fluck RJ, Taal MW, McIntyre CW. Automated peritoneal dialysis has significant effects on systemic hemodynamics. *Perit Dial Int.* 2006;26:328-335.

26. Davenport A. Neurogenic pulmonary edema post hemodialysis. *Nephrol Dial Transplant Plus.* 2008;1:41-44.

27. Davenport A, Will EJ, Davison AM. Rebound surges of intracranial pressure of a consequence of forced ultrafiltration used to control intracranial pressure. *Am J Kidney Dis.* 1989;14:516-519.

28. Mancini E, Mambelli E, Irpinia M, et al. Prevention of dialysis hypotension episodes using fuzzy

logic control system. *Nephrol Dial Transplant.* 2007;22:1420-1427.

29. Davenport A. Renal replacement therapy in the patient with acute brain injury. *Am J Kidney Dis.* 2001;37:457-466.

30. Davenport A, Will EJ, Losowsky MS, Swindells S. Continuous arteriovenous hemofiltration in patients with hepatic encephalopathy and renal failure. *Brit Med J.* 1987;295:1028.

31. Gondo GK, Fujitsu T, Kuwabara Y, et al. Comparison of five modes of dialysis in neurosurgical patients with renal failure. *Neurol Med Chir (Tokyo).* 1989;29:1125-1131.

32. Davenport A. Replacement and dialysate fluids for patients with acute renal failure treated by continuous veno-venous hemofiltration and/or hemodiafiltration. *Contrib Nephrol.* 2002;144: 317-328.

33. Davenport A. Potential adverse effects of replacing high volume hemofiltration exchanges on electrolyte balance and acid-base status using the current commercially available replacement solutions in patients with acute renal failure. *Int J Artif Organs.* 2008;31:3-5.

34. Karnad V, Thakar M. Continuous renal replacement therapy may aid recovery after cardiac arrest. *Resuscitation.* 2006;68:417-419.

35. Laurent I, Adrie C, Vinsonneau C, et al. High volume hemofiltration after out of hospital cardiac arrest, a randomized study. *J Am Coll Cardiol.* 2005;46:432-437.

36. Po HN, Senozan NM. Henderson-Hasselbalch equation: its history and limitations *J Chem Educ.* 2001;78:1499-1504.

37. Davenport A, Cox C, Thuraisingham R. Achieving blood pressure targets during dialysis improves control but increases intradialytic hypotension. *Kidney Int.* 2008;73:759-764.

38. Vinsonneau C, Camus C, Combes A, et al.; Hemodiafe Study Group. Continuous venovenous hemodiafiltration versus intermittent hemodialysis for acute renal failure in patients with multiple-organ dysfunction syndrome: a multicentre randomized trial. *Lancet.* 2006;368:379-385.

39. Munoz SJ, Rajender Reddy K, Lee W; Acute Liver Failure Study Group. The coagulopathy of acute liver failure and implications for intracranial pressure monitoring. *Neurocrit Care.* 2008;9:103-107.

40. Chanard J, Lavaud S, Maheut H, Kazes I, Vitry F, Rieu P. The clinical evaluation of low-dose heparin in hemodialysis: a prospective study using the heparin-coated AN69 ST membrane. *Nephrol Dial Transplant.* 2008;23:2003-2009.

41. Davenport A, Will EJ, Davison AM. Adverse effects on cerebral perfusion pressure of prostacyclin administered directly into patients with fulminant hepatic and acute renal failure. *Nephron.* 1991;59:449-454.

42. Kutsogiannis DJ, Gibney RT, Stollery D, Gao J. Regional citrate versus systemic heparin anticoagulation for continuous renal replacement in critically ill patients. *Kidney Int.* 2005;67:2361-2367.

43. Monchi M, Berghmans D, Ledoux D, Canivet JL, Dubois B, Damas P. Citrate vs. heparin for anticoagulation in continuous venovenous hemofiltration: a prospective randomized study. *Intensive Care Med.* 2004;30:260-265.

44. van der Wetering J, Westendorp RGJ, van der Hoeven JG, Stolk B, Feuth JD, Chang PC. Heparin use in continuous renal replacement therapies: the struggle between filter coagulation and patient hemorrhage. *J Am Soc Nephrol.* 1996;7:145-150.

45. Joannidis M, Kountchev J, Rauchenzauner M, et al. Enoxaparin vs. unfractionated heparin for anticoagulation during continuous veno-venous hemofiltration: a randomized controlled crossover study. *Intensive Care Med.* 2007;33:1571-1579.

46. Kishimoto TK, Viswanathan K, Ganguly T, et al. Contaminated heparin associated with adverse clinical events and activation of the contact system. *N Engl J Med.* 2008;358:2457-2467.

47. Murray PT, Reddy BV, Grossman EJ, et al. A prospective comparison of three argatroban treatment regimens during hemodialysis in end-stage renal disease. *Kidney Int.* 2004;66:2446-2453.

48. Brain Trauma Foundation, American Association of Neurological Surgeons, Joint Section on Neurotrauma and Critical Care. Methodology. *J Neurotrauma.* 2000;17:561-562.

49. Renagel-Castillo L, Gopinath S, Robertson CS. Management of intracranial hypertension. *Neurol Clin.* 2008;26:521-541.

50. Stevens RD, Lazaridis C, Chalela JA. The role of mechanical ventilation in acute brain injury. *Neurol Clin.* 2008;26:543-563.

51. Murphy N, Auzinger G, Bernel W, Wendon J. The effect of hypertonic sodium chloride on intracranial pressure in patients with acute liver failure. *Hepatology.* 2004;39:464-470.

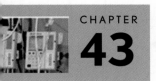

CHAPTER

43

Renal and Electrolyte
Disorders

Disorders of Water Homeostasis: Hypo- and Hypernatremia

Lawrence S. Weisberg, MD

Critically ill patients are prone to a wide variety of fluid, electrolyte, and acid-base disorders. Two of those disorders are of particular relevance to patients with critical neurologic illness: hyponatremia and hypernatremia. These are by far the most common electrolyte abnormalities in patients with central nervous system disease and have the most pressing diagnostic and therapeutic implications. This chapter therefore will focus exclusively on these disorders. Interested readers will find a recent, more comprehensive discussion of fluid, electrolyte, and acid-base abnormalities in critically ill patients elsewhere.[1]

Hypo- and hypernatremia are manifestations of impaired water homeostasis. They occur frequently in patients with central nervous system disease[2] and are associated with increased morbidity and mortality rates.[3,4]

Plasma sodium concentration (P_{Na}) normally varies very little. This tight regulation of the P_{Na} depends on the following elements: (1) modulation of pituitary secretion of arginine vasopressin (AVP; also known as antidiuretic hormone, or ADH) over a wide range in response to physiologic stimuli, (2) kidneys that are capable of responding to circulating AVP by varying the urine concentration, (3) intact thirst, and (4) access to water.

The normal response to water ingestion (of sufficient magnitude to lower the plasma osmolality even slightly) is the excretion of maximally dilute urine (urine osmolality < 100 mOsm/kg). The underlying physiologic sequence is as follows: the plasma hypo-osmolality is sensed by the cells comprising the hypothalamic osmostat. These hypothalamic nuclei then proportionately reduce their synthesis of AVP, leading to diminished AVP release into the circulation by the posterior pituitary. The lower circulating AVP concentration causes less vasopressin receptor type 2 (V_2 receptor) stimulation of the epithelial cells lining the renal collecting duct. This, in turn, results in the insertion of proportionately fewer water channels into the collecting duct, creating a more water-impermeable conduit, which allows excretion of the dilute urine elaborated by the more proximal segments of the nephron.[5]

Conversely, plasma hyperosmolality leads to higher circulating AVP concentration and proportionately higher water permeability of the collecting duct, and the excretion of a concentrated urine.[5]

Figure 43-1 shows the relationship between plasma osmolality, plasma AVP concentration, and urine osmolality. The normal "set point" is a plasma osmolality of about 285 mOsm/kg. Notice that the minimum urine osmolality is about 50 mOsm/kg, and the maximum about 1200 mOsm/kg.[6] When plasma osmolality rises beyond 290 to 295 mOsm/kg, the *thirst* center of the hypothalamus is stimulated. At that point, neurologically intact individuals with access to water will drink until the plasma osmolality returns to normal.[6]

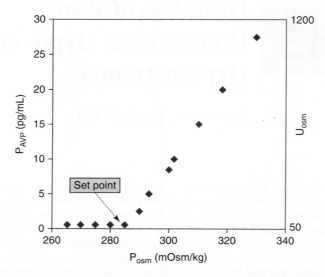

Figure 43-1. Relationship between plasma osmolality, plasma adenosine vasopressin concentration, and urine osmolality. P_{AVP}, plasma arginine vasopressin concentration; P_{osm}, plasma osmolality; U_{osm}, urine osmolality.

It is important to recognize that plasma osmolality is not the only determinant of AVP synthesis and release. Low arterial blood pressure and low effective arterial volume powerfully stimulate AVP release.[6] This *baroreceptor-mediated AVP release* is teleologic, since water retention is an important component in the defense against hypovolemia. So primal is this circulatory defense that the baroreceptor stimulation predominates over any osmolal effect on AVP release.[6] Thus, a volume-contracted or hypotensive individual will have high circulating AVP levels even if his or her plasma osmolality is low. In addition, circulating AVP levels rise with *pain, stress, nausea, hypoxia, hypercapnia*, and a variety of *medications*.[6]

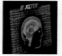 A 55-year-old man is admitted to the intensive care unit with a subarachnoid hemorrhage (SAH). The P_{Na} is 141 mmol/L. The patient is intubated and mechanically ventilated. The initial increase in intracranial pressure is effectively controlled (see Chapter 1). On the fifth hospital day, he is extubated. The P_{Na} is noted to have fallen to 134 mmol/L. The following day, it is 128 mmol/L.

What are the possible causes of the hyponatremia?

Hyponatremia (P_{Na} < 135 mmol/L) is seen in approximately 3% of hospitalized patients and as many as 30% of patients in intensive care units.[3] Among neurosurgical patients, the incidence of significant hyponatremia (P_{Na} < 130 mmol/L) is about 14%, with subarachnoid hemorrhage patients having the highest incidence (almost 20%).[2]

Although sodium is the vastly predominant solute in the extracellular space, hyponatremia may coexist with a normal, high, or low plasma osmolality.

Isotonic hyponatremia (also known as *factitious* or *pseudohyponatremia*) is a laboratory artifact seen in the setting of marked hypertriglyceridemia or paraproteinemia, when the sodium measurement method involves a predilution step.[7] The hyponatremia per se is of no clinical importance except as a clue to its pathogenesis.

Hypertonic hyponatremia results from the presence in extracellular fluid of abnormal amounts of osmotically effective solutes other than sodium (eg, glucose, mannitol, or glycerol). The osmotic pressure exerted by the nonsodium solute leads to redistribution of water from the intracellular to the extracellular fluid compartment, resulting in dilution of the extracellular sodium mass and resultant hyponatremia. The hyponatremia is real (not pseudo-), but it is accompanied by *hyper*tonicity and a *decrease* in cellular volume due to cellular dehydration, and thus carries no pathophysiologic importance in itself.

Hypotonic hyponatremia, by far the most common type of hyponatremia, is caused by an inability of the kidney to excrete sufficient electrolyte-free water to match water intake. It is this form of hyponatremia in which the hyponatremia itself is of clinical concern, for reasons detailed below.

Based on this differential diagnosis, the diagnostic algorithm for hyponatremia (Figure 43-2) begins with an assessment of the plasma osmolality (P_{osm}). This may be estimated by the following formula:

$$\text{estimated } P_{osm} = (2 \times P_{Na}) + \frac{P_{gluc}}{18} + \frac{BUN}{2.8}$$

where P_{gluc} is the plasma glucose concentration and BUN is blood urea nitrogen concentration, both in mg/dL. If there is a suspicion that an unmeasured, osmotically effective solute may be present in the plasma (eg, mannitol or glycerol), the P_{osm} should be measured directly.

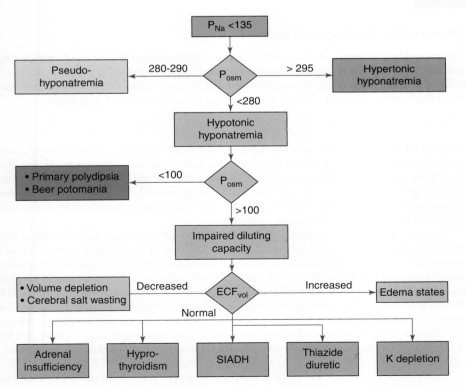

Figure 43-2. Diagnostic algorithm for hyponatremia. ECF_{vol}, extracellular fluid volume; P_{Na}, plasma sodium concentration; P_{osm}, plasma osmolality; SIADH, syndrome of inappropriate secretion of antidiuretic hormone.

The glucose concentration is 101 mg/dL and the BUN 14 mg/dL. The patient had never received mannitol or glycerol. Thus, the estimated P_{osm} is 267 mOsm/kg. To be sure, the patient's physician repeats the basic chemistry panel and measures the P_{osm}. The P_{Na} is now 125 mmol/L and the P_{osm} is 261 mOsm/kg.

What is the patient's diagnosis?

The normal P_{osm} is 280 to 285 mOsm/kg. This patient thus has hypotonic hyponatremia. This occurs either because the normal diluting capacity of the kidney is overwhelmed by excessive water intake or because the diluting capacity of the kidney is impaired. The former condition is characterized by excretion of a maximally dilute urine (U_{osm} < 100 mOsm/kg H_2O), and the latter is not. The classic example of the former condition is primary polydipsia, seen most commonly in patients with schizophrenia.[8] There are no reported cases of primary polydipsia in association with stroke, either hemorrhagic or ischemic.

The U_{osm} is 450 mOsm/kg, and the urine electrolytes (in mmol/L) are as follows: Na 180, K 40, Cl 220.

Can we refine the diagnosis further?

This patient clearly has impaired urinary diluting capacity. The concentrated urine usually reflects a high circulating AVP level, which is clearly inappropriate for the P_{osm} (see Figure 43-1). But since AVP release is affected by systemic hemodynamics as well as osmolality (see above), assessment of the patient's extracellular fluid volume status and hemodynamics is crucial at this juncture (see Figure 43-2).

Euvolemic Hyponatremia

Patients with hyponatremia as a result of pure (electrolyte-free) water excess appear clinically euvolemic because the excess water distributes throughout the total body water space; only one-third of total body water is extracellular, and only one-twelfth is intravascular. Thus, an adult patient whose total body water is expanded by 6 L, and thus has a P_{Na} of 122 mmol/L, will have expanded the intravascular volume by only 500 mL. The only evidence of the mild intravascular volume expansion is low blood urea nitrogen and plasma uric acid concentration.[9]

The paradigm of euvolemic hyponatremia with a concentrated urine is the *syndrome of inappropriate secretion of antidiuretic hormone (SIADH)*. SIADH is by far the most common cause of hyponatremia in patients with neurosurgical disease, accounting for over 70% of cases.[2] It is characterized by elevated circulating AVP (ADH) levels that are inappropriate to vasopressin's two physiologic stimuli (ie, osmotic or hemodynamic).[10] Hypotonic hyponatremia in patients with SIADH develops to the extent that water ingestion exceeds water elimination by insensible (sweat and perspiration; respiratory), gastrointestinal, and renal routes. Because the normal response to extracellular hypotonicity is the elaboration of maximally dilute urine (urine osmolality < 100 mOsm/kg), the urine need only be inappropriately concentrated (ie, > 100 mOsm/kg) to be compatible with a diagnosis of SIADH.

Because hypothyroidism[11] and glucocorticoid insufficiency[12] may impair urinary dilution even with suppressed AVP, patients in whom a diagnosis of SIADH is entertained should undergo appropriate tests of thyroid and adrenocortical function (see Chapter 52).

Once a diagnosis of SIADH is made, its cause must be established: just because a patient with SAH is found to have SIADH does not mean that the SAH is the cause. There may be another more easily remediable cause. Table 43-1 lists important causes of SIADH. They fall into five major categories: intracranial abnormalities, intrathoracic abnormalities, tumors, drugs, and idiopathic. Important adjunctive causes of SIADH in any hospitalized patient include pain, nausea, psychological stress, and, most commonly, medications.

Hypovolemic Hyponatremia

The urinary diluting impairment in hypovolemia is mediated both by decreased delivery of fluid to the diluting segments of the nephron and by baroreceptor stimulation of vasopressin release. Thus, the volume-contracted patient cannot excrete electrolyte-free water normally, and even in the face of modest water ingestion may become hyponatremic.

The cause of the volume contraction (negative sodium balance) usually is obvious (eg, hemorrhage, vomiting, diarrhea, diuretics). When it is not, the urine sodium concentration can be helpful in distinguishing between renal and extrarenal solute losses. *Renal losses* (eg, as a result of diuretic medications) are usually reflected by sodium wasting, and *extrarenal (gastrointestinal, skin, "third space," or hemorrhagic) losses* are usually accompanied by sodium conservation (urine sodium concentration < 10 mmol/L). Exceptions occur in the recovery phase after diuretic therapy, when the kidney has regained its capacity to respond to the volume depletion, and in metabolic alkalosis due to vomiting. In the latter situation, urinary sodium excretion is obligated by the bicarbonaturia, but the urine chloride concentration tends to be very low and is the best indicator of extracellular volume depletion.[13,14]

Renal salt wasting—in this setting more commonly called *cerebral salt wasting (CSW)*—may be responsible for hypovolemic hyponatremia in some patients with intracranial pathology (eg, tumors, hemorrhage).[15,16] The proposed underlying pathogenesis is a failure of the kidneys to adequately reabsorb sodium, leading to volume depletion. The mechanism of hyponatremia, then, is similar to that of other hypovolemic states. The pathogenesis of the renal salt wasting is incompletely understood: putative mechanisms include impaired sympathetic efferent pathways to the kidneys from the damaged central nervous system, and excessive secretion of a circulating natriuretic factor (eg, B-type natriuretic peptide [BNP]).[17] As a hyponatremic syndrome in patients with central nervous system disease, CSW is difficult to distinguish from SIADH, for several reasons. First, both are characterized by high urinary sodium excretion. Second, and particularly vexing, patients who have been diagnosed with CSW have *hypo*uricemia, in contrast to most volume-depleted patients, who have *hyper*uricemia. The hypouricemia is thought to reflect a generalized impairment of solute reabsorption in the proximal tubule.[17] Thus, the distinction of CSW from SIADH hinges completely on documentation of volume depletion. This seemingly simple determination is in fact quite complex and fraught with error.[15,18-20] Indeed, so controversial is the syndrome of CSW that some investigators think it accounts for the majority of hyponatremia in patients with central nervous system disease,[15,21] while others question its existence altogether.[18-20]

The hyponatremia associated with *diuretic treatment* is multifactorial in origin. Insofar as diuretics produce overt volume depletion, they can cause hyponatremia by the mechanisms discussed above. Thiazide diuretics in particular have been associated with the development of acute severe, symptomatic hyponatremia, particularly in small, elderly women, in the absence of overt signs of volume depletion.[22] The cause of this often precipitous syndrome remains uncertain,[23] although subtle volume depletion, hypokalemia, increased thirst,[24] and upregulation of aquaporin-2 water channels[25] have been implicated.

Hypervolemic Hyponatremia

Hypervolemic hyponatremia generally is seen in patients who cannot excrete sodium normally because they have either severe renal failure or one of the pathologic edema-forming states (eg, congestive heart failure, hepatic cirrhosis, nephrotic syndrome). Patients with advanced chronic kidney disease are

Table 43-1. Causes of SIADH

Intracranial abnormalities
Infection
Stroke
Hemorrhage
Tumor
Intrathoracic abnormalities
Malignancy
Pulmonary abscess
Pneumonia
Pleural effusion
Pneumothorax
Chest wall deformity
Drugs
Antidiuretic drugs (vasopressin, DDAVP, oxytocin)
Antidepressant medications
Amiodarone
Major antipsychotic medications
Chlorpropamide and other sulfonylurea drugs
Carbamazepine
Cyclophosphamide
Extracranial tumors
Small cell lung carcinoma
Pancreatic cancer
Others
HIV/AIDS
Hereditary
Gain-of-function mutation of vasopressin-2 receptor
Miscellaneous
Guillain-Barré syndrome
Nausea
Stress
Pain
Acute psychosis
Idiopathic

Abbreviations: DDAVP, desmopressin; SIADH, syndrome of inappropriate secretion of antidiuretic hormone.

predisposed to hyponatremia.[26] Acute oliguric renal failure or end-stage (dialysis-dependent) renal failure will be accompanied by hyponatremia to the extent that water intake exceeds insensible and gastrointestinal water elimination.

Hyponatremia is common in the pathologic edema states, especially congestive heart failure and hepatic cirrhosis. The hormonal milieu of such patients is typical of intravascular volume depletion, even though the absolute intravascular volume typically is increased. Thus, these disorders are said to be characterized by reduced effective circulating volume.[27] Because of the perceived intravascular volume depletion, renal diluting ability is compromised for reasons similar to those in hypovolemic hyponatremia.

The patient is afebrile and breathing at 18 breaths/min. His fluid volume status is equivocal: the blood pressure is 126/68 mm Hg; the heart rate is 96 bpm at rest; there is no jugular venous distention and no dependent edema. In view of the copious urinary sodium and the possibility of subtle volume depletion, his physician entertains the diagnosis of CSW. He gives him intravenous normal saline solution at a rate of 120 mL/h. The patient is incapable of taking anything by mouth. The next day, the P_{Na} has fallen to 118 mmol/L. The patient's mental status, which had been improving over the past few days, has now declined.

Why did the P_{Na} fall after infusing 3 L of normal saline solution (sodium concentration 154 mmol/L)?

The magnitude of the decline in the patient's P_{Na} implies that there was a gain of electrolyte-free water of about 2 L. By definition, normal saline solution contains no electrolyte-free water. The kidney, however, is capable of generating electrolyte-free water and returning it to the circulation, a process that has been called *desalination*.[28] This happens when the patient is excreting a large amount of electrolyte in a concentrated urine (under the influence of high circulating AVP)—exactly the case with our patient. In essence, the patient receives an isotonic saline solution, excretes a hypertonic saline solution, and returns the reabsorbed water to the circulation, further diluting his plasma sodium. In our patient's case, this could have been predicted by the recognition that his urine electrolyte concentration greatly exceeded his plasma electrolyte concentration.[29]

Why did the mental status decline?

The clinical manifestations of hyponatremia are largely attributed to intracellular volume expansion (*cellular edema*), which occurs only when hyponatremia is associated with hypotonicity. Intracellular volume expansion is of greatest consequence in the brain, where it is translated into increased intracranial pressure because of the rigid calvarium.[30]

The pathophysiology of hypotonic hyponatremia has important implications for its management. Most cells—especially brain cells—have adaptive mechanisms for mitigating tonicity-related volume changes.[30] Cell volume peaks 1 to 2 hours after the onset of acute hypotonicity. Thereafter, solute and water are lost from cells, and cell volume returns toward normal. After several days of sustained hypotonicity, cell volume is restored nearly to normal.[30]

The morbidity and mortality associated with hypotonic hyponatremia are influenced by several factors, including the magnitude and rate of development of the hyponatremia, the patient's age and gender, and the nature and severity of any underlying diseases.[30] The very young and very old, women, and alcoholics appear to be at particular risk.[31] Cell-volume adaptation to hypotonicity may be deficient in premenopausal women, who suffer more frequent and more severe neurologic consequences than men with equivalent degrees of hypotonicity.[32]

Neurologic symptoms usually do not occur until the P_{Na} falls below 125 mmol/L, although death from acute hyponatremia has been reported at 128 mmol/L.[33] The earliest symptoms include anorexia, nausea, and malaise. Between 120 and 110 mmol/L, headache, lethargy, confusion, agitation, and obtundation may be seen. More severe symptoms (seizures, coma) may occur with levels below 110 mmol/L.[34] Focal neurologic findings are unusual but do occur, and cerebral herniation has been described in severe cases, especially in young women following surgery.[32] In that setting, hypoxemia is common and often is associated with noncardiogenic pulmonary edema.[35] Hypoxia appears to exacerbate the cerebral damage in hyponatremia.[36]

Although symptoms generally resolve with correction of the hypotonicity, permanent neurologic deficits may occur, particularly in acute severe hypotonicity, when the brain's volume-regulatory defenses may be overwhelmed.[32] Profound hypotonicity that develops in less than 24 hours may be associated with residual neurologic deficits and has a 50% mortality rate in some populations.[32] In contrast, when hypotonicity develops more gradually, symptoms are both less common and less severe. Indeed, patients with chronic hyponatremia, even in the range of 115 to 120 mmol/L, may be completely asymptomatic.[30] Recent evidence suggests, however, that even chronic, mild, asymptomatic hyponatremia is associated with inattention, gait disturbances, falls, and fractures.[37-39] Thus, if hyponatremia is present upon presentation of a patient with traumatic brain injury after a fall, the hyponatremia may have led to the fall.

What should be done now?

Our patient's mental status has deteriorated as his P_{Na} has fallen. In this situation, a causal link should be presumed. Indeed, there is some evidence that hyponatremia in patients with SAH increases the risk of cerebral infarction, presumably by exacerbating cerebral edema.[40] Thus, the hyponatremia should be treated urgently.

The therapy of symptomatic hyponatremia, irrespective of cause, is directed at raising extracellular fluid tonicity to shift water out of cells, thereby ameliorating cerebral edema. Severe symptomatic hypotonic hyponatremia can be treated in two ways. The traditional treatment uses *hypertonic (3%) saline* (sodium concentration 513 mmol/L). The volume of 3% saline required can be estimated by the following formula:

$$\text{Volume of 3\% saline (liters/24 hours)} = \text{target change } P_{Na} \text{ (mmol/L/24 hours)} \times \text{TBW (L)} \div 513$$

where TBW is the total body water. Our patient weighs 70 kg and thus is estimated to have a total body water volume of 42 L (60% of body weight). If we want to raise the P_{Na} by 8 mmol/L over the next 24 hours (to 126 mmol/L), then the amount of sodium we need to administer is 8×42, or 336 mmol. Therefore, $336 \div 513$ or 0.66 L of 3% saline would be required in the first 24 hours, or 27 mL/h. It is important to recognize that the calculation provides only a very rough guideline. It does not account for other gains or losses of sodium or water. The P_{Na} must, therefore, be monitored frequently during treatment to adjust the rate of correction. If the rate of correction begins to exceed the target rate, the hypertonic saline infusion should be stopped; rarely, it may be necessary to administer water (enterally or intravenously [IV]) or even desmopressin in order to prevent overly rapid correction or overcorrection.[41] Rapid extracellular volume expansion with hypertonic saline may precipitate pulmonary edema, particularly in patients with underlying heart disease. Thus, patients receiving 3% saline should be assessed frequently for evidence of volume overload. One may administer a loop diuretic if necessary, recognizing that this will enhance electrolyte-free water clearance and accelerate the correction.

Conivaptan may be considered an alternative treatment for severe, symptomatic hyponatremia, although it has never been studied for this indication.[42] Conivaptan is a vasopressin receptor antagonist with both the V_{1A} and V_2 receptor antagonist effects. V_{1A} receptors mediate AVP-induced vasoconstriction, and V_2 receptors mediate AVP-induced water reabsorption in the renal collecting duct, thus augmenting electrolyte-free water excretion (aquaresis).[43] Conivaptan was the first *aquaretic* agent approved for use in the United States. It is approved for intravenous infusion in patients with euvolemic hyponatremia, and it causes an increase in electrolyte-free water excretion in a high percentage of treated patients.[44] When given in the recommended dosage (20 mg IV over 30 minutes, followed by 20 to 40 mg/d to a maximum of 40 mg/d), the average rate of rise in the P_{Na} is about 4 mmol/L in the first 24 hours.[44] Side effects, including hypotension, appear to be no more common than in the placebo group, except for mild infusion-site reactions. Despite its theoretical appeal, its use has several drawbacks. First, it is metabolized by, and competitively inhibits, hepatic CYP3A4, creating the opportunity for numerous drug interactions. Second, it is quite expensive (over $300 per 20 mg[45]), especially when compared with the nominal cost of hypertonic saline. Finally, and most important, if there is any possibility of CSW, the underlying volume depletion will only be exacerbated by conivaptan. *Particularly in view of this last consideration, I strongly recommend using hypertonic saline to treat symptomatic hyponatremia in patients with intracranial pathology.*

The rate of correction of the P_{Na} in severe hyponatremia must be carefully regulated. Overly rapid correction, particularly in patients with chronic hyponatremia (2-3 days' duration) in whom cell volume adaptations may be complete, can lead to the *osmotic demyelination syndrome,*[46,47] presumably as a result of cellular dehydration. The osmotic demyelination syndrome is associated with a variety of sometimes irreversible neurologic deficits (eg, dysarthria, dysphagia, behavioral disturbances, ataxia, quadriplegia, coma), which typically develop 3 to 10 days after treatment.[48] Additional risk factors for osmotic demyelination include hypokalemia, malnutrition, alcoholism, advanced age, and female sex.[49] The recommended maximum rate of correction, based on numerous studies over decades, is about 0.5 mmol/L per hour, 10 to 12 mmol/L in the first 24 hours, and no more than 18 mmol/L in the first 48 hours.[42] In profound, symptomatic hyponatremia, one may target a rate of correction in the first hour or two of 1 mmol/L per hour, but the 24- and 48-hour targets should not be exceeded.

 The patient is given 3% saline at a rate predicted to increase the P_{Na} by 8 mmol/L over 24 hours. Indeed, the result is 127 mmol/L 24 hours later. An enteral feeding regimen is begun, and over the next 3 days, the patient's P_{Na} drifts down to 121 mmol/L. The patient appears euvolemic. The repeat U_{osm} is 355 mOsm/kg, the urine sodium concentration is 92 mmol/L, and the urine potassium 40 mmol/L.

What can be done to normalize the patient's P_{Na} over the long term?

Because euvolemic hyponatremia represents pure water excess, treatment depends on inducing negative water balance: restricting water intake to less than the daily water output. Water output includes renal and extrarenal losses. Patients with SIADH excrete little or no electrolyte-free water in the urine. Indeed, sometimes (and in our patient's case) the kidney generates electrolyte-free water (essentially increasing water intake) by extracting it from the glomerular filtrate and returning it to the circulation, such desalination signaled by the fact that the sum of the cation concentration in the urine exceeds that in the plasma.[29] In this situation, even limiting water intake to less than the amount of insensible water losses (approximately 10 mL/kg body weight per day) will be unlikely to cause the P_{Na} to rise. Thus, most patients with SIADH require interventions to increase their urinary electrolyte-free water excretion.

A high-protein diet may enhance electrolyte-free water excretion in patients with SIADH by increasing urinary excretion of urea. Enforcing a high-protein diet in ill patients is difficult, but it is possible if they are fed by enteral tube. Similarly, oral administration of urea has been shown to normalize the P_{Na} over the long term in patients with SIADH,[50] but urea for this purpose is unavailable in the United States.

Demeclocycline is a tetracycline antibiotic that incidentally causes nephrogenic diabetes insipidus in about 70% of patients, increasing electrolyte-free water excretion by inhibiting vasopressin-mediated water reabsorption in the collecting duct.[42] Onset of action is 3 to 5 days with a dose of 300 mg two to four times daily. Demeclocycline is contraindicated in patients with renal disease, hepatic cirrhosis, or congestive heart failure because drug-related renal insufficiency has been described in these situations.[51]

Conivaptan (see earlier) is for short-term (4 days) parenteral use only, and is therefore not useful for long-term management of patients with SIADH. Tolvaptan, a selective V_2 receptor blocker, is available for long-term oral use, and is efficacious in a majority of patients with hyponatremia of various causes, including SIADH.[52] The starting dose is 15 mg daily, and the dose may be increased to 30 mg on day 2 and 60 mg on day 3. Clinical trials lasting 30 days showed that about 2% of patients exceeded the recommended rate of correction of P_{Na}.[52,53] This may be of particular concern in patients who cannot sense thirst or who have limited access to water, so the P_{Na} must be monitored daily when initiating therapy. No cases of osmotic demyelination syndrome were reported.[52,53] Like conivaptan, tolvaptan is metabolized by CYP3A4, so many drug interactions are possible. The current average wholesale cost of tolvaptan is about $300 a day.

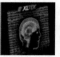

A 65-year-old woman with a history of hypertension, diabetes mellitus, and bipolar affective disorder is brought to the emergency department by ambulance after falling at home. According to the family, she was taking insulin, amlodipine, and lithium carbonate. She was comatose upon arrival. Initial P_{Na} was 141 mmol/L. A computed tomography scan showed a large subdural hematoma. The hematoma was evacuated and the patient was admitted to the intensive care unit (ICU). Hypertonic (3%) saline was given as a bolus injection. Urine output was 160 to 200 mL/h overnight. The next morning the P_{Na} was 155 mmol/L.

What are the possible causes of hypernatremia in this case?

Hypernatremia is common in critically ill patients, being present on admission in about 9% of patients and developing during the course of the ICU stay in another 6%.[54] Sustained hypernatremia develops in patients whose water output exceeds their input. Water ingestion can defend against the development of hypernatremia even when water losses are prodigious. For that reason, hypernatremia occurs most commonly in patients who are incapacitated: those who have impaired thirst sensation, who cannot access water, or who cannot express their need for water (eg, infants and patients with neurologic impairments). Thus, the development of hypernatremia in hospitalized patients is considered to be iatrogenic, reflecting an incomplete understanding of the factors that lead to hypernatremia.[54] The increased mortality rate seen in patients with hypernatremia[54] may be due to their underlying vulnerabilities[55] or an effect of the hypernatremia itself.[56] In patients in the neurologic ICU, severe hypernatremia ($P_{Na} > 160$ mmol/L) appears to be an independent predictor of death.[57]

The P_{Na} reflects the ratio of body sodium content to total body water. Thus, hypernatremia ($P_{Na} > 145$ mmol/L) can result from loss of pure water alone, loss of *hyponatric*[i] fluid, or a gain of sodium or *hypernatric* fluid. These will tend to be associated with euvolemia, hypovolemia, and hypervolemia, respectively. It is important to distinguish among these paths to hypernatremia since they have diagnostic and therapeutic implications (Figure 43-3).

Euvolemic Hypernatremia

Hypernatremic patients who appear euvolemic most likely have pure water loss as an explanation for their hypernatremia. This is because the water is lost from all body compartments proportionately; only one-twelfth of the water loss is intravascular. For example, a 60-kg woman with a 3-L pure water loss would experience an intravascular loss of only 250 mL (clinically imperceptible), but would develop a P_{Na} of 155 mmol/L.[ii] Pure water can be lost either through the skin and respiratory tract (so-called *insensible* losses) or in urine.

---

i. Hyponatric and hypernatric are used here to refer to a fluid with a sodium concentration less than or greater than that of plasma, respectively.

ii. The expected change in the serum sodium concentration is calculated as follows: [initial total body water volume] × [initial sodium concentration] ÷ [final total body water volume]; 30 L × 140 mmol/L ÷ 27 L = 155 mmol/L.

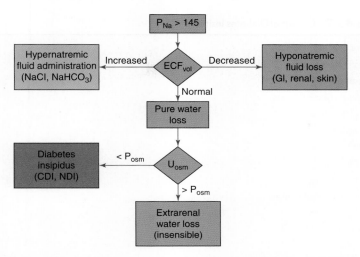

Figure 43-3. Paths to hypernatremia. CDI, central diabetes insipidus; ECF_{vol}, extracellular fluid volume; GI, gastrointestinal; NDI, nephrogenic diabetes insipidus; P_{Na}, plasma sodium concentration; U_{osm}, urine osmolality.

Insensible losses amount to about 10 mL/kg body weight per day under normal environmental conditions in an afebrile individual with a normal respiratory rate. A hot environment, fever, or rapid respiratory rate may double that rate.[6] Note that a patient on a mechanical ventilator using humidified gas will lose no water through the respiratory tract.

The loss of large amounts of dilute, electrolyte-free water in the urine is typical of *diabetes insipidus* (DI). Diabetes insipidus may be central (CDI) or nephrogenic (NDI) depending on whether the defect is in vasopressin release from the posterior pituitary or in the renal response to circulating vasopressin, respectively. The causes of DI are shown in Table 43-2. Most cases of CDI, especially those following trauma or intracranial surgery, are self-limited, lasting 3 to 5 days. Of special interest to neurointensivists is a classic triphasic syndrome that may be seen following severe head trauma or pituitary surgery[58,59]:

1. Initially, there is abrupt cessation of vasopressin release from the posterior pituitary, accompanied by polyuria.

2. About a week later, an antidiuretic phase ensues, characterized by urinary concentration and water retention with a tendency toward hyponatremia, lasting 2 to 14 days. This appears to result from the release of stored vasopressin from the degenerating hypothalamic neurons.

3. Persistent CDI recurs when the vasopressin stores are depleted.

Regardless of the cause, conscious and competent patients with DI of either type usually have a P_{Na} within the normal range because their water ingestion matches their urinary water output. They develop hypernatremia only with water deprivation, owing to mental or physical incapacity and/or neglect. An awareness of the causes of DI, a careful history, and familiarity with the differential diagnosis of polyuria will prevent hypernatremia in these circumstances.

Hypovolemic Hypernatremia

The loss of salt and water, with the water loss greater than the sodium loss, will lead to hypernatremia and volume depletion, manifested by orthostatic or persistent hypotension and tachycardia, and evidence of organ underperfusion (eg, acute renal failure, lactic acidosis). For example, if the 60-kg woman whose P_{Na} rose to 155 mmol/L (see above) had lost the equivalent of half-isotonic saline

Table 43-2. Causes of Diabetes Insipidus

Central Diabetes Insipidus
  Posthypophysectomy
  Posttraumatic
  Granulomatous diseases
    Histiocytosis
    Sarcoidosis
  Infections
    Meningitis
    Encephalitis
  Inflammatory/autoimmune
    Hypophysitis
  Vascular
    Hypoxia
    Thrombotic or embolic stroke
    Hemorrhagic stroke
  Neoplastic
    Craniopharyngioma
    Pituitary adenoma
    Lymphoma
    Meningioma
  Drugs or toxin
    Ethanol
    Snake venom
  Congenital/hereditary
Nephrogenic Diabetes Insipidus
  Drug induced
    Lithium
    Demeclocycline
    Cisplatin
    Ethanol
  Hypokalemia
  Hypercalcemia
  Vascular
    Sickle cell anemia
  Infiltrating lesions
    Sarcoidosis
    Multiple myeloma
    Amyloidosis
    Sjögren syndrome
Congenital
    Autosomal recessive: aquaporin-2 water channel gene mutations; X-linked recessive: arginine
  vasopressin V_2 receptor gene mutations

instead of pure water, her intravascular volume would have contracted by 750 mL, enough to cause at least orthostatic hypotension and tachycardia.

A common cause of hypovolemic hypernatremia is the loss of gastrointestinal fluids. Most gastrointestinal fluids have an electrolyte concentration below that of plasma: the concentration of sodium plus potassium in stool is roughly constant at 110 to 120 mmol/L over a wide range of stool volume.[60] Gastric fluid has an even lower electrolyte concentration: about 40 to 50 mmol/L total cation concentration.[61] Diuresis, either osmotic (glucose, mannitol, or urea induced) or medication induced, causes the loss of urine with an electrolyte concentration less than that of plasma, leading to volume contraction and hypernatremia. The loss of sweat, which contains some sodium, can cause hypovolemic hypernatremia in individuals who exercise vigorously in a hot environment. If the cause of the fluid loss is not apparent from the history or the physical examination, a urinary chloride concentration less than 10 mmol/L in the face of hypovolemic hypernatremia suggests that the electrolyte loss is extrarenal (cutaneous or gastrointestinal).

Hypervolemic Hypernatremia

Hypervolemic hypernatremia is relatively uncommon and often results from the administration of *hypertonic sodium salts* to patients without free access to water. Patients show signs of extracellular volume expansion (eg, hypertension, edema, congestive heart failure, and pulmonary edema). In infants, this syndrome has been caused by erroneous preparation of dietary formula using salt instead of sugar; in adult outpatients, it may be caused by ingestion of a concentrated salt solution, usually for its emetic effect.[62]

In hospitalized adults, hypervolemic hypernatremia is most often iatrogenic, caused by intravenous administration of undiluted sodium bicarbonate (formulated at 1 mEq/mL or 1000 mmol/L) or sodium chloride (3% [513 mmol/L] or 23.5% [4019 mmol/L]). In patients with neurosurgical disease, it is caused by parenteral administration of hypertonic saline solutions to reduce intracranial pressure and possibly decrease inflammation.[63,64]

The patient's vital signs were stable and normal. She had no edema.

What further test(s) might clarify the diagnosis?

The patient therefore appears euvolemic, so the most likely explanation for her hypernatremia is pure electrolyte-free water loss. (The amount of sodium in the hypertonic saline she received was 128 mmol, equivalent to about 830 mL of normal saline solution. This would be unlikely to cause significant fluid overload in a patient with normal heart and kidney function, although it exacerbated her hypernatremia.) The differential diagnosis at this point includes renal (DI) and extrarenal water loss (see Figure 43-3). The polyuria in her case suggests urinary water loss. A simple confirmatory test is the U_{osm}: if it is lower than the P_{osm} in the face of hyperosmolality, that would signal inappropriate urinary dilution (see Figure 43-1), consistent with DI. A high U_{osm} would be consistent with appropriate urinary concentration in the face of extrarenal water loss.

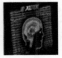

The patient's U_{osm} is 140 mOsm/kg.

What is the next step?

The patient has hypernatremia due to inadequate urinary concentration (DI). The differential diagnosis at this point includes inadequate circulating AVP levels (central or hypothalamic DI), in this setting due to the intracranial pathology, or renal resistance to appropriate concentrations of circulating AVP (nephrogenic or NDI). These can be distinguished by observing the effect of exogenous AVP on U_{osm}. The standard protocol consists of administering 5 units of aqueous vasopressin or 4 μg of desmopressin (DDAVP) subcutaneously, and measuring the U_{osm} every 30 minutes for 2 hours. Patients with NDI will show very little if any increase in U_{osm} (< 10% change), whereas patients with CDI will have a significant increase in U_{osm}, typically greater than 50%.[6] (The gray area between a 10% and 50% increase in U_{osm} may be seen in patients with partial central DI.)

Two hours after administration of DDAVP, there was no change in the urine volume, and the final U_{osm} was 138 mOsm/kg.

The patient apparently has NDI. In this setting, the most likely underlying cause is the patient's use of lithium. Twenty to 85% of patients taking lithium long-term will develop NDI.[65,66] As long as they have intact thirst and access to water, patients with DI (central or nephrogenic) typically have P_{Na} in the normal range since they drink enough to match their urinary water losses. When deprived of water, such patients will quickly dehydrate, as our patient did.

Is the hypernatremia itself of any concern?

The clinical manifestations of hypernatremia are attributable to osmotically driven intracellular volume contraction and are proportional to the magnitude and rate of rise of the P_{Na}. To counteract cellular volume contraction, cells begin to adapt within minutes by allowing the influx of electrolytes, thus mitigating cell shrinkage. When hypernatremia lasts more than a few hours, brain cells generate new organic osmolytes. This leads to further water movement back into brain cells, restoring cell volume nearly to normal after about 3 days.[67] Thus, chronic progressive hypernatremia is associated with fewer and milder symptoms than acute severe hypernatremia. Patients with hypernatremia tend to present with weakness, lethargy, and confusion. Seizure and coma may supervene. Acute severe hypernatremia in infants and small children is associated with intracranial bleeding,[68] presumably caused by brain shrinkage and traction on the penetrating vessels. There is some controversy, however, as to whether the hypernatremia in that situation is the cause or the effect of the intracranial hemorrhage.[69]

Now that we have a diagnosis, how should we treat the patient?

For patients with pure water losses (euvolemic), therapy has two goals: (1) reduction and/or replacement of ongoing water losses and (2) replacement of the existing water deficit.

The reduction of the urinary water losses that accompany lithium-associated NDI is best accomplished with amiloride, with or without cyclooxygenase (COX) inhibitors.[66] Because amiloride and most COX inhibitors are orally administered, treatment of NDI in the critically ill patient often consists of water administration (see below) until he or she is able to take medications by mouth. (Furthermore, a COX inhibitor would be contraindicated in a patient such as ours with an intracranial hemorrhage.)

If the urinary water losses had been due to CDI and not NDI, an antidiuretic hormone preparation would be the treatment of choice to reduce ongoing water losses. Several formulations

Table 43-3. Pharmacologic Treatment of Central Diabetes Insipidus

Agent	Total daily dose	Frequency of administration	Onset of action (h)	Duration of action (h)	Comments
Arginine vasopressin, 20 units/mL	5-10 units subcutaneously	q2-4h	1-2	2-6	Intravenous route may cause vasoconstriction and coronary spasm
Desmopressin acetate (DDAVP)					
10 μg/0.1 mL intranasally	10-40 μg intranasally	Daily or bid	1-2	8-12	
4 μg/mL injection	2-4 μg intravenously or subcutaneously	Daily or bid	1-2	8-12	

(Adapted from Singer I, Oster JR, Fishman LM. The management of diabetes insipidus in adults. Arch Intern Med. 1997;157(12): 1293-1301.)

are available (Table 43-3). In the acute (postsurgical or posttraumatic) setting, L-arginine vasopressin may be used either subcutaneously or intravenously, although the latter route may be associated with hypertension and coronary spasm and should therefore be used with extreme caution.[70] The advantage of vasopressin in this setting is its short half-life, which allows the physician to repeatedly assess the need for continued hormone replacement, especially when the disorder may be self-limited. DDAVP is a synthetic analogue of vasopressin that has no vasoconstrictor properties, and thus avoids the risks of hypertension and myocardial ischemia.

Once the ongoing water losses have been addressed, the current body water deficit can be estimated by the following formula:

$$\text{Water deficit (liters)} = \text{TBW}\left(1 - \left[\frac{140}{\text{current } P_{Na}}\right]\right)$$

where TBW is total body water in liters (estimated as about $0.5 \times$ lean body weight [kg] in women and $0.6 \times$ lean body weight in men). For example, our patient is a 60-kg woman with a P_{Na} of 155 mmol/L. She is estimated to have a total body water deficit of 30 (1 − 0.90) or 3 L. This formula provides only a rough estimate of the water deficit.

The rate of water replacement should be proportional to the rapidity with which the hypernatremia developed.[67] Thus, if the hypernatremia had developed over only a few hours (such as in our patient, or in postsurgical or posttraumatic DI), it can be corrected just as quickly. On the other hand, hypernatremia of more than a day's duration (or of unknown duration) must be corrected slowly in order to avoid inducing cerebral edema. In that setting, one should aim to correct half the water deficit in the first 24 hours, and the remainder over the next 24 to 48 hours.

Water is best administered enterally, as tap water. If that route is unavailable, 5% dextrose in water (D5W) may be used, with the understanding that the capacity to metabolize glucose is limited to about 15 g/h in a critically ill adult.[71] Thus, even in nondiabetic patients, the administration of more than 300 mL/h of D5W is likely to result in hyperglycemia, which may be relatively resistant to insulin administration. The hyperglycemia will exacerbate urinary water losses by causing an osmotic diuresis. Half-normal (0.45%) saline may be a good alternative, as long as one recognizes that only half the administered volume is electrolyte-free water, and that the sodium load may cause unwanted volume expansion.

Renal and Electrolyte Disorders

For the hypernatremic patient who presents with obvious volume depletion—manifested by hypotension, tachycardia, and evidence of impaired tissue perfusion—normal (0.9%) saline should be given intravenously, regardless of the degree of hypernatremia. This is consistent with the first principles of emergency and critical care, prioritizing the adequacy of the circulation. Only after the extracellular volume deficit has been largely corrected may the clinician direct his or her attention to the total body water deficit (see earlier).

Patients with hypervolemic hypernatremia need reduction in their extracellular and intravascular volume before their water deficit can be corrected. Failure to do so will exacerbate the volume overload. For patients with adequate renal function, this may be accomplished with the use of diuretic drugs. Loop diuretics tend to cause the excretion of an isotonic urine. Replacement of that urine volume with pure water will allow correction of the hypervolemia and the hypernatremia simultaneously.

Because of the imprecision of the estimation formulas and the failure of the foregoing analysis to take account of other fluids and electrolytes both administered and lost, it is imperative that the plasma electrolytes be monitored frequently during the correction of hypernatremia, especially because cerebral edema may develop with overly rapid correction.

! CRITICAL CONSIDERATIONS

- Hyper- and hyponatremia are common in patients with neurologic critical illness and are associated with increased morbidity and mortality rates.
- Hyponatremia itself is important only when it is associated with a low P_{osm}, because it can cause cerebral edema.
- The most common cause of euvolemic, hypotonic hyponatremia in neurocritically ill patients is SIADH, accounting for over 70% of cases.
- Cerebral salt wasting remains a controversial cause of hyponatremia.
- The clinical consequences of hypotonic hyponatremia are proportional to both the rate and the magnitude of fall in P_{Na}.
- Correction of severe symptomatic hyponatremia is best accomplished with hypertonic (3%) saline solution.
- The rate of correction of hyponatremia depends on its duration because of cell volume adaptation.
- Both delay in correction and overly rapid correction may result in permanent neurologic damage or death.
- Like hyponatremia, hypernatremia may be seen with volume depletion, volume overload, or normal volume status.
- Hypernatremia always develops in patients whose access to water is limited.
- Euvolemic hypernatremia with a dilute urine is very likely to be due to some form of diabetes insipidus.
- Correction of hypovolemic hypernatremia starts with correction of the volume deficit, regardless of the water deficit.
- Correction of hypernatremia depends on replacing and/or reducing ongoing water losses and replacing the water deficit.
- Overly rapid correction of hypernatremia can cause cerebral edema because of cell volume adaptation.

REFERENCES

1. Faridi AB, Weisberg LS. Acid-base, electrolyte and metabolic abnormalities. In: Parrillo JE, Dellinger RP, eds. *Critical Care Medicine: Principles of Diagnosis and Management in the Adult*. 3rd ed. Philadelphia, PA: Mosby Elsevier; 2008.

2. Sherlock M, O'Sullivan E, Agha A, et al. Incidence and pathophysiology of severe hyponatremia in neurosurgical patients. *Postgrad Med J.* 2009;85(1002):171-175.

3. DeVita MV, Gardenswartz MH, Konecky A, Zabetakis PM. Incidence and etiology of hyponatremia in an intensive care unit. *Clin Nephrol.* 1990;34(4):163-166.

4. Polderman KH, Schreuder WO, Strack van Schijndel RJ, Thijs LG. Hypernatremia in the intensive care unit: an indicator of quality of care? *Crit Care Med.* 1999;27(6):1105-1108.

5. Knepper M, Gamba G. Urine concentration and dilution. In: Brenner B, ed. *Brenner and Rector's The Kidney*. 7th ed. Philadelphia, PA: Saunders; 2004.

6. Verbalis JG, Berl T. Disorders of water balance. In: Brenner B, ed. *Brenner & Rector's The Kidney*. 8th ed. Philadelphia, PA: Saunders; 2007.

7. Weisberg LS. Pseudohyponatremia: a reappraisal. *Am J Med.* 1989;86(3):315-318.

8. McKinley MJ, Cairns MJ, Denton DA, et al. Physiological and pathophysiological influences on thirst. *Physiol Behav.* 2004;81(5):795-803.

9. Beck LH. Hypouricemia in the syndrome of inappropriate secretion of antidiuretic hormone. *N Engl J Med.* 1979;301(10):528-530.

10. Verbalis JG. Disorders of body water homeostasis. *Best Pract Res Clin Endocrinol Metab.* 2003;17(4):471-503.

11. Schrier RW, Bichet DG. Osmotic and nonosmotic control of vasopressin release and the pathogenesis of impaired water excretion in adrenal, thyroid, and edematous disorders. *J Lab Clin Med.* 1981;98(1):1-15.

12. Diederich S, Franzen NF, Bahr V, Oelkers W. Severe hyponatremia due to hypopituitarism with adrenal insufficiency: report on 28 cases. *Eur J Endocrinol.* 2003;148(6):609-617.

13. Kamel KS, Ethier JH, Richardson RM, Bear RA, Halperin ML. Urine electrolytes and osmolality: when and how to use them. *Am J Nephrol.* 1990;10(2):89-102.

14. Kamel KS, Magner PO, Ethier JH, Halperin ML. Urine electrolytes in the assessment of extracellular fluid volume contraction. *Am J Nephrol.* 1989;9(4):344-347.

15. Maesaka JK, Imbriano LJ, Ali NM, Ilamathi E. Is it cerebral or renal salt wasting? *Kidney Int.* 2009;76:934-938.

16. Nelson PB, Seif SM, Maroon JC, Robinson AG. Hyponatremia in intracranial disease: perhaps not the syndrome of inappropriate secretion of antidiuretic hormone (SIADH). *J Neurosurg.* 1981;55(6):938-941.

17. Palmer BF. Hyponatremia in patients with central nervous system disease: SIADH versus CSW. *Trends Endocrinol Metab.* 2003;14(4):182-187.

18. Brimioulle S, Orellana-Jimenez C, Aminian A, Vincent JL. Hyponatremia in neurological patients: cerebral salt wasting versus inappropriate antidiuretic hormone secretion. *Intensive Care Med.* 2008;34(1):125-131.

19. Carlotti AP, Bohn D, Rutka JT, et al. A method to estimate urinary electrolyte excretion in patients at risk for developing cerebral salt wasting. *J Neurosurg.* 2001;95(3):420-424.

20. Singh S, Bohn D, Carlotti AP, Cusimano M, Rutka JT, Halperin ML. Cerebral salt wasting: truths, fallacies, theories, and challenges. *Crit Care Med.* 2002;30(11):2575-2579.

21. Maesaka JK, Gupta S, Fishbane S. Cerebral salt-wasting syndrome: does it exist? *Nephron.* 1999;82(2):100-109.

22. Sharabi Y, Illan R, Kamari Y, et al. Diuretic induced hyponatremia in elderly hypertensive women. *J Hum Hypertens.* 2002;16(9):631-635.

23. Spital A. Diuretic-induced hyponatremia. *Am J Nephrol.* 1999;19(4):447-452.

24. Gross P, Palm C. Thiazides: do they kill? *Nephrol Dial Transplant.* 2005;20(11):2299-2301.

25. Kim GH, Lee JW, Oh YK, et al. Antidiuretic effect of hydrochlorothiazide in lithium-induced nephrogenic diabetes insipidus is associated with upregulation of aquaporin-2, Na-Cl co-transporter, and epithelial sodium channel. *J Am Soc Nephrol.* 2004;15(11):2836-2843.

26. Taal M, Luyckx V, Brenner B. Adaptation to nephron loss. In: Brenner B, ed. *Brenner and Rector's The Kidney*. 7th ed. Philadelphia, PA: Saunders; 2004.

27. Schrier RW, Gurevich AK, Cadnapaphornchai MA. Pathogenesis and management of sodium and water retention in cardiac failure and cirrhosis. *Semin Nephrol* 2001;21(2):157-172.

28. Steele A, Gowrishankar M, Abrahamson S, Mazer CD, Feldman RD, Halperin ML. Postoperative hyponatremia despite near-isotonic saline infusion: a phenomenon of desalination. *Ann Intern Med.* 1997;126(1):20-25.

29. Furst HMD, Hallows KRMDP, Post JMD, et al. The urine/plasma electrolyte ratio: a predictive guide

to water restriction. *Am J Med Sci.* 2000;319(4): 240-244.

30. Verbalis JG. Adaptation to acute and chronic hyponatremia: implications for symptomatology, diagnosis, and therapy. *Semin Nephrol.* 1998;18(1):3-19.

31. Lauriat SM, Berl T. The hyponatremic patient: practical focus on therapy. *J Am Soc Nephrol.* 1997;8(10):1599-1607.

32. Arieff AI. Hyponatremia, convulsions, respiratory arrest, and permanent brain damage after elective surgery in healthy women. *N Engl J Med.* 1986;314(24):1529-1535.

33. Ayus JC, Wheeler JM, Arieff AI. Postoperative hyponatremic encephalopathy in menstruant women. *Ann Intern Med.* 1992;117(11):891-897.

34. Sterns RH. Severe symptomatic hyponatremia: treatment and outcome. A study of 64 cases. *Ann Intern Med.* 1987;107(5):656-664.

35. Ayus JC, Arieff AI. Pulmonary complications of hyponatremic encephalopathy. Noncardiogenic pulmonary edema and hypercapnic respiratory failure. *Chest.* 1995;107(2):517-521.

36. Ayus JC, Armstrong D, Arieff AI. Hyponatremia with hypoxia: effects on brain adaptation, perfusion, and histology in rodents. *Kidney Int.* 2006;69(8):1319-1325.

37. Gankam Kengne F, Andres C, Sattar L, Melot C, Decaux G. Mild hyponatremia and risk of fracture in the ambulatory elderly. *QJM.* 2008;101(7): 583-588.

38. Kinsella S, Moran S, Sullivan MO, Molloy MG, Eustace JA. Hyponatremia independent of osteoporosis is associated with fracture occurrence. *Clin J Am Soc Nephrol.* 2010;5(2):275-280.

39. Renneboog B, Musch W, Vandemergel X, Manto MU, Decaux G. Mild chronic hyponatremia is associated with falls, unsteadiness, and attention deficits. *Am J Med.* 2006;119(1):71.e1-e8.

40. Wijdicks EF, Vermeulen M, Hijdra A, van Gijn J. Hyponatremia and cerebral infarction in patients with ruptured intracranial aneurysms: is fluid restriction harmful? *Ann Neurol.* 1985;17(2): 137-140.

41. Adrogue HJ, Madias NE. Hyponatremia. *N Engl J Med.* 2000;342(21):1581-1589.

42. Zietse R, van der Lubbe N, Hoorn EJ. Current and future treatment options in SIADH. *NDT Plus.* 2009;2(Suppl 3):iii12-iii19.

43. Greenberg A, Verbalis JG. Vasopressin receptor antagonists. *Kidney Int.* 2006;69(12):2124-2130.

44. Ghali JK, Koren MJ, Taylor JR, et al. Efficacy and safety of oral conivaptan: a V_{1A}/V_2 vasopressin receptor antagonist, assessed in a randomized, placebo-controlled trial in patients with euvolemic or hypervolemic hyponatremia. *J Clin Endocrinol Metab.* 2006;91(6):2145-2152.

45. Conivaptan (Vaprisol) for hyponatremia. *Med Lett Drugs Ther.* 2006;48(1237):51-52.

46. Kleinschmidt-DeMasters BK, Norenberg MD. Rapid correction of hyponatremia causes demyelination: relation to central pontine myelinolysis. *Science.* 1981;211(4486):1068-1070.

47. Martin RJ. Central pontine and extrapontine myelinolysis: the osmotic demyelination syndromes. *J Neurol Neurosurg Psychiatry.* 2004; 75(Suppl 3):iii22-iii28.

48. Gross P. Treatment of severe hyponatremia. *Kidney Int.* 2001;60(6):2417-2427.

49. Gross P, Reimann D, Henschkowski J, Damian M. Treatment of severe hyponatremia: conventional and novel aspects. *J Am Soc Nephrol.* 2001;12(Suppl 17):S10-S14.

50. Decaux G. Long-term treatment of patients with inappropriate secretion of antidiuretic hormone by the vasopressin receptor antagonist conivaptan, urea, or furosemide. *Am J Med.* 2001;110(7):582-584.

51. Oster JR, Epstein M. Demeclocycline-induced renal failure. *Lancet.* 1977;1(8001):52.

52. Schrier RW, Gross P, Gheorghiade M, et al. Tolvaptan, a selective oral vasopressin V_2-receptor antagonist, for hyponatremia. *N Engl J Med.* 2006;355(20):2099-2112.

53. Madias NE. Effects of tolvaptan, an oral vasopressin V_2 receptor antagonist, in hyponatremia. *Am J Kidney Dis.* 2007;50(2):184-187.

54. Palevsky PM, Bhagrath R, Greenberg A. Hypernatremia in hospitalized patients. *Ann Intern Med.* 1996;124(2):197-203.

55. Snyder NA, Feigal DW, Arieff AI. Hypernatremia in elderly patients. A heterogeneous, morbid, and iatrogenic entity. *Ann Intern Med.* 1987;107(3): 309-319.

56. Lindner G, Funk GC, Schwarz C, et al. Hypernatremia in the critically ill is an independent risk factor for mortality. *Am J Kidney Dis.* 2007;50(6):952-957.

57. Aiyagari V, Deibert E, Diringer MN. Hypernatremia in the neurologic intensive care unit: how high is too high? *J Crit Care.* 2006;21(2):163-172.

58. Blevins LS Jr, Wand GS. Diabetes insipidus. *Crit Care Med.* 1992;20(1):69-79.

59. Loh JA, Verbalis JG. Disorders of water and salt metabolism associated with pituitary disease. *Endocrinol Metab Clin North Am.* 2008;37(1):213-234, x.

60. Fordtran JS, Dietschy JM. Water and electrolyte movement in the intestine. *Gastroenterology.* 1966;50(2):263-285.

61. Feldman M. Gastric secretion. In: Feldman M, ed. *Sleisinger & Fordtran's Gastrointestinal and Liver Diseases*. Philadelphia, PA: Elsevier; 2002:725.

62. Moder KG, Hurley DL. Fatal hypernatremia from exogenous salt intake: report of a case and review of the literature. *Mayo Clin Proc.* 1990;65(12):1587-1594.

63. Himmelseher S. Hypertonic saline solutions for treatment of intracranial hypertension. *Curr Opin Anaesthesiol.* 2007;20(5):414-426.

64. Rockswold GL, Solid CA, Paredes-Andrade E, Rockswold SB, Jancik JT, Quickel RR. Hypertonic saline and its effect on intracranial pressure, cerebral perfusion pressure, and brain tissue oxygen. *Neurosurgery.* 2009;65(6):1035-1041; discussion 41-42.

65. Markowitz GS, Radhakrishnan J, Kambham N, Valeri AM, Hines WH, D'Agati VD. Lithium nephrotoxicity: a progressive combined glomerular and tubulointerstitial nephropathy. *J Am Soc Nephrol.* 2000;11(8):1439-1448.

66. Timmer RT, Sands JM. Lithium intoxication. *J Am Soc Nephrol.* 1999;10(3):666-674.

67. De Petris L, Luchetti A, Emma F. Cell volume regulation and transport mechanisms across the blood-brain barrier: implications for the management of hypernatremic states. *Eur J Pediatr.* 2001;160(2):71-77.

68. Simmons MA, Adcock EW 3rd, Bard H, Battaglia FC. Hypernatremia and intracranial hemorrhage in neonates. *N Engl J Med.* 1974;291(1):6-10.

69. Handy TC, Hanzlick R, Shields LB, Reichard R, Goudy S. Hypernatremia and subdural hematoma in the pediatric age group: is there a causal relationship? *J Forensic Sci.* 1999;44(6):1114-1118.

70. Singer I, Oster JR, Fishman LM. The management of diabetes insipidus in adults. *Arch Intern Med.* 1997;157(12):1293-1301.

71. Marsden PA, Halperin ML. Pathophysiological approach to patients presenting with hypernatremia. *Am J Nephrol.* 1985;5(4):229-235.

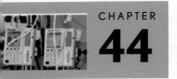

CHAPTER

44

Management of Systemic Blood Pressure in the NeuroICU

Samia Mian, MD
Thilagavathi Venkatachalam, MD
Christopher B. McFadden, MD

A 57-year-old man with a 5-year history of hypertension (HTN) presents to the emergency department with the assistance of family. They report progressive confusion and lethargy for 2 days. The patient has not been eating well or taking his home medications for 2 weeks. Home medications include clonidine 0.3 mg three times a day, atenolol 100 mg daily, escitalopram 20 mg daily, and hydrochlorothiazide 25 mg daily. The patient and his family deny any other symptoms including fevers, shortness of breath, slurring, or seizures. His initial vital signs include blood pressure (BP) of 186/104 mm Hg, pulse of 76 bpm, temperature of 36.5°C (97.6°F), and a respiratory rate of 18 breaths/min. He is not hypoxic. Initial neurologic examination and brain computed tomography (CT) do not reveal any motor deficits or acute anatomic abnormality.

Is uncontrolled hypertension responsible for the patient's acute change in mental status?

Mental status changes in the setting of poor cerebral blood flow are most often seen with low arterial BP. Cerebral perfusion pressure (CPP), the pressure gradient that influences blood flow to the brain, is the difference between mean arterial pressure (MAP) and intracranial pressure (ICP) and is represented by the formula:

$$CPP = CBF \times CVR$$

where CBF is cerebral blood flow and CVR is cerebrovascular resistance.

Cerebrovascular autoregulation maintains a constant blood flow over a wide range of CPPs. Normally, moderate changes in CPP have little effect on CBF. This is secondary to changes in CVR. An increase in CPP produces vasoconstriction and a decrease produces vasodilation. Typically for adults, CPP ranges between 50 and 100 mm Hg, though some research suggests 70 to 90 mm Hg to be a more accurate number.[1-3] In chronically hypertensive individuals, the cerebral arterioles develop medial hypertrophy and lose their ability to dilate effectively at lower pressures.[4] This can lead to decreased cerebral perfusion when systemic BP falls, even though BP may remain within a range that would provide adequate cerebral perfusion in patients without hypertension.

The mechanisms governing CBF autoregulation are controversial.[5] Most likely, the autoregulatory vessel caliber changes are influenced by arterial smooth muscle and metabolic mechanisms.[6,7] Perivascular nerves and the vascular endothelium may also play a role.[8-10] CBF autoregulation typically operates when mean systemic blood pressure is between 50 and 150 mm Hg[2] and can be modulated by sympathetic nervous activity and the renin-angiotensin system (RAS).

Central nervous system (CNS) trauma or acute ischemic stroke may impair CBF autoregulation, leaving surrounding CNS tissue vulnerable to over- or underperfusion. Likewise, autoregulation may be lost in the setting of a space-occupying brain lesion such as tumor or hematoma.[11] Autoregulation may be regained by hyperventilatory hypocapnia.[12] Patients with diabetes may have impaired CBF autoregulation, probably due to diabetic microangiopathy.[13] In summary, cerebral autoregulation is a dynamic process affected by a patient's medical condition and, in particular, previous blood pressure control.

Coming back to the case, our patient is neither diabetic nor having seizures. Could his impaired mental status represent hypertensive encephalopathy?

Hypertensive encephalopathy (HE) was first described by Oppenheimer and Fishberg in 1928 in the report of a patient with acute glomerulonephritis complicated by neurologic symptoms, convulsions, and severe hypertension.[14] It is a descriptive term referring to reversible cerebral disorders associated with high blood pressure in the absence of cerebral thrombosis or hemorrhage.

Hypertensive encephalopathy occurs most frequently when diastolic BP exceeds 120 mm Hg in a patient with chronic hypertension.[15] (Out-of-office BP control is known to be poor in most patients before they present with hypertensive emergency.[16,17]) At this level of diastolic BP, cerebral autoregulation cannot effectively limit blood flow to the brain and clinical symptoms develop.[18] Cerebral edema and microhemorrhages may occur. Hypertensive encephalopathy defines 16.3% of cases of hypertensive emergencies, more than intracranial hemorrhage or aortic dissection.[19] The syndrome is generally precipitated by a severe and rapid rise in BP. After BP reduction all signs and symptoms often resolve.

What is the pathogenesis of HE?

Two theories have been proposed to account for the clinical and radiologic abnormalities associated with hypertensive encephalopathy. The first proposes that HE results from spasm of the cerebral vasculature in response to acute hypertension; in other words, excessive autoregulation leads to ischemia and edema, particularly in the regions bordering the arterial blood supply.[20,21] A more recent hypothesis suggests the syndrome results from breakthrough of autoregulation.[22-24] This would result in interstitial extravasation of proteins and fluids, producing focal vasogenic edema in the peripheral vascular distribution of the involved vessel. Vascular injury, tissue ischemia, and the release of vasoconstrictive mediators worsen the condition.[17,25] Fibrinoid necrosis eventually occurs if the process is not interrupted. Figure 44-1 shows the renal arteriolopathy associated with hypertensive emergency, and Figure 44-2 shows changes associated with chronic hypertension.

Is there a role for imaging in diagnosing HE?

Magnetic resonance imaging (MRI) may now allow for a rapid and more specific diagnosis of HE. In uncomplicated cases, brain MRI shows areas of cerebral edema predominately in posterior white matter.[26] Lesions may be symmetric or asymmetric. Although not diagnostic, the terms *posterior reversible encephalopathy syndrome* or *reversible posterior leukoencephalopathy syndrome* have been adopted for this neuroradiologic finding. Flair imaging is the most sensitive sequence to detect areas of cerebral edema. The lesions are hyperintense on T2-weighted imaging and flair, and iso- to hypointense on T1-weighted imaging.[27] Diffusion-weighted imaging (DWI) with apparent diffusion coefficient (ADC) mapping shows the edema in HE to be vasogenic in origin.[26] Figure 44-3 demonstrates typical MRI findings of hypertensive encephalopathy.

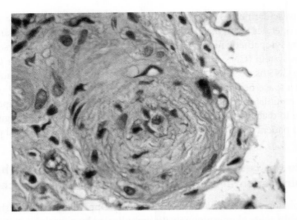

Figure 44-1. Small renal artery with severe mucinoid intimal inflammation and pinpoint lumen consistent with hypertensive emergency. *(Photo courtesy of I.B. Elfenbein, MD.)*

Do certain medications have a protective effect in maintaining cerebral autoregulation in patients with chronic hypertension?

Some drugs are cerebral vasodilators and have the potential for paralyzing autoregulation and raising intracranial pressure with systemic hypertension. This is seen most commonly with at least some calcium antagonists and hydralazine.[28,29] In particular, hydralazine has multiple cerebral hemodynamic effects. It raises ICP and thus, owing to its effect of also lowering systemic pressure, reduces CPP. Subsequently, CBF may increase, though not necessarily before cerebral underperfusion has occurred.[30]

Angiotensin-converting enzyme inhibitors improve autoregulation during hypotension, likely by reducing angiotensin II–dependent tone in cerebral resistance vessels. With chronic antihypertensive treatment, CBF autoregulation may return to normal. Angiotensin-converting enzyme inhibitors in particular, when given chronically, may maintain autoregulation at the lower limit of CPP. Apart from this, it is uncertain if there is a beneficial, class-specific pharmacologic effect of antihypertensive drugs directly on the cerebral circulation.

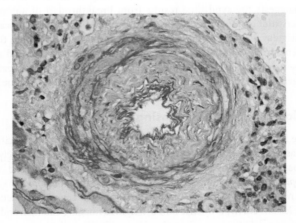

Figure 44-2. Intimal fibroelastic findings associated with chronic hypertension leading to a 70% lumen narrowing. *(Photo courtesy of I.B. Elfenbein, MD.)*

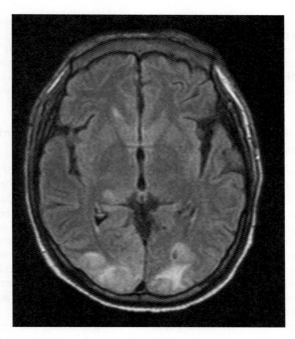

Figure 44-3. The typical findings associated with hypertensive encephalopathy are posterior reversible encephalopathy syndrome (PRES) as seen in this fluid-attenuated inversion recovery (FLAIR; long T2) sequence.

Can certain medications predispose to HE?

The development of uncontrolled hypertension associated with sudden discontinuation of antihypertensive medications has been described frequently in the medical literature and is referred to as *discontinuation syndrome, acute posttreatment syndrome, acute withdrawal syndrome,* and *rebound hypertension.*[31-33] This syndrome has been reported to occur with clonidine, methyldopa, propranolol, and rarely angiotensin-converting enzyme inhibitors.[34-41] Of the medications mentioned, clonidine has been studied the most in determining the mechanism responsible for rebound hypertension following discontinuation. Clonidine is a widely used antihypertensive drug that suppresses the sympathetic nervous system via a central mechanism by agonism of inhibitory α receptors. Sudden discontinuation of clonidine leads to rebound hypertension as a result of secretion of stored norepinephrine.[42] This effect is amplified in patients also taking propranolol (and possibly other β blockers) because of unopposed peripheral α-receptor activation.[43] Mirtazapine, which is a central α-receptor blocker, was reported to produce extreme hypertension in a patient maintained on clonidine, presumably by blocking clonidine's central effect.[44]

Does chronic hypertension have an effect on decline in cognitive function?

Hypertension is associated with impaired cognition, particularly executive functions, and is believed to play a causal role in cognitive decline above and beyond its relationship to stroke.[45,46] Pathologic changes in the brain associated with hypertension include vascular remodeling, impairment of cerebral autoregulation, white matter lesions, unrecognized lacunar infarcts, and Alzheimer-like changes such as amyloid angiopathy and cerebral atrophy.[47] Hypertension appears to affect the subcortical white matter in particular, and may affect a substantial volume of variably damaged tissue that is potentially salvageable through optimization of blood supply.

Based on the evidence above, it is probable that our patient presents with hypertensive encephalopathy in association with uncontrolled blood pressure secondary to withdrawal of high-dose clonidine, in the setting of atenolol use. This case emphasizes the importance of educating patients about the adverse effects of abrupt discontinuation of antihypertensive agents, particularly clonidine.

Consider now if this extremely hypertensive patient presented with acute stroke. How would this affect treatment?

Fairly strong evidence supports the deleterious effects of rapid reductions in BP in the early period following an acute stroke.[48-52] Immediately beyond the area of infarction, the *penumbra* is at high risk for ischemia and infarct extension.[53,54] A number of factors about BP in patients with a stroke are worth emphasizing. First, BP frequently rises immediately following cerebral ischemia.[54,55] (Proposed mechanisms for increases in blood pressure after stroke generally include excess sympathoadrenal tone from direct neural injury,[54] altered parasympathetic function, catecholamine release, and cytokine activation.[56-59]) BP typically begins to fall spontaneously within hours to days after stroke without intervention.[56,60] As a result, medication-induced reductions in BP may lead to CPP below a level that allows adequate cerebral perfusion to the penumbra. Exacerbating this tendency, patients with stroke typically have long-standing HTN and, thus, an autoregulatory curve that is shifted to the right.

Not all studies have shown deleterious effects of lowering BP acutely after stroke.[61,62] Small sample size may account for the inconsistent findings in this regard. Furthermore, it is important to recognize that low BP upon presentation may be a surrogate for independent cardiac disease, which may explain, in part, the worse outcomes seen with lower BP in this setting.[63] Most consensus guidelines recommend that BP not be treated acutely in the patient with ischemic stroke, except in the case of extreme hypertension (eg, systolic BP > 220 mm Hg or diastolic BP > 120 mm Hg) and end-organ damage. Typical examples of end-organ damage include hypertensive encephalopathy, aortic dissection, acute renal failure, acute pulmonary edema, and acute myocardial infarction. Ongoing studies are evaluating ideal BP control in the setting of acute stroke.[64]

When urgent BP reduction is needed in the setting of a stroke, limited data exist to guide selection of the optimal pharmacologic agent. Many agents have been tested without clear superiority.[1,65,66] Short-term, parenteral medications have the appeal of a quickly titratable effect. Nicardipine, esmolol, and labetalol are frequently used, and the use of these titratable agents is reasonable rather than the frequent bolus therapy. Alternative agents include enalaprilat or fenoldopam.[11] Sodium nitroprusside, a previous favorite in the management of HTN emergencies, may dilate both cerebral arterial and venous systems and lead to increased intracranial pressure.[67] When intravenous medications are used, particularly in states of altered consciousness, intra-arterial blood pressure should be continuously measured. When antihypertensive medication is given acutely to patients with ischemic stroke, MAP should be reduced by no more than 15% within the first 24 hours,[68,69] and reduction of BP should not occur during the acute phase of ischemic stroke. Parenteral antihypertensive agents and some of their properties are listed in Table 44-1.

Preliminary evidence suggests that *vasopressors* may have a role in maintaining CPP and thus limit infarct extension.[70-72] The use of a vasopressor in this setting is not standard of care, however, and has not yet been incorporated into guidelines. Volume expansion, with the goal of improving cerebral perfusion, does not have a role, unless polycythemia is present.[73,74] Many stroke patients are volume depleted on presentation, owing to BP-induced sodium excretion, a phenomenon known as *pressure natriuresis*. This volume depletion may exacerbate the fall in BP after antihypertensive agents are given.[75] Low BP in the setting of obvious hypovolemia warrants volume repletion, especially if it is

Table 44-1. Parenteral Agents for Hypertensive Emergencies

Drug	Type	Dose	Duration	Advantages	Disadvantages
Nicardipine hydrochloride	Vasodilator (CCB)	5-15 mg/h IV	15-30 min	Ease of dose	Tachycardia
Enalaprilat	Vasodilator (ACE-I)	1.25-5 mg every 6 h IV	6-12 h	Not IV drip	Duration of action long; potential large BP drop
Fenoldopam mesylate	Vasodilator (dopamine agonist)	0.1-1.6 μg/kg per min IV	30 min	Rapid onset	Reflex tachycardia; tachyphylaxis after 48 h
Sodium nitroprusside	Vasodilator (NO generator)	0.25-10 μg/kg per min[a]	1-2 min	Rapid onset	Thiocyanate toxicity, especially with renal failure
Nitroglycerin	Vasodilator (NO generator)	5-100 μg/min	5-10 min	Short duration	Headaches frequent
Phentolamine	α Blocker	5-15 mg IV bolus	10-30 min	Catecholamine excess	Pharmacy access
Esmolol hydrochloride	β Blocker	500 μg/kg (load) over 1 min	10-30 min	Aortic dissection	Contraindications to β blockade
Labetalol hydrochloride	α/β Blocker	20-80 mg IV bolus; infusion possible	3-6 h	Ease of access	Contraindications to β blockade

Abbreviations: ACE-I, angiotensin-converting enzyme inhibitor; BP, blood pressure; CCB, calcium channel blocker; IV, intravenous; NO, nitric oxide.

[a]Lower doses proposed to limit toxicity.[17]

Renal and Electrolyte Disorders

associated with neurologic deterioration in patients with acute stroke. Apart from volume depletion, other causes of hypotension one should consider include arrhythmias, sepsis, and aortic dissection.

Strokes qualifying for thrombolytic therapy have different blood pressure goals, in part because of the increased risk of bleeding with higher BP. Guidelines suggest initiating antihypertensive medications in eligible patients when systolic BP is above 185 mm Hg and diastolic BP is above 110 mm Hg. For the immediate 24 hours after thrombolytic agents are given, the target BP is below 180/105 mm Hg.

The optimal management of BP in hemorrhagic stoke is under active investigation. Initially, BP increases in the setting of intracranial hemorrhage (ICH).[76] While most patients with ICH have chronic HTN and a shifted autoregulatory curve, there is less of a concern for the ischemic penumbra seen in ischemic strokes.[77,78] Several clinical studies suggest that it is safe to reduce either the BP to less than 160/90 mm Hg or the MAP to less than 130 mm Hg within 24 hours.[79,80] Some studies even show reduction in hematoma growth with reduction in BP.[81,82] Current guidelines target a BP of 160/90 mm Hg or a MAP of 110 mm Hg in the acute management of intracerebral hemorrhage; as ICP may be elevated, ICP monitoring may be required to ensure CPP is maintained over 60 mm Hg.[83]

What other neurologic processes can affect blood pressure?

Blood pressure regulation is maintained in large part through autonomic regulation of blood vessel tone and sodium homeostasis. It is not surprising, then, that processes involving the central or peripheral nervous system can affect blood pressure. Brain and spinal cord injury frequently coexist with irregularities in blood pressure, both upward and downward. Beyond pain, proposed mechanisms include excess catecholamine release or sympathetic nervous system activation.[84,85]

Autonomic dysreflexia describes the phenomenon of vasoconstriction that occurs in spinal cord injuries above the level of T5. Specifically, a peripheral stimulus initiates a strong sympathetic nervous system discharge.[86,87] Often the stimulus is from the genitourinary tract, such as infection or urinary retention. Mechanisms include excess sympathetic drive, renal vasoconstriction, and an inability to dilate the splanchnic vessels. Flushing and bradycardia are frequent, caused by excess parasympathetic activity above the spinal lesion, mediated, in turn, by carotid baroreceptors.[88] Treatment of the offending stimulus (eg, urinary tract infection) should be the primary focus. Converting to an upright posture may mitigate the hypertension.[89] When pharmacotherapy is required, consideration should be given to the rapidity with which BP needs to be reduced, the concurrent presence of bradycardia, and the likelihood that the reflex vasoconstriction can be interrupted. Nifedipine has been shown to be effective in treating and preventing the hypertension of autonomic dysreflexia.[90]

The management of HTN in traumatic brain injury is similarly challenging. External factors including pain and stress may affect BP. Assessment of cerebral perfusion based on physical assessments may be limited by the patient's overall medical condition; as a result, CPP estimation through MAP and ICP monitoring is preferred.[11,91] Guidelines based on the best available evidence for BP therapy in various settings, including traumatic brain injury, are listed in Table 44-2. Tissue *hypoperfusion*, especially in patients whose BP is usually high, should always be considered as a possible complicating factor.

Table 44-2. Guidelines for BP Management in Neurocritical Care

Nonhemorrhagic Stroke[68]

Patient is not candidate for reperfusion therapy:
- No treatment unless systolic BP > 220 mm Hg or diastolic BP > 120 mm Hg, or target organ damage present (see text).

Patient is a candidate for reperfusion therapy:
- Treat systolic BP > 185 mm Hg or diastolic BP > 110 mm Hg.
- Keep BP < 180/105 mm Hg in first 24 h after reperfusion.

Hemorrhagic Stroke[83]

Presenting systolic BP > 200 mm Hg or MAP > 150 mm Hg:
- Reduce BP with IV medications.
- Goal is systemic BP of 160/90 mm Hg, unless CPP is reduced.

Presenting systolic BP > 180 mm Hg or MAP > 130 mm Hg, with increased ICP:
- Reduce BP while monitoring ICP.
- Keep CPP at 60-80 mm Hg.

Presenting systolic BP > 180 mm Hg or MAP > 130 mm Hg, without increased ICP:
- Goal is BP of 160/90 mm Hg or MAP of 110 mm Hg.
- Monitor for signs of cerebral hypoperfusion.

Traumatic Brain Injury[92,93]
- Avoid systolic BP < 90 mm Hg.
- Aim for CPP 50-70 mm Hg. A higher CPP may be tolerated in the setting of poor baseline BP control but active treatment should not be initiated to achieve this.

Abbreviations: BP, blood pressure; CPP, cerebral perfusion pressure; ICP, intracranial pressure; IV, intravenously; MAP, mean arterial pressure.

! CRITICAL CONSIDERATIONS

- The evaluation and management of hypertension in a neurocritical care environment is complex.
- BP may be affected by pain, high ICP, and even urinary tract infection.
- Catecholamine excess may lead to high BP despite intravascular volume depletion.
- Prior BP control has a dramatic effect on a patient's ability to tolerate reductions in BP. For this reason, it is important to try to ascertain the patient's typical premorbid BP control.
- A rapid reduction in BP, even within the normal range, can lead to underperfusion and permanent damage to otherwise viable brain tissue.
- Clinical assessment of cerebral perfusion should ultimately guide therapy.

Renal and Electrolyte
Disorders

REFERENCES

1. Steiner LA, Andrews PJ. Monitoring the injured brain: ICP and CBF. *Br J Anaesth.* 2006;97(1):26-38.
2. Powers WJ. Acute hypertension after stroke: the scientific basis for treatment decisions. *Neurology.* 1993;43(3 Pt 1):461-467.
3. Czosnyka M, Pickard JD. Monitoring and interpretation of intracranial pressure. *J Neurol Neurosurg Psychiatry.* 2004;75(6):813-821.
4. Varon J, Marik PE. Clinical review: the management of hypertensive crises. *Crit Care (London).* 2003;7(5):374-384.
5. Aoi M, Gremaud P, Tran HT, Novak V, Olufsen MS. Modeling cerebral blood flow and regulation. *Conf Pro IEEE Eng Med Biol Soc.* 2009;1:5470-5473.
6. Winn HR, Welsh JE, Rubio R, Berne RM. Brain adenosine production in rat during sustained alteration in systemic blood pressure. *Am J Physiol.* 1980;239(5):H636-H641.
7. Symon L, Held K, Dorsch NW. A study of regional autoregulation in the cerebral circulation to increased perfusion pressure in normocapnia and hypercapnia. *Stroke.* 1973;4(2):139-147.
8. McCarron RM, Chen Y, Tomori T, et al. Endothelial-mediated regulation of cerebral microcirculation. *J Physiol Pharmacol.* 2006;57(Suppl 11):133-144.
9. Edvinsson L, Hardebo JE, Owman C. Role of perivascular sympathetic nerves in autoregulation of cerebral blood flow and in blood-brain barrier functions. *Acta Neurol Scand Suppl.* 1977;64:50-51.
10. Wahl M, Schilling L. Regulation of cerebral blood flow—a brief review. *Acta Neurochir Suppl.* 1993;59:3-10.
11. Rose JC, Mayer SA. Optimizing blood pressure in neurological emergencies. *Neurocrit Care.* 2004;1(3):287-299.
12. Paulson OB, Olesen J, Christensen MS. Restoration of autoregulation of cerebral blood flow by hypocapnia. *Neurology.* 1972;22(3):286-293.
13. Pallas F, Larson DF. Cerebral blood flow in the diabetic patient. *Perfusion.* 1996;11(5):363-370.
14. Oppenheimer BS, Fishberg A. Hypertensive encephalopathy. *Arch Intern Med.* 1928;41(2):264-278.
15. Lenfant C, Chobanian AV, Jones DW, et al. Seventh report of the Joint National Committee on the Prevention, Detection, Evaluation, and Treatment of High Blood Pressure (JNC 7): resetting the hypertension sails. *Hypertension.* 2003;41(6):1178-1179.
16. Tisdale JE, Huang MB, Borzak S. Risk factors for hypertensive crisis: importance of out-patient blood pressure control. *Fam Pract.* 2004;21(4):420-424.
17. Marik PE, Varon J. Hypertensive crises: challenges and management. *Chest.* 2007;131(6):1949-1962.
18. Strandgaard S, Paulson OB. Cerebral blood flow and its pathophysiology in hypertension. *Am J Hypertens.* 1989;2(6 Pt 1):486-492.
19. Zampaglione B, Pascale C, Marchisio M, Cavallo-Perin P. Hypertensive urgencies and emergencies. Prevalence and clinical presentation. *Hypertension.* 1996;27(1):144-147.
20. Trommer BL, Homer D, Mikhael MA. Cerebral vasospasm and eclampsia. *Stroke.* 1988;19(3):326-329.
21. Coughlin WF, McMurdo SK, Reeves T. MR imaging of postpartum cortical blindness. *J Comp Assist Tomogr.* 1989;13(4):572-576.

22. Hauser RA, Lacey DM, Knight MR. Hypertensive encephalopathy. Magnetic resonance imaging demonstration of reversible cortical and white matter lesions. *Arch Neurol.* 1988;45(10):1078-1083.

23. Strandgaard S, Paulson OB. Cerebral autoregulation. *Stroke.* 1984;15(3):413-416.

24. Nag S, Robertson DM, Dinsdale HB. Cerebral cortical changes in acute experimental hypertension: an ultrastructural study. *Lab Invest.* 1977;36(2):150-161.

25. Ault MJ, Ellrodt AG. Pathophysiological events leading to the end-organ effects of acute hypertension. *Am J Emerg Med.* 1985;3(6 Suppl):10-15.

26. Schwartz RB, Mulkern RV, Gudbjartsson H, Jolesz F. Diffusion-weighted MR imaging in hypertensive encephalopathy: clues to pathogenesis. *Am J Neuroradiol.* 1998;19(5):859-862.

27. Casey SO, Sampaio RC, Michel E, Truwit CL. Posterior reversible encephalopathy syndrome: utility of fluid-attenuated inversion recovery MR imaging in the detection of cortical and subcortical lesions. *Am J Neuroradiol.* 2000;21(7):1199-1206.

28. Skinhoj E. The sympathetic nervous system and the regulation of cerebral blood flow in man. *Stroke.* 1972;3(6):711-716.

29. Luiten PG, de Jong GI, Schuurman T. Cerebrovascular, neuronal, and behavioral effects of long-term Ca^{2+} channel blockade in aging normotensive and hypertensive rat strains. *Ann N Y Acad Sci.* 1994;747:431-451.

30. Overgaard J, Skinhoj E. A paradoxical cerebral hemodynamic effect of hydralazine. *Stroke.* 1975;6(4):402-410.

31. Rupp H, Maisch B, Brilla CG. Drug withdrawal and rebound hypertension: differential action of the central antihypertensive drugs moxonidine and clonidine. *Cardiovasc Drugs Ther.* 1996;10(Suppl 1):251-262.

32. Cottrell JE, Illner P, Kittay MJ, et al. Rebound hypertension after sodium nitroprusside-induced hypotension. *Clin Pharmacol Ther.* 1980;27(1):32-36.

33. Lowenstein J. Drugs five years later: clonidine. *Ann Intern Med.* 1980;92(1):74-77.

34. Charalabopoulos K, Charalabopoulos A, Papalimneou V, et al. Consequences of the discontinuation of antihypertensive treatment in successfully treated patients. *Int J Clin Pract.* 2005;59(6):704-708.

35. Karachalios GN, Charalabopoulos A, Papalimneou V, et al. Withdrawal syndrome following cessation of antihypertensive drug therapy. *Int J Clin Pract.* 2005;59(5):562-570.

36. Takata Y, Yoshizumi T, Ito Y, et al. Comparison of withdrawing antihypertensive therapy between diuretics and angiotensin converting enzyme inhibitors in essential hypertensives. *Am Heart J.* 1992;124(6):1574-1580.

37. Ho GY, Blaufox MD, Wassertheil-Smoller S, et al. Plasma renin predicts success of antihypertensive drug withdrawal. *Am J Hypertens.* 1994;7(8):679-684.

38. Raftery EB. Cardiovascular drug withdrawal syndromes. A potential problem with calcium antagonists? *Drugs.* 1984;28(5):371-374.

39. Houston MC, Hodge R. Beta-adrenergic blocker withdrawal syndromes in hypertension and other cardiovascular diseases. *Am Heart J.* 1988;116(2 Pt 1):515-523.

40. Houston MC. Abrupt cessation of treatment in hypertension: consideration of clinical features, mechanisms, prevention and management of the discontinuation syndrome. *Am Heart J.* 1981;102(3 Pt 1):415-430.

41. Jennings GL, Reid CM, Sudhir K, Laufer E, Korner PI. Factors influencing the success of withdrawal of antihypertensive drug therapy. *Blood Press Suppl.* 1995;2:99-107.

42. Weber MA. Discontinuation syndrome following cessation of treatment with clonidine and other antihypertensive agents. *J Cardiovasc Pharmacol.* 1980;2(Suppl 1):S73-S89.

43. Neusy AJ, Lowenstein J. Blood pressure and blood pressure variability following withdrawal of propranolol and clonidine. *J Clin Pharmacol.* 1989;29(1):18-24.

44. Troncoso AL, Gill T. Hypertensive urgency with clonidine and mirtazapine. *Psychosomatics.* 2004;45(5):449-450.

45. Elias MF, Wolf PA, D'Agostino RB, Cobb J, White LR. Untreated blood pressure level is inversely related to cognitive functioning: the Framingham Study. *Am J Epidemiol.* 1993;138(6):353-364.

46. Knopman D, Boland LL, Mosley T, et al. Cardiovascular risk factors and cognitive decline in middle-aged adults. *Neurology.* 2001;56(1):42-48.

47. Kalaria RN. Small vessel disease and Alzheimer's dementia: pathological considerations. *Cerebrovasc Dis* 2002;13(Suppl 2):48-52.

48. Aslanyan S, Fazekas F, Weir CJ, et al. Effect of blood pressure during the acute period of ischemic stroke on stroke outcome: a tertiary analysis of the GAIN International Trial. *Stroke.* 2003;34(10):2420-2425.

49. Ahmed N, Nasman P, Wahlgren NG. Effect of intravenous nimodipine on blood pressure and outcome after acute stroke. *Stroke.* 2000;31(6):1250-1255.

50. O'Connell JE, Gray C. Treating hypertension after stroke. *BMJ.* 1994;308(6943):1523-1524.

51. Castillo J, Leira R, Garcia MM, et al. Blood pressure decrease during the acute phase of ischemic stroke is associated with brain injury and poor stroke outcome. *Stroke*. 2004;35(2):520-526.

52. Ahmed N, Wahlgren NG. Effects of blood pressure lowering in the acute phase of total anterior circulation infarcts and other stroke subtypes. *Cerebrovasc Dis*. 2003;15(4):235-243.

53. Heiss W-D. Ischemic penumbra: evidence from functional imaging in man. *J Cereb Blood Flow Metab*. 2000;20(9):1276-1293.

54. Qureshi AI, Ezzeddine MA, Nasar A, et al. Prevalence of elevated blood pressure in 563,704 adult patients with stroke presenting to the ED in the United States. *Am J Emerg Med*. 2007;25(1):32-38.

55. Willmot M, Leonardi-Bee J, Bath PM. High blood pressure in acute stroke and subsequent outcome: a systematic review. *Hypertension*. 2004;43(1):18-24.

56. Qureshi AI. Acute hypertensive response in patients with stroke: pathophysiology and management. *Circulation*. 2008;118(2):176-187.

57. Robinson TG, James M, Youde J, Panerai R, Potter J. Cardiac baroreceptor sensitivity is impaired after acute stroke. *Stroke*. 1997;28(9):1671-1676.

58. Rodriguez-Yanez M, Castellanos M, Blanco M, et al. New-onset hypertension and inflammatory response/poor outcome in acute ischemic stroke. *Neurology*. 2006;67(11):1973-1978.

59. Chamorro A, Amaro S, Vargas M, et al. Catecholamines, infection, and death in acute ischemic stroke. *J Neurol Sci*. 2007;252(1):29-35.

60. Wallace JD, Levy LL. Blood pressure after stroke. *JAMA*. 1981;246(19):2177-2180.

61. Rodriguez-Garcia JL, Botia E, de La Sierra A, Villanueva MA, Gonzalez-Spinola J. Significance of elevated blood pressure and its management on the short-term outcome of patients with acute ischemic stroke. *Am J Hypertens*. 2005;18(3):379-384.

62. Schrader J, Luders S, Kulschewski A, et al. The ACCESS study: evaluation of Acute Candesartan Cilexetil Therapy in Stroke Survivors. *Stroke*. 2003;34(7):1699-1703.

63. Leonardi-Bee J, Bath PM, Phillips SJ, Sandercock PA, Group ISTC. Blood pressure and clinical outcomes in the International Stroke Trial. *Stroke*. 2002;33(5):1315-1320.

64. Sare GM, Geeganage C, Bath PM. High blood pressure in acute ischemic stroke–broadening therapeutic horizons. *Cerebrovasc Dis*. 2009;27(Suppl 1):156-161.

65. Bath P. High blood pressure as risk factor and prognostic predictor in acute ischemic stroke: when and how to treat it? *Cerebrovasc Dis*. 2004;17(Suppl 1):51-57.

66. Chalmers J. Trials on blood pressure-lowering and secondary stroke prevention. *Am J Cardiol*. 2003;91(10A):3G-8G.

67. Cottrell JE, Patel K, Turndorf H, Ransohoff J. Intracranial pressure changes induced by sodium nitroprusside in patients with intracranial mass lesions. *J Neurosurg*. 1978;48(3):329-331.

68. Adams HP Jr, del Zoppo G, Alberts MJ, et al. Guidelines for the early management of adults with ischemic stroke: a guideline from the American Heart Association/American Stroke Association Stroke Council, Clinical Cardiology Council, Cardiovascular Radiology and Intervention Council, and the Atherosclerotic Peripheral Vascular Disease and Quality of Care Outcomes in Research Interdisciplinary Working Groups: the American Academy of Neurology affirms the value of this guideline as an educational tool for neurologists. [Erratum appears in *Circulation*. 2007;116(18):e515]. *Circulation* 2007;115(20):e478-e534.

69. Grossman E, Ironi AN, Messerli FH. Comparative tolerability profile of hypertensive crisis treatments. *Drug Saf*. 1998;19(2):99-122.

70. Rordorf G, Koroshetz WJ, Ezzeddine MA, Segal AZ, Buonanno FS. A pilot study of drug-induced hypertension for treatment of acute stroke. *Neurology*. 2001;56(9):1210-1213.

71. Rordorf G, Cramer SC, Efird JT, et al. Pharmacological elevation of blood pressure in acute stroke. Clinical effects and safety. *Stroke*. 1997;28(11):2133-2138.

72. Muzevich KM, Voils SA. Role of vasopressor administration in patients with acute neurologic injury. *Neurocrit Care*. 2009;11(1):112-119.

73. Adams HP Jr, del Zoppo G, Alberts MJ, et al. Guidelines for the early management of adults with ischemic stroke: a guideline from the American Heart Association/American Stroke Association Stroke Council, Clinical Cardiology Council, Cardiovascular Radiology and Intervention Council, and the Atherosclerotic Peripheral Vascular Disease and Quality of Care Outcomes in Research Interdisciplinary Working Groups: the American Academy of Neurology affirms the value of this guideline as an educational tool for neurologists. [Erratum appears in *Stroke*. 2007;38(6):e38. Erratum appears in *Stroke*. 2007;38(9):e96]. *Stroke*. 2007;38(5):1655-1711.

74. Pearson TC, Wetherley-Mein G. Vascular occlusive episodes and venous hematocrit in primary proliferative polycythaemia. *Lancet*. 1978;2(8102):1219-1222.

75. Bhalla A, Sankaralingam S, Dundas R, et al. Influence of raised plasma osmolality on clinical outcome after acute stroke. *Stroke*. 2000;31(9):2043-2048.

Renal and Electrolyte Disorders

76. Qureshi AI, Tuhrim S, Broderick JP, et al. Spontaneous intracerebral hemorrhage. *N Engl J Med.* 2001;344(19):1450-1460.

77. Qureshi AI, Wilson DA, Hanley DF, Traystman RJ. No evidence for an ischemic penumbra in massive experimental intracerebral hemorrhage. *Neurology.* 1999;52(2):266-272.

78. Powers WJ, Zazulia AR, Videen TO, et al. Autoregulation of cerebral blood flow surrounding acute (6 to 22 hours) intracerebral hemorrhage. *Neurology.* 2001;57(1):18-24.

79. Qureshi AI, Mohammad YM, Yahia AM, et al. A prospective multicenter study to evaluate the feasibility and safety of aggressive antihypertensive treatment in patients with acute intracerebral hemorrhage. *J Intens Care Med.* 2005;20(1):34-42.

80. Qureshi AI, Harris-Lane P, Kirmani JF, et al. Treatment of acute hypertension in patients with intracerebral hemorrhage using American Heart Association guidelines. *Crit Care Med.* 2006;34(7):1975-1980.

81. Anderson CS. Medical management of acute intracerebral hemorrhage. *Curr Opin Crit Care.* 2009;15(2):93-98.

82. Anderson CS, Huang Y, Wang JG, et al. Intensive blood pressure reduction in acute cerebral hemorrhage trial (INTERACT): a randomised pilot trial. *Lancet Neurol.* 2008;7(5):391-399.

83. Broderick J, Connolly S, Feldmann E, et al. Guidelines for the management of spontaneous intracerebral hemorrhage in adults: 2007 update: a guideline from the American Heart Association/American Stroke Association Stroke Council, High Blood Pressure Research Council, and the Quality of Care and Outcomes in Research Interdisciplinary Working Group. *Circulation.* 2007;116(16):e391-e413.

84. Karlsson AK, Friberg P, Lonnroth P, Sullivan L, Elam M. Regional sympathetic function in high spinal cord injury during mental stress and autonomic dysreflexia. *Brain.* 1998;121(Pt 9): 1711-1719.

85. Maiorov DN, Weaver LC, Krassioukov AV. Relationship between sympathetic activity and arterial pressure in conscious spinal rats. *Am J Physiol.* 1997;272(2 Pt 2):H625-H631.

86. Karlsson AK. Autonomic dysreflexia. *Spinal Cord.* 1999;37(6):383-391.

87. Karlsson AK. Overview: autonomic dysfunction in spinal cord injury: clinical presentation of symptoms and signs. *Prog Brain Res.* 2006;152:1-8.

88. Teasell RW, Arnold JM, Krassioukov A, Delaney GA. Cardiovascular consequences of loss of supraspinal control of the sympathetic nervous system after spinal cord injury. *Arch Phys Med Rehabil.* 2000;81(4):506-516.

89. Kirshblum SC, Priebe MM, Ho CH, et al. Spinal cord injury medicine. 3. Rehabilitation phase after acute spinal cord injury. *Arch Phys Med Rehabil.* 2007;88(3 Suppl 1):S62-S70.

90. Lindan R, Leffler EJ, Kedia KR. A comparison of the efficacy of an alpha$_1$-adrenergic blocker in the slow calcium channel blocker in the control of autonomic dysreflexia. *Paraplegia.* 1985;23(1):34-38.

91. Steiner LA, Johnston AJ, Czosnyka M, et al. Direct comparison of cerebrovascular effects of norepinephrine and dopamine in head-injured patients. *Crit Care Med.* 2004;32(4):1049-1054.

92. Brain Trauma Foundation, American Association of Neurological Surgeons, Congress of Neurological Surgeons, et al. Guidelines for the management of severe traumatic brain injury. I. Blood pressure and oxygenation. [Erratum appears in *J Neurotrauma.* 2008;25(3):276-278. Note: multiple author names added]. *J Neurotrauma.* 2007;24(Suppl 1):S7-S13.

93. Brain Trauma Foundation, American Association of Neurological Surgeons, Congress of Neurological Surgeons, et al. Guidelines for the management of severe traumatic brain injury. IX. Cerebral perfusion thresholds. *J Neurotrauma.* 2007;24:S59-S64.

Hematology

Section Editor: Louis Aledort, MD

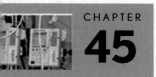

CHAPTER

45

Disseminated Intravascular Coagulation

Caroline Cromwell, MD
Louis M. Aledort, MD, MACP

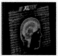

A 29-year-old man presented to the emergency department (ED) after a motorcycle accident. Upon arrival to the ED he was found to have suffered a crush injury to his left temple. He was intubated and underwent urgent evacuation of an epidural hematoma. The next day he developed progressive hypotension and spiking fevers. Oozing from multiple line and venipuncture sites was noted. His hemoglobin and platelet count began to decline and his prothrombin time (PT) and partial thromboplastin time (PTT), which were initially normal, started to rise. His liver function test showed a rise in transaminases.

What is the differential diagnosis?

The differential diagnosis includes the following:

- Thrombotic thrombocytopenic purpura
- Idiopathic thrombocytopenic purpura
- Disseminated intravascular coagulation
- Heparin-induced thrombocytopenia

The most likely diagnosis in this clinical setting is disseminated intravascular coagulation (DIC). DIC is a syndrome, not a diagnosis. It is an acquired state that occurs as a result of a number of underlying conditions (Table 45-1). For the purpose of this review, we will

Table 45-1. Etiology of Disseminated Intravascular Coagulation

Sepsis
Cancer: solid tumors, myeloproliferative disorders, lymphoproliferative disorders, leukemia
Obstetric complications: abruptio placentae, amniotic fluid embolism
Vascular disorders: large aneurysms, Kasabach-Merritt syndrome, atherosclerosis
Severe toxic reactions
Severe immunologic reactions
Transplant rejection
Severe trauma

focus on acute DIC. In the setting of DIC, there is global activation of the coagulation system with formation of fibrin within the circulation. Fibrin deposition leads to thrombosis and occlusion of small vessels, with subsequent end-organ damage. At the same time, depletion of platelets and clotting factors can also lead to bleeding.[1]

In the clinical scenario described above, DIC may be due to his traumatic brain injury as well as his sepsis. The brain has a high concentration of tissue thromboplastin, which has a tendency to become prothrombotic when released into systemic circulation.[2] He is also bacteremic. Sepsis may cause marked activity of the inflammatory system, and inflammation-induced activation of coagulation is a well-recognized phenomenon.[3] Severe sepsis may be complicated by DIC in about 35% of cases.[4]

What are the clinical manifestations of DIC?

DIC is a clinical diagnosis of a syndrome. Clinical manifestations include[5]:

- Thrombosis
- Bleeding
- Renal dysfunction
- Hepatic dysfunction
- Shock

On physical examination one may note cool, mottled extremities; petechiae; ecchymoses; or hemorrhages at the site of invasive procedures. From a laboratory standpoint, there is not one single laboratory test in isolation that can determine the diagnosis of DIC. Instead, DIC is a clinical syndrome, and laboratory data help support clinical suspicion (Table 45-2).

It is important to remember to monitor the trend in these parameters. As fibrinogen is an acute-phase reactant, it can be elevated in the setting of sepsis or inflammation. Therefore, evaluating serial measurements and analyzing the trend are essential. A review of the peripheral smear may reveal the presence of microangiopathic changes.

The subcommittee on DIC of the Scientific and Standardization Committee of the International Society of Thrombosis and Haemostasis (ISTH) has developed a scoring system based on the outcome of a combination of several laboratory tests (Table 45-3). A score of greater than or equal to 5 is compatible with the diagnosis of overt DIC.[6] Prospective studies have validated this scoring system.[4]

Table 45-2. Laboratory Characteristics of DIC

PT	Prolonged, normal, or (rarely) decreased
PTT	Prolonged, normal, or (rarely) decreased
Fibrinogen	Decreased
FDPs/D-dimers	Increased
Platelets	Decreased

Abbreviations: DIC, disseminated intravascular coagulation; FDPs, fibrin degradation products; PT, prothrombin time; PTT, partial thromboplastin time.

How would you treat DIC in this patient?

The first step is to treat the underlying diagnosis. Supportive care for DIC includes infusion of fresh-frozen plasma 10 mL/kg, platelet and blood transfusion,[7] and cryoprecipitate in order to improve abnormal coagulation and reduce active bleeding (Figure 45-1). Therapy is indicated in patients who are actively bleeding or who are at high risk of bleeding, but should not be used merely to "treat" abnormal laboratory values.

Heparin has been used in patients with thrombotic manifestations of DIC based on anecdotal evidence. Experimental studies have shown that heparin can at least partly inhibit the activation of coagulation in DIC.[8] There are no randomized controlled trials to demonstrate the use of heparin in patients with DIC leading to any improvement in clinical outcomes. Small uncontrolled studies have reported limited benefits with heparin use and have demonstrated that heparin infusion may improve laboratory abnormalities associated with DIC.[9-11] If it is used, a bolus is usually not needed and it should be initiated at 500 units/h as a starting dose. Patients must be monitored carefully for any bleeding.

Given the association of abnormal coagulation with systemic inflammation, substitution of coagulation products such as antithrombin III and protein C has been attempted in the setting of sepsis and DIC. However, results have been conflicting. The largest study using antithrombin III in patients with DIC demonstrated no benefit. Activated protein C has been shown in some studies to have a possible mortality benefit in patients with severe sepsis.[12-15]

Table 45-3. Scoring System for Diagnosis of Overt DIC

Does the patient have an underlying disorder associated with overt DIC?	(See Table 45-1.) If yes, proceed. If no, do not use this algorithm.
Coagulation tests	**Score**
Platelet count	> 100 = 0, < 100 = 1, < 50 = 2
Elevated fibrin-related marker (FDPs, D-dimers)	No increase = 0, moderate increase = 2, strong increase = 3
Prolonged PTT	< 3 s = 0, > 3 s but < 6 s = 1, > 6 s = 2
Fibrinogen level	> 1.0 g/L = 0, < 1.0 g/L = 1
Calculate score:	If ≥ 5, it is compatible with overt DIC; repeat labs daily. If < 5, it is suggestive but not affirmative of DIC; repeat in next 1-2 d

Abbreviations: DIC, disseminated intravascular coagulation; FDPs, fibrin degradation products; PTT, partial thromboplastin time.

Hematology

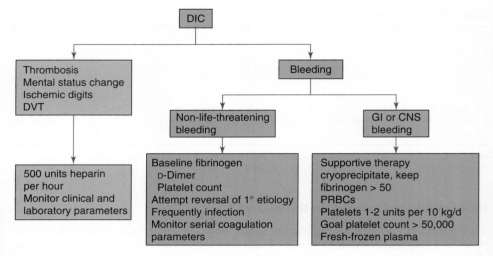

Figure 45-1. Algorithm for disseminated intravascular coagulation (DIC). CNS, central nervous system; DIC, disseminated intravascular coagulation; DVT, deep venous thrombosis; GI, gastrointestinal; PRBCs, packed red blood cells.

The overall prognosis of acute DIC is poor, with reported mortality rates ranging from 40% to 80% in patients with severe sepsis, trauma, or burn injuries.[16-18] Mortality is thought to be affected by the magnitude of underlying disease processes causing the DIC, rather than DIC per se. However, in a recent study of traumatic brain injury, patients with higher DIC scores were found to have increased likelihood of death or persistent vegetative state compared to patients with lower DIC scores, irrespective of their Glasgow Coma Scale scores.[19] In any event, early and prompt treatment of the underlying disease and providing hemodynamic support are the mainstays of DIC management.

! CRITICAL CONSIDERATIONS

- DIC is a clinical syndrome with an underlying etiology, not a diagnosis.
- The diagnosis of DIC is clinical, with laboratory values that may support your clinical suspicion.
- DIC is associated with a poor prognosis.
- DIC can present with thrombotic or hemorrhagic complications, or both simultaneously.
- First-line treatment of DIC is to treat the underlying diagnosis.
- Supportive care includes fresh-frozen plasma and blood and platelet transfusions.
- Consider low-dose heparin in patients with thrombotic manifestations, with close clinical monitoring for signs of bleeding.

REFERENCES

1. Levi M, Ten Cate H. Disseminated intravascular coagulation. *N Engl J Med.* 1999;341(8):586-592.

2. Goodnight SH, Kenoyer G, Rapaport SI, Patch MJ, Lee JA, Kurze T. Defibrination after brain-tissue destruction: a serious complication of head injury. *N Engl J Med.* 1974;290(19):1043-1047.

3. Levi M, van der Poll T. The role of natural anticoagulants in the pathogenesis and management of systemic activation of coagulation and inflammation in critically ill patients. *Semin Thromb Hemost.* 2008;34(5):459-468.

4. Bakhtiari K, Meijers JC, de Jonge E, Levi M. Prospective validation of the International Society of Thrombosis and Haemostasis scoring system for disseminated intravascular coagulation. *Crit Care Med.* 2004;32(12):2416-2421.

5. Siegal T, Seligsohn U, Aghai E, Modan M. Clinical and laboratory aspects of disseminated intravascular coagulation (DIC): a study of 118 cases. *Thromb Haemost.* 1978;39(1):122-134.

6. Taylor FB Jr, Toh CH, Hoots WK, Wada H, Levi M. Towards definition, clinical and laboratory criteria, and a scoring system for disseminated intravascular coagulation. *Thromb Haemost.* 2001;86(5):1327-1330.

7. Heim MU, Meyer B, Hellstern P. Recommendations for the use of therapeutic plasma. *Curr Vasc Pharmacol.* 2009;7(2):110-119.

8. Pernerstorfer T, Hollenstein U, Hansen J, et al. Heparin blunts endotoxin-induced coagulation activation. *Circulation.* 1999;100(25):2485-2490.

9. Corrigan JJ Jr, Jordan CM. Heparin therapy in septicemia with disseminated intravascular coagulation. *N Engl J Med.* 1970;283(15):778-782.

10. Audibert G, Lambert H, Toulemonde F, et al. Use of a low molecular weight heparin, CY 222, in the treatment of consumption coagulopathy. *J Mal Vasc.* 1987;12(Suppl B):147-151.

11. Feinstein DI. Treatment of disseminated intravascular coagulation. *Semin Thromb Hemost.* 1988;14(4):351-362.

12. Dhainaut JF, Yan SB, Joyce DE, et al. Treatment effects of drotrecogin alfa (activated) in patients with severe sepsis with or without overt disseminated intravascular coagulation. *J Thromb Haemost.* 2004; 2(11):1924-1933.

13. Aoki N, Matsuda T, Saito H, et al. A comparative double-blind randomized trial of activated protein C and unfractionated heparin in the treatment of disseminated intravascular coagulation. *Int J Hematol.* 2002;75(5):540-547.

14. Warren BL, Eid A, Singer P, et al. Caring for the critically ill patient. High-dose antithrombin III in severe sepsis: a randomized controlled trial. *JAMA.* 2001;286(15):1869-1878.

15. Dempfle CE. Coagulopathy of sepsis. *Thromb Haemost.* 2004;91(2):213-224.

16. Stephan F, Hollande J, Richard O, Cheffi A, Maier-Redelsperger M, Flahault A. Thrombocytopenia in a surgical ICU. *Chest.* 1999;115(5): 1363-1370.

17. Hulka F, Mullins RJ, Frank EH. Blunt brain injury activates the coagulation process. *Arch Surg.* 1996;131(9):923-927; discussion 927-928.

18. Gando S, Nanzaki S, Kemmotsu O. Disseminated intravascular coagulation and sustained systemic inflammatory response syndrome predict organ dysfunctions after trauma: application of clinical decision analysis. *Ann Surg.* 1999;229(1): 121-127.

19. Saggar V, Mittal RS, Vyas MC. Hemostatic abnormalities in patients with closed head injuries and their role in predicting early mortality. *J Neurotrauma.* 2009;26(10):1665-1668.

Hematology

CHAPTER
46

Bleeding Disorders and Coagulopathy Reversal

Caroline Cromwell, MD
Louis M. Aledort, MD, MACP

A 60-year-old white woman with a history of Crohn disease, factor V Leiden thrombophilia, and significant vascular and thrombotic disease in her left leg presents with headache. She has been maintained on 80 mg of Lovenox bid for years without a new thrombotic complication. One week prior to the admission, she fell and had minor head trauma. For the ensuing 3 days, she had headache, and on the fourth day she developed severe nausea and projectile vomiting. A noncontrast computed tomography (CT) scan of her brain showed acute hemorrhage in the right cerebellar hemisphere with minimal mass effect.

What are available antidotes for reversal of low-molecular-weight heparin (LMWH)?

The issue of LMWH use is commonly seen with patients and presents clinicians with a significant dilemma. It is common practice to stop all anticoagulation and antiplatelet agents once intracerebral hemorrhage (ICH) is detected. However, the diagnosis can sometimes be delayed, and the situation would be quite different if she had continued her LMWH. Reversal of anticoagulation, in the setting of continued, active bleeding, must be done on an emergent basis. The half-life of LMWH is 12 to 24 hours. There is no antidote that completely reverses the effect of LMWH, and such reversal reports are mostly anecdotal in the literature. Protamine sulfate is used intravenously to reverse unfractionated heparin and leads to full reversal. It is thought that protamine reverses approximately 60% of the effect of LMWH[1,2] based on in vitro studies.

It is unclear why protamine does not fully neutralize the anti-Xa activity of LMWH. One milligram of protamine is given for every 100 units of active unfractionated heparin, and per 1 mg of LMWH.[3] The maximum dose of protamine is 50 mg, with a maximum infusion rate of 5 mg/min. Hypotension, severe anaphylaxis, and death have been reported with protamine use.[4] These adverse reactions can often be minimized by premedication with antihistamines and steroids, as well as a slow rate of administration. If given in excess dose, protamine can have a paradoxical anticoagulant effect.

There are small studies describing recombinant activated factor VII (rFVIIa) for LMWH reversal, with some success. Doses in these studies ranged from 20 to 90 μg/kg.[5,6] The use of rFVIIa in the setting of spontaneous and warfarin-associated bleeding will be discussed later in this chapter.

When can anticoagulation therapy be resumed, as this patient could easily require amputation of her left leg if thrombosis occurs again?

A safe time to reinitiate full anticoagulation is determined on a case-by-case basis. If hematoma expansion does not occur and the patient doesn't receive decompressive surgery, in general, full anticoagulation may be resumed approximately 10 to 14 days after the bleeding episode. The decision as to when reinitiation of anticoagulation can occur in this setting must be decided with risk-benefit stratification.

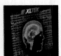 A 50-year-old right-handed white woman presents to the neurologic intensive care unit (ICU) with sudden onset of right arm and leg weakness. An emergency CT scan of the brain revealed a 40-mL (by ABC/2 calculation) left basal ganglia hemorrhage with a 3-mm midline shift. She has been on 5 mg of warfarin daily with international normalized ratios (INRs) of 2.5 to 2.8 for a long period of time. On admission, she has an INR of 2.5 and isn't on any other medications (aside from warfarin). She is on warfarin for factor V Leiden heterozygosity and a history of deep venous thrombosis (DVT) and pulmonary embolism (PE).

How would you reverse the warfarin-induced coagulopathy in this patient with deep brain hemorrhage?

The goal in this case would be rapid reversal of the underlying coagulopathy. For deep brain hemorrhages, neurosurgical intervention is usually not advocated. Warfarin functions as an anticoagulant by inhibiting the biosynthesis of vitamin K–dependent procoagulant factors II, VII, IX, and X.[7] Higher risk of intracranial hemorrhage is associated with the intensity of anticoagulation.[8] But often, as in this case, patients on warfarin present with ICH with an INR within therapeutic range.[9] In oral anticoagulant–associated ICH, the risk of continued bleeding is very high. In patients with ICH, the use of warfarin increases the risk of progressive bleeding and decompensation and doubles the risk of death.[10,11] It is imperative that reversal of coagulopathy is initiated immediately. Treatment consists of vitamin K, fresh-frozen plasma (FFP), and prothrombin-complex concentrates (PCCs).

Vitamin K

The patient should immediately receive vitamin K 10 mg intravenously (IV) over 10 minutes to begin the reversal of warfarin, which can take 6 to 24 hours. Vitamin K administration is necessary for the sustained reversal of the INR. American College of Chest Physicians guidelines recommend IV vitamin K in the face of life-threatening bleeding disorders.[12] While anaphylaxis reactions have been reported with intravenous administration of vitamin K, the overall incidence is rare, 3 per 10,000 doses.[13,14] Anaphylaxis reactions have also been reported with nonintravenous routes of administration.[15] In addition, the absorption of subcutaneous vitamin K can be unpredictable.[16] Therefore, intravenous vitamin K is the preferred route of administration in this setting.

Fresh-Frozen Plasma

FFP may be used at a dose of 15 mL/kg to achieve prompt reversal of warfarin by providing factors II, VII, IX, and X. These are the factors that are vitamin K dependent and those that warfarin suppresses. However, obtaining FFP can take quite some time. After the request arrives at the blood bank, the FFP must be blood-type matched and thawed, which can lead to an unacceptable delay in the face of a life-threatening hemorrhage. Volume status is also a concern, as the amount of FFP needed to fully and continuously reverse the coagulopathy may not be possible without infusing an unacceptably high volume intravenously.

The usual goal is to achieve an INR of less than 1.5, which reflects functioning of at least 40% of coagulation proteins, which is considered adequate for hemostasis.[17] A typical unit of FFP contains 200 to 250 mL, and 1 unit typically lowers the INR by approximately 10%. One unit of plasma will raise coagulation factors by 2.5%. Patients usually require 6 to 12 units of FFP and frequently even more, which leads to increased risk of volume overload and pulmonary edema. Severe allergic reactions, transfusion-associated circulatory overload, and transfusion-related acute lung injury (TRALI) can occur with FFP transfusion.[18]

Prothrombin-Complex Concentrate

PCCs are derived from large donor plasma pools and contain factors II, VII, IX, and X. They are highly concentrated coagulation factor replacement compounds. They were originally developed for the treatment of hemophilia patients with inhibitors. They are rapid, in small volume, with no need for typing and cross-matching. They have been found to normalize the INR more rapidly than vitamin K or FFP alone.[19,20] Large randomized trials comparing FFP to PCCs are currently ongoing.

While these products are licensed for warfarin reversal in Europe, none are licensed for this indication in the United States. Two PCCs are commercially available in the United States, and these products contain variable amounts of factor VII (Table 46-1). Clinicians need to be cautious when using PCCs in patients in whom there is a suspicion of disseminated intravascular coagulation (DIC) as thromboembolic events have been reported. While PCCs are generally considered safe to use, one should avoid the use in patients with DIC, hyperfibrinolysis, and a history of thromboembolism.

Recombinant Activated Factor VII

Factor VIIa is indicated for the treatment of hemophilia patients with inhibitors as well as patients with factor VII deficiency. Many studies have been published regarding the use of rFVIIa in the setting of spontaneous and warfarin-associated bleeding. Variable doses (10-90 μg/kg) have been used in studies attempting to reverse warfarin anticoagulation in the setting of ICH. These studies consist of case reports, case series, and retrospective cohort studies. Factor VIIa was found to lead to rapid reversal of the INR in these studies.[21-25] Due to the varied dosing, end points assessed make it difficult to draw any other conclusion. However, in the phase III Factor VII for Acute Hemorrhagic Stroke Treatment (FAST) trial, which assessed the use of rFVIIa in *spontaneous, noncoagulopathic* hemorrhage, there was a reduced hematoma expansion rate with the drug despite no improvement in long-term clinical outcomes (refer to Chapter 2, Intracranial Hemorrhage, for more detail). It is important to note that rFVIIa corrects the prothrombin time or INR, but this does not always correlate with cessation of bleeding.[26]

Thromboembolic complications have occurred in this setting and rVIIa use. In the FAST trial, a 5% absolute increase in the number of arterial thrombotic events was found in the group treated with the highest dose (80 μg/kg) of rFVIIa. Thus, particular caution should be used in patients with underlying thrombotic risk.

Table 46-1. Composition of Prothrombin-Complex Concentrates

Factor	Bebulin	Profilnine
II	120 units	148 units
VII	13 units	11 units
IX	100 units	100 units
X	139 units	64 units

(From Leissinger CA, Blatt PM, Hoots WK, Ewenstein B. Role of prothrombin complex concentrates in reversing warfarin anticoagulation: a review of the literature. Am J Hematol. 2008;83(2):137-143.)

A 60-year-old man with a history of hypertension and ischemic cardiomyopathy with a known left ventricular ejection fraction of 30% on chronic warfarin therapy presents with left-sided frontal lobe hemorrhage. INR is 3.5 at this time.

How would you reverse the coagulopathy in this patient?

This is an ideal scenario for considering the use of IV vitamin K 10 mg and PCC 50 units/kg (Table 46-2). PCC has been associated with thrombosis in recipients with hemophilia,[27] but in a review of PCC-treated patients, very few thrombotic episodes have been recorded.[28] In a 2008 publication,[29] Leissinger and colleagues reviewed the published evidence on the role of PCC in warfarin reversal. They identified 14 studies that included 460 patients, and 7 thrombotic complications were reported. There were no episodes of DIC. Overall, the thrombotic risk associated with the use of PCCs is reported to be low although not negligible.

A 59-year-old man is to undergo a spinal surgery. From preoperative screening, he is known to have an elevated partial thromboplastin time (PTT). There was no family history of bleeding disorder, but as a child he was told that following a tooth extraction he had bleeding that required multiple visits to the dentist to stop the bleeding.

What are the appropriate preoperative steps to take in order to minimize bleeding during a spine surgery?

Oral manipulation bleeding is a major clinical manifestation of a bleeding disorder as saliva contains a high concentration of fibrinolytic proteins. An appropriate workup includes mixing studies to rule out an inhibitor, a lupus anticoagulant, and an artifact, and if corrected factor deficiencies need to be ruled out. Factors VIII, IX, and XI are the most common.

Table 46-2. Coagulopathy Reversal

Agent	Reversal agent	Dose
Acetylsalicylic acid	DDAVP	0.3 μg/kg in 50 mL saline over 15 min
	Platelet transfusion	1 pack = 6 donors
Plavix	Platelet transfusion	2 packs = 12 donors
Heparin	Protamine	1 mg per 100 units of heparin
LMWH heparin	Protamine	1 mg per 1 mg of heparin
	rVIIa	20-90 μg/kg
NSAIDs	Platelets	1 pack = 6 donors
Coumadin without bleeding	Vitamin K	1-5 mg orally
Mild bleeding	Vitamin K	5-10 mg PO or IV
Severe bleeding	Vitamin K	10 mg IV
	PCC	50 units/kg
	Fresh-frozen plasma	15 mL/kg

Abbreviations: DDAVP, desmopressin; IV, intravenously; LMWH, low-molecular-weight heparin; NSAIDs, nonsteroidal anti-inflammatory drugs; PO, by mouth.

Hematology

Table 46-3. Bleeding Disorder Treatment Regimen

Hemophilia A	Factor VIII 40 units/kg to achieve 100% correction
	Half-life 12 h, 20 units/kg q12h thereafter
Hemophilia B	Factor IX 80 units/kg = 100%
	Half-life 24 h, 40 units/kg q24h thereafter
vW severe	Correct factor VIII to achieve 100% correction
	Correct ristocetin cofactor to > 50%
	Dose based on patient's baseline + product used
	Read label for content
vW mild	DDAVP 0.3 µg/kg in 50 mL saline over 15 min
XI	FFP 2 units night before
	2 units preoperation + 2 units postoperation and then 2 units every 2-3 d for a total of 14 d

Abbreviations: DDAVP, desmopressin; FFP, fresh-frozen plasma; vW, von Willebrand. High probability: 6-8 points; intermediate probability: 4-5 points; low probability: ≤ 3 points. *(From Lo GK, Juhl D, Warkentin TE, Sigouin CS, Eichler P, Greinacher A. Evaluation of pretest clinical score (4 T's) for the diagnosis of heparin-induced thrombocytopenia in two clinical settings. J Thromb Haemost. 2006;4(4):759-765.)*

Ensuring hemostasis after surgery would be the goal. An algorithm for the management of the different deficiencies, including von Willebrand, is shown in Table 46-3.

Preoperatively, one's goal is to reach 100% correction and never let the factor fall below 30% to maintain adequate hemostasis. It is important that aminosalicylic acid (ASA), nonsteroidal anti-inflammatory drugs (NSAIDs), and other antiplatelet agents not be used when levels are low, but they are acceptable during replacement therapy. Factor XI–deficient patients do not have available a concentrate in the United States, but do in many other countries. Therefore, we treat with FFP and do not need to achieve similar levels to achieve hemostasis.

 A 47-year-old woman undergoes a hemicraniotomy for removal of a ring-enhancing, high-grade glioma. In the neurologic ICU within 5 days postoperatively, where prophylactic subcutaneous heparin (5000 units q12h) on the third day was administered, swelling of the leg was noted. Venous Doppler revealed a proximal DVT.

What are the appropriate steps to address this proximal DVT?

The occurrence of DVT in postneurosurgic intervention is a well-known complication. Thrombosis in the setting of glioblastoma multiforme is particularly common, with an incidence rate of 20% to 24%.[30-33] As this case was a recurrence of a tumor that had been surgically resected 8 months prior and the patient had previously been exposed to heparin, one must be vigilant about the risk of development of heparin-induced thrombocytopenia (HIT) with thrombosis (Figure 46-1). As neoplastic disorders are frequently associated with DIC, one must rule out DIC as well (see Figure 45-1).

After ruling out DIC and HIT, full anticoagulation with intravenous heparin needs to be instituted. A bolus is usually not required. The recommended goal is 1000 units of heparin per hour, maintaining a PTT 2 to 2 1/2 times the normal value.

Treatment of most postoperative DVTs, regardless of other coexisting risk factors, consists of anticoagulation for 3 to 6 months. Transition to warfarin therapy should be undertaken while the patient is on heparin to prevent further clotting or skin necrosis by the reduction of proteins C and S by warfarin. In the subset of patients with malignancy, there may be a trend toward increased survival

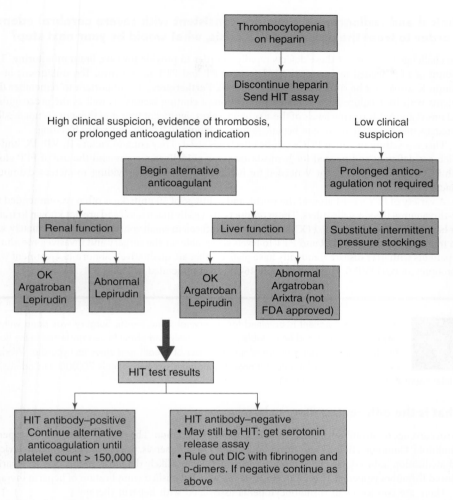

Figure 46-1. Algorithm for heparin-induced thrombocytopenia (HIT). DIC, disseminated intravascular coagulation; FDA, US Food and Drug Administration.

with the continued use of LMWH.[34-36] The current recommendation is to continue anticoagulation as long as the cancer is active.[37]

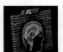
A 35-year-old woman is admitted for abdominal pain, jaundice, and fever. She rapidly deteriorates with the development of fulminant acute hepatitis A liver failure. As is frequently done to aid decision making regarding liver transplantation, an intracranial pressure (ICP)-monitoring probe device is requested and the patient is admitted to the neurologic ICU. In addition to being mildly pancytopenic, the patient has a prothrombin time (PT) of 35 seconds, INR of 6, and PTT of 70. Her hemoglobin was 9, white blood cell count was 3500, and platelet count was 80,000. Insertion of an ICP monitoring probe is not considered safe until the INR is less than at least 2.0 (most surgeons prefer a target of INR <1.4) and platelets are functioning.

Hematology

Clinical and radiographic signs are consistent with severe cerebral edema. In order to treat the presumed ICP crisis, what would be your next step?

The challenge is to correct these defects rapidly in order to provide invasive brain monitoring. The amount of FFP needed to correct these defects of PT and PTT is excessive. Ten milligrams of IV vitamin K would not be sufficient to lower the INR. Furthermore, it is important to remember that patients with liver failure have inhibited production of clotting factors, as well as the procoagulant proteins C and S. Measuring levels of these proteins takes significant time and therefore is not feasible in management of acute fulminant hepatic failure with both ICP crisis and active bleeding.

This is a setting in which PCCs can be effectively used. They contain factors II, VII, IX, and X, which are deficient and needed for hemostasis. Some guidelines recommend the use of FFP along with PCCs as it provides factor V needed for hemostasis, as well as providing an increased amount of factor VII.[38]

A variety of PCCs exist around the world, and a dosage of 50 units/kg is often recommended for life-threatening bleeding disorders. These products are virally inactivated and are not known to transmit hepatitis A, B, or C or HIV. PCCs can be rapidly infused in small volumes, work immediately, and can frequently reverse the INR and PTT to levels acceptable for the surgery and invasive procedures. As patients with liver disease frequently have platelets that are qualitatively abnormal, treatment with desmopressin (DDAVP, 0.3 µg/kg; see Table 46-2) is recommended as well.

 A 65-year-old patient is admitted for a cervical spine fusion. Surgery was done without any complications and he is stable postoperatively and about to be transferred to the floor. The following morning he develops shortness of breath and sinus tachycardia. Workup reveals right lower lobe PE. Of note, his morning platelet count is 70,000. His admission platelet count 4 days ago was 200,000.

What is the differential diagnosis?

The occurrence of thrombocytopenia in an ICU setting is common. The etiology of thrombocytopenia is multifold. Common etiologies for thrombocytopenia include sepsis, use of ventricular-assist devices, and medication induced. Given the clinical scenario, the most likely diagnosis in this case is heparin-induced thrombocytopenia. Thrombocytopenia is a well-established complication of heparin therapy.

There are two forms of thrombocytopenia associated with heparin therapy (Table 46-4). The first (type I) is a nonimmune form in which there is a moderate decrease in platelet count a few days after heparin initiation.[39] Type I HIT is not thought to be immune mediated. The second (type II) is the most important form of thrombocytopenia associated with heparin and is the focus of this chapter. Type II HIT, which we now refer to as HIT, is an immune-mediated reaction to heparin due to antibodies against the heparin/platelet factor 4 complex.[40] These antibodies lead to the activation of platelets, and subsequently the coagulation system, and may cause thrombosis and thrombotic multisystem complications.

Clinical features of HIT that help differentiate it from other causes of thrombocytopenia include the timing of onset, the degree of thrombocytopenia, and the presence of thrombosis. A scoring system is in use that helps assess the pretest probability of HIT. Clinical judgment must guide the diagnosis of HIT, as HIT testing results can take days to return.

Factors associated with an increased likelihood of the development of HIT include the following[41-43]:

- Use of unfractionated heparin more than LMWH
- Surgical more than medical patients
- Female more than male patients

Table 46-4. HIT Diagnosis Score

4 Ts	2 Points	1 Point	0 Point
Thrombocytopenia	Platelet count fall > 50% and platelet nadir ≥ 20 × 10⁹/L	Platelet count fall 30%-50% or platelet nadir 10-19 × 10⁹/L	Platelet count fall < 30% or platelet nadir < 10 × 10⁹/L
Timing of platelet count fall	Clear onset between days 5 and 14 or platelet fall ≤ 1 d (prior heparin exposure within 30 d)	Consistent with days 5-14 fall, but not clear, or onset after day 14 or fall ≤ 1 d (prior heparin exposure 30-100 d ago)	Platelet count fall ≤ 4 d without recent exposure
Thrombosis or other sequelae	New thrombosis (confirmed); skin necrosis at heparin injection sites; anaphylactoid reaction after IV heparin bolus	Progressive or recurrent thrombosis; nonnecrotizing (erythematous) skin lesions; suspected thrombosis (not confirmed)	None
Other causes of thrombocytopenia	None	Possible	Definite

It is important to recognize that HIT can occur in the setting of intravenous heparin therapy, subcutaneous heparin therapy, and heparin flushes.

HIT Assay Testing

Running a HIT assay can take time, and therefore treatment decisions are not based on test results. Laboratory testing for HIT falls into the category of either immunologic or functional assays. Immunologic tests, which are more readily available, assess for the presence of antibodies against the platelet factor 4/heparin complex but cannot assess their capacity to activate platelets. Functional assays assess the capacity of antibodies to activate platelets. However, this testing is not widely available and results may take many days. Therefore, the functional assays serve to merely confirm the diagnosis.

Treatment of HIT

One must make sure that all forms of heparin, including flushes, have been discontinued. As these patients continue to be at risk for thrombosis after the heparin is stopped, alternative anticoagulation should be initiated. Two nonheparin, direct thrombin inhibitors are approved for use in the United States.

Warfarin should then be initiated when the platelet count is greater than 150,000, with a 5-day overlap between treatment with an alternative anticoagulant and warfarin therapy. In a patient with HIT-associated thrombosis, anticoagulation should be continued for 3 to 6 months. In a patient with HIT but no evidence of thrombosis, the appropriate length of anticoagulation is unclear, but anticoagulation for at least 1 month should be considered. For every patient the risk-benefit of anticoagulation should be taken into account.

A 70-year-old man with hypertension and coronary artery disease presents to the ED with complaints of generalized weakness after a fall. A CT scan in the ED reveals acute, traumatic subarachnoid hemorrhage. He has been taking ASA 81 mg daily.

An increasing number of patients who have been taking chronic antiplatelet agents present to the ED with acute bleeding. Retrospective analyses suggest that prehospital antiplatelet therapy in trauma

Hematology

patients is associated with increased morbidity and mortality rates.[44,45] Reversal of these agents can be complex. The antiplatelet effect of aspirin is mediated by inhibition of cyclooxygenase 1 (COX-1) in platelets. Aspirin irreversibly inhibits COX-1 through protein acetylation.[46] Therefore, this effect lasts for the life of the platelets, which is approximately 5 to 10 days, after which a sufficient number of new platelets would be in systemic circulation.

DDAVP is a vasopressin analogue that increases release of von Willebrand factor and associated factor VIII from endothelial storage sites.[47] DDAVP may help overcome aspirin-induced platelet dysfunction and ameliorate hemostasis[48,49] based on retrospective and small case control studies.

DDAVP is known to improve hemostasis in von Willebrand disease and hemophilia,[47] as well as improving the acquired platelet dysfunction found in uremic or cirrhotic patients.[50] The usual dose of DDAVP is 0.3 µg/kg in 50 mL of normal saline administered over 30 minutes (a maximum of 20 µg is recommended). It works almost immediately. As DDAVP is a vasopressin analogue, it has antidiuretic properties, and hyponatremia can result after repeated dosing. Serum sodium must be monitored. A lower dose (0.15 µg/kg) is advised for patients with significant cardiovascular disease.

Platelet transfusion can also be used in this setting, as transfusion will provide normal platelets as long as aspirin is no longer in the system. Case reports in the literature also report successful use of DDAVP in clopidogrel-induced platelet dysfunction, as well as in patients on combination therapy, although there is not enough evidence to support this finding.

In order to ascertain which patients on aspirin and clopidogrel are at true risk for bleeding, rapid platelet-specific tests are available in certain institutions. Historically the bleeding time was used, but this test has fallen out of favor due to poor reproducibility of results. In place of bleeding times, platelet function tests are now used. These tests can assess the qualitative platelet dysfunction, and their use is spreading. They can rapidly provide valuable information about the degree of platelet inhibition occurring in a patient on aspirin or clopidogrel.[51,52] These tests can be particularly helpful in cases where the antiplatelet medication history is unclear, or in the setting of vague history while surgery and an invasive procedure are urgently indicated.

! CRITICAL CONSIDERATIONS

- The half-life of LMWH is 12 to 24 hours, and options for reversal include protamine sulfate and recombinant factor VIIa infusion.
- Treatment strategies for reversal of oral anticoagulant ICH include vitamin K 10 mg IV, FFP, and PCCs.
- Evaluation of a prolonged PTT begins with assessing for the presence of a factor deficiency, factor inhibitor, and lupus anticoagulant.
- Treatment of the hemophiliac patient should be performed in close coordination with a hematologist in order to ensure appropriate factor replacement.
- Postoperative DVT should be treated with anticoagulation for 3 to 6 months.
- In patients with malignancy, consider continued anticoagulation if the cancer is active.
- Suspect HIT in a patient initiated on heparin with a decrease in platelet count of 50% in the first 5 days, or sooner in a patient with prior exposure to heparin.
- HIT occurs more commonly with intravenous heparin, but can occur in the setting of LMWH and heparin flushes.
- Patients with HIT must be treated with a direct thrombin inhibitor because the risk of thrombosis after cessation of heparin continues.

- All heparin (including heparin flushes) must be stopped if HIT is suspected.
- While laboratory studies are confirmatory, decisions must be made based on clinical judgment, as a direct thrombin inhibitor should be initiated as soon as possible in order to avoid potential thrombotic complications.

REFERENCES

1. Crowther MA, Berry LR, Monagle PT, Chan AK. Mechanisms responsible for the failure of protamine to inactivate low-molecular-weight heparin. *Br J Haematol.* 2002;116(1):178-186.
2. Warkentin TE, Crowther MA. Reversing anticoagulants both old and new. *Can J Anaesth.* 2002;49(6):S11-S25.
3. Levi MM, Eerenberg E, Lowenberg E, Kamphuisen PW. Bleeding in patients using new anticoagulants or antiplatelet agents: risk factors and management. *Neth J Med.* 2010;68(2):68-76.
4. Weiler JM, Freiman P, Sharath MD, et al. Serious adverse reactions to protamine sulfate: are alternatives needed? *J Allergy Clin Immunol.* 1985;75(2):297-303.
5. Ingerslev J, Vanek T, Culic S. Use of recombinant factor VIIa for emergency reversal of anticoagulation. *J Postgrad Med.* 2007;53(1):17-22.
6. Firozvi K, Deveras RA, Kessler CM. Reversal of low-molecular-weight heparin-induced bleeding in patients with pre-existing hypercoagulable states with human recombinant activated factor VII concentrate. *Am J Hematol.* 2006;81(8):582-589.
7. Ansell J, Hirsh J, Poller L, Bussey H, Jacobson A, Hylek E. The pharmacology and management of the vitamin K antagonists: the Seventh ACCP Conference on Antithrombotic and Thrombolytic Therapy. *Chest.* 2004;126(3 Suppl):204S-233S.
8. Hylek EM, Singer DE. Risk factors for intracranial hemorrhage in outpatients taking warfarin. *Ann Intern Med.* 1994;120(11):897-902.
9. Wintzen AR, de Jonge H, Loeliger EA, Bots GT. The risk of intracerebral hemorrhage during oral anticoagulant treatment: a population study. *Ann Neurol.* 1984;16(5):553-558.
10. Hart RG, Boop BS, Anderson DC. Oral anticoagulants and intracranial hemorrhage. Facts and hypotheses. *Stroke.* 1995;26(8):1471-1477.
11. Neau JP, Couderq C, Ingrand P, Blanchon P, Gil R. Intracranial hemorrhage and oral anticoagulant treatment. *Cerebrovasc Dis.* 2001;11(3):195-200.
12. Ansell J, Hirsh J, Hylek E, Jacobson A, Crowther M, Palareti G. Pharmacology and management of the vitamin K antagonists: American College of Chest Physicians evidence-based clinical practice guidelines (8th edition). *Chest.* 2008;133(6 Suppl):160S-198S.
13. Riegert-Johnson DL, Volcheck GW. The incidence of anaphylaxis following intravenous phytonadione (vitamin K1): a 5-year retrospective review. *Ann Allergy Asthma Immunol.* 2002;89(4):400-406.
14. Shields RC, McBane RD, Kuiper JD, Li H, Heit JA. Efficacy and safety of intravenous phytonadione (vitamin K1) in patients on long-term oral anticoagulant therapy. *Mayo Clin Proc.* 2001;76(3):260-266.
15. Fiore LD, Scola MA, Cantillon CE, Brophy MT. Anaphylactoid reactions to vitamin K. *J Thromb Thrombolysis.* 2001;11(2):175-183.
16. Whitling AM, Bussey HI, Lyons RM. Comparing different routes and doses of phytonadione for reversing excessive anticoagulation. *Arch Intern Med.* 1998;158(19):2136-2140.
17. Heit JA. Perioperative management of the chronically anticoagulated patient. *J Thromb Thrombolysis.* 2001;12(1):81-87.
18. MacLennan S, Williamson LM. Risks of fresh frozen plasma and platelets. *J Trauma.* 2006;60(6 Suppl):S46-S50.
19. Yasaka M, Sakata T, Minematsu K, Naritomi H. Correction of INR by prothrombin complex concentrate and vitamin K in patients with warfarin related hemorrhagic complication. *Thromb Res.* 2002;108(1):25-30.
20. Makris M, Greaves M, Phillips WS, Kitchen S, Rosendaal FR, Preston EF. Emergency oral anticoagulant reversal: the relative efficacy of infusions of fresh frozen plasma and clotting factor concentrate on correction of the coagulopathy. *Thromb Haemost.* 1997;77(3):477-480.
21. Lin J, Hanigan WC, Tarantino M, Wang J. The use of recombinant activated factor VII to reverse warfarin-induced anticoagulation in patients with hemorrhages in the central nervous system: preliminary findings. *J Neurosurg.* 2003;98(4):737-740.
22. Sorensen B, Johansen P, Nielsen GL, Sorensen JC, Ingerslev J. Reversal of the international normalized ratio with recombinant activated factor VII in central nervous system bleeding during warfarin thromboprophylaxis: clinical and biochemical aspects. *Blood Coagul Fibrinolysis.* 2003;14(5):469-477.

Hematology

23. Freeman WD, Brott TG, Barrett KM, et al. Recombinant factor VIIa for rapid reversal of warfarin anticoagulation in acute intracranial hemorrhage. *Mayo Clin Proc.* 2004;79(12):1495-1500.

24. Brody DL, Aiyagari V, Shackleford AM, Diringer MN. Use of recombinant factor VIIa in patients with warfarin-associated intracranial hemorrhage. *Neurocrit Care.* 2005;2(3):263-267.

25. Bartal C, Freedman J, Bowman K, Cusimano M. Coagulopathic patients with traumatic intracranial bleeding: defining the role of recombinant factor VIIa. *J Trauma.* 2007;63(4):725-732.

26. Zupancic-Salek S. Rapid reversal of anticoagulant bleeding—rFVIIa an option? *J Postgrad Med.* 2007;53(1):3-4.

27. Gruppo RA, Bove KE, Donaldson VH. Fatal myocardial necrosis associated with prothrombin-complex concentrate therapy in hemophilia A. *N Engl J Med.* 1983;309(4):242-243.

28. Makris M, van Veen JJ, Maclean R. Warfarin anticoagulation reversal: management of the asymptomatic and bleeding patient. *J Thromb Thrombolysis.* 2010;29(2):171-181.

29. Leissinger CA, Blatt PM, Hoots WK, Ewenstein B. Role of prothrombin complex concentrates in reversing warfarin anticoagulation: a review of the literature. *Am J Hematol.* 2008;83(2):137-143.

30. Brandes AA, Scelzi E, Salmistraro G, et al. Incidence of risk of thromboembolism during treatment high-grade gliomas: a prospective study. *Eur J Cancer.* 1997;33(10):1592-1596.

31. Dhami MS, Bona RD, Calogero JA, Hellman RM. Venous thromboembolism and high grade gliomas. *Thromb Haemost.* 1993;70(3):393-396.

32. Marras LC, Geerts WH, Perry JR. The risk of venous thromboembolism is increased throughout the course of malignant glioma: an evidence-based review. *Cancer.* 2000;89(3):640-646.

33. Quevedo JF, Buckner JC, Schmidt JL, Dinapoli RP, O'Fallon JR. Thromboembolism in patients with high-grade glioma. *Mayo Clin Proc.* 1994;69(4):329-332.

34. Kakkar AK, Levine MN, Kadziola Z, et al. Low molecular weight heparin, therapy with dalteparin, and survival in advanced cancer: the Fragmin advanced malignancy outcome study (FAMOUS). *J Clin Oncol.* 2004;22(10):1944-1948.

35. Lee AY, Levine MN. Venous thromboembolism and cancer: risks and outcomes. *Circulation.* 2003;107(23 Suppl 1):I17-I21.

36. Lee AY, Rickles FR, Julian JA, et al. Randomized comparison of low molecular weight heparin and coumarin derivatives on the survival of patients with cancer and venous thromboembolism. *J Clin Oncol.* 2005;23(10):2123-2129.

37. Khorana AA, Streiff MB, Farge D, et al. Venous thromboembolism prophylaxis and treatment in cancer: a consensus statement of major guidelines panels and call to action. *J Clin Oncol.* 2009;27(29):4919-4926.

38. Baker RI, Coughlin PB, Gallus AS, Harper PL, Salem HH, Wood EM. Warfarin reversal: consensus guidelines, on behalf of the Australasian Society of Thrombosis and Haemostasis. *Med J Aust.* 2004;181(9):492-497.

39. Warkentin TE, Greinacher A, Koster A, Lincoff AM. Treatment and prevention of heparin-induced thrombocytopenia: American College of Chest Physicians evidence-based clinical practice guidelines (8th edition). *Chest.* 2008;133(6 Suppl): 340S-380S.

40. Warkentin TE, Kelton JG. Temporal aspects of heparin-induced thrombocytopenia. *N Engl J Med.* 2001;344(17):1286-1292.

41. Warkentin TE, Sheppard JA, Sigouin CS, Kohlmann T, Eichler P, Greinacher A. Gender imbalance and risk factor interactions in heparin-induced thrombocytopenia. *Blood.* 2006;108(9):2937-2941.

42. Smythe MA, Koerber JM, Mattson JC. The incidence of recognized heparin-induced thrombocytopenia in a large, tertiary care teaching hospital. *Chest.* 2007;131(6):1644-1649.

43. Warkentin TE, Eikelboom JW. Who is (still) getting HIT? *Chest.* 2007;131(6):1620-1622.

44. McMillian WD, Rogers FB. Management of prehospital antiplatelet and anticoagulant therapy in traumatic head injury: a review. *J Trauma.* 2009;66(3):942-950.

45. Ohm C, Mina A, Howells G, Bair H, Bendick P. Effects of antiplatelet agents on outcomes for elderly patients with traumatic intracranial hemorrhage. *J Trauma.* 2005;58(3):518-522.

46. Vane JR, Bakhle YS, Botting RM. Cyclooxygenases 1 and 2. *Annu Rev Pharmacol Toxicol.* 1998;38: 97-120.

47. Mannucci PM. Desmopressin (DDAVP) in the treatment of bleeding disorders: the first 20 years. *Blood.* 1997;90(7):2515-2521.

48. Mannucci PM, Vicente V, Vianello L, et al. Controlled trial of desmopressin in liver cirrhosis and other conditions associated with a prolonged bleeding time. *Blood.* 1986;67(4):1148-1153.

49. Reiter RA, Mayr F, Blazicek H, et al. Desmopressin antagonizes the in vitro platelet dysfunction induced by GPIIb/IIIa inhibitors and aspirin. *Blood.* 2003;102(13):4594-4599.

50. Franchini M. The use of desmopressin as a hemostatic agent: a concise review. *Am J Hematol.* 2007;82(8):731-735.

51. Bidet A, Jais C, Puymirat E, et al. VerifyNow and VASP phosphorylation assays give similar results for patients receiving clopidogrel, but they do not always correlate with platelet aggregation. *Platelets.* 2010;21(2):94-100.

52. Varenhorst C, James S, Erlinge D, et al. Assessment of P2Y(12) inhibition with the point-of-care device VerifyNow P2Y12 in patients treated with prasugrel or clopidogrel coadministered with aspirin. *Am Heart J.* 2009;157(3):562.e1-9.

Infectious Disease

Section Editor: Fred Rincon, MD, MSc, FACP

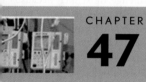

CHAPTER

47

Severe Sepsis and Septic Shock

Sergio L. Zanotti-Cavazzoni, MD, FCCM

Infectious Disease

A 32-year-old man was admitted to the neurologic intensive care unit (ICU) after presenting to the hospital with complaints of difficulty walking and numbness in the lower extremities. Initial workup supported a diagnosis of Guillain-Barré syndrome. The patient was started on treatment with intravenous immunoglobulin (IVIG) and on day 2 of his ICU stay was intubated and placed on mechanical ventilation because of worsening vital capacity measurements. The patient completed a 5-day course of IVIG treatments. One week after admission the patient remained intubated on mechanical ventilation.

On day 7 of the ICU admission the patient developed a new fever with tachycardia, and increased oxygen requirements on the ventilator. Vital signs were temperature 38.9°C (102.1°F), heart rate 120 bpm, respiratory rate 22 breaths/min, and blood pressure 100/65 mm Hg. Ventilator settings at the time included the following: assist-control mode at a rate of 14 with a set tidal volume of 450 mL, and the fraction of inspired oxygen (FIO_2) increased to 60% from 30% to maintain an arterial oxygen saturation (SaO_2) greater than or equal to 92%. On examination, the patient has an endotracheal tube and is on mechanical ventilation. Neurologic assessment is as follows: the patient is lethargic but arousable and able to follow simple commands. Strength is decreased in the upper extremities (2/5 bilaterally) and lower extremities (2/5 right, 3/5 left). Cardiac examination shows tachycardia with a regular rate and no gallops, rubs, or murmurs. Lung auscultation reveals coarse breath sounds bilaterally. The abdominal examination is unremarkable. The patient has a left subclavian triple-lumen catheter with mild erythema around the insertion site, which is nontender on palpation, and a urinary Foley catheter. Laboratory data obtained that day were significant for a white blood cell (WBC) count of 17,000/mm³ with 80% neutrophils, a platelet count of 120,000/mm³, a creatinine level of 2.1 mg/dL (increased from 1.1 mg/dL), and an international normalized ratio (INR) of 1.7. A chest radiograph shows a possible infiltrate in the right lower lobe and that the endotracheal tube and central line are in good position.

Does this patient have sepsis?

Sepsis is one of the most important causes of morbidity and mortality in patients admitted to the intensive care unit.[1,2] Early recognition of sepsis has important therapeutic implications, as there are multiple time-sensitive interventions that ultimately have a significant impact on patient outcomes. However, finding a clinically "fool-proof" definition of sepsis has been a challenge, most likely because of the platitude of signs and symptoms associated with the sepsis syndrome. In order to resolve this issue, a consensus conference was convened to create standardized definitions and formulate a blue-print to guide research on sepsis.[3] The term *systemic inflammatory response syndrome* (SIRS) was introduced. SIRS can occur in response to a variety of severe clinical insults and is defined by the presence of two or more of the following conditions: (1) temperature greater than 38°C (100.4°F) or less than 36°C (96.8°F); (2) heart rate greater than 90 bpm; (3) respiratory rate greater than 20 breaths/min or a $Paco_2$ less than 32 mm Hg; and (4) WBC count greater than 12,000 cells/mm³. *Sepsis* occurs when SIRS is caused by infection. *Severe sepsis* is sepsis with associated organ dys-function, hypoperfusion, or hypotension. Hypoperfusion and perfusion abnormalities may include, but are not limited to, lactic acidosis, oliguria, and an acute alteration in mental status. *Septic shock* is defined by the presence of sepsis-induced hypotension (systolic blood pressure < 90 mm Hg or a reduction ≥ 40 mm Hg from baseline in the absence of other causes for hypotension), despite adequate fluid resuscitation, along with the presence of perfusion abnormalities.[3] These definitions established a common language to describe patients with sepsis, and although they helped standard-ize inclusion criteria for clinical trials, they still did not provide clinicians with a perfect definition to use at the bedside.[4,5] Recognizing that the definitions proposed by the consensus conference had limitations, in 2001 a second consensus conference with a broader representation was convened to revisit these definitions.[6] The conference recommended keeping the 1992 definitions unchanged secondary to lack of new evidence to support new definitions. However, the consensus conference recommended expanding the diagnostic criteria for sepsis in an effort to enhance recognition at the bedside (Table 47-1). Our patient's presentation is consistent with an infection; in addition, he fulfills all the criteria for SIRS, making sepsis the likely diagnosis. Furthermore, our patient has evidence of new organ dysfunction (see Figure 47-1 for organ dysfunction associated with severe sepsis), mean-ing that at this point our patient meets criteria for the diagnosis of severe sepsis. Sepsis, severe sepsis, and septic shock constitute a continuum of disease that results from the host response to an infection. As patients progress in this continuum (from sepsis to severe sepsis and from severe sepsis to septic shock), their mortality risk increases.[7] The acute clinical syndrome of sepsis identifies a patient at risk for clinical deterioration and death. A diagnosis of sepsis, severe sepsis, or septic shock must prompt physicians to implement a time-sensitive therapeutic plan in order to prevent further organ dysfunc-tion and minimize mortality.

How would you approach the management of this patient?

Our patient has severe sepsis, most likely caused by an infection originating in his lungs (ventilator-induced pneumonia) or in his bloodstream (catheter-related bloodstream infection). Severe sepsis should be treated as a medical emergency and institution of appropriate therapeutic interventions should not be delayed. A simplified model of severe sepsis (Figure 47-2) includes the following com-ponents: (1) infection, (2) hemodynamic abnormalities, (3) host response to infection, and (4) organ

Table 47-1. Diagnostic Criteria for Sepsis

Infection, documented or suspected plus some of the following findings:

Clinical findings
 Temperature > 38.3°C or < 36°C
 Heart rate > 90 bpm or > 2 SD above normal value for age
 Arterial hypotension (SBP < 90 mm Hg, MAP < 70 mm Hg, or an SBP decrease > 40 in adults or < SD below
  normal for age)
 Tachypnea
 Decreased capillary refill or mottling
 Altered mental status
 Significant edema or positive fluid balances

Hemodynamic or laboratory findings
 Mixed venous oxygen saturation (SvO_2) > 70%
 Cardiac index > 3.5 L/min per m^2
 Hyperglycemia in the absence of diabetes
 WBC count > 12,000/μL or < 4000/μL
 Normal WBC with > 10% immature forms
 Plasma C-reactive protein > 2 SD above the normal value
 Plasma procalcitonin > SD above the normal value
 Hyperlactatemia (> 1 mmol/L)

Evidence of organ dysfunction
 Arterial hypoxemia (PaO_2/FIO_2 < 300)
 Acute oliguria
 Creatinine increase > 0.5 mg/dL
 Coagulation abnormalities (INR > 1.5 or PTT > 60 s)
 Ileus
 Thrombocytopenia
 Hyperbilirubinemia

Abbreviations: INR, international normalized ratio; MAP, mean arterial pressure; PTT, partial thromboplastin time; SBP, systolic blood pressure; SD, standard deviation; WBC, white blood cell.

dysfunction. Our treatment approach should be based on these factors: (1) antibiotics and source control for the infection, (2) fluids and vasoactive drugs for hemodynamic support, (3) novel therapies to modulate the host response, and (4) supportive care for prevention and treatment of organ dysfunction. The *Surviving Sepsis Campaign*, an international initiative supported by multiple medical professional societies, has published comprehensive evidence-based guidelines on treatment for patients with severe sepsis and septic shock.[8] Although these evidence-based guidelines are an invaluable resource to the clinician, they are not sufficient to change behavior at the bedside. In order to ensure that all patients with severe sepsis receive optimal care, more than published updated clinical guidelines are likely necessary. Recognizing this problem, the Surviving Sepsis Campaign partnered with the Institute for Healthcare Improvement (http://www.ihi.org/IHI/Topics/CriticalCare/Sepsis) and created a performance improvement program for severe sepsis and septic shock. At the core of the program are the Sepsis Bundles (Resuscitation Bundle and Management Bundle, Table 47-2).[9] The Sepsis Bundles represent a group of interventions that when implemented together are likely to have a greater impact on patients than when implemented individually and inconsistently. The elements within these bundles should occur within a specified time frame in every patient with a diagnosis of severe sepsis. The Sepsis Resuscitation Bundle includes the initial evaluation and hemodynamic interventions for patients with severe sepsis. These interventions must be implemented within the first 6 hours of recognition of the syndrome. This short time frame means that often implementation of these interventions might occur outside of the intensive care unit (ie, emergency department or

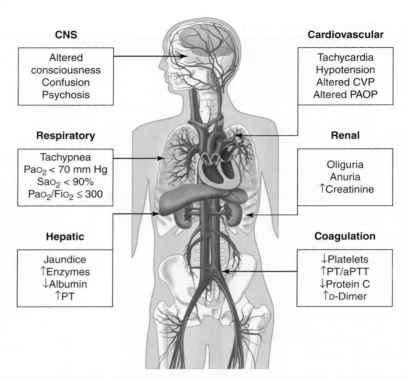

Figure 47-1. Identification of organ failure in severe sepsis. Clinical and laboratorial criteria to identify organ failure are shown for each organ system. aPTT, activated partial thromboplastin time; CVP, central venous pressure; PAOP, pulmonary artery occlusion pressure; PT, prothrombin time. *(Adapted from Balk RA. Pathogenesis and management of multiple organ dysfunction or failure in severe sepsis and septic shock. Crit Care Clin. 2000;16:337-352.)*

general hospital floors). The Sepsis Management Bundle addresses four management considerations that must occur within the first 24 hours after recognition of severe sepsis when the patient is in an intensive care unit setting. It is important to emphasize that the Sepsis Management Bundle does not mandate administration of corticosteroids or recombinant human activated protein C (APC); it instructs clinicians to properly evaluate every individual patient and based on current evidence and local protocols make a decision on whether use of one of these agents is appropriate. As new scientific evidence is developed, the merits and place of individual components of these bundles can be debated.

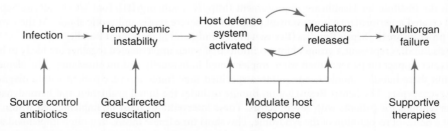

Figure 47-2. Simplified sepsis model and approach to treatment.

Table 47-2. Sepsis Bundles

Sepsis Resuscitation Bundle: to be started immediately and completed within 6 h
Serum lactate measured
Blood cultures obtained prior to antibiotic administration
From the time of presentation, broad-spectrum antibiotics administered within 3 h for ED admissions and 1 h for non-ED ICU admissions
In the event of hypotension and/or lactate > 4 mmol/L (36 mg/dL):
• Deliver an initial minimum of 20 mL/kg of crystalloid (or colloid equivalent)
• Apply vasopressors for hypotension not responding to initial fluid resuscitation to maintain mean arterial pressure ≥ 65 mmHg
In the event of persistent hypotension despite fluid resuscitation (septic shock) and/or lactate > 4 mmol/L (36 mg/dL):
• Achieve central venous pressure of ≥ 8 mm Hg[a]
• Achieve central venous oxygen saturation ($ScvO_2$) of ≥ 70%[b]
Sepsis Management Bundle: to be started immediately and completed within 24 h
Low-dose steroids administered for septic shock in accordance with a standardized hospital policy
Drotrecogin alfa (activated) administered in accordance with a standardized hospital policy
Glucose control maintained at or above lower limit of normal, but > 150 mg/dL (8.3 mmol/L)
Inspiratory plateau pressures maintained at < 30 cm H_2O for mechanically ventilated patients

Abbreviations: ED, emergency department; ICU, intensive care unit.

[a] Dynamic parameters such as pulse pressure, stroke volume variations, and stroke volume index monitoring by the use of pulse contour analysis, and echocardiographic assessment of both inferior vena cava and superior vena cava variability may be used in order to improve the reliability of fluid responsiveness.

[b] Achieving an SvO_2 of 65% is an acceptable alternative.

However, it is important to understand that what is most valuable regarding these bundles is the consistent application of a systematic approach to providing time-sensitive care to patients with severe sepsis and septic shock. Compliance with the Sepsis Bundles has been associated with significant reductions in mortality rate. A multicenter Spanish study in a before-and-after trial design evaluated the impact of implementing the Sepsis Bundles in a large group of ICUs.[10] This study demonstrated that a national educational program to promote the utilization of the Sepsis Bundles was associated with increased compliance and with lower patient mortality rate (preintervention cohort 44% versus postintervention cohort 39.7%; $P = .04$).[10] In a post hoc analysis, administration of antibiotics within 1 hour and the use of APC in patients with multiorgan failure were significant independent factors associated with lower mortality rate.[11] More recently the Surviving Sepsis Campaign published the results of its international guideline-based performance improvement program targeting severe sepsis with the implementation of the Sepsis Bundles.[12] In this cohort study that included over 15,000 patients and over 165 international sites, implementation of the Sepsis Bundles was associated with an unadjusted decrease in mortality rate from 37% to 30.8% over 2 years ($P = .01$).[12] The adjusted odds ratio for mortality rate improved the longer the site was participating in the campaign. The following bundle targets had a significant risk-adjusted impact on hospital mortality: initiation of broad-spectrum antibiotics, blood cultures prior to antibiotic administration, tight glucose control, and achievement of low plateau pressures.[12] It is important to point out that in both the Spanish and the Surviving Sepsis Campaign studies, even after implementation of the educational program/ Sepsis Bundles Campaign, there was still significant room for improvement in the overall compliance with achieving all targets. Although not necessarily cause and effect, the results of these and

Infectious Disease

other similar studies seem to consistently show a reduction in hospital mortality rate with improved compliance with the Sepsis Bundles. Returning to the question posed on how to approach the management of our patient, it would seem that a systematic approach targeting the main components of sepsis (infection, hemodynamic abnormalities, the host response, and organ dysfunction), utilizing the Sepsis Bundles as a road map, would constitute a sound clinical approach.

The patient is diagnosed with severe sepsis most likely due to pneumonia or a line-related bloodstream infection. As recommended by the Sepsis Resuscitation Bundle, a lactate level is measured and blood cultures are sent prior to antibiotic administration, and antibiotics are promptly initiated. The patient's lactate level is 5.2 mmol/L (normal range < 2.1 mmol/L).

What is the significance of the increased lactate in this patient?

An increased lactate level in a patient with sepsis is an indicator of severity and increased mortality. Several studies have shown an association between increased lactate levels and mortality in patients presenting to the hospital with infection.[13-15] Studies have also shown that in addition to the initial lactate level, lactate clearance over time has prognostic implications.[13] In sepsis, lactate is most likely a nonspecific marker of sepsis-induced tissue hypoxia. It remains unclear if the increased lactate levels are mostly due to regional hypoperfusion with the resultant increase in anaerobic metabolism or if other factors play an important role. It is critical to emphasize that lactate is not specific to sepsis and therefore cannot and should not be utilized as a diagnostic marker in patients with suspected sepsis. Lactate should be used as a marker of severity and can be helpful in triaging patients with sepsis and/or initiating aggressive goal-directed hemodynamic support. An increased serum lactate level is particularly useful in the setting of a patient who does not manifest overt hypotension. Studies have suggested that these patients most likely have what has been labeled "cryptic shock" and clearly represent a high-risk patient population that, based on their risk for mortality, should be treated aggressively in an ICU setting. In our patient the increased lactate level is an important indicator of severity. Since our patient is already in an ICU setting, the increased lactate level would be most helpful in triggering aggressive goal-directed hemodynamic support interventions as outlined in the Sepsis Resuscitation Bundle.

What are the most important considerations regarding antibiotic therapy in this patient?

Antibiotic therapy is the cornerstone in our efforts to treat the infection as the cause of the septic syndrome. Although, as discussed above, many of the clinical manifestations seen in sepsis are related to the host response to this infection, it is a priority to target the infectious source as early as possible. Probably the most important considerations regarding antibiotic use in the early phase of treatment for severe sepsis include (1) time to administration, (2) proper antibiotic selection, and (3) evaluation of a need for source control. If we accept that sepsis is SIRS caused by an infection, it would make sense that early administration of antibiotics would be better for patients than late administration of antibiotics. Results from a large multicenter retrospective study of patients with septic shock suggested that for every hour appropriate antibiotics are delayed after onset of hypotension, the odds ratio for mortality increases in a stepwise manner.[16] In this study, administration of appropriate antibiotics (those that covered the pathogens eventually grown in cultures) within the first hour of documented hypotension was associated with a survival rate of 79.9%. Each hour of delay in antimicrobial administration over the ensuing 6 hours was associated with an average decrease in survival of 7.6%.[16] The median time from onset of hypotension to administration of appropriate antibiotics was 6 hours, illustrating a common problem in the delivery of appropriate care for patients with severe sepsis.

The goal should be to administer appropriate antibiotics as soon as possible in patients with severe sepsis. In order to accomplish this goal, hospitals must examine their particular challenges and devise systems to optimize antibiotic administration. The next consideration is the selection of appropriate antibiotics. Studies have demonstrated that the appropriateness of initial antibiotic therapy has a significant impact on patient outcomes.[17,18] In one study, factors associated with administration of inadequate antibiotics included prior administration of antibiotics, bloodstream infections, increasing Acute Physiology and Chronic Health Evaluation (APACHE II) scores, and decreasing age.[19] Considering the detrimental effect on mortality, it is evident that in patients with severe sepsis one cannot afford to miss potential causative organisms when selecting an empiric antimicrobial regimen. Choice of antibiotics can be based on the following factors: (1) probable pathogens based on clinical diagnosis and source of infection (eg, pneumonia, bloodstream infection, abdominal source, etc.), (2) individual patient factors (eg, location when infection developed, previous antibiotic treatments, comorbidities), and (3) resistance patterns of local and hospital bacterial flora. Initial antibiotic therapy for severe sepsis should be broad in spectrum and progressively narrowed as microbiologic data become available. In culture-negative patients de-escalation of antibiotics may become challenging. In these cases clinical evolution can be used to guide decisions. A detailed discussion of specific antibiotic regimens is beyond the scope of this chapter; for further discussion on antibiotics please see Chapter 48. Finally, identifying potential sources amenable to source control measures should be part of the initial evaluation of patients with sepsis. Source control interventions can be divided into three broad categories: (1) drainage of an abscess, (2) debridement/drainage/incision of infected tissue, and (3) removal of an infected foreign body.[20] The timing of intervention depends on several factors. When source interventions are simple, such as removal of an infected central venous catheter, they should be implemented immediately. In cases of unstable patients where surgery might be required, delaying source control while optimizing hemodynamic status may be appropriate. However, in cases such as necrotizing fasciitis, in which delays carry a significant risk of increasing mortality, one must proceed to surgery as early as possible. Examples of specific source control measures in patients with sepsis are shown on Table 47-3.

Table 47-3. Source Control Techniques

Drainage	Intra-abdominal abscess
	Thoracic empyema
	Septic arthritis
	Pyelonephritis, cholangitis
Debridement	Necrotizing fasciitis
	Infected pancreatic necrosis
	Intestinal infarction
	Mediastinitis
Device removal	Infected vascular catheter
	Urinary catheter
	Colonized endotracheal tube
	Infected intrauterine contraceptive device
Definitive control	Sigmoid resection for diverticulitis
	Cholecystectomy for gangrenous cholecystitis
	Amputation for clostridial myonecrosis

Infectious Disease

The most likely sources for infection in this patient are the lungs (ventilator-associated pneumonia) and the bloodstream (catheter related). Potential pathogens this patient would be at risk for include gram negatives (including resistant gram negatives) and methicillin-resistant *Staphylococcus aureus* (MRSA). Accordingly, the patient is started on cefepime and vancomycin. In addition, the left subclavian central catheter is removed (source control) and a new central line (capable of measuring continuous central venous oxygen saturation [$ScvO_2$]) is inserted in the right internal jugular vein. The patient is started on intravenous fluids. Vital signs at this point are temperature 38.5°C (101.2°F), heart rate 125 bpm, respiratory rate 26 breaths/min, and blood pressure 82/55 mm Hg.

How would you treat this patient's hypotension?

Our patient has several signs suggesting sepsis-induced tissue hypoperfusion (high lactate level, hypotension, tachycardia). Early and aggressive hemodynamic optimization is indicated to decrease the progression of organ failure and improve overall outcome. The hemodynamic profile of severe sepsis and septic shock is characterized by components of hypovolemic, cardiogenic, and distributive shock.[21] Early in sepsis, increased capillary leak and increased venous capacitance will result in effective hypovolemia with decreased venous return to the heart and a depressed cardiac output. Administration of intravascular fluids can alter this early phase of sepsis. The importance of early intervention in patients with sepsis-induced tissue hypoperfusion has been highlighted by the results of an early goal-directed therapy (EGDT) clinical trial by Rivers et al.[22] In this study patients with sepsis-induced hypoperfusion (lactate > 4 mmol/L and/or hypotension after fluids) were randomized to receive either standard resuscitation or an EGDT protocol during the first 6 hours of admission to the emergency department. In both groups end points of resuscitation included central venous pressure (CVP) greater than or equal to 8 to 12 mm Hg, mean arterial pressure (MAP) greater than or equal to 65 mm Hg, and urine output greater than or equal to 0.5 mL/kg per hour. In order to achieve these goals patients were treated with intravenous crystalloids and vasopressors. The EGDT group had as an additional end point an $Scvo_2$ greater than or equal to 70%, which was continuously measured from a subclavian or jugular central venous catheter. $Scvo_2$ was used as an index for oxygen delivery. If $Scvo_2$ was less than 70% after reaching targets for CVP and MAP, patients received packed red blood cells for a hematocrit ≤ 30, or dobutamine infusion for a hematocrit was ≥ 30. Patients in the EGDT group received more fluids, dobutamine, and transfusions in the first 24 hours. In-hospital mortality rate was significantly lower in the EGDT group when compared to the standard therapy group (30.5% versus 46.5%, respectively; $P = .009$). Although the specific merits of each treatment within the EGDT protocol can be discussed, the results of this study strongly support early intervention with predefined hemodynamic settings and protocolized care. A recent study showed that within the context of early goal-directed resuscitation for severe sepsis/septic shock, an end point of lactate clearance (decrease in lactate ≥ 10% over first 6 hours) was noninferior to management targeting $Scvo_2$.[23] The Surviving Sepsis Campaign's recommendations for the Sepsis Resuscitation Bundle are based on the Rivers study and others that have shown the benefits of early intervention with predefined goals.[22,24-26]

The initial step in optimizing hemodynamics in our patient should be aggressive fluid resuscitation. Although experts agree on the value of early and aggressive volume replacement, controversy persists over the optimal type of fluid. This debate revolves around the use of crystalloids (saline, Ringer lactate) versus colloids (albumin, hydroxyethyl starches). Meta-analyses of clinical studies performed in general critical care populations have demonstrated no difference in outcomes between patients treated with crystalloids and those treated with colloids.[27-29] The Saline versus Albumin Fluid Evaluation (SAFE) study prospectively randomized 7000 critically ill patients to receive 4% albumin or 0.9% saline for fluid resuscitation.[30] There were no significant differences between groups in mortality and other secondary outcomes. A subgroup analysis conducted in patients with sepsis revealed a trend toward improved outcomes in patients treated with albumin, although this difference did not achieve statistical significance. We believe that achieving end points of resuscitation is more important than the type of fluid utilized. In North America consideration for cost differences has made crystalloids the fluid of choice for resuscitating patients with severe sepsis. How much fluid should be given? Patients with severe sepsis may present with significant intravascular volume depletion. Aggressive fluid boluses are usually required to restore tissue perfusion. An initial bolus of at least 20 mL/kg of crystalloid (or colloid equivalent) is currently recommended.[8] This may be supplemented with more fluids in repeated boluses of 300 to 500 mL based on markers of perfusion.[8,31] Current guidelines recommend a target CVP greater than or equal to 8 to 12 mm Hg as an initial end point for volume resuscitation during the first 6 hours of treatment.[8,31] After the initial hours of treatment, determining the need for further fluid administration may be challenging. Although CVP has been used for many years, static parameters (such as CVP) have been shown to be poor surrogates for volume responsiveness. Ideally, dynamic measures such as those measured by arterial pulse pressure variation, changes in stroke volume/cardiac output, or echocardiography should be utilized in addition to initial CVP measurements.

Septic shock is defined by hypotension refractory to fluid resuscitation. If after administration of fluids a patient with severe sepsis remains hypotensive, vasopressors targeted at raising the MAP should be initiated. Catecholamines such as dopamine, epinephrine, norepinephrine, and phenylephrine have traditionally been used to raise blood pressure in patients with septic shock (Table 47-4). The vasopressor of choice for septic shock is still an unresolved discussion, mostly because of the lack of convincing clinical data showing improved mortality rate with a specific agent. Additional considerations include agent-specific effects, individual patient characteristics, and effects on regional vascular beds (eg, splanchnic and renal circulations).[32] Dopamine and epinephrine are more likely to cause or exacerbate tachycardia than norepinephrine and phenylephrine. Dopamine, epinephrine, and norepinephrine will increase cardiac output via stimulation of β-adrenergic receptors. Phenylephrine is a pure α-receptor antagonist, and its vasoconstricting effects can be associated with a drop in cardiac index. With regards to effects of individual vasopressors on regional vascular beds, it is important to emphasize that there is no renal protection provided by "low-dose" dopamine. Studies have shown

Infectious Disease

Table 47-4. Vasoactive Drugs Utilized in Treating Septic Shock

Drug	Dosage	Comments
Dobutamine	1-40 µg/kg/min	Strong inotropic effect may produce vasodilation; utilized as a pure inotrope agent. Causes tachycardia
Dopamine	1-20 µg/kg/min	Effects vary with dose. Predominantly vasoconstrictor with inotropic effects. Causes tachycardia. Effects on renal vasculature not protective against renal failure
Epinephrine	1-20 µg/min	Strong inotropic, chronotropic, and vasoconstrictor. Can produce increased lactate and has unfavorable profile on splanchnic circulation
Norepinephrine	0.03-1.5 µg/kg/min	Strong vasoconstrictor with modest effect on contractility. Does not produce tachycardia
Phenylephrine	0.5-8 µg/kg/min	Pure vasoconstrictor. No direct effect on contractility or heart rate
Vasopressin	0.01-0.04 U/min	Not recommended as first-line agent. Increases blood pressure; may cause splanchnic and cardiac ischemia

that low-dose dopamine targeting stimulation of dopaminergic receptors in the renal vasculature is not associated with any beneficial effects on renal function.[33,34] Ultimately, the most important factor determining our choice of vasopressors in septic shock should be clinical effect on patient outcomes. Human and animal studies suggest a potential benefit of norepinephrine and dopamine over epinephrine (epinephrine is associated with more tachycardia, increased lactate, and worse effects on the splanchnic circulation). There is, however, no clear evidence that epinephrine is harmful to patients with septic shock. Furthermore, a recent prospective randomized trial comparing norepinephrine plus dobutamine to epinephrine in patients with septic shock found no significant difference in the primary outcome of 28-day mortality rate.[35] The largest study to date (> 1600 patients) enrolled patients with shock (the majority with septic shock) and randomized them to dopamine or norepinephrine.[36] There was no significant difference in the primary outcome of 28-day mortality rate (dopamine 52.5% versus norepinephrine 48.5%; $P = 0.10$). However, there were more arrhythmic events among patients treated with dopamine than among those treated with norepinephrine (dopamine 24.1% versus norepinephrine 12.4%; $P < .001$).[36] In recent years there has been increased interest in the use of vasopressin to raise blood pressure in septic shock. Studies have found that patients with septic shock have lower vasopressin levels than patients with other types of shock.[37] This phenomenon has been labeled "relative vasopressin deficiency." Studies have shown that low-dose vasopressin may be effective in raising blood pressures in patients refractory to other vasopressors.[38,39] The VASST trial, a randomized controlled trial, compared norepinephrine alone to norepinephrine plus vasopressin (0.03 units/h). There was no significant difference in mortality rate at 28 days between groups.[40] The trial had two predefined subgroups for analysis: a group with less-severe shock (patients receiving < 15 μg/min of norepinephrine) and a high-severity group (patients receiving < 15 μg/min of norepinephrine). The pretrial hypothesis was that vasopressin would improve mortality rate in the sickest group of patients. However, what the results showed was an improvement in mortality rate with vasopressin in patients with low-severity shock (norepinephrine 35.7% versus vasopressin 26.5%; $P = .05$).[40] The clinical significance of this finding is unclear. Current guidelines recommend that (1) norepinephrine or dopamine should be used as first-line vasopressors in septic shock, (2) epinephrine should be added in patients who remain hypotensive on the first-line agents, and (3) low-dose vasopressin can be utilized in cases refractory to catecholamines.[8] Titration of vasopressors should target MAP and patients ideally should have an arterial line for monitoring. Titration of vasopressors to a MAP of 65 mm Hg has been shown to preserve tissue perfusion.[41,42] In addition, preexisting conditions should be considered when defining the most appropriate target MAP for an individual patient. In patients who are chronically hypertensive, a higher MAP may be indicated; conversely, in a young normotensive patient a lower MAP may be appropriate. Current guidelines recommend a target MAP greater than or equal to 65 mm Hg.[8] It is important to supplement this end point with other markers of global and regional perfusion as well as clinical considerations that may apply to individual patients.

The final components in the hemodynamic optimization of patients with severe sepsis and septic shock are the evaluation and treatment of myocardial depression. Most patients will have adequate cardiac output (CO) after adequate fluid resuscitation. However, in early unresuscitated sepsis and in a subgroup of patients later in the disease process, there is evidence of low or inadequate CO. The CO can be measured using various techniques, most commonly in the ICU via a pulmonary artery catheter or from echocardiographically derived measurements. In addition, the measurement of venous oxygen saturation (Svo_2) or the $Scvo_2$ can be utilized as surrogates for adequate global oxygen delivery (and by proxy, adequate CO). In patients with low CO after achieving volume and perfusion targets, inotropes such as dobutamine can be utilized. Ideally, the cardiac index (CO/body surface area) should be greater than or equal to 2.5 L/min per m^2, the Svo_2 greater than or equal to 65%, or the $Scvo_2$ greater than or equal to 70%.

In summary, the hemodynamic support of patients with severe sepsis and septic shock should be implemented early and should be guided by predefined hemodynamic end points. The Sepsis

Resuscitation Bundle includes the following end points: CVP 8 to 12 mm Hg (may be higher in mechanically ventilated patients); MAP greater than or equal to 65 mm Hg; and Scvo$_2$ greater than or equal to 70%. These end points should be achieved as a group within the first 6 hours of treatment. At our institution we have adopted a protocol that is implemented in all patients with evidence of sepsis-induced hypoperfusion as soon as they are identified in the emergency department or medical ward; this protocol is then used as a guide for resuscitation once the patient is transferred to the intensive care unit (Figure 47-3).[43]

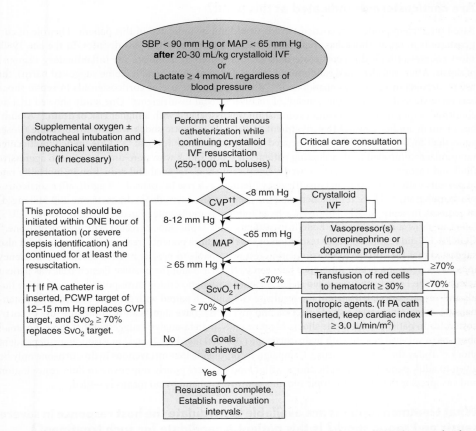

Figure 47-3. Sepsis hemodynamic support protocol. The early goal-directed therapy (EGDT) protocol utilized at Cooper University Hospital (an adaptation of the protocol by Rivers et al.). Clinical criteria for triggering the protocol include a clinical suspicion of sepsis plus one of the following: (1) systolic blood pressure (SBP) < 90 mm Hg or mean arterial pressure (MAP) < 65 mm Hg (despite a 20- to 30-mL/kg crystalloid intravenous fluid [IVF] bolus), or (2) lactate ≥ 4 mmol/L. IVF is administered to achieve a central venous pressure (CVP) ≥ 8 mm Hg, vasopressors (preferably norepinephrine or dopamine) are administered as needed to achieve a MAP ≥ 65 mm Hg, and packed red blood cells (PRBCs) and/or dobutamine are administered as needed in order to achieve a central venous oxygen saturation (Scvo$_2$) ≥ 70%. Our protocol differs slightly from the Rivers protocol in that (after initiation in the emergency department) it is intended to continue into the intensive care unit phase of patient care, where the monitoring device may be changed to a pulmonary artery (PA) catheter based on individual clinician preference. If a PA catheter is utilized, a target for pulmonary capillary wedge pressure (PCWP) replaces the target for CVP, and mixed venous oxygen saturation (Svo$_2$) replaces Scvo$_2$. (*Adapted from Trzeciak S, Dellinger RP, Abate NL, et al. Translating research to clinical practice: a 1-year experience with implementing early goal-directed therapy for septic shock in the emergency department. Chest. 2006;129(2):225-232.*)

After aggressive fluid resuscitation, norepinephrine (10 μg/min) and dobutamine (5 μg/min) are initiated. At this point the patient has the following hemodynamic parameters: CVP 10 mm Hg, MAP 68 mm Hg, and $ScvO_2$ 75%. The patient remains on the same ventilator settings and is now on a midazolam continuous infusion for sedation. Blood cultures that were sent last night are reported as growing gram-positive cocci.

Are corticosteroids indicated at this point?

Based on current guidelines, corticosteroids would not be indicated in this patient. The role of corticosteroids in septic shock has changed in a pendular way over the past decades. In the late 1980s short courses of high-dose corticosteroids were proposed to modulate the inflammatory response of sepsis. After well-designed randomized studies failed to show benefit (some suggested harm), the use of steroids in sepsis was abandoned.[44] More recently the use of corticosteroids in septic shock was reconsidered based on the concept of relative adrenal insufficiency. One study showed that an abnormal response to corticotropin stimulation was associated with a higher risk of death.[45] A number of small studies showed that treatment of patients in septic shock with hydrocortisone (doses equivalent to 200-300 mg/d) was associated with quicker shock reversal.[46,47] One French multicenter randomized controlled trial evaluating patients in septic shock who were unresponsive to aggressive fluid and vasopressor treatment showed a significant shock reversal and reduction in mortality rate in patients with relative adrenal insufficiency (defined as a rise in cortisol ≤ 9 μg/dL after corticotropin stimulation).[48] These results increased the use of corticosteroids (hydrocortisone 200-300 mg/d) in patients in septic shock. However, a large follow-up multicenter European study (CORTICUS) failed to show a mortality rate benefit in patients with septic shock treated with hydrocortisone.[49] CORTICUS did report a quicker resolution of shock in those patients treated with steroids and it also suggested that the corticotropin stimulation test was unable to predict relative adrenal insufficiency in patients.[49] An important difference between CORTICUS and the positive French trial was patient selection (the French study enrolled sicker patients, with hypotension unresponsive to aggressive fluids and vasopressors). Ultimately, the results of CORTICUS paired with genuine concerns for potential side effects (increased risk of infection and myopathy) have significantly limited the use of corticosteroids in patients with septic shock. Most recently, a meta-analysis suggested that there is a small short-term survival benefit with hydrocortisone (200-300 mg/d for 7 days) in vasopressor-dependent shock.[50] Today the Surviving Sepsis Campaign recommends that intravenous hydrocortisone only be given to adult patients with septic shock with blood pressure poorly responsive to fluid resuscitation and vasopressor therapy.[8] This topic remains controversial and by no means is settled.

What treatment options are available to modulate the host response in severe sepsis and septic shock? Is this patient a candidate for such treatment?

Currently the only drug approved by the US Food and Drug Administration (FDA) for targeting the host response in severe sepsis is recombinant human APC. APC is a protein with anticoagulant and anti-inflammatory properties. In addition, APC has been reported to inhibit nitric oxide–induced vascular dysfunction, apoptosis of lymphocytes and endothelial cells, and activation of neutrophils.[51] The seminal study with APC was PROWESS, a multicenter randomized controlled study in which patients with severe sepsis were randomized to APC (24 μg/kg per hour infused intravenously for 96 hours) or placebo.[52] Treatment with APC was associated with a lower mortality rate at 28 days than placebo (24.7% versus 30.8%; $P = .005$). The main complication associated with APC is bleeding. Serious bleeding episodes were higher in the APC group than in the placebo group (3.5% versus 2.0%; $P = .06$).[52] Subsequent subgroup analyses revealed that most of the benefit with APC was seen in the patients with the highest risk of death (failure of two or more organs and APACHE II scores ≥ 25).[53] Based on these results the FDA and its European counterpart approved APC for use in patients

Table 47-5. Use of Recombinant Human Activated Protein C in Severe Sepsis

Indication
Adult patients with severe sepsis (sepsis associated with acute organ dysfunction) who have a high risk of death (eg, as determined by APACHE II score or need for vasopressors)

Contraindications
Active internal bleeding
Recent (within 3 mo) hemorrhagic stroke
Recent (within 2 mo) intracranial or intraspinal surgery, or severe head trauma
Trauma with increased risk of life-threatening bleeding
Presence of epidural catheter
Intracranial neoplasm or mass lesion or evidence of cerebral herniation

Warnings
Coagulopathy (platelet count < 30,000 or INR > 3.0)
Concurrent use of heparin
Recent use of thrombolytics, acetylsalicylic acid, glycoprotein IIb/IIIa platelet inhibitors, or other anticoagulants
Recent (within 6 wk) gastrointestinal bleed
Recent (within 3 mo) ischemic stroke
Chronic severe hepatic disease
Known bleeding diathesis
Any condition in which bleeding poses a significant hazard of difficulty to manage secondary to its location

Abbreviation: INR, international normalized ratio.

with severe sepsis and a high risk of death. A subsequent study, ADDRESS, evaluated APC in patients with severe sepsis with a low risk of death (APACHE II < 25 and/or single-organ dysfunction).[54] This study did not show benefits with APC and was stopped prematurely due to futility. Criticism and controversy regarding this novel therapy have centered around the fact that it was approved based on one single positive study, it is approved for a patient population that has not been studied prospectively, and the risk of bleeding in clinical practice is likely higher, raising questions of the risk-benefit ratio of this therapy.[55-59] Currently a second randomized controlled trial targeting patients with septic shock and a high risk of death is ongoing. Pending the results of this study, APC is still approved for patients with severe sepsis at high risk of death with no contraindications related to the risk of bleeding (Table 47-5). The current recommendation from the Surviving Sepsis Campaign regarding APC is to consider APC in adult patients with sepsis-induced organ dysfunction associated with a clinical assessment of high risk of death (most of whom will have APACHE II scores ≥ 25 or multiple organ failure).[8] The patient presented in this chapter would certainly fall into the category of high risk of death (septic shock on vasopressors and multiple organ failure) and there are no obvious contraindications for APC. Therefore, to answer the question posed above, yes, this patient is eligible for treatment with APC.

The patient is started on APC at 24 μg/kg per hour; he continues to receive norepinephrine and dobutamine drips (titrated to hemodynamic end points). Mechanical ventilator settings remain unchanged. A new set of laboratory data is available and shows a blood glucose level of 197 mg/dL.

How would you manage this patient's glucose?

Hyperglycemia and insulin resistance are commonly present in patients with severe sepsis and other critical illnesses. There is evidence suggesting that hyperglycemia related to critical illness is associated with poor outcomes.[60-64] Proposed deleterious effects of critical illness–associated hyperglycemia include impaired neutrophil function, increased risk of infection, poor wound healing, and a procoagulant state.[65] Treatment of hyperglycemia in critically ill patients was greatly advocated based on the results of a study by Van den Berghe et al in a large group of mechanically ventilated surgical critical care patients.[66] This study showed that a tight glycemic control strategy (intravenous insulin targeting blood glucose levels of 80-110 mg/dL) was associated with a significant improvement in mortality rate, organ failure, and length of stay. These findings prompted many hospitals to adopt similar protocols and aggressively target high blood glucose levels in critically ill patients. A subsequent study by the same group evaluated the same protocol in a medical intensive care population.[67] In this study tight glycemic control was not associated with an overall mortality benefit, but was associated with a decreased hospital and ICU length of stay and less time on mechanical ventilation. In the subgroup of patients who remained more than 3 days in the ICU, mortality was reduced with tight glycemic control. However, the investigators were unsuccessful in predicting which patients would require more than 3 days of ICU care. In this second study the incidence of documented hypoglycemia was significantly higher in the tight glycemic control group than in the conventional glycemic control group (18% versus 6.2%).[67] The VISEP trial evaluated the use of tight glycemic control and pentastarch in patients with severe sepsis.[68] The study was stopped prematurely because of safety concerns. There was no significant difference in mortality rate or mean score for organ failure between the group treated with intensive insulin therapy and the conventional therapy group. The rate of severe hypoglycemia (glucose level ≤ 40 mg/dL [2.2 mmol/L]) was higher in the intensive therapy group than in the conventional therapy group (17.0% versus 4.1%; $P < .001$), as was the rate of serious adverse events (10.9% versus 5.2%; $P = .01$).[68] Finally, the NICE-SUGAR trial, the largest study to date, enrolled more than 6000 patients and randomized them to either intensive glucose control (target glucose 81-108 mg/dL) or conventional glucose control (target blood glucose < 180 mg/dL).[69] Mortality rate was higher in the intensive glucose control group when compared to the conventional glucose control group (27.5% versus 24.9%; $P = .02$). Severe hypoglycemia (blood glucose level ≤ 40 mg/dL) was higher in patients in the intensive glucose control group when compared to patients in the conventional glucose control group (6.8% versus 0.5%; $P < .001$).[69] The results of the latest trials have raised many questions regarding the tight glycemic control in critically ill patients. It seems most experts would agree that keeping blood glucose below 180 mg/dL based on the results of the NICE-SUGAR study is advisable. Furthermore, a recent cerebral microdialysis study revealed that intense glycemic control (systemic glucose 80-120 mg/dL as the target), compared to an intermediate range (121-180 mg/dL as the target), was associated with an increased risk of brain energy crisis and higher mortality rate at hospital discharge.[70] Based on the current literature, many experts recommend targeting blood sugars around 150 mg/dL by making use of an insulin protocol and monitoring glucose closely to prevent severe hypoglycemia.

What are other important therapeutic measures to consider in this patient?

Patients with severe sepsis, like other critically ill patients, require a host of general supportive therapies (Table 47-6). Improvement in critical care supportive therapy probably plays an important role in the observed decrease in mortality rate over the past decades in processes such as severe sepsis and acute respiratory distress syndrome (ARDS). Mechanical ventilation is often required in patients with

Table 47-6. Supportive Therapies for Patients with Severe Sepsis and Septic Shock

Mechanical ventilation
Deep vein thrombosis prophylaxis
Gastrointestinal ulcer prophylaxis
Nutrition
Glucose control
Sedation and analgesia

severe sepsis. Studies in patients with ARDS have demonstrated that protective lung ventilation strategies utilizing low tidal volume (6 mL/kg) are associated with significantly lower mortality rate than ventilation with more traditional tidal volumes (12 mL/kg).[71] This is most likely because of a decrease in ventilator-induced lung injury. Current guidelines recommend the use of a protective lung strategy (low tidal volume; inspiratory plateau pressure < 30 cm H_2O) in mechanically ventilated patients with severe sepsis.[8] Goals for oxygen saturation should be an Sao_2 greater than or equal to 90%; this can be achieved by increasing the Fio_2 and/or application of positive end-expiratory pressure (PEEP). Patients on mechanical ventilation who are clinically improving should be evaluated on a daily basis for weaning from mechanical ventilation. Patients with severe sepsis on mechanical ventilation should be managed with appropriate sedatives and analgesics (see Chapter 18 for more details).

Patients with severe sepsis should receive prophylaxis for the development of deep vein thrombosis (DVT). In the absence of contraindications patients should receive pharmacologic DVT prophylaxis. Treatment with low-dose unfractionated heparin (UFH), adjusted-dose UFH, or low-molecular-weight heparin (LMWH) is recommended.[72] Treatment for DVT prophylaxis with UFH or LMWH is not contraindicated during infusion of APC. Stress ulcer prophylaxis is recommended for all patients with severe sepsis. Histamine-2 receptor antagonists are more effective than sucralfate in decreasing bleeding risk and transfusion requirements.[73] Proton pump inhibitors have not been assessed in a direct comparison with histamine-2 receptor antagonists but do demonstrate equivalency and ability to increase gastric pH.[72]

Severe sepsis is a catabolic state. Metabolic alterations in patients with severe sepsis include breakdown of proteins, carbohydrates, and lipids; negative nitrogen balance; and hyperglycemia with insulin resistance. As with other critically ill patients, those with severe sepsis require adequate nutritional support. Enteral nutrition offers several advantages including lower cost, preservation of gastric mucosa integrity, decreased incidence of infections, and avoidance of parenteral nutritional catheters and their potential complications.[74] In patients who cannot tolerate enteral nutrition, parenteral nutrition should be utilized.[75] Finally, patients with severe sepsis and septic shock should receive early physical and occupational therapy as their clinical state starts to improve.

! CRITICAL CONSIDERATIONS

- Sepsis is the result of a systemic inflammatory response to infection. Severe sepsis is defined as sepsis with organ failure. Septic shock is defined by the presence of hypotension despite adequate fluid resuscitation.
- Severe sepsis is frequent and is associated with high morbidity and mortality rates.
- Severe sepsis is a medical emergency and requires clinicians to rapidly implement time-sensitive therapeutic interventions in order to maximize the impact on patient outcomes.
- An increased serum lactate in a patient with sepsis is a marker of severity and can identify patients who may benefit from more aggressive care.
- The approach for treatment of sepsis is based on the following components:
  - Management of the infection
  - Hemodynamic support
  - Modulation of the host response
  - General supportive care
- Infection management includes the early administration of appropriate antibiotics and institution of source control measures.

Infectious Disease

- Hemodynamic support consists of early and aggressive fluid resuscitation and maintenance of predefined hemodynamic end points. Studies have shown that early goal-directed therapy for hemodynamic support can improve mortality rate in patients with severe sepsis.

- Administration of corticosteroids (hydrocortisone 200-300 mg/d intravenously) should be considered in adult patients with septic shock with blood pressure poorly responsive to fluid resuscitation and vasopressor therapy.

- Administration of APC should be considered in patients with severe sepsis at a high risk of death with contraindications.

- To maximize patient outcomes, appropriate supportive therapy must be provided in the ICU. These include protective lung ventilation, glucose control, proper nutrition, gastrointestinal prophylaxis, and DVT prophylaxis.

- Implementation of a performance improvement program for patients with severe sepsis and septic shock based on the Surviving Sepsis Campaign Sepsis Bundles has been associated with improved process of care and significant reductions in mortality rate.

REFERENCES

1. Angus DC, Linde-Zwirble WT, Lidicker J, Clermont G, Carcillo J, Pinsky MR. Epidemiology of severe sepsis in the United States: analysis of incidence, outcome, and associated costs of care. *Crit Care Med.* 2001;29(7):1303-1310.

2. Annane D, Aegerter P, Jars-Guincestre MC, Guidet B. Current epidemiology of septic shock: the CUB-Rea Network. *Am J Respir Crit Care Med.* 2003;168(2):165-172.

3. Bone RC, Balk RA, Cerra FB, et al. Definitions for sepsis and organ failure and guidelines for the use of innovative therapies in sepsis. The ACCP/SCCM Consensus Conference Committee. American College of Chest Physicians/Society of Critical Care Medicine. *Chest.* 1992;101(6):1644-1655.

4. Trzeciak S, Zanotti-Cavazzoni S, Parrillo JE, Dellinger RP. Inclusion criteria for clinical trials in sepsis: did the American College of Chest Physicians/Society of Critical Care Medicine consensus conference definitions of sepsis have an impact? *Chest.* 2005;127(1):242-245.

5. Vincent JL. Dear SIRS, I'm sorry to say that I don't like you. *Crit Care Med.* 1997;25(2):372-374.

6. Levy MM, Fink MP, Marshall JC, et al. 2001 SCCM/ESICM/ACCP/ATS/SIS International Sepsis Definitions Conference. *Crit Care Med.* 2003;31(4):1250-1256.

7. Brun-Buisson C. The epidemiology of the systemic inflammatory response. *Intensive Care Med.* 2000;26(Suppl 1):S64-S74.

8. Dellinger RP, Levy MM, Carlet JM, et al. Surviving Sepsis Campaign: international guidelines for management of severe sepsis and septic shock: 2008. *Crit Care Med.* 2008;36(1):296-327.

9. Townsend SR, Schorr C, Levy MM, Dellinger RP. Reducing mortality in severe sepsis: the Surviving Sepsis Campaign. *Clin Chest Med.* 2008;29(4):721-733, x.

10. Ferrer R, Artigas A, Levy MM, et al. Improvement in process of care and outcome after a multicenter severe sepsis educational program in Spain. *JAMA.* 2008;299(19):2294-2303.

11. Ferrer R, Artigas A, Suarez D, et al. Effectiveness of treatments for severe sepsis: a prospective, multicenter, observational study. *Am J Respir Crit Care Med.* 2009;180(9):861-866.

12. Levy MM, Dellinger RP, Townsend SR, et al. The Surviving Sepsis Campaign: results of an international guideline-based performance improvement program targeting severe sepsis. *Crit Care Med.* 2010;38(2):367-374.

13. Arnold RC, Shapiro NI, Jones AE, et al. Multicenter study of early lactate clearance as a determinant of survival in patients with presumed sepsis. *Shock.* 2009;32(1):35-39.

14. Green JP, Berger T, Garg N, Shapiro NI. Serum lactate is a better predictor of short-term mortality when stratified by C-reactive protein in adult emergency department patients hospitalized for a suspected infection. *Ann Emerg Med.* 2011;57(3):291-295.

15. Shapiro NI, Howell MD, Talmor D, et al. Serum lactate as a predictor of mortality in emergency

department patients with infection. *Ann Emerg Med.* 2005;45(5):524-528.

16. Kumar A, Roberts D, Wood KE, et al. Duration of hypotension before initiation of effective antimicrobial therapy is the critical determinant of survival in human septic shock. *Crit Care Med.* 2006;34(6):1589-1596.

17. Ibrahim EH, Sherman G, Ward S, Fraser VJ, Kollef MH. The influence of inadequate antimicrobial treatment of bloodstream infections on patient outcomes in the ICU setting. *Chest.* 2000;118(1):146-155.

18. Leibovici L, Shraga I, Drucker M, Konigsberger H, Samra Z, Pitlik SD. The benefit of appropriate empirical antibiotic treatment in patients with bloodstream infection. *J Intern Med.* 1998;244(5):379-386.

19. Kollef MH, Sherman G, Ward S, Fraser VJ. Inadequate antimicrobial treatment of infections: a risk factor for hospital mortality among critically ill patients. *Chest.* 1999;115(2):462-474.

20. Jimenez MF, Marshall JC. Source control in the management of sepsis. *Intensive Care Med.* 2001;27(Suppl 1):S49-S62.

21. Parrillo JE, Parker MM, Natanson C, et al. Septic shock in humans. Advances in the understanding of pathogenesis, cardiovascular dysfunction, and therapy. *Ann Intern Med.* 1990;113(3):227-242.

22. Rivers E, Nguyen B, Havstad S, et al. Early goal-directed therapy in the treatment of severe sepsis and septic shock. *N Engl J Med.* 2001;345(19):1368-1377.

23. Jones AE, Shapiro NI, Trzeciak S, et al. Lactate clearance vs central venous oxygen saturation as goals of early sepsis therapy: a randomized clinical trial. *JAMA.* 24;303(8):739-746.

24. Lin SM, Huang CD, Lin HC, Liu CY, Wang CH, Kuo HP. A modified goal-directed protocol improves clinical outcomes in intensive care unit patients with septic shock: a randomized controlled trial. *Shock.* 2006;26(6):551-557.

25. Otero RM, Nguyen HB, Huang DT, et al. Early goal-directed therapy in severe sepsis and septic shock revisited: concepts, controversies, and contemporary findings. *Chest.* 2006;130(5):1579-1595.

26. Varpula M, Tallgren M, Saukkonen K, Voipio-Pulkki LM, Pettila V. Hemodynamic variables related to outcome in septic shock. *Intensive Care Med.* 2005;31(8):1066-1071.

27. Choi PT, Yip G, Quinonez LG, Cook DJ. Crystalloids vs. colloids in fluid resuscitation: a systematic review. *Crit Care Med.* 1999;27(1):200-210.

28. Cook D, Guyatt G. Colloid use for fluid resuscitation: evidence and spin. *Ann Intern Med.* 2001;135(3):205-208.

29. Schierhout G, Roberts I. Fluid resuscitation with colloid or crystalloid solutions in critically ill patients: a systematic review of randomised trials. *BMJ.* 1998;316(7136):961-964.

30. Finfer S, Bellomo R, Boyce N, French J, Myburgh J, Norton R. A comparison of albumin and saline for fluid resuscitation in the intensive care unit. *N Engl J Med.* 2004;350(22):2247-2256.

31. Hollenberg SM, Ahrens TS, Annane D, et al. Practice parameters for hemodynamic support of sepsis in adult patients: 2004 update. *Crit Care Med.* 2004;32(9):1928-1948.

32. Zanotti Cavazzoni SL, Dellinger RP. Hemodynamic optimization of sepsis-induced tissue hypoperfusion. *Crit Care.* 2006;10(Suppl 3):S2.

33. Bellomo R, Chapman M, Finfer S, Hickling K, Myburgh J. Low-dose dopamine in patients with early renal dysfunction: a placebo-controlled randomised trial. Australian and New Zealand Intensive Care Society (ANZICS) Clinical Trials Group. *Lancet.* 2000;356(9248):2139-2143.

34. Kellum JA, Decker JM. Use of dopamine in acute renal failure: a meta-analysis. *Crit Care Med.* 2001;29(8):1526-1531.

35. Annane D, Vignon P, Renault A, et al. Norepinephrine plus dobutamine versus epinephrine alone for management of septic shock: a randomised trial. *Lancet.* 2007;370(9588):676-684.

36. De Backer D, Biston P, Devriendt J, et al. Comparison of dopamine and norepinephrine in the treatment of shock. *N Engl J Med.* 2010;362(9):779-789.

37. Landry DW, Levin HR, Gallant EM, et al. Vasopressin deficiency contributes to the vasodilation of septic shock. *Circulation.* 1997;95(5):1122-1125.

38. Holmes CL, Patel BM, Russell JA, Walley KR. Physiology of vasopressin relevant to management of septic shock. *Chest.* 2001;120(3):989-1002.

39. Patel BM, Chittock DR, Russell JA, Walley KR. Beneficial effects of short-term vasopressin infusion during severe septic shock. *Anesthesiology.* 2002;96(3):576-582.

40. Russell JA, Walley KR, Singer J, et al. Vasopressin versus norepinephrine infusion in patients with septic shock. *N Engl J Med.* 2008;358(9):877-887.

41. Bourgoin A, Leone M, Delmas A, Garnier F, Albanese J, Martin C. Increasing mean arterial pressure in patients with septic shock: effects on oxygen variables and renal function. *Crit Care Med.* 2005;33(4):780-786.

42. LeDoux D, Astiz ME, Carpati CM, Rackow EC. Effects of perfusion pressure on tissue perfusion in septic shock. *Crit Care Med.* 2000;28(8):2729-2732.

Infectious Disease

43. Trzeciak S, Dellinger RP, Abate NL, et al. Translating research to clinical practice: a 1-year experience with implementing early goal-directed therapy for septic shock in the emergency department. *Chest*. 2006;129(2):225-232.

44. Bone RC, Fisher CJ Jr, Clemmer TP, Slotman GJ, Metz CA, Balk RA. A controlled clinical trial of high-dose methylprednisolone in the treatment of severe sepsis and septic shock. *N Engl J Med*. 1987;317(11):653-658.

45. Annane D, Sebille V, Troche G, Raphael JC, Gajdos P, Bellissant E. A 3-level prognostic classification in septic shock based on cortisol levels and cortisol response to corticotropin. *JAMA*. 2000;283(8):1038-1045.

46. Bollaert PE, Charpentier C, Levy B, Debouverie M, Audibert G, Larcan A. Reversal of late septic shock with supraphysiologic doses of hydrocortisone. *Crit Care Med*. 1998;26(4):645-650.

47. Briegel J, Forst H, Haller M, et al. Stress doses of hydrocortisone reverse hyperdynamic septic shock: a prospective, randomized, double-blind, single-center study. *Crit Care Med*. 1999;27(4):723-732.

48. Annane D, Sebille V, Charpentier C, et al. Effect of treatment with low doses of hydrocortisone and fludrocortisone on mortality in patients with septic shock. *JAMA*. 2002;288(7):862-871.

49. Sprung CL, Annane D, Keh D, et al. Hydrocortisone therapy for patients with septic shock. *N Engl J Med*. 2008;358(2):111-124.

50. Annane D, Bellissant E, Bollaert P-E, et al. Corticosteroids in the treatment of severe sepsis and septic shock in adults: a systematic review. *JAMA*. 2009;301(22):2362-2375.

51. Toussaint S, Gerlach H. Activated protein C for sepsis. *N Engl J Med*. 2009;361(27):2646-2652.

52. Bernard GR, Vincent JL, Laterre PF, et al. Efficacy and safety of recombinant human activated protein C for severe sepsis. *N Engl J Med*. 2001;344(10):699-709.

53. Ely EW, Laterre PF, Angus DC, et al. Drotrecogin alfa (activated) administration across clinically important subgroups of patients with severe sepsis. *Crit Care Med*. 2003;31(1):12-19.

54. Abraham E, Laterre PF, Garg R, et al. Drotrecogin alfa (activated) for adults with severe sepsis and a low risk of death. *N Engl J Med*. 2005;353(13):1332-1341.

55. Bertolini G, Rossi C, Anghileri A, Livigni S, Addis A, Poole D. Use of drotrecogin alfa (activated) in Italian intensive care units: the results of a nationwide survey. *Intensive Care Med*. 2007;33(3):426-434.

56. Eichacker PQ, Danner RL, Suffredini AF, Cui X, Natanson C. Reassessing recombinant human activated protein C for sepsis: time for a new randomized controlled trial. *Crit Care Med*. 2005;33(10):2426-2428.

57. Poole D, Bertolini G, Garattini S. Errors in the approval process and post-marketing evaluation of drotrecogin alfa (activated) for the treatment of severe sepsis. *Lancet Infect Dis*. 2009;9(1):67-72.

58. Sweeney DA, Natanson C, Eichacker PQ. Recombinant human activated protein C, package labeling, and hemorrhage risks. *Crit Care Med*. 2009;37(1):327-329.

59. Warren HS, Suffredini AF, Eichacker PQ, Munford RS. Risks and benefits of activated protein C treatment for severe sepsis. *N Engl J Med*. 2002;347(13):1027-1030.

60. Finney SJ, Zekveld C, Elia A, Evans TW. Glucose control and mortality in critically ill patients. *JAMA*. 2003;290(15):2041-2047.

61. Malmberg K, Norhammar A, Wedel H, Ryden L. Glycometabolic state at admission: important risk marker of mortality in conventionally treated patients with diabetes mellitus and acute myocardial infarction: long-term results from the Diabetes and Insulin-Glucose Infusion in Acute Myocardial Infarction (DIGAMI) study. *Circulation*. 1999;99(20):2626-2632.

62. Michaud LJ, Rivara FP, Longstreth WT Jr, Grady MS. Elevated initial blood glucose levels and poor outcome following severe brain injuries in children. *J Trauma*. 1991;31(10):1356-1362.

63. Norhammar AM, Ryden L, Malmberg K. Admission plasma glucose. Independent risk factor for long-term prognosis after myocardial infarction even in nondiabetic patients. *Diabetes Care*. 1999;22(11):1827-1831.

64. Zindrou D, Taylor KM, Bagger JP. Admission plasma glucose: an independent risk factor in nondiabetic women after coronary artery bypass grafting. *Diabetes Care*. 2001;24(9):1634-1639.

65. Nylen ES, Muller B. Endocrine changes in critical illness. *J Intensive Care Med*. 2004;19(2):67-82.

66. van den Berghe G, Wouters P, Weekers F, et al. Intensive insulin therapy in the critically ill patients. *N Engl J Med*. 2001;345(19):1359-1367.

67. Van den Berghe G, Wilmer A, Hermans G, et al. Intensive insulin therapy in the medical ICU. *N Engl J Med*. 2006;354(5):449-461.

68. Brunkhorst FM, Engel C, Bloos F, et al. Intensive insulin therapy and pentastarch resuscitation in severe sepsis. *N Engl J Med*. 2008;358(2):125-139.

69. Finfer S, Chittock DR, Su SY, et al. Intensive versus conventional glucose control in critically ill patients. *N Engl J Med*. 2009;360(13):1283-1297.

70. Oddo M, Schmidt JM, Carrera E, et al. Impact of tight glycemic control on cerebral glucose

metabolism after severe brain injury: a microdialysis study. *Crit Care Med.* 2008;36(12): 3233-3238.

71. Ventilation with lower tidal volumes as compared with traditional tidal volumes for acute lung injury and the acute respiratory distress syndrome. The Acute Respiratory Distress Syndrome Network. *N Engl J Med.* 2000;342(18):1301-1308.

72. Trzeciak S, Dellinger RP. Other supportive therapies in sepsis: an evidence-based review. *Crit Care Med.* 2004;32(11 Suppl):S571-S577.

73. Cook D, Guyatt G, Marshall J, et al. A comparison of sucralfate and ranitidine for the prevention of upper gastrointestinal bleeding in patients requiring mechanical ventilation. Canadian Critical Care Trials Group. *N Engl J Med.* 1998;338(12):791-797.

74. Heyland DK. Nutritional support in the critically ill patients. A critical review of the evidence. *Crit Care Clin.* 1998;14(3):423-440.

75. Heyland DK, MacDonald S, Keefe L, Drover JW. Total parenteral nutrition in the critically ill patient: a meta-analysis. *JAMA.* 1998;280(23):2013-2019.

Infectious Disease

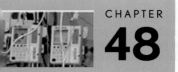

CHAPTER
48

Antimicrobial Therapies in the ICU

Quinn A. Czosnowski, PharmD, BCPS
Jomy M. George, PharmD, BCPS

 J.L., a 28-year-old man, was admitted with a severe traumatic brain injury following a motor vehicle crash. He required intubation and mechanical ventilation upon arrival at the hospital. He had no significant past medical or social history. His admission height and weight were 72 inches and 85 kg, respectively.

The patient progressed without complication until the morning of hospital day 6. During rounds it is identified that J.L. has an increasing white blood cell count (from 11.4 to 15.1 cells/mm^3), was febrile overnight (39°C), and has macroscopically purulent sputum on examination. His morning chest radiograph shows that he has a new right-sided infiltrate. Arterial blood gases (ABGs) on an inspiratory oxygen concentration of 40% are as follows: PaO$_2$ 76 mm Hg, PaCO$_2$ 36 mm Hg, HCO$_3^-$ 20 mEq/L, and pH 7.31. Blood pressure (BP) is 130/80 mm Hg and heart rate (HR) is 90 bpm. The team suspects late-onset ventilator-associated pneumonia and conducts a bronchoscopic bronchoalveolar lavage (BAL), along with blood and urine cultures. Following the sample collection empiric antibiotics are to be started.

What steps are involved prior to the initiation of antimicrobial therapies in this patient?

The clinical and radiographic presentation is consistent with late-onset ventilator-associated pneumonia. The goals of therapy include eradication of the causative organism and symptom resolution. Initiation of appropriate antibiotic therapy is essential in achieving these goals for all infections including ventilator-associated pneumonia. Prior to antibiotic initiation, samples for culture should be drawn from any suspected sources. It is important to obtain cultures prior to antibiotic therapy, as failure to do so has been shown to decrease the yield of the causative organism.[1] Current guidelines by the Infectious Diseases Society of America recommend that at least two sets of blood cultures and a lower respiratory tract sample be obtained to aid in the diagnosis of pneumonia.[2] Cultures are critical in helping to identify the causative organism(s), which will dictate the choice of antibiotics as well as the duration of therapy. Culture data also help to determine the duration of therapy as certain bacterial species have been shown to respond better to shorter durations of antibiotics than have other species.[3] Negative lower respiratory tract samples at 72 hours in the absence of antibiotic changes can be used to discontinue antibiotic therapy, limiting unnecessary drug exposure.[2] If the samples are positive, they help in the identification of the causative organism and its in vitro susceptibility profile. This information is essential for antibiotic de-escalation and tailoring of antibiotic therapy to ensure appropriate treatment while minimizing the risk for the development of resistance.

While culture data are extremely important in the delivery of an optimal antibiotic regimen, it is imperative that the collection of cultures not delay the initiation of the empiric antibiotic regimen. If cultures cannot be obtained in a timely manner, then antibiotics should not be withheld simply to increase the yield of cultures. The time to initiation of appropriate empiric therapy is vital in patients with suspected infection. This has been demonstrated in multiple types of infections including sepsis, pneumonia, and meningitis. A recent study assessing time from onset of hypotension to the delivery of appropriate antibiotics demonstrated an increase in mortality rate of 7% per hour for every hour in delay of antibiotic administration.[4] This was not an isolated finding, as several studies of sepsis due to varying infections have shown similar results.[5-7] These findings have led to consensus guidelines for sepsis to recommend antibiotic administration within 1 hour of onset of severe sepsis or septic shock.[8] Similar recommendations are made regarding timing of antibiotic administration in other guideline statements based on these or similar data.[2,9,10]

The important thing to remember with these data is that the key is delivery of appropriate antibiotics. An antibiotic regimen with poor or no in vitro activity against the causative organism is termed *inadequate* or *inappropriate empiric antibiotic therapy* (IEAT). The administration of IEAT has been shown to be an independent risk factor for mortality in critically ill patients with various infections, including bacteremia and pneumonia.[11,12] When deciding on an empiric regimen that will minimize IEAT and the associated mortality, there are multiple drug-, hospital-, infection-, and patient-specific factors that must be taken into account (Figure 48-1). These factors are highly dependent on one another and must all be addressed in order to select the most appropriate empiric antibiotic regimen.

What drug-specific factors need to be taken into consideration when selecting an empiric antibiotic regimen?

When providing an optimal antibiotic regimen, one must consider the drug's pharmacokinetic and pharmacodynamic parameters in order to maximize bactericidal or bacteriostatic activity and prevent antimicrobial resistance. Pharmacokinetics includes the processes of absorption, distribution, metabolism, and elimination of a given drug. A list of pharmacokinetic parameters and their definitions is given in Table 48-1. These factors along with the dose and administration frequency determine the amount of drug in the serum or body tissue and the duration of the drug's availability in those areas. Critical illness adds another level of complexity as critically ill patients undergo a number of physiologic changes that affect these pharmacokinetic parameters.

Absorption and Distribution

Some common changes in critical illness include decreases in gastrointestinal perfusion and motility, intestinal atrophy, and physical incompatibilities with enteral nutrition or other medications. These parameters are important to consider as they can significantly decrease the bioavailability of oral antibiotics, thereby limiting their role during critical illness. Changes in bioavailability can then affect the following pharmacokinetic parameters: maximum concentration (C_{max}) achieved in serum, steady-state or plateau serum concentration (C_{ss}), area under the curve (AUC), and time to peak concentration (T_{max}) seen after drug administration. Because of the aforementioned limitations, it is recommended to avoid the use of oral antibiotics in favor of intravenous antibiotics, particularly if there is a question of gastrointestinal function and/or motility. Drug distribution to tissues is also significantly affected in critical illness. Factors such as pH, fluid shifts, and hypoalbuminemia may have a significant effect on volume of distribution changes (V_d), resulting in varying concentrations at the site of infection. Physiochemical characteristics such as hydrophilicity and lipophilicity also

Infectious Disease

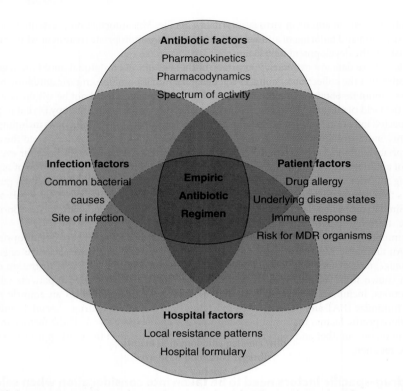

Figure 48-1. Venn diagram demonstrating the relationship of antibiotic-, hospital-, infection-, and patient-specific factors in selecting an empiric antibiotic regimen. MDR, multidrug-resistant.

Table 48-1. Pharmacokinetic Parameters and Definitions

Parameter	Definition
F	Bioavailability—amount of drug absorbed into systemic circulation
C_{max}	Maximum concentration in serum following a dose; also commonly referred to as the peak
C_{min}	Minimum concentration in serum during dosing regimen
Css	Steady-state concentration in plasma—concentration by which the rate of drug administration is equal to the rate of elimination; the concentration typically associated with maximal efficacy and toxicity
T_{max}	Time to reach the maximum serum concentration after administration
V_d	Volume of distribution—a measure of the distribution of drug throughout the body
Cl	Rate of drug clearance or elimination
$t_{1/2}$	Elimination half-life—time required to reduce plasma concentrations by 50%
AUC	Area under the concentration vs time curve

play a role in determining a drug's volume of distribution and clearance.[12] Blood levels achieved by hydrophilic antibiotics such as aminoglycosides, β-lactams, colistin, and linezolid are largely affected by increased volumes of distribution as commonly seen in critically ill patients. Lipophilic antibiotics such as fluoroquinolones, lincosamides, macrolides, and tigecycline distribute well into fat tissue and therefore have a largely unchanged V_d. All of these factors need to be taken into consideration when deciding on an antibiotic dosing regimen to ensure efficacy and avoid drug toxicity.

Metabolism and Excretion

In the critically ill, alterations in hepatic blood intrinsic clearance and protein binding can significantly affect the metabolism of antibiotics, possibly resulting in the need for dosage modifications.

The clearance of antibiotics is often unpredictable and can either be increased or decreased depending on the renal function. Renal clearance is the most common elimination pathway for antibiotics; therefore, renal dysfunction or failure encountered with critical illness can have a significant impact on a patient's elimination half-life ($t_{1/2}$).[13]

Pharmacodynamics

Pharmacodynamics demonstrates the relationship between the pharmacologic effect and drug concentrations and has been used to determine microbiologic and/or clinical outcomes. Pharmacodynamics predicts the ability of antibiotics to exert their bactericidal (ie, kill the bacteria) or bacteriostatic (ie, inhibit the growth of the bacteria) effects. The minimum inhibitory concentration (MIC) is the minimum concentration of an antimicrobial that will inhibit the growth of bacteria and is a good predictor of the efficacy of an antibiotic against a given pathogen. However, it does not take into account the duration or extent of antimicrobial activity. The time course of antimicrobial activity varies greatly from class to class and correlates with different pharmacodynamic parameters. A list of the commonly encountered antibiotic classes and the optimal pharmacodynamic parameters that correlate with efficacy is given in Table 48-2. A graphical representation of the interaction between pharmacokinetic and pharmacodynamic parameters is depicted in Figure 48-2.

In order to maximize efficacy and minimize toxicity, antibiotics will exert their action in one of two killing methods: time-dependent killing or concentration-dependent killing. In antibiotics that possess time-dependent kill, namely, β-lactams, maximal killing relies on the time antibiotic serum concentrations remain consistently above the MIC (T > MIC). It is important to note that time-dependent antibiotics do not rely on the peak concentration achieved in serum but, instead, on how long these concentrations remain above the MIC. Once the serum concentration drops below the MIC for time-dependent antibiotics, bacterial regrowth will occur, potentially resulting in therapeutic failure. Therefore, the goal with these agents should be to maximize the time of exposure. Among the time-dependent antibiotics, the goals to achieve maximum antimicrobial activity can vary greatly. For example, to maximize their antimicrobial effects, cephalosporins, penicillins, and carbapenems must spend 60% to 70%, 50%, and 40% of the dosing interval above the MIC, respectively.[14]

There are several drug classes that exhibit concentration-dependent or time-independent killing effects. For these antibiotics, maximal bactericidal activity is achieved when optimal concentrations are above the MIC. It is not dependent on how long they remain above the MIC; instead, it is dependent on the concentration achieved after a single dose. Aminoglycosides and fluoroquinolones are examples of two drug classes whose effects are concentration dependent. The peak/MIC and AUC/MIC ratios are the pharmacodynamic parameters that correlate with the efficacy of aminoglycosides and fluoroquinolones, respectively. Aminoglycosides must achieve a maximum concentration of greater than 10 times the MIC, while fluoroquinolones must achieve an AUC/MIC ratio of greater than 125.[14,15]

Table 48-2. Antibiotics and Pharmacodynamic Parameters Associated with Efficacy[14,16-20]

	Time dependent	Concentration dependent	Concentration and time dependent
Optimal PD parameter	T > MIC	C_{max}/MIC	AUC/MIC
Antibiotics	Carbapenems	Aminoglycosides	Aminoglycosides
	Cephalosporins	Daptomycin	Fluoroquinolones
	Clarithromycin	Fluoroquinolones	Glycopeptides
	Linezolid	Metronidazole	Ketolides
	Lincosamides	Polymyxins	Linezolid
	Penicillins	Quinupristin/ dalfopristin	Macrolides
			Polymyxins
			Quinupristin/dalfopristin
			Sulfamethoxazole/trimethoprim
			Tetracyclines
			Tigecycline

Abbreviations: AUC, area under the concentration curve; C_{max}, maximum concentration in serum; MIC, minimum inhibitory concentration; T > MIC, time above MIC.

Ideally, all antibiotic dosing should be determined by routine measurement of drug concentrations at the site of infection in order to ensure that the aforementioned pharmacodynamic parameters are met. Unfortunately, this is not routinely performed with all antibiotics. Serum levels are routinely monitored when aminoglycosides and glycopeptides are administered. However, there is a lack of

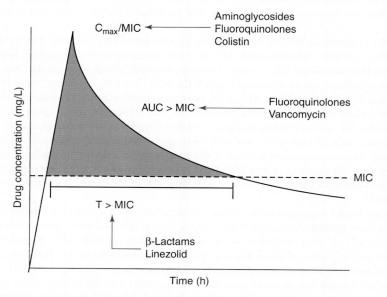

Figure 48-2. Pharmacokinetic and pharmacodynamic parameters on a concentration versus time curve. AUC, area under the serum concentration curve; C_{max}, peak serum drug concentration; MIC, minimum inhibitory concentration; T > MIC, time for which the serum concentration is above the MIC during a given dosing period.

data and experiences addressing measurable drug concentrations at all potential sites of infection. This dearth of information limits the degree to which pharmacodynamic parameters (AUC/MIC, T > MIC, C_{max}/MIC) can be calculated at the site of infection.

In addition to pharmacodynamic properties of a given antibiotic, the antibiotic spectrum of activity is extremely important. A basic understanding of a given antibiotics spectrum of activity is crucial to select an antibiotic that will cover the most likely causative pathogens from a suspected source. Failure to consider spectrum of activity can lead to an increased risk for administering IEAT, potentially increasing patient mortality rate.

What patient-specific factors need to be taken into consideration when selecting an empiric antibiotic regimen?

Patient-specific factors that need to be taken into account include drug allergies and/or intolerances, risk for resistant organisms, and concomitant disease states. Allergies to antibiotics are commonly reported in hospitalized patients. Of these reported allergies, immunoglobulin E (IgE)–mediated allergic reactions are of the most concern. Signs and symptoms of IgE-mediated reactions may include but are not limited to anaphylaxis, urticarial rash, pruritus, angioedema, hyperperistalsis, broncho spasm, hypotension, and arrhythimas.[21] Patients reporting these types of allergies to a given antibiotic or antibiotic class should receive alternative therapy with another antibiotic class that does not possess cross-reactivity. However, in circumstances where a patient has limited options and must receive a drug to which he or she is allergic, antibiotic desensitization should be conducted. Desensitization is the process of administering small amounts of drug in doubling amounts every 10 to 15 minutes until a therapeutic dose can be administered.[22] This is a time-consuming process that requires several hours before being able to administer the first full dose of an antibiotic. As was discussed previously, current data demonstrate that delays in antibiotic administration of greater than 1 hour increase mortality rates by about 7% compared to the previous hour.[4] Therefore, an alternative antibiotic class should be considered before undergoing the timely process of desensitization. Patients with a history of a non–IgE-mediated reaction to a drug should be challenged with that drug if it is the drug of choice for the given infection.

Antimicrobial resistance has become a significant problem in critically ill patients. Multiple patient-specific parameters may increase a patient's risk for developing a multidrug-resistant (MDR) infection. Infections caused by *Pseudomonas aeruginosa*, *Acinetobacter baumannii*, extended-spectrum β-lactamase (ESBL)-producing Enterobacteriaceae species, vancomycin-resistant *Enterococcus* species (VRE), and methicillin-resistant *Staphylococcus aureus* (MRSA) are of particular concern. A general list of factors that increase the risk for infection with resistant organisms is included in Table 48-3. Of note, a growing body of evidence reports that previous exposure to various antibiotics is related to the rise in infections caused by ESBL-producing Enterobacteriaceae species, VRE, and MRSA.[23,24] Initial assessment of a patient should include identification of these risk factors and consideration when selecting an empiric antibiotic regimen. Of note, antibiotics that have been administered within the past 2 weeks should be avoided in the empiric regimen as the causative organisms may have developed resistance.[2] Failure to identify patients with these risk factors increases the likelihood of providing inadequate empiric antibiotic therapy, potentially increasing the risk of mortality.

Concomitant disease states are an extremely important factor when selecting and dosing an empiric antibiotic regimen. Figure 48-3 lists disease states commonly encountered in critically ill patients and the impact on pharmacodynamic parameters and drug dosing requirements. Critical illness typically encompasses one or more of these disease states.

The most common reason antibiotics are adjusted in the critically ill is because many currently available antibiotics are renally eliminated. Common causes of reduced renal clearance include age and acute or chronic renal failure. Failure to adjust doses of renally eliminated antibiotics can result in accumulation to supra-therapeutic levels, thereby increasing the risk of concentration-dependent adverse effects. Examples of these adverse effects include seizures secondary to use of β-lactams,

Infectious Disease

Table 48-3. Risk Factors for Multidrug-Resistant (MDR) Infections

Antimicrobial therapy in the preceding 90 d
Current hospitalization of ≥ 5 d
High prevalence of resistance in community
Hospitalization of ≥ 2 d in the last 90 d
Residence in long-term care facility
Chronic hemodialysis
Home wound care
Exposure to others with MDR organisms
Immunosuppression (drug or disease related)
Chronic alcoholism
Structural lung diseases

(From Guidelines for the management of adults with hospital-acquired, ventilator-associated, and healthcare-associated pneumonia. Am J Respir Crit Care Med. 2005;171(4):388-416; and Mandell LA, Wunderink RG, Anzueto A, et al. Infectious Diseases Society of America/American Thoracic Society consensus guidelines on the management of community-acquired pneumonia in adults. Clin Infect Dis. 2007;44(Suppl 2):S27-S72.)

carbapenems, and fluoroquinolones, and further renal insult after aminoglycoside use.[25,26] Depending on the agent chosen, a reduction in dose for concentration-dependent or in dosing interval for time-dependent antibiotics may be the optimal adjustment. Another complicating factor is the initiation of hemodialysis in patients with acute or chronic renal failure. Different modes of dialysis remove

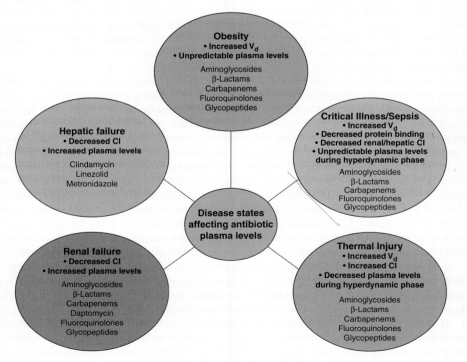

Figure 48-3. Common ICU disease states, effects on pharmacokinetic parameters, and antibiotic classes affected. Cl, clearance; V_d, volume of distribution changes.

varying amounts of drug, and therefore specific references regarding dosage adjustments should be sought out for patients in renal failure receiving hemodialysis.[27,28] It is important to assess the need for antimicrobial dosage adjustment in any patient with unstable renal function, renal dysfunction, or failure.

Much like the kidneys, the liver also plays an important role in the absorption, distribution, and elimination of many drugs. Hepatic impairment and subsequent alterations in hepatic drug clearance are much more difficult to quantify than changes in drug clearance observed with renal disease. The pharmacokinetic alterations seen in hepatic impairment are not consistent or are not well defined, making it difficult to assess the need for drug dosage adjustment. The semiquantitative Child-Pugh score can be used to assess the degree of liver dysfunction, but this only offers minimal guidance for drug adjustment as it does not take into account the ability to metabolize drugs.[29] In drugs eliminated through both renal and hepatic routes, a decrease in hepatic clearance may be partially compensated for by increases in renal clearance. Owing to large variations in pharmacokinetics in liver disease, specific dosage recommendations are generally lacking, particularly in severe liver disease. Most sources simply recommend reducing the dose without giving specific dosing recommendations, or avoiding the drug in severe hepatic disease.[30-32]

Obesity is extremely prevalent in our society today and may impact as many as one in four patients in the intensive care unit (ICU).[33] Unfortunately, there is a paucity of data regarding antibiotic dosing in patients who are obese, and even less in those who are critically ill. Obesity is most likely to affect an antibiotic's V_d, and therefore dosage adjustments may be necessary. Further complicating matters is that estimation of creatinine clearance (CrCl) is difficult in these patients as many of the calculations used for this purpose include weight. In fact, these calculations have been shown to overestimate CrCl when using total body weight (TBW) and underestimate CrCl when using ideal body weight (IBW). As a result, it is difficult to determine an appropriate antibiotic dosing regimen in obese patients.[34,35] More recent data suggest that the use of lean body weight or fat-free weight may better predict CrCl in morbidly obese patients.[36] Aminoglycoside antibiotics have the most data in regards to dosing in obesity, partially because of their narrow therapeutic index. The V_d of aminoglycosides in obese patients is increased. However, the degree of increase seen varies based on the study.[37] Dosing based on TBW tends to overshoot the desired concentration, while dosing based on IBW tends to underdose obese patients. Therefore, an adjusted body weight (ABW) calculation [ABW = IBW + 0.4 (TBW − IBW)] is typically used for dosing with close therapeutic drug monitoring. Vancomycin dosing appears to correlate best with TBW and should be dosed using this weight with careful therapeutic drug monitoring.[38] Despite β-lactams being the largest class of antibiotics, there are relatively few data for dosing in the obese patient population. Available data suggest that increased doses may be warranted for cephalosporins and penicillins.[37] The data for carbapenems are minimal, and therefore it is difficult to make dosing recommendations.[37] The data on fluoroquinolones are variable, but higher doses may be required because of their concentration-dependent activity.[37] Current data for linezolid suggest that no dosage adjustments are necessary.[39,40] Data for daptomycin suggest that it should be dosed on TBW.[41,42] While these provide us some direction on dosage requirements in obese patients, there are few data in critically ill obese patients. This makes it difficult to determine the most appropriate doses for these patients. These patients will likely require higher doses than patients of normal body weight, but to what degree is unknown.

Patients who have experienced thermal injury undergo significant changes in pharmacokinetics, resulting in dramatic increases in V_d and clearance for most antibiotics. These patients tend to have an acute phase, lasting for approximately 48 hours following injury, which is marked by increased capillary permeability and hypovolemia. These patients then enter the hyperdynamic phase of their injury with increased cardiac output, protein loss, and fluid shifts. This hyperdynamic phase varies based on the extent of injury but typically persists for 7 to 10 days.[43] For nearly all antibiotics studied, increases in dose and frequency of administration are required in patients with thermal injury.[43-46] Patients with traumatic injuries are often thought to be most similar to patients with thermal injuries in that they tend to be younger and hypermetabolic. However, there are very few studies evaluating the effects of traumatic injury on dosage requirements. The available data are highly variable, showing increased, decreased, and no change in clearances for various drugs.[13]

What infection-specific factors need to be taken into consideration when selecting an empiric antibiotic regimen?

In addition to underlying disease states and organ dysfunction, the site of infection plays a significant role in selection of an antibiotic regimen. For antimicrobials to be effective they must be able to reach the site of infection at concentrations high enough to exert their bacteriostatic or bactericidal effects. Antibiotic penetration into tissues is determined by passive diffusion, active transport, lipid solubility, molecular weight, and protein binding. These factors are of particular importance when selecting an antibiotic regimen for the treatment of meningitis, osteomyelitis, and pneumonia in particular.

In the treatment of meningitis, the degree of lipid solubility of the antibiotic must be taken into consideration. Lipid solubility is a major factor in determining an antibiotic's ability to cross the blood-brain barrier. Drugs that are lipophilic and nonpolar penetrate the cerebrospinal fluid (CSF) most readily and include fluoroquinolones, rifampin, and metronidazole.[47] β-Lactams are the antibiotic class used most frequently in the treatment of CSF infections despite the fact that they are hydrophilic and highly polarized. They are used frequently because of their wide therapeutic index and the ability of patients to tolerate large systemic doses. However, their use may be largely limited by their inability to achieve significant concentrations at the site of infection when treating infections caused by organisms with high MICs. Aminoglycosides are often also used in the treatment of CSF infections. However, intravenous therapy is discouraged due to inadequate penetration into the site of infection. In these cases, direct or local instillation into the CSF via intraventricular or intrathecal administration ensures drug delivery to the site of infection.

The treatment of osteomyelitis poses a challenge as clinical evidence is lacking and differs between the stages (acute versus chronic) and location of the infection. Data from drug penetration studies into bone matrix are evolving.[48-50] For these reasons, the treatment of osteomyelitis often requires larger than normal doses and a longer duration of treatment—often a minimum of 6 to 8 weeks. Generally antibiotics that possess a moderate to large V_d may be used to treat such invasive infections. Commonly used antibiotics include β-lactams, trimethoprim-sulfamethoxazole, clindamycin, rifamycins, and vancomycin. There is a growing body of evidence in the use of local instillation of antibiotic-impregnated cement beads with drugs such as aminoglycosides for the treatment of chronic osteomyelitis.[51-53]

Hospital-acquired pneumonia accounts for approximately 25% of all ICU-acquired infections in the United States.[2] Inadequate antimicrobial therapy has been identified as the most significant predictor of patient mortality. It is imperative that the antimicrobial treatment chosen possesses adequate lung penetration ability in order to ensure treatment success while decreasing the potential for future antibiotic resistance. Antibiotics such as β-lactams, macrolides, fluoroquinolones, linezolid, rifamycins, and trimethoprim-sulfamethoxazole penetrate well into the lungs, especially in the setting of inflammation. Drugs such as intravenous vancomycin and aminoglycosides have low to moderate penetration into the lungs and are dependent on the level of inflammation. It is therefore important to maximize the doses of these agents to avoid potential therapeutic failure and antimicrobial resistance. While daptomycin possesses a large volume of distribution, the parent compound is inactivated by lung surfactant and should not be used for the treatment of pneumonia. Optimization of these antimicrobial regimens must consider the pharmacokinetic/pharmacodynamic parameters of each antibiotic (time- versus concentration-dependent killing). Broad-spectrum agents should be administered as empiric treatment in order to prevent IEAT in a patient with MDR organisms. Culture results are usually finalized within the first 48 to 72 hours, at which time the antibiotic regimen should be de-escalated. De-escalation or narrowing the spectrum of activity and/or decreasing the number of antibiotics should be individualized and culture/pathogen guided. For recommendations on empiric and pathogen-guided therapy as well as antibiotic dosage recommendations, please refer to the guidelines published by the Infectious Diseases Society of America and the American Thoracic Society.[2]

What hospital-specific factors need to be taken into consideration when selecting an empiric antibiotic regimen?

The most important factors to take into consideration when prescribing an empiric antibiotic regimen are the patient and hospital microbiologic flora as well as local and institutional resistance patterns. This information is typically available in a hospital setting in the form of a hospital antibiogram. An antibiogram is simply a report of the antimicrobial susceptibility profile of an organism or bacterial species to a group of antimicrobial agents. Table 48-4 shows an example of a hospital antibiogram. While patient-specific cultures are pending, the antibiogram can be used to guide empirical antibiotic therapy based on the likely pathogens and the susceptibilities to anti-infectives available at a given institution. Antibiograms report data as a percent of susceptibilities and are usually updated annually to evaluate resistance trends. A common mistake encountered when interpreting the hospital antibiogram is the assumption that if two different antibiotics possess activity against 90% of *Pseudomonas aeruginosa* isolates, then the combination of both antibiotics will possess activity against 100% of these isolates. This is an incorrect assumption and the selection of the appropriate antibiotic therapy should be carefully considered. For example, looking at the antibiogram in Table 48-4, the selection of cefepime would cover 94% of *P aeruginosa* isolates and amikacin would cover 93% of these isolates. However, if given as combination therapy you can only assume that you will cover 94% of isolates as the 6% of isolates that are resistant to cefepime may also be resistant to amikacin. When used correctly to determine a patient's empiric regimen, antibiograms can be extremely helpful in minimizing inadequate empiric antibiotic therapy, but they are not without their limitations.

Table 48-4. Example of Hospital Antibiogram

Organisms	No. of Isolates	Antibiotics and Susceptibilities Reported as %						
		Amikacin	Cefepime	Ceftriaxone	Ciprofloxacin	Imipenem/ Cilastatin	Piperacillin/ Tazobactam	Tobramycin
Acinetobacter baumannii	13	100	17	0	25	85		100
Enterobacter cloacae	19	100	100	84	84	100	89	100
Escherichia coli	58	100	90	90	55	100	98	88
Klebsiella pneumoniae	73	57	64	61	61	87	75	61
Pseudomonas aeruginosa	62	93	94	0	77	84	94	88

Infectious Disease

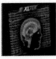

Immediately following the BAL an empiric antibiotic regimen of cefepime 2 g intravenously (IV) every 12 hours, ciprofloxacin 400 mg IV every 8 hours, and vancomycin 1750 mg IV every 12 hours is started. Over the next few days J.L.'s clinical condition continues to worsen. On the morning of hospital day 8, examination findings include the following: temperature, 39.4°C; white blood cell count, 25.8 cells/mm^3; BP, 80/40 mm Hg; HR, 105 bpm; ABG on 80% FIO$_2$, positive end-expiratory pressure (PEEP) 10 cm H$_2$O (PaO$_2$, 60 mm Hg; PacO$_2$, 50 mm Hg; HCO$_3^-$, 28 mEq/L; and pH, 7.2). He has received 4 L of normal saline over the last 2 hours; however, he remains hypotensive. Your preliminary BAL results show *P aeruginosa* 100,000 colony-forming units/mL with susceptibilities pending.

Later in the day the susceptibilities for the *P. aeruginosa* species isolated on BAL are available and are reported as follows (where S, sensitive; R, resistant; I, intermediate):

Antibiotic	Minimum inhibitory concentration	Susceptibility
Amikacin	16	S
Aztreonam	32	R
Cefepime	32	R
Ciprofloxacin	4	R
Imipenem/cilastatin	4	S
Piperacillin/tazobactam	32	I
Tobramycin	16	R

How do you evaluate an antibiotic susceptibility panel and select the most appropriate therapy?

An antibiotic susceptibility panel is a report provided by the microbiology laboratory. A susceptibility panel will commonly include a selection of antibiotics, the MIC against the isolated organism, and susceptibility to that antibiotic. Once a causative organism is identified, it is imperative that the patient receive an antibiotic regimen to which the organism is sensitive. This may require modification of the initial empiric regimen. Often times you must wait for susceptibilities to be finalized by the laboratory before adjusting your empiric regimen. The susceptibilities are determined by comparing the concentrations to the established MIC breakpoints set by the US Food and Drug Administration and Clinical Labs Standards Institute. These susceptibilities are then reported as sensitive, intermediate, or resistant. If an organism is resistant to a listed antibiotic, the use of it will result in therapeutic failure and should be avoided. If an organism is reported to be intermediate, successful eradication of the infection will be largely dependent on the location of the infection and the ability to achieve that concentration at the site. In general, antibiotics that are reported as having intermediate activity should be avoided.

When an organism is reported as being susceptible to an antibiotic, the MIC should be evaluated. Treatment success is dependent on whether the chosen antibiotic can achieve concentrations above the MIC at the site of infection. However, one cannot simply compare the MICs between antibiotics and choose the one with the lowest MIC. For example, in the above susceptibility panel example, both imipenem/cilastatin and amikacin were tested for susceptibility against *P aeruginosa* and the reported MICs were 4 μg/mL and 16 μg/mL, respectively. One cannot assume imipenem/cilastatin is the better option simply because the MIC is lower. Each organism has a different MIC breakpoint and therefore a different threshold for resistance to tested antibiotics. Instead, one should compare the MICs of the isolated organism to the known MIC breakpoints for an antibiotic. This information is typically found along with the antibiogram. An example of MIC breakpoints can be found in Table 48-5. Rather than directly comparing the concentrations, a better method would be to compare how many dilutions the MIC is from its respective breakpoint. The closer the MIC is to its breakpoint, the less favorable the antibiotic option.

Once susceptibilities have been reported, the next step is to evaluate the appropriateness of the antibiotic therapy. It is at this point that the decision should be made to either broaden or narrow therapy as indicated. There are many situations in which broad-spectrum antibiotics should be continued—particularly when the source of the infection is not identified or controlled. However, it is important to consider that one of the leading causes of antimicrobial resistance is the inappropriate continuation of broad-spectrum antibiotics and failure to narrow therapy when a susceptibility panel

Table 48-5. MIC Breakpoints for Commonly Used Antibiotics

Antibiotic	Organism	2009 MIC Breakpoints (μg/mL)		
		S	I	R
Amikacin	GNR	≤16	32	≥64
Ampicillin	Enterococci	≤8	–	≥16
	Haemophilus spp	≤1	2	≥4
Ampicillin/sulbactam	GNR	≤8/4	16/8	≥32/16
Cefazolin	GNR/*Staphylococcus* spp	≤8	16	≥32
Cefepime	GNR	≤8	16	≥32
Ceftriaxone	GNR	≤8	16-32	≥64
	Streptococcus pneumoniae (meningitis)	≤0.5	1	≥2
	S pneumoniae	≤1	2	≥4
	Haemophilus spp	≤2	–	–
Imipenem	GNR	≤4	8	≥16
Levofloxacin	GNR	≤2	4	≥8
Linezolid	Staph spp	≤4	–	–
	Enterococci	≤2	4	≥8
Penicillin	*S pneumoniae* (CSF)	≤0.06	–	≥0.12
	S pneumoniae (non-CSF infection)	≤2	4	≥8
Piperacillin/tazobactam	GNR	≤16/4	32/4-64/4	≥128/4
Tobramycin	GNR	≤4	8	≥16
Vancomycin	*Staphylococcus aureus*	≤2	4-8	≥16
	Enterococci	≤4	8-16	≥32

Abbreviations: GNR, gram-negative rod; I, intermediate; MIC, minimum inhibitory concentration; R, resistant; S, sensitive.

Infectious Disease

is available. Narrowing of therapy, also referred to as de-escalation, is often defined as switching to a regimen with a narrower spectrum of activity or decreasing the total number of antibiotics. This approach to antibiotic therapy can also help in decreasing the development of future infection with MDR organisms.[54,55]

In the above patient case, *P aeruginosa* was isolated, which was sensitive to only amikacin and imipenem/cilastatin. When comparing the MICs of the isolated organism to the known breakpoints for those drugs, the isolate had an MIC to amikacin of 16, which is 1 dilution from being intermediate (32), while the MIC to imipenem was 4, which is also 1 dilution from being intermediate (8). To ensure treatment success and decrease the development of antimicrobial resistance, antibiotic concentrations must reach at least the MIC, but preferentially four to five times the MIC, at the site of infection. These concentrations are not only difficult to quantify but they will also be difficult to achieve as high concentrations increase the risk for drug-related toxicities. The choice between imipenem/cilastatin and amikacin should be made based on patient-specific factors such as drug allergies, intolerances, drug interactions, and organ dysfunction and the ability of the chosen agent to adequately penetrate the site of infection.

With high-MIC organisms, how can you maximize the drugs' bactericidal effects?

Inadequate dosing and inappropriate and/or untimely administration of antibiotics are known risk factors for the increase in mortality rate observed in critically ill patients.[11,56] Increasing antibiotic resistance in recent years has led to a renewed interest in ways to maximize the pharmacodynamic parameters of antibiotics.[17,57-59] Areas of interest and research have included once-daily dosing of aminoglycosides, prolonged and continuous infusions of time-dependent antibiotics, and aerosolized antibiotics. Pharmacodynamics is influencing the mode of administration for both time- and concentration-dependent antibiotics. For time-dependent antibiotics, several studies have demonstrated continuous (total daily dose administered over 24 hours) or extended infusion (intermittent dose administered over 3-4 hours) as alternative dosing schemes for β-lactams.[60-64] These dosing schemes recommend an initial loading dose prior to the continuous or extended-interval infusion. The initial loading dose is given to increase the probability of attaining the pharmacodynamic target sooner. Population studies of pharmacokinetics and distribution of MIC values have demonstrated a higher probability of achieving the goal percentage of time above the MIC with continuous or extended infusions when compared to the conventional 30- or 60-minute intermittent infusions at similar daily doses. Attaining consistent concentrations above the MIC has been shown to correlate to better clinical cure rates as demonstrated by several retrospective reviews conducted by Lorente et al. These studies suggested that continuous infusions of meropenem, ceftazidime, and piperacillin/tazobactam resulted in higher clinical cure rates in patients with ventilator-associated pneumonia due to gram-negative bacilli compared to when these same agents were given intermittently (30-minute infusions).[65,66] Limitations to the continuous or extended-interval administration include drug-drug compatibility, intravenous access, and drug stability at room temperature.

For concentration-dependent antibiotics, namely, aminoglycosides, once-daily administration of these agents is also guided by pharmacodynamic concepts.[67,68] Maximal concentration achieved above the MIC ($C_{max} > MIC$) or the AUC/MIC ratio ensures optimal bactericidal activity when these antibiotics are administered once daily (eg, tobramycin 5-7 mg/kg daily) compared to the conventional thrice-daily dosing (eg, tobramycin 2 mg/kg q8h). Once-daily administration of aminoglycosides does not pose a greater risk for toxicities, specifically nephrotoxicity and ototoxicity, compared to the conventional dosing scheme. The clinical efficacy of once-daily aminoglycosides has been demonstrated in a variety of different patient populations including those with intra-abdominal infections, pneumonia, and bacteremia. However, patient populations such as those with significant and/or unpredictable alterations in pharmacokinetic parameters of volume of distribution and drug clearance have not been adequately studied. These populations include patients receiving renal replacement therapy; patients with renal failure, ascites, or burns; pregnant women; and neonatal/pediatric patients.[67,68]

These modes of administration allow for optimization of microbiologic coverage, and thus the practical and cost advantages of their applications are important for treating complex infections (eg, severe nosocomial pneumonia) involving difficult-to-treat organisms with higher MIC values (eg, *P aeruginosa*, *Acinetobacter* species).[69,70]

Local instillation of antibiotics, namely via aerosolization, plays a unique role in the treatment of MDR organisms. Aerosolized antibiotics (eg, aminoglycosides, colistin) distribute almost exclusively into the lungs with minimal systemic exposure. Most of the literature on the clinical utility of aerosolized antibiotics exists in patients with cystic fibrosis. However, there is a growing body of evidence in their utility for the adjunctive treatment of ventilator-associated pneumonia. The current Infectious Diseases Society of America and American Thoracic Society pneumonia guidelines recommend considering adjunctive aerosolized antibiotic therapy when treating MDR pathogens, most commonly *P aeruginosa* and *A baumannii*.[2] A recent retrospective study of aerosolized aminoglycosides and colistin, in addition to intravenous therapy, had a notable clinical response (73%) in critically ill trauma patients with MDR ventilator-associated pneumonia.[71] In addition, several other case series of aerosolized antibiotics have reported high levels of clinical success with difficult-to-treat infections.[72-74]

Because of the highly resistant strain of *P aeruginosa* that was isolated in the patient case, the ability to maximize your pharmacodynamic target for imipenem (T > MIC) with traditional dosing would be difficult, if not impossible. If traditional dosing were chosen for this patient, it would not be unreasonable to select the highest dose of imipenem/cilastatin approved per the package insert (1000 mg IV q6h) in an attempt to maximize the T > MIC. Another option in this patient would be to give imipenem as a 1-g loading dose followed by either a continuous infusion of 2 g over 24 hours or inter-mittent prolonged infusions of 1 g over 3 to 4 hours given every 8 hours. In general, aminoglycosides should never be used as monotherapy for gram-negative infections. However, due to the high MIC to amikacin and the relatively poor penetration of aminoglycosides into the lung, IV amikacin would likely be of little benefit owing to an inability to maximize the pharmacodynamic goal (C_{max}/MIC).

Once the antibiotic sensitivities are reported, is coverage with two antibiotics active against the organism still necessary?

As previously discussed, the practice of administering an empiric antibiotic regimen containing more than one antibiotic with activity against a given organism to minimize the risk of IEAT is a widely utilized practice. Empiric double coverage is of particular benefit when infections due to *P aeruginosa* or other nosocomial pathogens are suspected. However, once the susceptibility profile is available, the use of more than one antibiotic with activity against the causative organism is a topic of much debate. The argument for the use of combination therapy is based on two potential benefits: synergy against the causative organism and prevention of the development of resistance. However, these arguments are based primarily on in vitro results, which cannot be assumed to also occur in vivo. Potential disadvantages of the continued use of combination therapy include the possibility for antagonism, increased cost, and adverse effects, as well as potential for selection of MDR bacteria.

Numerous studies have compared monotherapy to combination therapy with varied results. In an effort to control for the differences between these studies, several meta-analyses have been conducted. The largest of these meta-analyses included 64 studies comparing β-lactam monotherapy with β-lactam/aminoglycoside combination therapy in the treatment of sepsis. The authors demonstrated no differences in mortality outcomes between the treatment groups. However, monotherapy resulted in significantly less nephrotoxicity.[75] A meta-analysis evaluating the same question in ventilator-associated pneumonia demonstrated similar results with no mortality rate differences between monotherapy and combination therapy.[76] Despite these meta-analyses, some practitioners will continue to treat specific organisms (*P aeruginosa*) and infections (endocarditis) with combination therapy. Various guideline recommendations actually make differing recommendations on continued combination therapy after organism identification based on site and causative organism. Therefore, current guideline recommendations should be referenced when deciding on monotherapy or combination therapy at this stage in treatment.[2,8-10,77] In general, once a causative organism is identified, monotherapy based on the susceptibility profile is adequate for most patients and most infections. Patients who would be the most likely to benefit from continued combination therapy are patients with MDR infections or those with infections due to high MIC organisms where the susceptible antibiotics have limited penetration into the site of infection. However, there are few available data to support this practice.

In the patient case discussed above, the causative organism for the ventilator-associated pneumonia was an MDR *P aeruginosa* susceptible to only amikacin and imipenem/cilastatin. In this patient it would be reasonable to consider combination intravenous therapy because both drugs have limited penetration into the lung parenchyma and the MIC for the organism is relatively high. This limited penetration could potentially result in an increased risk for clinical failure with antibiotic monotherapy. To overcome this limited penetration you would likely need to give very high doses of IV amikacin, potentially increasing the risk of nephrotoxicity and ototoxicity associated with this drug. Adjunctive therapy with aerosolized amikacin at a dose of 1000 mg inhaled every 12 hours would provide not only local delivery of drug to the site of infection but also double coverage while potentially limiting the risk of systemic adverse effects.

What is the optimal duration of antibiotic therapy?

The optimal duration of antibiotic treatment is highly variable based on the site of infection, the causative organism, concomitant disease states, and the patient's clinical response to therapy. Guideline-recommended treatment durations range from as little as 3 days in asymptomatic catheter-associated urinary tract infections to as many as 8 weeks for some etiologies of endocarditis.[77,78] Traditionally the majority of these recommendations for optimal duration are based on expert opinions rather than data supporting one duration over another. For example, the traditional duration of therapy for pneumonia was 14 to 21 days. However, recent data demonstrated that as few as 8 days of therapy results in therapeutic resolution without any differences in mortality rate, ventilator-free days, or recurrent infections compared to 15 days of therapy. In addition, patients who received 15 days of therapy had higher rates of recurrent infections due to more resistant organisms. Similar data are available for selected forms of endocarditis as well. It is important to realize that these durations are simply starting points and that each individual patient may respond differently and require shorter or longer durations of therapy.

! CRITICAL CONSIDERATIONS

- Prior to antibiotic initiation, samples for culture should be drawn from all suspected sources provided it does not delay time to antibiotic delivery.
- Time from suspicion of infection to delivery of antibiotics should be minimized to decrease infection-related mortality rate.
- Numerous patient-, hospital-, infection-, and drug-specific factors should be taken into consideration when selecting an appropriate empiric antibiotic regimen.
- Pharmacokinetics is the processes of absorption, distribution, metabolism, and elimination.
- Pharmacodynamics is the relationship between drug concentrations and pharmacologic effects.

- Critical illness leads to numerous pharmacokinetic and dynamic changes in patients, affecting responses to antibiotics.
- Different classes of antibiotics have different pharmacodynamic parameters correlating with efficacy, and a basic understanding of these is required to select the most appropriate regimen.
- Patients with IgE-mediated allergic reactions (eg, anaphylaxis, urticarial rash, angioedema, hyperperistalsis, etc.) to a given antibiotic can undergo antibiotic desensitization if necessary. However, alternative agents should be considered first, as desensitization can be a time-consuming and expensive process.
- Antibiotic resistance is a widespread problem and all patients should be assessed for risks of infection with an MDR organism.
- Renal failure, liver failure, obesity, traumatic injury, thermal injury, and sepsis can all affect antibiotic dosage requirements in patients.
- Antibiotic penetration into the site of infection needs to be considered when selecting an appropriate antibiotic. This is of particular importance in the treatment of meningitis, osteomyelitis, and pneumonia.
- Every hospital has different bacterial flora with different susceptibilities. Therefore, a hospital-specific antibiogram should be utilized when selecting an empiric regimen.
- Susceptibility profiles should be utilized to narrow or broaden therapy as necessary.
- MICs reported on a susceptibility profile cannot be compared to one another, but must be compared to the standard (MIC breakpoint) for that drug.
- Continuous infusions, prolonged intermittent infusions, or locally instilled antibiotics are all potential methods to maximize the pharmacodynamic properties of a given antibiotic.
- Upon identification of an organism, continued coverage with two antibiotics to which the organism is susceptible is a topic of much debate. Expert panel recommendations vary based on infection.
- Data supporting the optimal duration of antibiotics are unknown for most infectious diseases and therefore should be based on infection and patient response to therapy.

Infectious Disease

REFERENCES

1. Souweine B, Veber B, Bedos JP, et al. Diagnostic accuracy of protected specimen brush and bronchoalveolar lavage in nosocomial pneumonia: impact of previous antimicrobial treatments. *Crit Care Med.* 1998;26(2):236-244.
2. Guidelines for the management of adults with hospital-acquired, ventilator-associated, and healthcare-associated pneumonia. *Am J Respir Crit Care Med.* 2005;171(4):388-416.
3. Chastre J, Wolff M, Fagon JY, et al. Comparison of 8 vs 15 days of antibiotic therapy for ventilator-associated pneumonia in adults: a randomized trial. *JAMA.* 2003;290(19):2588-2598.
4. Kumar A, Roberts D, Wood KE, et al. Duration of hypotension before initiation of effective antimicrobial therapy is the critical determinant of survival in human septic shock. *Crit Care Med.* 2006;34(6):1589-1596.
5. Meehan TP, Fine MJ, Krumholz HM, et al. Quality of care, process, and outcomes in elderly patients with pneumonia. *JAMA.* 1997;278(23):2080-2084.
6. Vergis EN, Hayden MK, Chow JW, et al. Determinants of vancomycin resistance and mortality rates in enterococcal bacteremia: a prospective multicenter study. *Ann Intern Med.* 2001;135(7):484-492.
7. Miner JR, Heegaard W, Mapes A, Biros M. Presentation, time to antibiotics, and mortality of patients

with bacterial meningitis at an urban county medical center. *J Emerg Med.* 2001;21(4):387-392.

8. Dellinger RP, Levy MM, Carlet JM, et al. Surviving Sepsis Campaign: international guidelines for management of severe sepsis and septic shock: 2008. *Crit Care Med.* 2008;36(1):296-327.

9. Mandell LA, Wunderink RG, Anzueto A, et al. Infectious Diseases Society of America/American Thoracic Society consensus guidelines on the management of community-acquired pneumonia in adults. *Clin Infect Dis.* 2007;44(Suppl 2): S27-S72.

10. Tunkel AR, Hartman BJ, Kaplan SL, et al. Practice guidelines for the management of bacterial meningitis. *Clin Infect Dis.* 2004;39(9):1267-1284.

11. Kollef MH, Sherman G, Ward S, Fraser VJ. Inadequate antimicrobial treatment of infections: a risk factor for hospital mortality among critically ill patients. *Chest.* 1999;115(2):462-474.

12. Ibrahim EH, Sherman G, Ward S, Fraser VJ, Kollef MH. The influence of inadequate antimicrobial treatment of bloodstream infections on patient outcomes in the ICU setting. *Chest.* 2000;118(1):146-155.

13. Boucher BA, Wood GC, Swanson JM. Pharmacokinetic changes in critical illness. *Crit Care Clin.* 2006;22(2):255-271, vi.

14. Roberts JA, Lipman J. Pharmacokinetic issues for antibiotics in the critically ill patient. *Crit Care Med.* 2009;37(3):840-851; quiz 59.

15. Lodise TP, Lomaestro BM, Drusano GL. Application of antimicrobial pharmacodynamic concepts into clinical practice: focus on beta-lactam antibiotics: insights from the Society of Infectious Diseases Pharmacists. *Pharmacotherapy.* 2006;26(9): 1320-1332.

16. Maglio D, Nicolau DP, Nightingale CH. Impact of pharmacodynamics on dosing of macrolides, azalides, and ketolides. *Infect Dis Clin North Am.* 2003;17(3):563-577, vi.

17. Craig WA. Basic pharmacodynamics of antibacterials with clinical applications to the use of beta-lactams, glycopeptides, and linezolid. *Infect Dis Clin North Am.* 2003;17(3):479-501.

18. Nation RL, Li J. Colistin in the 21st century. *Curr Opin Infect Dis.* 2009;22(6):535-543.

19. Ambrose PG, Bhavnani SM, Owens RC Jr. Clinical pharmacodynamics of quinolones. *Infect Dis Clin North Am.* 2003;17(3):529-543.

20. Wisell KT, Kahlmeter G, Giske CG. Trimethoprim and enterococci in urinary tract infections: new perspectives on an old issue. *J Antimicrob Chemother.* 2008;62(1):35-40.

21. Robinson JL, Hameed T, Carr S. Practical aspects of choosing an antibiotic for patients with a

reported allergy to an antibiotic. *Clin Infect Dis.* 2002;35(1):26-31.

22. Castells M. Rapid desensitization for hypersensitivity reactions to medications. *Immunol Allergy Clin North Am.* 2009;29(3):585-606.

23. Falagas ME, Karageorgopoulos DE. Extended-spectrum beta-lactamase-producing organisms. *J Hosp Infect.* 2009;73(4):345-354.

24. Charbonneau P, Parienti JJ, Thibon P, et al. Fluoroquinolone use and methicillin-resistant *Staphylococcus aureus* isolation rates in hospitalized patients: a quasi experimental study. *Clin Infect Dis.* 2006;42(6):778-784.

25. Wallace KL. Antibiotic-induced convulsions. *Crit Care Clin.* 1997;13(4):741-762.

26. Rougier F, Claude D, Maurin M, Maire P. Aminoglycoside nephrotoxicity. *Curr Drug Targets Infect Disord.* 2004;4(2):153-162.

27. Heintz BH, Matzke GR, Dager WE. Antimicrobial dosing concepts and recommendations for critically ill adult patients receiving continuous renal replacement therapy or intermittent hemodialysis. *Pharmacotherapy.* 2009;29(5):562-577.

28. Trotman RL, Williamson JC, Shoemaker DM, Salzer WL. Antibiotic dosing in critically ill adult patients receiving continuous renal replacement therapy. *Clin Infect Dis.* 2005;41(8):1159-1166.

29. Pugh RN, Murray-Lyon IM, Dawson JL, Pietroni MC, Williams R. Transection of the oesophagus for bleeding oesophageal varices. *Br J Surg.* 1973;60(8):646-649.

30. Lau AH, Evans R, Chang CW, Seligsohn R. Pharmacokinetics of metronidazole in patients with alcoholic liver disease. *Antimicrob Agents Chemother.* 1987;31(11):1662-1664.

31. *Zyvox [package insert].* New York: Pharmacia & Upjohn Company; 2008.

32. Avant GR, Schenker S, Alford RH. The effect of cirrhosis on the disposition and elimination of clindamycin. *Am J Dig Dis.* 1975;20(3):223-230.

33. Joffe A, Wood K. Obesity in critical care. *Curr Opin Anaesthesiol* 2007;20(2):113-118.

34. Snider RD, Kruse JA, Bander JJ, Dunn GH. Accuracy of estimated creatinine clearance in obese patients with stable renal function in the intensive care unit. *Pharmacotherapy.* 1995;15(6):747-753.

35. Spinler SA, Nawarskas JJ, Boyce EG, Connors JE, Charland SL, Goldfarb S. Predictive performance of ten equations for estimating creatinine clearance in cardiac patients. Iohexol Cooperative Study Group. *Ann Pharmacother.* 1998;32(12):1275-1283.

36. Demirovic JA, Pai AB, Pai MP. Estimation of creatinine clearance in morbidly obese patients. *Am J Health Syst Pharm.* 2009;66(7):642-648.

37. Pai MP, Bearden DT. Antimicrobial dosing considerations in obese adult patients. *Pharmacotherapy.* 2007;27(8):1081-1091.

38. Rybak M, Lomaestro B, Rotschafer JC, et al. Therapeutic monitoring of vancomycin in adult patients: a consensus review of the American Society of Health-System Pharmacists, the Infectious Diseases Society of America, and the Society of Infectious Diseases Pharmacists. *Am J Health Syst Pharm.* 2009;66(1):82-98.

39. Meagher AK, Forrest A, Rayner CR, Birmingham MC, Schentag JJ. Population pharmacokinetics of linezolid in patients treated in a compassionate-use program. *Antimicrob Agents Chemother.* 2003; 47(2):548-553.

40. Stein GE, Schooley SL, Peloquin CA, et al. Pharmacokinetics and pharmacodynamics of linezolid in obese patients with cellulitis. *Ann Pharmacother.* 2005;39(3):427-432.

41. Dvorchik BH, Damphousse D. The pharmacokinetics of daptomycin in moderately obese, morbidly obese, and matched nonobese subjects. *J Clin Pharmacol.* 2005;45(1):48-56.

42. Pai MP, Norenberg JP, Anderson T, et al. Influence of morbid obesity on the single-dose pharmacokinetics of daptomycin. *Antimicrob Agents Chemother.* 2007;51(8):2741-2747.

43. Boucher BA, Kuhl DA, Hickerson WL. Pharmacokinetics of systemically administered antibiotics in patients with thermal injury. *Clin Infect Dis.* 1992;14(2):458-463.

44. McKinnon PS, Davis SL. Pharmacokinetic and pharmacodynamic issues in the treatment of bacterial infectious diseases. *Eur J Clin Microbiol Infect Dis.* 2004;23(4):271-288.

45. Mohr JF 3rd, Ostrosky-Zeichner L, Wainright DJ, Parks DH, Hollenbeck TC, Ericsson CD. Pharmacokinetic evaluation of single-dose intravenous daptomycin in patients with thermal burn injury. *Antimicrob Agents Chemother.* 2008;52(5):1891-1893.

46. Lovering AM, Le Floch R, Hovsepian L, et al. Pharmacokinetic evaluation of linezolid in patients with major thermal injuries. *J Antimicrob Chemother.* 2009;63(3):553-559.

47. Andes DR, Craig WA. Pharmacokinetics and pharmacodynamics of antibiotics in meningitis. *Infect Dis Clin North Am.* 1999;13(3):595-618.

48. Schintler MV, Traunmuller F, Metzler J, et al. High fosfomycin concentrations in bone and peripheral soft tissue in diabetic patients presenting with bacterial foot infection. *J Antimicrob Chemother.* 2009;64(3):574-578.

49. Yin LY, Calhoun JH, Thomas TS, Wirtz ED. Efficacy of telavancin in the treatment of methicillin-resistant *Staphylococcus aureus* osteomyelitis: studies with a rabbit model. *J Antimicrob Chemother.* 2009;63(2):357-360.

50. Rasyid HN, van der Mei HC, Frijlink HW, et al. Concepts for increasing gentamicin release from handmade bone cement beads. *Acta Orthop.* 2009;80(5):508-513.

51. Dagum AB, Park DJ, Lau KN, Khan SU. Antibiotic-impregnated polymethylmethacrylate beads and cement in the treatment of posttraumatic infections of the frontal sinus. *Plast Reconstr Surg.* 2009;123(6):193e-194e.

52. Sancineto CF, Barla JD. Treatment of long bone osteomyelitis with a mechanically stable intramedullar antibiotic dispenser: nineteen consecutive cases with a minimum of 12 months follow-up. *J Trauma.* 2008;65(6):1416-1420.

53. Efstathopoulos N, Giamarellos-Bourboulis E, Kanellakopoulou K, et al. Treatment of experimental osteomyelitis by methicillin resistant *Staphylococcus aureus* with bone cement system releasing grepafloxacin. *Injury.* 2008;39(12):1384-1390.

54. Niederman MS. De-escalation therapy in ventilator-associated pneumonia. *Curr Opin Crit Care.* 2006;12(5):452-457.

55. Ibrahim EH, Ward S, Sherman G, Schaiff R, Fraser VJ, Kollef MH. Experience with a clinical guideline for the treatment of ventilator-associated pneumonia. *Crit Care Med.* 2001;29(6):1109-1115.

56. Pea F, Viale P. Bench-to-bedside review: appropriate antibiotic therapy in severe sepsis and septic shock–does the dose matter? *Crit Care.* 2009;13(3):214.

57. Nicasio AM, Kuti JL, Nicolau DP. The current state of multidrug-resistant gram-negative bacilli in North America. *Pharmacotherapy.* 2008;28(2):235-249.

58. Craig WA. Interrelationship between pharmacokinetics and pharmacodynamics in determining dosage regimens for broad-spectrum cephalosporins. *Diagn Microbiol Infect Dis.* 1995; 22(1-2):89-96.

59. Ambrose PG, Bhavnani SM, Rubino CM, et al. Pharmacokinetics-pharmacodynamics of antimicrobial therapy: it's not just for mice anymore. *Clin Infect Dis.* 2007;44(1):79-86.

60. Craig WA. Pharmacokinetic/pharmacodynamic parameters: rationale for antibacterial dosing of mice and men. *Clin Infect Dis.* 1998;26(1):1-10; quiz 1-2.

61. Burgess DS, Frei CR. Comparison of beta-lactam regimens for the treatment of gram-negative pulmonary infections in the intensive care unit based on pharmacokinetics/pharmacodynamics. *J Antimicrob Chemother.* 2005;56(5):893-898.

Infectious Disease

62. Lorente L, Lorenzo L, Martin MM, Jimenez A, Mora ML. Meropenem by continuous versus intermittent infusion in ventilator-associated pneumonia due to gram-negative bacilli. *Ann Pharmacother.* 2006;40(2):219-223.

63. Kasiakou SK, Lawrence KR, Choulis N, Falagas ME. Continuous versus intermittent intravenous administration of antibacterials with time-dependent action: a systematic review of pharmacokinetic and pharmacodynamic parameters. *Drugs.* 2005;65(17):2499-2511.

64. Roberts JA, Paratz J, Paratz E, Krueger WA, Lipman J. Continuous infusion of beta-lactam antibiotics in severe infections: a review of its role. *Int J Antimicrob Agents.* 2007;30(1):11-18.

65. Lorente L, Jimenez A, Palmero S, et al. Comparison of clinical cure rates in adults with ventilator-associated pneumonia treated with intravenous ceftazidime administered by continuous or intermittent infusion: a retrospective, nonrandomized, open-label, historical chart review. *Clin Ther.* 2007;29(11):2433-2439.

66. Lorente L, Jimenez A, Martin MM, Iribarren JL, Jimenez JJ, Mora ML. Clinical cure of ventilator-associated pneumonia treated with piperacillin/tazobactam administered by continuous or intermittent infusion. *Int J Antimicrob Agents.* 2009;33(5):464-468.

67. Freeman CD, Nicolau DP, Belliveau PP, Nightingale CH. Once-daily dosing of aminoglycosides: review and recommendations for clinical practice. *J Antimicrob Chemother.* 1997;39(6):677-686.

68. Nicolau DP, Freeman CD, Belliveau PP, Nightingale CH, Ross JW, Quintiliani R. Experience with a once-daily aminoglycoside program administered to 2,184 adult patients. *Antimicrob Agents Chemother.* 1995;39(3):650-655.

69. Florea NR, Kotapati S, Kuti JL, Geissler EC, Nightingale CH, Nicolau DP. Cost analysis of continuous versus intermittent infusion of piperacillin-tazobactam: a time-motion study. *Am J Health Syst Pharm.* 2003;60(22):2321-2327.

70. Richerson MA, Ambrose PG, Bui KQ, et al. Pharmacokinetic and pharmacoeconomic evaluation of piperacillin/tazobactam administered as either continuous or intermittent infusion with once-daily gentamicin. *Infect Dis Clin Pract.* 1999;8:195-200.

71. Czosnowski QA, Wood GC, Magnotti LJ, et al. Adjunctive aerosolized antibiotics for treatment of ventilator-associated pneumonia. *Pharmacotherapy.* 2009;29(9):1054-1060.

72. Kwa AL, Loh C, Low JG, Kurup A, Tam VH. Nebulized colistin in the treatment of pneumonia due to multidrug-resistant *Acinetobacter baumannii* and *Pseudomonas aeruginosa. Clin Infect Dis.* 2005;41(5):754-757.

73. Berlana D, Llop JM, Fort E, Badia MB, Jodar R. Use of colistin in the treatment of multiple-drug-resistant gram-negative infections. *Am J Health Syst Pharm.* 2005;62(1):39-47.

74. Mohr AM, Sifri ZC, Horng HS, et al. Use of aerosolized aminoglycosides in the treatment of Gram-negative ventilator-associated pneumonia. *Surg Infect (Larchmt).* 2007;8(3):349-357.

75. Paul M, Silbiger I, Grozinsky S, Soares-Weiser K, Leibovici L. Beta lactam antibiotic monotherapy versus beta lactam-aminoglycoside antibiotic combination therapy for sepsis. *Cochrane Database Syst Rev.* 2006;(1):CD003344.

76. Aarts MA, Hancock JN, Heyland D, McLeod RS, Marshall JC. Empiric antibiotic therapy for suspected ventilator-associated pneumonia: a systematic review and meta-analysis of randomized trials. *Crit Care Med.* 2008;36(1):108-117.

77. Baddour LM, Wilson WR, Bayer AS, et al. Infective endocarditis: diagnosis, antimicrobial therapy, and management of complications: a statement for healthcare professionals from the Committee on Rheumatic Fever, Endocarditis, and Kawasaki Disease, Council on Cardiovascular Disease in the Young, and the Councils on Clinical Cardiology, Stroke, and Cardiovascular Surgery and Anesthesia, American Heart Association: endorsed by the Infectious Diseases Society of America. *Circulation.* 2005;111(23):e394-e434.

78. Hooton TM, Bradley SF, Cardenas DD, et al. Diagnosis, prevention, and treatment of catheter-associated urinary tract infection in adults: 2009 international clinical practice guidelines from the Infectious Diseases Society of America. *Clin Infect Dis.* 2010;50:625-663.

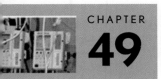

CHAPTER

49

Catheter-Related Bloodstream Infections

Rose Kim, MD
Daniel K. Meyer, MD
Annette C. Reboli, MD

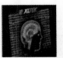

A 69-year-old man with a history of diabetes mellitus, hypertension, coronary artery disease, and ventricular arrhythmias was admitted after a witnessed collapse at home. The patient underwent cardiac resuscitation and intubation by emergency medical services (EMS); upon admission he was found to have an inferior wall myocardial infarction. There was also some concern that the patient had seizure activity noted upon arrival in the emergency department. He underwent cardiac catheterization and was found to have diffuse three-vessel disease, with a 90% occlusion in the posterolateral (PL) segment of the right coronary artery (RCA). He underwent successful coronary angioplasty of the RCA lesion and was transferred to the intensive care unit (ICU) for further monitoring. A right internal jugular central venous catheter (CVC) and right radial arterial line were placed on hospital day 2. On hospital day 5 the patient was noted to have fever, with his temperature measured as high as 39.3°C (102.7°F), and tachycardia. He remained normotensive. Cultures were obtained, including two sets of blood cultures drawn within 10 minutes of each other. One set of blood cultures was drawn peripherally, and one set was drawn through the CVC. Broad-spectrum antibiotics, including vancomycin and cefepime, were started empirically. Within 6 hours, the microbiology lab reported positive growth from one of the two bottles that was drawn via the CVC.

Given this clinical scenario, how would you go about diagnosing catheter-related bloodstream infection (CRBSI)?

Positive microbiologic results of paired blood cultures drawn from the CVC and peripheral vein support the diagnosis of CRBSI, with particular emphasis on the differential time to positivity. CVC catheter tip cultures showing the same organism as found in the blood are also useful in identifying the line as the source of bloodstream infection.[1]

The differential diagnosis for infections causing fever in the ICU setting is broad, and CRBSIs are the third most common infection diagnosed in the ICU, following pneumonia and sinusitis.[2] About 5% of patients with central venous catheters develop CRBSIs, and the incidence increases with the duration of catheter use and number of lumens.

Diagnosis of CRBSI includes both examination of the catheter site, looking for overt signs of infection such as purulence, erythema, or tenderness, and the use of blood cultures.[3] Blood cultures must always be obtained before initiating antimicrobial therapy, one set from the catheter and one from a peripheral vein. The blood culture sets must be labeled with the source and time to assist in diagnosis. In CRBSI, the cultures drawn from the

Infectious Disease

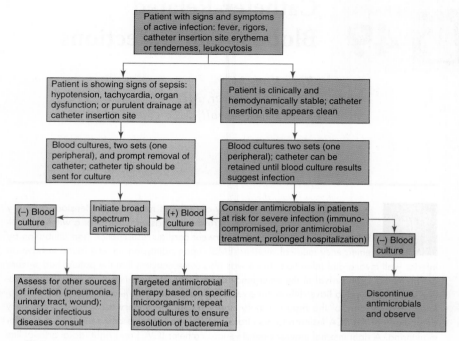

Figure 49-1. Initial approach in patients with suspected catheter-related bloodstream infections.

catheter will often become positive before the peripheral blood culture, reflecting the higher burden of organisms on the catheter.[4]

If there are signs of infection at the catheter insertion site or tenderness over the subcutaneous portion of the catheter, the catheter must be removed and the catheter tip submitted for quantitative culture. Positive catheter tip cultures are considered clinically significant when greater than 15 colony-forming units (CFU) of the same organism isolated from the blood culture are also isolated from the catheter tip.[1] Figure 49-1 delineates the initial approach to patients with CRBSI.

Catheters commonly used in ICU settings include both short-term and long-term catheters. Short-term catheters include peripheral intravenous (IV) lines, arterial lines, peripherally inserted central catheters (PICCs), and central venous catheters such as subclavian lines and pulmonary arterial catheters. Long-term catheters are surgically implanted lines including Hickman-type catheters and subcutaneous ports. In most cases of suspected CRBSI, short-term catheters are removed and the catheter tip sent for culture. Long-term catheters often require removal as well, particularly in cases of *Staphylococcus aureus, Candida*, and multidrug-resistant (MDR) infections.[1] Long-term catheters may be retained for treatment of coagulase-negative *Staphylococcus* species and *Enterococcus* species, unless there are overt signs of catheter-site infection or complicated infection such as endocarditis or osteomyelitis are present.

The next day, the blood culture results were reported as two of four bottles with gram-positive cocci in clusters (one from each set). The blood cultures drawn from the CVC were reported to be positive several hours before the peripheral culture. The CVC was removed promptly based on the positive blood culture results, and the catheter tip was sent for culture.

What types of organisms are of concern in CRBSI?

S aureus and *Candida* species are of particular concern. Other common pathogens are coagulase-negative *Staphylococcus* species and enteric gram-negative organisms, particularly MDR gram-negative rods.

Organisms identified with CRBSI in the ICU include coagulase-negative *Staphylococcus* species (36%), *S aureus* (17%), *Candida* species (10%), and *Enterococcus* species (10%). Enteric gram-negative organisms, including *Escherichia coli, Klebsiella, Pseudomonas,* and *Enterobacter*, collectively account for 15% to 20% of CRBSIs in the ICU.[5]

S aureus and *Candida* species are of particular concern because of the possibility of causing complicated bloodstream infection, including sepsis syndromes, endocarditis, and osteomyelitis. *Candida* species may cause endophthalmitis. Additional evaluation is warranted when *S aureus* and *Candida* are isolated to identify potential complications that will impact on the selection of the appropriate antimicrobial agent and duration of treatment. These evaluations may include the use of transesophageal echocardiography (TEE) to exclude endocarditis in patients with *S aureus*, venous Doppler ultrasound to evaluate for venous thrombosis, computed tomography to look for occult abscesses, and ophthalmologic examination to assess for endophthalmitis in the case of *Candida* infection.[1]

Enteric gram-negative organisms are of concern in the ICU because of the increasing prevalence of MDR organisms, including extended-spectrum β-lactamase (ESBL)-producing organisms and carbapenemase-producing organisms, making selection of appropriate antibiotics for both empirical and directed therapy a challenge. Knowledge of one's local ICU epidemiology will assist in selecting appropriate empirical antimicrobial therapy, particularly the prevalence of methicillin-resistant *S aureus* (MRSA) and MDR gram-negative bacteria.

Common empirical regimens include an antibiotic effective for gram-positive organisms, including *Staphylococcus* species, such as vancomycin or daptomycin, with a broad-spectrum antibiotic for gram-negative organisms, such as a fourth-generation cephalosporin or an aminoglycoside.[6,7] Therapy is then tailored to the specific organism isolated from the blood cultures and the results of susceptibility testing.[1]

The initial blood cultures eventually grew methicillin-sensitive *S aureus* (MSSA), and the catheter tip also grew greater than 15 CFU of MSSA. The patient's medication allergies were reviewed; he had a history of an allergic reaction to penicillin, which manifested as hives.

What treatment would be optimal for this patient?

β-Lactam antibiotics, such as nafcillin and cefazolin, are the preferred agents for MSSA. Alternative agents for penicillin-allergic patients include vancomycin and daptomycin.

MSSA is best treated with antistaphylococcal penicillins such as nafcillin or oxacillin. Cefazolin, a first-generation cephalosporin, is also effective.[8] In vitro data suggest that β-lactam antibiotics are more bactericidal than alternatives.

For penicillin-allergic patients, clarifying the allergy history is important. For less severe or remote allergies such as skin rashes, the use of cefazolin is often tolerated, given the reported cross-reactivity of 10% to penicillins. Vancomycin and daptomycin may be used in the highly allergic patient, such as those with a history suggestive of immediate hypersensitivity reactions, such as hives; tongue, lip, or facial swelling; and shortness of breath. Higher failure rates are reported with vancomycin.[9] For highly allergic individuals, consultation with an allergist is helpful to obtain

Infectious Disease

skin testing and provide desensitization to the β-lactam antibiotic when indicated for complicated infections with MSSA.

In addition to β-lactam allergies, clinicians need to be aware that β-lactam antimicrobials also lower the seizure threshold. This patient with seizure activity reported on presentation must be monitored closely for the precipitation of seizures.

For MRSA, vancomycin or daptomycin are effective. Daptomycin is preferred when the minimum inhibitory concentration (MIC) to vancomycin is greater than 2 µg/mL.[1] Linezolid appears less effective for MRSA bloodstream infections, and resistance has been reported.[1] Table 49-1 delineates preferred and alternate antimicrobial therapies for MSSA, MRSA, and other gram-positive organisms.

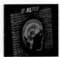 Once the patient was desensitized to nafcillin, he was started on specific therapy with nafcillin 2 g every 4 hours; vancomycin and cefepime were discontinued.

What other tests should be ordered to ensure that the patient is responding to treatment?

Follow-up blood cultures to document clearance of infection and additional testing to eliminate the possibility of endocarditis, which would lengthen the antimicrobial course, should be done. In cases of persistent fever or hypotension, repeated blood cultures are essential both to ensure the current infection is adequately treated and to eliminate the possibility of new pathogens. Figure 49-2 outlines the approach to *S aureus* CRBSI.

Follow-up blood cultures should be drawn after the patient is started on antimicrobial therapy to confirm clearance of the organisms and establish the start date for the antimicrobial course. In all cases of *S aureus* CRBSI, the catheter should be removed if not done on the first day. If follow-up cultures are positive or if fever persists, further testing to evaluate for endovascular or metastatic foci of infection must be performed. This would include TEE to evaluate the endocardium and rule out endocarditis, venous ultrasounds to rule out venous thrombophlebitis, or computed tomography of the abdomen to look for occult abscesses and other sites of infection.

 Repeat blood cultures were negative for growth. The patient had resolution of fever and was weaned off the ventilator. A PICC line was placed for treatment of the MSSA bloodstream infection.

How would you determine the duration of treatment?

In cases of *S aureus* CRBSI, a minimum of 4 weeks of antimicrobial therapy is indicated, unless signs and symptoms resolve quickly after the initiation of antibiotics and line removal, there is no evidence of complicated infection, and the patient does not have diabetes or immunocompromise elevating the risk for complications. A negative TEE is essential if a 2-week course of antibiotics is considered.[1]

Four weeks of antimicrobial therapy is generally indicated in cases of *S aureus* CRBSI.[10] The antibiotic course is extended to 6 weeks or longer for patients with complicated bloodstream infections, prolonged periods of bacteremia, endocarditis, or other sites of infection. The duration of therapy is counted from the date when follow-up blood cultures have documented sterility.

Table 49-1. Antimicrobial Therapy for Select Microorganisms Commonly Recovered in Uncomplicated Catheter-Related Bloodstream Infections

Microorganism	Preferred antimicrobial regimen/dosing[a]	Alternate antimicrobial regimen/dosing[a]	Duration of treatment[b]	Comments
Methicillin-sensitive *Staphylococcus aureus* (MSSA)	Nafcillin or oxacillin, 2 g q4h Or Cefazolin 2 g q8h	Vancomycin 15 mg/kg q12h Daptomycin 6-8 mg/kg daily	2-4 wk	
Methicillin-resistant *S aureus* (MRSA)	Vancomycin 15 mg/kg q12h	Daptomycin 6-8 mg/kg daily	2-4 wk	
Coagulase-negative *Staphylococcus*				
Methicillin susceptible	Nafcillin or oxacillin, 2 g q4h Or Cefazolin 2 g q8h	Vancomycin 15 mg/kg q12h Daptomycin 6-8 mg/kg daily	5-7 d	• If catheter is retained, treat for 10-14 d through the catheter lumen
Methicillin resistant	Vancomycin 15 mg/kg q12h	Daptomycin 6-8 mg/kg daily Linezolid 600 mg q12h	5-7 d	• If catheter is retained, treat for 10-14 d through the catheter lumen
Enterococcus species				
Ampicillin susceptible	Ampicillin 2 g q4h or q6h ± Gentamicin 1 mg/kg q8h	Vancomycin 15 mg/kg q12h	7-14 d	
Ampicillin resistant, vancomycin susceptible	Vancomycin 15 mg/kg q12h ± Gentamicin 1 mg/kg q8h	Linezolid 600 mg q12h Daptomycin 6-8 mg/kg daily	7-14 d	
Ampicillin and vancomycin resistant	Linezolid 600 mg q12h Daptomycin 6-8 mg/kg daily	Quinupristin/dalfopristin 7.5 mg/kg q8h	7-14 d	• Quinupristin/dalfopristin not effective against *E faecalis*

(Continued)

Table 49-1. Antimicrobial Therapy for Select Microorganisms Commonly Recovered in Uncomplicated Catheter-Related Bloodstream Infections (*Continued*)

Microorganism	Preferred antimicrobial regimen/dosing[a]	Alternate antimicrobial regimen/dosing[a]	Duration of treatment[b]	Comments
ESBL-negative gram-negative organisms	Third-generation cephalosporin: Ceftriaxone 1 g daily	Quinolone: Levofloxacin IV/PO 500 mg daily Ciprofloxacin IV 400 mg q12h Ciprofloxacin PO 500 mg q12h	7-14 d	• Target-specific therapy based on susceptibilities
ESBL-producing organisms (ie, *Escherichia coli*, *Klebsiella* species)	Carbapenem: Ertapenem 1 g daily Doripenem 500 mg q8h Imipenem 500 mg q6h Meropenem 1 g q8h	Aztreonam 2 g q8h Or Aminoglycoside: Gentamicin 5 mg/kg daily Amikacin 15 mg/kg daily Tobramycin 5 mg/kg daily Or Colistin 5 mg/kg in 2-4 divided doses	7-14 d	• Target-specific therapy based on susceptibilities
Pseudomonas aeruginosa	Cefepime 2 g q8h Or Pip/tazo 4.5 g q6h Or Carbapenem (see above) ± Aminoglycoside: Amikacin 15 mg/kg daily Tobramycin 5-7 mg/kg daily	Aztreonam 2 g q8h Or Quinolone: Levofloxacin IV/PO 500 mg daily Ciprofloxacin IV 400 mg q12h Ciprofloxacin PO 500 mg q12h	2 wk	• Target therapy based on susceptibilities • For severe illness, may want to add aminoglycoside to β-lactam • Ertapenem is the only carbapenem that is not effective in *P aeruginosa* infection

Candida species			
C albicans, C tropicalis, C parapsilosis	Fluconazole 800 mg loading dose, then 400 mg daily	2 wk	• Drug-drug interaction may preclude the use of fluconazole
	Echinocandin: Anidulafungin 200 mg loading dose, then 100 mg daily Caspofungin 70 mg loading dose, then 50 mg daily Micafungin 100 mg daily		• Echinocandins are administered intravenously only. Oral fluconazole has 100% bioavailability if GI tract functional
C glabrata, C krusei	Echinocandin: Anidulafungin 200 mg loading dose, then 100 mg daily Caspofungin 70 mg loading dose, then 50 mg daily Micafungin 100 mg daily	2 wk	• If susceptibility to azoles is demonstrated for C glabrata isolate, then can be transitioned to oral fluconazole or voriconazole
	Amphotericin B formulations		• C krusei are inherently resistant to fluconazole, voriconazole may be used instead

Abbreviations: ESBL, extended-spectrum β-lactamase; IV, intravenous; Pip/tazo, piperacillin/tazobactam; PO, orally.

[a]Dosing is based on adult patients without renal or liver dysfunction.

[b]Treatment duration contingent upon first negative blood culture.

Infectious Disease

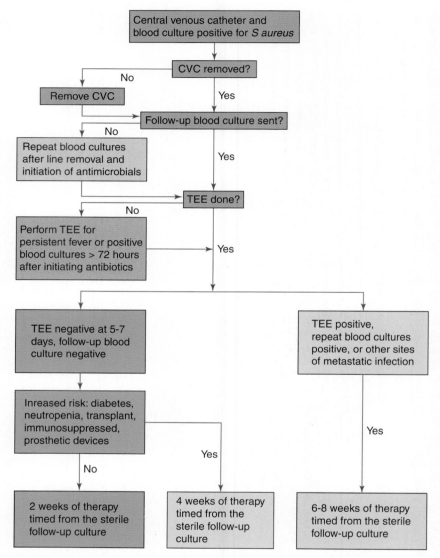

Figure 49-2. Approach to *Staphylococcus aureus* catheter-related bloodstream infection. CVC, central venous catheter; TEE, transesophageal echocardiography.

A 14-day course may be considered in patients who defervesce quickly with therapy and catheter removal, and whose follow-up blood cultures are negative and who do not have signs or symptoms of complicated infections such as endocarditis or thrombophlebitis. Patients with diabetes, immunocompromised states, or permanent intravascular devices such as pacemakers are excluded from short-course therapy.[11]

In cases where the patient is found to have a catheter tip colonized with *S aureus* with negative blood cultures, a very short (5- to 7-day) course of antibiotics is warranted to ensure more complicated infection does not result.[12]

On hospital day 12, the patient was noted to be febrile to 39.4°C (102.9°F), with rigors, tachycardia, and hypotension. Two sets of blood cultures were drawn, one set through the PICC and the other set peripherally. Twenty-four hours later, the microbiology lab reports both sets of cultures positive for yeast.

How should this new infection be managed? How would your management be different from the first episode of CRBSI?

The PICC line was removed promptly, and the tip was sent for culture. Intravenous caspofungin was started (70-mg loading dose, then 50 mg daily), and repeat blood cultures were drawn. A dilated funduscopic examination was performed; endophthalmitis was not detected.

Candida ranks fourth as a cause of nosocomial bloodstream infections in the United States, and third in the ICU.[5] Risk factors for candidemia include the following: use of broad-spectrum antibiotics, parenteral nutrition, or immunosuppressive agents; neutropenia; bone marrow or solid organ transplantation; major abdominal surgery; femoral catheterization; or colonization with *Candida* at multiple anatomic sites.[1,13] Common species that are recovered, in order of frequency, are *C albicans, C glabrata, C parapsilosis, C tropicalis,* and *C krusei.*[14] Speciation and, in some cases, susceptibility testing are important for determining which antifungal treatment is optimal. Three major classes of antifungal therapy are commonly used. The triazoles, which include fluconazole, voriconazole, and posaconazole, have excellent efficacy against *C albicans, C parapsilosis,* and *C tropicalis,* but less predictable activity against *C glabrata*, and fluconazole has no activity against *C krusei.*[15] Because of its excellent oral bioavailability and ease of dosing, fluconazole is the agent of choice for *C albicans, C parapsilosis,* and *C tropicalis.* The echinocandins, which include anidulafungin, caspofungin, and micafungin, are efficacious in treating almost all *Candida* species. The echinocandins have been shown to have decreased in vitro activity against *C parapsilosis*, and are not recommended as primary therapy for infection with this organism. However, clinical studies have not shown a significant failure rate with use of echinocandins in *C parapsilosis* candidemia. Thus, patients started empirically on an echinocandin can complete a treatment course with this agent in the setting of *C parapsilosis* infection if they show an appropriate clinical response to therapy.[13] Advantages of echinocandins include once-daily dosing and few drug interactions; however, echinocandins can only be administered intravenously.[16] Finally, amphotericin B preparations are also effective in treating most *Candida* species. However, given the increased rates of side effects and drug toxicity, use of amphotericin B preparations should be limited to resource-limited environments or specific situations, such as central nervous system or endovascular disease.[13] Specific antifungal therapies and dosing for commonly encountered *Candida* species are listed in Table 49-1.

In patients with presumptive candidemia, prompt initiation of an antifungal agent is crucial.[17] In cases where there is evidence for moderate to severe disease, hemodynamic instability, or recent azole use, an echinocandin is the recommended initial empiric therapy.[13] For patients with presumptive candidemia but with less severe illness and no recent azole exposure, fluconazole may be utilized as initial therapy. This particular patient did show signs of hemodynamic instability; as such, initiation of an echinocandin was appropriate.

Similar to *S aureus* CRBSI, prompt removal of indwelling catheters should be performed in patients with candidemia. This is because of the higher rates of failure, longer duration of therapy, and increased mortality rate associated with catheter retention.[18,19] Once the catheter is removed, the tip should be sent for microbiologic evaluation to confirm catheter-related infection. After catheter removal and initiation of antifungal therapy, repeat blood cultures need to be done to document clearance of fungemia. Given the increased risk of endophthalmitis associated with candidemia and the potentially devastating consequences of this complication, patients should have a dilated funduscopic examination within a week of fungemia.[13] This has important implications for duration of treatment and therapeutic choice, as well as possible need for surgical intervention.[20] Figure 49-3 illustrates the general approach to patients with CRBSI caused by *Candida* species.

Infectious Disease

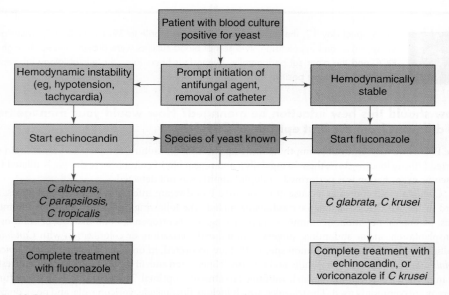

Figure 49-3. Approach to patients with catheter-related bloodstream infection due to *Candida* species.

The initial blood cultures eventually grew *C albicans*, and the repeat blood cultures were negative for growth.

Would you change the patient's treatment based on this information? How long would this patient need therapy?

If blood cultures reveal a *Candida* species that is susceptible to fluconazole, patients can be safely switched from the echinocandin to fluconazole.[13,21] Since the isolate was *C albicans*, transition from caspofungin to fluconazole is appropriate and cost-effective. Alternative agents can be considered if there are significant medication interactions with fluconazole, adverse events, or chronic conditions that increase the potential for adverse events such as end-stage liver disease and transaminitis. Duration of treatment in uncomplicated candidemia is 2 weeks from the time of the first negative blood culture.[1,13] If the patient has persistently positive blood cultures, an evaluation for metastatic foci of infection is needed; this would include a TEE to assess for infective endocarditis.

If the blood cultures grew a gram-negative bacteria instead, how would your management have been different?

Although less commonly seen in patients, CRBSI due to gram-negative organisms is routinely encountered in the ICU setting. In hospitalized patients, infections due to highly virulent MDR organisms, such as *Pseudomonas aeruginosa*, ESBL-producing gram-negative bacteria, and *Acinetobacter* species, are becoming more prevalent.[22] Empiric initiation of a broad-spectrum antibiotic that targets these gram-negative organisms is necessary, especially in patients who are critically ill and show signs of sepsis. Because bacteremia due to gram-negative organisms can be attributed to other causes, such as a urinary tract infection, pneumonia, or intra-abdominal abscess, assessing for other sources of infection is usually warranted. If the patient has a known history of colonization or infection with an MDR organism, targeted empiric therapy using two agents from different classes should be started.[1] Once the gram-negative organism is identified and susceptibilities are performed, antibiotic therapy can be narrowed to a single specific agent. Unlike *S aureus* and *Candida* species, gram-negative organisms tend not to cause metastatic foci of infection or endocarditis unless there is prosthetic material present; thus, further evaluation is indicated only if the patient has persistent bacteremia. Catheters can be salvaged if there is prompt response to antibiotic therapy; however, catheter removal is urged for highly virulent organisms such as *P aeruginosa* and MDR organisms.[1] Specific therapies and duration of treatment for select gram-negative organisms are listed in Table 49-1. Of note, carbapenems such as imipenem, meropenem, doripenem, and ertapenem are the antibiotics of choice for ESBL-producing organisms. Imipenem has the potential to lower seizure threshold and should be avoided in patients with risk factors for seizures.

If the patient initially had a long-term catheter (eg, Hickman, port, hemodialysis), how would management be different?

Tunneled catheters and totally implantable ports are commonly used for patients who require long-term therapy. These catheters tend to have lower rates of bloodstream infection as compared to non-tunneled catheters and may be kept in place for an extended period of time. Extraction of some of these catheters requires surgical intervention, which could create issues for patients with limited vascular access. Studies have shown that catheters can be salvaged with antibiotic-lock therapy and systemic antibiotics in select bloodstream infections.[23] Antibiotic-lock therapy consists of instilling an appropriate antibiotic solution in the lumen of the catheter while not in use, allowing the solution to dwell through the length of the catheter. Systemic antibiotics should be administered through the catheter, and the duration of treatment generally is about 2 weeks.[1] Removal of long-term catheters is indicated in patients who have persistent bacteremia despite 72 hours of appropriate antibiotic therapy, severe sepsis, tunnel infection, pocket infection, thrombophlebitis, or metastatic foci of infection. For *S aureus, P aeruginosa,* mycobacteria, or *Candida* CRBSI, removal of the catheter is strongly recommended. This is because of the increased risk of metastatic foci of infection that is associated with these organisms, which may lead to complications such as osteomyelitis, septic arthritis, and endovascular infection.[10,13] For this particular patient, removal of a long-term catheter would have been warranted for either infection.

What can be done to avoid CRBSI, especially in patients who require indwelling catheters?

Given the increased risk of morbidity and mortality, as well as excess hospital costs associated with CRBSI, prevention of these infections, particularly in the ICU, has become a priority in the health care setting. Implementing specific evidence-based interventions has been shown to be effective in decreasing the rates of infection; together, these interventions are commonly referred to as a "bundle."[24,25] The use of a checklist documenting appropriate steps is beneficial for ensuring proper catheter placement. Prior to catheter insertion, thorough hand hygiene should always be performed, as this has been shown to decrease rates of health care–associated infection.[26] Maximal barrier protection, including a mask, cap, sterile gloves, and gown, should be used, and a full-body sterile drape that completely covers the patient should be placed to minimize contamination.[27] Chlorhexidine-containing solutions have been shown to be more effective in preventing infection than povidone-iodine, and should be used routinely for sterilization of the skin prior to catheter insertion.[28] If there is a contraindication to using chlorhexidine, povidone-iodine can be used; however, povidone-iodine requires 2 minutes

Infectious Disease

to dry before its antiseptic properties are in effect. One study also showed a decrease in CRBSI when ICU patients were bathed daily with a 2% chlorhexidine-impregnated washcloth.[29] In terms of types of catheters, both antimicrobial- and antiseptic-impregnated catheters have been shown to decrease infection rates, a consideration when CRBSI rates are high, despite all other appropriate measures.[30] Use of topical antibiotic ointments at insertion sites is not recommended, as this may encourage MDR bacteria and/or fungal colonization and risk of invasive disease. Location of catheter placement also influences risk of infection. Higher rates of infection are associated with jugular and femoral veins versus subclavian vein cannulation; likewise, lower extremity sites (ie, femoral) have increased risk versus upper extremity sites.[31] A multicenter prospective study demonstrated that implementation of these preventative measures yielded a significant decrease in CRBSI in the ICU by as much as 66%.[24] Indwelling catheters should be removed promptly when they are no longer needed, and routine replacement of catheters should not be done unless there is concern for active infection.

! CRITICAL CONSIDERATIONS

- In evaluating a febrile ICU patient, obtain two sets of blood cultures, one from the CVC and one from a peripheral site, before initiating antibiotic therapy.

- Remove short-term CVCs and culture the catheter tip for seriously ill unstable patients and for all patients with documented bloodstream infection.

- Empiric antibiotic choices are tailored to the local ICU microbiologic epidemiology and should include an antistaphylococcal agent and a broad-spectrum antibiotic for gram-negative organisms.

- Use β-lactam antibiotics to treat MSSA. Consider desensitization for patients with β-lactam allergies.

- Pursue a TEE in patients with *S aureus* when they are not responding to therapy or if a 2-week course is anticipated (see Figure 49-2).

- Always obtain follow-up blood cultures to document sterility and to provide the start date in timing antibiotic duration.

- *Candida* is the third most common cause of CRBSI in the ICU setting. In patients with risk factors for candidemia and clinical and laboratory findings consistent with *Candida* CRBSI, prompt initiation of an antifungal agent is imperative.

- Initiation of an echinocandin is indicated in patients with presumptive candidemia in the following scenarios: moderate to severe disease, hemodynamic instability, or recent azole use.

- Identification of *Candida* species is important for determining optimal antifungal therapy.

- Given the risk of complications, catheters should be removed and a dilated funduscopic examination should be performed in cases of candidemia. Repeat blood cultures should be done to document clearance of infection.

- If an echinocandin is used initially for empiric antifungal coverage, patients can be switched to an azole, such as fluconazole, if the *Candida* isolate is susceptible.

- Although less common, CRBSIs due to gram-negative organisms are encountered in the ICU setting. Broad-spectrum empiric therapy should be considered in patients with risk factors for MDR gram-negative organisms and suspected CRBSI.

- For long-term catheters, preservation of the catheter can be attempted with antibiotic-lock therapy and systemic antibiotics. However, long-term catheter removal is recommended in patients with the following: persistent bacteremia despite 72 hours of appropriate antibiotic therapy, severe sepsis, tunnel infection, pocket infection, thrombophlebitis, metastatic foci of infection, or infection with *S aureus, P aeruginosa,* mycobacteria, or *Candida* species.
- CRBSI rates have been shown to decrease when specific interventions, known as a "bundle," have been implemented during catheter placement in the ICU. Bundles include the use of a checklist, meticulous hand hygiene, maximum barrier protection for the patient and health care worker, and use of chlorhexidine-containing solution for skin antisepsis.

REFERENCES

1. Mermel LA, Allon M, Bouza E, et al. Clinical practice guidelines for the diagnosis and management of intravascular catheter-related infection: 2009 update by the Infectious Diseases Society of America. *Clin Infect Dis.* 2009;49(1):1-45.
2. Marik PE. Fever in the ICU. *Chest.* 2000;117(3): 855-869.
3. Brun-Buisson C, Abrouk F, Legrand P, Huet Y, Larabi S, Rapin M. Diagnosis of central venous catheter-related sepsis. *Arch Intern Med.* 1987;147(5):873-877.
4. Martinez JA, DesJardin JA, Aronoff M, Supran S, Nasraway SA, Snydman DR. Clinical utility of blood cultures drawn from central venous or arterial catheters in critically ill surgical patients. *Crit Care Med.* 2002;30(1):7-13.
5. Wisplinghoff H, Bischoff T, Tallent SM, Seifert H, Wenzel RP, Edmond MB. Nosocomial bloodstream infections in US hospitals: analysis of 24,179 cases from a prospective nationwide surveillance study. *Clin Infect Dis.* 2004;39(3):309-317.
6. Moise PA, Sakoulas G, Forrest A, Schentag JJ. Vancomycin in vitro bactericidal activity and its relationship to efficacy in clearance of methicillin-resistant *Staphylococcus aureus* bacteremia. *Antimicrob Agents Chemother.* 2007;51(7):2582-2586.
7. Blot SI, Depuydt P, Annemans L, et al. Clinical and economic outcomes in critically ill patients with nosocomial catheter-related bloodstream infections. *Clin Infect Dis.* 2005;41(11):1591-1598.
8. Corey GR. *Staphylococcus aureus* bloodstream infections: definitions and treatment. *Clin Infect Dis.* 2009;48(S4):254-259.
9. Chang FY, Peacock JE, Musher DM, et al., *Staphylococcus aureus* bacteremia: recurrence and the impact of antibiotic treatment in a prospective multicenter study. *Medicine.* 2003;82(5):333-339.
10. Fowler VG, Justice A, Moore C, et al. Risk factors for hematogenous complications of intravascular catheter-associated *Staphylococcus aureus* bacteremia. *Clin Infect Dis.* 2005;40(5):695-703.
11. Pigrau C, Rodriguez D, Planes AM, et al. Management of catheter-related *Staphylococcus aureus* bacteremia: when may sonographic study be unnecessary? *Eur J Clin Microbiol Infect Dis.* 2003;22(12):713-719.
12. Ekkelenkamp MB, van der Bruggen T, van de Vijver DA, Wolfs TF, Bonten MJ. Bacteremic complications of intravascular catheters colonized with *Staphylococcus aureus. Clin Infect Dis.* 2008;46(1):114-118.
13. Pappas PG, Kauffman CA, Andes D, et al. Clinical practice guidelines for the management of candidiasis: 2009 update by the Infectious Diseases Society of America. *Clin Infect Dis.* 2009;48(5): 503-535.
14. Horn DL, Neofytos D, Anaissie EJ, et al. Epidemiology and outcomes of candidemia in 2019 patients: data from the prospective antifungal therapy alliance registry. *Clin Infect Dis.* 2009;48(12):1695-1703.
15. Espinel-Ingroff A, Barchiesi F, Cuenca-Estrella M, et al. International and multicenter comparison of EUCAST and CLSI M27-A2 broth microdilution methods for testing susceptibilities of *Candida* spp. to fluconazole, itraconazole, posaconazole, and voriconazole. *J Clin Microbiol.* 2005;43(8):3884-3889.
16. Kim R, Khachikian D, Reboli A. A comparative evaluation of properties and clinical efficacy of the echinocandins. *Expert Opin Pharmacother.* 2007;8(10):1479-1492.
17. Garey KW, Rege M, Pai MP, et al. Time to initiation of fluconazole therapy impacts mortality in patients with candidemia: a multi-institutional study. *Clin Infect Dis.* 2006;43(1):25-31.
18. Nguyen MH, Peacock JE Jr, Tanner DC, et al. Therapeutic approaches in patients with candidemia:

Infectious Disease

evaluation in a multicenter, prospective, observational study. *Arch Intern Med.* 1995;155(22):2429-2435.

19. Rex JH, Bennett JE, Sugar AM, et al. Intravascular catheter exchange and duration of candidemia. NIAID Mycoses Study Group and the Candidemia Study Group. *Clin Infect Dis.* 1995;21(4): 994-996.

20. Rex JH, Bennett JE, Sugar AM, et al. A randomized trial comparing fluconazole with amphotericin B for the treatment of candidemia in patients without neutropenia. Candidemia Study Group and the National Institute. *N Engl J Med.* 1994;331(20):1325-1330.

21. Reboli AC, Rotstein C, Pappas PG, et al. Anidulafungin versus fluconazole for invasive candidiasis. *N Engl J Med.* 2007;356(24):2472-2482.

22. National Nosocomial Infections Surveillance (NNIS) System Report, data summary from January 1992 through June 2004, issued October 2004. *Am J Infect Control.* 2004;32(8):470-485.

23. Fortún J, Grill F, Martín-Dávila P, et al. Treatment of long-term intravascular catheter-related bacteraemia with antibiotic-lock therapy. *J Antimicrob Chemother.* 2006;58(4):816-821.

24. Pronovost P, Needham D, Berenholtz S, et al. An intervention to decrease catheter-related bloodstream infections in the ICU. *N Engl J Med.* 2006;355(26):2725-2732.

25. Warren DK, Cosgrove SE, Diekema DJ, et al. A multicenter intervention to prevent catheter-associated bloodstream infections. *Infect Control Hosp Epidemiol.* 2006;27(7):662-669.

26. Doebbeling BN, Stanley GL, Sheetz CT, et al. Comparative efficacy of alternative hand-washing agents in reducing nosocomial infections in intensive care units. *N Engl J Med.* 1992;327(2):88-93.

27. Lee DH, Jung KY, Choi YH. Use of maximal sterile barrier precautions and/or antimicrobial-coated catheters to reduce the risk of central venous catheter-related bloodstream infection. *Infect Control Hosp Epidemiol.* 2008;29(10):947-953.

28. Chaiyakunapruk N, Veenstra DL, Lipsky BA, et al. Chlorhexidine compared with povidone-iodine solution for vascular catheter-site care: a meta-analysis. *Ann Intern Med.* 2002;136(11):792-801.

29. Bleasdale SC, Trick WE, Gonzalez IM, Lyles RD, Hayden MK, Weinstein RA. Effectiveness of chlorhexidine bathing to reduce catheter-associated bloodstream infections in medical intensive care unit patients. *Arch Intern Med.* 2007;167(19):2073-2079.

30. O'Grady NP, Alexander M, Dellinger P, et al; for the Healthcare Infection Control Practices Advisory Committee. Guidelines for the prevention of intravascular catheter-related infections. *Infect Control Hosp Epidemiol.* 2002;23(12):759-769.

31. Merrer J, De Jonghe B, Golliot F, et al. Complications of femoral and subclavian venous catheterization in critically ill patients: a randomized controlled trial. *JAMA.* 2001;286(6):700-707.

CHAPTER	**Common Infections**
50	**in the ICU**

Constantine Tsigrelis, MD
Annette C. Reboli, MD

A 66-year-old man with no known medical history was admitted after a fall while working at a silo on his farm. On physical examination, he had aphasia and right upper and lower extremity weakness. Computed tomography of the head revealed a large left intracerebral hemorrhage. He was intubated on hospital day 1 because of a depressed level of consciousness.

On hospital day 7, he developed fever with a temperature of 39.1°C (102.3°F), heart rate of 99 bpm, blood pressure of 146/53 mm Hg, and respiratory rate of 16 breaths/minute. He required an increase in inspired oxygen concentration from 40% to 60%. He had a moderate amount of thick, tan-colored tracheal secretions from the endotracheal tube. He did not have diarrhea. On physical examination, there were decreased breath sounds at the left lung base. There were no signs of exit-site erythema or drainage at the central venous catheter and right radial artery catheter insertion sites. A urinary catheter was in place. Peripheral blood leukocyte count was 17,600 cells/mm³. Chest imaging revealed a new left lower lung field opacity (Figure 50-1).

What is the differential diagnosis of a new fever in an intensive care unit (ICU) patient?

The evaluation of a new fever in an ICU patient should always begin with a thorough review of the patient's history and a focused physical examination, rather than automatic ordering of microbiologic studies.[1] After a differential diagnosis is formulated based on the history and physical examination, pertinent laboratory and radiologic studies should then be performed.

The differential diagnosis of a new fever in an ICU patient includes both infectious and noninfectious etiologies (Table 50-1).[1-3] The most common infectious etiologies include hospital-acquired pneumonia (including ventilator-associated pneumonia), intravascular catheter-related bloodstream infection, catheter-associated urinary tract infection, surgical site infection, and *Clostridium difficile* infection. Infections unique to a neurologic/neurosurgical ICU include (1) superficial and deep surgical site infections that occur after neurosurgical procedures (eg, superficial wound infection after laminectomy or deep abscess after craniotomy) and (2) bacterial meningitis occurring after placement of internal and external ventricular catheters and lumbar catheters. Drug-related fever and intracranial hemorrhage are common noninfectious etiologies of fever in a neurologic/neurosurgical ICU.

Infectious Disease

877

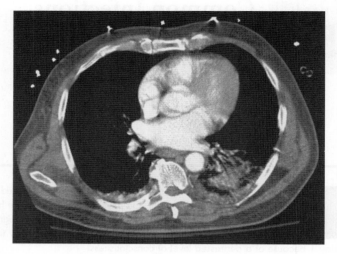

Figure 50-1. Computed tomography of the chest showing left lower lobe consolidation.

Ventilator-associated pneumonia was suspected as the etiology of the patient's new fever. How are hospital-acquired pneumonia and ventilator-associated pneumonia diagnosed?

Hospital-acquired pneumonia (HAP) is defined as the development of pneumonia 48 hours or longer after hospital admission. Ventilator-associated pneumonia (VAP) is a subtype of HAP that occurs more than 48 to 72 hours after endotracheal intubation.[4] The diagnosis of HAP/VAP is initially suspected on the basis of clinical findings, including fever, peripheral blood leukocyte count, quality and quantity of tracheal secretions, changes in oxygenation, and chest radiography.[4] The development of a new or progressive radiographic pulmonary infiltrate combined with two of three clinical crite-

Table 50-1. Common Etiologies of New Fever in a Patient in the Intensive Care Unit

Infectious etiologies
1. Hospital-acquired pneumonia (*discussed in this chapter*)
2. Intravascular catheter-related bloodstream infection (*Chapter 49*)
3. Catheter-associated urinary tract infection (*discussed in this chapter*)
4. Surgical site infection (*Chapter 24*)
5. *Clostridium difficile*–associated disease (*discussed in this chapter*)
6. Ventricular catheter-associated meningitis (*Chapters 7 and 22*)
7. Nosocomial sinusitis

Noninfectious etiologies
1. Drug-related fever
2. Intracranial hemorrhage
3. Acalculous cholecystitis
4. Blood product transfusion reaction
5. Aspiration pneumonitis without infection
6. Pancreatitis
7. Venous thrombosis

ria—(1) fever higher than 38°C (100.4°F), (2) purulent tracheal secretions, and (3) leukocytosis—has been shown to have a good balance of sensitivity and specificity for the diagnosis of HAP/VAP.[5]

Cultures of lower respiratory tract secretions help determine the microbial etiology of HAP/VAP and should be collected prior to starting or changing antibiotic therapy.[6] Lower respiratory tract secretion samples may be cultured either (1) semiquantitatively (typically via an endotracheal aspirate sample), which is usually reported as heavy, moderate, light, or no growth; or (2) quantitatively (via bronchoalveolar lavage [BAL], protected specimen brush [PSB], or endotracheal aspirate), where a specific colony count is reported. For quantitative cultures, growth above a certain threshold may help distinguish infection from colonization. The following thresholds are commonly used to diagnose infection, assuming antibiotic therapy was not started or changed in the 24 to 72 hours before obtaining the culture: greater than or equal to 10^4 colony-forming units (CFU)/mL for BAL samples, greater than or equal to 10^3 CFU/mL for PSB samples, and greater than or equal to 10^6 CFU/mL for endotracheal aspirate samples.[4,7-9] These thresholds may be lowered if recent antibiotic changes were made or if the pretest probability of HAP/VAP is very high.[6]

Is there a benefit of obtaining quantitative cultures of lower respiratory tract secretions over semiquantitative cultures for the diagnosis of HAP/VAP?

There is controversy regarding which culture method (semiquantitative or quantitative culture) is preferred. The benefits of obtaining a semiquantitative culture include rapid sampling (via an endotracheal aspirate) and lack of need for specialized microbiology techniques. Although semiquantitative cultures are more sensitive than quantitative cultures, they are less specific because tracheal secretions rather than deeper respiratory tract secretions are sampled and a specific colony count is not reported.[4] This makes it more difficult to distinguish between colonization and infection. The benefit of obtaining quantitative cultures is that they are more specific, thus decreasing the rate of false-positive culture results.[4] The disadvantages of quantitative cultures are that bronchoscopy is generally required, specialized microbiologic techniques are needed, and in some cases lower sensitivity may lead to a false-negative result.[4]

Clinical trial data comparing the two methods have not shown a difference in mortality or length of ICU or hospital stay.[4,10-12] The data are conflicting whether obtaining quantitative cultures influences the overall number of days of antibiotic use.[10-12] We generally reserve obtaining quantitative cultures for patients with a low severity of illness who have a low to intermediate pretest probability of HAP/VAP. In these instances, assuming empiric antibiotic therapy is not given, the information gained from quantitative cultures is more likely to influence whether antibiotic therapy is ultimately administered or witheld.[13] On the other hand, when the pretest probability of HAP/VAP is high or when a patient is clinically unstable, empiric antibiotic therapy is typically initiated, and a quantitative culture is less likely to influence discontinuation of antibiotic therapy.

Infectious Disease

An endotracheal aspirate was obtained for semiquantitative culture to assist with defining the microbial etiology.

What is the approach to initial empiric antibiotic therapy for HAP/VAP?

Unless there is low suspicion for HAP/VAP, empiric antibiotic therapy should be initiated as soon as possible after a lower respiratory tract sample is obtained for culture.[4] The rationale for prompt treatment is that a delay in appropriate antibiotic therapy has been associated with a higher attributable mortality rate from HAP/VAP.[14,15] In order to increase the probability of administering appropriate antibiotic therapy, the initial empiric antibiotic regimen should be based on the patient's risk for multidrug-resistant (MDR) pathogens (Figures 50-2 and 50-3).[4,16-23] For patients at risk for MDR

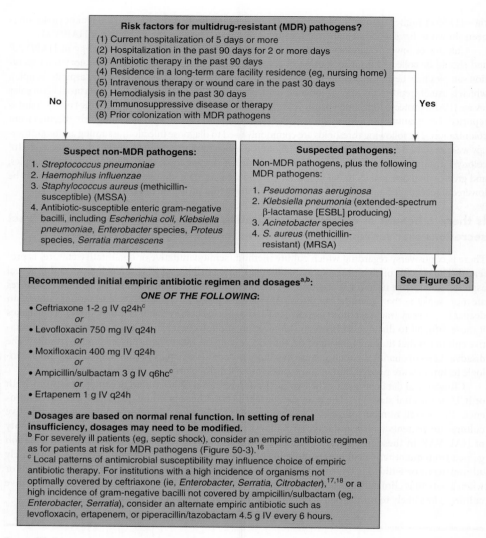

Risk factors for multidrug-resistant (MDR) pathogens?
(1) Current hospitalization of 5 days or more
(2) Hospitalization in the past 90 days for 2 or more days
(3) Antibiotic therapy in the past 90 days
(4) Residence in a long-term care facility residence (eg, nursing home)
(5) Intravenous therapy or wound care in the past 30 days
(6) Hemodialysis in the past 30 days
(7) Immunosuppressive disease or therapy
(8) Prior colonization with MDR pathogens

No   Yes

Suspect non-MDR pathogens:
1. *Streptococcus pneumoniae*
2. *Haemophilus influenzae*
3. *Staphylococcus aureus* (methicillin-susceptible) (MSSA)
4. Antibiotic-susceptible enteric gram-negative bacilli, including *Escherichia coli, Klebsiella pneumoniae, Enterobacter* species, *Proteus* species, *Serratia marcescens*

Suspected pathogens:
Non-MDR pathogens, plus the following MDR pathogens:

1. *Pseudomonas aeruginosa*
2. *Klebsiella pneumonia* (extended-spectrum β-lactamase [ESBL] producing)
3. *Acinetobacter* species
4. *S. aureus* (methicillin-resistant) (MRSA)

Recommended initial empiric antibiotic regimen and dosages[a,b]:

ONE OF THE FOLLOWING:

• Ceftriaxone 1-2 g IV q24h[c]
  or
• Levofloxacin 750 mg IV q24h
  or
• Moxifloxacin 400 mg IV q24h
  or
• Ampicillin/sulbactam 3 g IV q6hc[c]
  or
• Ertapenem 1 g IV q24h

[a] **Dosages are based on normal renal function. In setting of renal insufficiency, dosages may need to be modified.**
[b] For severely ill patients (eg, septic shock), consider an empiric antibiotic regimen as for patients at risk for MDR pathogens (Figure 50-3).[16]
[c] Local patterns of antimicrobial susceptibility may influence choice of empiric antibiotic therapy. For institutions with a high incidence of organisms not optimally covered by ceftriaxone (ie, *Enterobacter, Serratia, Citrobacter*),[17,18] or a high incidence of gram-negative bacilli not covered by ampicillin/sulbactam (eg, *Enterobacter, Serratia*), consider an alternate empiric antibiotic such as levofloxacin, ertapenem, or piperacillin/tazobactam 4.5 g IV every 6 hours.

See Figure 50-3

Figure 50-2. Initial empiric antibiotic regimen for hospital-acquired pneumonia/ventilator-associated pneumonia. *(Adapted in part from American Thoracic Society, Infectious Diseases Society of America. Guidelines for the management of adults with hospital-acquired, ventilator-associated, and healthcare-associated pneumonia. Am J Respir Crit Care Med. 2005;171(4):388-416.)*

pathogens, initial combination therapy for gram-negative bacilli is recommended to maximize the chance of appropriate antibiotic therapy.

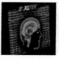

Since the patient was hospitalized for 7 days, he was considered to be at risk for MDR pathogens and was empirically started on vancomycin, cefepime, and levofloxacin.

Recommended initial empiric antibiotic regimen and dosages[a,b] for patients with risk factors for multidrug-resistant (MDR) pathogens:

ONE OF THE FOLLOWING:

• Cefepime 1-2 g IV q8-12h

or

• Ceftazidime 2 g IV q8h

or

• Piperacillin/tazobactam 4.5 g IV q6h

or

• Imipenem 500 mg IV q6h or 1 g IV q8h

or

• Meropenem 1 g IV q8h

or

• Doripenem 500 mg IV q8h (via 1-hour or 4-hour infusion)[19,20]

or

• Aztreonam 1-2 g IV q6-8h (if β-lactam allergy)

PLUS

ONE OF THE FOLLOWING:

• Gentamicin 7 mg/kg IV q24h[c]

or

• Tobramycin 7 mg/kg IV q24h[c]

or

• Amikacin 20 mg/kg IV q24h[c]

or

• Levofloxacin 750 mg IV q24h

or

• Ciprofloxacin 400 mg IV q8h

PLUS

ONE OF THE FOLLOWING:

• Vancomycin 15-20 mg/kg IV q12h[d]

or

• Linezolid 600 mg IV q12h

[a] **Dosages are based on normal renal function. In setting of renal insufficiency, dosages may need to be modified.**

[b] Local patterns of antimicrobial susceptibility may influence choice of empiric antibiotic therapy.
[c] For gentamicin and tobramycin, a trough level of <1 is suggested. For amikacin, a trough level of <4-5 is suggested.[4] Consider infectious diseases or pharmacy consultation for dosing recommendations.
[d] Suggested vancomycin trough level is 15-20 μg/mL.[4,21] Every-8-hour dosing interval may be needed in certain patients.[21] Loading dose of 25-30 mg/kg can be considered in seriously ill patients to attain target serum concentration.[21] Dose based on actual body weight (suggested maximum dose for each infusion is 2000 mg).[21]

Figure 50-3. Initial empiric antibiotic regimen for hospital-acquired pneumonia/ventilator-associated pneumonia. *(Adapted in part from American Thoracic Society, Infectious Diseases Society of America. Guidelines for the management of adults with hospital-acquired, ventilator-associated, and healthcare-associated pneumonia. Am J Respir Crit Care Med. 2005;171(4):388-416.)*

Infectious Disease

What are the recommendations for modification of the initial empiric antibiotic regimen for HAP/VAP?

After initiating appropriate empiric antibiotic therapy for HAP/VAP, clinical improvement (based on peripheral blood leukocyte count, temperature, oxygenation, and quantity of tracheal secretions) typically begins to occur by 48 to 72 hours.[24,25] By this point in time, the results of lower respiratory tract culture data may be available, and the initial empiric antibiotic therapy regimen can usually be modified by either narrowing treatment or adding treatment for an organism not being covered. Narrowing antibiotic therapy (ie, de-escalation) is important to minimize the emergence of antibiotic resistance.[26]

Modification of the empiric antibiotic regimen should be based on results of lower respiratory tract culture data. The interpretation of a positive lower respiratory tract culture is influenced by a number of factors, including whether semiquantitative or quantitative cultures are performed (eg, when quantitative cultures are obtained, growth above a predefined threshold may support infection over colonization) and the level of suspicion that that organism is causing HAP/VAP (eg, certain organisms are not considered pulmonary pathogens, such as coagulase-negative staphylococci and enterococci). A negative lower respiratory tract culture in an intubated patient may be clinically useful, as it has a strong negative predictive value for HAP/VAP in the absence of a recent change in antibiotic therapy in the preceding 72 hours.[4,6,27] In addition, in an intubated patient, a lower respiratory tract culture that does not grow an MDR pathogen, in the absence of a recent change in antibiotic therapy in the preceding 72 hours, suggests that these pathogens are not causing HAP/VAP and antibiotic therapy can be narrowed accordingly.[4,25]

There was improvement in the patient's fever, leukocytosis, and oxygenation after 48 hours. A semiquantitative endotracheal aspirate culture subsequently grew moderate *Klebsiella pneumoniae* (susceptible to levofloxacin and cefazolin) and blood cultures were negative. Vancomycin and cefepime were discontinued, and levofloxacin was continued.

Should combination antibiotic therapy (ie, "double coverage") be given for the full treatment course for HAP/VAP caused by *Pseudomonas aeruginosa*?

The rationale for using empiric combination antibiotic therapy for HAP/VAP while awaiting culture data is to maximize the chance of administering appropriate antibiotic therapy. Once antimicrobial susceptibility data return, therapy can usually be narrowed to a single agent. However, for cases where *P aeruginosa* is found to be the etiologic agent of HAP/VAP and antibiotic susceptibility data are known, a common question is whether combination antibiotic therapy with two antibiotics active against *P aeruginosa* should be given for the full treatment course (ie, definitive combination therapy).

Proposed theoretical reasons to support the use of definitive combination therapy for *P aeruginosa* pneumonia include the potential for (1) synergy, (2) prevention of emergence of resistance, and (3) change in clinical outcome. In vitro synergy has not been consistently established and improved outcome has not been demonstrated for patients receiving synergistic antibiotic combinations for *P aeruginosa* pneumonia as compared with combinations not synergistic in vitro.[4,28] Furthermore, prevention of emergence of resistance has also not been documented with the use of definitive combination therapy for *P aeruginosa* pneumonia.[4,29,30] Lastly, definitive combination therapy for pseudomonal pneumonia has not been associated with a difference in mortality,[30-32] clinical treatment failure,[29,31,32] length of ICU and hospital stay,[30,31] or recurrence of VAP[30] and it may lead to increased nephrotoxicity when aminoglycoside combination therapy is used.[29] An exception is that combination therapy may have a survival benefit in patients with pseudomonal pneumonia and bacteremia.[28]

For select patients with severe pseudomonal HAP/VAP or pseudomonal pneumonia and bacteremia, we consider the use of combination antibiotic therapy for at least the first 5 to 7 days of treatment, although this decision should ultimately be individualized based on the specific clinical scenario.

Is there an advantage of using linezolid over vancomycin for HAP/VAP due to methicillin-resistant *Staphylococcus aureus* (MRSA)?

There are insufficient data to suggest an advantage of linezolid over vancomycin for the treatment of HAP/VAP caused by MRSA. Two initial clinical trials did not show an advantage of linezolid over vancomycin for patients with HAP due to MRSA.[33,34] A retrospective analysis of data from these two clinical trials showed increased survival and clinical cure for patients treated with linezolid as compared with vancomycin[35]; however, this study was criticized for methodologic issues (lack of randomization leading to unmeasured confounding, and lack of modification of a significant *P* value in the setting of multiple comparisons).[36] A subsequent clinical trial failed to show a difference in microbiologic cure, clinical cure, or survival between linezolid and vancomycin for the treatment of VAP due to MRSA; however, the sample size was small.[37] A larger clinical trial to further address this question is currently in progress.[37]

An additional factor that may influence the treatment of MRSA HAP/VAP is the minimum inhibitory concentration (MIC) of MRSA to vancomycin. For patients with MRSA HAP/VAP where the vancomycin MIC is greater than or equal to 2 µg/mL, use of an alternate agent has been suggested (eg, linezolid) because of a concern for treatment failure if vancomycin is used; however, further data are needed to address this question.[21,38] In addition, for patients with HAP/VAP due to MRSA, suggested vancomycin trough levels are 15 to 20 µg/mL,[4,21] although clinical data documenting improved outcome with higher trough levels are lacking.[38,39]

What is the recommended duration of antibiotic therapy for HAP/VAP?

In the past, the recommended duration of antibiotic therapy for HAP/VAP was as high as 14 to 21 days.[4] However, prolonged antibiotic treatment (ie, more than 7 days of treatment) has been associated with newly acquired tracheal colonization with organisms such as *P aeruginosa*, Enterobacteriaceae, and *S aureus*.[4,25]

In a clinical trial comparing 8 days versus 15 days of antibiotic treatment for VAP, there was no difference in mortality rate or recurrent infections between the two groups.[40] Furthermore, among patients who developed recurrent VAP and received 15 days of antibiotic treatment, there was a higher rate of emergence of MDR pathogens as compared with patients who received 8 days of treatment. In a subgroup of patients who developed VAP due to nonfermenting gram-negative bacilli (ie, *P aeruginosa* and *Acinetobacter* species), there was a higher VAP recurrence rate in patients who received 8 days of antibiotic treatment as compared with 15 days of treatment.

Based on these data, a shorter duration (7-8 days) of antibiotic therapy for HAP/VAP is recommended for patients who clinically respond to treatment and who are not infected with nonfermenting gram-negative bacilli.[4] For patients infected with nonfermenting gram-negative bacilli, 14 days of antibiotic treatment should be considered.

In this patient, 8 days of treatment with levofloxacin was given for the diagnosis of VAP due to *K pneumoniae*.

Infectious Disease

What are the recommended strategies for reducing the risk of HAP/VAP?

Infection control measures to prevent transmission of microorganisms from one patient to another via health care worker contact are critical; these include (1) strict compliance with hand hygiene, (2) strict compliance with isolation precautions for MDR pathogens, and (3) staff education.[4]

Mechanical ventilation is one of the most important risk factors for HAP, and the following measures are recommended to reduce the risk of HAP/VAP: (1) avoiding intubation if possible, (2) minimizing the duration of mechanical ventilation by using protocols that accelerate weaning and improve sedation use, (3) avoiding reintubation if possible, and (4) use of noninvasive positive pressure ventilation as an alternative to intubation when indicated.[4]

Preventing aspiration of gastric and oropharyngeal contents into the lower respiratory tract also reduces the risk of HAP/VAP. Maintaining intubated patients in the semirecumbent position (ie, 30- to 45-degree elevation of the head of the bed) and avoiding the supine position (ie, 0-degree elevation) reduces the risk of aspiration of gastric contents, especially during enteral feeding.[4] The endotracheal tube cuff pressure should be maintained at greater than 20 cm H_2O to reduce the risk of aspiration of oropharyngeal bacteria around the cuff and into the lower respiratory tract.[4] Continuous aspiration of subglottic secretions can be considered via a specially designed endotracheal tube, although these tubes are not readily available.[4]

Selective decontamination of the digestive tract with oral and/or intravenous antibiotics may reduce the risk of HAP/VAP; however, this strategy is not recommended because of the potential for selecting for antibiotic-resistant microorganisms.[4]

 An 82-year-old woman with severe aortic stenosis was admitted to the intensive care unit from a long-term care facility with dyspnea. She did not complain of fever, chills, rigors, or lethargy. Her temperature was 37.1°C (98.8°F). Physical examination revealed diffuse bilateral rales on lung examination and bilateral lower extremity edema. Mental status examination was normal. A chronic indwelling urinary catheter was present on admission. The peripheral blood leukocyte count was normal at 8500 cells/mm³ without a left shift. Her serum creatinine was elevated at 1.5 mg/dL. Chest radiography showed findings consistent with pulmonary edema. She was given low-dose diuretic therapy and her dyspnea improved.

Because of the elevated serum creatinine, a urinalysis was performed, which showed 10 to 25 leukocytes per high-power field. Although the patient did not have any symptoms or signs compatible with catheter-associated urinary tract infection, a urine culture was performed on a catheterized urine specimen, which grew greater than or equal to 100,000 CFU/mL of penicillin-susceptible *Enterococcus faecalis*. Antibiotic treatment was not administered. During the rest of her hospital stay, she did not display any symptoms or signs of symptomatic urinary tract infection.

What is the natural history of bacteriuria and urinary tract infection after placement of a urinary catheter?

Bacteriuria (ie, significant growth of bacteria in urine) is a very common finding in patients with indwelling urinary catheters, and the majority of patients are asymptomatic.[41] It is estimated that the incidence of bacteriuria is between 3% and 8% per day of urinary catheterization.[41-45] The duration of catheterization is the most important risk factor for the development of catheter-associated bacteriuria, and almost all patients develop bacteriuria after 1 month of catheterization.[41,46]

The majority of patients with bacteriuria do not develop symptoms or signs of infection (Figure 50-4). The proportion of patients with catheter-associated bacteriuria that develop symptomatic infection

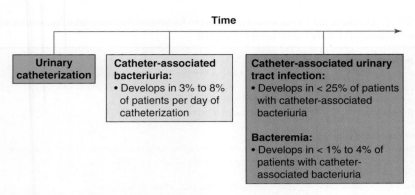

Figure 50-4. Natural history of bacteriuria and urinary tract infection after urinary catheterization.

is less than 25%.[42,43,47,48] The proportion of patients with catheter-associated bacteriuria that develop bacteremia is even lower, ranging between less than 1% and 4%.[41,47-50] The reason for the low rates of symptomatic infection in patients with catheter-associated bacteriuria is unclear; however, it has been hypothesized that decompression of the urinary tract with a urinary catheter prevents obstruction, which is known to predispose to symptomatic urinary tract infection and bacteremia.[47]

 The patient had catheter-associated asymptomatic bacteriuria in the setting of an indwelling urinary catheter.

How are catheter-associated asymptomatic bacteriuria (CA-ASB) and catheter-associated urinary tract infection (CA-UTI) diagnosed?

Guidelines for the diagnosis and treatment of CA-UTI in adults have recently been published, and the importance of distinguishing between CA-ASB and CA-UTI is emphasized, since they are managed differently (ie, CA-ASB does not require antibiotic treatment except in certain clinical scenarios, while CA-UTI should be treated).[41]

CA-ASB is defined by growth of greater than or equal to 100,000 CFU/mL of one or more bacterial species from a catheterized urine specimen (either from an indwelling urinary catheter, suprapubic catheter, or intermittent catheterization) in a patient who does not have symptoms or signs compatible with CA-UTI (Tables 50-2 and 50-3).[41,51] Obtaining a screening urine culture in an asymptomatic patient is only recommended in the setting of pregnancy and in patients undergoing urologic procedures where visible mucosal bleeding is anticipated.[41,51] Other than these clinical scenarios, obtaining a urine culture is not recommended unless there are signs or symptoms compatible with CA-UTI.

CA-UTI is defined as a patient with symptoms and signs compatible with CA-UTI, with growth of greater than or equal to 1000 CFU/mL of one or more bacterial species from a catheterized urine specimen (either from an indwelling urinary catheter, suprapubic catheter, or intermittent catheterization) or from a midstream voided urine specimen from a patient whose catheter was removed in the preceding 48 hours (see Tables 50-2 and 50-3).[41] The diagnosis of CA-UTI can often be challenging, since patients with urinary catheters do not have typical symptoms of UTI (ie, dysuria, frequency, or urgency) that are seen in noncatheterized patients.[41,47] In addition, many ICU patients are intubated and/or sedated and soliciting symptoms is difficult or impossible.

Infectious Disease

Table 50-2. Diagnosis and Management of Catheter-Associated Asymptomatic Bacteriuria and Catheter-Associated Urinary Tract Infection (CA-UTI)

Catheter-associated asymptomatic bacteriuria
• Presence of > 100,000 CFU/mL of ≥ 1 bacterial species from a catheterized urine specimen
Plus
• No symptoms or signs compatible with CA-UTI (see Table 50-3)
Management: No antibiotic therapy indicated, except in select situations (see text)

- -

Catheter-associated urinary tract infection
• Presence of ≥ 1000 CFU/mL of ≥ 1 bacterial species from a catheterized urine specimen or from a midstream voided urine specimen if a catheter was removed in the preceding 48 h
Plus
• Symptoms compatible with CA-UTI with no other identified source (see Table 50-3)
Management: Antibiotic therapy indicated

(Adapted from Hooton TM, Bradley SF, Cardenas DD, et al. Diagnosis, prevention, and treatment of catheter-associated urinary tract infection in adults: 2009 International Clinical Practice Guidelines from the Infectious Diseases Society of America. Clin Infect Dis. 2010;50(5):625-663.)

 The patient had CA-ASB, since she had significant bacteriuria (ie, growth of ≥ 100,000 CFU/mL of *Enterococcus faecalis*), but no symptoms or signs suggestive of CA-UTI. The trigger for obtaining a urinalysis in this patient was renal insufficiency in the setting of congestive heart failure. The urinalysis showed 10 to 25 leukocytes per high-power field; however, as discussed below (see "Can pyuria distinguish between CA-ASB and CA-UTI?"), pyuria is not specific for infection in catheterized patients. This led to obtaining a urine culture, despite no symptoms or signs of infection. One of the important lessons to learn from this case is that obtaining a urine culture in an asymptomatic patient is not recommended, except in certain scenarios (eg, pregnancy, prior to urologic procedures).

Does growth of greater than or equal to 100,000 CFU/mL of an organism from a catheterized urine specimen indicate CA-UTI, regardless of whether the patient has symptoms compatible with infection?

As discussed above, the quantity of growth of an organism in urine culture does not distinguish symptomatic from asymptomatic infection in catheterized patients (see Tables 50-2 and 50-3). The

Table 50-3. Symptoms and Signs Compatible with Catheter-Associated Urinary Tract Infection

New onset or worsening of any of the following (with no other identified cause):
• Fever, rigors, altered mental status, malaise, or lethargy

Any of the following:
• Flank pain, costovertebral angle tenderness, acute hematuria, or pelvic discomfort

For patients whose catheters have been removed:
• May also have dysuria, urinary frequency or urgency, or suprapubic pain or tenderness, in addition to above

For patients with spinal cord injury:
• May also have increased spasticity, autonomic dysreflexia, or sense of uneasiness, in addition to above

Other:
• Malodorous or cloudy urine alone should not be used to differentiate infection from asymptomatic bacteriuria

(Adapted from Hooton TM, Bradley SF, Cardenas DD, et al. Diagnosis, prevention, and treatment of catheter-associated urinary tract infection in adults: 2009 International Clinical Practice Guidelines from the Infectious Diseases Society of America. Clin Infect Dis. 2010;50(5):625-663.)

quantitative count of greater than or equal to 100,000 CFU/mL has only been validated for use as a cutoff for the diagnosis of UTI in patients with symptoms of UTI who do not have a urinary catheter and provide a midstream voided sample.[51-53] This quantitative count has been shown to be able to reliably distinguish true bacteriuria from contamination by periurethral flora when a midstream voided sample is obtained.[51-53]

However, for patients with urinary catheters, there is no standard definition for significant bacteriuria.[41] The specific quantitative count of bacterial growth required to differentiate contamination from true bladder bacteriuria is recommended to be lower than the traditional cutoff of greater than or equal to 100,000 CFU/mL for noncatheterized patients.[41] There are several reasons why a lower quantitative culture cutoff (ie, ≥ 1000 CFU/mL) is likely to reflect true bladder bacteriuria in catheterized patients and is suggested for the diagnosis of CA-UTI.[41] First, catheterized urine specimens are less likely to be contaminated by periurethral flora, as are voided urine specimens; therefore, lower colony counts are more likely to represent true bladder bacteriuria.[41] Second, patients with symptomatic UTI have been shown to have colony counts considerably below 100,000 CFU/mL, and as low as 100 CFU/mL.[52,53] Last, almost all catheterized patients with colony counts as low as 1000 cfu/mL progress rapidly to concentrations greater than or equal to 100,000 CFU/mL, usually within 72 hours, if antimicrobial therapy is not given.[52]

What are the issues with obtaining a urine culture in a patient with a long-term urinary catheter (in place for ≥ 30 days)?

With respect to collection of urine specimens for patients with long-term catheters (ie, catheters in place for ≥ 30 days), it may be useful to obtain a urine culture after removing and placing a new catheter.[41] The reason for this is that some organisms (eg, staphylococci, enterococci, *P aeruginosa*, and *Proteus* species) are more likely to adhere to the urinary catheter rather than to uroepithelial cells; this is in contrast to other organisms (eg, *E coli* and *Klebsiella* species) that are more likely to adhere to uroepithelial cells and persist after catheter exchange.[54] Therefore, urine specimens obtained from a freshly placed catheter in patients with long-term catheters may be a better reflection of organisms present in the bladder.

Can pyuria distinguish between CA-ASB and CA-UTI?

Pyuria (commonly defined as > 5 leukocytes per high-power field) is common in patients with CA-ASB and CA-UTI and cannot reliably distinguish between asymptomatic and symptomatic infection.[51] This is in contrast to patients without a urinary catheter who provide a midstream voided specimen, where pyuria has been shown to have high sensitivity and specificity for the diagnosis of UTI.[55,56] For patients with a urinary catheter, pyuria has a low positive predictive value for CA-UTI (32% in one prospective study of 761 catheterized patients).[55] Thus, in a catheterized patient, presence of pyuria is not diagnostic of CA-UTI. The negative predictive value of pyuria for CA-UTI appears to be high (94% in that same study)[55]; therefore, the absence of pyuria makes the diagnosis of CA-UTI less likely.[41]

What are the recommendations for management of CA-ASB?

Screening for or treating CA-ASB is not recommended, except in select clinical scenarios.[41,51] Studies have shown that catheter-associated bacteriuria may be transiently cleared with antimicrobial therapy; however, bacteriuria recurs in the majority of patients.[45,57,58] Antibiotic therapy has not been shown to reduce the incidence of future episodes of bacteriuria or urinary tract infection, since bacteriuria rapidly recurs, especially if the catheter is still in place.[41,51,57-59] Furthermore, in patients with CA-ASB who are treated with antibiotic therapy, recurrence of bacteriuria typically occurs with resistant microorganisms.[41,51,57,58]

The exceptions are that asymptomatic bacteriuria is recommended to be screened for and treated in (1) pregnant women, since treatment has been shown to decrease the risk of pyelonephritis, and

(2) patients undergoing urologic procedures associated with mucosal bleeding, where the risk of post-procedure bacteremia is high.[51] Other patient groups where treatment of ASB may be considered include renal transplant patients and patients with ureteral stents or nephrostomy tubes, although evidence is limited to support this recommendation. Another group where treatment of ASB may be considered is in catheterized women with asymptomatic bacteriuria that persists 48 hours after catheter removal. A clinical trial in this population showed that treatment with antibiotic therapy reduced the risk of subsequent development of a symptomatic UTI as compared with women who did not receive antibiotic therapy.[60]

The patient had CA-ASB and antibiotic therapy appropriately withheld. Unfortunately, inappropriate treatment of CA-ASB, especially with fluoroquinolones, is not uncommon. This frequently results in antimicrobial resistance and can predispose to *C difficile* infection, particularly since fluoroquinolones are now one of the most likely antibiotic agents to predispose to *C difficile* infection.[61,62]

What are the recommendations for treatment of CA-UTI?

To help guide antibiotic therapy, obtaining a urine culture prior to initiating antibiotic therapy is recommended. Microorganisms that frequently cause CA-UTI include *E coli*, *Klebsiella* species, *Serratia* species, *Citrobacter* species, and *Enterobacter* species.[63] Of the nonfermenting gram-negative bacilli, *P aeruginosa* is also commonly isolated.[63] Enterococci and coagulase-negative staphylococci are also commonly isolated, but are less virulent and more commonly lead to asymptomatic bacteriuria.[63] For patients with long-term urinary catheters (ie, catheters in place for ≥ 30 days), CA-UTI is frequently polymicrobial, and in addition to the above listed organisms, the following organisms may be seen: *Proteus* species, *Morganella* species, and *Providencia* species.[63] If antibiotic coverage for CA-UTI is desired prior to availability of culture results, empiric coverage for the most likely pathogens is recommended. Prior culture results may affect empiric antibiotic choice (eg, recent isolation of fluoroquinolone-resistant *E. coli* should prompt empiric use of a different antibiotic other than a fluoroquinolone). The antibiotic treatment should subsequently be modified based on identification of the pathogen and antimicrobial susceptibility results.

Does changing the urinary catheter prior to treatment for CA-UTI affect outcome?

Prior to initiating therapy for CA-UTI, it may be reasonable to change the catheter if it has been in place for 2 weeks or longer.[41] A clinical trial in nursing home residents who had urinary catheters in place for at least 2 weeks showed that changing the urinary catheter prior to treatment led to a greater proportion of patients with clearance of bacteriuria at 72 hours and a lower recurrence rate of bacteriuria 28 days after treatment was completed.[64]

What is the recommended duration of treatment for CA-UTI?

The optimal duration of therapy for CA-UTI is not known. Recommended duration of therapy varies from 7 to 14 days.[41,63,65] A shorter duration is desired to limit the emergence of antibiotic resistance. For patients with milder infection and those who respond to treatment promptly, a 7-day course of antibiotic therapy is recommended.[41,63] For patients with a delayed response to treatment, a 10- to 14-day course is recommended.[41] For CA-UTI with bacteremia and/or pyelonephritis, a 14-day course of antibiotic therapy is suggested.

What are the recommendations for the diagnosis and management of candiduria?

Catheter-associated (CA) candiduria can be divided into CA asymptomatic candiduria and CA symptomatic candiduria. CA candiduria is most commonly asymptomatic[47,65,66,]; however, it can rarely lead to complications such as bladder fungus ball or ascending infection.[65] The diagnostic approach is similar to CA-ASB and CA-UTI, in that a positive urine culture for *Candida* does not distinguish symptomatic from asymptomatic infection in catheterized patients. Thus, the diagnosis of CA symptomatic candiduria can be challenging, since typical symptoms of UTI (ie, dysuria, frequency, or urgency) are not seen and symptoms and signs compatible with CA-UTI (see Table 50-3) may be difficult to attribute to the candiduria.

Treatment of CA asymptomatic candiduria is not recommended, except in certain clinical scenarios.[67,68] In a clinical trial of 316 patients with candiduria (over 95% were asymptomatic, and about half had a urinary catheter), there was a higher eradication rate of candiduria in catheterized patients receiving 14 days of fluconazole (50% versus 29%); however, the rates of candiduria 2 weeks after therapy was completed were similar in both groups (61% versus 56%), pointing out the difficulty of eradicating candiduria in patients with an indwelling urinary catheter.[68] Treatment of CA asymptomatic candiduria is only recommended in certain high-risk patient groups including patients undergoing urologic procedures, neutropenic patients, and infants with low birth weight.[67] Other patient groups where treatment may be considered include renal transplant patients and patients with ureteral stents or nephrostomy tubes, although further data are needed to support this recommendation.

Treatment of CA symptomatic candiduria is recommended. The preferred agent for fluconazole-susceptible *Candida* species (eg, *Candida albicans*) is fluconazole (200 mg daily for 2 weeks for cystitis; 200-400 mg daily for 2 weeks for pyelonephritis; and 400 mg daily for 2 weeks for patients with disseminated candidiasis).[67] For fluconazole-resistant *Candida* species, infectious diseases consultation is recommended, where intravenous amphotericin B deoxycholate may be considered.[67] Echinocandins, such as caspofungin, have been used for cases of symptomatic UTI caused by fluconazole-resistant *Candida* species; however, clinical trial data are lacking.[69]

What are the recommended strategies for reducing the risk of CA-UTI?

The most important strategy for reducing the risk of CA-UTI is to minimize the inappropriate use of urinary catheters. Indwelling urinary catheters should only be placed for acceptable indications and they should be removed as soon as they are no longer necessary.[41] Urinary catheters should be placed using aseptic technique and sterile equipment.[41] A closed catheter drainage system should be used and the drainage bag and connecting tube should always be kept below the level of the bladder; disconnection of the catheter junction should be minimized.[41,45] Prophylaxis with systemic antimicrobials and catheter irrigation with antimicrobials are not recommended, and addition of antimicrobials or antiseptics to the drainage bag should be avoided.[41] Daily meatal cleansing with povidone-iodine solution, silver sulfadiazine, or antibiotic creams is not recommended.[41]

A 49-year-old woman with severe osteoarthritis of the knees underwent a right total knee joint replacement. On hospital day 2, she developed fever with a temperature of 38.2°C (100.8°F). Urinalysis performed on a catheterized urine specimen showed 10 to 25 leukocytes per high-power field. She was presumptively diagnosed with CA-UTI and was given empiric oral ciprofloxacin, although a urine culture that was obtained prior to starting antibiotic therapy subsequently showed no growth. She did not have further fever. Ciprofloxacin was discontinued after

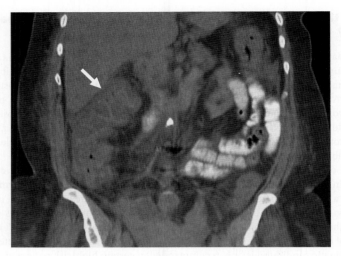

Figure 50-5. Computed tomography of the abdomen/pelvis (coronal view) showing extensive thickening of the wall of the ascending colon with pericolonic infiltration (*white arrow*).

the urine culture result returned, although she received a total of 3 days of antibiotic therapy. She was discharged to an acute rehabilitation facility on hospital day 5.

Four days later, she developed watery diarrhea. The following day, she developed fever with a temperature of 38.3°C (101°F), profuse diarrhea (> 10 watery bowel movements), severe abdominal pain, and altered mental status. A stool enzyme immunoassay for *C difficile* toxin A/B was positive. She was started on oral metronidazole and was admitted to the intensive care unit. She had a temperature of 38.8°C (101.8°F), blood pressure of 79/45 mm Hg, and heart rate of 118 bpm. She required 5 L of intravenous fluids. The peripheral blood leukocyte count was 25,500 cells/mm³, with 34% band forms. The serum creatinine was elevated at 2.5 mg/dL. Computed tomography of the abdomen and pelvis showed extensive thickening of the wall of the ascending colon with pericolonic infiltration, and thickening of the transverse, descending, and sigmoid colon as well (Figure 50-5). There was no free intraperitoneal air, bowel wall pneumatosis, or toxic megacolon.

What are the clinical features that suggest severe *C difficile*-associated disease?

There is currently no standard definition for severe *C difficile*–associated disease (CDAD). In one study of risk factors for complicated CDAD (defined as presence of toxic megacolon, perforation, requirement for colectomy, shock requiring vasopressor therapy, or death) in Quebec, age 65 years or older, an elevated creatinine level greater than 1.1 mg/dL, immunosuppression, and a peripheral blood leukocyte count greater than 20,000 cells/mm³ were predictive of complicated CDAD.[70] When the creatinine was above 2.3 mg/dL, the risk of complicated CDAD was even greater.[70]

In a clinical trial comparing metronidazole versus vancomycin for CDAD, variables used to define severity of disease included age older than 60 years, temperature greater than 38.3°C (101°F), albumin less than 2.5 mg/dL, peripheral blood leukocyte count greater than 15,000 cells/mm³, endoscopic evidence of pseudomembranous colitis, and intensive care unit admission.[71] In a subsequent clinical trial comparing metronidazole, vancomycin, and tolevamer for CDAD, severe CDAD was defined as one of the following: 10 or more bowel movements per day, peripheral blood leukocyte count greater than 20,000 cells/mm³, or severe abdominal pain due to CDAD.[72]

Table 50-4. Clinical Features and Management of Severe Clostridium difficile–Associated Disease (CDAD)

Clinical features suggestive of severe CDAD
• Blood leukocyte count > 15,000-20,000 cells/mm^3
• Acute renal failure
• Profuse diarrhea (eg, ≥ 10 bowel movements per day)
Management of severe CDAD
• Vancomycin 125-500 mg orally every 6 h
+/–
• Metronidazole 500 mg intravenously every 6-8 h^a

^{a}Consider intravenous metronidazole for patients with severe CDAD associated with ileus or for patients with complicated CDAD (eg, shock, perforation, or toxic megacolon).

Deciding whether a patient has severe CDAD should be based on clinical judgment; however, most patients with severe disease will have an elevated peripheral blood leukocyte count greater than 15,000 to 20,000 cells/mm^3 (which is likely a marker of the severity of colonic inflammation) and/or severe diarrhea that may be complicated by acute renal failure (Table 50-4). Severe CDAD can progress to complicated CDAD, where shock, perforation, or toxic megacolon may be seen.

 The patient initially had findings suggestive of severe CDAD, including profuse diarrhea (≥ 10 bowel movements per day), acute renal failure, and increased peripheral blood leukocyte count greater than 20,000 cells/mm^3.

What is the recommended management for severe *C. difficile*-associated disease?

There are two recent clinical trials comparing oral metronidazole versus oral vancomycin for the treatment of CDAD.[71,72] Both trials showed no difference in clinical success or cure rate between metronidazole and vancomycin for mild or moderate CDAD; however, for patients with severe CDAD, vancomycin was superior to metronidazole. Based on these data, oral vancomycin has been recommended by many experts as the preferred treatment for patients with severe CDAD (see Table 50-4).[62,73] Treatment duration should be 10 to 14 days.[62] Doses of oral vancomycin that have been used include 125 mg, 250 mg, or 500 mg orally every 6 hours. It appears that 125 mg every 6 hours may be as efficacious as 500 mg every 6 hours, although more data are needed.[74]

For patients with severe infection associated with ileus or for patients with complicated CDAD, metronidazole 500 mg intravenously every 6 to 8 hours may be combined with oral vancomycin (if patient is able to take medications enterally).[62] The rationale for this is that if there is delayed passage of oral vancomycin to the colon, intravenous metronidazole may have activity as it has been shown to have adequate fecal concentrations.[62,75] Use of intracolonic vancomycin via retention enema may be considered in select situations, although data are limited.[76] Although cases of intravenous immunoglobulin (IVIG) being used for severe CDAD have been reported,[77,78] a recent small retrospective cohort study with propensity matching did not show a benefit of IVIG for severe CDAD.[79] Other treatments, including probiotics, rifaximin, cholestyramine, and fecal bacteriotherapy, do not play a role in the treatment of severe CDAD, but may be beneficial in patients with recurrent CDAD.[62] For patients with signs of complicated CDAD including perforation, shock, or toxic megacolon, antibiotic

Infectious Disease

coverage for bowel flora, including enteric gram-negative bacilli, should be considered. Lastly, early surgical consultation is recommended for patients with severe CDAD, since early subtotal colectomy may be required if complicated CDAD develops.[62,80]

Oral vancomycin 250 mg orally every 6 hours and metronidazole 500 mg intravenously every 8 hours were initiated. Despite this, her peripheral blood leukocyte count increased to 44,800 cells/mm^3, with 54% band forms, and she required vasopressor support. She was taken to the operating room for exploratory laparotomy, where ischemia of the colon was identified, necessitating subtotal colectomy. Important points to learn from this case include avoiding unnecessary antibiotic use, clinical features that suggest severe CDAD, and treatment considerations for severe CDAD.

! CRITICAL CONSIDERATIONS

- Evaluation of a new fever in an ICU patient should always begin with a thorough review of the patient's history and a focused physical examination, rather than automatic ordering of microbiologic studies.
- The differential diagnosis of a new fever in an ICU patient includes both infectious and noninfectious etiologies.
- Cultures of lower respiratory tract secretions help determine the microbial etiology of HAP/VAP and should be collected prior to starting or changing antibiotic therapy.
- Unless there is low suspicion for HAP/VAP, empiric antibiotic therapy should be initiated as soon as possible after a lower respiratory tract sample is obtained for culture.
- In order to increase the probability of achieving appropriate antibiotic therapy for HAP/VAP, the initial empiric antibiotic regimen should be based on the patient's risk for multidrug-resistant pathogens.
- Narrowing antibiotic therapy (ie, de-escalation) for HAP/VAP is important to minimize the emergence of antibiotic resistance.
- A shorter duration (7-8 days) of antibiotic therapy for HAP/VAP is recommended for patients who clinically respond to treatment and who are not infected with nonfermenting gram-negative bacilli.
- Bacteriuria is a very common finding in patients with indwelling urinary catheters, and the majority of patients are asymptomatic.
- Symptoms or signs compatible with CA-UTI are required for the diagnosis of CA-UTI.
- Screening for or treating CA-ASB is not recommended, except in select clinical scenarios.
- A shorter duration of treatment for CA-UTI is desired to limit the emergence of antibiotic resistance. For patients with milder infection and those who respond to treatment promptly, a 7-day course of antibiotic therapy is recommended.
- Patients with severe CDAD may have an elevated leukocyte count greater than 15,000 to 20,000 cells/mm^3 and/or severe diarrhea that may be complicated by acute renal failure.
- Oral vancomycin is recommended for patients with severe CDAD, which may be combined with intravenous metronidazole for patients with ileus or complicated infection.
- Early surgical consultation is recommended for patients with severe CDAD.

REFERENCES

1. O'Grady NP, Barie PS, Bartlett JG, et al.; American College of Critical Care Medicine; Infectious Diseases Society of America. Guidelines for evaluation of new fever in critically ill adult patients: 2008 update from the American College of Critical Care Medicine and the Infectious Diseases Society of America. *Crit Care Med.* 2008;36(4):1330-1349.

2. Commichau C, Scarmeas N, Mayer SA. Risk factors for fever in the neurologic intensive care unit. *Neurology.* 2003;60(5):837-841.

3. Marik PE. Fever in the ICU. *Chest.* 2000;117(3): 855-869.

4. American Thoracic Society, Infectious Diseases Society of America. Guidelines for the management of adults with hospital-acquired, ventilator-associated, and healthcare-associated pneumonia. *Am J Respir Crit Care Med.* 2005;171(4):388-416.

5. Fàbregas N, Ewig S, Torres A, et al. Clinical diagnosis of ventilator associated pneumonia revisited: comparative validation using immediate post-mortem lung biopsies. *Thorax.* 1999;54(10):867-873.

6. Souweine B, Veber B, Bedos JP, et al. Diagnostic accuracy of protected specimen brush and bronchoalveolar lavage in nosocomial pneumonia: impact of previous antimicrobial treatments. *Crit Care Med.* 1998;26(2):236-244.

7. Torres A, El-Ebiary M. Bronchoscopic BAL in the diagnosis of ventilator-associated pneumonia. *Chest.* 2000;117(4 Suppl 2):198S-202S.

8. Cook D, Mandell L. Endotracheal aspiration in the diagnosis of ventilator-associated pneumonia. *Chest.* 2000;117(4 Suppl 2):195S-197S.

9. Marquette CH, Georges H, Wallet F, et al. Diagnostic efficiency of endotracheal aspirates with quantitative bacterial cultures in intubated patients with suspected pneumonia. Comparison with the protected specimen brush. *Am Rev Respir Dis.* 1993;148(1):138-144.

10. Fagon JY, Chastre J, Wolff M, et al. Invasive and noninvasive strategies for management of suspected ventilator-associated pneumonia. A randomized trial. *Ann Intern Med.* 2000;132(8):621-630.

11. Canadian Critical Care Trials Group. A randomized trial of diagnostic techniques for ventilator-associated pneumonia. *N Engl J Med.* 2006;355(25):2619-2630.

12. Berton DC, Kalil AC, Cavalcanti M, Teixeira PJ. Quantitative versus qualitative cultures of respiratory secretions for clinical outcomes in patients with ventilator-associated pneumonia. *Cochrane Database Syst Rev.* 2008;(4):CD006482.

13. Baker AM, Bowton DL, Haponik EF. Decision making in nosocomial pneumonia. An analytic approach to the interpretation of quantitative bronchoscopic cultures. *Chest.* 1995;107(1):85-95.

14. Alvarez-Lerma F. Modification of empiric antibiotic treatment in patients with pneumonia acquired in the intensive care unit. ICU-Acquired Pneumonia Study Group. *Intensive Care Med.* 1996;22(5): 387-394.

15. Iregui M, Ward S, Sherman G, Fraser VJ, Kollef MH. Clinical importance of delays in the initiation of appropriate antibiotic treatment for ventilator-associated pneumonia. *Chest.* 2002;122(1):262-268.

16. Craven DE, Chroneou A. Nosocomial pneumonia. In: Mandell GL, Bennett JE, Dolin R, eds. *Mandell, Douglas, and Bennett's Principles and Practice of Infectious Diseases.* 7th ed. Philadelphia, PA: Churchill Livingstone Elsevier; 2010:3717-3724.

17. Kaye KS, Fraimow HS, Abrutyn E. Pathogens resistant to antimicrobial agents. Epidemiology, molecular mechanisms, and clinical management. *Infect Dis Clin North Am.* 2000;14(2):293-319.

18. Chow JW, Fine MJ, Shlaes DM, et al. *Enterobacter* bacteremia: clinical features and emergence of antibiotic resistance during therapy. *Ann Intern Med.* 1991;115(8):585-590.

19. Chastre J, Wunderink R, Prokocimer P, Lee M, Kaniga K, Friedland I. Efficacy and safety of intravenous infusion of doripenem versus imipenem in ventilator-associated pneumonia: a multicenter, randomized study. *Crit Care Med.* 2008;36(4):1089-1096.

20. Réa-Neto A, Niederman M, Lobo SM, et al. Efficacy and safety of doripenem versus piperacillin/tazobactam in nosocomial pneumonia: a randomized, open-label, multicenter study. *Curr Med Res Opin.* 2008;24(7):2113-2126.

21. Rybak MJ, Lomaestro BM, Rotschafer JC, et al. Therapeutic monitoring of vancomycin in adults summary of consensus recommendations from the American Society of Health-System Pharmacists, the Infectious Diseases Society of America, and the Society of Infectious Diseases Pharmacists. *Pharmacotherapy.* 2009;29(11):1275-1279.

22. Trouillet JL, Vuagnat A, Combes A, Kassis N, Chastre J, Gibert C. *Pseudomonas aeruginosa* ventilator-associated pneumonia: comparison of episodes due to piperacillin-resistant versus piperacillin-susceptible organisms. *Clin Infect Dis.* 2002;34(8):1047-1054.

23. Namias N, Samiian L, Nino D, et al. Incidence and susceptibility of pathogenic bacteria vary between intensive care units within a single hospital: implications for empiric antibiotic strategies. *J Trauma.* 2000;49(4):638-646.

24. Luna CM, Blanzaco D, Niederman MS, et al. Resolution of ventilator-associated pneumonia:

prospective evaluation of the clinical pulmonary infection score as an early clinical predictor of outcome. *Crit Care Med.* 2003;31(3):676-682.

25. Dennesen PJ, van der Ven AJ, Kessels AG, Ramsay G, Bonten MJ. Resolution of infectious parameters after antimicrobial therapy in patients with ventilator-associated pneumonia. *Am J Respir Crit Care Med.* 2001;163(6):1371-1375.

26. Niederman MS. De-escalation therapy in ventilator-associated pneumonia. *Curr Opin Crit Care.* 2006; 12(5):452-457.

27. Kirtland SH, Corley DE, Winterbauer RH, et al. The diagnosis of ventilator-associated pneumonia: a comparison of histologic, microbiologic, and clinical criteria. *Chest.* 1997;112(2):445-457.

28. Hilf M, Yu VL, Sharp J, Zuravleff JJ, Korvick JA, Muder RR. Antibiotic therapy for *Pseudomonas aeruginosa* bacteremia: outcome correlations in a prospective study of 200 patients. *Am J Med.* 1989;87(5):540-546.

29. Cometta A, Baumgartner JD, Lew D, et al. Prospective randomized comparison of imipenem monotherapy with imipenem plus netilmicin for treatment of severe infections in nonneutropenic patients. *Antimicrob Agents Chemother.* 1994;38(6):1309-1313.

30. Garnacho-Montero J, Sa-Borges M, Sole-Violan J, et al. Optimal management therapy for *Pseudomonas aeruginosa* ventilator-associated pneumonia: an observational, multicenter study comparing monotherapy with combination antibiotic therapy. *Crit Care Med.* 2007;35(8):1888-1895.

31. Heyland DK, Dodek P, Muscedere J, Day A, Cook D; Canadian Critical Care Trials Group. Randomized trial of combination versus monotherapy for the empiric treatment of suspected ventilator-associated pneumonia. *Crit Care Med.* 2008;36(3):737-744.

32. Aarts MA, Hancock JN, Heyland D, McLeod RS, Marshall JC. Empiric antibiotic therapy for suspected ventilator-associated pneumonia: a systematic review and meta-analysis of randomized trials. *Crit Care Med.* 2008;36(1):108-117.

33. Rubinstein E, Cammarata S, Oliphant T, Wunderink R; Linezolid Nosocomial Pneumonia Study Group. Linezolid (PNU-100766) versus vancomycin in the treatment of hospitalized patients with nosocomial pneumonia: a randomized, double-blind, multicenter study. *Clin Infect Dis.* 2001;32(3):402-412.

34. Wunderink RG, Cammarata SK, Oliphant TH, Kollef MH; Linezolid Nosocomial Pneumonia Study Group. Continuation of a randomized, double-blind, multicenter study of linezolid versus vancomycin in the treatment of patients with nosocomial pneumonia. *Clin Ther.* 2003;25(3):980-992.

35. Wunderink RG, Rello J, Cammarata SK, Croos-Dabrera RV, Kollef MH. Linezolid vs vancomycin: analysis of two double-blind studies of patients with methicillin-resistant *Staphylococcus aureus* nosocomial pneumonia. *Chest.* 2003;124(5):1789-1797.

36. Powers JH, Ross DB, Lin D, Soreth J. Linezolid and vancomycin for methicillin-resistant *Staphylococcus aureus* nosocomial pneumonia: the subtleties of subgroup analyses. *Chest.* 2004;126(1):314-315.

37. Wunderink RG, Mendelson MH, Somero MS, et al. Early microbiological response to linezolid vs vancomycin in ventilator-associated pneumonia due to methicillin-resistant *Staphylococcus aureus.* *Chest.* 2008;134(6):1200-1207.

38. Hidayat LK, Hsu DI, Quist R, Shriner KA, Wong-Beringer A. High-dose vancomycin therapy for methicillin-resistant *Staphylococcus aureus* infections: efficacy and toxicity. *Arch Intern Med.* 2006;166(19):2138-2144.

39. Jeffres MN, Isakow W, Doherty JA, et al. Predictors of mortality for methicillin-resistant *Staphylococcus aureus* health-care-associated pneumonia: specific evaluation of vancomycin pharmacokinetic indices. *Chest.* 2006;130(4):947-955.

40. Chastre J, Wolff M, Fagon JY, et al.; PneumA Trial Group. Comparison of 8 vs 15 days of antibiotic therapy for ventilator-associated pneumonia in adults: a randomized trial. *JAMA.* 2003;290(19):2588-2598.

41. Hooton TM, Bradley SF, Cardenas DD, et al. Diagnosis, prevention, and treatment of catheter-associated urinary tract infection in adults: 2009 International Clinical Practice Guidelines from the Infectious Diseases Society of America. *Clin Infect Dis.* 2010;50(5):625-663.

42. Garibaldi RA, Burke JP, Dickman ML, Smith CB. Factors predisposing to bacteriuria during indwelling urethral catheterization. *N Engl J Med.* 1974;291(5):215-219.

43. Hartstein AI, Garber SB, Ward TT, Jones SR, Morthland VH. Nosocomial urinary tract infection: a prospective evaluation of 108 catheterized patients. *Infect Control.* 1981;2(5):380-386.

44. Classen DC, Larsen RA, Burke JP, Stevens LE. Prevention of catheter-associated bacteriuria: clinical trial of methods to block three known pathways of infection. *Am J Infect Control.* 1991;19(3):136-142.

45. Kunin CM, McCormack RC. Prevention of catheter-induced urinary-tract infections by sterile closed drainage. *N Engl J Med.* 1966;274(21):1155-1161.

46. Maki DG, Tambyah PA. Engineering out the risk for infection with urinary catheters. *Emerg Infect Dis.* 2001;7(2):342-347.

47. Tambyah PA, Maki DG. Catheter-associated urinary tract infection is rarely symptomatic: a prospective

study of 1,497 catheterized patients. *Arch Intern Med.* 2000;160(5):678-682.

48. Saint S. Clinical and economic consequences of nosocomial catheter-related bacteriuria. *Am J Infect Control.* 2000;28(1):68-75.

49. Bryan CS, Reynolds KL. Hospital-acquired bacteremic urinary tract infection: epidemiology and outcome. *J Urol.* 1984;132(3):494-498.

50. Krieger JN, Kaiser DL, Wenzel RP. Urinary tract etiology of bloodstream infections in hospitalized patients. *J Infect Dis.* 1983;148(1):57-62.

51. Nicolle LE, Bradley S, Colgan R, Rice JC, Schaeffer A, Hooton TM; Infectious Diseases Society of America; American Society of Nephrology; American Geriatric Society. Infectious Diseases Society of America guidelines for the diagnosis and treatment of asymptomatic bacteriuria in adults. *Clin Infect Dis.* 2005;40(5):643-654.

52. Stark RP, Maki DG. Bacteriuria in the catheterized patient. What quantitative level of bacteriuria is relevant? *N Engl J Med.* 1984;311(9):560-564.

53. Stamm WE, Counts GW, Running KR, Fihn S, Turck M, Holmes KK. Diagnosis of coliform infection in acutely dysuric women. *N Engl J Med.* 1982;307(8):463-468.

54. Tenney JH, Warren JW. Bacteriuria in women with long-term catheters: paired comparison of indwelling and replacement catheters. *J Infect Dis.* 1988;157(1):199-202.

55. Tambyah PA, Maki DG. The relationship between pyuria and infection in patients with indwelling urinary catheters: a prospective study of 761 patients. *Arch Intern Med.* 2000;160(5):673-677.

56. Steward DK, Wood GL, Cohen RL, Smith JW, Mackowiak PA. Failure of the urinalysis and quantitative urine culture in diagnosing symptomatic urinary tract infections in patients with long-term urinary catheters. *Am J Infect Control.* 1985;13(4):154-160.

57. Warren JW, Anthony WC, Hoopes JM, Muncie HL Jr. Cephalexin for susceptible bacteriuria in afebrile, long-term catheterized patients. *JAMA.* 1982;248(4):454-458.

58. Alling B, Brandberg A, Seeberg S, Svanborg A. Effect of consecutive antibacterial therapy on bacteriuria in hospitalized geriatric patients. *Scand J Infect Dis.* 1975;7(3):201-207.

59. Leone M, Perrin AS, Granier I, et al. A randomized trial of catheter change and short course of antibiotics for asymptomatic bacteriuria in catheterized ICU patients. *Intensive Care Med.* 2007;33(4):726-729.

60. Harding GK, Nicolle LE, Ronald AR, et al. How long should catheter-acquired urinary tract infection in women be treated? A randomized controlled study. *Ann Intern Med.* 1991;114(9):713-719.

61. Pépin J, Saheb N, Coulombe MA, et al. Emergence of fluoroquinolones as the predominant risk factor for *Clostridium difficile*-associated diarrhea: a cohort study during an epidemic in Quebec. *Clin Infect Dis.* 2005;41(9):1254-1260.

62. Kelly CP, LaMont JT. *Clostridium difficile*—more difficult than ever. *N Engl J Med.* 2008;359(18):1932-1940.

63. Nicolle LE. Catheter-related urinary tract infection. *Drugs Aging.* 2005;22(8):627-639.

64. Raz R, Schiller D, Nicolle LE. Chronic indwelling catheter replacement before antimicrobial therapy for symptomatic urinary tract infection. *J Urol.* 2000;164(4):1254-1258.

65. Warren JW. Catheter-associated urinary tract infections. *Infect Dis Clin North Am.* 1997;11(3):609-622.

66. Kauffman CA, Vazquez JA, Sobel JD, et al. Prospective multicenter surveillance study of funguria in hospitalized patients. The National Institute for Allergy and Infectious Diseases (NIAID) Mycoses Study Group. *Clin Infect Dis.* 2000;30(1):14-18.

67. Pappas PG, Kauffman CA, Andes D, et al.; Infectious Diseases Society of America. Clinical practice guidelines for the management of candidiasis: 2009 update by the Infectious Diseases Society of America. *Clin Infect Dis.* 2009;48(5):503-535.

68. Sobel JD, Kauffman CA, McKinsey D, et al. Candiduria: a randomized, double-blind study of treatment with fluconazole and placebo. The National Institute of Allergy and Infectious Diseases (NIAID) Mycoses Study Group. *Clin Infect Dis.* 2000;30(1):19-24.

69. Sobel JD, Bradshaw SK, Lipka CJ, Kartsonis NA. Caspofungin in the treatment of symptomatic candiduria. *Clin Infect Dis.* 2007;44(5):e46-e49.

70. Pépin J, Valiquette L, Alary ME, et al. *Clostridium difficile*-associated diarrhea in a region of Quebec from 1991 to 2003: a changing pattern of disease severity. *CMAJ.* 2004;171(5):466-472.

71. Zar FA, Bakkanagari SR, Moorthi KM, Davis MB. A comparison of vancomycin and metronidazole for the treatment of *Clostridium difficile*-associated diarrhea, stratified by disease severity. *Clin Infect Dis.* 2007;45(3):302-307.

72. Louie T, Gerson M, Grimard D, et al. Results of a phase III trial comparing tolevamer, vancomycin and metronidazole in *Clostridium difficile*-associated diarrhea (CDAD) [abstract K-425a]. In: *Program and Abstracts of the 47th Interscience Conference on Antimicrobial Agents and Chemotherapy (Chicago, IL).* Washington, DC: American Society for Microbiology; 2007.

Infectious Disease

73. Bartlett JG. The case for vancomycin as the preferred drug for treatment of *Clostridium difficile* infection. *Clin Infect Dis.* 2008;46(10):1489-1492.

74. Fekety R, Silva J, Kauffman C, Buggy B, Deery HG. Treatment of antibiotic-associated *Clostridium difficile* colitis with oral vancomycin: comparison of two dosage regimens. *Am J Med.* 1989;86(1):15-19.

75. Bolton RP, Culshaw MA. Faecal metronidazole concentrations during oral and intravenous therapy for antibiotic associated colitis due to *Clostridium difficile. Gut.* 1986;27(10):1169-1172.

76. Apisarnthanarak A, Razavi B, Mundy LM. Adjunctive intracolonic vancomycin for severe *Clostridium difficile* colitis: case series and review of the literature. *Clin Infect Dis.* 2002;35(6):690-696.

77. Salcedo J, Keates S, Pothoulakis C, et al. Intravenous immunoglobulin therapy for severe *Clostridium difficile* colitis. *Gut.* 1997;41(3):366-370.

78. McPherson S, Rees CJ, Ellis R, Soo S, Panter SJ. Intravenous immunoglobulin for the treatment of severe, refractory, and recurrent *Clostridium difficile* diarrhea. *Dis Colon Rectum.* 2006;49(5):640-645.

79. Juang P, Skledar SJ, Zgheib NK, et al. Clinical outcomes of intravenous immune globulin in severe *clostridium difficile*-associated diarrhea. *Am J Infect Control.* 2007;35(2):131-137.

80. Lamontagne F, Labbé AC, Haeck O, et al. Impact of emergency colectomy on survival of patients with fulminant *Clostridium difficile* colitis during an epidemic caused by a hypervirulent strain. *Ann Surg.* 2007;245(2):267-272.

Nutrition and Endocrinology

Section Editor: Neeraj Badjatia, MD, MSc

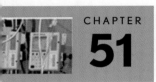

CHAPTER

51

Nutrition and Metabolic Support

Dongwook Kim, MD
David S. Seres, MD

A 71-year-old Caucasian man was brought to the emergency department (ED) for left-sided weakness and confusion. According to his wife, he was found on the floor in his bathroom at home with a paralyzed left arm and leg and slurred speech. This was 6 hours before he came to the ED. The patient has a history of non–insulin-dependent diabetes, hypertension, and hyperlipidemia. On arrival to the ED, he was confused and was noted to have left hemiparesis and left facial droop with aphasia. The vital signs revealed a blood pressure of 119/60 mm Hg, pulse of 119 beats per minute (bpm), respiratory rate of (RR) 33 breaths/min, and arterial oxygen saturation (SaO$_2$) of 85%. He was intubated and ventilated after appropriate sedation and chemical paralysis. A noncontrast computed tomography (CT) scan of the head was performed, which showed a dense right middle cerebral artery sign and no evidence of acute intracranial hemorrhage. The electrocardiogram revealed atrial fibrillation. The radiograph of the chest revealed appropriate endotracheal tube position and a right lower lobe infiltrate.

On his arrival in the neurologic intensive care unit (ICU), his vital signs showed a temperature of 36.4°C (97.5°F), pulse of 132 bpm (sinus), respirations (ventilated) at 14 breaths/min, blood pressure of 113/47 mm Hg, and oxygen saturation of 100%. On physical examination, he appeared acutely ill and cachectic. The carotid pulses were equal, and there were no bruits. A pulmonary examination demonstrated right lower lobe crackles. The heart sounds were

Table 51-1. Laboratory Values on Admission

Laboratory test	Value	Normal range
Sodium	149 mEq/L	136-145 mEq/L
Potassium	5.0 mEq/L	3.6-4.9 mEq/L
Cl	114 mEq/L	101-111 mEq/L
CO_2	20 mEq/L	23-31 mEq/L
Blood urea nitrogen	31 mg/dL	23-31 mg/dL
Creatinine	1.3 mg/dL	0.6-1.0 mg/dL
Glucose	233 mg/dL	80-120 mg/dL
Albumin	2.5 g/dL	4.0-5.5 g/dL
C-reactive protein	25 mg/L	<5 mg/L
White blood cell count	$15 \times 10^3/\mu L$	$4.5-11.0 \times 10^3/\mu L$
Hematocrit	35%	41%-53%
Platelets	$552 \times 10^3/\mu L$	$150-350 \times 10^3/\mu L$

normal. The limbs were well perfused, and the abdomen revealed diminished bowel sounds with a soft and nondistended abdomen. A musculoskeletal examination showed moderate diffuse muscle wasting. The neurologic examinations were not informative because of deep sedation. The results of laboratory tests are shown in Table 51-1.

According to his wife, he retired a year ago from his previous occupation as a taxicab driver for 40 years. He had been smoking 1 pack of cigarettes per day on average for 35 years and drank alcohol occasionally. For the last 5 months, his appetite has been decreased and he has been eating small portions at 2 to 3 meals per day. He lost 15 lb (6.8 kg) during the past 5 months and his most recently measured weight was 115 lb (52 kg). His height was 5 feet and 8 inches (172 cm).

What is your nutritional assessment of this patient? How would you calculate his metabolic requirements?

The severity of his ischemic stroke and pneumonia, which resulted in low serum albumin concentration, puts him at risk for prolonged admission and a potentially poor outcome.

He has had significant weight loss (12% over 5 months). Subsequent to his weight loss, the patient's body mass index (BMI) was 17.6 kg/m². Based on the clinical status, his significant weight loss, and his underweight status, he is considered at nutritional risk and has malnutrition (Table 51-2).

Critical illness is typically associated with a catabolic stress state and a systemic inflammatory response, which increases intravascular permeability and suppresses the production of transport proteins such as albumin and transthyretin (prealbumin).[2] A patient who was previously well nourished may develop severe hypoalbuminemia due to critical illness within hours to days. Therefore, traditional nutrition assessment markers (serum albumin, prealbumin, transferrin) are not validated in critically ill patients because these protein markers vary, depending on vascular permeability, catabolic rate, and hepatic protein synthesis,[3] and not on nourishment.[4]

Table 51-2. Nutritional Assessment for Neurologic Intensive Care Unit Patients

Severity of illness	Severity of neurologic injury
	History of trauma
	Sepsis
	Seizure
	Systemic organ function
Weight history	Body mass index, recent weight changes, ideal body weight
	Significant weight loss[1,a]
	5% over 1 mo, 7.5% over 3 mo, 10% over 6 mo
	Malnutrition[1,a]
	> 5% weight loss based on usual body weight
	< 90% of ideal body weight
Physical examination	Neurologic functionality
	Fat and muscle mass
	Gastrointestinal function
	Volume status
	Body composition
Laboratory data interpretation	Urinary urea protein for nitrogen balance
	Serum transport protein[b]
	Albumin, prealbumin, transferrin
	Systemic inflammatory markers[b]
	C-reactive protein, interleukin 6, tumor necrosis factor
	Acid-base balance, electrolyte, liver function, cholesterol

[a]While commonly used, these criteria have never been validated.

[b]These are not impacted by nourishment. Rather, they reflect severity of illness and are useful to assess risk.

Indirect calorimetry may be used to determine this patient's energy requirement. It is difficult to estimate his caloric requirements accurately because of his acute respiratory failure, neurologic injury, and malnutrition (Table 51-3). When indirect calorimetry is not an option, energy requirements may be calculated either through simplistic formulas (20-30 kcal/kg per day) or published predictive equations. Many of these predictive equations have been published in the literature (Harris-Benedict, Scholfield, Owen, Mifflin-St. Jeor, Swinamer, Ireton-Jones, etc.).[5] The calculation of energy requirements using kilocalories per kilogram is, however, more often used and widely accepted by clinicians than the published predictive equations because of convenience and practicality. Consultation with a nutrition clinician is strongly recommended.

When would you initiate feeding? Which method of feeding, enteral feeding or parenteral feeding, is more suitable to this patient?

You should initiate nutrition support therapy in the form of enteral nutrition as soon as possible, preferably within the first 48 hours after injury. Early feeding of patients who have had a cerebral vascular accident (CVA) has been proved to shorten the hospital length of stay.[7] A large multicenter, randomized, controlled clinical trial showed a reduction in mortality risk when tube feedings were initiated

Table 51-3. Clinical Indications for Indirect Calorimetry

Indication	Example
Unable to estimate caloric requirements accurately[6,a]	Acute respiratory distress syndrome, sepsis, malnutrition, neurologic injury, multisystem organ failure, use of paralytic or barbiturate
Inadequate clinical response in the patient with the use of predictive equations[b]	Poor wound healing, failure to wean from mechanical ventilator
The presence of clinical signs suggesting either underfeeding or overfeeding[b]	Underfeeding: decreased respiratory muscle strength, poor wound healing, immunosuppression
	Overfeeding: hyperglycemia, hepatic steatosis, electrolyte imbalance

[a]Clinical outcomes resulting from providing nourishment based on predictive equations vs calorimetry vs kcal/kg have not been compared.

[b]These may also result from persistent systemic inflammatory response, and not be reflective of nutritional adequacy.

within the first 7 days following a CVA ($P = .09$).[8] Early enteral feeding in patients with severe brain injury has resulted in decreasing infectious complications and an inflammatory response after injury. Neurologic recovery may also be accelerated in patients who are given an adequate amount of calories within the first 48 hours after injury.[9]

Enteral feeding may have benefits beyond providing nourishment. These include maintenance of gut integrity, preservation of a systemic immune response (especially mucosal immunity), and attenuation of the severity of an inflammatory response. Enteral feeding is the preferred method over parenteral feeding, except in the presence of prolonged and severe gut dysfunction or where the risk of obtaining enteral access exceeds the risk of malnourishment for an extended period. This comparison has not been done in neurologically injured patients; however, in general, enteral feeding is the preferred method of feeding over parenteral nutrition for critically ill patients who require nutrition support therapy.[10-12]

Enteral feeding of the hemodynamically compromised patient may increase the risk of ischemic bowel. Therefore, if patients require significant hemodynamic support, including high-dose catecholamine agents and large-volume fluid or blood product resuscitation, to maintain cellular perfusion, enteral nutrition should be withheld until the patient is resuscitated or stabilized.[13]

The patient developed diarrhea 24 hours after continuous enteral tube feeding is initiated. What would you do differently with regard to his feeding method?

You should continue feeding. Before making a change in the feeding formula, you should conduct an investigation and determine whether the diarrhea was caused by an excessive intake of hyperosmolar medications, such as liquid medications delivered in sorbitol; use of broad-spectrum antibiotics; *Clostridium difficile* pseudomembranous colitis; or another infectious etiology. If you are using calorically dense formula, it may cause or exacerbate diarrhea because of its osmotic density. Therefore, it would be reasonable to consider changing the feeding formula to one that is isotonic. Most products designed for use in tubes that are 1 kcal/mL are isotonic.

In hemodynamically stable patients with diarrhea, you may utilize soluble fiber-containing or small peptide feeding formulations. While expert opinions support the use of the small peptide enteral formulations, large prospective trials are not available to justify a strong recommendation for these products, which may cost 15 times that of a standard feed product.[3] Fiber should be avoided in hemodynamically unstable patients and those with hypoperistaltic states because of the risk of bezoar formation. See Figure 51-1.

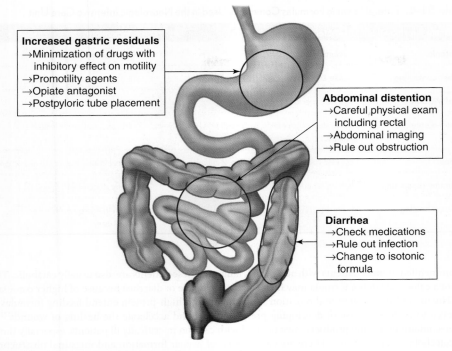

Increased gastric residuals
→Minimization of drugs with
    inhibitory effect on motility
→Promotility agents
→Opiate antagonist
→Postpyloric tube placement

Abdominal distention
→Careful physical exam
    including rectal
→Abdominal imaging
→Rule out obstruction

Diarrhea
→Check medications
→Rule out infection
→Change to isotonic
    formula

Figure 51-1. Strategy for evaluating enteral nutrition intolerance.

 The patient developed septic shock, became hemodynamically compromised, and developed ischemic hepatic and acute renal failure. Tube feeding was stopped because of high lactic acid and possible intestinal ischemia. He was treated with multiple antibiotics and large-volume intravenous fluid resuscitation. He stabilized over the next few days, the lactic acid level normalized, urine output increased, and the requirements for catecholamine agents decreased significantly. He continued to require ventilator support, and liver enzyme levels remained high.

When tube feeding is resumed, what is the best feeding formula in this situation? What are the characteristics of enteral feeding formulas that can be used in the neurologic ICU?

A standard isotonic feeding product is recommended for this patient; this is also sufficient for most patients who are critically ill.

Patients with liver failure have high plasma aromatic amino acids (AAAs) and low branched-chain amino acids (BCAAs) because of impaired hepatic deamination. A decrease in the BCAA/AAA ratio and high AAAs are believed to be factors in the pathogenesis of hepatic encephalopathy.[14] Specialized enteral formulations that contain increased BCAAs and reduced AAAs were promoted for patients with acute and chronic hepatic failure. There is, however, no evidence to suggest that these specialized formulas for hepatic failure improve patient outcomes compared to standard isotonic formulas.[3]

In the setting of significant renal dysfunction, a calorically dense formula (usually 2 kcal/mL) may be helpful if fluid restriction is desired. A renal formula may be useful if electrolyte restriction is also needed. Some renal formulas are also severely protein restricted. Protein restriction is no longer

Table 51-4. Enteral Feeding Formulas Commonly Used in the Neurologic Intensive Care Unit

Category (formula)	Characteristics	Indications
Isotonic	Standard (≈1 cal/mL)	Most patients, long-term use
Fiber containing	Soluble and insoluble fiber (1-1.5 cal/mL)	Long-term use, bolus feeding
Calorie dense	High fat, hypertonic (2 cal/mL)	Fluid restriction
Semi-elemental	Predigested, oligopeptide, high medium-chain fatty acid (1 cal/mL)	Malabsorption, chyle leak
Renal	Low electrolyte, fiber, high fat (1.8-2 cal/mL)	Renal failure, electrolyte restriction
Immune supporting	High fat, omega-3 supplemented (1.5 cal/mL)	Early stage of ARDS and ALI
Wound healing	High protein (1-1.3 cal/mL)	Protein energy malnutrition, pressure ulcer

Abbreviations: ALI, acute lung injury; ARDS, acute respiratory distress syndrome.

recommended in most patients with acute renal failure as these patients are also usually catabolic. The use of a calorically dense formula may increase the incidence of diarrhea because of higher osmolarity. The use of high-protein oral nutrition supplements and high-protein enteral feeding formulas is believed to reduce the risk of developing pressure ulcers and accelerate the healing of wounds.[15,16] Fiber-containing feeding products must be used with caution in critically ill patients, especially those on catecholaminergic agents. There are case reports of bezoar formation and intestinal obstruction related to the use of fiber in these patients.[17,18]

Inflammation-modulating formulas enriched with eicosapentaenoic acid (EPA) and γ-linolenic acid (GLA) are currently recommended for patients with acute respiratory distress syndrome (ARDS) and acute lung injury (ALI) based on three clinical trials with questionable controls.[3] These products have not been studied in neurologically injured patients, but the use of products high in omega-3 fatty acids and higher levels of antioxidants may help reduce the inflammatory response while promoting vasodilation and oxygen delivery.[19] See Table 51-4.

The patient develops an ileus, which is predicted to last for more than 1 week. How should he be fed?

This patient presented with protein-calorie malnutrition, and complete nourishment via the intestine is not expected for more than 1 week. For these reasons, it is appropriate to start parenteral nutrition.[3] See Figure 51-2.

It is not clear when parenteral nutrition should be started in neurologically critically ill patients who were previously well nourished. The European Society for Clinical Nutrition and Metabolism (ESPEN) guidelines for parenteral nutrition recommend that all critically ill patients (both previously well nourished and malnourished) receiving less than the targeted enteral feeding after 2 days should be considered for parenteral nutrition.[20] The American Society for Parenteral and Enteral Nutrition (ASPEN) and the Society of Critical Care Medicine (SCCM) recommend that parenteral nutrition be reserved until attempts at enteral nutrition for 7 days have failed in a patient who was previously healthy prior to critical illness with no evidence of protein-calorie malnutrition.[3] There is a meta-ana-lysis comparing standard therapy and parenteral nutrition in critically ill patients, which recommended starting parenteral nutrition if enteral feeding cannot be initiated within a 14-day period.[21] The timing of when to start parenteral nutrition in previously well-nourished critically ill patients still remains controversial. Observational studies suggest that an absence of nutrition therapy for more than 14 days of hospitalization was associated with significantly greater mortality rate (21% versus 2%; $P < .05$) and a longer hospital length of stay (36.3 days versus 23.4 days; $P < .05$) when compared retrospectively to

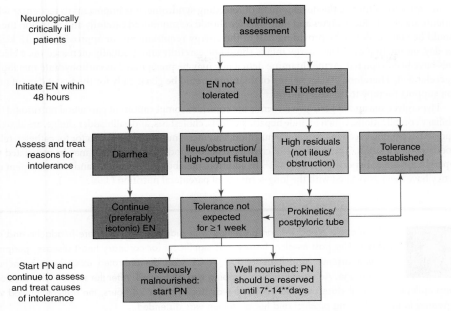

Figure 51-2. Strategy for nutritional support in neurologically critically ill patients. EN, enteral nutrition; PN, parenteral nutrition. *ASPEN/SCCM guidelines (*McClave SA, Martindale RG, Vanek VW, et al. Guidelines for the provision and assessment of nutrition support therapy in the adult critically ill patient: Society of Critical Care Medicine [SCCM] and American Society for Parenteral and Enteral Nutrition [A.S.P.E.N.]. J Parenter Enteral Nutr. 2009;33:277*). **Our current practice.

use of parenteral nutrition,[22] but sicker patients are harder to feed. It is our practice to start parenteral nutrition after 14 days in previously well-nourished patients when enteral feeding is not possible.

 The patient's calorie intake was minimal for a couple of days because of persistently high nasogastric tube output. A postpyloric tube was placed and the feeding goal achieved. The following day, he developed hypokalemia, hypophosphatemia, and hypomagnesemia.

What is the diagnosis and how can you minimize this electrolyte imbalance? What are general complications of artificial nutrition?

The patient developed refeeding syndrome. Refeeding syndrome most often occurs when enteral or parenteral feeding is initiated in a malnourished patient. It may even result from intravenous fluids containing as little as 5% dextrose. The syndrome is characterized by hypophosphatemia, hypokalemia, hypomagnesemia, fluid shifts, and occasionally Wernicke encephalopathy, all of which may develop within hours. Delivery of carbohydrates stimulates insulin secretion, which causes an intracellular shift of these electrolytes. Refeeding syndrome may adversely affect the cardiac, respiratory, hematologic, hepatic, and neuromuscular systems, leading to clinical complications and occasionally death.[23] A patient with malnutrition, especially with greater than 10% recent weight loss, has a high risk of developing refeeding syndrome,[24] as do patients with chronic electrolyte losses. Patients at high risk of developing refeeding syndrome include individuals with evidence of stress and depletion from not being fed for 7 to 10 days, chronic alcoholics, those with anorexia nervosa, oncology patients, and postoperative patients.

Nutrition and Endocrinology

In order to minimize the development of refeeding syndrome, it is important to recognize which patients are at risk. Electrolytes and fluid balance should be monitored carefully and nutrition therapy should be started slowly by providing half of the energy requirements, or approximately 15 kcal/kg per day, on the first day. The energy intake should be carefully and gradually increased once electrolytes have been repleted. Acute thiamine deficiency may be precipitated as carbohydrate metabolism is accelerated. Therefore, 200 to 300 mg of thiamine should be given daily for the first 3 days of nutrition support therapy for at-risk patients.[23]

Hyperglycemia and hypertriglyceridemia are common complications of parenteral nutrition. Hepatobiliary complications, which include hepatic steatosis, cholestasis, and gallbladder sludge, are also often reported in patients receiving parenteral nutrition. Parenteral nutrition is a risk factor for catheter-related bloodstream infection. The incidence of catheter-related bloodstream infection may be associated with hyperglycemia and hypertriglyceridemia.[25] In addition, metabolic bone disease and micronutrient deficiency have been associated with the long-term use of parenteral nutrition (Table 51-5).

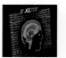

A 55-year-old Asian woman presented with sudden onset of severe headache and neck stiffness. Her past medical history was significant for coronary heart disease, peripheral vascular disease, and hypertension. A CT scan demonstrated extensive subarachnoid hemorrhage. An urgent surgical clipping was performed. After the surgery, she developed status epilepticus. A high-dose pentobarbital drip was started. After 24 hours, the patient vomited what appeared to be the feeding product and her abdomen was distended.

Table 51-5. Complications of Parenteral Nutrition

Complications	Etiology	Prevention and management
Hyperglycemia	Excess carbohydrate	Insulin therapy
	Most common complication	
Hypersensitivity reaction	IVFE	Discontinue parenteral nutrition (severe case)
	Multivitamins	Discontinue IVFE or vitamins
Hypertriglyceridemia	Excess IVFE	Restrict IVFE to < 30% of total calories
Refeeding syndrome	Insulin secretion and intracellular shift of electrolytes and minerals	Restrict total calories (initial dose)
		Replete electrolytes and minerals
Hepatic steatosis	Overfeeding	Decrease calories
	Excess carbohydrate	Decrease dextrose
Cholestasis	Phytosterols in IVFE	Decrease IVFE, cycle parenteral nutrition
	Lack of gut stimulation	Increase enteral intake
Infection	Line-related infection	Antibiotics and antifungal
		Discontinue parenteral nutrition
Metabolic bone disease	Vitamin D deficiency	Extra vitamin D
	Long-term parenteral nutrition related	Sun exposure

Abbreviation: IVFE, intravenous fat emulsion.

How does the use of pentobarbital affect the nutrition regimen? How would you manage this patient's feeding intolerance? What are the other commonly used drugs in the neurologic ICU that have nutritional implications?

The use of pentobarbital is associated with feeding intolerance due to reduced peristalsis, but it also causes a concurrent decrease in the metabolic demand. Induction of a barbiturate coma for treatment of severely elevated intracranial pressure or refractory status epilepticus may decrease gastrointestinal muscle tone and contraction. When a barbiturate coma results in delayed gastric emptying and a reduction in lower esophageal sphincter tone, which are already present in patients with increased intracranial pressure, feeding intolerance may occur. The use of barbiturates to decrease cerebral metabolism also results in decreased systemic metabolic needs.[26] Indirect calorimetry may be useful in determining the patient's requirements for total calories.

An aggressive cathartic bowel regimen and promotility agents (metoclopramide, erythromycin) may be initiated for the patients with diminished gastrointestinal motility. Postpyloric tube placement should be considered. Parenteral nutrition may be considered if the feeding intolerance persists for an extended period.

Narcotic analgesics may also cause feeding intolerance because of a decrease in bowel motility. For patients receiving continuous nasogastric feeding, absorption of phenytoin may decrease by as much as 70%.[27] The mechanism of interaction between phenytoin and enteral feeding products has not yet been elucidated, but it is thought to be related to protein binding.

Propofol, a short-acting anesthetic and sedative, is used to decrease cerebral metabolic activity. The 1% propofol product is formulated in a 10% egg phospholipid emulsion providing 1.1 kcal/mL. These calories should be considered when calculating the nutrition regimen (Table 51-6).

If the patient needs long-term enteral nutrition because of severe dysphagia after having a stroke, when should gastrostomy be performed?

Placement of percutaneous endoscopic gastrostomy (PEG) devices for enteral nutrition support has been reported to be associated with a higher risk of poor outcome and death compared to nasogastric feeding in patients with acute dysphagic stroke.[8] If enteral nutrition support is necessary 2 to 3 weeks

Table 51-6. Medications Commonly Used in the Neurologic Intensive Care Unit That Affect Nutritional Status

Medication	Nutritional effects
Barbiturates	Decreased gastrointestinal muscle tone, feeding intolerance, decreased systemic metabolic rate
Corticosteroids	Hyperglycemia, muscle atrophy, hyperlipidemia
Demeclocycline	Binds to cations (calcium, iron, and magnesium) and decreases absorption. Should not be taken concurrent with feeding products
Narcotic analgesics	Constipation, ileus, feeding intolerance
Phenytoin	Decreased absorption with continuous feeding
Propofol	Formulated in a 10% egg phospholipid emulsion providing 1.1 kcal/mL
Catecholamine agents	Hypoperistalsis, gastric emptying dysfunction, bezoar formation with fiber-containing feeding products

Nutrition and Endocrinology

after the onset of stroke, the use of a PEG device is generally preferred to the chronic presence of a nasogastric tube, but outcome studies comparing them are lacking.

Should you continue parenteral or enteral nutrition support when death is expected?

Nutrition support, in the short term, does not improve the outcomes of patients with untreatable disease, particularly those associated with significant systemic inflammation. One pilot study showed that for dying patients, there is no sign of suffering attributable to starvation and dehydration.[28] Specialized nutrition therapy is generally not recommended in end-of-life situations. However, family members may be under the impression that any lack of nutrition would result in more suffering for the dying patients. Therefore, it is important to inform the family members of the correct medical principles in advance.

! CRITICAL CONSIDERATIONS

- Nutrition assessment is global and includes both nutritional status and the severity of illness (see Table 51-1). Traditional nutrition markers (serum albumin, transthyretin [prealbumin], transferrin) are not validated in critically ill patients because these protein markers vary based on vascular permeability, catabolic rate, and hepatic protein synthesis, and not nutritional adequacy.

- It is difficult to accurately estimate caloric requirements in the neurologically critically ill. Indirect calorimetry may be helpful. Consultation with a nutrition professional is strongly recommended.

- Early enteral feeding of patients after CVA may shorten the hospital length of stay and reduce mortality rate. Enteral feeding is the preferred method to parenteral feeding. Enteral feeding, itself may help to maintain gut integrity, preserve the immune response, and attenuate the systemic inflammatory response.

- Disease-specific enteral feeding products have limited usefulness. Renal formulas are fluid and electrolyte restricted. There may be improved clinical outcomes for ventilated patients with ALI/ARDS given inflammation-modulating formula enriched with EPA and GLA.

- If there is evidence of protein-calorie malnutrition and enteral nutrition is not available, it is appropriate to start parenteral nutrition if it is expected that enteral nutrition will not be possible for more than a week. The timing of when to start parenteral nutrition in a previously well-nourished critically ill patient still remains controversial. It is our practice that parenteral nutrition be started in a previously well-nourished patient after attempting to feed enterally for 14 days has failed.

- Refeeding syndrome results from initiation of enteral or parenteral feeding and may occur as a result of dextrose-containing intravenous solutions in malnourished patients; it results in hypophosphatemia, hypokalemia, and hypomagnesemia. A patient with malnutrition, especially with greater than 10% recent weight loss, or chronic electrolyte losses has a high risk of developing refeeding syndrome.

- The use of barbiturates is associated with feeding intolerance and a decrease in the metabolic demand.

- Specialized nutrition therapy is generally not recommended in cases of end-of-life situations.

REFERENCES

1. Blackburn GL, Bistrian BR, Maini BS, Schlamm HT, Smith MF. Nutritional and metabolic assessment of the hospitalized patient. *J Parenter Enteral Nutr.* 1977;1(1):11-22.

2. Don BR, Kaysen G. Serum albumin: relationship to inflammation and nutrition. *Semin Dial.* 2004;17(6):432-437.

3. McClave SA, Martindale RG, Vanek VW, et al. Guidelines for the provision and assessment of nutrition support therapy in the adult critically ill patient: Society of Critical Care Medicine (SCCM) and American Society for Parenteral and Enteral Nutrition (A.S.P.E.N.). *J Parenter Enteral Nutr.* 2009;33:277.

4. Koretz RL. Death, morbidity and economics are the only end points for trials. *Proc Nutr Soc.* 2005;64(3):277-284.

5. Foster GD, Knox LS, Dempsey DT, Mullen JL. Caloric requirements in total parenteral nutrition. *J Am Coll Nutr.* 1987;6:231-253.

6. Wooley JA, Sax HC. Indirect calorimetry: applications to practice. *Nutr Clin Pract.* 2003;18(5):434-439.

7. Nyswonger GD, Helmchen RH. Early enteral nutrition and length of stay in stroke patients. *J Neurosci Nurs.* 1992;24:220-223.

8. Dennis MS, Lewis SC, Warlow C. Effect of timing and method of enteral tube feeding for dysphagic stroke patients (FOOD): a multicentre randomised controlled trial. *Lancet.* 2005;365:764-772.

9. Taylor SJ, Fettes SB, Jewkes C, Nelson RJ. Prospective, randomized, controlled trial to determine the effect of early enhanced enteral nutrition on clinical outcome in mechanically ventilated patients suffering head injury. *Crit Care Med.* 1999;27(11):2525-2531.

10. Kang W, Kudsk KA. Is there evidence that the gut contributes to mucosal immunity in humans? *J Parenter Enteral Nutr.* 2007;31:246-258.

11. Windsor AC, Kanwar S, Li AG, et al. Compared with parenteral nutrition, enteral feeding attenuates the acute phase response and improves disease severity in acute pancreatitis. *Gut.* 1998;42:431-435.

12. Hermsen JL, Sano Y, Kudsk KA. Food fight! Parenteral nutrition, enteral stimulation and gut-derived mucosal immunity. *Langenbecks Arch Surg.* 2009;394:17-30.

13. Zaloga GP, Roberts PR, Marik P. Feeding the hemodynamically unstable patient: a critical evaluation of the evidence. *Nutr Clin Pract.* 2003;18:285-293.

14. Dejong CH, van de Poll MC, Soeters PB, Jalan R, Olde Damink SW. Aromatic amino acid metabolism during liver failure. *J Nutr.* 2007;137:1579S-1585S.

15. Stratton RJ, Ek AC, Engfer M, et al. Enteral nutritional support in prevention and treatment of pressure ulcers: a systematic review and meta-analysis. *Ageing Res Rev.* 2005;4:422-450.

16. Chernoff RS, Milton KY, Lipschitz DA. The effect of a high protein formula (Replete) on decubitus ulcer healing in long-term tube fed institutionalized patients. *J Am Diet Assoc.* 1990;90:A130.

17. McIvor AC, Meguid MM, Curtas S, Warren J, Kaplan DS. Intestinal obstruction from cecal bezoar; a complication of fiber-containing tube feedings. *Nutrition.* 1990;6(1):115-117.

18. O'Neil HK, Hibbein JF, Resnick DJ, Bass EM, Aizenstein RI. Intestinal obstruction by a bezoar from tube feedings. *Am J Roentgenol.* 1996;167(6):1477-1478.

19. Pacht ER, DeMichele SJ, Nelson JL, Hart J, Wennberg AK, Gadek JE. Enteral nutrition with eicosapentaenoic acid, gamma-linolenic acid, and antioxidants reduces alveolar inflammatory mediators and protein influx in patients with acute respiratory distress syndrome. *Crit Care Med.* 2003;31:491-500.

20. Singer P, Berger MM, Van den Berghe G, et al. ESPEN guidelines on parenteral nutrition *Clin Nutr.* 2009;28(4):387-400.

21. Heyland DK, MacDonald S, Keefe L, Drover JW. Total parenteral nutrition in the critically ill patient: a meta-analysis. *JAMA.* 1998;280:2013-2019.

22. Sandstrom R, Drott C, Hyltander A, et al. The effect of postoperative intravenous feeding (TPN) on outcome following major surgery evaluated in a randomized study. *Ann Surg.* 1993;217:185-195.

23. Stanga Z, Brunner A, Leuenberger M, et al. Nutrition in clinical practice—the refeeding syndrome: illustrative cases and guidelines for prevention and treatment. *Eur J Clin Nutr.* 2008;62(6):687-694.

24. Crook MA, Hally V, Panteli JV. The importance of the refeeding syndrome. *Nutrition.* 2001;17:632-637.

25. Ziegler TR. Parenteral nutrition in the critically ill patient. *N Engl J Med.* 2009;361:1088-1097.

26. Magnuson B, Hatton J, Zweng TN, Young B. Pentobarbital coma in neurosurgical patients: nutrition considerations. *Nutr Clin Pract.* 1995;9(4):146-150.

27. Saklad JJ, Graves RH, Sharp WP. Interaction of oral phenytoin with enteral feedings. *JPEN J Parenter Enteral Nutr.* 1986;10(3):322-323.

28. Van der Riet P, Brooks D, Ashby M. Nutrition and hydration at the end of life: pilot study of a palliative care experience. *J Law Med.* 2006;14:182-198.

Nutrition and Endocrinology

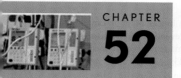

CHAPTER

52

Endocrine Disorders in Critical Illness

Kiwon Lee, MD, FACP, FAHA, FCCM

A 42-year-old woman with past medical history of hyperthyroidism who had radioactive iodine treatment 2 years prior now presents to the emergency department with high fever, sweating, and confusion. These symptoms were preceded by coughing, sore throat, and body aches for 3 days. Shortly after arriving at the hospital, the patient started to have a partial-onset seizure with secondary generalization leading to generalized tonic-clonic jerks for a duration of 30 seconds followed by a period of postictal confusion. Two hours later, the patient is admitted to the neurologic intensive care unit (ICU) with a working diagnosis of "rule out status epilepticus" and is being hooked up to continuous electroencephalography. The initial vital signs are as follows: blood pressure (BP) 190/104 mm Hg, heart rate (HR) 105 to 110 beats per minute (bpm) in sinus rhythm, temperature 38.8°C (102°F), and O_2 saturation 98% in room air. On examination, the patient's eyes are closed and she is arousable to nonpainful tactile stimulation; she is lethargic and diaphoretic, with hyperpyrexia, sinus tachycardia, tachypnea, mild resting tremors, and delirium. The patient's family reports normal diet and adequate hydration up until she started feeling ill this morning. While being examined, the patient develops a narrow QRS-complex supraventricular tachycardia with HR of 120 bpm, which subsided with an intravenous (IV) esmolol drip at 50 µg/kg per minute, which was given without the typical 0.5 mg/kg loading dose.

Given this patient's past medical history significant for hyperthyroidism, a working diagnosis of thyroid storm is made, which was believed to be triggered by an upper respiratory viral infection.

Describe the syndrome, mechanism, and typical clinical features.

Thyroid Crisis

Also known as thyroid storm or thyrotoxic crisis, it is an uncommon, acute, life-threatening manifestation of hyperthyroidism. If treatment is delayed, mortality rate exceeds 90%. Even with prompt diagnosis and treatment, commonly reported mortality rates range from 20% to 30%.[1,2]

Mechanism

Thyroid storm is secondary to excessive thyroid hormones leading to hypermetabolic states. Common etiologies including trauma, perioperative surgical trauma to the thyroid glands, severe infection and sepsis, diabetic ketoacidosis, anesthesia induction, drug induced (chemotherapy, nonsteroidal anti-inflammatory drugs [NSAIDS], etc.), and partially treated hyperthyroidism with radioactive iodine for people with known hyperthyroidism have been reported to trigger this illness. Multinodular goiter and thyroid tumor with hypersecretion of thyroid-stimulating hormone (TSH) have been associated with this illness. In children, thyroid storm typically occurs in the setting of Graves disease.

Clinical features

Clinical features include high fever/hyperpyrexia, diarrhea, diaphoresis, hypertension (although the patient may be hypotensive in the late stage with heart failure or shock), sinus tachycardia, both supraventricular (more common) and ventricular tachyarrhythmia, high-output heart failure, tremors, convulsions, delirium, and coma.

The patient suddenly develops supraventricular tachyarrhythmia with a rapid ventricular response of 160 bpm and the BP drops to 60/30 mm Hg. She is in a stupor and is minimally responsive to painful stimulation. A synchronized shock of 100 joules is given, which immediately converts the rhythm to sinus at a rate of 65 bpm.

What are the next steps in treating thyroid storm in order to avoid recurrent complications?

Diagnosis and Treatment

Diagnosing thyroid storm is based on clinical findings, and one should not delay treatment while waiting for laboratory results. Elevated triiodothyronine (T_3), thyroxine (T_4), and free T_4 with low TSH and elevated iodine 24-hour uptake are common laboratory findings. The following outlines the key therapies:

1. Airway, breathing, circulation (ABC): Full ICU support and monitoring, securing the airway; providing adequate oxygen, breathing, and circulatory support; and addressing any unstable cardiac arrhythmia
2. Hyperpyrexia/high fever treatment: Cooling with conventional or advanced temperature modulation, acetaminophen, IV hydration
3. Address hypersympathomimetic symptoms with propranolol 1 to 2 mg IV q4h or 40 to 120 mg by mouth (PO) q4-6h: caution—heart failure
4. Glucocorticoids reduce T_4 to T_3 conversion: Either hydrocortisone 50 mg IV q6h or Decadron 2 to 4 mg IV q6h, which should be tapered as the symptoms improve
5. Address underlying hyperthyroidism illness: Administer antithyroid medication
6. Saturated solution of potassium iodide 5 drops (250 mg of potassium iodide) PO q6h, sodium iodide 0.25 g IV q6h, or strong iodine (Lugol solution) 10 drops PO q8h mixed in juice
7. Avoid aspirin (may increase free T_4 level by freeing up T_4 from thyroid-binding globulin)
8. Methimazole (Tapazole): Inhibits thyroid hormone synthesis but does not inhibit peripheral T_4 to T_3 conversion; only available in PO formulation; should try this before propylthiouracil as there is no known side effects of liver injury: 15 to 25 mg PO q6h

9. Propylthiouracil (PTU): Has been used with popularity as it inhibits thyroid hormone synthesis as well as peripheral T_4 to T_3 conversion, but it is now considered a second-line agent as US Food and Drug Administration (FDA) has released a black box warning: potentially fatal hepatic failure cases have been reported after the use of PTU—use with caution and immediately stop with any signs/symptoms of liver injury; for thyroid storm, 200 to 400 mg via nasogastric tube/PO q6h

10. Definitive treatment of the hyperthyroidism with surgery or radioactive iodine after clinical stabilization

Describe myxedema coma.

Myxedema Coma

In contrast to thyrotoxic crisis, myxedema coma is a rare but highly fatal exacerbation of hypothyroidism triggered by acute illnesses such as infection/sepsis and any factor that may lead to hypoventilation resulting in hypercapnia and hypoxemia. A variety of drugs may precipitate such hypoventilation including narcotics, sedatives, anxiolytics, anesthetics, and antidepressants, and when these medications are used in patients with known hypothyroidism a severe exacerbation of the hypothyroidism may occur. Other common precipitating factors include sepsis, bacteremia, congestive heart failure exacerbation with pulmonary edema, pneumonia, myocardial infarction, stroke, bleeding disorders, and trauma. Clinically, hypothermia, hyponatremia, hypoglycemia, hypoxia, and obtunded mental status are commonly seen. This syndrome is most commonly seen in the elderly population.

How do you treat myxedema coma?

1. ABC: Full ICU support and monitoring, securing the airway; providing adequate oxygen, breathing, and circulatory support; and addressing any unstable cardiac arrhythmia.

2. IV levothyroxine loading dose 400 to 500 µg × 1, followed by maintenance dose of 50 to 100 µg/d IV.

3. Potentially fatal arrhythmia may occur for body temperature less than 30°C (86°F), so external, passive, slow rewarming is important; follow serum potassium (cellular shift of potassium may lead to hyperkalemia) and avoid rapid rewarming to prevent arrhythmia during rewarming.

4. Hydrocortisone 100 mg IV loading dose followed by maintenance dose of 50 mg IV q6h: Treat adrenal insufficiency in the setting of severe hypothyroidism.

5. Treat any underlying infections with antibiotics if necessary.

What is sick euthyroid syndrome?

This syndrome refers to abnormal thyroid function without any defect in the hypothalamic-pituitary-thalamic axis or underlying disease in the thyroid gland occurring in acute illnesses. Patients are "sick" but their thyroid gland is not dysfunctional despite abnormal hormonal status. It is important to remember that any critical illness may significantly alter thyroid function, and there may be multiple patterns in hormonal secretion. Diagnosis is presumptive and speculative, as thyroid function testing is not reliable in diagnosing this syndrome in acute critical illness. There are no symptoms that are specific to this syndrome, and often symptoms are absent. Acutely ill patients are ill because of their underlying acute illness but may also present with symptoms that are similar to hypothyroidism. After the underlying illness is resolved, complete normalization of thyroid function occurs. Any acute and severe illnesses including trauma, infection/sepsis, burns, and surgical stress may lead to this syndrome. Multiple mechanisms for this syndrome have been proposed, including cytokines such as interleukin 6 and tumor necrosis factor α, which might disrupt hypothalamic and pituitary function.

How do you differentiate low T_3 syndrome from low T_4 syndrome?

There are two major patterns of thyroid function abnormality that may be seen in sick euthyroid syndrome. These patterns are true in general, and may not be specific for each syndrome.

1. Low T_3 syndrome:
   Low total T_3
   Low free T_3
   Normal total T_4
   Normal free T_4
   Normal TSH
   High reverse T_3 (rT_3) due to impaired T_4 to T_3 conversion and decreased clearance
2. Low T_4 syndrome:
   In addition to low total and free T_3:
   Low T_4
   Fluctuating TSH levels
   Usually more severe form than low T_3 syndrome version
   Changed function in binding to thyroxine-binding globulin contributes to low T_4

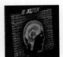

A 34-year-old woman who goes to church decides to fast at the chapel for 3 days while praying. She is brought to the emergency department after another church member found her on the floor in lethargic mental status and with hypothermia. On arrival, her BP is 90/62 mm Hg, HR is 56 bpm, temperature is 35.5°C (96°F), and O_2 saturation is 98% in room air. The patient is lethargic but arousable to loud verbal stimulation; oriented to person, place, and time; and generally weak but able to follow commands. There is 4/5 motor strength throughout with give-out weakness, negative Babinski signs, and hyporeflexia.

What laboratory tests do you need to order? Would you give thyroid hormone for suspected hypothyroidism in this patient?

Patients who are suspected to have sick euthyroid syndrome should be distinguished from those having true underlying hypothyroidism as the syndrome can mimic signs and symptoms of hypothyroidism.

There are no specific symptoms for this syndrome, however. Laboratory tests should include free and total T_3, T_4, TSH, and rT_3. Despite there being some classically described variations of this syndrome, diagnosis is challenging as there are no specific signs or symptoms and the laboratory findings may vary. In the absence of large prospective randomized trial data, whether to treat sick euthyroid syndrome with thyroid hormones continues to be a debatable topic, and it is generally recommended to only monitor the thyroid function (and not give thyroid hormones) and expect full recovery as the underlying nonthyroidal illness resolves.

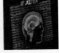

A 53-year-old man is admitted to the ICU after experiencing urosepsis. The patient is lethargic and complaining of abdominal pain, nausea, vomiting, and diarrhea. The initial vital signs are as follows: BP 80/42 mm Hg, HR sinus tachycardia at 120 bpm, and temperature 38.3°C (101°F). On examination, the patient has dry skin with decreased skin turgor, oliguria, a tender abdomen, sinus tachycardia, persistently low central venous pressure of 2 mm Hg, stroke volume variation of 22% on a PiCCO2 monitor (Pulsion Medical Systems, Germany), and cardiac output of 4.6 L/min; he is hypotensive and having frequent vomiting and diarrhea. Laboratory data reveal serum hyperkalemia, metabolic acidosis on arterial blood-gas analysis, and hypoglycemia and hyponatremia. A 500-mL 0.9% NaCl saline infusion has been given as a bolus via an 18-gauge peripheral IV line, but hypotension continues.

How do you diagnose adrenal crisis?

This is an acute, severe adrenocortical insufficiency and should be distinguished from Addison disease, which is a chronic, primary adrenocortical insufficiency. The problem is lack of cortisol, and this can be due to either (1) exacerbation of primary insufficiency (more common) or (2) a problem in pituitary-adrenal axis (secondary) insufficiency. Adrenal crisis may occur in patients who are being treated with glucocorticoid replacement (and when withdrawal of such long-term replacement therapy occurs rapidly) or as the initial presenting illness for someone who has not been diagnosed with adrenal insufficiency in the past. Common risk factors include significant general stress such as sepsis/infection (eg, *Staphylococcus* and *Streptococcus* species, viral or fungal etiologies), trauma, surgery, burn injury, and direct injury of the adrenal glands such as adrenal tumor, removal of the adrenal glands, direct trauma to the adrenal gland, or adrenal hemorrhage/infarction.

Clinical presentation may include lethargy, high fever (or hypothermia), abdominal (flank) pain, nausea/vomiting, diarrhea, skin hyperpigmentation, dehydration, and hypovolemic shock. Laboratory findings typically include serum hyperkalemia (peaked T waves on electrocardiography may be seen), metabolic acidosis, hyponatremia, hypoglycemia, and less commonly hypercalcemia. Often, systemic hypotension is not responsive to colloid or crystalloid fluid resuscitation.

Diagnosis and Workup

Normally, severe stress such as major trauma or sepsis would lead to a normal rise in the serum cortisol level. The same rise should also be seen after the adrenocorticotropic hormone (ACTH) stimulation test. In adrenal crisis, the cosyntropin (synthetic ACTH 1-24) stimulation test fails to elevate the serum cortisol level greater than 20 μg/dL or at least produce a 9-μg/dL increase compared to baseline. Cosyntropin 0.25 mg IV is given and the serum cortisol level is checked 30 to 60 minutes after the stimulation injection. In order to avoid false-negative results, it is important to make sure that patients do not take glucocorticoid (hydrocortisone) before the ACTH stimulation test. If steroid needs to be given to support otherwise refractory frank hypotension, then use of IV dexamethasone (4-6 mg IV bolus) can be given instead of hydrocortisone. A computed axial tomography scan of the chest and abdomen should be performed in order to rule out underlying etiologies and risk factors mentioned above. Sepsis/bacteremia needs to be at the top of the differential diagnoses as a trigger because infection is one of the most common causes. Panculture, complete blood count, thyroid panel test, and serum chemistry should be obtained initially.

Describe the treatment steps for adrenal crisis.

1. Airway, breathing, and circulation stabilization
2. Once adrenal crisis is suspected, immediate treatment with IV normal saline infusion and hydrocortisone 100 mg IV q6h must begin without checking the cortisol response level after the ACTH stimulation test; after a couple of days, IV hydrocortisone may be switched to PO hydrocortisone
3. IV normal saline is appropriate as it would replace both sodium and free water deficits:

Free water deficit = Normal total body water × [(Current Na/140) − 1]

Sodium deficit = Normal total body water × (Target Na − Current Na)

An accurate assessment of intravascular volume status is important, and as such, additional hemodynamic parameters may be used such as stroke volume, stroke volume variation, pulse pressure variation for preload, and preload/volume responsiveness in order to adequately resuscitate the patients.

! CRITICAL CONSIDERATIONS

- Thyroid storm is secondary to excessive thyroid hormones leading to hypermetabolic states.
- Common etiologies including trauma, perioperative surgical trauma to the thyroid glands, severe infection and sepsis, diabetic ketoacidosis, anesthesia induction, drug induced (chemotherapy, NSAIDS, etc), and partially treated hyperthyroidism with radioactive iodine for people with known hyperthyroidism have been reported to trigger this illness.
- Diagnosing thyroid storm is based on clinical findings, and one should not delay treatment while waiting for laboratory results. Elevated T_3, T_4, and free T_4 with low TSH and elevated iodine 24-hour uptake are common findings.
- Myxedema coma is a rare but highly fatal exacerbation of hypothyroidism triggered by acute illnesses such as infection/sepsis and any factor that may lead to hypoventilation resulting in hypercapnia and hypoxemia. IV levothyroxine and hydrocortisone are useful treatments.
- Sick euthyroid syndrome presents with an abnormal thyroid function without any defect in the hypothalamic-pituitary-thalamic axis. There is no underlying disease in the thyroid gland and the syndrome occurs in the setting of acute, severe illnesses. Treatment with thyroid hormone (despite low T_3 and T_4) is generally not recommended and full normalization of thyroid function is expected when the underlying illness is resolved.
- Adrenal crisis is an acute, severe adrenocortical insufficiency, and treating physicians should make an effort to distinguish it from Addison disease, which is a chronic, primary adrenocortical insufficiency. Typically refractory hypotension despite volume resuscitation, hyponatremia, hyperkalemia, hypoglycemia, hypercalcemia, and metabolic acidosis are commonly seen. Lack of cortisol should be supplemented by IV hydrocortisone. The ACTH stimulation test may confirm the diagnosis, and it is important not to use hydrocortisone prior to administering ACTH in order to not confound the results. Dexamethasone may be used prior to or during the ACTH stimulation test if necessary. Correcting electrolyte imbalances, providing aggressive volume resuscitation with dextrose, containing normal saline, and treating the underlying illness are critical steps for treatment.

REFERENCES

1. Fauci AS, Braunwald E, Kasper DL, et al. *Harrison's Principles of Internal Medicine.* 17th ed. New York: McGraw-Hill; 2008(II):2236-2237.

2. Misra M, Singhal A, Campbell DE. Thyroid storm. *www.emedicine.com.* Accessed April 23, 2010.

Ethics and End-of-Life Issues

Section Editor: Kiwon Lee, MD, FACP, FAHA, FCCM

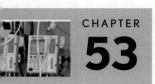

CHAPTER

53

Brain Death and Organ Donation

Guillermo Linares, MD
Mireia Anglada, MD
Kiwon Lee, MD, FACP, FAHA, FCCM

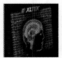

A 55-year-old right-handed woman presents to the emergency department (ED) because of sudden loss of consciousness. The patient has a history of tobacco smoking as well as poorly controlled hypertension for which she takes metoprolol and captopril. She is brought into the ED by emergency medical services (EMS), who transported her from a grocery store near her home. She is accompanied by her husband, who describes the sudden onset of headache quickly followed by paralysis of the right face, arm, and leg while they were shopping for food. EMS personnel report that during transport she stopped moving her left side, lost consciousness, developed dilated and unresponsive pupils, and had to undergo orotracheal intubation for airway protection. She received a neuromuscular blocking agent as well as propofol during the procedure. Intubation occurred 12 minutes prior to arrival in the ED.

She is evaluated immediately upon arrival and found to have a blood pressure (BP) of 212/123 mm Hg, respiratory rate (RR) of 12 breaths/min, heart rate (HR) of 121 beats per minute (bpm), temperature of 37.3°C (99.1°F), and O_2 saturation of 98%. She is promptly placed on telemetry, two large-bore intravenous (IV) lines are placed, and a set of laboratory values is drawn. On physical examination, she is found to be unresponsive to painful stimuli. The orotracheal tube is at 23 cm to the lip and secured. Thoracic auscultation reveals clear breath sounds in both lung fields,

S_1, S_2, and a loud S_4. The point of maximal impulse (PMI) is displaced and pulses are palpable without difficulty. Funduscopy reveals retinal changes consistent with malignant hypertensive retinopathy. The abdomen is soft and nontender and there are no skin findings or stigmata. Neurologic examination performed off sedation shows no motor response to nasal tickle or deep sternal rub. The pupils are 7 mm and nonreactive to light. Corneal reflexes are absent on both sides. There are no spontaneous breaths and no gag response on manipulation of the endotracheal tube. Oculocephalic reflexes are absent and no "doll's-eye" responses are noted. Deep tendon reflexes are absent and no plantar response was elicited. The charge nurse in the ED has secured the patient's possessions including her wallet and driver's license.

As you prepare to transport the patient for a computed tomography (CT) scan, you ask her husband about the presence of advanced directives and find out that there is no written living will or oral advanced directives. Her husband asks you to "please save her no matter what." You inform him that she will be transported to the neurologic intensive care unit (ICU) immediately after the CT scan. The nonenhanced head CT scan is shown in Figure 53-1.

Laboratory results become available shortly afterward and reveal a normal comprehensive metabolic panel, complete blood count, toxicology screen, arterial blood gases (ABGs), cardiac ischemia markers, and coagulation tests.

When you return from radiology, the medical student assigned to the case asks you if it would be appropriate to limit medical interventions given the absence of neurologic response.

What is the most appropriate answer?

Immediate interventions are indicated to improve hemodynamic parameters. In this case, the presence of a large hemorrhage and severe hypertension mandate blood pressure control. At this point, no

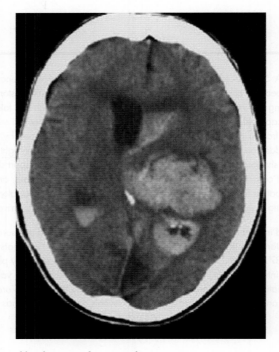

Figure 53-1. Nonenhanced head computed tomography scan.

medical care should be withheld on the basis of the physical examination since the patient was recently exposed to neuromuscular blocking agents as well as sedatives. Coupled with cardiovascular interventions, "brain resuscitation" with hyperosmolar therapy is indicated since increased intracranial pressure (ICP) is likely and cannot be adequately assessed on clinical grounds. If other physiologic derangements are present such as coagulation abnormalities, these should be promptly corrected. Insertion of an external ventricular drain (EVD) by an appropriately credentialed physician such as a neurosurgeon or neurointensivist should be considered at this point. An EVD would allow the intensivist to diagnose increased ICP, trigger hyperosmolar therapy use, directly reduce ICP by removal of cerebrospinal fluid, and adequately titrate blood pressure medications in order to ensure adequate brain perfusion.

Limiting clinical interventions early in this case may be premature since the neurologic examination is confounded by sedative medications and neuromuscular junction–blocking agents. In addition, the patient has no advanced directives guiding the physicians to limit care in a situation such as this one and her husband has asked you to continue to deliver full medical care. At this point, safe and expedited transfer to the neurologic ICU is indicated.

Twenty-five minutes has elapsed and the patient is now in the neurologic ICU. The resident assigned to the case prepares for his initial evaluation.

What should the main focus of the neurologic examination be if brain death is suspected?

The first part of the systemic coma examination begins with the careful assessment of coma and brainstem reflexes. This is accomplished by testing and documenting the presence and quality of motor responses to noxious or painful stimuli. Gentle stimulation of the nares and periorbital area with a cotton swab is frequently all that is necessary to elicit a motor response. When deeper coma states exist, it is best to use standardized maneuvers that elicit pain such as supraorbital nerve, temporomandibular joint, or nail bed pressure.[1]

The next step in the assessment of the comatose patient involves direct testing of brainstem function. Optimal tests assess the pathways of all three main parts of the brainstem: the midbrain, pons, and medulla. The classically described rostral-to-caudal progression of brainstem dysfunction is frequently observed; however, other patterns are also observed. Frequently the medulla is the last part of the brainstem to cease to function and in some cases respiratory drive, mediated by the medullary respiratory centers, persists for prolonged periods of time.[2] A less frequently performed medullary function test is monitoring of heart rate after the administration of atropine. Increased heart rate suggests function of the medullary vagal centers.[3,4] This test is not routinely performed in many institutions but should be familiar to neurointensivists. Table 53-1 presents commonly tested brainstem reflexes. When testing by the bedside whether the patient is apneic, one of the common mistakes made is simply switching the ventilation mode from assist-control ("AC") to spontaneous setting ("PSV") and seeing whether the patient's respiratory rate goes down. This is not a sensitive test, as the modern ventilators are extremely sensitive to minimal respiratory changes, and depending on the sensitivity setting on the pressure or flow trigger mode, brain-dead patients may or may not become apneic even on spontaneous mode. The best method is simply to disconnect the patient and carefully observe for any chest rise or listen to the chest for any breath sounds.

The motor examination is performed jointly with the sensory examination, since the stimuli used to elicit movement must be processed before a response occurs. Noncortically mediated movements such as extensor and flexor posturing and triple flexion are frequently observed. The differentiation of reflex stereotyped movements from complex cortically mediated movements can be complicated and requires repeated testing with different noxious stimuli.

Table 53-1. Tested Brainstem Reflexes

- **Pupils:**
  Response to bright light
  Size and shape
- **Ocular movement:**
  Oculocephalic reflex (testing only when no fracture or instability of the cervical spine or skull base is apparent)
  Oculovestibular: Provoked eye movements must be confirmed by testing with cold caloric stimulation
- **Facial sensation and facial motor response**
  Gentle nasal and periorbital tickle
  Corneal reflex
  Jaw reflex
  Grimacing to deep pressure on nail bed, supraorbital ridge, or temporomandibular joint
- **Pharyngeal and tracheal reflexes**
  Response after stimulation of the posterior pharynx
  Response to deep tracheal suctioning

The on-call resident finishes his initial evaluation and documents lack of response to all stimuli and absence of brainstem reflexes.

Does this patient meet criteria for brain death?

No. This patient was exposed to neuromuscular-blocking agents and sedatives, which may confound the neurologic examination. A commonly used way of testing for the presence of neuromuscular blockade is the train-of-four test. In this test, a series of four consecutive electrical stimuli are applied along the path of a peripheral nerve and the resulting contraction of the innervated muscles is measured. Absence or diminished response to electrical stimulation suggests the presence of neuromuscular-blocking agents. This test should be performed before repeating the neurologic examination. It should be noted that until confounding metabolic or pharmacologic factors are ruled out, the documented neurologic examination should not be used in the determination of brain death. In this case, the elimination half-life of propofol is short and any meaningful pharmacologic effect should disappear within minutes to hours. It should be noted that given propofol's lipophilic nature, continued infusion may lead to deposition and accumulation in fatty tissue and the pharmacologic effects can be longer lasting. The clinical examination can be performed once a drug level (eg, barbiturates used to treat high ICP) is below the therapeutic range.[5,6] When levels are unavailable, a waiting period of 4 to 5 half-lives of the agent is necessary. If high suspicion of confounding due to pharmacologic effects remains despite an appropriate waiting period, an ancillary test may be performed. Documentation of specific testing for confounding conditions is an important part of brain death evaluation. Table 53-2 lists common conditions that must be excluded before performing a brain death examination.

Two hours later, a train-of-four test confirms the absence of neuromuscular blockade. Serum testing rules out the presence of a metabolic derangement confounding the clinical picture and vital signs are within the limits of normal including blood pressure and temperature. As the neurointensivist assigned to the case, you ask the on-call fellow to show the rest of the team how to perform vestibular cold caloric testing while you supervise the procedure.

Table 53-2. Common Conditions That Must Be Excluded Before Brain Death Examination

- **Exclusion of complicating medical conditions that may confound clinical assessment**
  Electrolyte disturbances
  Acid-base disturbances
  Endocrine disturbances
- **Lack of significant hypothermia**
  Core temperature: $\geq 32°C$ (89.6°F)
- **Lack of significant hypotension**
  Systolic blood pressure: ≥ 90 mm Hg
- **Exclusion of drug intoxication or poisoning**

What should the fellow's examination consist of?

Although both warm and cold caloric testing are possible, cold caloric testing is the most commonly performed test at the bedside. In this test the absence of provoked eye movements must be confirmed. The tympanum should be irrigated with ice water after the head has been tilted 30 degrees. There should be no tonic deviation of gaze or an individual eye toward the cold stimulus. The unfortunate mnemonic "COWS" (cold other warm same) has been used by medical students to memorize the response to caloric stimuli. The COWS mnemonic refers to the fast component of nystagmus in a patient who is conscious, not comatose. In a comatose patient, the expected normal response is tonic gaze deviation toward the side irrigated with cold water. Performing otoscopy prior to irrigation of the tympanum is an important step since a ruptured membrane should not be irrigated because of risk of infection. Otoscopy should rule out the presence of clotted blood or cerumen in the ear canals, which may diminish the response in a person who is not brain dead. No deviation of the eyes to irrigation in each ear with 50 mL of cold water is considered a positive test. One minute of observation should be allowed after irrigation. The clinician should wait 5 minutes before testing the contralateral vestibular apparatus.

Vestibulo-ocular examination including cold caloric testing shows absence of any response.

What is the next clinical test that should be performed to test for brainstem function?

An apnea test can be performed. Although frequently performed during the second neurologic assessment for brain death, an apnea test can be performed at any point after confounding metabolic and pharmacologic factors have been ruled out. When this test is performed, hypoventilation is induced by discontinuing mechanical ventilation with the goal of increasing the amount of CO_2 in arterial blood. The test is considered positive when no respiratory movements are observed after adequate increase in CO_2. As a matter of convention, the threshold of maximal stimulation for the medullary respiratory centers has been set at a partial pressure of carbon dioxide ($Paco_2$) of 60 mm Hg. In chronic carbon dioxide retainers, an increase of 20 mm Hg from baseline in the $Paco_2$ is considered an acceptable stimulus.[7]

Preoxygenation is mandatory to perform this test safely and also helps eliminate the stores of respiratory nitrogen. To achieve this, the fraction of inspired oxygen (Fio_2) is set at 100% on the ventilator for a few minutes prior to discontinuation of mechanical ventilation. After mechanical ventilation is discontinued, a catheter is introduced through the endotracheal tube to infuse oxygen. The infusion rate of oxygen should not be too high to avoid unintended ventilation of CO_2. The mechanical ventilator must be disconnected in order to obtain an appropriate assessment, since the ventilator's sensors may be triggered inappropriately, providing false-negative results.[8] An increase in CO_2 usually occurs at a predictable rate of 3 mm Hg per minute. A baseline ABG is used to assess the increase in CO_2 and confirm adequate oxygenation. Repeat blood gases are obtained periodically during the test, which can last for several minutes as long as hemodynamic stability and adequate oxygenation determined by pulse oximetry are maintained. The test is considered positive and consistent with brain death when no respiratory movements are observed and an adequate rise in the $Paco_2$ is documented.[1,9,10] Figure 53-2 is a flow diagram of a commonly followed protocol for apnea testing. It should be noted that protocols may vary in different institutions and that close collaboration with respiratory therapists is essential. Apnea testing is an essential component of brain death evaluation.

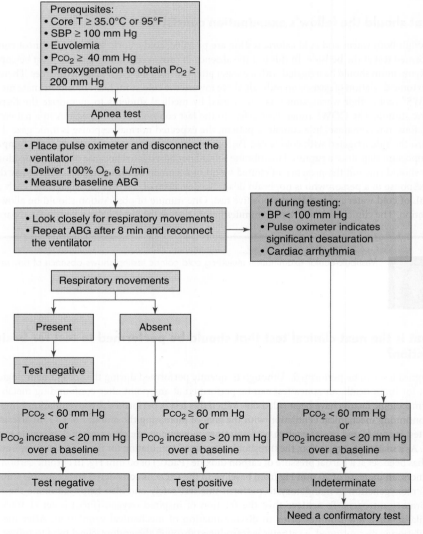

Figure 53-2. Flow diagram of a commonly followed protocol for apnea testing. ABG, arterial blood gas; BP, blood pressure; SBP, systolic blood pressure; T, temperature.

Your complete neurologic evaluation at this time remains unchanged and the apnea test fails to elicit respiratory movements. You find the patient's husband in the waiting room and suggest that a family meeting may be appropriate at this time.

Who should be present at this meeting?

At this time brain death has not been diagnosed. The purpose of a family meeting at this point is not to focus on brain death. Sudden-onset neurologic conditions with devastating consequences such as the one illustrated in this case frequently leave family members stunned and unable to adequately understand the situation. Establishing an open line of communication with families early on in the course of illness is essential. Except for rare occasions, family meetings should include all available close members of the family. In this case, it would be helpful to ask the patient's husband who he thinks should be present at a family meeting. It should be emphasized that the term *family* is used to denote anyone who is designated as such by a health care agent, in this case, the husband. When a family is composed of a large group of people, it is helpful to designate a spokesperson. Communications outside of the context of a family meeting can then be directed to the family spokesperson and he or she can disseminate the information. This method can help avoid misunderstandings and most efficiently utilizes the clinician's time. It is worth mentioning that on occasion a health care agent (in this case the patient's husband) may designate someone else as the family spokesperson, such as a sibling or close family friend. These requests should be honored as much as permitted by hospital policy and individual states' laws.

Successful family meetings are often attended by different members of the health care team including nurses, residents, intensivists, and social workers. At the start of the meeting it is important to introduce the members of the health care team as well as their roles and to inquire about the individual members of the family.

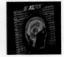

At the family meeting, the patient's husband tells you that he has witnessed movements of the patient's arms and legs, sweating, flushing, and chest movements.

Are these observations incompatible with brain death?

No. The following manifestations are occasionally seen and should not be misinterpreted as evidence for brain function[11-14]:

- Spontaneous movements of limbs other than pathologic flexion or extension response
- Respiratory-like movements (shoulder elevation and adduction, back arching, intercostal expansion without significant tidal volumes)
- Sweating, flushing, tachycardia
- Normal blood pressure without pharmacologic support or sudden increases in blood pressure
- Absence of diabetes insipidus
- Deep tendon reflexes; superficial abdominal reflexes; triple flexion response
- Babinski reflex

You inform the patient's husband and family that you don't expect any change in the patient's neurologic status but that you wish for a colleague of yours, also a neurologist, to perform a second examination to be absolutely certain of the severity of the condition.

How much time should elapse before the second examination is performed?

Arbitrary recommendations for the length of observation periods have varied extensively throughout the world and the United States. There are no detailed studies on serial examinations in adult patients who have been declared brain dead. Although there is insufficient evidence to determine the minimally acceptable observation period, it is generally considered that a 6-hour period between the two examinations is sufficient. It should be noted that at different institutions, the waiting period may vary according to arbitrary reasons and that there is no standard waiting period based on scientific data.[1,15-18]

A second complete examination is performed and documented in the chart by your colleague. No brainstem response was elicited.

Is further ancillary testing necessary for the diagnosis of brain death?

No. In this case there is no need for ancillary testing for the diagnosis of brain death. Performing ancillary tests when unnecessary can occasionally lead to difficult situations in which contradictory information is present. Although savvy clinicians can usually interpret this contradictory information, it can lead to confusion among family members and the health care team. The most sensitive and specific tool for the diagnosis of brain death is the clinical examination including cold caloric and apnea testing.

In which situations is ancillary testing most useful in the evaluation of brain death?

The following conditions may interfere with the clinical diagnosis of brain death, so that the diagnosis cannot be made with certainty on clinical grounds alone. In such instances, confirmatory tests are helpful.

- Severe facial or cervical spine trauma
- Preexisting pupillary abnormalities
- Toxic levels of any sedative drugs, tricyclic antidepressants, anticholinergics, antiepileptic drugs, chemotherapeutic agents, or neuromuscular-blocking agents
- Sleep apnea or severe pulmonary disease resulting in chronic retention of CO_2
- Formal apnea testing cannot be done because patient's hemodynamic status becomes unstable before completing the test

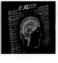

The medical student who saw the patient in the ED comes to the neurologic ICU to follow up on the patient's status. After speaking with the resident and fellow in the unit, he asks you if there are any official guidelines he could look up for the diagnosis of brain death that are commonly accepted in the United States.

What is your answer?

The American Academy of Neurology (AAN) published in 1995 a practice parameter for the diagnosis of brain death in adults. In 2010, an evidence-based guideline update was published by the AAN evaluating the most relevant literature regarding ancillary testing for brain death, the most adequate length of observation, the relevance of complex motor movements in brain-dead patients, and the comparative safety of different apnea testing modalities. Both of these documents can be found on the AAN's Web site. Table 53-3 provides a sample checklist for determination of brain death criteria.[1,19]

Table 53-3. Checklist for Determination of Brain Death

Prerequisites (all must be checked)
- Coma, irreversible and cause known
- Neuroimaging explains coma
- CNS depressant drug effect is absent
- No evidence of residual paralytics (electrical stimulation if paralytics used)
- Absence of severe acid-base, electrolyte, and endocrine abnormalities
- Normothermia or mild hypothermia (core temperature $\geq 36°C$)
- Systolic blood pressure ≥ 100 mm Hg
- No spontaneous respirations

Examination (all must be checked)
- Pupils nonreactive to bright light
- Corneal reflex absent
- Oculocephalic reflex absent (tested only if cervical spine integrity ensured)
- Oculovestibular reflex absent
- No facial movement to noxious stimuli at supraorbital nerve, temporomandibular joint
- Gag reflex absent
- Cough reflex absent to tracheal suctioning
- Absence of motor response to noxious stimuli in all four limbs (spinally mediated reflexes are permissible)

Apnea testing (all must be checked)
- Patient is hemodynamically stable
- Ventilator adjusted to provide normocarbia ($PaCO_2$ 34-45 mm Hg)
- Patient preoxygenated with 100% FiO_2 for ≥ 10 min to $PaO_2 \geq 200$ mm Hg
- Patient well oxygenated with a PEEP of 5 cm H_2O
- Provide oxygen via a suction catheter to the level of the carina at 6 L/min or attach T-piece with CPAP at 10 cm H_2O
- Disconnect ventilator
- Spontaneous respirations is absent
- Arterial blood gas drawn at 8-10 min, patient reconnected to ventilator
- $PCO_2 > 60$ mm Hg, or 20 mm Hg rise from normal baseline value

Or
- Apnea test aborted

Ancillary testing (only one needs to be performed; to be ordered only if clinical examination cannot be fully performed because of patient factors, or if apnea testing inconclusive or aborted)
- Cerebral angiogram
- HMPAO SPECT
- EEG
- TCD

Time of death (DD/MM/YY) _____

Name of physician and signature _____

Abbreviations: CNS, central nervous system; CPAP, continuous positive airway pressure; EEG, electroencephalography; HMPAO SPECT, technetium 99m hexametazime single-photon emission computed tomography; PEEP, positive end-expiratory pressure; TCD, transcranial Doppler. (*Report of the Quality Standards Subcommittee of the American Academy of Neurology, 2010.*)

Ethics and End-of-Life Issues

Table 53-4. Methods of Ancillary Testing for the Determination of Brain Death

---

Cerebral angiography
- The contrast medium should be injected in the aortic arch under high pressure and reach both anterior and posterior circulations.
- No intracerebral filling should be detected at the level of entry of the carotid or vertebral artery to the skull.
- The external carotid circulation should be patent.
- The filling of the superior longitudinal sinus may be delayed.

Electroencephalography
- A minimum of 8 scalp electrodes should be used.
- Interelectrode impedance should be between 100 and 10,000 Ω.
- The integrity of the entire recording system should be tested.
- The distance between electrodes should be at least 10 cm.
- The sensitivity should be increased to at least 2 μV for 30 min with inclusion of appropriate calibrations.
- The high-frequency filter setting should not be set below 30 Hz, and the low-frequency setting should not be above 1 Hz.
- Electroencephalography should demonstrate a lack of reactivity to intense somatosensory or audiovisual stimuli.

Transcranial Doppler (TCD) ultrasonography
- TCD is useful only if a reliable signal is found. The abnormalities should include either reverberating flow or small systolic peaks in early systole. A finding of a complete absence of flow may not be reliable owing to inadequate transtemporal windows for insonation. There should be bilateral insonation and anterior and posterior insonation. The probe should be placed at the temporal bone, above the zygomatic arch and the vertebrobasilar arteries, through the suboccipital transcranial window.
- Insonation through the orbital window can be considered to obtain a reliable signal. TCD may be less reliable in patients with a prior craniotomy.

Cerebral scintigraphy (technetium Tc 99m hexametazime [HMPAO])
- The isotope should be injected within 30 min after its reconstitution.
- Anterior and both lateral planar image counts (500,000) of the head should be obtained at several time points: immediately, between 30 and 60 min later, and at 2 h.
- A correct IV injection may be confirmed with additional images of the liver demonstrating uptake (optional).
- No radionuclide localization in the middle cerebral artery, anterior cerebral artery, or basilar artery territories of the cerebral hemispheres (hollow skull phenomenon).
- No tracer in superior sagittal sinus (minimal tracer can come from the scalp).

(Report of the Quality Standards Subcommittee of the American Academy of Neurology, 2010.)

What are the most commonly used ancillary tests for the diagnosis of brain death?

Cerebral angiography,[20,21] electroencephalography (EEG),[22,23] transcranial Doppler (TCD) ultrasound,[24] and cerebral scintigraphy[25] are the most commonly utilized ancillary tests in confirming brain death. Table 53-4 lists the most relevant aspects of these diagnostic modalities. Other imaging modalities such as magnetic resonance angiography (MRA)[26-29] and computed tomography angiography (CTA)[30-34] have been utilized in the diagnosis of brain death; however, there is insufficient information regarding their specificity or sensitivity and their use is not recommended at this time. Electrophysiologic tests such as somatosensory evoked potentials[35,e1] and bispectral index[e2] with a limited EEG montage have been described in small case series; however, because of a high risk of bias and inadequate statistical precision, they are not currently recommended as aids in the diagnosis of brain death at this time.

If a transcranial Doppler ultrasound test were performed, what would be the most likely result of this test?

Transcranial Doppler sonography is a practical, noninvasive method for the diagnosis of arrest of the cerebral circulation. It is an operator-dependent test that requires appropriate training, certification, and skill. The most likely finding in this patient is reverberating flow or small systolic peaks in early

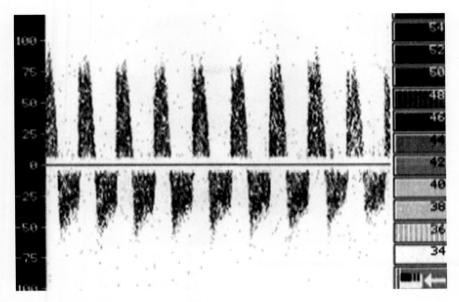

Figure 53-3. Waveform consistent with circulatory arrest.

systole.[36,37] Figure 53-3 shows an example of a waveform consistent with circulatory arrest. Transcranial Doppler is most useful in the evaluation of brain death when a baseline study has previously shown the presence of adequate bone windows and has mapped the vascular anatomy. If a change in waveform morphology from normal low-resistance flow is noted to change to a reverberant flow pattern, this test can be very useful. Absence of flow on TCD should be interpreted with care in cases in which no baseline study is available since cranial hyperostosis can lead to a false-positive test with complete absence of blood flow signals.

If a cerebral angiogram were performed, what would be the most likely result of this test?

After injection of contrast into the aortic arch, no intracranial enhancement of the intracranial vessels should be observed. A high-pressure injection is required for this test. The cerebral venous sinuses should not enhance with contrast, although the superior sagittal sinus may show some delayed enhancement. Figure 53-4 shows an angiogram consistent with brain death.

If an EEG were performed, what would be the most likely result of this test?

Guidelines for the use of EEG as an ancillary test for brain death are available from the American Electroencephalographic Society. The most relevant aspects of these recommendations are listed in Table 53-4. Figure 53-5 shows an example of electrocerebral silence recorded from an EEG in a brain-dead patient.

If cerebral scintigraphy with technetium 99m hexametazime (HMPAO) were performed, what would be the most likely result of this test?

After injection of a radioactive isotope, no radionuclide localization should be found in the intracranial circulation. This result is also known as the "empty skull phenomenon." Figure 53-6 shows an example of a radionuclide study in a brain-dead patient. Radionuclide uptake should be visualized in other organs such as the liver.

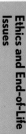

Ethics and End-of-Life Issues

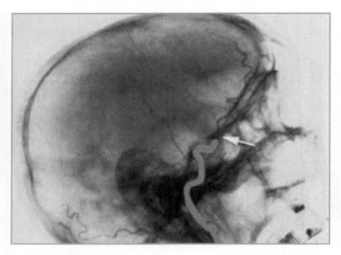

Figure 53-4. Angiogram consistent with brain death.

 You gather the family again and, along with the rest of the medical team as well as your colleague who performed the second evaluation, you inform them of the sad news.

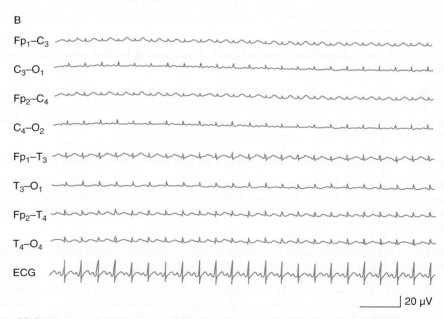

Figure 53-5. Electrocerebral silence recorded from an electroencephalogram in a brain-dead patient.

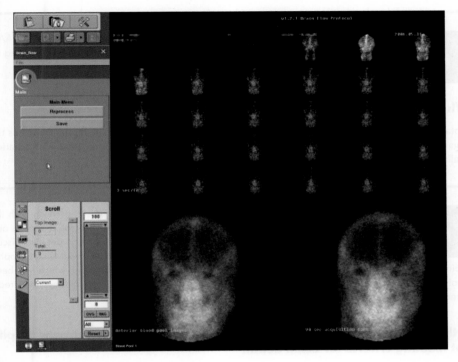

Figure 53-6. Radionuclide study in a brain-dead patient.

Is this a good time to discuss organ donation?

Discussing organ donation is complex and delicate. Physicians should not be prohibited from discussing any subject relevant to patient care. If questions regarding organ donation are posed by family members at this point, they should be addressed with honesty. The medical team should make an effort to differentiate itself from the organ donation team and establish its main goal as the care provider for the patient. Whenever possible, organ donation specialists, who are not a part of the clinical team, should be allowed to discuss organ donation with family members. It is best not to jump to the topic of organ donation prematurely. The best result is obtained when the treating physicians and nursing staff who have built a good physician-family relationship introduce the organ donation team, rather than having the organ donation team introduce themselves.

What is the best time to involve organ donor specialists?

Organ donation specialists should be alerted of possible cases as early as possible. Their specialized training prepares them for conversations with families as well as complex medical decision making. It is important to note that organ donation specialists do not approach family members without consulting with the medical team, and not before the family has had a chance to discuss treatment plans and prognosis. However, when involved early in a case, they can initiate the evaluation of potential donors. This strategy avoids coercive conversations or acting against patient and family member wishes and maximizes success.

The medical student from the ED returns to the neurologic ICU and distributes the AAN 2010 guideline update to the residents and fellows. He asks you if there is anything he could do to find out about the patient's attitudes toward organ donation.

What do you ask him to do?

Obtaining the patient's wallet and looking for her driver's license may help the family as well as the organ donor team elucidate the patient's known wishes toward organ donation. Any documentation available to aid the family in decision making should be sought out.

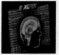

The family meeting was an emotionally charged and cathartic event in which both the medical team and family members were able to discuss the certainty of the diagnosis and express their feelings regarding the unfortunate events. The patient had detailed discussions with her husband urging him to consider organ donation in the event of catastrophic brain injury and had also stated this on her driver's license. The organ donation team, which had been involved from the beginning, was able to coordinate donation of heart, lungs, liver, kidneys, pancreas, cornea, bone, and skin, helping 11 different patients improve their health.

Is there is a way for a brain-injured patient to donate his or her organs despite not meeting criteria for brain death?

Yes. Donation after cardiac death protocols are available in many institutions. These protocols allow patients in whom withdrawal of care is planned because of known wishes or substituted judgment to donate their organs. Life-sustaining measures are withdrawn under controlled circumstances, often in the operating room. After cardiac function ceases, a physician pronounces the patient dead and the transplant team may begin the procurement procedure. To avoid conflicts of interest, the surgeon who recovers the organs and the rest of the transplant team may not be involved in end-of-life care for these patients.[38]

! CRITICAL CONSIDERATIONS

- To correctly diagnose brain death, it is essential for clinicians to adhere to a uniform methodology.
- Ancillary tests are not required for the diagnosis of brain death but may be helpful in select circumstances.
- Essential findings in brain death are coma or unresponsiveness, clinically confirming absence of brainstem reflexes typically by two independent physicians, and formal apnea testing, confirming lack of any spontaneous breathing.
- Organ donation has a tremendous impact on society and should be thought of early in the course of illness for patients with severe neurologic injury. The best result is obtained when the medical team who has built a good relationship with the patient's family members introduces the organ donation team and conveys a positive note: a notion of the gift of life.

REFERENCES

1. Report of the Quality Standards Subcommittee of the American Academy of Neurology. Practice parameters for determining brain death in adults (Summary statement). *Neurology.* 1995;45:1012-1014.

2. Wijdicks EFM. The diagnosis of brain death. *N Engl J Med.* 2001;344:1215-1221.

3. Wijdicks EFM, Atkinson JLD, Okazaki H. Isolated medulla oblongata function after severe traumatic brain injury. *J Neurol Neurosurg Psychiatry.* 2001;70:127-129.

4. Danzl DF, Pozos RS. Accidental hypothermia. *N Engl J Med.* 1994;331:1756-1760.

5. Grattan-Smith PJ, Butt W. Suppression of brainstem reflexes in barbiturate coma. *Arch Dis Child.* 1993;69:151-152.

6. Goldfrank LR, Flomenbaum NE, Lewin NA, Weisman RS, Howland MA, Hoffman RS, eds. *Goldfrank's Toxicologic Emergencies.* 6th ed. Stamford, CT: Appleton & Lange; 1998.

7. Wijdicks EFM. Determining brain death in adults. *Neurology.* 1995;45:1003-1011.

8. Willatts SM, Drummond G. Brainstem death and ventilator trigger settings. *Anesthesia.* 2000;55:676-677.

9. Brain Death Task Force. Guidelines for the diagnosis of brain death. *Can Med Assoc J.* 1987;136:200A-200B.

10. Medical Consultants on the Diagnosis of Death to the President's Commission. Guidelines for the determination of death. *JAMA.* 1981;246:2184-2185.

11. Ropper AH. Unusual spontaneous movements in brain-dead patients. *Neurology.* 1984;34:1089-1092.

12. Saposnik G, Bueri JA, Maurino J, Saizar R, Garretto NS. Spontaneous and reflex movements in brain death. *Neurology.* 2000;54:221-223.

13. Martí-Fàbregas J, López-Navidad A, Caballero F, Otermin P. Decerebrate-like posturing with mechanical ventilation in brain death. *Neurology.* 2000;54:224-227.

14. Christie JM, O'Lenic TD, Cane RD. Head turning in brain death. *J Clin Anesth.* 1996;8:141-143.

15. Haupt WF, Rudolf J. European brain death codes: a comparison of national guidelines. *J Neurol.* 1999;246:432-437.

16. Wang M, Wallace P, Gruen JP. Brain death documentation: analysis and issues. *Neurosurgery.* 2002;51:731-736.

17. Wijdicks EFM. Brain death worldwide: accepted fact but no global consensus in diagnostic criteria. *Neurology.* 2002;58:20-25.

18. Real Decreto 2070/1999, de 30 de diciembre, por el que se regulan las actividades de obtención y utilización clínica de órganos humanos y la coordinación territorial en materia de donación y trasplante de órganos y tejidos. BOE 3/2000 de 4-1-2000, p. 179-90.

19. Wijdicks EF, Varelas PN, Gronseth GS, Greer DM; American Academy of Neurology. Evidence-based guideline update: determining brain death in adults. Report of the Quality Standards Subcommittee of the American Academy of Neurology. *Neurology.* 2010;74:1911-1918.

20. Bradac GB, Simon RS. Angiography in brain death. *Neuroradiology.* 1974;7:25-28.

21. Ames AD, Wright RL, Kowada M, Thurston JM, Majno G. Cerebral ischemia: II. The no-reflow phenomenon. *Am J Pathol.* 1968;52:437-453.

22. American Electroencephalographic Society. Guideline three: minimum technical standards for EEG recording in suspected cerebral death. *J Clin Neurophysiol.* 1994;11:10-13.

23. Silverman D, Saunders MG, Schwab RS, Masland RL. Cerebral death and the electroencephalogram: report of the ad hoc committee of the American Electroencephalographic Society on EEG Criteria for determination of cerebral death. *JAMA.* 1969;209:1505-1510.

24. Assessment: transcranial Doppler: report of the American Academy of Neurology, Therapeutics and Technology Assessment Subcommittee. *Neurology.* 1990;40:680-681.

25. Bonetti MG, Ciritella P, Valle G, Perrone E. 99mTc HM-PAO brain perfusion SPECT in brain death. *Neuroradiology.* 1995;37:365-369.

26. Karantanas AH, Hadjigeorgiou GM, Paterakis K, Sfiras D, Komnos A. Contribution of MRI and MR angiography in early diagnosis of brain death. *Eur Radiol.* 2002;12:2710-2716.

27. Ishii K, Onuma T, Kinoshita T, Shiina G, Kameyama M, Shimosegawa Y. Brain death: MR and MR angiography. *AJNR Am J Neuroradiol.* 1996;17:731-735.

28. Matsumura A, Meguro K, Tsurushima H, et al. Magnetic resonance imaging of brain death. *Neurol Med Chir.* 1996;36:166-171.

29. Lovblad KO, Bassetti C. Diffusion-weighted magnetic resonance imaging in brain death. *Stroke.* 2000;31:539-542.

30. Quesnel C, Fulgencio J-P, Adrie C, et al. Limitations of computed tomography in the diagnosis of brain death. *Intensive Care Med.* 2007;33:2129-2135.

31. Combes JC, Chomel A, Ricolfi F, d'Athis P, Freysz M. Reliability of computed tomographic angiography in the diagnosis of brain death. *Transplant Proc.* 2007;39:16-20.

32. Frampas E, Videcoq M, de Kerviler E, et al. CT angiography for brain death diagnosis. *Am J Neuroradiol.* 2009;30:1566-1570.

33. Escudero D, Otero J, Marques L, et al. Diagnosing brain death by CT perfusion and multislice CT angiography. *Neurocrit Care.* 2009;11:261-271.

34. Greer DM, Strozyk D, Schwamm LH. False positive CT angiography in brain death. *Neurocrit Care.* 2009;11:272-275.

35. Wagner W. Scalp, earlobe and nasopharyngeal recordings of the median nerve somatosensory evoked P14 potential in coma and brain death. *Brain.* 1996;119:1507-1521

36. Petty GW, Mohr JP, Pedley TA, et al. The role of transcranial Doppler in confirming brain death: sensitivity, specificity, and suggestions for performance and interpretation. *Neurology.* 1990;40:300-303.

37. Ropper AH, Kehne SM, Wechsler L. Transcranial Doppler in braindeath. *Neurology.* 1987,37:1733-1735.

38. Steinbrook R. Organ donation after cardiac death. *N Engl J Med.* 2007:357;3.

e1. Roncucci P, Lepori P, Mok MS, Bayat A, Logi F, Marino A. Nasopharyngeal electrode recording of somatosensory evoked potentials as an indicator in brain death. *Anaesth Intensive Care.* 1999;27:20-25.

e2. Misis M, Raxach JG, Molto HP, Vega SM, Rico PS. Bispectral index monitoring for early detection of brain death. *Transplant Proc.* 2008;40:1279-1281.

Index

Note: Page numbers referencing figures are followed by an "*f*". Page numbers referencing tables are followed by a "*t*".